Contents

Preface   xv

Acknowledgments   xvii

Contributors   xix

SECTION I   **Historical and Work Perspectives** **1**

Chapter 1   **The Lactation Consultant:**
                Roles and Responsibilities **3**

   History   3

   Do Lactation Consultants Make a Difference?   4

   Certification: International Board of Lactation Consultant Examiners   5

   Professional Association: International Lactation Consultant Association   6

   Gaining Clinical Experience   6

   Lactation Consultant Education   8

   Hospital Lactation Programs   8

   The Unique Characteristics of Counseling Breastfeeding Women   15

   Roles and Responsibilities   15

   Lactation Consultants in the Community Setting   16

   Worksite Lactation Programs   17

   Medical Clinics/Offices   17

   Professional Lactation Care and Volunteer Counselors   17

   Mentoring and Networking   18

   Documentation   19

   Legal Concerns   21

   Confidentiality   23

   Intellectual Property Rights   23

   Ethics   24

   Reimbursement   27

   Private Practice   33

Acknowledgments   35
Summary   35
Key Concepts   35
Internet Resources   36
References   36

Chapter 2   Tides in Breastfeeding Practice **41**

Evidence About Breastfeeding Practices   41
The Biological Norm in Infant Feeding   48
Infant Feeding: Alternatives to Maternal Breastfeeding   49
Technological Innovations in Infant Feeding   52
The Prevalence of Breastfeeding   57
The Cost of Not Breastfeeding   59
The Promotion of Breastfeeding   62
Summary   68
Key Concepts   69
References   70

SECTION II   Anatomic and Biological Imperatives **77**

Chapter 3   Anatomy and Physiology of Lactation **79**

Introduction   79
Mammogenesis   79
Breast Structure   80
Pregnancy   85
Lactogenesis   86
Clinical Implications: Mother   95
Newborn Oral Development   97
Sucking   100
Frequency of Feedings   107
Summary   108
Key Concepts   108
References   110
Appendix 3-A: Suck Training for Breastfeeding   116
Basic Suck-Training Technique   117
La Leche League Technique   119
Sensorial Oral Stimulation in Infants with Suck Feeding Disabilities   119
Suck-Training Methods for Specific Dysfunctions   119
Suck-Training Method for Infants with Neurologic Dysfunction   120
Internet Resources   120
References   120

Chapter 4   The Biological Specificity of Breastmilk **121**

Milk Synthesis and Maturational Changes   122
Energy, Volume, and Growth   123
Nutritional Values   129
Preterm Milk   137
Anti-infective Properties   137
The Immune System   146
Bioactive Components   153
Implications for Clinical Practice   156
Summary   157
Key Concepts   158
References   159
Appendix 4-A: Composition of Human Colostrum and Mature Breastmilk   170

Chapter 5   Drug Therapy and Breastfeeding **171**

Introduction   171
The Alveolar Subunit   172
Drug Transfer into Human Milk   173
Calculating Infant Exposure   177
Effect of Medications on Milk Production   180
Review of Selected Drug Classes   183
Drugs of Abuse   195
Radioactive Agents   197
Summary   197
Key Concepts   199
References   199

Chapter 6   Viral Infections and Breastfeeding **207**

Introduction   207
Human Immunodeficiency Virus   208
Herpes Simplex Virus   212
Varicella-Zoster Virus (Chickenpox/Varicella/Zoster/Shingles)   214
Cytomegalovirus   215
Rubella   216
Hepatitis B   217
Hepatitis C   218
Human T-Cell Lymphotropic Viruses   219
West Nile Virus   219
Implications for Practice   220
Acknowledgments   220

Summary   221
Key Concepts   221
Internet Resources   222
References   222

SECTION III   Prenatal, Perinatal, and Postnatal Periods 225
Chapter 7   Perinatal and Intrapartum Care 227

Breastfeeding Preparation   227
Early Feedings   228
Epidurals and Other Birth Practices   232
Postbirth Care of the Newborn   233
Normal Newborn Sleep and Eating Patterns   234
Pain Medications   237
Feeding Positions   238
The Infant Who Has Not Latched On   240
Late-Preterm Infants   246
Feeding Methods   247
Nipple Shields   249
Hypoglycemia   251
Cesarean Birth   253
Breast Engorgement   254
Breast Edema   255
Hand Expression   256
Clinical Implications   256
The Baby-Friendly Hospital Initiative   261
Acknowledgment   262
Summary   262
Key Concepts   263
Internet Resources   264
References   264
Appendix 7-A: Research and Scholarly Papers on the Newborn's Reactions to the
    Smell of Mother's Milk or Secretions from the Montgomery Glands on the Areola   271

Chapter 8   Postpartum Care 273

Immediate Postbirth Events   273
First Weeks: Principles and Expectations   273
Common Problems in the Early Days and Weeks   276
Supplementation Guidelines and Cautions   279
Nipple Pain   280
Engorgement + Milk Stasis = Involution   285
Milk Supply/Milk Production   287
Breast Massage   291
Nausea and Other Negative Feelings During the Milk-Ejection   291
Clothing, Leaking, Bras, and Breast Pads   293

Infant Concerns   294
Multiple Infants   299
Breastfeeding During Pregnancy and Tandem Nursing   304
Sleeping, SIDS, and Bedsharing   305
Clinical Implications   307
Acknowledgments   308
Summary   309
Key Concepts   309
Internet Resources   310
References   310

Chapter 9   Breast-Related Problems 319

Introduction   319
Nipple Variations   319
Plugged Ducts   321
Mastitis   323
Breast Abscess   328
Dermatoses of the Breast   328
Candidiasis (Thrush)   330
Other Breast Pain   335
Milk Blister   336
Mammoplasty   336
Breast Lumps and Surgery   342
Galactoceles   343
Fibrocystic Changes of the Breast   344
Bleeding from the Breast   345
Breast Cancer   346
Clinical Implications   350
Acknowledgement   350
Summary   350
Key Concepts   351
Internet Resources   353
References   353

Chapter 10   Low Intake in the Breastfed Infant: Maternal and Infant Considerations 359

Introduction   359
Global Standards for Optimal Growth: The WHO Child Growth Standards   362
The Relationship of Newborn Weight Loss to Onset of Lactation   367
Initial Newborn Weight Loss and Early Weight Gain   370
Low Intake and Low Milk Supply: Definitions and Incidence of Occurrence, Confusing
    Terminology, Limited Data, and Nonstandardized Research   371
Abnormal Patterns of Growth: The Baby Who Appears Healthy   373
Abnormal Patterns of Growth: The Baby with Obvious Illness   384
Maternal Considerations: The Mother Who Appears Healthy   384

Maternal Considerations: Obvious Illness   389
History, Physical Exam, and Differential Diagnosis   389
Clinical Management   390
Special Techniques for Management of Low Intake or Low Supply   395
Summary   399
Key Concepts   399
Internet Resources   400
References   401

Chapter 11   Jaundice and the Breastfed Baby 405

Neonatal Jaundice   406
Assessment of Jaundice   407
Postnatal Pattern of Jaundice   408
Evaluation of Jaundice   412
Diagnostic Assessment   412
Management of Jaundice   413
Acknowledgment   415
Summary   415
Key Concepts   416
Internet Resources   416
References   416

Chapter 12   Breast Pumps and Other Technologies 419

Concerns of Mothers   421
Hormonal Considerations   425
Pumps   428
A Comparison of Pumps   430
Simultaneous and/or Sequential Pumping   437
Flanges   439
Pedal Pumps   441
Clinical Implications Regarding Breast Pumps   441
Cleaning Pumps   443
Maternal Concerns and Education Needs   443
When Pumps Cause Problems   444
Sample Guidelines for Pumping   444
Common Pumping Problems   446
Nipple Shields   447
Breast Shells   454
Feeding-Tube Devices   454
Summary   457
Key Concepts   457
Resources for Mothers   461
Resources for Healthcare Providers   461
Internet Resources   461

References   462
Appendix 12-A: Manufacturers and Distributors of Breast Pumps and Feeding
   Equipment   467

Chapter 13   The Use of Human Milk and Breastfeeding in the Neonatal Intensive Care Unit 469

Introduction   469
Informed Decision: Human Milk as a Medical Intervention   469
Mothers of Preterm Infants   472
Rates of Breastfeeding Initiation and Duration   473
Evidence-Based Lactation Support Services   474
Initiation and Maintenance of Milk Supply   476
Maintaining Maternal Milk Volume   479
Human Milk Management   482
Optimization of Human Milk for Feeding 486
Methods of Milk Delivery   489
Non-nutritive Sucking at the Breast   491
Measuring Milk Transfer   497
Discharge Planning for Postdischarge Breastfeeding   504
Postdischarge Breastfeeding Management   506
Acknowledgment   507
Summary   507
Key Concepts   507
Internet Resources   508
References   508
Appendix 13-A: The Preterm Infant Breastfeeding Behavior Scale (PIBBS)   520

Chapter 14   Donor Milk Banking 523

Introduction   523
Use of Donor Milk   523
History of Donor Milk Banking   526
Donor Milk Today   527
Safety   532
Availability   532
Milk Banking Procedures   533
Informed Decision Making   537
Wet-Nursing, Informal Sharing, and Sale of Milk   538
For-Profit and Not-for-Profit Milk Banking   539
Research Findings on Donor Milk   539
Selected Case Studies   542
A Tribute to Mary Rose Tully   542
Summary   542
Key Concepts   545

Internet Resources   545
References   545
Appendix 14-A: Expressing, Storing, and Handling Human Milk   549

SECTION IV   Beyond Postpartum 551

Chapter 15   Women's Health and Breastfeeding 553

Postpartum Health and Care   553
Lactation, Fertility, Sexuality, and Contraception   556
Fertility   556
Postpartum Well-Being and Sexual Health   565
Women's Health Across the Childbearing Years   570
Acute Illnesses and Infections   588
Chronic Illnesses   594
Mood Disorders During Lactation   603
Autoimmune Diseases   608
Physically Challenged Mothers   613
Surgery   618
Transplants   619
Donating Blood   619
The Impact of Maternal Illness and Hospitalization   619
Acknowledgment   620
Summary   620
Key Concepts   620
Internet Resources   623
References   623

Chapter 16   Maternal Employment and Breastfeeding 635

Introduction   635
Historical Perspective and Statistics on Maternal Employment   635
The Effect of Work on Breastfeeding   636
Facilitators and Barriers to Breastfeeding in the Workplace   637
Individual Strategies to Manage Breastfeeding and Work   638
Special Issues Related to Returning to Work   642
Workplace Strategies to Support Breastfeeding and Work   649
Community Strategies to Support Breastfeeding and Work   654
National and Global Strategies in Promoting and Supporting Breastfeeding   655
Clinical Implications   658
Summary   660
Key Concepts   660
Internet Resources   661
References   662

Chapter 17   Child Health 667

Developmental Outcomes and Infant Feeding   667
Oxytocin and Breastfeeding   672
Growth and Development   673
Theories of Development   678
Clinical Implications   691
Immunizations   692
Vitamin D and Rickets   696
Dental Health and Orofacial Development   697
Solid Foods   699
Obesity   704
Long-Term Breastfeeding   706
Weaning   707
Implications for Practice   707
Acknowledgment   708
Summary   708
Key Concepts   708
Internet Resources   709
References   709

Chapter 18   The Ill Child: Breastfeeding Implications 717

Team Care for the Child with Feeding Difficulties   717
Feeding Behaviors of the Ill Infant/Child   719
What to Do If Weight Gain Is Inadequate   719
Pain Management Concerns   725
Breastfeeding Care of the Hospitalized Infant   725
Perioperative Care of the Breastfeeding Infant/Child   726
Emergency Room   728
Care of Children with Selected Conditions   728
Alterations in Neurologic Functioning   735
Congenital Heart Disease   740
Oral/Facial Anomalies   741
Gastrointestinal Anomalies and Disorders   747
Metabolic Dysfunction   753
Allergies   759
Food Intolerance   761
Psychosocial Concerns   762
Acknowledgment   765
Summary   765
Key Concepts   765
Internet Resources   766
References   767

Chapter 19 Infant Assessment 775

Introduction 775
Perinatal History 775
Gestational Age Assessment 775
Indicators of Effective Breastfeeding and Assessment Scales 780
Physical Assessment 788
Behavioral Assessment 800
Summary 807
Key Concepts 807
References 808
Appendix 19-A: Infant Breastfeeding Assessment Tool (IBFAT) 810
Appendix 19-B: LATCH Assessment Tool 811
Appendix 19-C: Mother–Baby Assessment Scale 812

SECTION V   Sociocultural and Research Issues 813

Chapter 20   Research, Theory, and Lactation 815

Introduction 815
Theories Related to Lactation Practice 815
Origins of Research Methodologies 821
Types of Research Methods 822
Elements of Research 828
Application of Methods to Qualitative Approaches 836
Application of Methods to Quantitative Approaches 838
Evaluating Research for Use in Practice 848
Using Research in Clinical Practice 850
Summary 851
Key Concepts 853
Acknowledgment 853
Internet Resources 853
References 854

Chapter 21   Breastfeeding Education 859

Introduction 859
Factors Creating the Need for Breastfeeding and Lactation Education 859
The Changing Landscape for Breastfeeding Education 860
Breastfeeding Programs for Healthcare Professionals 870
The Breastfeeding Team 872
Parent Education 875
Adult Learning Principles and Education 880
Curriculum Development 883
Teaching Strategies 885
Educational Materials 887
Summary 889

Key Concepts   889
Resources   891
References   891

Chapter 22   The Cultural Context of Breastfeeding 895

Introduction   895
The Dominant Culture   896
Ethnocentrism Versus Relativism   897
Cultural Competence   897
Assessing Cultural Practices   898
Language Barriers   898
The Effects of Culture on Breastfeeding   899
Maternal Foods   906
Weaning   908
Implications for Practice   909
Summary   910
Key Concepts   911
Internet Resources   911
References   911

Chapter 23   The Familial and Social Context of Breastfeeding 915

Family Forms and Functions   915
Family Theory   916
Social Factors That Influence Breastfeeding   917
Fathers   920
The Adolescent Mother   923
The Adoptive Mother and Family   926
The Low-Income Family   927
The Downside of Family Experience   929
Summary   935
Key Concepts   935
Internet Resources   936
Other Resources   936
References   937

Index   943

Preface

It is with great pride that I assume the lead editor position for *Breastfeeding and Human Lactation, Fifth Edition*. This is the final edition of the book that Dr. Jan Riordan, the book's founding editor and honorary editor of this edition, will participate in. I gratefully acknowledge Dr. Riordan's historic efforts and accomplishments in making this textbook the classic resource that it has come to be. I personally am grateful to Jan for her long-time mentoring and recognition of me as worthy of "taking over the book."

Changes to this *Fifth Edition* are plentiful and hopefully useful to our readers. We now have 23 chapters in the book, down from 25. Some content from the two deleted chapters has been incorporated elsewhere. Extensive changes and revisions were made to some chapters, while fewer revisions/changes were made to others. We are fortunate that the evidence underlying the science of breastfeeding and human lactation continues to grow, and we have done our best to include such evidence in the chapters. We welcome several new contributors to the book and we acknowledge those who took on chapters previously authored by Dr. Riordan. Our goal was to include knowledgeable experts, and we believe we have done so. On a sad note, we mourn the passing of Mary Rose Tully, and at the same time, laud Frances Jones's sole authorship of the chapter on human milk banking.

Since the last edition of the book, many advances have been made in the promotion and support of breastfeeding in the United States and around the world. For example, in the United States the *Healthy People 2020* goals expanded to further support breastfeeding and exclusive breastfeeding by including goals related to increasing breastfeeding support in the workplace, reducing formula supplementation in the hospital in the first two days of life, and increasing the proportion of births that occur in facilities that provide recommended care and support of lactating mothers and their infants. The *Surgeon General's 2011 Call to Action to Support Breastfeeding* brought additional attention to how breastfeeding women can be supported by the healthcare community (including lactation consultants), employers, community leaders, family and friends, and policy makers. The Patient Protection and Affordable Care Act (ACA) of 2010 incorporated provisions to reimburse costs for lactation care and breast pumps. The act also amended the Fair Labor Standards Act (FLSA) to require employers to provide break time and a private location to express breastmilk for non-exempt employees. In 2011, the Centers for Disease Control and Prevention (CDC) and the National Institute for Child Health Quality (NICHQ), in collaboration with Baby-Friendly USA and the United States Breastfeeding Committee, collaborated in Best Fed Beginnings, a first-of-its-kind, nationwide quality improvement initiative to help 89 hospitals improve maternity care and increase the number of Baby-Friendly-designated hospitals in the United States. In 2013, the CDC published the *CDC Guide to Strategies to Support Breastfeeding Mothers and Babies*. All of these efforts demonstrate our government's recognition of the health value of breastfeeding.

As lactation care providers, educators, and researchers, we have an obligation to do our part in enhancing support for breastfeeding mothers. We hope our book provides the evidence and information on practical application of that evidence in support of breastfeeding mothers.

Birth practices affect lactation. Thus, this edition again contains considerable content on obstetrical issues, especially the importance of skin-to-skin care and keeping mothers and babies together 24 hours a day during the birth hospitalization. Maternity practices and obstetrical intervention that impact breast-feeding have gained considerable attention from professional healthcare organizations. This is good news for efforts to support breastfeeding initiation and continuation. Examples include the American College of Obstetrics and Gynecology efforts to reduce cesarean section and the Association of Women's Health, Obstetric and Neonatal Nursing campaign to reduce elective induction of labor prior to 39 weeks' gestation.

As is true of earlier editions, the fifth edition of this text has a clear clinical focus. Nearly every chapter contains a clinical implications section. Important concepts discussed in chapters are summarized at the end of each chapter—a feature that makes studying easier. Throughout the book are new references deemed by the authors to be the most important from the vastly expanded research and clinical literature. Some older references—which introduced then-new ideas that are now accepted common knowledge—have been removed to make room for the new.

Section 1 contrasts the past and present. Chapter 1, with three new esteemed authors, concentrates on the work of the present-day healthcare worker who specializes in lactation and breastfeeding, and it addresses work-related issues of lactation consulting, such as staffing. Chapter 2 presents the history of breastfeeding by placing lactation and breastfeeding in its historical context.

Section 2 focuses on basic anatomic and biologic imperatives of lactation. Researchers continue to find amazing properties in breastmilk, such as stem cells. Clinical application of techniques must be based on a clear understanding of the relationships between form, function, and biological constructs. Chapter 3 has a section on basic suck-training technique for infants with suckling problems. This section, too, provides the background upon which to understand other aspects of lactation and breastfeeding behavior.

Section 3 is the clinical "heart" of the book, and describes the basics of what to do, when to do it, and how to do it when one assists the lactating mother. Section 3 thus concerns itself with the perinatal period in the birth setting and concerns during the postpartum period following the family's return home—notably breast problems, neonatal jaundice, and infant weight gain. This section also addresses special needs of preterm and ill babies and their mothers, and it critically evaluates breastfeeding devices and recommends how and when they are most appropriately used. It concludes with a review of the development and current activities of human milk banking.

The first part of Section 4 focuses on the mother: the mother's health and returning to work. The topics then turn to the infant's health and special health needs. The techniques of infant assessment are explained and demonstrated with photographs.

Section 5 begins with a careful look at research—how it is conducted, why ongoing research is needed, how research findings can be applied in clinical settings, and what theories are related to lactation practice. The principles of education, the cornerstone of clinical practice, are explored next. The book concludes with chapters on culture's effect on breastfeeding and the sociological context of the breastfeeding family functions.

To avoid linguistic confusion, the book uses the following conventions. The masculine pronoun has been used to denote the infant or child throughout the text as a matter of convenience to distinguish the child from the breastfeeding mother. Nurses, lactation consultants, and other healthcare workers are referred to by feminine pronouns, although we recognize that men serve in all healthcare professions.

Acknowledgments

We gratefully acknowledge the contributions to this book made by the following individuals:

Mary Margaret Coates, MS, IBCLC, TECH Edit, Wheat Ridge, Colorado
Nancy Powers, MD, FAAP, FABM, University of Kansas School of Medicine, Wichita
Miriam Labbok, MD, MPH, Director, Carolina Global Breastfeeding Institute, University of North Carolina, Chapel Hill

University of Kansas School of Nursing graduate students:

Sandi Hudson
Genevieve Barrett
Mandy McKinley
Tiffany Lemanski
Liza Murray
Alicia Reeves
Colleen Britt

We are grateful to La Leche League International for providing the foundation for our breastfeeding knowledge and to those institutions that encouraged and supported us in writing the book over the years: The University of Kansas School of Nursing in Kansas City, Kansas, as well as the Wichita State University School of Nursing and Via Christi Regional Medical Center, both of Wichita, Kansas.

Finally, we would like to thank our families for their help and encouragement over the years:

The Wambach family: Bill; Jackie, Brian, and Brianne; and Nathan, Sugar, Logan, and Samantha.
The Riordan family: Michael, Neil, and Shirley; Brian, Quinn, and Rika; Teresa, Renee, and Don Olmstead; and 12 grandchildren.

Contributors

Heather Baker, MSN, APRN, PNP
Clinical Educator, Retired
School of Nursing
Wichita State University
Wichita, Kansas

Teresa E. Baker, MD, FACOG
Associate Professor
Department of Obstetrics and Gynecology
Texas Tech University Health Sciences Center
Amarillo, Texas

Elizabeth C. Brooks, JD, IBCLC, FILCA
Private Practice Lactation Consultant
Wyndmoor, Pennsylvania

E. Stephen Buescher, MD
Professor of Pediatrics
Eastern Virginia Medical School
Norfolk, Virginia

Mary-Margaret Coates, MS
Technical Editor
TECH Edit
Wheat Ridge, Colorado

Jolynn Dowling, MSN, APRN, NNP-BC, IBCLC
Instructor
School of Nursing
Wichita State University
Wichita, Kansas

Lawrence M. Gartner, MD, FAAP
Professor Emeritus
Department of Pediatrics and Obstetrics
and Gynecology
University of Chicago
Chicago, Illinois

Catherine Watson Genna, BS, IBCLC
Private Lactation Consultant Practice,
New York City
Woodhaven, New York

Thomas W. Hale, PhD
Professor
Department of Pediatrics
Texas Tech University Health Sciences Center
Amarillo, Texas

Kay Hoover, MEd, IBCLC, FILCA
Lactation Consultant
Morton, Pennsylvania

Frances Jones, RN, MSN, IBCLC
Coordinator Lactation Services and Provincial
Milk Bank
BC Women's Hospital and Health Centre
Vancouver, British Columbia, Canada

Mary Koehn, PhD, APRN, FACCE
Associate Professor
School of Nursing
Wichita State University
Wichita, Kansas

Rebecca Mannel, BS, IBCLC, FILCA
Clinical Instructor and Lactation Manager
Department of Obstetrics and Gynecology
University of Oklahoma Health Sciences Center
Oklahoma City, Oklahoma

Barbara Morrison, PhD, CNM
Janice M. Riordan Distinguished Professor in
Maternal Child Health
School of Nursing
Wichita State University
Wichita, Kansas

Sallie Page-Goertz, MN, APRN, IBCLC, FILCA
Clinical Associate Professor
University of Kansas School of Medicine
Department of Pediatrics
Kansas City, Kansas

Nancy G. Powers, MD, FAAP, IBCLC, FABM
Clinical Associate Professor
Pediatric Hospitalist
Department of Pediatrics
University of Kansas School of Medicine
Wichita, Kansas

Jan Riordan, EdD, IBCLC, FAAN, FILCA
Professor Emeritus
School of Nursing
Wichita State University
Wichita, Kansas

Wilaiporn Rojjanasrirat, PhD, RNC, IBCLC
Associate Professor
School of Nursing
Graceland University
Independence, Missouri

Hilary Rowe, BSc(Pharm), PharmD, ACPR
Clinical Pharmacy Specialist Maternal Fetal
Medicine
Fraser Health Authority
Surrey, British Columbia, Canada

Linda J. Smith, MPH, IBCLC, FACCE, FILCA
Owner and Director
Bright Future Lactation Resource Centre, Ltd.
Dayton, Ohio

Diane L. Spatz, PhD, RN, FAAN
Professor of Perinatal Nursing and Helen
M. Shearer Professor of Nutrition
University of Pennsylvania School of Nursing
Nurse Researcher and Manager of the Lactation
Program
Children's Hospital of Philadelphia
Philadelphia, Pennsylvania

Marsha Walker, RN, IBCLC
Executive Director
National Alliance for Breastfeeding Advocacy
Weston, Massachusetts

Karen Wambach, PhD, RN, IBCLC, FILCA
Professor
School of Nursing
University of Kansas
Kansas City, Kansas

Section One

Historical and Work Perspectives

CHAPTER 1   The Lactation Consultant: Roles and Responsibilities

CHAPTER 2   Tides in Breastfeeding Practice

Just as the course of breastfeeding flows and ebbs in a woman's life, so breastfeeding has experienced flows and ebbs through many millennia. It takes a village to return to breastfeeding, and community-based programs that promote breastfeeding are working to increase the rate of breastfeeding around the world.

Until breastfeeding is again the unremarkable norm, the increasing numbers of mothers who begin breastfeeding will continue to prompt a need for increasing numbers of specialists who can help those mothers continue breastfeeding. The visibility and acceptance of lactation consulting as an allied health profession offers opportunities for practice in hospitals, the community, private practice, and public health. Randomized clinical trials conducted around the globe during the past 20 years have consistently demonstrated that lactation consultant services can lengthen a mother's breastfeeding course and result in healthier mothers and babies.

Chapter 1

The Lactation Consultant: Roles and Responsibilities

Elizabeth C. Brooks
Catherine Watson Genna
Rebecca Mannel

A lactation consultant (LC) is a specialist trained to focus on the needs and concerns of the breastfeeding mother–baby pair and to prevent, recognize, and solve breastfeeding difficulties. LC services do not replace those of other healthcare workers; instead, the LC is an extender of maternal–child services. Lactation consultants work with the public in many settings: hospitals, clinics, private medical practices, community health departments, home health agencies, and private practices. Almost all lactation specialists are women; many have educational and clinical backgrounds in the health professions or mother-to-mother support. Many are registered nurses, although physicians, dietitians, speech therapists, and other health professionals practice as lactation specialists as well. A growing interest in the profession is also attracting many candidates who study and work to enter directly into the lactation consulting field.

Lactation consulting is a rapidly growing healthcare specialty. Prior to recognition of the LC as a paid specialist in 1985, individuals serving breastfeeding women did so as volunteers or as unrecognized practitioners. Over time, the lack of standardization of skills and minimal competencies prompted formal development of the specialty practice. This occurred in part through a certification examination administered by the International Board of Lactation Consultant Examiners (IBLCE), and through the establishment of the International Lactation Consultant Association (ILCA), which publishes the peer-reviewed *Journal of Human Lactation* and other documents relating to lactation consultant education and practice. In 1994, the Academy of Breastfeeding Medicine, an international physician organization, was formed. Its official journal, *Breastfeeding Medicine*, also publishes peer-reviewed articles and helpful clinical protocols. In addition, La Leche League International and the Australian Breastfeeding Association publish professional materials that teach and support the LC as well as patient/family information. This chapter traces the historical roots of lactation professionals and discusses work-related issues.

History

In a cultural setting in which nearly all mothers breastfed, help with breastfeeding was available through the shared knowledge of other family members, neighbors, and friends. As childbirth came to be managed by health professionals in hospital settings and formula-feeding became the cultural norm, however, knowledge of lactation—which a mother formerly shared with her daughters or a sister with her younger siblings—was set aside or even lost.

Thus, during the 1960s (at the nadir of breastfeeding) in the United States and shortly thereafter in other countries (such as Australia and

Scandinavia), volunteer mother-to-mother breast-feeding support groups became a major source of assistance and information about how to breast-feed (Phillips, 1990). As the number of breastfeeding mothers increased, healthcare providers at first ignored these groups; later they came to appreciate them for the important role they played in helping mothers and in forcing the medical profession to consider lactation as a missing piece of prenatal and postpartum care.

As these volunteers promoted the art of breastfeeding, they also sought more knowledge of the science of lactation. La Leche League responded by providing research information to its group leaders, who serve as mother-to-mother helpers, and by publishing a quarterly newsletter, *Breastfeeding Abstracts*, which focuses exclusively on the scientific literature. Through La Leche League's professional liaison department, key individuals sought to cultivate and maintain communication links to health providers in local communities.

Out of this context, some experienced breastfeeding support group members began to look beyond what they could accomplish as volunteers. Many of these women sought to apply in a paid work setting what they had learned from many years of helping breastfeeding mothers. In 1982, La Leche League formed its Lactation Consultant Department. From this beginning grew the concept of the need for a new healthcare worker, and in 1985 the independent certification board, IBLCE, was formed. Shortly thereafter, the *Journal of Human Lactation* (*JHL*) began. Edited by Kathleen Auerbach from 1985 to 1996, by Jane Heinig from 1996 to 2012, and currently by Anne Merewood, *JHL* is peer reviewed, professionally published, and cited on international indices with a competitive Impact Factor score (Bailey, 2005; *Journal of Human Lactation*, 2013).

Do Lactation Consultants Make a Difference?

In this day of cost containment in health care, administrators want to know if lactation consultants are effective. Put simply, do interventions by lactation specialists and other healthcare providers make a difference in breastfeeding outcomes? Randomized controlled trials of breastfeeding interventions worldwide, most of which were conducted in developed countries, that were published in a meta-analysis commissioned by the U.S. Preventive Services Task Force (USPSTF) can be accessed at http://www.uspreventiveservicestaskforce.org/uspstf08/breastfeeding/brfdartfig3txt.htm (USPSTF, 2008). In the meta-analysis, breastfeeding promotion interventions significantly increased both short- and long-term exclusive breastfeeding rates. In a subgroup analysis, combining prenatal and postpartum interventions had a greater effect on these rates, and including some form of lay or peer support increased breastfeeding rates even more.

In addition to this meta-analysis, a Cochrane review—the "gold standard" of medical research—studied the effect of any extra support given to breastfeeding women. Lay and professional support together extended duration of breastfeeding, especially that of exclusive breastfeeding (Britton et al., 2007). Face-to-face counseling (Figure 1-1) is the most effective intervention in increasing not only exclusive breastfeeding rates but also the total duration of breastfeeding (Albernaz et al., 2003; Andaya et al., 2012; Witt et al., 2012).

If the data from the randomized controlled trials included in the meta-analysis and Cochrane review were translated to healthcare costs saved by

Figure 1-1 EARLY ASSISTANCE PROMOTES CONFIDENCE.

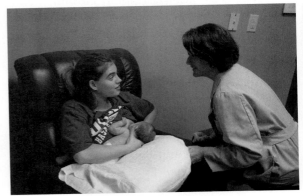

breastfeeding, the result would show that lactation services save the healthcare system enormous amounts of money through reduction in illnesses in both baby and mother. When rates of breastfeeding at hospital discharge were compared between facilities that employed certified lactation consultants and those that did not, those having LCs had a 2.28 times increase in the odds of breastfeeding at hospital discharge. Among women receiving Medicaid, there was a 4.13 increase (Castrucci et al., 2006).

Studies show that peer counselor interventions are also effective. Clearly, lactation services improve the health of the United States, but we have yet to document the extent of this effect in terms of money savings. We do know the estimated cost to U.S. society when medical recommendations for breastfeeding are not met: $13.6 billion for 10 infant illnesses and infections and 911 additional infant deaths per year (Bartick & Reinhold, 2010). In terms of maternal impact, 4981 excess cases of breast cancer, 13,946 heart attacks, and 53,847 cases of hypertension are estimated to occur when these recommendations are not met, compared to a cohort of 1.88 million U.S. women who optimally breastfed, leading to $17.4 billion in costs to society resulting from premature maternal deaths (Bartick et al., 2013).

Certification: International Board of Lactation Consultant Examiners

In 1981, experienced La Leche League leaders JoAnne Scott and Linda Smith were asked to develop a certification and training program for lactation consultants. This need derived from (1) an awareness that many healthcare providers discredited the value of the volunteer counselor because she was unpaid, (2) a need to establish minimum standards for individuals who were already providing LC services for a fee, and (3) the need for a knowledgeable healthcare team member who was responsible for lactation and breastfeeding care. A certification program was viewed as a way to recognize the important role of the volunteer and to provide a credential that identified knowledge and experience.

Scott and Smith assembled a small group of breastfeeding experts who had come to the field of lactation consulting through voluntary service, mostly through La Leche League. In 1984, these individuals gathered at a conference and concluded that legitimacy of the field would be heightened if minimal standards of knowledge and skills were recognized through a certification examination. Subsequently, a 62-member panel of experts was recruited and selected to serve as the respondent population for the first practice analysis and to develop the first exam blueprint with the guidance of a psychometrician. The work of this expert panel represented a broad-based practitioner and professional assessment of practice in the emerging profession of lactation consulting (Smith, personal communication, 2013).

The first examination was administered in July 1985 by the IBLCE. Since 1985, a psychometrically reviewed certification examination has been given annually to applicants who meet eligibility criteria for education and clinical training. To date, more than 26,000 candidates have been certified as International Board Certified Lactation Consultants (IBCLCs), the majority of whom live in Australia, Canada, Japan, South Korea, and the United States. Table 1-1 summarizes the number and regional

Table 1-1 NUMBER AND DISTRIBUTION OF IBCLCs

Year	World-wide	Americas Region	Asia Pacific Region	Europe/Middle East Region
2005	14,705	9305	3184	2216
2006	15,726	9726	3083	2917
2007	17,026	10,229	3464	3333
2008	18,032	10,554	3695	3783
2009	21,200	11,903	4754	4543
2010	22,736	12,827	4843	5066
2011	25,737	14,972	5076	5689
2012	26,815	15,929	5047	5839

Data from International Board of Lactation Consultant Examiners (IBLCE) www.iblce.org

distribution of completed IBLCE exams over 2005–2012 (IBCLE, 2013). In 2013, IBLCE administered the exam to 3660 candidates in 945 locations across 52 countries and territories in several languages. Recertification as an IBCLC is required every 5 years through the acquisition of continuing education credits or reexamination, and every 10 years by required reexamination. This dual-recertification option increases the likelihood that the IBCLC will stay current in knowledge and practice.

The IBCLC is the only international certification in breastfeeding and human lactation, awarded by an independently accredited organization. It has been accredited by the National Commission for Certifying Agencies (NCCA) since 1988—a mark of distinction for certification organizations (NCCA, 2013). IBLCE maintains a registry of IBCLCs who are currently certified. Employers, regulators, and the public, therefore, can confirm that an individual is currently certified. For more information on IBCLC certification, go to the International Board of Lactation Consultant Examiners' website at www.iblce.org.

Certification—a process by which an individual demonstrates advanced knowledge and/or experience in a specialty—is especially popular in the United States. More than 40 specialty certifications exist in the field of nursing alone, despite the fact that certification is a voluntary credential. Certified nurses and healthcare workers from across a wide variety of specialties consistently place a high value on certification (Niebuhr & Biel, 2007). Nurses in the United States and Canada who earned certification in a specialty area report feeling more confident and experiencing fewer errors in patient care since they were certified; thus certification may be a marker for excellence (Cary, 2000; Raudonis & Anderson, 2002).

Professional Association: International Lactation Consultant Association

About the same time that IBLCE certification began, the International Lactation Consultant

Association (ILCA) formed as the professional organization for IBCLCs and others supporting the member association's mission (ILCA, 2005). ILCA has played a vital role in professional development of the IBCLC and in promoting policies to protect and support breastfeeding, IBCLCs, and the IBCLC profession worldwide (Bailey, 2005). ILCA arose primarily through the grassroots vision and creativity of its founding members; by 2013, there were nearly 6000 individual members from 85 countries worldwide (Brooks, 2013).

ILCA's website is a rich and current source of information and resources of interest to lactation professionals; many items are translated into several languages. In addition, ILCA hosts an annual international conference, serves as a nongovernmental organization (NGO) in official relations with the World Health Organization (WHO), and publishes the peer-reviewed research periodical *Journal of Human Lactation*. Directories list IBLCE-certified ILCA members who (1) provide lactation care to mothers (searchable by location, anywhere in the world), (2) offer support to employers/workplaces with breastfeeding employees, and (3) are speakers/writers for educational or conference settings (ILCA, home page, n.d.).

In addition to individual members, ILCA has affiliates organized primarily by country, focusing on IBCLC issues of particular geopolitical interest. For example, the United States Lactation Consultant Association (USLCA) is the professional organization for ILCA members living in the United States; it publishes the journal *Clinical Lactation*. The Canadian Lactation Consultant Association and the Lactation Consultants of Australia and New Zealand represent the interests of ILCA members in those countries.

Gaining Clinical Experience

IBLCE certification requires a considerable number of clinical hours in direct care of the breastfeeding dyad: from 300 to 1000 clinical hours, preferably supervised by an experienced IBCLC. For specific criteria on qualifying under the IBLCE Pathways, go to http://iblce.org/certify/preparing-for-ibclc-certification/.

A healthcare professional who needs clinical hours to qualify to take the IBLCE certification examination under Pathway 1 should seek out a job where he or she will work with breastfeeding mothers. Working on a mother–baby unit in a hospital or in a community clinic setting are examples. Other candidates for Pathway 1 come from a mother-to-mother support background, meet the education requirements, and have acquired clinical experience through peer mentoring. Examples include La Leche League leaders, Australian Breastfeeding Association counselors, and peer counselors in the U.S. federal Women, Infants, and Children (WIC) program.

Not everyone who desires to work as a lactation consultant wishes to become a nurse or other type of health professional. Thus Pathway 2 covers direct-entry applicants who are in an academic lactation program that includes the required clinical training. Pathway 3 covers direct-entry applicants who come from other backgrounds, meet the educational requirements, and acquire their clinical experience in a formal arrangement supervised by experienced IBCLCs. Some of these arrangements are available at local hospitals or community settings or with IBCLCs in private practice. Box 1-1 provides general guidelines on mentoring lactation consultants, available on the ILCA website along with numerous other documents for clinical training programs: http://www.ilca.org/i4a/pages/index.cfm?pageid=3488.

BOX 1-1 MENTORING AND PRECEPTING LACTATION CONSULTANTS

Desired Qualities of a Mentor/Preceptor

- Acts as a role model and advocate
- Has leadership experience
- Is available and responsive
- Is willing to share expertise and insight
- Believes in the capabilities of the mentee/intern
- Motivates, supports, and enhances the mentee's/intern's development
- Has vision
- Is current in the knowledge of the field
- Knows how to access professional networks
- Seeks to enhance political awareness

Desired Qualities of a Mentee/Intern

- Has a desire to learn
- Has a capacity to accept constructive feedback and coaching
- Has an ability to identify personal and professional career goals
- Has a willingness to take risks
- Exhibits a desire for professional success
- Seeks challenging assignments and new responsibilities
- Actively seeks the advice and counsel of an experienced mentor/preceptor

Source: Modified from Lauwers, J. Mentoring and Precepting Lactation Consultants, International Lactation Consultant Association: http://www.ilca.org/i4a/pages/index.cfm?pageid=3488

Lactation Consultant Education

Because the IBCLC certification is relatively new (established in 1985), formalized lactation education programs, with approved curricula offered by independently accredited institutions of higher education, are not yet widely available. The Lactation Education Approval and Accreditation Review Committee (LEAARC) provides approval for individual short-term courses and classes on breastfeeding management and formulates recommendations to the Commission on Accreditation of Allied Health Education Programs (CAAHEP) for accreditation of an academic program (LEAARC, n.d.). LEAARC approval of short-term courses serves as a "reliable indicator of educational quality to employers, insurers, counselors, educators, governmental officials, and the public" (LEAARC, n.d., para. 2). LEAARC also has developed *Standards and Guidelines for the Accreditation of Lactation Education Programs*, available at www.leaarc.org.

Healthcare providers seeking to learn more about supporting breastfeeding families in their care can seek out the many other short-term courses in breastfeeding management that are available. For example, facilities seeking designation under the Baby-Friendly Hospital Initiative (BFHI) require all healthcare workers in maternal–child health to take a 20-hour course in basic breastfeeding management (WHO & UNICEF, 2009). Short-term courses may also be taken by those individuals seeking to provide mother-to-mother support, such as WIC peer counselors trained by the U.S. Department of Agriculture Food and Nutrition Service's Special Supplemental Nutrition Program for Women, Infants and Children (WIC) (U.S. Department of Agriculture, n.d.). In addition, IBCLC aspirants seeking to meet IBLCE examination requirements in lactation-specific education may seek out excellent short-term courses offering evidence-based information on breastfeeding support.

Ideally, every woman giving birth will receive timely and appropriate lactation care delivered by qualified providers. Clinicians and nurses working in maternal–child health will have education and training in basic breastfeeding management

(e.g., Association of Women's Health, Obstetric and Neonatal Nurses [AWHONN], 2008; also see United States Breastfeeding Committee [USBC] website http://www.usbreastfeeding.org/HealthCare /TrainingforHealthCareProfessionals/tabid/96 /Default.aspx for listing of several sources of healthcare professional training). Mothers will have timely access to IBCLCs when needed—for example, in higher-acuity situations (Mannel, 2011)—and will also have community support from experienced breastfeeding mothers, such as La Leche League leaders.

Hospital Lactation Programs

A New York state law mandated in 1984 that any institution providing care for new mothers and babies had to have at least one person on staff who was designated to serve as a resource for other staff members and to provide breastfeeding assistance to patients. The need for skilled lactation support in the hospital during the perinatal period and for any other hospital admission of a breastfeeding mother or child has been recognized by many healthcare organizations including the World Health Organization (2003), the U.S. Department of Health and Human Services (2011), the European Union (EU Project on Promotion of Breastfeeding in Europe, 2004), and the Australian Health Ministers' Conference (2009).

The 1990s could be characterized as the decade for widespread emergence of breastfeeding programs and clinics (Figure 1-2). Only a small number of hospitals in the United States had a lactation program in the early 1990s, but over the past two decades lactation programs have proliferated rapidly. Today, most hospitals and birth centers have lactation services staffed by certified lactation specialists, who have thus grown in numbers and visibility (Figure 1-3). Although some lactation expertise has long been integrated into midwifery practice in countries where midwives predominate, IBCLCs are now available in many countries.

Developing a Hospital Lactation Service

Providing quality lactation and breastfeeding care is an essential part of a hospital's maternal–newborn

Figure 1-2 BREASTFEEDING CLINIC.

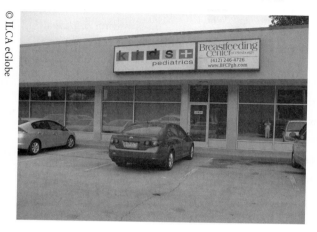

Figure 1-3 HOSPITAL LACTATION SERVICE.

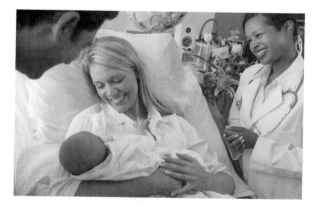

© Monkey Business Images/ShutterStock, Inc.

service. The Baby-Friendly Hospital Initiative provides the evidence-based guidelines for quality hospital care (WHO, 1998), and Baby-Friendly designated hospitals demonstrate improved breastfeeding outcomes across all racial and ethnic groups. (DiGirolamo, Grummer-Strawn, & Fein, 2008). The U.S. Surgeon General's Call to Action to Support Breastfeeding compels the healthcare system to ensure that maternity care practices are supportive of breastfeeding and to provide access to IBCLC services. The Joint

Commission (TJC) in the United States has adopted a quality core measure on exclusive breastfeeding that hospitals with greater than 1100 births per year will be required to report beginning in 2014 (TJC, 2013). The European Union's Blueprint for Action on Breastfeeding (EU Project of Promotion of Breastfeeding in Europe, 2004) expects all mothers to have affordable access to qualified lactation consultants. ILCA and IBLCE now award recognition to hospitals and community-based agencies that employ IBCLCs and provide training in breastfeeding management for other healthcare professionals. For a list of organizations that have received the IBCLC Care Award or for more information on the criteria, go to http://www.ibclccare.org/.

A key element in quality hospital lactation care is appropriate policy development and staff training. IBCLCs are ideally suited to work with a hospital's leadership team to develop evidence-based policies and education for nursing staff, including clinical competencies. Hospitals are particularly concerned with patient safety and risk management issues, both of which are increased when inadequate lactation care is provided, especially in high-acuity lactation situations (Table 1-2). Identifying mothers and children who are at higher risk for poor breastfeeding outcomes enables a hospital to allocate appropriate resources in a more timely fashion (Mannel, 2011, 2013).

Department heads particularly critical to securing support for a lactation program include the director of maternity nursing (who may oversee labor and delivery, mother–baby care, and sometimes the intensive care nursery), the director of the pediatric unit, and the chairman or medical director for obstetrics, pediatrics, and family medicine. If the institution has a midwifery service, the support of its director should also be sought.

Physicians remain influential figures in the hospital, although their power has diminished since the adoption of managed care; therefore, maintaining positive relations with physicians is critical for LCs. Even with managed care, the physician as "gatekeeper" plays a major role in the fiscal health of a hospital. If the physician's patients do not want to go to a particular hospital because it lacks certain amenities—such as a lactation service—the

Table 1-2 LACTATION ACUITY LEVELS FOR DETERMINING LACTATION RESOURCES

Acuity Level I	Level I acuity patients can be cared for by nursing staff who have basic breastfeeding knowledge and competency.
Maternal Characteristics	Basic breastfeeding education, routine management
	Latch/milk transfer appear optimal
	Maternal decision to routinely supplement
	Maternal decision to pump and feed expressed breastmilk (EBM)
	Maternal indecision regarding breastfeeding
	Mother can latch baby with minimal assistance
	Multiparous mother with healthy term baby and prior breastfeeding experience
Acuity Level II	Level II acuity patients should be cared for by RLC staff as soon as possible, or referral made to RLCs in the community. Early follow-up after discharge is critical.
Maternal Characteristics	Antenatal admission with increased risk of preterm delivery
	Cesarean section delivery
	Delayed breastfeeding initiation (defined as after 1 hour with routine vaginal delivery and after 2 hours with routine cesarean section)
	Maternal acute illnesses/conditions (e.g., preeclampsia, cardiomyopathy, postpartum depression, postpartum hemorrhage)
	Maternal age (mother < 18 years or > 35 years)
	Maternal chronic conditions (e.g., rheumatoid arthritis, systemic lupus erythematosus, hypertension, cancer, history of gastric bypass, obesity)
	Maternal cognitive impairment (e.g., mental retardation, Down syndrome, autism)
	Maternal endocrine disorders (e.g., polycystic ovary syndrome, infertility, thyroid disorders, diabetes)
	Maternal medication concerns
	Maternal physical disability (e.g., paraplegic, cerebral palsy, visual impairment, psychiatric)
	Maternal readmission (breastfeeding well established/noncritical issues)
	Maternal request
	Multiparous mother with history of breastfeeding difficulty
	Primiparous mother or first-time breastfeeding mother with healthy term baby
	Social/cultural issues (e.g., communication barriers, domestic/sexual abuse)
Infant Characteristics	Consistent LATCH score < 6 at day of discharge
	Breastfeeding Assessment Score ≤ 5
	Latch difficulties (e.g., pain)
	Infant readmission (breastfeeding well established/noncritical issues)
	Newborn birth trauma (e.g., cephalohematoma, shoulder dystocia)
	Suboptimal/inadequate milk transfer leading to medical recommendation to supplement

Table 1-2 LACTATION ACUITY LEVELS FOR DETERMINING LACTATION RESOURCES (CONTINUED)

Acuity Level III	Level III acuity patients need to be cared for by RLC staff while in hospital. These patients will require in-depth assessment and ongoing management. Early follow-up after discharge is critical.
Maternal Characteristics	Abscess/mastitis
	High maternal anxiety
	Induced lactation
	Maternal breast conditions (e.g., breast/nipple anomalies, glandular insufficiency, history of breast surgery)
	Maternal illness/surgery
	Maternal readmission (breastfeeding not well established and/or critical issues)
	Pathologic engorgement
Infant Characteristics	High-risk infant on mother–baby unit (e.g., late preterm, small or large for gestational age, multiple gestation)
	Hyperbilirubinemia
	Hypoglycemia
	Infant admission to neonatal intensive care unit
	Infant congenital anomalies
	Infant illness/surgery
	Infant oral/motor dysfunction (e.g., tight frenulum, hypotonia, or hypertonia)
	Infant readmission (breastfeeding not well established and/or critical issues)
	Infant weight loss > 7% of birth weight before discharge

Note: Acuity levels can change based upon assessment by the RLC or other healthcare team members.
Source: Modified from Mannel, R. J Hum Lact. 2011; 27, 163–170. Defining lactation acuity to improve patient safety and outcomes.

birthing service administrator, with the backing of physicians, may create such a program rather than lose patients to a competing institution. Supportive physicians are more likely to be mothers who breastfed, fathers of breastfed children, those building a new practice, and those from countries where breastfeeding is the norm.

If the institution has an employee health service or a women's health clinic, their supervisors should be informed of the proposal and asked for their support. Written proposals or documents that highlight how the new program will assist and support the services that are already being provided will help ensure their acceptance. For example, the head of employee health may be particularly interested in learning that the lactation program will include services to employees, such as a special place where employees returning to work after the birth of a baby can express milk or nurse their babies during work hours (Dodgson & Duckett, 1997). Many countries are now requiring employers to provide support for working breastfeeding mothers (International Labour Office, 2010; U.S. Department of Labor, 2010).

Resources

Determining the resources needed for a quality lactation program depends on the level of service provided by the hospital in other areas (Mannel & Mannel, 2006) and the goals of the lactation services. For example, does the hospital

Figure 1-4 OUTPATIENT
BREASTFEEDING CLINIC.

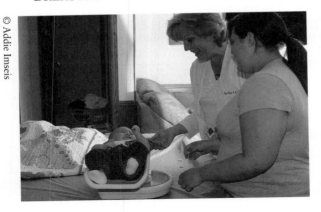

© Addie Imseis

have a neonatal intensive care unit, provide high-risk antepartum care, or have inpatient pediatric units? Does the hospital want a lactation service that provides telephone follow-up, outpatient care, or prenatal education (see Figure 1-4)? All of these services need to be factored into the equation when determining the necessary resources.

Jan Riordan has estimated three visits (one 20-minute initial visit and two 15-minute follow-ups) from a lactation consultant are needed, for a total of 50 minutes per dyad per day. Given these numbers, a lactation specialist would spend at least 8 hours each day to see 9 dyads on a mother–baby unit. This figure does not take into account time spent charting, having lunch, meetings, planning, and so on. Daily rounds on breastfeeding women may be feasible in a hospital in which the LC sees fewer than 9 patients per day; it may not be feasible if more than 9 breastfeeding mothers are housed in the maternity unit on a given day—unless there is more than one specialist in the service or staff members providing other care are trained to provide optimal lactation-related care as well, thus reserving the LC for mothers and babies needing additional help and as a resource for the staff (Angeron & Riordan, 2007).

Another author reported 2.6 full-time equivalent (FTE) LC positions (about 90 hours) were required for a hospital with 1600 deliveries (Hinson, 2000). These lactation consultants saw each breastfeeding mother every day but later, to keep up with the

demand for their services, they saw each breastfeeding mother once, and again only if there was a referral. In an effort to meet patient needs, it is not uncommon for LCs to volunteer additional time for which they are unpaid. Heinig (1998) addressed this issue as "closet consulting," warning that when the caseload is invisible to the employer, the LC's professional time is undervalued and may result in further limits on LC time.

The two reports cited previously relied on "educated guesses." Mannel and Mannel (2006) collected data from the lactation program's productivity reports at a tertiary care teaching hospital (4200 births per year). They measured actual hours worked by LCs over a 2-year period, allocated the hours to their respective activities, and developed ratios for optimal IBCLC staffing for each component of service. Optimal IBCLC staffing was calculated as follows:

- Mother–baby inpatient care requires 1 FTE per 783 breastfeeding couplets.
- Neonatal intensive care unit (NICU) inpatient care requires 1 FTE per 235 infant admissions.
- Mother–baby outpatient care requires 1 FTE per 1292 breastfeeding couplets discharged.
- NICU outpatient care requires 1 FTE per 818 breastfeeding infants discharged.
- Telephone follow-up requires 1 FTE per 3915 breastfeeding couplets or infants discharged.
- Education requires 0.1 FTE per 1000 deliveries.
- Program development and administration requires 0.1 FTE per 1000 deliveries.
- Research requires 0.1 to 0.2 FTE total.

Using these ratios, IBCLC staffing needs can be calculated for hospital staffing according to number of deliveries (Box 1-2). All three hospitals have inpatient service, follow-up telephone service and education, administration, and research. Table 1-3 is a calculation of the staffing needs for a hospital with 3000 births per year using the Mannel and Mannel (2006) model. A similar table for hospitals with 1000 and 6000 births per year can be found in their article in the *Journal of Human Lactation*. These data were utilized in the staffing recommendations released by the USLCA (2010) and the Association of Women's Health, Obstetric and Neonatal Nurses (2010).

Box 1-2 IBCLC Staffing Guidelines from the United States Lactation Consultant Association

Hospital with Level I Neonatal Service

The hospital with level I neonatal service would require 1.3 FTEs per 1000 deliveries per year for the inpatient setting. To include the breastfeeding rate in this calculation, multiply the FTEs calculated times the percentage of breastfeeding mothers in that facility.

Hospital with Level II Neonatal Service

The hospital with level II neonatal service would require 1.6 FTEs per 1000 deliveries per year for the inpatient setting. To include the breastfeeding rate in this calculation, multiply the FTEs calculated times the percentage of breastfeeding mothers in that facility.

Hospital with Level III (Tertiary Care) Neonatal Service

Based on the standard of a 20% preterm delivery rate (Mannel & Mannel, 2006), the tertiary care facility would require 1.9 FTEs per 1000 deliveries per year for the inpatient setting. To include the breastfeeding rate in this calculation, multiply the FTEs calculated times the percentage of breastfeeding mothers in that facility.

Source: Reproduced from United States Lactation Consultant Association IBCLC Staffing Recommendations. http://www.ilca.org/files/USLCA/Resources/Publications/IBCLC_Staffing_Recommendations_July_2010.pdf

---

Managing a Hospital Lactation Service

A quality lactation service requires dedicated positions for lactation consultants to ensure timely access to care. Some hospitals hire only IBCLCs who are also RNs and plan to use them in nursing staffing. When it is not busy in labor and delivery, then the IBCLC/RN can "do lactation." Unfortunately, this type of service leads to inconsistent access to care and increases risk management concerns. When census is higher and no lactation consultants are available, mothers are more likely to be discharged with inadequate knowledge of breastfeeding management or even knowledge of how to identify if their baby is feeding adequately (Centers for Disease Control and Prevention [CDC], 2011; Martens, Derksen, & Gupta, 2004; Paul et al., 2006).

In other hospitals that have dedicated lactation positions, nursing staff may stop providing basic breastfeeding care based on their belief that all breastfeeding care is handled by the lactation

consultant (Spatz, 2010). This type of environment is not effective either. As Spatz (2010, p. 500) said, "Educated nurses should be the first level of intervention for all breastfeeding women and their infants. If this occurred in all institutions, the burden on the LC would decrease, and the LC could focus on complex breastfeeding cases. Educated nurses can change institutional and community breastfeeding cultures."

In 2010, Mannel described an effective lactation service where the IBCLCs make lactation rounds each morning to identify high-acuity patients, using a daily lactation census and scripted rounding questions (see Box 1-3). Low-acuity breastfeeding couplets (level I) are managed by nursing staff, all of whom have training in basic breastfeeding management. The IBCLCs are then able to focus more effectively on higher-acuity breastfeeding couplets/patients (level II or III). This system represents a change from the hospital's previous method of relying only on referrals from physicians, nurses, and patients—a common practice in many hospitals.

Table 1-3 BREAKDOWN OF STAFFING FOR HOSPITAL LACTATION PROGRAM WITH 3,000 BIRTHS PER YEAR

Approx. number of births/yr = 3000 (68% initiate breastfeeding)

Approx. number of NICU admissions/yr = 400 (85% initiate breastfeeding)

One FTE =

1900 work hours (excluding vacations, sick days, etc.)

1292 hours direct consult time

608 hours indirect clinical time

FTE ratio is number of available direct consult work hours divided by the amount of hours per dyad.

For example, 1292 hours/FTE divided by 1.65 hrs of direct consult with each dyad = 783 dyads per LC FTE.

2040 births (68% breastfeeding of 3000) divided by 783 = the number of LC FTEs that are needed for direct consult inpatient care.

Category	FTE Ratio	Calculation	Number	FTEs
Inpatient	1:783	3000 × .68 = 2040	2040/783 =	2.6
Outpatient	1:1292	120 couples 120 hours (1 hr each)	1292/120 =	0.1
Telephone	1:3915	3000 × .60	1800/3915 =	0.45
NICU inpatient	1:235	400 × .85 85% initiate BF	340/235 =	1.44
Education	0.1:1000	3000 × .68	2040/1000 =	0.2
Program admin	0.1:1000	3000 × .68	2040/1000 =	0.2
Research/QA	0.2:1000	3000 × .68	2040/1000 =	0.4
Total				about 5.4

Source: Adapted from Mannel R, Mannel RS. Staffing for hospital lactation programs: recommendations from a tertiary care teaching hospital. J Hum Lact. 2006;22:409–417.

BOX 1-3 LACTATION ROUNDING SCRIPT FOR THE LACTATION CONSULTANT

Introduction	"Hi, Ms. Jones, I'm Paula, one of the registered lactation consultants here at OUMC and I'll just be in here for one or two minutes. I'm checking on all the new moms to see who is breastfeeding or wanting to breastfeed and who might need some extra help from us. Were you planning to breastfeed?" [or: "I see you've been doing some breastfeeding already…"]
Mother says, "I'm bottle-feeding" (i.e., exclusively formula-feeding)	"Well, you have a great nurse to help you with that. You know, your body will still make milk to feed your baby so you will have some breast fullness in 1–2 days. You can apply ice packs and take acetaminophen or ibuprofen if the swelling gets uncomfortable. It should get better in a couple of days. Here's one of our brochures in case you ever need to call us."

Mother says, "I'm breastfeeding"	"Great, then I have just a few quick questions to help us decide who might need a visit from us later today…"
Questions for breastfeeding mothers	"Is this your first baby?"
	If multiparous: "Have you breastfed any of your others?"
	"Have you had to give any formula?" (i.e., Has her baby been EBF so far?)
	"Have you had any nipple or breast pain when your baby is nursing?" If yes, rate on pain scale. (Pain scale = 1–10, with 10 being most severe.)

Results from rounding and identifying high-acuity patients have improved quality of care, lactation staff productivity, and employee satisfaction on the lactation team. As one IBCLC said, "Rounds make us more efficient… I know where to start." This model has been adopted by many hospital lactation programs.

The Unique Characteristics of Counseling Breastfeeding Women

There are unique aspects of working with breast-feeding women that differ from other aspects of health care. Breastfeeding is an emotion-laden subject for almost anyone who has had a child, whether the new mother or the healthcare provider. Some professionals remain concerned about making mothers feel guilty by encouraging breastfeeding, so they abdicate this important responsibility completely. Others counsel mothers by relating their own personal experiences, whether positive or negative. Mothers deserve objective, evidence-based information to help them make informed decisions, such as whether to breastfeed at all, or whether to supplement with formula when the mother is not sure if her baby is getting enough sustenance. Mothers who do not reach their breastfeeding goals tend to blame themselves, when often it is the lack of timely and skilled support that made breastfeeding difficult, if not impossible.

This emotional context makes breastfeeding counseling, like sex counseling or childbirth education,

unusually sensitive. Healthcare workers assisting breastfeeding families must be especially intuitive, caring listeners and advisors. For more information on communication and counseling skills, see other sources such as Lauwers and Swisher's (2010) *Counseling the Nursing Mother: A Lactation Consultant's Guide* or Lauwers's (2012) chapter in *ILCA's Core Curriculum for Lactation Consultant Practice*.

Roles and Responsibilities

The LC is responsible to the mothers she sees to provide up-to-date, accurate information and appropriate assistance. Quality practice and service are core responsibilities of any profession in regard to the public. ILCA standards of practice are measures or levels of quality that are models for the conduct and evaluation of practice (ILCA, 2013).

LCs report that the majority of their time is spent in direct care of clients. The role of the LC may closely parallel that of the clinical nurse specialist, in that it requires in-depth clinical knowledge and expertise in a particular area. Gibbins et al. (2000) describe a model of the nurse practitioner (NP) or clinical nurse specialist (CNS) in the role as a lactation consultant in a breastfeeding clinic. This advanced practice role encompasses key dimensions of the advanced practice model: research, leadership, education, and clinical practice. Like the clinical specialist, the LC does the following:

- Gives direct care
- Teaches
- Consults
- Conducts or assists in conducting research

Giving breastfeeding mothers consistent breast-feeding information is vital. Many times mothers identify support received from healthcare providers as the single most important intervention in the healthcare system in helping them breastfeed (Taveras et al., as cited in Shealy et al., 2005, p. 15). The patient takes for granted that the healthcare professional advising her is giving her accurate information and "new mothers rarely request care different from that offered them by health professionals" (Shealy et al., 2005, p. 1). If confusion or controversy is found among the staff, healthcare providers cannot expect the patient to become knowledgeable and comfortable with learning mother–infant tasks. Staff and clinician training in basic breastfeeding management increases the likelihood that the healthcare team will provide consistent information.

A leadership function of the LC, whether based in a hospital or the community, is policy development. Identifying needed policies related to breastfeeding and ensuring they are evidence based is an important element that lays the foundation for a breastfeeding/family-friendly environment and optimal patient care (ILCA, n. d.; WHO, 2003).

Stages of Role Development

Roles of health professionals have been extensively studied and shown to progress through stages of development. For example, Benner (1984) used the Dreyfus and Dreyfus (1980) model of skill acquisition to describe the progression of skills and competencies of nurses in the clinical setting. This model—which outlines a structure for the metamorphosis that occurs as nurses persevere in their practice—can also apply to lactation consultants. According to Benner (1984), there are five stages of role acquisition:

- Novice: Develops technical skills, has a narrow scope of practice, needs a mentor
- Advanced beginner: Enhances clinical competencies, develops diagnostic reasoning and clinical decision-making skills, begins to incorporate research findings into practice
- Competent: Expands the scope of practice, becomes competent in diagnostic reasoning and clinical skills, senses nuances, develops organizational skills

- Proficient: Achieves the highest level of clinical expertise, conducts or directs research projects, acts as a change agent, uses a holistic approach, interprets nuances
- Expert: Global scope of practice, consults widely, empowers patients and families, serves as a mentor

In following Benner's progression from novice to expert, LCs will spend more time as consultants and in scholarly work as they gain experience in the field (Auerbach, Riordan, & Gross, 2000). Because the role of the lactation consultant is relatively new, other health providers may be unclear about what to expect of this healthcare team member. Some nursing managers may be unclear as to the competency of an IBCLC versus an RN/IBCLC. All IBCLCs should be clinically competent as outlined in the IBLCE's (2012a) *Clinical Competencies for the Practice of International Board Certified Lactation Consultants*. This document is suitable for verifying the competency of any IBCLC during orientation to a clinical position (available at http://iblce.org/resources/professional-standards/).

Lactation Consultants in the Community Setting

Breastfeeding is a public health imperative. It was identified by the U.S. Surgeon General in her 2011 *Call to Action to Support Breastfeeding* as "the best source of infant nutrition and immunologic protection, [providing] remarkable health benefits to mothers as well" (U.S. Department. of Health and Human Services, 2011, p. v). The CDC's Division of Nutrition, Physical Activity, and Obesity "is committed to increasing breastfeeding rates throughout the United States and to promoting and supporting optimal breastfeeding practices toward the ultimate goal of improving the public's health" (CDC, n.d. para. 1). The Baby-Friendly Hospital Initiative's *Ten Steps to Successful Breastfeeding* have been shown to increase breastfeeding initiation and duration; Step 10 says, "Foster the establishment of breastfeeding support groups and refer mothers to them on discharge from the hospital or birth center" (Baby-Friendly USA, n.d.).

Because of this heightened awareness of the importance of breastfeeding support, both access to highly skilled lactation care in the community and ongoing breastfeeding support for mothers are important. Women's preventive healthcare protections outlined in the 2010 Affordable Care Act are intended to provide, at no out-of-pocket expense to U.S. women with health insurance, "comprehensive lactation support and counseling, by a trained provider during pregnancy and/or in the postpartum period, and costs for renting breastfeeding equipment (U.S. Department of Health and Human Services, Human Resources and Services Administration, n.d., para. 4). This community-based health care differs from hospital-based care in that the healthcare provider works with the mother over the long term—throughout her pregnancy, childbirth, and postpartum course; thus community-based healthcare workers have an advantage over those working in the hospital in that they see the mother and her family in their total environment. Someone once described this as seeing a whole movie, whereas in the hospital the healthcare provider sees only one frame. Being in the family home gives a much wider perspective on the mother's needs that might not otherwise be apparent. Moreover, community-based services are organized around a system of interdisciplinary resources. A community health nurse may work with low-income mothers who are eligible for many different programs of assistance besides breastfeeding support.

Worksite Lactation Programs

Corporate lactation programs pay off. Women prefer to work at jobs where the breastfeeding woman is welcomed. Not only that, but breastfeeding mothers miss less work than mothers who are formula-feeding (Cohen, Mrtek, & Mrtek, 1995). As a result, many corporate offices are becoming "breastfeeding friendly," offering pumping rooms and multiuser pumps. Mothers working full-time spend less than 1 hour over the course of one workday expressing breastmilk. The *Business Case for Breastfeeding* published by the Office on Women's Health (2008) is an excellent resource for employers and employees and is available online.

Medical Clinics/Offices

A growing number of physicians are emphasizing breastfeeding in their practices. For some, this entails advocating for breastfeeding among patients in their general practice (family practice, obstetrics, or pediatrics) and providing staff to assist mothers to be successful. For other physicians, their general practice also becomes a consulting practice for more complex breastfeeding problems referred by lactation consultants or other physicians. A small number of physicians are developing breastfeeding and lactation specialty clinics or programs either in an academic setting or as a private practice. The specialty clinics serve as tertiary referral practices for complicated medical conditions of mother and baby, for conditions that require prescription medications, or for minor procedures that may be indicated (e.g., frenulotomy for tongue-tie). Such tertiary centers often rely upon the close working relationships of the physicians with other non physician lactation consultants.

Physicians, especially pediatricians, realize the value of having staff who are knowledgeable about breastfeeding and can quickly and effectively work with breastfeeding women in their practice; thus many lactation consultants are employed in the medical office. Their responsibilities include answering phone calls from breastfeeding women, making home visits, and working with the physician during postpartum visits to the medical office and while making hospital rounds. The physician office usually pays the lactation consultant a salary; however, some IBCLCs may do their own billing, particularly if they are also advanced practice nurses.

Professional Lactation Care and Volunteer Counselors

Breastfeeding support does not always require professional lactation care. The mother/client will obtain the best in comprehensive care when IBCLCs, volunteer breastfeeding support counselors, and other healthcare or program service providers all work together to provide support.

While volunteer counselors and IBCLCs can offer general support to mothers, the scope of practice and clinical competencies for the IBCLC include skill at assessing both mother- and infant-related lactation issues, as well as an ethical duty to protect the breastfeeding relationship (IBLCE, 2011, 2012a, 2012b). Volunteer counselors are an excellent source of general support for mothers, offering preventive healthcare information pertaining to breastfeeding and lactation. They also spend more time giving long-term assistance as the child ages, whereas the IBCLC may see clients/patients only in a clinic or hospital setting. It is not uncommon for a mother to continue to receive assistance and caring concern from a volunteer counselor throughout the entire lactation course; only rarely will an IBCLC meet with a client regularly during that entire period. Instead, IBCLC contact may be sporadic, initiated by the client/patient when a question or concern requiring specific clinical skills to assess or resolve a problem arises.

Volunteer breastfeeding helpers and lactation specialists can assist one another (Thorley, 2000). The volunteer may have seen a certain mother in her own home and, therefore, may be able to alert the IBCLC working in a hospital, doctor's office, or clinic to elements of the mother's home life that may bear on her lactation course. The IBCLC, in turn, may serve as a referral source for persons with complex problems. When the IBCLC works in a medical center where ongoing research is part of this role, he or she helps generate new knowledge. Both the volunteer and the paid IBCLC can review materials written for clients/patients. The volunteer may be sensitive to ongoing issues that crop up after the mother has left the hospital, including those that the mother may choose not to mention to her healthcare providers. The IBCLC may be aware of aspects of the healthcare system that influence breastfeeding.

Mentoring and Networking

Mentoring plays a major role in any clinically based profession, especially a new specialty. A mentor (whether serving by informal or formal arrangement) is a trusted counselor, guide, or coach for the student/intern, and fills this role over a long period of time. Mentors nurture the novice's growth with advice, information, and support (Altman, 2010;

ILCA, 2012; Lauwers, 2007). The early pioneers in this relatively new field are now the teachers and mentors of novice IBCLCs (Wiessinger, 2003). Educational programs with a clinical component are rare at this early stage in the evolution of LCs, and supervised clinical preceptorships are difficult to obtain. Shadowing experienced lactation specialists in one's area, however, is an excellent way to hone clinical skills. Students in rural areas with fewer qualified mentors may need to travel to visit the work setting of a colleague for mentoring purposes. The IBLCE defines the stages of training that a student will achieve during supervised clinical mentoring: observation, supervised practice, and independent practice with mentor nearby. See Pathway 3 in the *Plan Approval Guide 2013*, at http://www.iblce.org /preparing-for-ibclc-certification#Description%20 of%20the%20Pathways.

Networking, whereby members of a group exchange information and get help in solving problems, is a valuable mechanism for gaining and sharing expertise. When a difficult case arises, IBCLCs can use local in-person gatherings, telephone, and e-mail lists to gain insight from colleagues (while being careful, of course, to protect client/patient privacy). Networking can identify job openings, colleagues who will cover for one another, and referrals for clients needing equipment or specialized help. Networking also enhances advocacy efforts that seek to change systems and improve methods of providing care.

Opportunities to communicate with others also abound on the Internet, especially with social media networks, which are, in the early 21st century, a predominant means of fact gathering and communication. A forerunner of such interactions was LACT-NET, a worldwide breastfeeding e-mail list with more than 3000 subscribers in English, and a sister list in German (LACTNET-DE). Electronic communication is inexpensive and connects professionals in far-flung parts of the world with diverse cultural perspectives. Being able simply to vent and obtain sympathetic commiseration provides validation for the hard-working but perhaps isolated practitioner. The Internet has allowed for an explosion in the availability of valuable, evidence-based practice-guiding websites, research articles, and other resources.

Documentation

It is the responsibility of the lactation specialist, regardless of where he or she practices, to chart each contact with clients and to provide complete reports to referring physicians and other healthcare providers (IBLCE, 2010; Williams, 1995). Almost all record keeping involves using a computer; thus computer skills are a necessity for healthcare workers. As in other healthcare practices, computers can be used to generate records, reports, and charts that do the following:

- Provide other health workers with valuable information
- Reflect quality of care delivered (quality assurance, continuous quality improvement)
- Highlight sometimes subtle observations or findings
- Validate health services for insurance companies to determine reimbursement
- Provide data that can be used for research
- Serve as evidence in a legal dispute

In the hospital, the mother's and infant's charts are clinical records that contain information about the hospital stay and all contacts with everyone involved in their care. Because the mother and infant usually have separate charts, it is often necessary to "double chart." At the same time, care plans tend to be geared toward the mother, because it is she who is taught and the baby who is the recipient of her learning.

Health professionals use computers or smart phones to look up medical information and to document their interventions. Free and fee-based software and applications ("apps") for coding, charting, and medication information are available online. The most commonly used methods of charting are narrative charting and problem-oriented charting. Flow sheets and standard care plans that are individualized are becoming more popular, however, as they reduce paperwork and save time (and money).

Narrative Charting

Narrative documentation uses a diary or story format to document client-care events. A simple paragraph describes the client's status and the care that was given. Narrative notes, sometimes called progress notes, are used less frequently now, owing to the adoption of flow sheets and clinical care plans that capture the routine aspects of care. Narrative notes (Box 1-4) can be easily combined with flow sheets or any other client record.

Problem-Oriented Charting

Charting based on a problem uses a structured problem list and logical format for each entry in the medical record. The format used in problem-oriented charting is called the SOAP or SOAPIE method. Each letter stands for a different phase of the process: subjective data, objective data,

BOX 1-4 AN EXAMPLE OF A NARRATIVE NOTE

Date	Time	Progress note
05–22–03	0800	Infant alert. Rooting and suckling movements noted. Infant latched on breast and suckled effectively until asleep. Breastfeeding assessment score 9/10.
05–22–03	1500	Discussed basic breastfeeding information including normal infant elimination patterns to watch for after discharge. Mother given written materials on sore nipples, engorgement, use of breast pump, and breastmilk storage.
05–23–03	1100	Explained that a follow-up call will be made 2 to 3 days after discharge. Mother will have the option of a home visit.

BOX 1-5 EXAMPLE SOAP NOTE

1. Subjective = what mother tells you
   a. For example: *Mom c/o nipple pain and not sure if baby is getting enough.*

2. Objective = what LC saw and did, and information from medical record (e.g., interventions, education, mother return demonstration)
   a. For example: *P2B2 mom, term infant <48 hrs old, output WNL to date (2 voids, 4 stools), baby is 8% below birth weight. Maternal pain = 8 out of 10.*
   b. *Baby latched with areolar compression, rhythmic sucking, audible swallowing. Adjusted positioning and latch to decrease pain and increase milk removal. Mom needed moderate assistance with positioning and latch.*
   c. *LATCH Score = 8 (L2A2T2C1H1).*
   d. *Breasts: full, heavy, milk easily expressed.*
   e. *Nipples: everted, compressible, midline cracks.*
   f. *Educated re: s/s adequate infant intake, position and latch, newborn nutrition in 1st 48 hrs, milk production.*

3. Assessment = identify the problem; YOUR assessment of what the situation is (a lactation diagnosis)
   a. Example for a normal mother–baby couplet, IF you assessed the mother's breasts or baby at breast: *Transitioning to Lactogenesis II. Effective breastfeeding with milk transfer.*
   b. For a NICU mother: *Lactogenesis I apparent, at risk for compromised milk production due to lactation risk factors: preterm delivery, PIH, GDM, late initiation of milk expression.*

4. Plan = what is the goal and plan to get there
   a. With a normal breastfeeding couplet with effective breastfeeding: *EBF on cue of baby or at least 8×/day, monitor output, call (community resources) prn.*
   b. For a NICU mother: *Express milk 8–10×/day, use hand expression/hands-on pumping, monitor milk volume collected, practice kangaroo care with baby daily as possible, acquire pump for use after discharge, request LC support when baby ready to initiate direct breastfeeding. Call prn.*

assessment, plan, interventions, and evaluation of care (see Box 1-5). When the LC functions as a consultant, problem-oriented charting is more appropriate.

In private practice, the completeness of reports also assists the referring healthcare worker to understand the "how" as well as the "why" of an LC's practice and methods. Reporting provides a database for all types of information (e.g., an increase in the number of referrals from a particular physician's practice). Early referrals may be for one or two common problems, whereas tracking over an extended time period may reveal that later referrals deal with a wider variety of problems.

Electronic Health Records

A patient's lactation information is usually incorporated into existing information systems (IS) in clinics and hospitals. Lactation professionals need to work closely with IS technicians to make sure that the format employed for electronic healthcare records accommodates breastfeeding information, especially if mother–infant care is involved. Transition to such a system takes significant amounts of time and resources, and often engenders a great deal of staff frustration. Each facility, outpatient lactation clinic, private lactation practice, medical office, and hospital will have unique needs.

The Cincinnati Children's Center for Breastfeeding Medicine developed a lactation-friendly electronic health record (EHR) at its pediatric facility, which has a breastfeeding clinic. New forms specific to breastfeeding are (1) maternal history, (2) maternal exam, (3) infant feeding history, and (4) breastfeeding assessment. This organization's computer system includes electronic prescriptions, printed patient handouts, and telephone notes (List et al., 2008). LCs will find the computer pages and drop-down lists in this article to be helpful for developing their own computerized records.

Clinical Care Plans

A clinical care plan provides basic information about client assessment, diagnosis, and planned interventions. It also offers a guide for care, establishes continuity of care, and represents a means of communication among all caregivers. Two types of care plans may be created: individual and standard. Individual care plans are developed "from scratch" for each client based on her specific needs. A standard care plan is a preprinted plan of care for a group of patients within the same diagnosis. Because each standard care plan must be tailored according to the needs of a particular client, they are designed to include space for adding information.

The Joint Commission requires a care plan for each patient in the hospital as a necessity for accreditation; however, the plan of care can be computer generated, be preprinted, or appear in progress notes or standards of care (American Nurses Association, 1991). Care plans are legal requirements of practice and may also serve as protocols or standards of care.

Traditionally, individual care plans are divided into columns. Column headings change over the years to reflect new ideas in nursing, and some column labels are preferred over others. In this text, for instance, the clinical care plans include assessment, interventions, and rationale. Other commonly used labels are "problem," "evaluation," "nursing diagnosis," "patient outcomes," "nursing action," or simply "intervention-evaluation." Box 1-6 provides an example of a nursing diagnosis and nursing care plan. The critical care path or clinical path is a commonly used type of care plan in hospitals. These paths, which are abbreviated care plans that focus on the client's length of stay in the hospital, integrate infant feeding into the overall care plan.

Legal Concerns

As credentialed allied healthcare providers, IBCLCs will take care to use best practices in clinical care, to abide by the ethical rules of their profession, to stay within their scope of practice and clinical competencies as lactation professionals, and to follow the legal requirements of the workplace setting. Liability may result when the mother or baby is placed at risk, even if the IBCLC is following a physician's order. While no caregiver is immune from litigation (even excellent clinicians can be named in a specious lawsuit), excellence in professional practice is the best way to reduce such risks (Miller, 2006).

The following guidelines suggest ways to avoid liability:

- Carry professional liability (or malpractice) insurance, covering all of your practice settings. If you are named in a suit, the insurance entitles you to legal counsel and advice.
- Keep up-to-date on new research findings and clinical practices. Read current relevant articles, network with respected colleagues, attend live or online conferences.
- Use mother-centered care with all of your patients/clients, meeting each woman's needs and supporting her choice after she has been offered evidence-based information and consultation. People tend to sue healthcare providers when they feel they were not treated with respect and dignity.
- Thorough documentation, as close to the time of the intervention/assessment as possible, will verify your excellence in care. Document development of the care plan, suggested interventions, and the rationale for doing so. Methodically record updates and revisions to the plan, based on follow-up contacts (often made by phone).
- In the newborn period at the hospital or birthing center, a latch and feed by the infant

Box 1-6 Nursing Interventions • Nursing Care Plan *Lactation Counseling*

COUNTY OF ORANGE • HEALTH CARE AGENCY • FIELD NURSING
NURSING INTERVENTIONS • NURSING CARE PLAN

Client's Name:_____   Client's Number:_____

Lactation Counseling — 5244

DEFINITION: Use of an interactive helping process to assist in maintenance of successful breastfeeding.

ACTIVITIES:	DATE:						
Determine knowledge base about breastfeeding							
Educate parent(s) about infant feeding for informed decision making							
Provide information about advantages and disadvantages of breastfeeding							
Correct misconceptions, misinformation, and inaccuracies about breastfeeding							
Determine mother's desire and motivation to breastfeed							
Provide support of mother's decisions							
Give parent(s) recommended education material, as needed							
Inform parent(s) about appropriate classes or groups for breastfeeding (e.g., La Leche League)							
Evaluate mother's understanding of infant's feeding cues (e.g., rooting, sucking, and alertness)							
Determine frequency of feedings in relationship to baby's needs							
Monitor maternal skill with latching infant to the nipple							
Evaluate newborn suck/swallow pattern							
Demonstrate suck training, as appropriate							
Teach mother about:							
• Relaxation techniques, including breast massage							
• Ways of increasing rest, including delegation of household tasks and ways of requesting help							
• Record keeping of length and frequency of nursing sessions							
• Infant stool and urination patterns							
• Adequacy of breast emptying with feeding							
• Quality and use of breastfeeding aids							
• Appropriateness of breast pump use							
• Formula information for temporary low supply problems							
• Skin integrity of nipples							
• Nipple care							
• Relieving breast congestion							
• Applying warm compresses							
• Signs of problems to report to health care practitioner							
• How to relactate							
• Continuing lactation upon return to work or school							
• Signs of readiness to wean							
• Options for weaning							
• Alternative methods of feeding							
• Contraception							

Source: Reproduced from Parris KM. Integrating nursing diagnosis, interventions, and outcomes in public health nursing practice. Nurs Diag. 1999;10:49–56.

at the breast should be assessed and documented before the mother and baby are discharged. If this has not occurred, the IBCLC should make certain the baby's primary healthcare provider is apprised of the situation. The mother and baby may be allowed to stay a day or two longer; if not, the discharge care plan should describe how the mother can know when breastfeeding is going well and how she can access support and expert care if she is unsure about its effectiveness. Immediate follow-up care by the IBCLC might include a daily phone call, helping the mother to schedule an early visit to the baby's physician, or an outpatient consult or home visit—or all three.

• Refer to someone else if the situation calls for expertise you do not have in special situations.

People tend to become disenchanted with their healthcare providers (and are more likely to sue) not because of clinical actions, but rather because the patient/client felt uninformed, ignored, or rudely treated. Therefore, the most effective protection against such actions is establishing clinical rapport and forging a mutually respectful relationship (Miller, 2006). The lactation specialist's pattern of practice should seek to avoid causing the mother, the baby, or any other member of the client's family any emotional distress as a result of words said, reports written, or other actions taken.

A clearly written, detailed record of the healthcare provider's actions, initial recommendations, and follow-up assistance is one of the most effective ways of avoiding legal scrutiny. Well-written, complete reports will allow the other healthcare providers in your community to become familiar with your standards of excellence. Information that is sent in a timely and professional manner may lead to future client/patient referrals to the IBCLC. While charts and client records are considered admissible in the case of a lawsuit, clear records can also prevent cases from going beyond the discovery phase and into the courthouse. Lawsuits often are won or lost based on what appears in the written or digitized record.

The IBCLC who works in a doctor's office, clinic, or hospital may be considered an employee who is covered in an "umbrella" professional liability policy for the office/institution. The IBCLC in private practice must obtain her own insurance policy coverage. Members of CLCA and USLCA have access to professional liability insurance coverage at a reasonable cost as a membership benefit. Although legal action against an IBCLC is rare, it does occur; therefore, all individual practitioners need to consider how they will protect themselves (and their personal/family assets) against protracted litigation, and even a judgment.

Confidentiality

Maintaining confidentiality and protecting the privacy of the mother, baby, and family is a primary healthcare provider responsibility. It is part of the IBCLC's professional conduct code, clinical competencies, and scope of practice (IBLCE, 2011, 2012a, 2012b) and is identified by the professional association as a standard of best practices (ILCA, 2013). To fail to preserve confidentiality is an invasion of privacy and a tort (wrongful act) that occurs when information is revealed without permission to someone not entitled to know it.

Privacy obligations are also imposed by federal regulatory law in the United States, enforceable by civil and criminal sanctions. The Health Insurance Portability and Accountability Act (HIPAA) of 1996, and the subsequent requirements under the 2009 Health Information Technology for Economic and Clinical Health (HITECH) Act, are intended to standardize and protect the communication of electronic health information between healthcare providers and health insurers. The regulations are very clear: protect the privacy and security of the patient/client (Health Insurance Portability and Accountability Act, 2002; Omnibus Final Rule [HITECH], 2013).

Intellectual Property Rights

The IBLCE Code of Professional Conduct (IBLCE CPC) contains a principle specifically mandating IBCLC respect for intellectual property rights (IBLCE, 2011). While all people around the world should respect all laws, the IBLCE CPC provision means that IBCLCs can be sanctioned under the disciplinary procedures of their profession in addition to whatever liability they may assume under the laws of their country. Intellectual property covers patents, trademarks (including certification marks and service marks), trade secrets, and copyright law. For IBCLCs, copyright is the form of intellectual property law most likely to affect professional practice, as these consultants typically rely heavily on written, audio, and visual images in education and support of breastfeeding families. Unless materials created by others are clearly marked as available for redistribution, permission *must* be sought from the creator *before* the material can be reproduced, distributed, performed, displayed, licensed, communicated, or broadcast (Brooks, 2013).

Note that copyright law is not concerned with assembling proper citations in professional or scholarly writing. Academic, clinical, and professional rigor require appropriate attribution, in a bibliography, of any materials used to help inform the knowledge, thoughts, and conclusions of the practitioner. It is important to acknowledge the original creator or provider of written material, slides/photographs, video clips, Internet sites, blogs, illustrations, online courses, and other materials.

Note, too, that the IBCLC has the additional requirement, also unrelated to copyright law, under IBLCE CPC Principle 3.1, to obtain *prior, written consent* from the mother for *any* photograph, recording, or taping of her or her baby. Even if the image will be stored and viewed only by the IBCLC (perhaps to measure how interventions are helping to promote healing of nipple trauma), prior written consent is required.

The following basic concepts apply when using other people's original, copyright-protected materials:

- Seek authorization (permission) of the creator/source to reproduce, present, record, broadcast, translate, or adapt materials protected by copyright. A work is considered copyright-protected as soon as it exists in tangible form. The copyright-holder does not have to file it with the U.S. Copyright Office (although doing so fixes in time the creator's rights—a critical element when enforcing rights).
- There is no official form or format for seeking permission to reuse another person's materials. A phone call, e-mail, letter, or fax may be used for this purposes, but the requestor should always keep a record of the contact. Indicate who you are, the conditions under which reproduction is sought and will be used, and whether there is any commercial aspect to the reuse.
- Credit summaries of research findings or ideas to the original authors or copyright owners; indicate when adaptations have been made.
- Users of another's work are generally limited to one photocopy or download per person; making several copies even for educational, noncommercial purposes is not allowed.
- Quote directly from the original source, citing the exact page or paragraph where the quote is found. Use the citation style required of your workplace or academic institution; often a quotation of five or fewer typewritten lines should be enclosed in quotation marks, followed by a reference. Some styles require quotations of lengthier material to be indented in addition to having adequate citation (U.S. Copyright Office, 2012).

Legal issues for IBCLCs are discussed generally by Priscilla Bornmann (2013) in *Core Curriculum for Lactation Consultant Practice*, third edition, and by Elizabeth Brooks (2013) in *Legal and Ethical Issues for the IBCLC*.

Ethics

Ethical decisions are a routine, inherent part of lactation practice. Legal requirements for the IBCLC (and all healthcare providers) may be characterized as black-and-white, applicable to all practitioners equally. Ethics analysis looks at the gray: the considerations and evaluations of what is "right and wrong" differ with each instance, as the facts and players change (Brooks, 2013; Noel-Weiss, Cragg, & Woodend, 2013). The IBLCE Code of Professional Conduct (2011) is a "must," describing mandatory professional behaviors by the practitioner, whereas the ILCA Standards of Practice (2013) are a "should," describing voluntary best practices. The purpose of these documents, along with the mandatory ("must") IBLCE Scope of Practice (2012b) and Clinical Competencies (2012a), is to provide guidance to IBCLCs in their professional practice. The IBLCE Code of Professional Conduct is an ethical code built on the premise that it is in the best interests of the IBCLC profession, and serves to protect the health, welfare, and safety of the public, to have required minimum standards of acceptable conduct. IBCLC certificants agree to abide by these principles, and are subject to disciplinary action for failure to do so (IBLCE, 2011).

Ethical Questions in Lactation Practice

Different personalities, ethical obligations, and value systems may come into play in the LC's practice, complicating judgment or limiting neutrality. Many times there is no clear right or wrong course of action in trying to resolve ethical dilemmas. Consider the following issues:

- Whether to attend a continuing education lunch sponsored and paid for by a formula company. Attendees may also receive other free products.

- Whether to distribute free samples of formula or coupons to breastfeeding women who are being discharged from the birth setting. Do IBCLCs employed at the facility have a right to refuse to distribute these items?
- Whether to file a complaint against a colleague who transferred client files out of the health agency without prior consent, thereby failing to protect privacy and security under HIPAA/HITECH regulations. What are the circumstances surrounding this incident? Was it intentional? Was the offender aware of privacy regulations ? Did any harm come of the action—that is, was, in fact, any client/ patient's privacy compromised?
- How to offer evidence-based information and support for the breastfeeding mother who is a smoker, who is a user of illicit drugs, who seeks to informally share breastmilk with her friend, or who does not want to express milk for her hospitalized, premature baby.
- Whether to write an article with evidence-based information about breastfeeding for mothers that will be published in a magazine or on a website that also carries ads for formula, bottles, and teats.

Ethics considerations are relevant for lactation specialists, in part because this is a relatively new profession in health care. As such, the public is just now becoming aware of LCs, their special knowledge and skills, and the role they play and the impact they have in the maternal–child and public health fields (ILCA & Henderson, 2011). Our professional behaviors contribute to IBCLC acceptance by the public as a welcomed, respected discipline.

The nature of IBCLC practice involves assessment of the mother (including touching her breasts) and assessment of the infant (including touching the mother's precious baby). The birth of a child is a major family and life event. The circumstances surrounding it will be remembered (for good or ill) by the mother and her family for years to come. Further, a mother is emotionally vulnerable during and after childbirth. The IBCLC holds a place of great privilege and honor to be welcomed into this close circle of family members celebrating a birth, and struggling perhaps with normal concerns of parenthood. Technologies used in lactation practice have expanded dramatically in the last quarter century. New families need guidance, free from conflict of interest on the part of the healthcare provider, as to the appropriate use of such devices.

International Code of Marketing of Breast-milk Substitutes ("WHO Code")

Predating the IBCLC profession and the IBLCE examination, WHO's 1981 *International Code of Marketing of Breast-milk Substitutes*, in conjunction with the 18 relevant World Health Assembly resolutions passed since then (WHO, n.d.; WHO & UNICEF, 2009), is a model policy against predatory marketing practices that could reduce optimal breastfeeding by mothers and children worldwide. It recognizes the public health imperative of breastfeeding promotion and support. It seeks to limit commercial marketing of infant formula, bottles, teats (called bottle nipples in the United States), and baby foods or juices meant to replace breastfeeding at the breast. Sales and purchases of those products are allowed.

For the IBCLC, or any other healthcare provider, the principles of the WHO Code can be easily met and supported, regardless of the status of legislative enactment in one's country. The practitioner should refuse any free gifts, samples, or other financial inducements from product marketers. The practitioner should confine clinical or educational discussion of the use of WHO Code–covered products to a one-on-one setting. The practitioner should avoid the professional conflict of interest inherent in the use of pens, handouts, lanyards, tote bags, coffee mugs, or any other gadget bearing the logos and brand names of any commercial product manufacturer. The healthcare provider markets good health; commercial vendors market products (Brooks, 2013; International Baby Food Action Network [IBFAN] & International Code Documentation Centre, 2009).

Moral and Ethical Dilemmas

Moral dilemmas and ethical issues can be subtle and complex, and are intertwined in some situations. Often they entail simply a feeling that something is not quite right about a situation, and this uneasy feeling lasts for a long time. Most of us remember an incident in our childhood where a parent made it very clear that we were doing the wrong thing. Although it was painful at the time, our parents inculcated a moral sense that gave us a behavior compass so that we headed in the right direction as we grew up (Noel-Weiss et al., 2013; Noel-Weiss & Walters, 2006).

What should healthcare workers do when their job responsibilities conflict with their ethics—for example, when they are asked by a supervisor to distribute free samples of formula to a breastfeeding mother? When lactation specialists feel that they are being asked to do something outside their professional ethical code, an analysis can be conducted by looking at legal and ethical obligations, and flexibility within the workplace to explore other options. Sometimes the IBCLC will not be able to change the outcome of the situation at hand but can initiate a review of policy and procedure to form better options for future mothers (and colleagues).

Most hospitals and large clinics have an ethics or risk assessment committee to help in sorting out these types of issues. The committee may hold a forum for interdisciplinary review where discussion of the dilemma and answers to questions are addressed.

Principles of Bioethics

Ethics is the branch of philosophy that structures morality; morality concerns choosing actions perceived to be right or wrong, and bioethics is the study of ethics in healthcare (Noel-Weiss et al., 2013). Major principles of bioethics include the following (Paola, Walker, & Nixon, 2010):

- Autonomy
- Beneficence
- Nonmaleficence
- Justice

Autonomy

The principle of personal autonomy refers to self-governance; it is respect for self-determination and freedom to make one's own decisions.

Example. Autonomy includes the mother's right to choose whether to follow a treatment suggestion, or to refuse treatment or care plan options. Autonomy fits well with caring for breastfeeding families because we know so much about the advantages of breastfeeding that it is difficult for us sometimes to stand back and accept the well-informed mother who decides to supplement her baby when she goes back to work even after we suggest ways that she can exclusively breastfeed in this situation. Autonomy for the patient requires the IBCLC to recognize and appreciate the client and family's value choices.

Beneficence

Beneficence is the principle of the duty to do good. It may ask the IBCLC to prevent or remove harm. Beneficence is just what it sounds like: being kind, merciful, and caring about the welfare of others. It involves promoting the interests and well-being of others in one's sphere, including colleagues and clients/patients.

Example. Maintain nurturing relationships with your colleagues and your clients/patients. That includes those providers who are in training to become an IBCLC. Critical comments and gossip about other colleagues' skills do not promote a spirit of collaborative care by the healthcare team. Such behavior can undermine the confidence of the mother if she thinks the IBCLC has no trust in the abilities of other caregivers.

Nonmaleficence

Nonmaleficence is the duty to do no harm, and underlies the medical maxim "Above all, first do no harm" (Paola et al., 2010, p. 52). It must be balanced with the principles of beneficence.

Example. Giving an injection to a patient causes the harm of pain, but if it delivers medicine to cure disease, then it is justifiable. The rare mother who must take a powerful medication that is contraindicated during lactation can be counseled by the IBCLC about preventing harm to the baby through her breastmilk, or by discussing options to maintain lactation until the medication is no longer in the mother's bloodstream.

Justice

Justice speaks to the principles of fairness, and how social benefits and burdens should be distributed.

Example. Is the need for skilled expertise of an affluent breastfeeding mother who can access private, individualized care because she can afford to pay the IBCLC on an out-of-pocket basis, without regard to her health insurance coverage, any greater than that of the mother who must rely solely on her health insurance benefits? Or the mother with no insurance at all?

IBLCE Ethics and Discipline Committee

IBLCE has established an enforcement and sanctions procedure for its mandatory IBLCE Code of Professional Conduct, which is triggered by the filing of a complaint with the IBLCE Ethics and Discipline Committee (IBLCE, 2011). Once such a complaint is filed, a hearing process commences to review the allegations, with an opportunity for all parties to be heard and represented. Remedies can range from dismissal of the complaint to public censure and revocation of the IBCLC certification. Examples of matters brought before IBLCE include the following:

- An IBCLC was accused of contradicting a physician's order. There was not clear evidence to prove the accusation. The case was dismissed because it was unsubstantiated.
- An IBCLC suggested a potentially dangerous practice in a published article, which carried

her name and IBCLC certification. This was substantiated, but there were mitigating circumstances. Private reprimand was given.
- IBCLC certification was revoked for proof of theft of products while at a conference, and for making copies of the IBLCE certification exam in violation of testing protocols (IBLCE, 2010).

Reimbursement

In most countries, lactation services are a part of the national healthcare system, and reimbursement for these services occurs mainly through salaried positions paid for by government programs. In the United States, reimbursement for lactation services is extremely complex and depends on the setting where the services are provided, the educational qualifications of the provider, and the type of insurance. Reimbursement has also been made more complicated by recent changes in federal law requiring increased access to preventive care services; among those services listed for women are access to skilled lactation care and equipment to support breastfeeding (U.S. Department of Health and Human Services, Human Resources and Services Administration, n.d.).

Lactation specialists who work in a birthing center, hospital, or medical office are usually salaried employees reimbursed with a set hourly or weekly wage. Hospitals usually include lactation services as part of the total cost of the maternity "package." The cost package is an agreement between the insurance company and the hospital to charge a certain amount of money for healthcare coverage for each birth—a reimbursement mechanism known as capitation. Managed care companies compete through price bids to win the healthcare contract, with the lowest bid winning the contract.

If postpartum home visits are part of a maternity insurance package, breastfeeding assistance is given as part of a routine postpartum visit to the mother's home. Nurses providing these home visits are usually salaried employees of the home health company. Services above and beyond the packaged IBCLC services are paid for either by a separate insurance claim or by the family themselves.

For the IBCLC in private practice, cash payment for services rendered or for equipment may be requested from the client at the time of the service. The client, in turn, may seek reimbursement from her insurance company and provides the third-party payer with the information it needs, perhaps using forms supplied by the IBCLC for sending to the insurer in the hope of being reimbursed. Such a lactation consult bill with payment- and assessment-related codes is displayed in Box 1-7.

BOX 1-7 LACTATION SERVICES BILL

OU PHYSICIANS FOR WOMEN'S HEALTH

Department of Obstetrics and Gynecology

825 N.E. 10th Street, Suite 3300

Oklahoma City, OK 73104

(405) 271-9494 Scheduling (405) 271-5293 Billing

TAX ID# 73-1477155

Patient Name_____

Patient SSN_____

Patient DOB_____

Date of Service_____

Insurance_____

MRN#_____

Prenatal _____

Postpartum _____ Delivery Date / Baby's Date of Birth: _____

LACTATION CONSULTANT: _____

(PRINT NAME)

	SERVICE PROVIDED		Supplies to Be Charged for
S9443	Initial Lactation Consultation		
S9445	Follow-up Lactation Consultation		
	MATERNAL DIAGNOSIS - PRIMARY		**CHILD DIAGNOSIS - PRIMARY**
675.14	Abscess, Breast	783.2X	Abnormal or Rapid Weight Loss
676.44	Agalactia	796.1	Abnormal Reflex
676.34, 757.6	Anomaly of Breast or Nipple (Includes Breast Surgery)	750.1	Anomaly of Tongue
676.34, 757.6	Axillary Breast Tissue	767.9	Birth Trauma
649.24	Bariatric Surgery (Status Post) Complicating Puerperium	774.39	Breast Milk Jaundice
676.34	Breast Pain	771.7	Candidiasis / Thrush
675.84, 112.89	Candidiasis of Breast or Nipple	749.10	Cleft Lip, 749.00-Cleft Palate, 749.20-Cleft Palate w/Cleft Lip

676.14	Cracks or Fissures of Nipple	775.5	Dehydration, Newborn
676.84	Delayed Lactation	758.00	Down Syndrome
648.04	Diabetes, Mellitus	787.20	Dysphagia - Difficulty Swallowing
648.84	Diabetes, Gestational	783.41	Failure to Thrive
676.34	Ecchymosis of Breast or Nipple	783.3	Feeding Problem - Infant, 787.03 - Vomiting - Infant
676.34, 692.9	Eczema of Breast or Nipple	779.3	Feeding Problem or Vomiting - Newborn (Includes Prematurity)
676.24	Engorgement of Breast	780.91	Fussy Baby
676.84	Galactocele	779.89	Hypertonicity or Hypotonicity - Newborn or Infant
676.64	Galactorrhea	750.15	Macroglossia (Hypertrophy of Tongue)
676.34, 757.6	Hypoplasia of Breast	750.16	Microglossia (Hypoplasia of Tongue)
675.94	Infection Breast or Nipple Unspecified (Specified - 675.84)	524.06	Microgenia: Recessive/Small Chin
676.04	Inverted Nipple(s)	315.4	Oral Motor Dysfunction/Jaw Clench
675.24	Mastitis - Non-purulent (Interstitial)	750.0	Tongue-Tie/Ankyloglossia
675.14	Mastitis - Purulent (Infective)		**CHILD DIAGNOSIS - SECONDARY**
649.1, 278.00	Obesity	787.70	Abnormal Stools
676.84	Breastfeeding Difficulty	770.81	Apnea
676.34	Painful Nipple (No Apparent Trauma)	789.00	Colic
676.84	Plugged Duct	787.91	Diarrhea
676.84	Polygalactia	779.5	Drug Withdrawal
676.84	Relactation	754.0	Facial Assymetry
676.54	Suppressed Lactation	767.5	Facial Palsy
676.34	Trauma to Nipple	767.2	Fractured Clavicle
649.0	Tobacco Use Complicating Puerperium	693.1	Food Allergy
676.34	Ulceration of Nipple	530.81	GE Reflux
		750.26	High Arched Palate
		478.29	Hyperactive Gag Reflex
V24.1	Lactation Care / Exam	775.6	Hypoglycemia 775.0 - (IDM)
V67.59	Follow-up Exam (When the original reason for visit is resolved)	764.90	Intrauterine Growth Retardation
		774.6	Jaundice/Hyperbillirubinemia
		766.1	Large for Gestational Age

(continues)

BOX 1-7 (*CONTINUED*)

	MATERNAL DIAGNOSIS - SECONDARY	524.00	Micrognathia
304.90	Drug Dependency	315.9	Motor Retardation
244.90	Hypothyroidism (Unspecified)	769	Respiratory Distress Syndrome
761.5	Multiple Birth	764.00	Small for Gestational Age
642.44	Pre-eclampsia (Mild or unspecified)	520.7	Teething syndrome
V10.3	Unilateral Mastectomy	528.9	Ulceration of Oral Mucosa - Traumatic
		528.2	Ulceration of Oral Mucosa - Nontraumatic

Diagnosis Codes:

1. _____   2. _____   3. _____   4. _____

Return

Days: _____   Weeks: _____   Months: _____

LACTATION CONSULTANT _____   TIME SPENT _____
SIGNATURE

Form 2008-G Revised 10'08

Source: Reproduced from Oklahoma University Department of Obstetrics and Gynecology.

Insurance and Third-Party Payment

Insurance and third-party payment for lactation services is a complex issue. Third-party payment—insurance or payment by another entity besides the patient—varies according to the state (and country) where the services were given. In the United States, third-party payers can be divided into two general categories: government or public health insurance (Medicare, Medicaid) and managed care organizations (MCOs).

Medicare applies to individuals older than age 65 and is not applicable for breastfeeding except that insurance companies usually follow Medicare rules for payment. Medicaid is a federal program administered by the states, and state regulations apply to mothers and children who qualify on the basis of low income. The regulations in various states may differ in billing rules and regulations. Approximately one-third of U.S. births are paid for under Medicaid. Medicaid reimbursement for health care is further complicated by the fact that some Medicaid recipients are also enrolled in managed care plans. These plans' policies on reimbursement differ from the state and federal rules governing reimbursement when the patient is not enrolled in managed care. Medicaid requires a practitioner to be licensed to be eligible for reimbursement; no U.S. state licensed IBCLCs in 2013.

Insurance policies usually spell out by title who may be reimbursed with third-party payment. Physicians and midlevel providers such as nurse practitioners, certified nurse midwives, and physician assistants are recognized by third-party payers as providers who can receive direct payment for their services.

To receive reimbursement from Medicaid, the lactation consultant must be accepted as a Medicaid provider by his or her state Medicaid agency to be admitted to the provider panel of an MCO. Generally, providers are accepted on the basis of having a medical or medically related degree, state licensure, and national certification. Lactation consultants can receive direct reimbursement if they are also a licensed care provider (physician, nurse practitioner [NP], or certified nurse–midwife) who has graduated from an accredited educational program, is licensed, and is certified nationally in a specialty.

Physicians or nurse practitioners can apply for a provider number through the state Medicaid agency by filing a provider application. If accepted as a provider, they can bill the state Medicaid agency on an HCFA 1500 form using the patient's name and identifying information, the ICD-10 code, the Current Procedural Terminology (CPT) code, the charge, and the provider's name, number, and location for services. Fees for CPT codes vary according to locations and providers. For example, in many states to receive third-party payment, LC services must be provided in collaboration with a physician. A book by Carolyn Buppert (2008), *Nurse-Practitioner's Business Practice and Legal Guide*, third edition, is an excellent resource for learning about reimbursement. The USLCA also has a section on reimbursement on its website, available at http://uslca.org/resources. In addition, the U.S. Breastfeeding Committee has published a document giving guidance for third-party payers on implementing the lactation care provisions in the Affordable Care Act; this document is available at http://www.usbreastfeeding.org /NewsInfo/NewsRoom/201307ModelPayerPolicy /tabid/345/Default.aspx.

"Incident to" Billing

Lactation services that fall under the category "incident to" can be billed if they are an integral but incidental part of a physician's professional services; however, the physician must personally treat the client on the first visit to the practice and be on site when the service is rendered. Thus, if the IBCLC is a nurse practitioner working in a medical office, he or she can bill for services to the breastfeeding dyad offered "incident to" the physician also seeing the mother and baby, and also being on-site. Medicare requires that the claim form for an "incident to" service be filled out with the physician's name and provider number.

Rejection of Billing

If the company rejects a bill, the HCFA 1500 form is returned with a short explanation about why it is being rejected. Sometimes several letters back and forth are necessary before the bill will be paid. Persistence is the key, as many claims may not be paid on the first submission. Anyone in a medically related practice quickly learns from trial and error how to best file third-party insurance claims to maximize the number of paid claims.

Payers may require documentation to validate that the care was given, the site of the care, and the medical necessity and appropriateness of services provided. Fees for care of breastfeeding women on Medicaid are based on number and type of services provided using the CPT, published in the tenth edition of *International Classification of Diseases* (ICD10) (see Box 1-8).

Major barriers to third-party reimbursement for nonphysician healthcare workers such as lactation consultants have been lack of state licensure for IBCLCs, opposition by other medical professions, and third-party payers that fear expansion of provider eligibility. The 1997 passage of a provision in the budget bill Public Law 105-33 to expand Medicare reimbursement for NPs allows for reimbursement of NP services including lactation services; however, each state has the option of covering NP services. Since the law was passed, these nonphysician providers have continued to encounter difficulties in getting third-party payment.

Physicians in the United States are able to obtain reimbursement by using established ICD-10 medical codes for breastfeeding diagnoses, billing for both mother and baby as indicated, and submitting bills for insurance coverage. This type of reimbursement often falls under the constraints of contracted fees, managed care, and/or HMO contracts. The American Academy of Pediatrics' section on breastfeeding published *Breastfeeding and Lactation: The Pediatrician's Pocket Guide to Coding* in 2006. However, owing to the time-consuming nature of fully evaluating the breastfeeding dyad and observing a feeding, the physician's time will rarely be adequately

BOX 1-8 ICD-10 LACTATION DIAGNOSIS CODES

Maternal

091.21 Non-purulent mastitis associated with pregnancy

091.22 Non-purulent mastitis associated with puerperium

091.23 Non-purulent mastitis associated with lactation

091.11 Purulent mastitis; mammary abscess during pregnancy

091.12 Mastitis associated with puerperium

091.13 Mastitis associated with lactation

091.03 Infected nipple associated with lactation

092.03 Retracted nipple associated with lactation

092.13 Cracked nipple associated with lactation

092.3 Complete failure of lactation

092.4 Partial failure of lactation

092.5 Suppressed lactation

092.79 Other disorders of lactation

Q83.3 Supernumerary nipple

Q89.9 Breast or nipple deformity/anomaly, congenital

N64.82 Hypoplasia of breast

N64.89 Subinvolution (postlactational or postpuerperium); galactocele

L24.4 Irritant contact dermatitis due to skin contact with drugs (see list of drugs for fifth and sixth digits)

Infant

P92.5 Neonatal difficulty feeding at breast

P74.1 Dehydration of newborn

P37.5 Neonatal candida

M26.06 Microgenia (hypoplasia of chin)

M26.04 Micrognathia (hypoplasia of mandible)

M26.11 Maxillary asymmetry

M26.19 Retrognathia (other specified anomalies of jaw–cranial base relationship)

Q35 Isolated cleft palate (.1 hard palate, .3 soft palate, .5 hard and soft palate, .7 cleft uvula, .9 unspecified cleft palate)

Q36 Isolated cleft lip (.0 bilateral, .1 median, .9 unilateral)

Q37 Cleft palate with either bilateral (even fourth digit)/unilateral (odd fourth digit) cleft lip (.0/.1 cleft hard palate, .2/.3 cleft soft palate, .4/.5 cleft hard and soft palate)

Q 90.9 Down syndrome

Q38.1 Ankyloglossia (tongue-tie)

Q38.2 Macroglossia

R 13.10 Dysphagia (.11 oral phase, .12 oropharyngeal phase, .13 pharyngeal phase;)

P92.6 Failure to thrive in newborn (younger than 28 days)

R62.51 Failure to thrive in child (older than 28 days)

R68.12 Fussy infant (irritable infant)

Source: Reproduced with permission from ICD-10 Lactation Diagnosis Codes. ICD10Data.com.

compensated in full. Creative use of staff is often featured in the physician-led lactation clinic to allow effective time management for the physician.

Coding

Accurate and complete coding for services and supplies is vital to the financial success of a lactation program or service. Several resources related to coding, billing, and reimbursement, specific to skilled lactation care and frequently updated in light of fast-changing regulations in this area, are available from the United States Lactation Consultant Association (USLCA, n.d.)

Private Practice

The need to provide continuity of care in community-based settings has led to a rise in the number of private practitioners offering skilled care. Some physicians have built practices that specialize in breastfeeding medicine; others are making IBCLC care a regular part of their practice. Lactation consultants in private practice may have full- or part-time practices; they may partner with other IBCLCs or align themselves formally or informally with other healthcare practices (such as obstetricians or midwives, childbirth educators, pediatricians, chiropractors, and complementary or holistic practitioners). Some IBCLCs also offer a retail side to the business— perhaps renting breastfeeding equipment or offering classes. IBCLCs may do home visits (handling all clinical contact in the mother's home), have a home-based office, or rent or share office space.

The Business of Doing Business

A private practice is a small business, and there are important legal and business considerations that any IBCLC must take into account before deciding to open a practice. Each IBCLC must choose which business form the practice will take, run the practice, market it, and report income (and pay taxes) for fees earned as part of the practice. The IBCLC's insurance should cover business and professional liability contingencies, and consider the locations where the IBCLC conducts his or her clinical work (Smith, 2003).

Payment and Fees

Most clients pay for their lactation consultation services at the time of service. Practitioners can elect to waive or reduce their fees in light of exigent circumstances of mothers, but the IBCLC's professional responsibilities remain unchanged. Setting fees is an important part of establishing a thriving practice, taking into account what the market will bear for the location of the IBCLC practice as well as the IBCLC's particular level of experience and expertise. The prospective private-practice IBCLC can investigate the fees charged by comparable professionals in his or her community. Other factors to consider in setting fees are the anticipated length of visits, costs and time to travel and park, and providing single-user breastfeeding supplies during the consult. While visits to a physician's office may last only 15 to 20 minutes, a thorough IBCLC consult (involving assessment of the mother, the baby, and a full breastfeeding session) may run 60 to 120 minutes.

Phone consultations may also be considered in establishing IBCLC services. The risk in "answering a few questions" for the mother who calls is that the formalities of establishing a professional relationship are not evident. No consent forms have been signed, no histories have been taken or assessments noted, and no individualized care plan has been created with follow-up built in. This is bad for business, and bad for excellent clinical care. IBCLCs in private practice are most successful when they have ongoing, mutually respectful relationships with other healthcare providers in the community, who refer clients to them.

Private practice is clearly not for every lactation consultant. However, those who choose this practice model enjoy rewards not found in other practice settings. The independence also offers an opportunity to flexibly structure the workday, offering better work–life balance for some LCs. Linda Smith's (2003) book, *The Lactation Consultant in Private Practice: The ABCs of Getting Started,* is a valuable resource for the IBCLC thinking of opening a private practice. Box 1-9 lists some dos and don'ts suggested by IBCLCs in private practice—either when establishing a private practice or when initiating an office-, clinic-, or hospital-based lactation service.

BOX 1-9 DOS AND DON'TS OF LACTATION CONSULTING

DO . . .

- Insist on gaining credibility for the profession by passing the IBLCE examination. Ensure that people know this is the minimum credential for any person practicing as an LC in the community.
- From the very first client, behave with the utmost professionalism.
- Charge what you are worth; do not apologize for your fees.
- Set limits immediately, so that people know the boundaries of your availability.
- Establish your own knowledge and skills boundaries. Do not be afraid to ask for help.
- Develop a network of LCs in the community; they can serve as a sounding board for problems and as back-up when you are not available.
- Avoid repeating problems other LCs have experienced by learning from those with more experience than you have.
- Know what you are doing if you rent or sell equipment. Learn how the equipment works, and who should and should not use it. Be aware that its availability from you may influence what you tell a client to do.
- Use a computer to maintain a database of clients and practice documents and for maintaining your business.
- Learn as much as possible about running a business. It can take years to break even.
- Get a competent business advisor for accounting, marketing, and taxes. Ensure that those advisors understand exactly what you are trying to do.
- Bill the client directly for the service. The client then files a claim to her insurance company. Use standard forms for billing and a letter that the client can use to seek insurance coverage.
- Develop a specialization within the field and make your work visible to others through good care (Brimdyr, 2002).
- Document what you have done and send the original to the primary care provider, whether or not this individual made the initial referral.
- Recognize that this business is a labor of love. Do not expect to get rich.

DON'T . . .

- Don't get heavily involved in phone consultations, paid or unpaid, without having seen the mother and baby. An overall assessment is needed.
- Don't give away your time without reimbursement.
- Don't waste your money on a lot of expensive advertising. Advertise judiciously and be patient.
- Don't use someone else's opinion as a reason for doing something. Experiment; be creative. What works in one practice may not work in another one.
- Don't get too many partners at the beginning. Knowing how each partner works as an individual will not necessarily predict how each works as part of a group. The more partners one has, the greater the number of problems that can arise.
- Never forget that a happy mother and thriving baby are your best advertisements.

ACKNOWLEDGMENTS

The authors of this first chapter of the fifth edition of *Breastfeeding and Human Lactation* acknowledge, thank, and laud Jan Riordan. She served as editor on the first four editions of this seminal text in human lactation; she authored the first chapter of each of the four earlier editions of this publication. We all learned from Jan Riordan as we began our careers as International Board Certified Lactation Consultant certificants. We are honored to have been asked to write the introductory chapter to the fifth edition, and to carry on Jan's tradition of educating and mentoring the next generation of skilled lactation consultants.

SUMMARY

The field of lactation, now into its third decade, is an allied healthcare specialty. Most hospitals now offer lactation services, provided by IBCLCs or other licensed caregivers (e.g., nurses) who also have IBCLC certification. Some physicians are also starting breastfeeding specialty private practices. The opportunity to work with families and babies—and to enhance early parenting and maternal/child health—has made professional lactation care a popular, satisfying field. As this is a fairly young field of healthcare, there remains some confusion by families, and administrators who hire healthcare providers, about the range of expertise an IBCLC can bring to bear.

KEY CONCEPTS

- A lactation consultant (IBCLC) is a specialist trained to focus on the needs and concerns of the breastfeeding mother–baby pair in hospitals, clinics, private medical practice, health departments, home health agencies, and private practices. IBCLCs usually have educational and clinical backgrounds in the health professions.

- Randomized clinical trials consistently show that interventions by healthcare workers have a positive effect on breastfeeding. Translated to healthcare costs, these studies show that IBCLC services save the healthcare system enormous amounts of money through reduction in illnesses for both baby and mother.

- The number of candidates taking the IBLCE certification examination for lactation consultants has grown steadily since the exam's inception in 1985. Most candidates are from Australia, Canada, South Korea, Japan, and the United States. Periodic recertification is required.

- Opportunities to gain clinical experience working with breastfeeding dyads can be obtained through La Leche League; finding a preceptor arrangement with an experienced IBCLC, nurse, or physician; serving as a WIC peer counselor; and teaching prenatal classes.

- Certification by the IBLCE is the gold standard for working as a lactation consultant.

- Most hospitals have lactation services. These services usually include inpatient consults and may include telephone hotline and post-discharge telephone calls; prenatal classes on breastfeeding; outpatient postpartum consults; and continuing education for staff.

- A hospital with 3000 births per year should have at least five full-time LC positions, which can be split into part-time positions. The usual time per visit with mothers when doing daily rounds is 15 to 20 minutes. The majority of LC work time is spent in direct care of patients.

- A "prime mover" (e.g., a nursing director, administrator, or physician) who has institutional power is needed to develop a lactation program as well as to obtain the wide support of those who have influence in deciding budget allocations.

- The role of the LC is based on an advanced practice model. Roles develop sequentially according to experience, as follows: novice, advanced beginner, competent, proficient, and expert.

- A major responsibility of the LC is documentation through reports and charting. Narrative and problem-oriented charting and clinical care plans are popular methods to organize and chart clinical care. Computer skills are mandatory.

- Ethics is a set of principles that guide human conduct. Morals are specific behaviors based on beliefs. A situation in which an individual feels compelled to make a choice between two or more actions that he or she can reasonably and morally justify, or when evidence or arguments are inconclusive, is called an ethical dilemma.
- Physicians and midlevel providers such as nurse practitioners, certified nurse–midwives, and physician assistants are recognized by third-party payers as providers who can receive direct payment for their services. In the United States, IBCLCs are increasingly being recognized by third-party payers as providers who can receive direct payment for their services. Physicians and nurse practitioners, clinical nurse specialists, and certified midwives who are also IBCLCs can choose which role to claim reimbursement under for lactation services.

INTERNET RESOURCES

Academy of Breastfeeding Medicine: A worldwide organization of physicians dedicated to the promotion, protection, and support of breastfeeding and human lactation. Publishes numerous evidence-based clinical protocols related to breastfeeding. www.bfmed.org

International Board of Lactation Consultant Examiners: Provides information on how to qualify to take the certification exam to be awarded the credential of International Board Certified Lactation Consultant. Includes a worldwide registry of IBCLCs. www.iblce.org

International Lactation Consultant Association (ILCA): Educational, conference, and professional development resources including the *Journal of Human Lactation*. www.ilca.org

Canadian Lactation Consultant Association (CLCA): National Canadian affiliate.

Provides professional liability insurance and professional development opportunities.

Lactation Consultants of Australia and New Zealand (LCANZ): Multinational affiliate that provides professional development opportunities in Australia and New Zealand.

United States Lactation Consultant Association (USLCA): National U.S. affiliate that provides professional development opportunities, offers professional liability insurance, and publishes the *Clinical Lactation Journal*. www.uslca.org

Lactation Education Accreditation and Approval Review Committee (LEAARC): Reviews and grants formal recognition to education programs in lactation. LEAARC recognition is a formal, nongovernmental, peer-review process of voluntary self-evaluation. Approved/accredited programs can be found on its website. www.leaarc.org

United States Breastfeeding Committee: An independent nonprofit coalition of more than 40 nationally influential professional, educational, and governmental organizations that share a common mission to improve (U.S.) health by working collaboratively to protect, promote, and support breastfeeding. www.usbreastfeeding.org

Hale Publishing: Publishes books on breastfeeding and lactation consulting. www.ibreastfeeding.com

Jones and Bartlett Learning: Publishes books on breastfeeding. http://www.jblearning.com/

La Leche League International: Provides publications, seminars, and answers to breastfeeding questions. www.lalecheleague.org

REFERENCES

Albernaz E, Victora CG, Haisma H, et al. Lactation counseling increases breast-feeding duration but not breast milk intake as measured by isotopic methods. *J Nutr*. 2003;133:205–209.

Altman, D. *Clinics in human lactation: mentoring our future.* Amarillo, TX: Hale Publishing; 2010.

American Nurses Association (ANA). Has JCAHO eliminated care plans? *Am Nurse*. June 1991:6.

Andaya E, Bonuck K, Barnett J, Lischewski-Goel J. Perceptions of primary care-based breastfeeding promotion interventions: qualitative analysis of randomized controlled trial participant interviews. *Breastfeed Med.* 2012; 7(6):417–422. doi: 10.1089/bfm.2011.0151.

Angeron J, Riordan J. *Staffing for a lactation program* [Unpublished manuscript]. Wichita, KS: Via Christi Medical Center; 2007.

Association of Women's Health, Obstetric and Neonatal Nurses (AWHONN). Position statement: breastfeeding. 2008. Available at: http://www.awhonn.org /awhonn/content.do?name=07_PressRoom%2F07 _PositionStatements.htm. Accessed May 14, 2014.

Association of Women's Health, Obstetric and Neonatal Nurses (AWHONN). *Guidelines for professional registered nurse staffing for perinatal units.* Washington, DC: Author; 2010.

Auerbach KG, Riordan J, Gross A. The lactation consultant: an increasingly visible health care role. *Mother Baby J.* 2000;5(1):41–46.

Australian Health Ministers' Conference. *The Australian National Breastfeeding strategy 2010–2015.* Canberra, Australia: Australian Government Department of Health and Ageing; 2009.

Baby-Friendly USA. Ten steps to successful breastfeeding. n.d. Available at: http://www.babyfriendlyusa.org/about-us /baby-friendly-hospital-initiative/the-ten-steps. Accessed June 9, 2013

Bailey D. ILCA: 20 years of building a profession. *J Hum Lact.* 2005;21(3):239–242.

Bartick M, Reinhold A. The burden of suboptimal breastfeeding in the United States: a pediatric cost analysis. *Pediatrics.* 2010;125:e1048–e1056.

Bartick MC, Steube AM, Schwarz EB, et al. Cost analysis of maternal disease associated with suboptimal breastfeeding. *Obstet Gynecol.* 2013;122(1):111–119.

Benner P. *From novice to expert: excellence and power in clinical nursing practice.* Menlo Park, CA: Addison-Wesley; 1984.

Bornmann P. A legal primer for lactation consultants. In: International Lactation Consultant Association, Mannel R, Marten PJ, Walker M, eds. *Core curriculum for lactation consultant practice* (3rd ed.). Burlington, MA: Jones & Bartlett Learning; 2013:215–242.

Brimdyr K. Lactation management: a community of practice. In: Cadwell K, ed. Reclaiming Breastfeeding for the United States. Sudbury, Mass: Jones and Bartlett; 2002:51–63.

Britton C, McCormick FM, Renfrew MJ, et al. Support of breastfeeding mothers [Review]. Cochrane Collaboration. Available at: http://www.thecochranelibrary.com. Accessed July 28, 2007.

Brooks E. *Legal and ethical issues for the IBCLC.* Burlington, MA: Jones & Bartlett Learning; 2013.

Buppert C. *Nurse practitioner's business practice and legal guide* (3rd ed.). Sudbury, MA: Jones and Bartlett; 2008.

Cary AH. *International survey of certified nurses in the U.S. and Canada.* Washington, DC: Nursing Credentialing Center; 2000.

Castrucci BC, Hoover K, Lim S, et al. A comparison of breastfeeding rates in an urban birth cohort among women delivering infants at hospitals that employ and do not employ lactation consultants. *J Pub Health Manage Pract.* 2006;12:577–585.

Centers for Disease Control and Prevention. Breastfeeding. n.d. Available at: http://www.cdc.gov/breastfeeding /index.htm. Accessed January 2, 2014.

Centers for Disease Control and Prevention. Vital Signs: Hospital Practices to Support Breastfeeding—United States, 2007 and 2009. *Morbidity and Mortality Weekly Report.* 2011;60(30):1020–1025.

Cohen R, Mrtek MB, Mrtek RG. Comparison of maternal absenteeism and infant illness rates among breast-feeding and formula-feeding women in two corporations. *Am J Health Promotion.* 1995;10:148–153.

DiGirolamo AM, Grummer-Strawn LM, Fein SB. Effect of maternity-care practices on breastfeeding. *Pediatrics.* 2008;122(suppl 2):S43–S49. doi: 10.1542/peds.2008-1315e.

Dodgson JE, Duckett L. Breastfeeding in the workplace: building a support program for nursing mothers. *AAOHN J.* 1997;45:290–298.

Dreyfus SE, Dreyfus HO. *A five-stage model of the mental activities involved in directed skill acquisition* (USAF Contract No. F49620–79–C–0063). Berkeley, CA: University of California; 1980.

EU Project on Promotion of Breastfeeding in Europe. Protection, promotion and support of breastfeeding in Europe: a blueprint for action. European Commission, Directorate Public Health and Risk Assessment, Luxembourg, 2004. Available at: http://ec.europa .eu/health/ph_projects/2002/promotion/fp_promotion _2002_frep_18_en.pdf. Accessed May 14, 2014.

Gibbins S, Green PE, Scott PA, et al. The role of the clinical nurse specialist/neonatal nurse practitioner in a breastfeeding clinic: a model of advanced practice. *Clin Nurse Special.* 2000;14:56–59.

Health Insurance Portability and Accountability Act (HIPAA) of 1996, 45 C.F.R. 160, 162, 164 (2002).

Heinig MJ. Closet consulting and other enabling behaviors. *J Hum Lact.* 1998;14:181–182.

Hinson P. The business of clinical practice. In: Auerbach KG, ed. *Current issues in clinical lactation 2000.* Sudbury, MA: Jones and Bartlett; 2000:43–47.

International Baby Food Action Network, International Code Documentation Centre. *Code essentials 3: responsibilities of health workers under the international code of marketing of breastmilk substitutes and subsequent WHA resolutions* (Report No. 3). Penang, Malaysia: Author; 2009.

International Board of Lactation Consultant Examiners (IBLCE). Sanctions list. April 2010. Available at: http://iblce.org/wp-content/uploads/2013/08/sanctions -list.pdf. Accessed May 14, 2014.

International Board of Lactation Consultant Examiners (IBLCE). Code of professional conduct for IBCLCs. November 1, 2011. Available at: http://iblce.org/wp -content/uploads/2013/08/code-of-professional-conduct .pdf. Accessed May, 14, 2014.

International Board of Lactation Consultant Examiners (IBLCE). Examination data. Provided by IBLCE Executive Director, August 2013.

International Board of Lactation Consultant Examiners (IBLCE). Clinical competencies for the practice of international board certified lactation consultants (IB-CLCs). September 15, 2012a. Available at: http://iblce .org/wp-content/uploads/2013/08/clinical -competencies.pdf. Accessed May 14, 2014.

International Board of Lactation Consultant Examiners (IBLCE). Scope of practice for international board certified lactation consultant (IBCLC) certificants. September 15, 2012b. Available at: http://iblce.org /wp-content/uploads/2013/08/scope-of-practice.pdf. Accessed May 14, 2014.

International Labour Office, Conditions of Work and Employment Programme. Maternity at work: a review of national legislation. 2010. Available at: www.ilo.org /wcmsp5/groups/public/@dgreports/@dcomm/@publ /documents/publication/wcms_124442.pdf. Accessed July 13, 2013.

International Lactation Consultant Association (ILCA). Home page. n.d. Available at: http://www.ilca.org/i4a/pages /index.cfm?pageid=1. Accessed June 9, 2013.

International Lactation Consultant Association (ILCA). *Lactation consulting: the first twenty years a history. ILCA: 1985-2005 the birth of a profession and an association*, Lauwers J, ed. Raleigh, NC: Author; 2005.

International Lactation Consultant Association (ILCA), Henderson S. Position paper on the role and impact of the IBCLC. 2011. Available at: http://www.ilca.org/files /resources/ilca_publications/Role%20%20Impact%20 of%20the%20IBCLC-webFINAL_08-15-11.pdf. Accessed July 13, 2013.

International Lactation Consultant Association (ILCA). *Clinical instruction in lactation: teaching the next generation*, Kombol P, Kutner L, Barger J, comps.; Lauwers J, ed. Amarillo, TX: Hale Publishing; 2012.

International Lactation Consultant Association (ILCA). Standards of practice for International Board Certified Lactation Consultants. 2013. Available at: http://www. ilca.org/files/resources/ilca_publications/Standard_of_ Practice.pdf. Accessed January 2, 2014.

The Joint Commission (TJC). Specifications manual for national Joint Commission quality core measures. 2013. Available at: http://manual.jointcommission.org /releases/TJC2013B/. Accessed July 13, 2013.

Journal of Human Lactation. Available at: http://jhl.sagepub .com/. Accessed July 13, 2013.

Lactation Education Approval and Accreditation Review Committee (LEAARC). Home page. n.d. Available

at: http://www.leaarc.org/index.html. Accessed July 13, 2013.

Lauwers J. Mentoring and precepting lactation consultants. *J Hum Lact*. 2007;23:10–11.

Lauwers J. Communication and counseling skills. In: Mannel R, Martens P, Walker M, eds. *ILCA core curriculum for lactation consultant practice* (3rd ed.). Burlington, MA: Jones & Bartlett Learning; 2012:53–64.

Lauwers J, Swisher A. *Counseling the nursing mother: a lactation consultant's guide* (5th ed.). Sudbury, MA: Jones and Bartlett; 2010.

List BA, Ballard JL, Langworthy KS, et al. Electronic health records in an outpatient breastfeeding medicine clinic. *J Hum Lact*. 2008;24:58–68.

Mannel R. Lactation rounds: a system to improve hospital productivity. *J Hum Lact.* 2010;26:393–398.

Mannel R. Defining lactation acuity to improve patient safety and outcomes. *J Hum Lact.* 2011;27:163–170.

Mannel R. Developing and managing a hospital lactation service. In: International Lactation Consultant Association; Mannel R, Marten PJ, Walker M, eds. *Core curriculum for lactation consultant practice* (3rd ed.). Burlington, MA: Jones & Bartlett Learning; 2013:243–255.

Mannel R, Mannel RS. Staffing for hospital lactation programs: recommendations from a tertiary care teaching hospital. *J Hum Lact.* 2006;22:409–417.

Martens PJ, Derksen S, Gupta S. Predictors of hospital readmission of Manitoba newborns within six weeks postbirth discharge: a population-based study. *Pediatrics.* 2004;14(3):708–713.

Miller RD. Civil liability. In: Miller RD. *Problems in health care law* (9th ed.). Sudbury, MA: Jones and Bartlett; 2006:587–681.

National Commission for Certifying Agencies Standards (NCCA). Available at: http://www.credentialingexcel-lence.org/p/cm/ld/fid=66. Accessed July 13, 2013.

Niebuhr B, Biel M. The value of specialty certification. *Nurs Outlook.* 2007;55:176–181.

Noel-Weiss J, Cragg B, Woodend AK. Exploring how IBCLCs manage ethical dilemmas: a qualitative study. *BMC Med Ethic.* 2013;13(18):1–8. Available at: http://www.biomedcentral.com/1472-6939/13/18.

Noel-Weiss J, Walters GJ. Ethics and lactation consultants: developing knowledge, skills and tools. *J Hum Lact.* 2006;22(2):203–212.

Office on Women's Health, U.S. Department of Health and Human Services. Business case for breastfeeding. 2008. Available at: https://www.womenshealth.gov /breastfeeding/government-in-action/business-case .html. Accessed May 14, 2014.

Omnibus Final Rule, including Health Information Technology for Economic and Clinical Health Act (HITECH), 78 Fed. Reg. 5566 (January 25, 2013).

Paola FA, Walker R, Nixon LL. *Medical ethics and humanities*. Sudbury, MA: Jones and Bartlett; 2010.

Parris KM. Integrating nursing diagnosis, interventions, and outcomes in public health nursing practice. *Nurs Diag.* 1999;10:49–56.

Paul IM, Lehman EB, Hollenbeak CS, Maisels MJ. Preventable newborn readmissions since passage of the Newborns' and Mothers' Health Protection Act. *Pediatrics.* 2006;118(6):2349–2358.

Phillips V. The Nursing Mother's Association of Australia as a self-help organization. In: Katz AH, Bender EL, eds. *Helping one another: self-help groups in a changing world.* Oakland, CA: Third Party Publishing; 1990.

Raudonis BM, Anderson CM. A theoretical framework for specialty certification in nursing practice. *Nurs Outlook.* 2002;50:247–252.

Shealy KR, Li R, Benton-Davis S, Grummer-Strawn LM. *The CDC guide to breastfeeding interventions.* Atlanta, GA: U.S. Department of Health and Human Services, Centers for Disease Control and Prevention; 2005. Available at: http://www.cdc.gov/breastfeeding/resources/guide.htm. Accessed July 13, 2013.

Smith L. *The lactation consultant in private practice: the ABCs of getting started.* Sudbury, MA: Jones and Bartlett; 2003.

Spatz D. The critical role of nurses in lactation support. *JOGNN.* 2010;39:499–500.

Thorley V. Complementary and competing roles of volunteers and professionals in the breastfeeding field. *Int Self Help Self Care.* 2000;1(2):171–179.

U.S. Copyright Office. Copyright basics (Report No. Circular 1). Washington, DC: U.S. Copyright Office; 2012. Available at: http://www.copyright.gov/circs/circ01.pdf. Accessed February 19, 2014.

U.S. Department of Agriculture. WIC works resource system (Loving Support WIC peer counselor training). n.d. Available at: http://wicworks.nal.usda.gov/. Accessed June 7, 2013.

U.S. Department of Health and Human Services, Human Resources and Services Administration. Women's preventive services: required health plan coverage guidelines. n.d. Available at: http://www.hrsa.gov/womensguidelines/. Accessed June 9, 2013.

U.S. Department of Health and Human Services. *The Surgeon General's call to action to support breastfeeding.* Washington, DC: U.S. Department of Health and Human Services, Office of the Surgeon General; 2011. Available at: http://www.surgeongeneral.gov/library/calls/breastfeeding/calltoactiontosupportbreastfeeding.pdf. Accessed July 13, 2013.

U.S. Department of Labor, Wage and Hour Division. Fact sheet #73: break time for nursing mothers under the FLSA. 2010. Available at: http://www.dol.gov/whd/regs/compliance/whdfs73.htm. Accessed July 13, 2013.

U.S. Lactation Consultant Association (USLCA). Licensure and reimbursement. n.d. Available at: http://www.ilca.org/i4a/pages/index.cfm?pageid=4126. Accessed June 10, 2013.

U.S. Lactation Consultant Association (USLCA). International Board Certified Lactation Consultant staffing recommendations for the inpatient setting. 2010. Available at: http://uslca.org/resources/publications. Accessed July 13, 2013.

U.S. Preventive Services Task Force (USPSTF). Primary care interventions to promote breastfeeding: an evidence review for the U.S. Preventive Services Task Force. 2008. Available at: http://www.uspreventiveservicestaskforce.org/uspstf08/breastfeeding/brfdartfig3txt.htm. Accessed July 20, 2013.

Wiessinger D. Professional responsibility revisited. In: Smith L, ed. *The lactation consultant in private practice.* Sudbury, MA: Jones and Bartlett; 2003:214–226.

Williams EL. Increasing your credibility with physicians: strategies for lactation consultants [editorial]. *J Hum Lact.* 1995;11:3–4.

Witt AM, Smith S, Mason MJ, et al. Integrating routine lactation consultant support in to a pediatric practice. *Breastfeed Med.* 2012;7:38–42.

World Health Organization (WHO). The full code and subsequent WHA resolutions. n.d. Available at International Baby Food Action Network website: http://www.ibfan.org/issue-international_code-full.html. Accessed June 10, 2013.

World Health Organization, Division of Child Health and Development. *Evidence for the ten steps to successful breastfeeding.* Geneva, Switzerland: Author; 1998. Available at: http://whqlibdoc.who.int/publications/2004/9241591544_eng.pdf.

World Health Organization (WHO). *The global strategy for infant and young child feeding.* Geneva, Switzerland: Author; 2003.

World Health Organization (WHO) & United Nations Children's Fund (UNICEF). Baby-Friendly Hospital Initiative. Revised, updated and expanded for integrated care. Geneva, Switzerland: Author; 2009. Available at: http://www.who.int/nutrition/publications/infantfeeding/bfhi_trainingcourse/en/index.html

Chapter 2

Tides in Breastfeeding Practice

Mary-Margaret Coates

The news is mixed. Worldwide, about 38% of the world's infants younger than the age of 6 months were exclusively breastfed during 2010 (World Health Organization [WHO], 2012)—the same overall rate as in 1985 (WHO, 2011) but an increase from more-depressed rates around 1990 (Labbok et al., 2006), and certainly, in the United States, a higher rate than during the nadir of breastfeeding in the 1960s and early 1970s. Until the 1940s, the prevalence of breastfeeding was high in nearly all societies. Although the feeding of manufactured milk products (for general use or specifically for infants) had begun before the turn of the century in parts of Europe and North America, the practice spread slowly during the next several decades. It was still generally limited to segments of population elites (or for medical indications), and it involved only a small percentage of the world's people. During World War II and thereafter, however, the way in which most mothers in industrialized regions fed their infants began to change. Increasingly, breastfeeding was replaced by cow milk formulations, and the export of these new practices and associated products to developing regions gained speed (for one of many examples, see Schaefer, 1956).

Evidence About Breastfeeding Practices

How do we know what we "know" about the prevalence of breastfeeding? (The word *prevalence* is used here to mean the occurrence of any breastfeeding.) Before attempting to trace long-term trends in infant feeding practices, let us consider the nature of available evidence.

Large-Scale Surveys

During the latter part of the 1900s and earliest years of this century, reliable information about breastfeeding rates in the United States and elsewhere was difficult to obtain. National surveys that allow statistical evaluation of their results have become available only relatively recently anywhere in the world. It is a marker of the late interest in breastfeeding among public health officials, and the medical profession in general, that the earliest and longest continued survey of breastfeeding initiation rates in the United States began in 1955 to provide marketing information for the maker of manufactured substitutes for human milk. These surveys now consist primarily of national fertility, health, nutrition, or natality surveys, as well as marketing surveys conducted by manufacturers of baby milk products. By the new millennium, government-sponsored health surveys in the United States and other nations and surveys sponsored by international organizations had begun asking not only about any breastfeeding, but also about the age of the infant when foods other than breastmilk were introduced and the nature of those foods. More recently, surveys have begun to ask about the timing of the first breastfeeding. A brief description of national surveys conducted in the United States follows (Box 2-1).

BOX 2-1   BREASTFEEDING SURVEYS

United States

The federal government sponsors several health surveys that include questions about infant feeding.

Centers for Disease Control and Prevention

www.cdc.gov/breastfeeding/data/
This web address contains links to all CDC surveys listed below.

Breastfeeding Report Card

http://www.cdc.gov/breastfeeding/pdf/2013BreastfeedingReportCard.pdf
Breastfeeding Report Cards, which have been issued annually since 2007, provide state-by-state data on breastfeeding initiation, continuation, and exclusivity rates at 3, 6, and 12 months. Additional data show how each state encourages breastfeeding: number of births at Baby-Friendly hospitals, number of International Board Certified Lactation Consultants (IBCLCs) and number of La Leche League leaders per 1000 live births, and support of breastfeeding at childcare centers.

Infant Feeding Practices Survey II

http://www.cdc.gov/breastfeeding/data/infant_feeding.htm
This study has not been repeated since 2007, but information collected then may still be useful. By using a series of questionnaires administered from the mother's seventh month of pregnancy through the baby's first year of life, the study gathered information about the following:

- Maternal and infant diets
- Correlates of infant feeding, sleep practices, and long-term breastfeeding
- Mothers' labor and delivery experiences and postpartum depression
- How mothers manage employment and child care
- Related topics such as food allergies, use of breast pumps, and WIC participation

Maternity Care Practices Survey

http://www.cdc.gov/breastfeeding/data/mpinc/index.htm
Every two years, beginning in 2007, the Maternity Care Practices Survey collects nationwide data about maternity care that is associated with establishing breastfeeding. A questionnaire is completed in all birth centers and hospitals that routinely provide maternity services. These data reinforce the importance of certain maternity-care practices that support establishment of breastfeeding: immediate postpartum skin-to-skin contact; rooming-in and in-hospital teaching about breastfeeding; early,

frequent, and exclusive breastfeeding; and in-person follow-up visits after discharge to monitor the progress of breastfeeding.

National Health and Nutrition Examination Survey

http://www.cdc.gov/nchs/nhanes.htm

The National Health and Nutrition Examination Survey assesses the health and nutrition status of respondents to the survey. It is the only U.S. survey that includes a home interview and a physical examination. The population sampled includes blacks, whites, and Hispanics in several age categories from younger than 6 years to more than 60 years. Questions related to breastfeeding concern whether—and if not, why not—newborns were breastfed.

U.S. National Immunization Survey

http://www.cdc.gov/breastfeeding/data/NIS_data/index.htm

Although the primary purpose of this survey is to collect data on prevalence of vaccination in young children, since July 2001 questions pertaining to breastfeeding have also been asked. Data since 2000 are available on any breastfeeding postpartum and at 6 and 12 months; in addition, data since 2003 are available on exclusive breastfeeding through 3 and 6 months. Supplementation with manufactured milks for infants has also been tracked since 2003. Tables and maps present these data by social and demographic factors and by geographic location, although for fewer years; as of fall 2013, 2007 was the most recent year for which these presentations appear on the website.

National Survey of Family Growth

http://www.cdc.gov/nchs/nsfg.htm

The National Survey of Family Growth, which collects data on an irregular basis, samples women age 15–45 years about family life, fertility, and maternal and infant health. For breastfed infants, questions ask about addition of supplemental nutriment as well as infant age at complete weaning. The resulting information is used by federal agencies to plan health services and health education programs as well as to develop statistical studies of families, fertility, and health.

National Birth Certificate Data

http://www.cdc.gov/nchs/data/dvs/birth11-03final-ACC.pdf

In 2003, a revised U.S. Standard Certificate of Live Birth was released; several revised questions ask about labor, delivery, and the general health of parents and newborn. One new question asks if the newborn is being breastfed at the time of discharge. The new certificate has been adopted on a state-by-state basis, but all states are expected to be in compliance in 2014. For a discussion of data quality and validity, refer to http://www.cdc.gov/nchs/data/nvsr/nvsr62/nvsr62_02.pdf Martin JA, Wilson EC, Osterman MJK, et al. Assessing the quality of medical and health data from the 2003 birth certificate revision: results from two states. *National Vital Statistics Reports*. 2013;62(2):1–20.

Pediatric Nutrition Surveillance System
Pregnancy Nutrition Surveillance System

http://www.cdc.gov/pednss/

The Pediatric Nutrition Surveillance System and Pregnancy Nutrition Surveillance System collect information about the nutritional status of low-income pregnant and postpartum women and their children enrolled in federally funded programs such as Special Supplemental Nutrition Program

(continues)

BOX 2-1 (*CONTINUED*)

for Women, Infants, and Children (WIC) and Head Start. Data have been collected from more than 8 million children aged birth to 5 years. These data are used to plan, manage, and evaluate the programs serving these children, to develop nutrition education programs, and to monitor progress in achieving *Healthy People* objectives for the United States. The most recent summary of data from this survey, the Pediatric Nutrition Surveillance 2010 report, can be found at http://www.cdc.gov/pednss /pdfs/PedNSS_2010_Summary.pdf.

Pregnancy Risk Assessment Monitoring System

http://www.cdc.gov/PRAMS/index.htm

The CDC and state health departments collaborate to collect data on maternal and child health indicators from women who recently gave birth; topics addressed include unintended pregnancy, prenatal care, incidence and duration of breastfeeding, alcohol and tobacco use, and infant health. These data are published in a state-by-state format. As of 2013, 40 states and New York City participated in the systems, accounting for nearly 80% of live births in the United States. The data are used to implement and review state programs and policies that affect maternal and infant health.

Food and Nutrition Service of the U.S. Department of Agriculture

WIC Participant and Program Characteristics—Special Supplemental Nutrition Program for Women, Infants, and Children

http://www.fns.usda.gov/wic-program-and-participant-characteristics-2010

Data on breastfeeding are collected each even-numbered year by the U.S. Department of Agriculture about participants in the WIC program; data are submitted by state WIC agencies. In 2010, the year covered by the most recent report available in 2013, approximately 10 million women and children were enrolled in WIC; approximately one-fourth each were mothers and infants younger than 1 year of age, and about a half were children aged 1 through 4 years. In 2010, 63% of WIC mothers began breastfeeding. Overall median duration of any breastfeeding was 13 weeks, but in some states the median was considerably higher or lower. The estimated proportion of children receiving any breastmilk for at least 6 months is 21% to 29%.

Breastfeeding Data Local Agency Report—Special Supplemental Nutrition for Women, Infants, and Children

http://www.fns.usda.gov/sites/default/files/FY2011-BFdata-localagencyreport.pdf

In 2010, for the first time, WIC compiled and published breastfeeding performance data, a requirement of Public Law 111-296. Data are tabulated by state and local agencies. The 2011 report, the most recent year of coverage available in 2013, presents breastfeeding percentages by region and by degree of breastfeeding, partial or full; these data are compared with the previous year's data.

Surveys Sponsored Privately

Ross Laboratories Mothers Survey

The Ross Mothers Survey, used for marketing purposes, has been conducted since 1955 and was the chief source of statistical data about breastfeeding for many decades. Until 2006, the survey was the source of data used to monitor breastfeeding goals in the U.S. Surgeon General's *Healthy People* programs, the current version of which is *Healthy People 2020*. It is still the largest survey; as long ago as 2002, about 1.4 million questionnaires were mailed, and about 300,000 were returned.

Questionnaire recipients are part of a probability sample of mothers whose names are obtained from a large national database of pregnant or newly delivered women. Data about the type of milk or milk product fed, but not about exclusive breastfeeding, are collected monthly for up to 12 months for a given cohort and are published on an ad hoc basis. Neither Ross nor Abbot Laboratories (which owns Ross) has a website that discusses the Mothers Survey.

HealthStyles Survey

http://www.cdc.gov/breastfeeding/data/healthstyles_survey/survey_2012.htm
The HealthStyles survey, a proprietary national marketing survey, has collected data annually since 1995 in several categories. One of these categories is health beliefs and practices, to which the CDC has contributed questions about breastfeeding since 1999. The population sampled is structured so that it mirrors demographic categories and proportions of U.S. census data; thus the data acquired are considered to reflect current cultural norms. The CDC then licenses the data to use in its own health promotion activities.

Child Trends Data Bank

http://www.childtrends.org/?indicators=breastfeeding
Child Trends is a nonprofit, nonpartisan research center in the United States that collects and analyzes data about topics in family life, health, and child development in many countries; this information is used to improve policies and programs serving children. Some breastfeeding information is collected.

Around the World

World Health Organization

Global Data Bank on Infant and Young Child Feeding

http://www.who.int/nutrition/databases/infantfeeding/en/
The WHO Global Data Bank on Infant and Young Child Feeding, which came online about 2003, continues the work begun in 1991 by WHO's Global Data Bank on Breastfeeding. It pools data from national Ministries of Health, national research and academic institutions, nongovernmental organizations, organizations within the United Nations, and reports published online. About 145 countries are represented in its 2013 online database, approximately three-fourths of the nations of the world. Studies included in the database must have a population-based sample and use standard infant and young child feeding indicators. Information is updated continually as new data become available. The data bank can be searched by country or year, and with respect to breastfeeding, it contains information about initiation of breastfeeding, exclusive breastfeeding, and any breastfeeding.

Baby-Friendly Hospital Initiative

http://www.who.int/nutrition/topics/bfhi/en/
Although the purpose of the Baby-Friendly Hospital Initiative is to promote and support breastfeeding, the website listed above presents no statistical data about changes in rates of breastfeeding after adoption of the *Ten Steps to Successful Breastfeeding*, which help qualify a birthing location as "baby friendly." For that information, turn to the many articles that focus on a given region or hospital. A 2012 review of Baby-Friendly birth facilities in the United States finds some correlation between the increasing number of birth facilities qualifying for Baby-Friendly status and increasing

(continues)

BOX 2-1 (*CONTINUED*)

rates of breastfeeding initiation (Labbok MH. Global Baby-Friendly hospital initiative monitoring data: update and discussion. *Breastfeed Med.* 2012;7:210–222. doi: 10.1089/bfm.2012.0066; http://www.ncbi.nlm.nih.gov/pubmed/22861482).

UNICEF (United Nations International Children's Fund)

ChildInfo—Monitoring the Situation of Children and Women

http://www.childinfo.org/

UNICEF monitors the well-being of women and children worldwide and, to that end, collects and analyzes demographic information on many health topics. Statistical information about breastfeeding is placed under two headings in its 2013 webpage: Statistical tables—http://www.childinfo.org/breastfeeding_tables.php and Statistics by country—http://www.childinfo.org/country_list.php.

State of the World's Children 2009—Maternal and Newborn Health

http://www.unicef.org/cotedivoire/SOWC_2009_.pdf

The 2009 issue of *State of the World's Children*, an annual publication of the World Health Organization and UNICEF, reviews maternal and newborn health throughout the world (topics differ each year). Benefits of breastfeeding are discussed in the 2009 issue, and one figure and one appendix table provide statistical information relating to breastfeeding.

Demographic and Health Surveys

http://www.measuredhs.com/What-We-Do/Survey-Types/DHS.cfm

The Demographic and Health Surveys ("Measure DHS" surveys) are nationally representative household surveys with large sample sizes (usually between 5000 and 30,000 households); they typically are conducted in a given country every 5 years. The surveys are funded by a U.S. Agency for International Development program that collects and analyzes information on infant and young child nutrition in some 90 countries. Questionnaires used in 2012 contained questions on initiation and duration of breastfeeding and on attitudes toward transmission of HIV through breastfeeding. The data sets are available to the public for analysis.

Organization for Economic Cooperation and Development Family Database

Child Outcomes

http://www.oecd.org/els/family/43136964.pdf

The Organization for Economic Cooperation and Development works with governments to improve the economic and social well-being of people around the world. Four broad categories of interest focus on the structure of families, families and the job market, public policy related to families, and child outcomes. Child Outcome 1.5 (CO1.5) reviews breastfeeding. The webpage that was currently in place in 2013 was last updated in 2009, and some data presented look back as far as 2005.

World Breastfeeding Trends Initiative (WBTi) (IBFAN Asia)

http://worldbreastfeedingtrends.org/

The World Breastfeeding Trends Initiative, in 2008 and 2012, compiled assessments of breastfeeding from 82 countries total in Africa, the Arab world, Asia, Latin America, and Oceania. These assessments are provided to governments to inform policies on infant and young child feeding and to International Baby Food Action Network (IBFAN) as a way to monitor its activities, all with the goal of reducing young child mortality.

In the United States, various arms of the Centers for Disease Control and Prevention (CDC) have now added questions about breastfeeding to their data collection instruments. The National Immunization Survey now regularly collects information about breastfeeding. Other surveys have collected such data from time to time, such as the National Health Interview Survey, National Health and Nutrition Examination Survey, and National Survey of Family Growth. In addition, the Supplemental Nutrition for Women, Infants, and Children (WIC) program sponsors the Pediatric Nutrition Surveillance System.

With the notable exception of the National Health and Nutrition Examination Survey and the National Immunization Survey, questions in many surveys pertain to "any breastfeeding"; that is, they do not distinguish between initiation, mixed feeding, or exclusive breastfeeding, and they do not report the age of the infant when other liquids or foods were first regularly added to the child's diet. Thus our ability to calculate rates of exclusive breastfeeding and continuation rates for other breastfed infants lags well behind our ability to calculate initiation rates. Government- and United Nations–sponsored surveys in developing countries collected minimal data on breastfeeding prior to the 1970s but have added more questions since then. These data have been made available to the public on the ChildInfo website (United Nations International Children's Emergency Fund [UNICEF], 2013).

Other Evidence

Until the last several decades, breastfeeding was the unremarkable norm. Thus what we "know" about breastfeeding from much earlier times often must be inferred from evidence of other methods of feeding infants. Most historical material available in English-language literature derives from a limited geographic area: Western Europe, Asia Minor, the Middle East, and North Africa. More recently, English-language reviews of ancient breastfeeding practices in other regions and varied religious traditions have begun to fill this gap (Gartner & Stone, 1994; Laroia & Sharma, 2006; Shaikh & Ahmed, 2006). Written materials, although sparse, extend back to before 2000 BC and include verses, legal statutes, religious tracts, personal correspondence, inscriptions, and medical literature.

Some of the earliest existing medical literature addresses infant feeding, at least in passing. An Egyptian medical encyclopedia, the Papyrus Ebers (c. 1500 BC), contains recommendations for increasing a mother's milk supply (Fildes, 1986). The first writings to discuss infant feeding in detail are those of the physician Soranus, who practiced in Rome around AD 100; his views were widely repeated by other writers until the mid-1700s. It is not immediately apparent to what degree these early exhortations either reflected or influenced actual practice. Many writings before AD 1800 deal primarily with wet nurses or how to hand-feed infants.

Archeological evidence provides some information about infant feeding prior to 2000 BC. Some of the earliest artifacts are Middle Eastern pottery figurines that depict lactating goddesses, such as Ishtar of Babylon and Isis of Egypt. The abundance of this evidence suggests that lactation was held in high regard (Fildes, 1986). Such artifacts first appear in sites about 3000 BC, when pottery making first became widespread in that region. Information about infant feeding may also be derived from paintings, inscriptions, and infant feeding implements.

Today, modern ethnography documents the infant feeding practices of low-technology hunter-gatherer, herding, and farming societies. Ethnographers expand our knowledge of the range of normal breastfeeding practices, and they provide a richer appreciation of cultural practices that enhance the prevalence of breastfeeding. Such studies may serve as a window into those earlier breastfeeding practices that may be the biological norm for *Homo sapiens sapiens*.

In summary, the historical aspect of this chapter deals with limited data from a limited social stratum in a limited geographic region. However, the common threads of these data provide a useful context within which we may better understand modern breastfeeding practices, especially in Western cultures.

The Biological Norm in Infant Feeding

Early Human Evolution

The class Mammalia is characterized principally by the presence of breasts (mammae), which secrete and release a fluid, milk, that for a time provides the sole nourishment of the young. This manner of sustaining newborns is extremely ancient; it dates back to the late Mesozoic era, some 100 million years ago, when the first mammals appeared (see Figure 2-1). Hominids—the precursors of *Homo sapiens*—first appeared about 4 million years ago; the genus *Homo* has existed for about 2 million years. Fossil evidence shows that our species, *Homo sapiens*, has existed for approximately 200,000 years. Our species of

anatomically modern humans, *Homo sapiens sapiens*, first became differentiated about 130,000 years ago in Africa, were present in the Near East by 90,000 years ago, and first appeared in what is now southern Europe about 40,000 years ago. Although other information about Paleolithic societies that existed 10,000 or more years ago sheds some light on this subject, direct information about breastfeeding practices among our earliest ancestors is lacking.

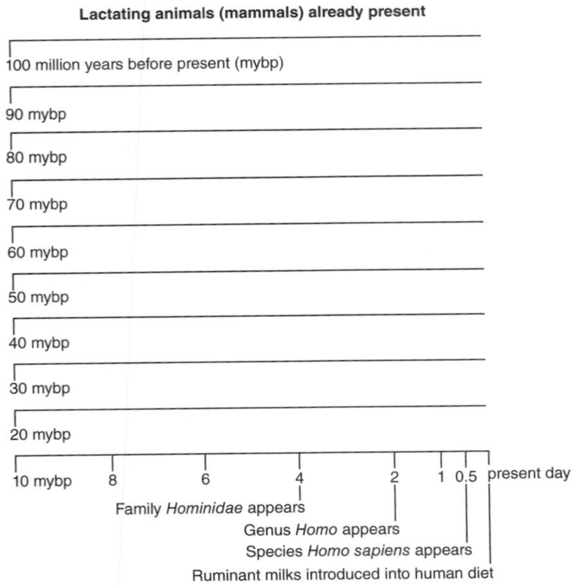

Early Breastfeeding Practices

Diets reconstructed by archeological methods reveal that the world of the Late Paleolithic era, roughly 40,000 to 10,000 years ago, was populated by hunter-gatherer peoples who ate a wide variety of fruits, nuts, vegetables, meat (both large and small game), and, where available, fish and shellfish (Eaton, 1992). This diet closely resembles that of 20th-century hunter-gatherer societies. Therefore, the infant-feeding practices of such societies today may reflect breastfeeding practices of much earlier (prehistoric) times. Consider the breastfeeding practices of the Kung of the Kalahari Desert in southern Africa (Konner & Worthman, 1980) and of hunter-gatherer societies of Papua New Guinea and elsewhere. Among these peoples, breastfeeding of young infants is frequent (averaging four feeds per hour) and short (about 2 minutes per feed). Young infants are carried much of the time, are commonly in skin-to-skin contact with their mother, and attach to the breast at will (Konnor, 2004). Breastfeeding is equally distributed throughout a 24-hour period and continues, tapering off gradually, for 2 to 6 years (Short, 1984).

Age of weaning (complete cessation of breastfeeding) in this ancient era is more difficult to pin down, but at least two lines of evidence suggest that 2 to 4 years was common in many cultures. First, weaning would be difficult before eruption of a full set of deciduous teeth, about 24 months, that allowed an infant to consume the family diet (Dettwyler, 1995). Second, as is true of other mammals, a human infant must produce lactase, the enzyme that cuts lactose (an otherwise indigestible disaccharide that is the principal sugar in milk) into

Figure 2-1 THE ANTIQUITY OF LACTATION. THE BOTTOM LINE SHOWS THE APPROXIMATE TIMES OF FIRST APPEARANCE OF LACTATING PRECURSORS OF MODERN HUMANS AND OF REGULAR USE OF NONHUMAN ANIMAL MILK BY HUMANS.

Lactating animals (mammals) already present

100 million years before present (mybp)

90 mybp

80 mybp

70 mybp

60 mybp

50 mybp

40 mybp

30 mybp

20 mybp

10 mybp   8   6   4   2   1 0.5 present day

Family *Hominidae* appears

Genus *Homo* appears

Species *Homo sapiens* appears

Ruminant milks introduced into human diet

easily digestible monosaccharides. In most mammals, the ability to produce lactase persists during the nursing interval but attenuates after weaning. In most modern human children who do not continue breastfeeding, this ability declines steadily after age 2 years and is rare by age 4 years (Dettwyler, 1995). These breastfeeding patterns are considered a direct inheritance of widely used practices that prevailed at the end of a long, and dietetically stable, evolutionary period before about 15,000 BC, after which the diffusion of agriculture brought new foods into both the adult and the infant diet. A similar pattern is seen in humans' closest primate relative, the chimpanzee, which secretes a milk quite similar to that of humans, suckles several times per hour, and sleeps with and nurses its young at night (Short, 1984).

Infant Feeding: Alternatives to Maternal Breastfeeding

To sustain their infants, most societies commonly mix breastfeeding, wet-nursing, and hand-feeding (also called dry-nursing) to one degree or another and at one time or another in the infant's life.

Wet-Nursing

Wet-nursing may not have been the only alternative to maternal breastfeeding, but it was the only one likely to enable the infant to survive. Wet-nursing is common, although not universal, in traditional societies of today and (by inference) among ancient human societies. An already-lactating woman may have been the most obvious choice for a wet nurse, but women who stimulate lactation without a recent pregnancy are also reported in descriptions of many traditional societies (Slome, 1976; Wieschhoff, 1940) and in today's literature on re-lactation (Newman & Goldfarb, 2002).

Wet-nursing for hire is mentioned in some of the oldest surviving texts, which implies that the practice was well established even in ancient times. The Babylonian Code of Hammurabi (c. 1700 BC) forbade a wet nurse to substitute a new infant for one who had died. The Old Testament Book of Exodus (Exodus 2:7–9; c. 1250 BC) records the hiring of a wet nurse for the foundling Moses (that the wet nurse was Moses's own mother is incidental). The epic poems of Homer, written down around 900 BC, contain references to wet nurses. A treatise on pediatric care in India, written during the 2nd century AD, contains instructions on how to qualify a wet nurse when the mother could not provide milk. The Koran, set in written form about AD 500, permits parents to "give your children out to nurse" (and also forbade children nursed by the same woman to marry).

Although the history of wet-nursing has continued virtually unbroken from the earliest times to the present, the popularity of the practice among the classes who used it most has waxed and waned (Stevens et al., 2009). In England during the 1600s and 1700s, as well as elsewhere in Europe, the middle classes began to employ wet nurses. The use of less attentive nurses and the sending of infants greater distances from home diminished maternal supervision of either nurse or infant. Infants might not be seen by their parents from the time they were given to the nurse until they were returned home after weaning (providing they lived). However, by the latter part of the 1700s, wet-nursing was on the decline in both North America and England, except in foundling hospitals, owing to increased public concern regarding the moral character of wet nurses—in the belief that character was transmitted through the milk—and the quality of the care they provided. In France, government officials and physicians led a campaign against wet-nursing.

Throughout this long period, wet nurses were used sometimes because of maternal debility but more often because of the social expectations of the class of women who could afford to hire a wet nurse. Thus the use of wet nurses by social elites foreshadows the demographic pattern later seen in the use of cow milk formulations to substitute for human milk.

Hand-Fed Foods

The Agricultural Revolution

The idea that animal milks are suitable foods for human infants is reflected in myths such as that of Romulus and Remus, the mythical founders of Rome, who are usually depicted as being suckled by a wolf. Surprisingly, the currently most popular hand-fed infant foods—animal milks and cereals— did not become part of the human diet until well along in human history. Cereal grains first appeared in the human diet in the Near East, only about 10,000 years ago (Eaton, 1992), and animal milks considerably later, perhaps 7000–5000 years ago (McCracken, 1971). The diffusion of agriculture and, later, animal husbandry permitted the widespread adoption of these foods.

Gruels

In much of the world, the soft foods added most commonly to the infant diet have been paps or gruels containing a liquid, a cereal or another starchy food, and other substances common in the family diet that added variety or nutritional value. The liquid might be water or cooking water, animal milk, or meat broth. The starch might be rice, wheat, or corn; or taro, cassava, or plantain. It might be boiled and mashed, ground and boiled, or—as in the case of bread crumbs—ground, baked, crushed, moistened, and reheated. In some cultures, eggs or butter products, or honey or oils, might also be added.

Animal Milks

The use of animal milk (directly or in household or commercial formulations) to nourish infants was unknown in the human diet for most of our history as a species, and animal milk is a food to which human physiology is incompletely adapted. This "newcomer" status is implied genetically, because children beyond weaning age commonly do not produce the enzyme lactase needed to digest the milk sugar lactose. In cultures that traditionally do not use animal milks, such as those in Mexico, Bangladesh, and Thailand, children may become lactose intolerant shortly after breastfeeding ceases. In other cultures that use animal milks abundantly, especially northern European societies, the onset of lactose intolerance occurs considerably later—in

Finland, for instance, after age 10 (Simoons, 1980). A young infant should be nourished by such a food only with greatest caution, as is attested by recent research into the relationship between celiac disease and a high-gluten diet early in life (Ivarsson et al., 2013).

Feeding Vessels

The earliest "vessel" used to hand-feed an infant was undoubtedly the human hand, and the foods so fed were probably soft or mashed, rather than liquid. The earliest crafted vessels for feeding liquids were probably animal horns pierced by a hole in the tip; such horns continued to be used into the 1900s in parts of Europe. The oldest pottery vessel thought to have been used for infant feeding, a small spouted bowl found in an infant's grave in France, is dated c. 2000–1500 BC (Lacaille, 1950). Small spouted or football-shaped bowls have been found in infant burial sites in Germany (c. 900 BC) and in the Sudan in North Africa (c. 400 BC) (Lacaille, 1950). These utensils suggest that hand-feeding of infants has been attempted for more than three millennia (see Figure 2-2).

Figure 2-2 AN ENGLISH STAFFORSHIRE SPODE NURSING BOTTLE, C. 1825.

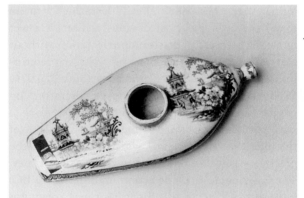

Courtesy of V. H. Brackett

Age of Infant at Introduction of Hand-Feeding

What archeological evidence cannot tell us is why or how much these infants were hand-fed. Neonates may be offered certain foods as prelacteal feeds; young infants may be offered occasional tastes of other foods, and they will be offered increasing amounts of soft foods as they slowly transition to the family diet in later infancy. Finally, infants may be reared from birth on non-human milks and other foods, whether homemade or manufactured.

Prelacteal Feeds

Many of the world's infants, even those who later will be fully breastfed, receive other foods as newborns. Of 120 traditional societies (and, by inference, many ancient preliterate societies) whose neonatal feeding practices have been described, 50 delay the initial breastfeeding more than 2 days, and some 50 others delay it 1 to 2 days. The stated reason is to avoid the feeding of colostrum, which is described as being dirty, contaminated, bad, bitter, constipating, insufficient, or stale (Morse et al., 1990). For instance, it is reported that as many as three-fourths of women in India discard colostrum for these reasons (Jethi & Shriwastava, 1987; McKenna & Shankar, 2009; Saha, 1991). The actual amount of milk discarded may range from none at all—rather, breastfeeding is delayed a day or two—to a small volume—only a few drops before the baby is put to breast—to expression of larger quantities (Bhale & Jain, 1999). Early medical writers in the eastern Mediterranean region (Greece, Rome, Asia Minor, and Arabia) and later in Europe—from Soranus through the authors of the 1600s—also discouraged the use of colostrum for feeding. These writers recommended avoiding breastfeeding for periods as short as 1 day (Avicenna, c. AD 1000) to as long as 3 weeks (Soranus, c. AD 100). Commonly, to promote the passage of meconium, the newborn was first given a "cleansing" food such as honey, sweet oils (e.g., almond), or sweetened water or wine. It is not clear why these traditions developed, because each day's delay in initiation of breastfeeding steadily increases the likelihood of neonatal death from infection (Edmond et al., 2007). Perhaps the health cost to the infant was outweighed by the social benefit that led more people to care for the newborn.

In Europe, the fear of feeding colostrum may have contributed to the undermining of maternal breastfeeding, at least among the upper classes, and helped to spread wet-nursing (Deruisseau, 1940)—wet nurses typically offered a newborn mature milk rather than colostrum. A modern version of this charge has been leveled at the prelacteal bottle feeds commonly given in Western (or Western-style) hospital nurseries; many studies show that day 1 or 2 bottle-feeds of manufactured milk products are associated with increased maternal use of manufactured substitutes for the mother's milk. (Ostensibly these practices allowed staff to check for esophageal patency and to protect against hypoglycemia; neither practice is considered an appropriate standard of care today.) One can only wonder if customary Western hospital practices, which have included delaying first breastfeeding and instead offering the neonate prelacteal feeds of water or artificial baby milk, are technological vestiges of this widespread traditional taboo.

Not all published work supports the idea that prelacteal feeds and a delay in initiating breastfeeding in and of themselves reduce the likelihood of continued lactation (see the *Anatomy and Physiology of Lactation* chapter). Some authors propose that the ensuing breastfeeding is associated with the maternal belief that prelacteal feeds are appropriate and, once breastfeeding is begun, that certain culturally approved maternal behaviors will lead to an uneventful breastfeeding course: nearly constant contact with or proximity to the infant, breastfeeding on an ad lib basis day and night, and no further use of feeding bottles (Nga & Weissner, 1986; Woolridge et al., 1985).

Mixed Feeds

Historically, early mixed feedings may have been the most common infant-feeding regimen (Dimond & Ashworth, 1987; Kusin et al., 1985; Latham et al., 1986). Mixed feeding is widely practiced today, even during the time when breastmilk forms the foundation of the infant diet. In regions such as Africa and Latin America, breastfeeding commonly continues into the second or third year of life, well after the infant has been introduced to family foods. In non-Western cultures, hand-fed foods include tea infusions, mashed fruits, and a variety of starchy gruels or pastes. Where the use of a particular food dominates a culture (such as rice in many parts of Asia), that food is usually the principal family food fed to an infant (Jelliffe, 1962). In some (mostly non-Western) cultures, such foods are offered to weaning infants in such a way that they complement, rather than replace, breastmilk (Greiner, 1996; Whitehead, 1985); thus they do not appreciably hasten complete cessation of breastfeeding. The use of feeding bottles, however, can shorten the weaning interval, that period between full sustenance by breastmilk and full sustenance by family foods (Winikoff & Laukaran, 1989). In the United States, even as the prevalence of any breastfeeding increased during the years 2000–2004, the prevalence of exclusive breastfeeding lagged. Fewer than 24% of breastfed infants were exclusively breastfed for 3 months by mothers who were still teenagers, who completed formal education at or before grade 12, who were unmarried, who lived in rural areas, or who were African American (Centers for Disease Control and Prevention [CDC], 2013b).

Hand-Feeding from Birth

In a few regions of northern Europe, a long history of dairy farming in a cool, dry climate allowed (long before the introduction of refrigeration) dairy milk to remain unspoiled for some useful interval. This happenstance permitted the survival of at least some infants who were fed cow milk nearly from birth. However, even in climatically optimal areas, lack of breastfeeding, combined with hand-feeding, was hazardous. In Iceland, infants were generally hand-fed from birth during the 1600s and 1700s despite disastrous results; married women bore as many as 30 infants because so few survived (Hastrup, 1992). In France, some foundlings and infants with syphilis were fed directly from goats; this practice was first described in writings in the 1500s, and it persisted until the early 1800s (Wickes, 1953a). Of necessity, foundling hospitals of the 1700s and 1800s in Europe and the United States hand-fed infants but with appalling death rates: as many as 100% died.

However, by the mid-1900s in many industrialized countries, hand-feeding from birth had become the norm and hand-fed infants survived and grew. How did that happen?

Technological Innovations in Infant Feeding

The Social Context

During the late 1800s and the early 1900s, high infant mortality, even among infants cared for at home, was a major public concern. Physicians and parents recognized that poorly nourished children were more susceptible to illness. Between 1910 and 1915, the newly created United States Children's Bureau sponsored several studies of infant mortality in major cities. Each study showed that babies fed any fluid other than mother's milk were three to five times as likely to die as those who were breastfed. The studies also documented that both the rate of breastfeeding and the rate of infant mortality were linked: each increased steadily as family income decreased. In summarizing these results, Williamson (1915) commented, "The disadvantages of a low income were sufficient to offset the greater prevalence of breastfeeding among the babies of the poorer families." During this same period, a similar observation was made in England, where high infant mortality prevailed among poor, working-class mothers, 80% of whom breastfed their infants (Levenstein, 1983). (However, we do not know the patterns of breastfeeding in this population, nor have we ascertained the prevalence of supplementary feeding.)

As women's aspirations for community service and commercial employment began rising, the logistics of integrating breastfeeding with regular absence from home increased the difficulty of long-term breastfeeding. Advertising that promoted bodily cleanliness may have led to associating breastmilk with body fluids that were unclean or noxious, a notion that persists to this day, at least in North America (Morse, 1989). Advances in the prevention of disease, largely through public health measures related to sanitation, extended an expanding faith in "modern science" in general to "modern medicine" in particular. Women's magazines developed a wide audience of readers interested in women's accomplishments outside the home, in modern attitudes, and in technological innovations. At the same time, these same magazines reinforced concerns about infant health and maternal adequacy. An 1880 issue of the *Ladies' Home Journal* contained this statement (Apple, 1986): "If fed from your breast, be sure that the quantity and quality supply his demands. If you are weak or worn out, your milk cannot contain the nourishment a babe needs."

The Technological Context

Between about 1860 and 1910, scientific advances and technological innovations created many new options in infant feeding that appeared to increase the survival of infants who were not breastfed. The upright feeding bottle and the rubber nipple, each of which could be cleaned thoroughly, made artificial feeding easier and somewhat safer. This equipment and the new commercial foods to be used with them were widely marketed as modern and better for mother and child. Large-scale dairy farming produced abundant supplies of cow milk which, when sold as canned evaporated milk and later in condensed (highly sweetened to retard spoilage) or dried forms, came with recipes for infant-food formulas.

This technological ferment, fueled both by the need for improved infant health care and by a popular belief in the ability of science and technology to provide answers, attracted analytical chemists. Around 1850, chemists had begun to turn their attention to food products. Early investigations (now viewed as rudimentary) into the composition of human and cow milk convinced them that "the combined efforts of the cow and the ingenuity of man" could construct a food the equal of human milk (Gerrard, 1974). Patented foods, such as Liebig's Food and Nestlé's Milk Food, were first marketed in Europe and the United States in the 1860s. The Nestlé's product was a mixture of flour, cow milk, and sugar that was to be dissolved in milk or water before feeding. Milk modifiers, such as Mellin's Food, and milk foods, such as Horlick's Malted Milk, were popular in the United States by the 1880s.

Extravagant claims for these foods (Liebig's Food was called "the most perfect substitute for mother's milk") were combined with artful advertising that played on fears for the health of the infant and faith in modern science (Apple, 1986) (Figure 2-3). A hundred years later, we see these advertising themes replayed again and again.

In the 1890s, physician Thomas Rotch developed a complex system for modifying cow milk so that it "more closely resembled human milk." Rotch observed that the composition of human milk varies, as do digestive capacities in infants. He devised mathematical formulas to denote the proportions of fat, sugar, and protein that some infants required at a particular age (Rotch, 1907). The result was an exceedingly complex system of feeding that required constant intervention by the physician, who often changed the "formula" weekly. Supervising infant feeding then became a principal focus of the newly emerging specialty of pediatrics—a situation that may continue to influence the field today.

Commercial advertising promoted the use of manufactured milk products for infant feeding to mothers and to health workers. Again, the basic themes—a mother's concern for her infant's welfare, the supposed difficulty of breastfeeding, and the "perfection" of the manufactured product—have persisted into the 21st century (Apple, 1986).

The Role of the Medical Community

Breastfeeding, in fact, may have become more onerous during the last 200 years, as women were increasingly impelled to give birth and then to feed according to externally generated ideas about how those activities should be accomplished.

Figure 2-3 AN ADVERTISEMENT FOR ARTIFICIAL INFANT MILK THAT APPEARED IN THE *LADIES' HOME JOURNAL* IN 1895.

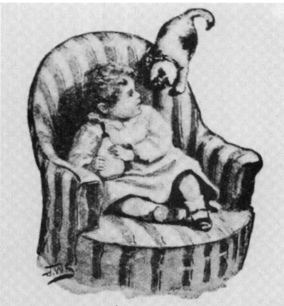

Nestlé's Food

Nestlé's Food is a complete and entire diet for babies. Over all the world Nestlé's Food has been recognized for more than thirty years as possessing great value as a protection against Cholera Infantum and all other forms of Summer Complaint.

Nestlé's Food is safe. It requires only the addition of water to prepare it for use. The great danger always attendant on the use of cow's milk is thus avoided.

Consult your doctor about Nestlé's Food, and send to us for a large sample can and our book, "The Baby," both of which will be sent free on application.

THOMAS LEEMING & CO.
73 Warren Street, New York

Regulation of Childbirth

During the early part of the 1900s, childbirth moved (for all but the most impoverished families) largely from home or midwife-attended births to hospitals. In these facilities, a birthing woman was separated from her family and friends (in part because of the fear of infection) and was attended by hospital staff. During the middle part of the 20th century, the widespread use of general anesthesia during labor and delivery and other hospital routines were instituted that separated mother and infant for much of the early postpartum period. Bottle-feeding by nursery staff, initially with hospital-produced formulas but later with manufactured milk products, became common. Normal postpartum hospital stays in the United States lengthened; during the 1930s and 1940s, they were sometimes as long as 2 weeks. This period, which was intended to permit the mother to recuperate from a commonly highly medicated childbirth, usually resulted in a return home with an impaired milk supply and a baby who was accustomed to feeding from bottle nipples. As long ago as the mid-1940s, Bain noted that babies who were older than 8 days at discharge were less apt to be breastfed than were younger ones (Bain, 1948).

Regulation of Breastfeeding

Underlying many changes in the feeding of infants was a "regulatory" frame of mind, the seeds of which had been sown in Europe as early as the 1500s. The advent of book printing about that time permitted a much wider dissemination of works on infant care. Their authors, male physicians, shared a concern for the high incidence of gastrointestinal illness in infants and for high infant mortality. For reasons not at all clear today, "overfeeding" was deemed a central factor in both conditions. Writers concerned with child care responded by advocating the regulation of feeding to prevent presumed overfeeding. Writing in the mid-1600s, Ettmuller (1703; cited in Wickes, 1953a) was not the first to recommend infrequent feedings: "Nothing is more apt to disorder the child than suckling it too often, since large quantities of milk stagnating in the stomach, must need corrupt ... especially if fresh milk be pour'd in before the preceding be digested." Some 250 years later in 1900, Pierre Budin (1907; cited in Wickes, 1953b), a French obstetrician famous for his early interest in caring for premature infants and for his advocacy of breastfeeding, was nonetheless typical of many others in recommending small feedings: "It is better at first to give too little than too much (for an underfed infant failed to gain weight but it was free from digestive troubles)."

Even early medical writers who strongly recommended breastfeeding also recommended highly regulated times for feedings—a fixed number of feedings at fixed times. William Cadogan (1749; cited in Kessen, 1965), whose firm endorsement of breastfeeding and largely sound advice prompted many privileged English women to breastfeed, advocated only four feeds per day at equal intervals, and no night feeds. A prototype mothercraft manual by Hugh Smith (1774; cited in Fildes, 1986) contains excellent advice: to feed colostrum and to allow the newborn to suckle frequently to stimulate lactation. However, it then instructs mothers to limit feeds (beginning at 1 month), to five per day between 7 A.M. and 11 P.M. (although how those feedings were timed in households that generally lacked clocks is difficult to imagine). About 50 years later, after recommending ad lib feeds for the first 10 days, Thomas Bull (1849; cited in Wickes, 1953a) instructed mothers to feed for the rest of the first month at regular 4-hour intervals day and night, because he also believed that irregular feeding harmed the infant. After 1 month, the night feed was to be eliminated.

These influential publications began to remove the management of infant feeding from the mother (and from the realm of women in general) and place it in the hands of (usually male) "authorities." Cadogan (1749; cited in Kessen, 1965) commended this change that put "men of sense rather than foolish unlearned women" in charge; Rotch, a century and a half later (1907), deplored the fact that "mothers and nurses ... dominated the physicians."

Despite earlier concern on the part of "authorities" about too much milk, the most common concern among all classes of women in the United States, at least since popular women's magazines became widely distributed in the late 1800s, was that the mother did not have enough milk. It has been observed that "not enough milk" corresponds closely with the widespread implementation of infant feeding schedules (Wolf, 2006). For far too long, women able to consult physicians were thus placed in a double bind, and—as they tried to satisfy both the baby and the physician who directed how the mother cared for her baby—breastfeeding oftentimes got left behind.

With respect to a newborn's first breastfeed, as late as the 1950s physicians in the United States ordered that newborns be given nothing by mouth for the first 24 hours after birth. In Australia, midwifery texts of the 1940s recommended that the baby not go to the breast until 12 hours after birth (Thorley, 2001). Today, immediate postpartum skin-to-skin contact between mother and neonate and encouragement to breastfeed are thought best. At a minimum, bringing baby to breast within the first hour after birth is recommended (WHO, 2009). One can only wonder which of today's standard recommendations to breastfeeding mothers will be shown, at some time in the future, to be counterproductive.

Many—and perhaps most—of our everyday decisions are influenced by the social norms of our culture, our civic community, and our immediate circle of family and friends (Baranowski et al., 1983; Matich & Sims, 1992; Saadeh et al., 1993; Tiedje et al., 2002). The long-standing need in the United States for breastfeeding "promotion" is rooted in the common perception (in the United States) that the breast is primarily for sexual gratification and, therefore, should not be exposed in public. Notwithstanding the fact that legislation in all states in the United States permits breastfeeding in public (CDC, 2013a), many mothers avoid doing so because of social censure. However, considerable regional and demographic variation in such attitudes exists in the United States (Hannan et al., 2005; Ryan et al., 2004). In general, New England, the mountain West, and Pacific regions appear to be most accepting of breastfeeding in public. In a survey conducted in the United States in 2004, 37% of people questioned agreed that mothers should breastfeed only in private; a nearly equal percentage favored allowing breastfeeding in public, and the remainder, about 27%, were undecided (CDC, 2004). Almost 10 years later, little had changed. A news story in 2013 reported that 40% of surveyed mothers were "concerned" (the term was not further defined) about breastfeeding in public (*Business Wire*, 2013). The same prejudice is present in some other countries. An Australian telephone survey found that almost 83% of respondents favored bottle-feeding rather than breastfeeding in public (McIntyre et al., 2001); discussion of that topic was still taking place in social media in 2013 (Parenting Central Australia, 2013).

Mass media may also influence perceptions of breastfeeding. One study in the United States found that after the number of commercial advertisements for manufactured infant food products increased in one widely circulated magazine geared toward parents, breastfeeding prevalence dropped during the following year (Foss & Southwell, 2006). Magazine illustrations depicting breastfeeding may produce a decidedly mixed reaction. In 2006, one popular magazine's cover photo depicted a portion of breast with a baby latched on (no nipple visible); in a poll of about 4000 readers, only about one-fourth objected to the photo, but those people objected strongly (*CBS News*, 2006).

Regulation and Industrialization

This "regulatory" frame of mind fit nicely with the needs of the growing industrial sector of the economy, which relied on efficiency best obtained through schedules governed by the clock. Societal perceptions of infants' innate characteristics and needs were interpreted in this light (Millard, 1990). Early in the 1900s, infants were seen as needing order imposed onto their characters from the outside (Rossiter, 1908): "An infant two days old may be forming either a good or a bad habit. A child that is taken up whenever it cries is trained into a bad habit; the same principle is true in reference to nursing a baby to stop its crying. Both these habits cultivate self-indulgence and lack of self-control." "Good mothering" thus drifted toward meeting the letter of schedules commonly imposed by the

medical profession rather than meeting the mutual needs of mother and infant as expressed by and interpreted within the dyad.

Although the use of rigid, externally imposed infant-care schedules began diminishing in the 1970s, much "how to" breastfeeding literature, even now, assumes that lactation functions better when mother and baby develop feeding routines—and the sooner those routines are settled, the better. The lack of some routine is usually perceived as abnormal by both mother and physician (Millard, 1990). Unfortunately, certain attitudes required of most employees, such as an awareness of time within a hierarchical authority structure, are least apt to enable a mother or a pediatrician to accommodate the normal irregularities of early breastfeeding.

Regulation of Contraception

During the late 1950s and early 1960s, the widespread acceptance of oral contraceptives may have hurried the decline in breastfeeding (Meyer, 1968). Contraceptives containing estrogen reduce milk volume and, therefore, contribute to lactation insufficiency, early supplementation, and early weaning from the breast. Moreover, women who planned to use combined estrogen and progestin oral contraceptives were discouraged from breastfeeding so as to avoid passing those hormones to the infant. During this period, several million women per year in the United States alone were thereby removed from the pool of potential breastfeeders. Concurrently, the widespread adoption of manufactured substitutes for human milk led to loss of the contraceptive benefit of lactation amenorrhea.

Although low-progestin contraceptives once were thought to pose fewer hazards to the maternal milk supply and the baby (Kelsey, 1996), a later review of the literature found the evidence on this point to be contradictory (Truitt et al., 2003). The Academy of Breastfeeding Medicine (2005) recommended that mothers be advised that all contraceptives that contain any exogenous hormone may reduce breastmilk supply. [A revision of the contraception protocol under way in 2013 continued to caution against estrogenic methods during lactation and against early progestogenic methods, because onset of lactation results from the decline in progestin levels following the delivery of the placenta. However, it will also include new CDC (2013c) recommendations that allow all methods during lactation by 4 weeks postpartum, with cautionary notes.]

As a result of the wide use of exogenous contraceptives for many decades, the understanding of how early full breastfeeding can serve as a reliable contraceptive has been lost by most laywomen and medical professionals alike.

Accommodation Between Physicians, Other Health Professionals, and Infant Milk Manufacturers

The relationship between physicians, other health professionals, and infant food manufacturers has in general promoted mothers' dependency on either the manufacturer or the physician for information on infant feeding. In the late 1800s as proprietary infant foods were being developed, manufacturers advertised to both groups. By the 1920s, some preparations were advertised to mothers but could be purchased only by prescription or used only after consulting a physician: the package contained no instructions for use. By 1932 the American Medical Association essentially required manufacturers of milk products for infants to advertise only to the medical profession (Greer & Apple, 1991). The mutual economic benefits of this policy were clearly spelled out in many advertisements placed by formula manufacturers in medical journals: "When mothers in America feed their babies by lay advice, the control of your pediatric cases passes out of your hands, Doctor. Our interest in this important phase of medical economics springs, not from any motives of altruism, philanthropy, or paternalism, but rather from a spirit of enlightened self-interest and cooperation because (our) infant diet materials are advertised only to you, never to the public" (Mead Johnson, 1930). For many decades, this unwritten agreement extended to medical education as well. Formula companies may spend as much as $10,000 per medical student during a student's education

(National Alliance for Breastfeeding Advocacy, 2007). Many nursing and dietetic professional organizations also accept money from formula companies to fund continuing education, grants, and other projects.

Despite several early studies that showed breastfed infants to be healthier than bottle-fed ones (Grulee et al., 1934; Howarth, 1905; Woodbury, 1922), for years many physicians advised mothers that there was little advantage to breastfeeding. This view was expressed consistently up through the 1960s. For instance, Aitken and Hytten (1960) reported that "with modern standards of hygiene, artificial feeding on simple mixtures of cow's milk, water, and sugar is a satisfactory substitute for breast feeding." Despite an overwhelming amount of research that shows that infants fed manufactured milk products have greater morbidity, hospitalization, and mortality (Raisler et al., 1999; Steube, 2009 [see also extensive references therein]), or the inverse, that breastfed infants enjoy better health (Ip et al., 2007), even in 2013 statements similarly dismissive of the crucial role of breastmilk in infant health could still be heard. On a more positive note, since 1997 many professional health organizations have endorsed breastfeeding as the superior way to feed infants (see a subsequent section, "Statements by Health Organizations").

The Prevalence of Breastfeeding

United States

1940–2000

Beginning in the 1940s, the net result of shifts in technology, commercial advertising, and social attitudes (discussed previously) was a rapid decline in the prevalence of breastfeeding in Western nations. In the United States, the proportion of newborns receiving any breastmilk at 1 week postpartum declined steadily to a low of 25% in 1970 (Martinez & Krieger, 1985). The proportion of newborns exclusively breastfed at hospital discharge was even lower: in 20 years, it declined from 38% in 1946

(Bain, 1948) to 21% in 1956 (Meyer, 1968) and to only 18% in 1966 (Meyer, 1968).

This period of sharpest decline of breastfeeding coincided with economic factors in the United States that encouraged major migrations from rural to urban areas, and those migrations may have contributed to the decline. For example, between 1945 and 1970, approximately 5 million African Americans, seeking greater opportunity and financial security, moved from the rural South to the urban North or far West (Coombs, 1972; Gregory, 2005). The association between internal migration from rural to urban areas and a decline in breastfeeding has been noted in other countries as well (Brockerhoff, 1994; Millman, 1986; Pasternak & Ching, 1985).

Current Breastfeeding Practices

In the United States, breastfeeding rates reversed in the 1970s and rose gradually until the mid-1980s. Breastfeeding prevalence then dipped for a few years but has slowly risen since the early 1990s. As of spring 2013, the provisional rate of any breastfeeding of children born in 2009 (the most recent year for which National Immunization Survey data had been analyzed) was 77%—five percentage points below the *Healthy People 2020* goal of 81.5%—of hospital-born infants initiating breastfeeding. The rate of any breastfeeding at 6 months of age rose to 47%—an encouraging trend but still lower than the 61% goal set by *Healthy People 2020* (CDC, 2013b; U.S. Department of Health and Human Services [DHHS], 2010a).

Various populations of women differ considerably in their breastfeeding practices. Notably, lower rates of initiation and continuation (especially for exclusive breastfeeding—nothing fed by mouth except human milk)—persisted among women who were younger, nonwhite, and unmarried; who had less formal education and low incomes; and who lived in rural areas (Grummer-Strawn & Shealy, 2009; Kogan et al., 2008). Geographic variations in the United States are also evident. In general, higher initiation rates and continuation rates at 6 months were found in the West and Northwest (Kogan et al., 2008). In 2013, about half of U.S. states collected "ever breastfed" data on the basis of information provided on a birth certificate. The birth certificate approach, however, does not include continued breastfeeding or exclusive breastfeeding, information that would add much to our understanding at the state level. All states are now collecting breastfeeding data on women within the WIC program.

Outside North America

The Role of Colonial Empires

Declines in the prevalence of breastfeeding were noted in non-Western regions somewhat later than in Europe and North America. Between World Wars I and II, British, French, and German colonial empires controlled fully one-fourth of the inhabited globe and one-fourth of the world's population. These empires served as vehicles for the expansion of markets for, among other things, manufactured milk products for infants.

Colonial ruling elites who followed the practices of their social class in their country of origin (a class that placed social distance between the ruling elites and the population ruled) were much more likely to feed their infants artificial milks than to breastfeed. The fact that most of these infants survived is due in large part to the larger roles played by the sanitation and medical care that their position in life afforded them. To some degree, these colonial elites served as unwitting models for indigenous peoples.

Concern for the health of indigenous peoples led many healthcare workers to transmit Western attitudes toward infant feeding to the populations they served by example, by direct recommendations, and by the training provided to indigenous healthcare providers. Westerners have traditionally assumed that foods good for them must be good for all people and have passed these notions to foreign nationals trained in Western schools (McCracken, 1971). Perhaps because Western medical personnel were successful in treating many other health problems, local populations were prepared to accept attitudes that encouraged the use of artificial baby-milk products. Healthcare personnel in hospitals who helped to introduce the use of those products reinforced the undermining of breastfeeding (Winikoff & Laukaran, 1989).

Colonial transportation and communication networks and health clinics and hospitals aided the advertisement and sale of manufactured milk products to this huge population. The decline in breastfeeding accelerated after World War II: contact increased between Western healthcare personnel and populations in developing countries; relief projects originating in the United States shipped to war-torn countries a surplus of skim milk, produced by the large dairy industry in the United States; and manufacturers of milk products for infants created large new markets. Later, their sales practices were damningly documented in the report *The Baby Killer* (War on Want & Muller, 1974; see also National Alliance for Breastfeeding Advocacy, 2007). Subsequently, the market for such milk products diminished somewhat in Europe and North America; in turn, manufacturers' intensive sales efforts were redirected toward Africa and Asia. Those efforts continue to reward manufacturers: in 2011, formula manufacturers spent $190 million on advertising in Indonesia alone; in return, they grossed $1.1 billion in sales (Prakasa, 2013).

Infant Feeding and Infant Mortality

The relationship between infant feeding and infant mortality is complex. Infant mortality has tended to be highest among populations in which breastfeeding was most common—the poor. The same relationship held in the United States as early as the early 1900s (Williamson, 1915).

Although artificial feeding has been associated with more illness (Steube, 2009)—especially gastrointestinal illness (Quigley et al., 2006)—and with poorer infant survival in all countries studied—developing nations (Habicht et al., 1988) and Western developed nations (Chen & Rogan, 2004) alike—the reverse is not always the case. The advent of primary health care for a large portion of a population may explain decreases in infant mortality in the face of declines in breastfeeding. The pervasive problems of poverty, in both Western and non-Western (Lartey, 2008) locales, continue to be at the root of the high infant mortality seen in many impoverished populations.

Current Breastfeeding Practices

During the 1970s, when breastfeeding initiation rates were generally rising in Western nations, the corresponding rates among developing countries fluctuated around post–World War II developing-country rates in response to societal adjustments such as advertising of substitutes for human milk, internal migration from rural to urban locales, and entry of greater numbers of women into the paid labor force (Millman, 1986). However, breastfeeding continued to be widely practiced in many countries studied in Africa, Asia, Europe, and Latin America. During the period 1999–2004, pooled data from demographic and health surveys showed that more than 95% of infants younger than 6 months old were breastfed, as were 88% of infants 6–12 months old. Although mixed feeds were the norm, manufactured infant milk products formed only a small portion of infant diets (Marriott et al., 2007). Detailed information for individual countries about rates of exclusive breastfeeding and of continuation after introduction of complementary feedings can be found in child nutrition statistics published by UNICEF (2009).

The Cost of Not Breastfeeding

> To see a world in a grain of sand
> And a heaven in a wild flower,
> Hold infinity in the palm of your hand
> And eternity in an hour.
>
> —William Blake,
> "Auguries of Innocence," c. 1803

Breastfeeding—or not—can be that grain of sand through which one can see various influences on the health of infant and mother, the costs of healthcare infrastructure, and the economics of infant feeding at many scales. Although isolated voices championed breastfeeding throughout its years of steady decline, not until the 1970s did the trend toward artificial feeding reverse. What prompted this change? The reasons are not clear but seem to reflect a widespread desire by many to include simpler, more natural practices in their lives—and, in the case of breastfeeding, a reliance on new scientific evidence. Existing lay organizations that promoted breastfeeding began to spread more widely. Basic, clinical, and demographic research increasingly demonstrated the benefits of human milk and breastfeeding to the infant and of lactation and breastfeeding to the mother. Later still, it was recognized that not only does breastfeeding promote better long-term health for infant and mother, but that *not* breastfeeding entails long-term physiological and financial costs.

Health Risks of Using Manufactured Substitutes for Human Milk

Risks to the Infant

It has been recognized since the advent of manufactured infant milks that infants fed these products suffer more acute illness than do breastfed infants (Cunningham et al., 1991; Grulee et al., 1934; Howarth, 1905; INFACT Canada, 2006; Quigley et al., 2006; Raisler et al., 1999; United States Breastfeeding Committee, 2002; Woodbury, 1922). Moreover, even in the United States, both black and white infants fed on manufactured infant milk products suffer 20% more deaths in their first year than do breastfed infants (Chen & Rogan, 2004). Artificially fed infants are denied the benefits of autoimmunization, whereby the breast produces antibodies to organisms to which the infant has been exposed. This observation is confirmed by more recent studies that are discussed in subsequent chapters of this text. At the time of the earlier studies, the immunological role of breastmilk was unclear; hence most of the deleterious effects of manufactured milk products for infants were attributed to contamination. In more recent decades, it has become established that artificial baby milks increase the risk of ill health by many pathways (Walker, 1993). Not only can manufactured infant milks be (or easily become) contaminated, but they also lack the immunological and other health-promoting factors present in human milk. In addition, they contain compounds that are either foreign to humans or are present in nonphysiologic proportions. Furthermore, the act of bottle-feeding differs from that of breastfeeding in ways that may contribute to cardiopulmonary problems in some infants. The effects of artificial feeding may extend well beyond infancy.

Risks to the Mother

Artificial feeding is also detrimental to maternal health. In the absence of lactation amenorrhea, additional pregnancies may ensue that adversely affect the mother's health. As discussed in a later chapter, mothers who artificially feed their infants are more likely than breastfeeding mothers to later develop health problems such as osteoporosis, premenopausal breast cancer, and ovarian cancer (INFACT Canada, 2006; Labbok, 2001). Bottle-feeding mothers who have diabetes will not enjoy the same amelioration of symptoms that may be experienced by breastfeeding mothers who have diabetes (Butte et al., 1987). Moreover, healthy mothers who use manufactured infant milk products to feed their infants (and those infants as well) are more likely to develop type 2 diabetes later in life (Stuebe et al., 2005).

Economic Costs of Using Manufactured Substitutes for Human Milk

The presence or absence of breastfeeding affects the economics of the family, the community, and the country at large. Some of these effects are more pronounced in less developed regions, but to some degree they affect all segments of populations in technologically advanced regions.

Costs to the Family

Although lactation imposes some metabolic demands on the mother—an extra 500 kcal/day is needed to synthesize human milk (Butte et al., 2001)—these demands are moderated by gastric changes that allow lactating women to metabolize foods more efficiently (Illingworth, 1986;

Uvnas-Moberg et al., 1987) and by the water-conserving effect of prolactin (Dearlove & Dearlove, 1981). Moreover, the contraceptive effect of full, unrestricted breastfeeding reduces a woman's physical and economic costs of childbearing (Jackson, 1988; Kennedy et al., 1989).

The direct monetary costs of rearing an infant who is breastfed are markedly lower than the costs of rearing one who is artificially fed (Ball & Bennett, 2001; Ball & Wright, 1999). Approximately 150 cans of ready-to-feed manufactured milk products for infants are used during the first 6 months of full artificial feeding (approximate 6-month cost, 2013, ready-to-feed: $1050–$2250). Even mothers who receive free manufactured infant milk from the WIC program (see the later discussion) must pay for it after their WIC eligibility expires. In industrial nations, the cost of manufactured baby milk may exceed the cost of additional food for the lactating mother by two or three times (Jarosz, 1993)—and by even more if a special mixture is required to minimize the baby's allergies or other health problems. In developing nations, this ratio is many times higher. In regions where one-third to one-half of those persons in large urban areas live in poverty, the cost of manufactured milk products required to provide adequate nutrition (and implements with which to feed them) represents a substantial portion of the family income (Serva et al., 1986). Other members of the family may eat more poorly because the baby is artificially fed.

An equally important consideration is the increased need for medical care by infants fed with manufactured milk products (Weimer, 2001). The frequency and severity of illnesses in a young infant is directly related to the proportion of the diet that comes from human milk substitutes (Cattaneo et al., 2006; Chen et al., 1988). As intake of manufactured milk products increases, infant intake of high-quality protein and a variety of other needed nutrients decreases, as compared with the intake of breastfed infants, and artificial feeding increases infant exposure to potential pathogens in other foodstuffs (Habicht et al., 1988). One study

calculated that if 90% of U.S. families breastfed exclusively for 6 months, as medical organizations now recommend (in 2013), $13 billion would be saved in excess medical costs of treating infants fed manufactured human milk substitutes (Bartick & Reinhold, 2010). A decade or more ago, it was estimated that insurers paid out $1.3 billion more for infants fed manufactured infant milks, as compared with breastfed infants, to treat only three conditions in the first year of life: respiratory infections, ear infections, and diarrhea (Riordan, 1997; Weimer, 2001). That sum is even larger now. These mind-boggling figures likely underestimate the total excess cost of caring for artificially fed infants because they account for the treatment of only a few types of childhood illness.

Because full breastfeeding that incorporates frequent feeds throughout a 24-hour period tends to delay resumption of ovulation (Chao, 1987; Lewis et al., 1991), spacing between births tends to increase. Births spaced less than 3 years apart tend to increase the mortality risk of both the older child and the younger infant (Retherford et al., 1989; Rutstein & Macro International, 2008). Especially in families living at subsistence level, the older a child is when he or she is displaced from the breast and the fewer the number of children in a family, the more likely each child is to be healthy. In malnourished communities, breastfeeding may substantially increase child survival up to 3 years of age (Briend et al., 1988; WHO & UNICEF, 2003).

Thus the breastfed infant stands a significantly greater likelihood of surviving. The mother's physical and emotional investment in pregnancy and lactation and the familial investment in time and money are repaid by the survival of a child; they are lost to the family when that child dies.

Cost to the Community and State

Community or national units that provide health care must respond to the local epidemiology of infant illness, in which feeding may play a major role. Morbidity is more prevalent in artificially fed infants regardless of location. The increase in the infant population resulting from the loss of the contraceptive effect of breastfeeding also serves to increase the need for pediatric health care.

The debate on the economic value of breastfeeding has tended to focus on health costs or on the cost of food for the mother rather than manufactured milks for the infant, but the value of the time and energy women expend on breastfeeding is rarely estimated. The value of time spent breastfeeding is neglected (along with other unwaged caring work women do, such as caring for children who fall ill as a result of not breastfeeding).

Another little-discussed aspect of the replacement of breastfeeding by use of manufactured products is that certain sectors of an economy can become economically dependent on the payrolls met and taxes paid by manufacturers of milk products for infants, especially if capital funds are obtained from outside the country. Once they become a financial presence in a country, those manufacturers may be politically and economically difficult to dislodge, despite increases in health costs elsewhere in the economy. Worldwide, revenues from the manufacture of infant milks, baby food, and ancillary products such as bottles and bottle nipples are projected to reach $23.8 billion by the year 2015 (Global Industry Analysts, 2010). In the process of developing this market, the industry creates a large payroll and tax revenues in communities where factories are located. Moreover, such manufactured milk products are subsidized by the diversion of resources (land and dairy cattle, and people to manage both) as well as by manufacturing capacity pulled from other possible uses. When one considers that more than 30 million babies are born annually in Africa alone (United Nations, 2011), it becomes apparent that providing adequate volumes of manufactured milks represents a staggering burden and a largely unnecessary diversion of human and monetary resources from other more beneficial programs. At a time when environmental issues have become paramount, these unnecessary uses of power and raw material, not to mention the disposal of discarded packaging, is an increasing concern. The benefits of breastfeeding, then, extend through a small environmental footprint to the society at large (DHHS, 2010b).

The Promotion of Breastfeeding

The many ways of encouraging mothers to breastfeed their own infants—breastfeeding promotion—may be considered to lie on a continuum. At one end, in societies where breastfeeding is the cultural norm, "promotion" consists of assuming that mother and infant will breastfeed. This assumption is combined with social arrangements, such as special foods for the mother or lightened duties, especially during the first few weeks after birth, to ensure that breastfeeding becomes well established. At the other end, in societies in which artificial feeding is the norm, promotion often consists of encouragement to breastfeed, sometimes offered by government officials and often by healthcare professionals or members of elite population groups. These "promoters," unfortunately, may be unable to cultivate in the general population more accepting attitudes toward breastfeeding or to remove social or workplace barriers to breastfeeding. It is now clear that promotion of breastfeeding without support and protection of the breastfeeding mother produces little long-term gain, and that the ways in which manufactured infant milks are inferior to human milk—rather than the reverse—need to become more generally understood.

Breastfeeding Promotion in the United States

"Healthy People" Statements

National health objectives were first formally defined in 1978 and published the following year as *Healthy People* (DHHS, 1979). The initial goal for breastfeeding stated that 75% of women should breastfeed at hospital discharge and 35% at 6 months, as opposed to the actual 1978 figures of 45% and 21%, respectively. The current report, *Healthy People 2020*, proposed increasing the percentage of ever-breastfed infants to 82% and those breastfed at 6 months to 60%, among other goals (DHHS, 2010a) (Table 2-1). Another document issued by

Table 2-1 BREASTFEEDING GOALS AND PREVALENCE IN THE UNITED STATES, 1990–2020 (PERCENT)[a]

Degree of Breastfeeding	Healthy People 2000[b]		Healthy People 2010[c]		Healthy People 2020[e]	
	Actual, 1990	Goal, 2000	Actual, 2001[c]	Goal, 2010	Actual, 2006[f]	Goal
Any breastfeeding						
Early postpartum	52	75	72	75	74	82
6 months	18	50	37	50	44	61
12 months		25	18	25	23	34
Exclusive breastfeeding						
3 months			31[d]	40	34	46
6 months			12[d]	17	14	26

[a] Percentages are rounded to the nearest whole number.

[b] *Source:* http://www.cdc.gov/nchs/data/hp2000/hp2k01.pdf (National Center for Health Statistics. *Healthy People 2000 final review.* Hyattsville, MD: Public Health Service; 2001).

[c] *Source:* http://wonder.cdc.gov/data2010/obj.htm (U.S. Department of Health and Human Services. DATA2010: the *Healthy People* 2010 database. 2011 edition. Updated August 2013).

[d] For year 2004, first year reported in DATA2010 website (as in note c).

[e] *Source:* http://www.healthypeople.gov/2020/topicsobjectives2020/objectiveslist.aspx?topicId=26#102124 (U.S. Department of Health and Human Services. *Healthy People 2020.* Maternal, infant, and child health objectives (MICH) 21: increase the proportion of infants who are breastfed. 2010a).

[f] Data for children born in 2006 as reported in 2007–2009; see *Healthy People 2020* website (as in note e).

the Department of Health and Human Services (2011) affirms the benefits of breastfeeding, recognizes barriers to breastfeeding, and recommends actions that will make it more likely that babies will be breastfed. However, it does not recommend specific legislation to support breastfeeding.

The WIC Program

Although other government agencies in the United States also work to improve infant nutrition, the Special Supplemental Nutrition Program for Women, Infants, and Children—the WIC program—probably directly affects the greatest number of people. Established in 1972, this program provides free nutrition counseling and food supplements, which may include manufactured infant milk products, to low-income mothers and their infants (U.S. Department of Agriculture, 2012a). Clients typically come from those population segments in the United States least likely to breastfeed (those of low income, less formal education, and black race) (CDC, 2006, 2013b).

The WIC program follows in the footsteps of U.S. infant welfare programs established in the 1890s and at the turn of the century, as well as in France, England, and elsewhere, that operated centers where infants could be weighed and examined weekly. These centers also provided cow milk ("fresh and clean" in some cases, sterilized in others) to nonbreastfeeding mothers in an effort to reduce infant illness and death caused by the use of contaminated milk. By 1903, such milk dispensaries were already being accused of discouraging breastfeeding because they seemed to endorse artificial feeding of infants (Wickes, 1953b). Even today, government-sponsored distribution of free milk has been considered one reason for the decline of breastfeeding (Ryan & Zhou, 2006; Sandiford et al.,

1991). The WIC program remains the largest purchaser (and distributor, at little cost to the manufacturers) of manufactured milk products for infants in the United States (Kent, 2006; Oliveira, 2011; Tuttle, 2000): in 2010 it served more than half of all infants born in the United States (Oliveira, 2011), of whom the majority were fed formula. As a result, the direct cost to WIC of supporting mothers who never breastfeed is nearly twice the cost of supporting breastfeeding mothers (United States Breastfeeding Committee, 2002).

The promotion of breastfeeding finally became a goal within WIC in the late 1980s. The Child Nutrition and WIC Reauthorization Act of 1989 required that a certain proportion of WIC's budget be spent on the promotion and support of breastfeeding and that each state health department establish a breastfeeding promotion coordinator. That budget proportion remains small, however. In 2005, only 0.6%—$34 million—of a $5.2 billion WIC budget was earmarked for promotion and support of breastfeeding (Ryan & Zhou, 2006); in 2011, a budget of $7.6 billion earmarked 1.1% —$83 million—for breastfeeding promotion (U.S. Department of Agriculture, 2011). Thus the dollar amount spent to promote breastfeeding is only a small fraction of the amount spent for manufactured infant milk. In 2013, breastfeeding women had a higher priority for enrollment in WIC programs than did nonbreastfeeding mothers: they were provided with more, and more varied, foods, and their benefits persist longer—1 year, as opposed to 6 months for nonbreastfeeders (U.S. Department of Agriculture, Food and Nutrition Service, 2012b).

Despite these efforts, the increases in breastfeeding rates of WIC enrollees have been minimal. Mothers enrolled in WIC not only initiate breastfeeding at a much lower rate (at least 20% lower at all time points; 2003 data) than mothers at large (Ryan & Zhou, 2006), but they also initiate breastfeeding at a lower rate than mothers who qualify for WIC aid but are not enrolled in this program (Li et al., 2005). Even women of Hispanic or Asian ethnicity, who traditionally breastfeed, do so at lower rates if they are enrolled in WIC. The conclusion, then, is that WIC participation lowers breastfeeding initiation and duration (Ryan & Zhou, 2006).

Breastfeeding advocates such as the American Academy of Nursing Expert Panel on Breastfeeding are speaking out on the disconnect between WIC's breastfeeding supportive policy and its practices that indicate "funding is overwhelmingly spent on formula with only a small fractional portion allocated toward peer counseling programs" (Baumgartel et al., 2013). The group is calling for the Food and Nutrition Service to adjust funding to more fully support peer counseling programs, which are known to increase breastfeeding rates and duration.

United States Breastfeeding Committee

In 1998, supported by the Maternal and Child Health Bureau of the Department of Health and Human Services, a national breastfeeding conference was convened to form a breastfeeding committee. The United States Breastfeeding Committee was established, composed of representatives from government and nongovernmental organizations and health professional associations. The committee's goals have been to expand awareness of the value of breastfeeding and to recommend policies to government and corporate organizations that increase breastfeeding prevalence (United States Breastfeeding Committee, 2001).

Legislation

Legislation intended to increase the prevalence of breastfeeding may mandate actions that encourage breastfeeding or discourage feeding of artificial baby milk (or use of wet nurses), or both. One of the earliest known examples was set in 350 BC by Lycurgus, the king of Sparta: he required not only that mothers nurse their own infants, but also that nursing mothers be shown kindness and respect (Hymanson, 1934).

Pressures external to the mother and infant have dictated not only when an infant should be breastfed, but also where. Social censure and in some places the interpretation of statutory laws regarding indecent exposure have often limited the public places in which a woman might breastfeed. Although the best situation would be a pervasive social acceptance of breastfeeding such that legislation permitting breastfeeding in public is not needed, legislation protecting the right to breastfeed is, at least for the moment, the next best thing. Beginning in 1984 in New York State, American women began to gain the legal right to breastfeed in public places. Ten years later, laws in five states addressed breastfeeding. In the United States, a 1999 federal law makes breastfeeding legal on all federal property where a woman has the right to be (United States Breastfeeding Committee, 2013). As of 2012, no state laws forbade breastfeeding in public. Laws of 48 states and the District of Columbia—but not Idaho or West Virginia—address breastfeeding in public, either by permitting a woman to breastfeed anyplace where she is entitled to be or by exempting a woman who is breastfeeding in public from charges of indecent exposure (National Conference of State Legislatures, 2012).

Statements by Health Organizations

In 1997, the American Academy of Pediatrics Work Group on Breastfeeding issued a policy statement endorsing breastfeeding; the current statement was published in 2012. The initial statement received considerable attention from the press, accelerating nationwide interest in breastfeeding. Other professional organizations have published similar endorsements of breastfeeding: the American College of Obstetricians and Gynecologists (2007),

the Association of Women's Health, Obstetric, and Neonatal Nurses (2007), the National Association of Pediatric Nurse Practitioners (2007), the American Dietetic Association (2009), the American College of Nurse–Midwives (2011), the Academy of Breastfeeding Medicine (2008), the American Public Health Association (2011), and the American Academy of Family Physicians (2013).

International Breastfeeding Promotion

The International Code of Marketing of Breast-Milk Substitutes

In the 1970s, as the deleterious effects of manufactured baby milk products on infant health and survival became better appreciated, the role of advertising in spreading the use of these products became increasingly suspect. In 1981, the World Health Organization, by a vote of 118 to 1 (the United States cast the sole dissenting vote), approved the International Code of Marketing of Breast-Milk Substitutes. This code provides a model of marketing practices that permits the availability of manufactured baby milk products but forbids advertisement or free distribution directly to consumers (Box 2-2).

BOX 2-2 WHO CODE OF MARKETING OF BREAST-MILK SUBSTITUTES

- No advertising of these products to the public.
- No free samples to mothers.
- No promotion of products in healthcare facilities.
- No company mothercraft nurses to advise mothers.
- No gifts or personal samples to health workers.
- No words or pictures idealizing artificial feeding, including pictures of infants, on the products.
- Information to health workers should be scientific and factual.
- All information on artificial feeding, including the labels, should explain the benefits of breastfeeding, and the costs and hazards associated with artificial feeding.
- Unsuitable products, such as condensed milk, should not be promoted for babies.
- All products should be of a high quality and take into account the climatic and storage conditions of the country where they are used.

Source: Reproduced, with permission of the publisher, from International Code of Marketing of Breast-milk Substitutes http://whqlibdoc.who.int/publications/9241541601.pdf, page16
ISBN/WHO Reference Number 92 4 154160 1, Geneva, World Health Organization, 1981.

The code also seeks to balance the information provided by manufacturers of milk products for infants, in both written "educational" material and in the text or pictures on containers of the product (Armstrong, 1988; International Baby Food Action Network, 1985). In 1996, the World Health Assembly of the World Health Organization passed six resolutions that further clarify the intent of the international code. Of these six, one reaffirms the use of local family foods to complement the diet of breastfeeding infants beyond about 6 months of age. Another reaffirms the need to end the free or low-cost (subsidized) distribution of manufactured baby-milk products to newly parturient women in the hospital. Two other resolutions proscribe receipt of funds from manufacturers or distributors of artificial baby milk or feeding supplies to be used for professional training in infant and child health, or for financial support of any organization that monitors compliance with the international code (World Health Organization 1996). As of 2011, of 168 countries surveyed, exactly half had enacted into law many or all of the provisions of the international code: 37 had adopted all or substantially all of the provisions, and 47 had enacted many of the provisions. Most others had enacted some of the provisions. Only 6 countries—including the United States—have not adopted any of the provisions of the code (UNICEF, Nutrition Section, 2011).

The international code focuses attention on ways in which the infant formula industry influences both consumers and professionals to increase the use of its products. Direct advertising to consumers may be the most obvious method, but what Jelliffe and Jelliffe (1978) called "manipulation by assistance" is also effective. For example, formula manufacturers not only provide free formula to hospital nurseries, but also assist in the design of those nurseries (usually leading to greater separation of mothers and infants), donate equipment and supplies to hospitals and individual physicians (bottles of formula and sterile water, for example), support conferences (including some dealing with breastfeeding), and even entertain hospital staff at company-sponsored events. Gift bags containing formula or coupons for formula for many years have been presented to new mothers at hospital discharge. These gift bags are given to the hospitals by manufacturers of baby-milk products; mothers who receive such bags are less likely to breastfeed exclusively during the first 10 weeks postpartum (Merewood, 2008). Such "gifts" have received greater publicity from watchdog organizations since 2006, and such publicity has led some hospitals to eliminate this practice. These "gifts" are treated by the baby-milk manufacturers as marketing expenses. As individuals and institutions become financially dependent on such gifts and enmeshed in social relationships with company salespeople, they are more likely to tacitly endorse, or even recommend, artificial baby milks. By highlighting such practices as marketing ploys, the international code may make healthcare professionals more aware of the intent behind them and, in turn, perhaps more resistant to their allure. Lactation consultants should be watchful to avoid succumbing to such "manipulation by assistance" banned by the international code.

Innocenti Declaration

In 1990, the World Health Organization and the United Nations International Children's Emergency Fund (UNICEF) were instrumental in the development of the Innocenti Declaration, which restated the importance of breastfeeding for maternal and child health. It set forth four goals to be met by 1995: (1) the establishment of national breastfeeding coordinators and a national breastfeeding committee, (2) the practice of *Ten Steps to Successful Breastfeeding* by maternity services (Box 2-3), (3) the implementation of the WHO International Code of Marketing of Breast-Milk Substitutes, and (4) enactment of enforceable laws for protecting the breastfeeding rights of employed women (UNICEF, 1990).

An offshoot organization, the World Alliance for Breastfeeding Action (WABA), was founded in 1991; it is a multinational coalition of individuals and private organizations active in research and promotion of breastfeeding (WABA, 2013). It works to ensure that the goals of the Innocenti Declaration are met, and it annually supports activities presented during World Breastfeeding Week, the first

---

Box 2-3 Ten Steps to Successful Breastfeeding

Every facility providing maternity services and care for newborn infants should:

1. Have a written breastfeeding policy that is routinely communicated to all healthcare staff.
2. Train all healthcare staff in skills necessary to implement this policy.
3. Inform all pregnant women about the benefits and management of breastfeeding.
4. Help mothers initiate breastfeeding within 30 minutes after birth.
5. Show mothers how to breastfeed, and how to maintain lactation even if they should be separated from their infants.
6. Give newborn infants no food or drink other than breastmilk, unless medically indicated.
7. Practice rooming-in—that is, allow mothers and infants to remain together 24 hours a day.
8. Encourage breastfeeding on demand.
9. Give no artificial teats or pacifiers (also called dummies or soothers) to breastfeeding infants.
10. Foster the establishment of breastfeeding support groups and refer mothers to them on discharge from the hospital or clinic.

Source: Reproduced, with permission of the publisher, from Evidence for the ten steps to promote successful breastfeeding - http://whqlibdoc.who.int/publications/2004/9241591544_eng.pdf, p. 5. Protecting, Promoting, and Supporting Breastfeeding: The Special Role of Maternity Services. [A joint WHO/UNICEF statement]. Geneva, Switzerland: World Health Organization, 1989.

Note: These steps and the complete elimination of free and low-cost supplies of breastmilk substitutes, bottles, and teats from healthcare facilities form the basis for the Baby-Friendly Hospital Initiative.

See also: World Health Organization, Evidence for the Ten Steps to Promote Successful Breastfeeding, 1998.

---

week in August—an opportunity for people worldwide to celebrate and support breastfeeding.

Baby-Friendly Hospital Initiative

The World Health Organization and UNICEF launched the Baby-Friendly Hospital Initiative (BFHI) in 1991 to encourage specific birth-center practices in all countries that promote exclusive breastfeeding. To be designated "Baby-Friendly," a hospital must demonstrate to an external review board that it practices each of the 10 steps to successful breastfeeding outlined in the Innocenti Declaration. With the major exception of the Scandinavian countries, industrialized nations have moved more slowly than developing nations. Of some 20,000 maternity facilities worldwide that have been designated as Baby-Friendly, 170 are in the United States (Baby-Friendly USA, 2013). The principal stumbling block has been the political and financial difficulty of the requirement that hospitals not accept free infant milk products from manufacturers. Breastfeeding advocates in the industrialized world continue to struggle against

three impediments: a manufactured-milk industry that is powerful enough, both financially and politically, to avoid most regulation; a pervasive bottle-feeding culture that does not consider breastfeeding important to child or maternal health; and the lack of much precedence for government-mandated health programs. As a result, all industrialized nations together can claim only a small percentage of all Baby-Friendly hospitals.

Several studies have examined the degree to which the "Ten Steps" are being implemented and their effect on hospital practices and breastfeeding outcomes (Broadfoot et al., 2005; DiGirolamo et al., 2008; Merewood et al., 2005; Merten et al., 2005). Without exception, these studies have shown that implementation of the "Ten Steps" leads to higher rates of initiation and longer duration of breastfeeding, even in hospitals that have implemented only half of the steps, and even among populations less likely to breastfeed. A high proportion of mothers delivering in a hospital or birthing center designated as Baby-Friendly are able to breastfeed because of the consistent support they receive from the staff and from their birth experience in a breast-feeding-friendly environment.

Private Support Movements

In the 1950s and 1960s, during the nadir of breast-feeding in the United States, the first voluntary groups to offer information and support to women interested in breastfeeding were formed: La Leche League International (LLLI) in the United States, Nursing Mothers' Association of Australia, and Ammehjelpen of Sweden. Such groups assist individual women and have focused national attention on the benefits of breastfeeding. La Leche League is officially recognized as a nongovernmental organization qualified to consult on breastfeeding to organizations such as the United Nations and the United States Agency for International Development. As of 2012, it had a presence—accredited leaders or other ongoing source of LLLI information—in 70 countries (La Leche League International, 2013). Members of groups such as these, by their demonstration that even "modern" mothers can breastfeed, and by their requests to medical personnel for information about medical practices that support breastfeeding, have been a major force behind the dissemination of technical information concerning lactation, human milk, and breastfeeding.

To better reach low-income women, who are not commonly La Leche League members, LLLI has trained more than 3000 peer counselors—low-income women who have breastfed and have completed a training program. Offering breastfeeding advice and support in clinics that serve low-income populations, such counselors can be very effective.

SUMMARY

Humans evolved within the mammalian lineage, which has provided a species-specific milk for the nourishment and protection of the young of each species. For millennia, the staple of the human infant's diet has been human milk obtained directly from the human breast, commonly in situations where no other food was suitable. Within the last century or so, as breastfeeding became associated with restrictive aspects of women's lives, as breastmilk was thought by some to be inferior to increasingly available manufactured infant milk products, and as use of manufactured milks became a hallmark of privileged segments of society, large portions of both lay and healthcare populations came to believe that there was little reason to persist in traditional breastfeeding practices.

Since the early 1990s, however, it has become increasingly clear that breastfeeding confers health, cognitive, and psychological advantages both on the breastfeeding infant and on the child and adult into which that infant will grow. Breastfeeding enhances aspects of maternal health as well. Breastfeeding is economically frugal and ecologically sound. Breastfeeding is important at both the family and the community level. The promotion efforts outlined in this chapter are needed because, to some degree in most countries (and particularly in the United States), the most important requirements are missing: acceptance by society at large of the need for a mother and child to be together, and the right of the breastfeeding dyad to participate in social, civic, and commercial activities outside the home. For many women, the ultimate barrier to breastfeeding is not sore nipples, night-time nursing, or employment outside the home, but rather the disapproval they encounter for "wasting" their education and career skills by staying home with their breastfeeding infants, or for being considered disruptive or even obscene for taking their breastfeeding infant with them to work or to worship, or perhaps to a city council or parent–teacher meeting, or simply to a restaurant or to a park. A goal for all women should be to empower mothers so that they are able to attend to all of their duties, maternal as well as civic, religious, and professional.

Those who breastfeed or who promote the reestablishment of breastfeeding as the norm in infant feeding do so not because there are no alternatives, but because the alternatives are inferior. Unfortunately, the belief that breastfeeding is the optimal way to nourish an infant may not be enough to empower a woman to breastfeed. Knowledge of beneficial breastfeeding practices and society's acceptance of those practices are also required. Currently, the prevalence of breastfeeding reflects the importance that society places on it, as measured by the degree to which breastfeeding mothers and infants are accepted within the life of the community at large. Returning breastfeeding wisdom to the public domain and reintegrating breastfeeding into the social fabric so that women who wish to breastfeed may do so without hindrance is the challenge that awaits.

KEY CONCEPTS

- The class Mammalia is characterized by breasts (mammae) that secrete and release a fluid that for a time is the sole nourishment of the young; breastfeeding dates back some 100 million years.
- Among modern hunter-gatherers, whose breastfeeding practices may be very ancient, breastfeeds tend to be frequent (on average 4 of per hour), short (about 2 minutes), and equally distributed throughout a 24-hour day, and they persist for 2 to 6 years.
- Beginning in the 1700s, mothercraft manuals began to shift the management of infant feeding from the mother (or women in general) to "authorities," usually male. By the early part of the 1900s, "good mothering" had drifted toward following the feeding and infant-care schedules advocated by those authorities.
- Before about 1900, information about breastfeeding incidence, prevalence, and practices came from indirect sources; since the mid-1900s, national surveys and World Health Organization data have been available.
- Before about 1900, wet-nursing was the only alternative to breastfeeding that was likely to allow the infant to survive.
- The currently typical hand-fed infant foods did not become part of the human diet until late in human history; cereal grains were domesticated only about 10,000 years ago and animal milks only about 5000 years ago.
- In the 1890s, physician Thomas Rotch developed a complex system of progressive modifications of cow milk to make it more digestible by infants of various ages; this system required constant intervention by the physician, who might change an infant's "formula" on a weekly basis.
- In the decades around 1900, high infant mortality was a major public concern, standards of modesty strictly limited breastfeeding outside the home, and advances in science and technology led to the creation of dry or tinned artificial infant foods.
- In the United States, the proportion of newborns receiving any breastfeeding declined steadily after 1940 to a low of 25% in 1970; the trend then reversed and, despite a dip in the late 1980s, rose steadily until it generally plateaued in the first decade of the 21st century.
- Infants fed manufactured milk products experience more illness because such milks lack the nutritive and immunologic qualities of breastmilk. Mothers who use manufactured infant milks are more susceptible to osteoporosis, premenopausal breast cancer, and ovarian cancer.
- Infants who are fed manufactured milk products are more costly to raise, in part because of the considerable cost of the formula and in part because they commonly suffer more, and more severe, illness as compared with breastfed infants.
- The diversion of land, power, and raw material to the manufacture of milk products for infants and the disposal of discarded packaging are sources of increasing ecological concern.
- Especially after World War II, the United States and Western Europe exported hand-feeding practices to countries that they colonized or otherwise influenced.
- Voluntary groups dedicated to promoting breastfeeding, such as La Leche League International in the United States, Nursing Mothers' Association of Australia, and Ammehjelpen in Sweden, began in the 1960s and 1970s and paved the way for governmental efforts to promote and support breastfeeding.

- In the United States, national breastfeeding goals were first stated in 1979 in *Healthy People: The Surgeon General's Report on Health Promotion and Disease Prevention*.
- During the 1980s, the promotion of breastfeeding in the United States became a goal within the Women, Infants, and Children (WIC) program. However, only a small percentage of that program's budget goes for breastfeeding promotion and support, and breastfeeding rates of WIC enrollees, who typically come from population segments less likely to breastfeed, are low.
- The International Code of Marketing of Breast-Milk Substitutes was approved in 1981 by the World Health Organization; it permits manufactured infant milks to be available but forbids their advertisement or free distribution directly to consumers.
- The Innocenti Declaration was approved in 1990 by the World Health Organization and the United Nations International Children's Emergency Fund; it encourages specific hospital perinatal practices that promote exclusive breastfeeding.
- Breastfeeding promotion efforts in 2013 recognize that promotion must also include support and protection of the breastfeeding mother and that the harmful outcomes of feeding manufactured infant milks must be addressed as well as the many health benefits of breastfeeding to infant and mother.

References

Academy of Breastfeeding Medicine. Contraception during breastfeeding: clinical protocol 13. Available at: http://www.bfmed.org/ace-files/proto col/finalcontraceptionprotocolsent2.pdf. 2005. Accessed August 4, 2013.

Academy of Breastfeeding Medicine. Position on breastfeeding. *Breastfeeding Medicine*. 2008;8(4):267–270.

Aitken FC, Hytten FE. Infant feeding: comparison of breast and artificial feeding. *Nutr Abstr Rev.* 1960;30:341–371.

American Academy of Family Physicians. Breastfeeding [Policy statement]. 2013. Available at: http://www.aafp.org/about/policies/all/breastfeeding.html. Accessed August 2013.

American Academy of Pediatrics, Section on Breastfeeding. Policy statement: breastfeeding and the use of human milk. *Pediatrics.* 2012;129:e827–e841.

American Academy of Pediatrics, Work Group on Breastfeeding. Breastfeeding and the use of human milk. *Pediatrics.* 1997;100:1035–1039.

American College of Nurse–Midwives. Position statement on breastfeeding. 2011. Available at: http://www.midwife.org/ACNM/files/ACNMLibraryData/UPLOADFILENAME/000000000248/Breastfeeding%20statement%20May%202011.pdf. Accessed August 2013.

American College of Obstetricians and Gynecologists. Breastfeeding: maternal and infant aspects. 2007. Available at: http://www.acog.org/Resources%20And%20Publications/Committee%20Opinions/Committee%20on%20Health%20Care%20for%20Underserved%20Women/Breastfeeding%20Maternal%20and%20Infant%20Aspects.aspx. Accessed July 2013.

American Dietetic Association. Promoting and supporting breastfeeding. *J Am Dietetic Assoc.* 2009;109(11):1926–1942. Available at: http://www.eatright.org/About/Content.aspx?id=8377. Accessed August 2013.

American Public Health Association. APHA endorses the Surgeon General's call to action to support breastfeeding. 2011. Available at: http://www.apha.org/advocacy/policy/policysearch/default.htm?id=1422. Accessed August 2013.

Apple RD. "Advertised by our loving friends": the infant formula industry and the creation of new pharmaceutical markets, 1870–1910. *J Hist Med Allied Sci.* 1986;41:3–23.

Armstrong H. The International Code of Marketing of Breast-Milk Substitutes (Part 2). *J Hum Lact.* 1988;4:194–199.

Association of Women's Health, Obstetric and Neonatal Nurses (AWHONN). Breastfeeding. 2007. Available at: https://www.awhonn.org/awhonn/binary.content.do;jsessionid=18DC4DFDA7A95EA82E7AFB308008EF63?name=Resources/Documents/pdf/5_Breastfeed.pdf

Baby-Friendly USA. Baby-friendly hospitals and birth centers. 2013. Available at: http://www.babyfriendlyusa.org/find-facilities. Accessed November 2013.

Bain K. The incidence of breast feeding in hospitals in the United States. *Pediatrics.* 1948;2:313–320.

Ball TM, Bennett DM. The economic impact of breastfeeding. *Pediatr Clin North Am.* 2001;48:253–262.

Ball TM, Wright AL. Health care costs of formula-feeding in the first year of life. *Pediatrics.* 1999;103:870–876.

Baranowski T, Bee DE, Rassin DK, et al. Social support, social influence, ethnicity and the breastfeeding decision. *Soc Sci Med.* 1983;17:1599–1611.

Bartick M, Reinhold A. The burden of suboptimal breastfeeding in the United States: a pediatric cost analysis. *Pediatrics.* 2010;125(5):e1048–e1056.

Baumgartel, KL, Spatz, DL, American Academy of Nursing Expert Breastfeeding Panel. WIC (the Special Supplemental Nutrition Program for Women, Infants, and Children): policy versus practice regarding breastfeeding. *Nurs Outlook.* 2013;61:466–470.

Bhale P, Jain S. Is colostrum really discarded by Indian mothers? *Indian Pediatrics.* 1999;36:1069–1070.

Briend A, Wojtyniak B, Rowland MGM. Breast feeding, nutritional state, and child survival in rural Bangladesh. *Br Med J.* 1988;296:879–882.

Broadfoot M, Britten J, Tappin DM, MacKenzie JM. The Baby Friendly Hospital Initiative and breast feeding rates in Scotland. *Arch Dis Child Fetal Neonat Ed.* 2005;90:F114–F116.

Brockerhoff M. The impact of rural–urban migration on child survival. *Health Transition Review.* 1994;4:127–149.

Business Wire. Lansinoh study reveals nearly half of U.S. moms uncomfortable breastfeeding in public. Available at: http://www.businesswire.com/news/home /20130110006362/en/Lansinoh-Study-Reveals-U.S.-Moms-Uncomfortable-Breastfeeding. Accessed 24 June 2013.

Butte NF, Garza C, Burr R, et al. Milk composition of insulin-dependent diabetic women. *J Pediatr Gastroenterol Nutr.* 1987;6:936–941.

Butte NF, Wong WW, Hopkinson JM. Energy requirements of lactating women derived from doubly labeled water and milk energy output. *J Nutr.* 2001;131:53–58.

Cattaneo A, Ronfani L, Burmaz T, et al. Infant feeding and cost of health care: a cohort study. *Acta Paediatrica.* 2006;95:540–546.

CBS News. Eyeful of breast-feeding mom sparks outrage. July 28, 2006. Available at: http://www.cbsnews.com /stories/2006/07/28/national/main1844454_page2. shtml. Accessed September 21, 2007.

Centers for Disease Control and Prevention (CDC). HealthStyles Survey: breastfeeding practices, 2004. Available at: http://www.cdc.gov/breastfeeding/data /healthstyles_survey/survey_2004.htm#2004. Accessed September 21, 2007.

Centers for Disease Control and Prevention (CDC). Racial and socioeconomic disparities in breastfeeding—United States, 2004. *MMWR.* 2006;55:335–339. Accessed June 1, 2013.

Centers for Disease Control and Prevention (CDC). Breastfeeding among U.S. children born 2000–2010, CDC National Immunization Survey. 2013a. Available at: http://www.cdc.gov/breastfeeding/data/nis_data/. Accessed August 2013.

Centers for Disease Control and Prevention (CDC). Progress in increasing breastfeeding and reducing racial/ethnic differences—United States, 2000–2008 births. *MMWR.* 2013b;62(5):77–80.

Centers for Disease Control and Prevention (CDC). U.S. selected practice recommendations for contraceptive use, 2013 (adapted from the World Health Organization selected practice recommendations for contraceptive use, 2nd edition). *MMWR.* 2013c;62. Available at: http://www.cdc.gov/mmwr/pdf/rr/rr62e0614.pdf. Accessed December 9, 2013.

Chao S. The effect of lactation on ovulation and fertility. *Clin Perinatol.* 1987;14(1):39–50.

Chen A, Rogan WJ. Breastfeeding and the risk of postneonatal death in the United States. *Pediatrics.* 2004;113(5):e435–e439.

Chen Y, Yu S, Li W. Artificial feeding and hospitalization in the first 18 months of life. *Pediatrics.* 1988;81:58–62.

Coombs N. The new Negro, immigration and migration. In: *The black experience in America.* 1972. Available at: http:// www.gale.cengage.com. Accessed September 15, 2007.

Cunningham AS, Jelliffe DB, Jelliffe EFP. Breast-feeding and health in the 1980s: a global epidemiologic review. *J Pediatr.* 1991;118:659–666.

Dearlove JC, Dearlove BM. Prolactin fluid balance and lactation. *Br J Obstet Gynaecol.* 1981;88:652–654.

Deruisseau LG. Infant hygiene in the older medical literature. *Ciba Symposia.* 1940;2:530–560.

Dettwyler KA. A time to wean: the hominid blueprint for the natural age of weaning in modern human populations. In: Stuart-Macadam P, Dettwyler KA, eds. *Breastfeeding: biocultural perspectives.* New York, NY: Aldine de Gruyter; 1995:39–73.

DiGirolamo AM, Grummer-Strawn LM, Fein S. Effect of maternity care practices on breastfeeding. *Pediatrics.* 2008;122(suppl 2):543–549.

Dimond HJ, Ashworth A. Infant feeding practices in Kenya, Mexico and Malaysia: the rarity of the exclusively breastfed infant. *Hum Nutr Appl Nutr.* 1987;41A:51–64.

Eaton SB. Humans, lipids and evolution. *Lipids.* 1992;27(10):814–820.

Edmond KM, Kirkwood BR, Amenga-Etego S, et al. Effect of early infant feeding practices on infection-specific neonatal mortality: an investigation of the causal links with observational data from rural Ghana. *Am J Clin Nutr.* 2007;86(4):1126–1131.

Fildes VA. *Breasts, bottles, and babies: a history of infant feeding.* Edinburgh, Scotland, UK: Edinburgh University Press; 1986.

Foss KA, Southwell BG. Infant feeding and the media: the relationship between *Parents' Magazine* content and breastfeeding, 1972–2000. *Intl Breastfeeding J.* 2006;1:10. Available at: http://www.international-breastfeedingjournal.com/content/1/1/10. Accessed August 15, 2007.

Gartner LM, Stone C. Two thousand years of medical advice on breastfeeding: comparison of Chinese and western texts. *Sem Perinatol.* 1994;18(6):532–536.

Gerrard JW. Breast-feeding: second thoughts. *Pediatrics.* 1974;54:757–764.

Global Industry Analysts, Inc. Baby foods and infant formula: a global strategic business report. San Jose, CA, June 15, 2010. Available at: http://www.prweb.com

/releases/baby_foods_market/infant_formula_market
/prweb4123354.htm. Accessed July 15, 2013.

Greer FR, Apple RD. Physicians, formula companies, and advertising: a historical perspective. *Am J Dis Child.* 1991;145:282–286.

Gregory JN. *The Southern diaspora.* Chapel Hill, NC: University of North Carolina Press; 2005.

Greiner T. The concept of weaning: definitions and their implications. *J Hum Lact.* 1996;12:123–128.

Grulee CG, Sanford HN, Herron PH. Breast and artificial feeding: influence on morbidity and mortality of twenty thousand infants. *JAMA.* 1934;103:735–739.

Grummer-Strawn L, Shealy K. Progress in protecting, promoting, and supporting breastfeeding, 1984–2009. *Breastfeed Med.* 2009;4(suppl 1):S31–S39.

Habicht J-P, DaVanzo J, Butz WP. Mother's milk and sewage: their interactive effect on infant mortality. *Pediatrics.* 1988;88:456–461.

Hannan A, Li R, Benton-Davis S, Grummer-Strawn L. Regional variation in public opinion about breastfeeding in the United States. *J Hum Lact.* 2005;21(3):284–288.

Hastrup K. A question of reason: breastfeeding patterns in seventeenth and eighteenth-century Iceland. In: Maher V, ed. *The anthropology of breast-feeding: natural law or social construct.* Oxford, UK: Berg; 1992:91–108.

Howarth WJ. The influence of feeding on the mortality of infants. *Lancet.* July 22, 1905;2:210–213.

Hymanson A. A short review of the history of infant feeding. *Arch Pediatr.* 1934;51:1–10.

Illingworth PJ. Diminution in energy expenditure during lactation. *Br Med J.* 1986;292:437–441.

INFACT Canada. *Risks of not breastfeeding: a brief annotated bibliography,* 2nd rev. (prepared by Sterken E). Toronto, Canada: INFACT Canada; 2006.

International Baby Food Action Network/International Organization of Consumers Unions (IBFAN/IOCU). *Protecting infant health: a health worker's guide to the International Code of Marketing of Breast-Milk Substitutes.* Penang, Malaysia: IBFAN/IOCU; 1985.

Ip S, Chung M, Raman G, et al. *Breastfeeding and maternal and infant health outcomes in developed countries.* Evidence Report/Technology Assessment 153 (prepared by Tufts–New England Medical Center, Evidence-Based Practice Center, under Contract No. 290-02-0022). AHRQ Publication No. 07-E007. Rockville, MD: Agency for Healthcare Research and Quality; 2007. Available at: http://citeseerx.ist.psu.edu/viewdoc/download?doi=10.1.1.182.8429&rep=rep1&type=pdf. Accessed March 11, 2014.

Ivarsson A, Myléus A, Norström F, et al. Prevalence of childhood celiac disease and changes in infant feeding. *Pediatrics.* 2013;131(3):e687–e694. doi: 10.1542/peds.2012-1015. E-pub February 18, 2013.

Jackson RI. Ecological breastfeeding and child spacing. *Clin Pediatr.* 1988;27:373–377.

Jarosz LA. Breast-feeding versus formula: cost comparison. *Hawaii Med J.* 1993;52:14–16.

Jelliffe DB. Culture, social change and infant feeding: current trends in tropical regions. *Am J Clin Nutr.* 1962;10:19–45.

Jelliffe DB, Jelliffe EFP. *Human milk in the modern world.* Oxford, UK: Oxford University; 1978.

Jethi SC, Shriwastava DK. Knowledge, attitudes and practices regarding infant feeding among mothers. *Indian Pediatr.* 1987;24:921–924.

Kelsey JJ. Hormonal contraception and lactation. *J Hum Lact.* 1996;12:315–318.

Kennedy K Rivera R, McNeilly AS. Consensus statement on the use of breastfeeding as a family planning method. *Contraception.* 1989;39:447–496.

Kent G. WIC's promotion of infant formula in the United States. *Intl Breastfeed J.* 2006;1(8). Available at: http://www.international breastfeedingjournal.com/content/1/1/8. Accessed October 14, 2007.

Kessen W. *The child.* New York, NY: Wiley; 1965.

Kogan MD, Singh GK, Dee DL, et al. Multivariate analysis of state variation in breastfeeding rates in the United States. *Am J Public Health.* 2008;98(10):1872–1880. Available at: http://www.ncbi.nlm.nih.gov/pmc/articles/PMC2636475/. Accessed March 11, 2014.

Konnor M. Hunter-gatherer infancy and childhood. 2004:19–64. Available at: http://anthro.vancouver.wsu.edu/media/Course_files/anth-302-barry-hewlett/melkonner.pdf. Accessed December 7, 2013.

Konner M, Worthman C. Nursing frequency, gonadal function, and birth spacing among Kung hunter-gatherers. *Science.* 1980;207:788–791.

Kusin JA, Kardjati S, van Steenbergen W. Traditional infant feeding practices: right or wrong? *Soc Sci Med.* 1985;21:283–286.

Labbok MH. Effects of breastfeeding on the mother. *Pediatr Clin North Am.* 2001;48:143–158.

Labbok MH, Wardlaw T, Blanc A, et al. Trends in exclusive breastfeeding: findings from the 1990s. *J Hum Lact.* 2006;22(2):272–276.

Lacaille AD. Infant feeding-bottles in prehistoric times. *Proc R Soc Med.* 1950;43:565–568.

La Leche League International. Annual report 2011–2012. Available at: http://www.llli.org/docs/00000000000000001AnnualReport/2011-2012annual_report.pdf. Accessed July 29, 2013.

Laroia N, Sharma D. The religious and cultural bases for breastfeeding practices among the Hindus. *Breastfeed Med.* 2006;1(2):94–98.

Lartey A. Maternal and child nutrition in sub-Saharan Africa: challenges and interventions. *Proc Nutr Soc.* 2008;(67(1):105–108.

Latham MC, Elliott TC, Winikoff B, et al. Infant feeding in urban Kenya: a pattern of early triple nipple feeding. *J Trop Pediatr.* 1986;32:276–280.

Levenstein H. "Best for babies" or "preventable infanticide"? The controversy over artificial feeding of infants in America, 1880–1920. *J Am Hist.* 1983;70:75–94.

Lewis PR, Brown JB, Renfree MB, Short RV. The resumption of ovulation and menstruation in a well-nourished population of women breastfeeding for an extended period of time. *Fertil Steril.* 1991;55:529–536.

Li R, Darling N, Maurice E, et al. Breastfeeding rates in the United States by characteristics of the child, mother, or family: the 2002 National Immunization Survey. *Pediatrics.* 2005;115(1):e31–e37.

Marriott BM, Campbell L, Hirsch E, Wilson D. Preliminary data from demographic and health surveys on infant feeding in 20 developing countries. *J Nutr.* 2007;137:518S–523S.

Martinez GA, Krieger FW. 1984 Milk-feeding patterns in the United States. *Pediatrics.* 1985;76:1004–1008.

Matich JR, Sims LS. A comparison of social support variables between women who intended to breast or bottle-feed. *Soc Sci Med.* 1992;34:919–927.

McCracken RD. Lactase deficiency: an example of dietary evolution. *Curr Anthrop.* 1971;12:479–517.

McIntyre E, Hiller JE, Turnbull D. Community attitudes to infant feeding. *Breastfeed Rev.* 2001;9(3):27–33.

McKenna KM, Shankar RT. The practice of prelacteal feeding to newborns among Hindu and Muslim families. *J Midwifery Women's Health.* 2009:54(1):78–81.

Mead Johnson [advertisement]. *JAMA.* 1930;95:22.

Merewood A. Ban the bags: a national movement to eliminate take-home formula sample packs from the hospital. Winter 2008. Available at: http://www.apha.org/membergroups/newsletters/sectionnewsletters/food/winter08/banthebags.htm. Accessed December 9, 2013.

Merewood A, Mehta SD, Chamberlain LB, et al. Breastfeeding rates in US baby-friendly hospitals: results of a national survey. *Pediatrics.* 2005;116(3):628–634.

Merten S, Dratva J, Ackermann-Liebrich U. Do baby-friendly hospitals influence breastfeeding duration on a national level? *Pediatrics.* 2005;116:702–708.

Meyer HF. Breastfeeding in the United States: report of a 1966 national survey with comparable 1946 and 1956 data. *Clin Pediatr.* 1968;7:708–715.

Millard AV. The place of the clock in pediatric advice: rationales, cultural themes, and impediments to breastfeeding. *Soc Sci Med.* 1990;31:211–221.

Millman S. Trends in breastfeeding in a dozen developing countries. *Intl Family Plan Perspect.* 1986;12(3):91–95.

Morse JM. "Euch, those are for your husband!" Examination of cultural values and assumptions associated with breastfeeding. *Health Care Women Intl.* 1989;11:223–232.

Morse JM, Jehle C, Gamble D. Initiating breastfeeding: a world survey of the timing of postpartum breastfeeding. *Intl J Nurs Stud.* 1990;27:303–313.

National Alliance for Breastfeeding Advocacy. *Still selling out mothers and babies: marketing of breast milk substitutes in the USA.* Weston MA: National Alliance for Breastfeeding Advocacy; 2007.

National Association of Pediatric Nurse Practitioners. Position paper on breastfeeding. 2007. Available at: http://www.napnap.org/PNPResources/Practice/PositionStatements.aspx. Accessed August 2013.

National Center for Health Statistics. *Healthy People 2000 final review.* Public Health Service; 2001. Available at: http://www.cdc.gov/nchs/data/hp2000/hp2k01.pdf. Accessed August 2013.

National Conference of State Legislatures. State breastfeeding laws. 2012. Available at: http://www.ncsl.org/research/health/breastfeeding-state-laws.aspx. Accessed July 29, 2013.

Nestlé's Food [advertisement]. *Ladies' Home Journal.* 1892;9:26.

Newman J, Goldfarb L. The protocols for induced lactation: a guide for maximizing breastmilk production. 2002. Available at: http:// www.asklenore.info/. Accessed December 7, 2013.

Nga NT, Weissner P. Breast-feeding and young child nutrition in Uong Bi, Quang Ninh Province, Vietnam. *J Trop Pediatr.* 1986;32:137–139.

Oliveira V. Winner takes (almost) all: how WIC affects the infant formula market. U.S. Department of Agriculture Economic Research Service; 2011. Available at: http://www.ers.usda.gov/amber-waves/2011-september/infant-formula-market.aspx. Accessed July 17, 2013.

Parenting Central Australia. Breastfeeding in public. 2013. Available at: http://parentingcentral.com.au/bfeeding-in-public/. Accessed June 24, 2013.

Pasternak B, Ching W. Breastfeeding decline in urban China: an exploratory study. *Human Ecol.* 1985;13(4):433–466.

Prakasa E. No formulaic stand on breastfeeding. 2013. Available at: ttp://www.youtube.com/watch?v=qioqB7IKRlI. Accessed June 30, 2013.

Quigley MA, Cumberland P, Cowden JM, Rodrigues LC. How protective is breast feeding against diarrhoeal disease in infants in 1990s England? A case-control study. *Arch Dis Child.* 2006;91:245–250.

Raisler J, Alexander C, O'Campo P. Breast-feeding and infant illness: a dose-response relationship? *Am J Public Health.* 1999;89(1):25–30.

Retherford RD, Choe MK, Thapa S, Gubhaju BB. To what extent does breastfeeding explain birth-interval effects on early childhood mortality? *Demography.* 1989;26:439–450.

Riordan J. Cost of not breastfeeding: a commentary. *J Hum Lact.* 1997;13:93–97.

Rossiter FM. *The practical guide to health: a popular treatise on anatomy, physiology, and hygiene, with a scientific description of diseases, their causes and treatment, designed for nurses and home use.* Mountain View, CA: Pacific Press Publishing; 1908. (Reprinted in part in *J Hum Lact.* 1991;7:89–91.)

Rotch TM. An historical sketch of the development of percentage feeding. *NY Med J.* 1907;85:532–537.

Rutstein SO, Macro International. Further evidence of the effects of preceding birth intervals on neonatal, infant, and under-five-years mortality and nutritional status in developing countries. Measure DHS (Demographic and

Health Surveys) working paper WP41. 2008. Available at: http://www.measuredhs.com/publications /publication-WP41-Working-Papers.cfm. Accessed July 15, 2013.

Ryan AS, Zhou W. Lower breastfeeding rates persist among the Special Supplemental Nutrition for Women, Infants, and Children participants, 1978–2003. *Pediatrics.* 2006;117(4):1136–1146.

Ryan AS, Zhou W, Gaston MH. Regional and sociodemographic variation of breastfeeding in the United States. *Clin Pediatr.* 2004;43:815–824.

Saadeh RJ, ed., with Labbok MH, Cooney KA, Koniz-Booher P. *Breast-feeding: the technical basis and recommendations for action: role of mother support groups.* Geneva, Switzerland: World Health Organization; 1993:62–74. Available at: http://apps.who.int/iris/bitstream/10665/58728 /2/WHO_NUT_MCH_93.1_(part2).pdf. Accessed August 2013.

Saha K. Studies on colostrum: nutrients and immunologic factors. *Nutr Foundation India Arch.* 1991. Available at: http://nutritionfoundationofindia.res.in/pdfs /BulletinArticle/Pages_from_nfi_10_91_2.pdf. Accessed August 2, 2007.

Sandiford P, Morales P, Gorter A, et al. Why do child mortality rates fall? An analysis of the Nicaraguan experience. *Am J Public Health.* 1991;81:30–37.

Schaefer O. The impact of culture on breastfeeding patterns. *J Perinatology.* 1956;6(1):62–65.

Serva V, Karim H, Ebrahim GJ. Breast-feeding and the urban poor in developing countries. *J Trop Pediatr.* 1986;32:127–129.

Shaikh U, Ahmed O. Islam and infant feeding. *Breastfeed Med.* 2006;1(3):164–167.

Short RV. Breast feeding. *Sci Am.* 1984;250:35–41.

Simoons FJ. Age of onset of lactose malabsorption. *Pediatrics.* 1980;66:646–648.

Slome C. Nonpuerperal lactation in grandmothers. *J Pediatr.* 1976;49:550–552.

Stevens EE, Patrick TE, Pickler R. A history of infant feeding. *J Perinatal Educ.* 2009:18(2):32–39.

Steube A. The risks of not breastfeeding for mothers and infants. *Rev Obstet Gynecol.* 2009;2(4):222–231.

Stuebe AM, Rich-Edwards JW, Willett WC, et al. Duration of lactation and incidence of type 2 diabetes. *JAMA.* 2005;294(20):2601–2610.

Thorley V. Initiating breastfeeding in postwar Queensland. *Breastfeed Rev.* 2001;9(3):21–26.

Tiedje LB, Schiffman R, Omar M, et al. An ecological approach to breastfeeding. *Am J Matern Child Nurs.* 2002;27:154–161.

Truitt ST, Fraser AB, Grimes DA, et al. Combined hormonal versus nonhormonal versus progestin-only contraception in lactation. *Cochrane Database Syst Rev.* 2003;2:CD003988.

Tuttle CR. An open letter to the WIC program: the time has come to commit to breastfeeding. *J Hum Lact.* 2000;16:99–103.

United Nations. Annual number of births, 2011. In: UNICEF, State of the world's children. Available at: http://data.un.org/Data.aspx?d=SOWC&f=inID %3A75. Accessed July 15, 2013.

United Nations International Children's Emergency Fund (UNICEF). *Innocenti declaration on the protection, promotion and support of breastfeeding, Florence, Italy, August 1990.* New York, NY: UNICEF, Nutrition Cluster (H-8F); 1990.

United Nations International Children's Emergency Fund (UNICEF). ChildInfo: statistics by area/child nutrition: infant and young child feeding (2000–2007). Last update January 2009. Available at: http://www.childinfo.org /breastfeeding_countrydata.php. Accessed June 1, 2013.

United Nations International Children's Emergency Fund (UNICEF), Nutrition Section. *National implementation of the International Code of Marketing of Breastmilk Substitutes.* New York, NY: UNICEF; April 2011. Available at: http://www.unicef.org/nutrition/files /State_of_the_Code_by_Country_April2011.pdf. Accessed July 29, 2013.

United States Breastfeeding Committee. *Breastfeeding in the United States: a national agenda.* Rockville, MD: Health Resources and Services Administration, Maternal and Child Bureau; 2001.

United States Breastfeeding Committee. *Economic benefits of breastfeeding* [Issue paper]. Raleigh, NC: United States Breastfeeding Committee; 2002. Available at: http://www.breastfeedingmadesimple.com /EconomicsofBF.pdf.

United States Breastfeeding Committee. Right to breastfeed on federal property. 2013. Available at: http://www .usbreastfeeding.org/LegislationPolicy/ExistingLegislation/tabid/233/Default.aspx. Accessed August 2013.

U.S. Department of Agriculture. FY 2011 budget summary and annual performance plan—US Department of Agriculture. 2011. Available at: http://www.obpa .usda.gov/budsum/FY11budsum.pdf. Accessed July 20, 2013.

U.S. Department of Agriculture. National survey of WIC participants II. Vol. 1. Participant characteristics (final report). 2012a. Available at: http://www.fns.usda.gov /Ora/menu/Published/WIC/FILES/NSWP-II.pdf. Accessed July 2013.

U.S. Department of Agriculture, Food and Nutrition Service. WIC: the supplemental nutrition program for women, infants, and children. 2012b. Available at: http://www .fns.usda.gov/sites/default/files/WIC-Fact-Sheet.pdf Accessed July 2013.

U.S. Department of Health and Human Services (DHHS). Healthy people: the Surgeon General's report on health promotion and disease prevention. 1979. Available at: http://profiles.nlm.nih.gov/NN/B/B/G/K/

U.S. Department of Health and Human Services (DHHS). Healthy people 2020. Maternal, infant, and child health objectives (MICH) 21: increase the proportion of infants who are breastfed. 2010a. Available at: http://healthypeople.gov/2020/topicsobjectives2020 /overview.aspx?topicid=26. Accessed July 2013.

U.S. Department of Health and Human Services (DHHS), Office on Women's Health. Why breastfeeding is important. 2010b. Available at: http://www .womenshealth.gov/breastfeeding/why-breastfeeding -is-important/. Accessed July 2013.

U.S. Department of Health and Human Services (DHHS). *Healthy people: the Surgeon General's call to action to support breastfeeding.* Washington, DC: DHHS; 2011. Available at: http://www.surgeongeneral.gov/library /calls/breastfeeding/index.html. Accessed July 2013.

U.S. Department of Health and Human Services (DHHS). DATA2010: the Healthy People 2010 database. 2011 edition. Updated August 2013. Available at: http: //wonder.cdc.gov/data2010/obj.htm. Accessed August 2013.

Uvnas-Moberg K, Widström AM, Marchini G, Winberg J. Release of GI hormones in mother and infant by sensory stimulation. *Acta Paediatr Scand.* 1987;76:851–860.

Walker M. A fresh look at the risks of artificial infant feeding. *J Hum Lact.* 1993;9:97–107.

War on Want, Muller M. *The baby killer.* London, UK: War on Want; 1974.

Weimer JP. *The economic benefits of breastfeeding: a review and analysis.* Food Assistance and Nutrition Research Report No. 13. Washington DC: Food and Rural Economics Division, Economic Research Service, U.S. Department of Agriculture; March 2001.

Whitehead RG. The human weaning process. *Pediatrics.* 1985;75(suppl 1):189–193.

Wickes IG. A history of infant feeding: III. Eighteenth and nineteenth century writers. *Arch Dis Child.* 1953a;28:332–340.

Wickes IG. A history of infant feeding: V. Nineteenth century concluded and twentieth century. *Arch Dis Child.* 1953b;28:495–502.

Wieschhoff HA. Artificial stimulation of lactation in primitive cultures. *Bull Hist Med.* 1940;8:1403–1415.

Williamson MA. *Infant mortality: Montclair, NJ. A study of infant mortality in a suburban community.* Washington, DC: U.S. Department of Labor, Children's Bureau; 1915.

Winikoff B, Laukaran VH. Breast feeding and bottle feeding controversies in the developing world: evidence from a study in four countries. *Soc Sci Med.* 1989;29:859–868.

Wolf JH. The first generation of American pediatricians and their inadvertent legacy to breastfeeding. *Breastfeed Med.* 2006;1(3):172–177.

Woodbury RM. The relation between breast and artificial feeding and infant mortality. *Am J Hyg.* 1922;2:668–687.

Woolridge MW, Greasley V, Silpisornkosol S. The initiation of lactation: the effect of early versus delayed contact for suckling on milk intake in the first week postpartum. A study in Chiang Mai, northern Thailand. *Early Hum Dev.* 1985;12:269–278.

World Alliance for Breastfeeding Action (WABA). 2013. Who we are. Available at: http://www.waba.org.my /aboutus.htm. Accessed July 29, 2013.

World Health Organization (WHO). World Health Assembly Resolutions WHA49.15. Infant and young child nutrition. Geneva, Switzerland. 20-25 May 1996. Accessed at http://www.who.int/nutrition/topics/WHA49.15 _iycn_en.pdf?ua=1. Accessed March 11, 2014.

World Health Organization (WHO). *International code of marketing breastmilk substitutes.* Geneva, Switzerland: WHO; 1981.

World Health Organization (WHO). Protecting, promoting, and supporting breastfeeding: the special role of maternity services [A joint WHO/UNICEF statement]. Geneva, Switzerland: WHO; 1989.

World Health Organization. Division of Child Health and Development. Evidence for the Ten Steps to Successful Breastfeeding. Geneva, Switzerland: World Health Organization. 1998. Available at http://whqlibdoc .who.int/publications/2004/9241591544_eng.pdf

World Health Organization (WHO). Maternal, infant and young child nutrition: draft comprehensive implementation plan, global target 5. Geneva, Switzerland: WHO; 2011.

World Health Organization (WHO). World Breastfeeding Week 2013: breastfeeding support close to mothers. Geneva, Switzerland: WHO; 2012.

World Health Organization (WHO), UNICEF. *Global strategy for infant and young child feeding.* Geneva, Switzerland: WHO, UNICEF; 2003.

World Health Organization (WHO), UNICEF. Baby-Friendly Hospital Initiative 2009: revised, updated, and expanded for integrated care. Geneva, Switzerland: WHO; 2009.

Section Two

Anatomic and Biological Imperatives

CHAPTER 3   Anatomy and Physiology
             of Lactation

CHAPTER 4   The Biological Specificity of
             Breastmilk

CHAPTER 5   Drug Therapy and
             Breastfeeding

CHAPTER 6   Viral Infections and
             Breastfeeding

After pregnancy, the mother continues to nourish and support the development of her child through her milk. Energy and trophic (tissue-building) factors, immune factors, and cells are gathered by or synthesized in and stored in the breast. Human milk—a living fluid that benefits infants, mothers, and society—changes throughout lactation to meet the infant's nutriment, developmental, and immunologic needs. No human-made substitute nourishes the infant as well. Which drugs and viral infections pose a risk to the breastfeeding baby? Most drugs are compatible with breastfeeding, as this section shows. Viruses and bacteria stimulate antibodies in the mother's body, which, except for HIV, protect the vulnerable infant through mother's milk. Scientists are attempting to catch the elusive thread that unravels the tragedy of AIDS and the mystery of the HIV virus within breastmilk cells.

Chapter 3

Anatomy and Physiology of Lactation

Karen Wambach
Catherine Watson Genna

Introduction

It is essential that healthcare providers understand the anatomy of the human female breast and the physiological mechanisms of milk production. It is equally necessary to recognize the unique anatomy of the infant's oral structures and the physiological mechanisms of suckling. Anatomy is not supposed to change, but our perception and knowledge of it has changed considerably since high-resolution ultrasound has allowed us to look inside the breast.

This chapter is divided into two parts: the first focuses on the mother, the second on the infant. In lactation, as in all human biological systems, there is a working relationship between anatomy (form) and physiology (function). Although function changes as form changes, the functional capacity of the human breast is not wholly dictated by form. Breast size, for instance, is a poor predictor of lactational capability. It is the infant's appetite (and milk removal) that determines milk yield, rather than the mother's capacity to produce milk. Ultrasound—a simple noninvasive method to observe and measure the lactating breast—has opened the functioning and anatomy of the breast to our examination and allows us to look inside. The developmental cycle of the mammary gland has four phases: mammogenesis, lactogenesis (stages I [secretory differentiation] and II [secretory activation]), galactopoiesis, and involution.

Mammogenesis

The mammary system is unlike other organ systems. From birth through puberty, pregnancy, and lactation, no other human organ displays such dramatic changes in size, shape, and function as does the breast. The Latin term for breasts, *mammae*, developed from the infant's hunger cry, "mamma." In some cultures, female breasts serve more than one function: they attract the sexual attention of the male adult and then give nourishment and nurturing to the suckling infant. The first part of this chapter, which focuses on the mother, describes breast development from embryo to adulthood, breast anatomy, changes during pregnancy and lactation, and hormones that influence the course of lactogenesis.

Breast development begins early, by the fourth or fifth week of gestation when two parallel primitive milk streaks develop from axilla to groin on the trunk of the embryo. These streaks become the mammary ridge or milk line by the fifth week of embryonic life. This ridge or line is actually a thickening of epithelial cells in a localized ventrolateral area on the embryo (the "milk hill" stage) that continues through weeks 7 and 8 and is accompanied by inward growth into the chest wall. Between 12 and 16 weeks' gestation, these specialized cells differentiate further into the smooth muscle of the nipple and areola. Also during this period, epithelial cells continue to develop into mammary buds and then, in a treelike pattern, proliferate to form the epithelial branches that will eventually become alveoli (Dawson, 1934; Gusterson & Stein, 2012; Russo & Russo, 2004; Vorherr, 1974).

Placental sex hormones enter the fetal circulation and stimulate formation of channels (canalization) of the branched epithelial tissue. This process continues until the fetus is 32 weeks old. From 32 to 40 weeks' gestation, lobular–alveolar structures containing colostrum develop. During this time, the mass of the fetal mammary gland increases to four times its original mass, and the nipple and areola develop further and become pigmented. After birth, the neonate's mammary tissue may secrete colostral milk (so-called witch's milk) for as long as 3 or 4 weeks (Russo & Russo, 2004).

Mammary gland development during childhood is limited to general growth. However, at puberty, estrogen, prolactin, luteinizing hormone, follicle stimulating hormone, and growth hormone influence breast growth in a girl when, at 10 to 12 years of age, primary and secondary ducts grow and divide and form club-shaped terminal end buds that are associated with beginning function of the hypothalamus–pituitary–ovarian axis. These buds develop into new branches and small ductules of areolar buds, which later become the acini or alveoli in the mature female breast, also known as terminal ductule lobular units (TDLU/acini) (Sternlicht et al., 2006). During each menstrual cycle, proliferation and active growth of duct tissue occurs during the follicular and ovulatory phases, reaching a maximum in the late luteal phase and then regressing. During each ovulatory cycle, peaks of ovarian steroids, primarily progesterone, foster further mammary development that never regresses to its former state of the preceding cycle (Russo & Russo, 2004; Vorherr, 1974). Trauma, incisions, or radiation therapy to the breast bud in the prepubertal era can trigger maldevelopment with hypoplasia of the vestigial breast that has future consequences for lactation. For example, radiation during childhood can be associated with an inadequate breastmilk supply as an adult.

Complete development of mammary function occurs only in pregnancy, when the breasts increase in size and the nipple pigment darkens. Except for the uterus, no other organ changes so dramatically as the breast does during pregnancy and lactation. New budding of structures continues until about age 35. In addition to progesterone, prolactin or human placental lactogen is thought to be necessary for the final stages of mammary growth and differentiation (Neville, 2001).

Breast Structure

The basic units of the mature glandular tissue are the alveoli, which are composed of secretory acinar units in which the ductules terminate. Each cluster of secretory cells of an alveolus is surrounded by myoepithelial cells, a contractile unit responsible for ejecting milk into the ductules. Ducts grow inward from the ectodermal layer and canalize by 32 weeks' gestation. Each ductule then merges, without communicating with its neighbors, into a larger duct (Figure 3-1). Figure 3-2 shows an ultrasound image of a lactating breast, where ducts filled with milk can be clearly seen. These ducts intertwine erratically much like tree roots, making it difficult to separate them surgically.

Each breast has duct openings, sometimes called nipple "pores." The ducts are lined with stratified squamous epithelium near the nipple, with columnar epithelium at more distal areas, and with highly vascular connective tissue.

The alveolus or milk-secreting unit is a single layer of epithelial cells that is surrounded by supporting structures: myoepithelial cells, contractile cells for milk ejection, and connective tissue. Milk is continuously secreted into the alveolar lumina, where it is stored until the letdown reflex triggers the myoepithelial cells to contract and eject the milk (Neville, 2001).

Mammary ducts do not widen into sinuses located behind the nipple and the areola (as was previously thought). Figure 3-3, which shows contrast

Figure 3-1 SCHEMATIC DIAGRAM OF THE BREAST.

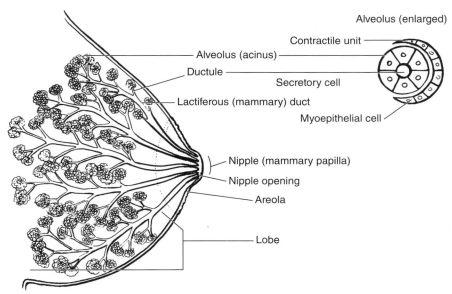

Alveolus (enlarged)

Contractile unit

Alveolus (acinus)

Ductule

Secretory cell

Lactiferous (mammary) duct

Myoepithelial cell

Nipple (mammary papilla)

Nipple opening

Areola

Lobe

Figure 3-2 ULTRASOUND IMAGE SHOWING MILK-FILLED DUCTS. MOTHER LACTATING 10 MONTHS.

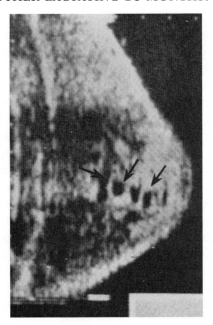

Source: Reproduced from Telles, NC, ed. Atlas of breast ultrasound. Philadelphia, Pa: Department of Radiology and Department of Pathology, Thomas Jefferson University Medical College and Hospital; 1980:121.

Figure 3-3 CONTRAST OPACIFICATION OF A SINGLE LACTIFEROUS DUCT DEMONSTRATES A BRANCHING NETWORK THAT DEFINES A SINGLE LOBE OF THE BREAST.

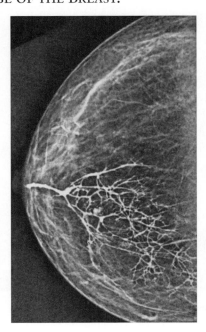

Source: Reproduced from Kopans DB. Breast imaging. Philadelphia, Pa: Lippincott; 1989:20.

opacification of a single lactiferous duct, confirms that the duct does not widen before it branches in mammary ducts. In each breast, there are 15 to 25 interwoven lobes (Geddes, 2007), each containing between 10 and 100 alveoli.

Between and around the uneven edges of the lobes is a thick layer of fat. The amount of adipose tissue present differs considerably among women—in some, fat composes as much as half of the breast. The amount of adipose tissue does not affect either the breast storage capacity or the milk production (Ramsay, Kent, et al., 2005).

Attaching the deep layer of the subcutaneous tissue to the dermis of the skin are the suspensory ligaments, or Cooper's ligaments (Figure 3-4). The breast's

Figure 3-4 CURVILINEAR DENSITIES REPRESENT COOPER'S LIGAMENTS.

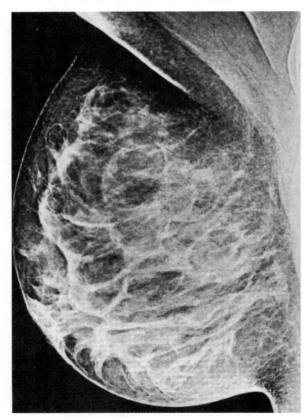

Source: Reproduced from Kopans DB. Breast imaging. Philadelphia, Pa: Lippincott; 1989:20.

structure is mainly the result of the fibrous tissues that surround and course through it. Glandular tissue that extends toward the axilla partly under the lateral border of the pectoralis majora is known as the axillary tail (Figure 3-5). Each breast of an adult woman weighs, on average, 150 to 200 g; it doubles in weight to 400 to 500 g (approximately 1 pound) during lactation. Between 6 and 9 months after the beginning of lactation, breast size decreases slightly. Whether this results from mobilization of breast fatty tissue or greater breast tissue efficiency in making milk, milk production remains constant (Hartmann et al., 1995).

The breast is highly vascularized. Blood is supplied to it through the internal mammary (60%) and lateral thoracic (30%) arteries. The lymph vessels of the breast are numerous and, for the most part, join the lymph nodes of the axilla. The majority of lymph vessels follow the lactiferous ducts and, therefore, converge toward the nipple, where they join a plexus situated beneath the areola (subareolar plexus).

The nerve supply of the breast is derived from the second to the sixth intercostal nerves. The fourth intercostal nerve penetrates the posterior aspect of the breast (left breast at 4 o'clock, right breast 8 o'clock) and supplies the greatest amount of sensation to the nipple and to the areola. The breast has uneven patterns of sensation: the areola is the most sensitive part of the breast, the skin adjacent to the areola is less sensitive, and the nipple itself is the least sensitive. Women with larger breasts report less sensation than women with smaller breasts. Among women with small or moderate-sized breasts, those who have never been pregnant report greater sensation in their nipples and areolae. Midway to the nipple and areola, the fourth intercostal nerve becomes more superficial. As it reaches the areola, it divides into five branches: one central, two upper, and two lower. The lowermost branch consistently pierces the areola at 5 o'clock on the left side and 7 o'clock on the right side. Any trauma to this nerve will cause some loss of sensation in the breast (Courtiss & Goldwyn, 1976). If the lowermost nerve branch is severed, the mother will lose sensation to the nipple and areola (Farina et al., 1980).

Figure 3-5 ANTERIOR PECTORAL DISSECTION SHOWING THE LOBULAR NATURE OF THE MAMMARY GLAND EXTENDING TOWARD THE AXILLA AND ITS LOCATION ANTERIOR TO THE PECTORALIS MAJOR MUSCLE. INCLUDES THE SUPERFICIAL AXILLARY LYMPH AND SWEAT GLANDS.

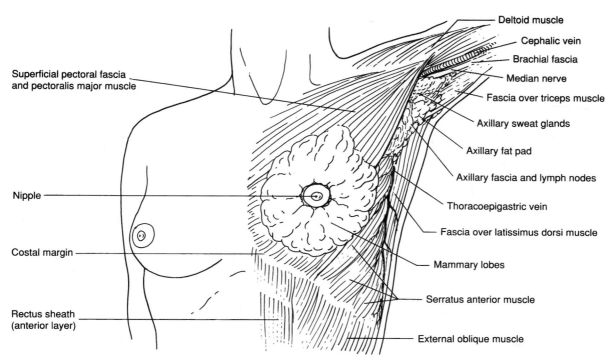

Source: Adapted from Clemente, 1978.

The covering smooth skin is modified at the center of each breast to form a mammary papilla, or nipple, into which the ducts open. Some of these ducts join so that about nine openings appear on the nipple surface. It is not known whether these ducts are all open to the outside or patent. Some ducts may be "blind" and not open to the outside. For example, Cooper (1840) found 7–12 patent ducts in a cadaver dissection of a breast from a woman who was lactating before death, although he could cannulate up to 22 ducts.

Milk ducts are small, superficial, easily compressed, and increase in diameter at milk ejection (Geddes, 2007). The nipple projects as a small cylindrical body with pigmented wrinkled skin slightly below the center of each breast at about the level of the fourth intercostal space. Surrounding the nipple is the areola. The nipple and areola contain erectile smooth muscles. Hair follicles surround the nipple and areola but are not within the nipple and areola proper. Contraction of bundles of smooth muscles beneath the nipple and areola cause the nipple to be firm and protruding. These structures are seen in Color Plates 1–3.

Nipple Size

In a lactating mother, the average diameter of the areola is 6.4 cm. The size of the areola increases significantly in the first few days postpartum, especially on day 3 with lactogenesis. The average diameter of the erectile portion of the nipple is 1.6 cm and the length is 0.7 cm (Ziemer, 1993). The diameter of the nipple increases during pregnancy approximately from 9.5 mm to 11.5 mm, although the nipple cannot be measured exactly because it varies with the degree of erection. However, studies of nipple diameter of breastfeeding women show that the sizes are fairly consistent: Ziemer (1993) found an average diameter of 16 mm, Ramsay, Kent, et al. (2005) 16 mm, and Hoover 17.5 mm (Wilson-Clay & Hoover, 2013). Wilson-Clay and Hoover (2013) noted that women with extra-large nipples seem to have more problems with breastfeeding, specifically low milk supply supposedly related to early latch problems that factor into milk supply calibration.

Areolar Glands

Within the areola lie Montgomery's tubercles, which consist of mammary milk glands and sebaceous glands; together they are called areolar glands (AG) (Doucet et al., 2012; Schaal et al., 2006; Smith, 1982). Long a focus of anatomic debate, some of the AG (Figure 3-6) are true mammary glands whose ducts and secretory parenchyma are the same as those of the mammary glands that open at the tip of the nipples. As such, they are an integral part of the mammary structure and total breast tissue (MacPherson & Montagna, 1974). From an evolutionary standpoint, it is of interest that the rhesus monkey does not have AGs (MacPherson & Montagna, 1974).

The number of AG present on the areola varies widely among women. Schaal et al. (2006) found that all but one woman in their study (*n* = 29) had AG and Doucet et al. (2012) found four women without AG in their study (*n* = 121). The mean number of glands per each areola was 8.9 (range 0–38) in the Schaal et al. study, and 10.39 (range 0–48.5) in the Doucet et al. study. In both of these studies, the number of AG was unrelated to the size of the areola and was similar between the left and right breasts. More AGs were located on the upper, lateral section of the areola (Doucet et al., 2012; Schaal et al., 2006), generally the area in which the baby's nose is most frequently directed. Approximately one in five lactating women reports seeing a visible fluid

Figure 3-6 (A) PHOTOGRAPH OF AN AREOLA (LEFT BREAST, POSTPARTUM DAY 3), SHOWING (ARROWS) SKIN STRUCTURES (REVEALED BY RELATIVE ELEVATION AND PIGMENTAL HETEROGENITY RELATIVE TO SURROUNDING SKIN), WHICH WERE COUNTED AS AREOLAR GLANDS. (B) ENLARGED (2.5X) VIEW OF AN AREOLAR GLAND. (C) AN AREOLAR GLAND GIVING OFF A MILK-LIKE SECRETION DURING A BREASTFEED. (D) ENGLARGED (3X) REPRESENTATION OF A SECRETORY DROP FROM AN AREOLAR GLAND.

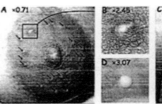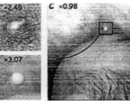

Source: From Schaal et al., 2006. Human breast areolae as scent organs: morphological data and possibel involvement in maternal-neonatal coadaptation. *Dev Psychobiol.* 2006;18(2):100–110. Reprinted with permission of John Wiley & Sons, Inc.

emission from their areolar glands in the Schaal et al. study while 34 of the 121 women in Doucet et al. sample visibly emitted fluid (see Figure 3-6).

The presence and number of AG may play a more important role in breastfeeding than was previously thought. Infants whose mothers have more areolar glands had greater weight gain in the first few days, tended to latch on more rapidly, and suckled more actively after latching (Schaal et al., 2006). Additionally, lactogenesis occurred more rapidly and parity influences were present; infants of primiparae with the fewest number of AG lost the most weight in the first 3 days (Doucet et al., 2012). It is possible to conclude that the AG is a scent organ and the fluid from the AG provides a sensory stimulation to the newborn that not only helps guide him to the nipples, especially among primiparae who are not as assistive as multiparae, but also stimulates the nipples more effectively, increases colostrum intake, and ultimately increases chances for survival.

Variations

From woman to woman, breasts vary in color, size, shape, and placement on the chest wall; these variations are genetically influenced. Lobular size varies within a single breast, from one breast to another, and from woman to woman. Moreover, breast asymmetry is common; the left breast is often larger than the right. Areola and nipple color vary according to complexion: pink in blonds, browner in brunettes, and black in dark-skinned women.

Polymastia occurs frequently (in 1% to 5% of women) because of the way mammary tissues develop along paired "milk lines" of multiple sites in all mammals. In humans, usually all but the upper thoracic pair of breasts regress during development. Persistence of mammary tissue at other sites (from the axilla to the groin) is responsible for the finding of additional nipples (polythelia, or supernumerary nipples), breast tissue (polymastia), or both. Occasionally, polythelia is associated with kidney and urinary tract anomalies (Berman & Davis, 1994). Only rarely does a complete accessory mammary gland develop (Grossl, 2000). Accessory nipples are most common on the axilla and thorax (see Color Plate 21).

Lack of full protraction of the nipple on the pinch test (see Figure 3-12, later in this chapter) is fairly common in primigravid women. The rate of poor nipple protractility in women during their first pregnancy has been reported to range from 10% to 35% (Alexander et al., 1992; Blaikeley et al., 1953; Hytten & Baird, 1958; Waller, 1946). Protractility of the nipple gradually improves during pregnancy and, by puerperium, most women have good nipple protraction. Generally, nipple protraction continues to improve with each subsequent pregnancy and lactation experience. The relationship between protractility and subsequent breastfeeding difficulty is minimal. Because the infant makes a teat not from the nipple alone but from the surrounding breast

tissue, the actual shape of the nipple may be a secondary consideration.

Nipple inversion is found in approximately 3% of women and is usually bilateral (87%) (Park et al., 1999). Of the total number of inverted nipples, 96% are umbilicated and only 4% are invaginated (true inversion). Although true inversion is uncommon, its treatment can be difficult. If the inversion affects one breast only, the mother can breastfeed from a single breast and use a silicone breast shield on the other breast. Placing a silicone breast shield over the inverted nipple allows the infant to grasp on to the breast and suckle effectively. Supple Cups (www.supplecups.com) can be used between pregnancies, from 37 weeks' gestation onward, and during lactation to produce gentle traction to gradually correct inverted or flat nipples. Occasionally, severe nipple inversion is associated with reduced ability to transfer milk, in which case the affected mother may need to supplement her infant. The mother's first breastfeeding experience may be more difficult than subsequent ones—frequent suckling by the infant helps to evert the previously inverted tissue. See the *Breast-Related Problems* chapter for further information on nipple variations.

Pregnancy

During pregnancy, the breasts grow larger, the skin appears thinner, and the veins become more prominent. The diameter of the areola increases from about 34 mm in early pregnancy to 50 mm postpartum (Hytten, 1954), although there is a wide range of areolar width in any population. As the nipples become more erect, pigmentation of the areola increases and the Montgomery's glands enlarge.

Serum hormones stimulate breast growth during pregnancy: nipple growth is related to serum prolactin levels; areolar growth is related to serum placental lactogen (Cregan & Hartmann, 1999). Estrogen and progesterone also exert their specific effects on the breast during pregnancy; the ductal system proliferates and differentiates under the influence of estrogen, whereas progesterone promotes an increase in size of the lobes, lobules, and alveoli.

Adrenocorticotropic hormone (ACTH) and growth hormone combine synergistically with prolactin and progesterone to promote mammary growth.

Breast growth during pregnancy varies among women. In a study of eight pregnant women, most had a gradual increase in breast growth throughout their pregnancy. However, one mother had a spurt of breast growth between 10 and 15 weeks' gestation, but afterward experienced very little growth; another had little or no breast growth (Cregan & Hartmann, 1999).

Lactogenesis

The transition from pregnancy to lactation is called lactogenesis. Growth and proliferation of the ductal tree and further formation of lobules characterize the first half of pregnancy. During the second half of pregnancy, secretory activity accelerates and the acini or alveoli become distended by accumulating colostrum (Russo & Russo, 1987). After 16 weeks of pregnancy, lactation occurs even if the pregnancy does not progress. An accessory breast may also swell. Just before and during childbirth, a new wave of mitotic activity increases the total DNA of the mammary gland (Salazar & Tobon, 1974; Vorherr, 1974).

The developing capacity of the mammary gland to secrete milk from midpregnancy to late pregnancy is called lactogenesis, stage I (or lactogenesis I) (Table 3-1). During lactogenesis I (secretory differentiation), breast size increases as epithelial cells of the alveoli differentiate into secretory cells for milk production. Fat droplets accumulate in these cells, and the plasma concentrations of lactose and α-lactalbumin increase. The milk droplets move through the cell membrane and into the ductules (Figure 3-7).

The onset of copious milk secretion after birth is lactogenesis, stage II (days 2 or 3 to 8 postpartum). During lactogenesis II (secretory activation), milk volume increases rapidly from 38 to 98 hours postpartum and then abruptly levels off. Lactogenesis II is triggered by a rapid drop of serum progesterone (and possibly estrogen) after the delivery of the placenta. It is also accompanied by a significant decline

Figure 3-7 **MILK IS SECRETED FROM THE ALVEOLAR CELLS, WHERE SMALL DROPLETS FFORM AND MIGRATE THROUGH THE CELL MEMBRANE AND INTO THE ALVEOLAR DUCTULES.**

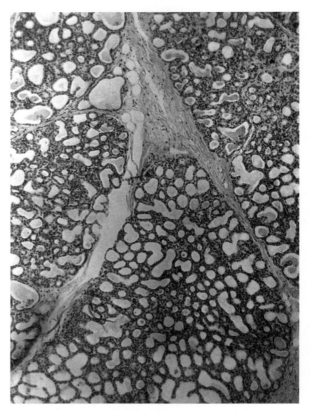

Source: With permission, Victor B. Eichler, PhD.

in breastmilk levels of sodium, chloride, and protein, and a rise in lactose and milk lipids levels. These changes in cellular metabolism result from closure of the tight junction complexes between alveolar cells. Before lactogenesis (first 3 to 4 days), large gaps are present between the alveolar cells. During full lactation, the passage of substances between alveolar cells is stopped by a gasketlike protein structure called the desmosome, which joins the epithelial cells tightly to one another (Figure 3-8).

Table 3-1 STAGES OF LACTATION

Mammogenesis	• Mammary (breast) growth; increased size and weight of breast • Proliferation of ducts and glandular system under estrogen and progesterone
Lactogenesis, stage I (midpregnancy to day 2 postpartum)	• Initiation of milk synthesis from midpregnancy to late pregnancy • Differentiation of alveolar cells into secretory cells • Prolactin stimulates mammary secretory epithelial cells to produce milk
Lactogenesis, stage II (day 3 to day 8)	• Closure of tight junctions in alveolar cell (Figure 3-8) • Triggered by rapid drop in mother's progesterone levels • Onset of copious secretion of milk • Fullness and warmth in breasts • Switch from endocrine to autocrine control
Galactopoiesis (day 9 to beginning of involution)	• Maintenance of established secretion • Control by autocrine system (supply–demand) • Breast size decreases between 6 and 9 months postpartum
Involution (average 40 days after last breastfeeding)	• Additions of regular supplementation • Decreased milk secretion from build-up of inhibiting peptides • High sodium levels

Figure 3-8 (A) FIRST 4 DAYS POSTPARTUM. GAPS BETWEEN ALVEOLAR CELLS BEFORE LACTOGENESIS. (B) AFTER 14 DAYS POSTPARTUM. INTRACELLULAR GAPS CLOSE TIGHTLY TO ONE ANOTHER FOLLOWING LACTOGENESIS.

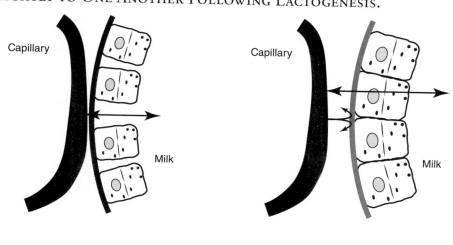

Source: Used with permission from Hale TW. Medications and mother's milk. 9th ed. Amarillo, TX: Pharmasoft; 2000:6.

The closure of these tight junctions precedes the onset of copious milk secretion (Neville, 2001).

As secretory activation (full lactation) begins, these hormonal changes are essential:

- Drop in progesterone levels
- Release of prolactin from the anterior pituitary, which stimulates lactogenesis and initiates milk secretion
- Removal of breastmilk by the infant or pump
- Release of oxytocin from the posterior pituitary (at least by day 3)

Involution of the mammary gland is a process that removes the milk-producing epithelial cells when they become superfluous at weaning. This two-step process involves the death of the secretory epithelium and its replacement by adipocytes. The awesome capacity of the breast to produce milk is matched by the mechanism of apoptosis, a form of programmed cell death (Watson, 2006).

Delay in Lactogenesis II/ Secretory Activation

Not all women experience the coming in of the milk on the third or fourth day postpartum. A delay or diminishment in lactogenesis II, which is common in certain situations (listed in Table 3-2), invites us to gain a better understanding of the specific biochemical or hormonal nature of lactogenesis that may lead to a delay in secretory activation. We do know that high breastmilk sodium levels on or before the third day after birth are significant for impending breastfeeding problems and for involution (Humenick et al., 1998; Morton, 1994). Delayed lactogenesis II has been associated with maternal obesity (Nommsen-Rivers et al., 2010) and maternal–infant separation. In settings where infants are held constantly, secretory activation begins significantly earlier than in most U.S. postpartum units.

Table 3-2 MATERNAL CONDITIONS THAT CAN DELAY OR IMPAIR LACTOGENESIS

Factor	Evidence Sources
Primiparity	Chapman & Perez-Escamilla, 1999, 2000; Chen et al., 1998; Dewey et al., 2003
Cesarean birth	Dewey et al., 2003; Sozmen, 1992
Long stage II of labor	Chen et al., 1998; Dewey et al., 2003; Neville et al., 2001
Maternal fluid loads in labor	Chantry et al., 2011
Diabetes, type I	Hartmann & Cregan, 2001; Neubauer et al., 1993; Oliveira et al, 2008
Labor analgesia	Hildebrandt, 1999; Riordan et al., 2000
Obesity	Nommsen-Rivers et al., 2010; Rasmussen et al., 2001; Rasmussen & Kjolhede, 2004
Polycystic ovary syndrome	Marasco et al., 2000; Vanky et al., 2008
Gestational ovarian theca lutein cysts	Betzold et al., 2004; Hoover et al., 2002
Placental retention	Anderson, 2001; Neifert, 1981
Sheehan's syndrome/ischemic pituitary necrosis as result of postpartum hemorrhage	Dökmetaş et al., 2006; Sert et al., 2003
Stress	Chen et al., 1998; Grajeda & Perez-Escamilla, 2002
Isolated prolactin (PRL) deficiency	Iwama et al., 2013
Breast surgery, especially reduction mammoplasty	See the *Breast-Related Problems* chapter. Thibaudeau et al., 2010.

Hormonal Influences

Lactogenesis II is triggered following the expulsion of the placenta by a fall in progesterone levels and the continued presence of prolactin. The functions of these hormones during lactation have been examined and elucidated through radioimmunoassay studies.

A programmed transformation of the mammary epithelium mediated by a cascade of hormonal changes leads to a rapid synthesis of milk by day 4 following birth. The postpartum period is characterized hormonally by a drop in progesterone and elevated levels of prolactin, which act synergistically with cortisol, thyroid-stimulating hormone, prolactin-inhibiting factor, and oxytocin to establish and maintain lactation. If the delicate interplay of these hormones is disturbed—for example, by high testosterone levels in the woman with gestational ovarian theca lutein cysts (Betzold et al., 2004; Hoover et al., 2002) or polycystic ovary syndrome (Marasco et al., 2000; Vanky et al., 2008), lactogenesis II may be delayed and possibly suppressed.

Progesterone

Progesterone is required to maintain pregnancy, and its concentration remains high throughout pregnancy. Lactation during pregnancy is inhibited by high levels of progesterone, which interfere with prolactin action at the alveolar cell receptor level. The inhibiting influence of progesterone is so powerful that secretory activation is delayed if placental fragments are retained after birth (Neifert et al., 1981). Following birth, progesterone decreases about tenfold during the first 4 days. This rapid decline in the progesterone level in the presence of maintained prolactin levels triggers lactogenesis. Once lactation is initiated, the principal hormone in maintaining milk biosynthesis is prolactin.

Prolactin

Prolactin is essential for both initiating and maintaining milk production. Although the action of oxytocin appears to be keyed more closely to milk ejection, milk is not made if prolactin is lacking. During pregnancy, prolactin, which is secreted by the anterior pituitary gland, has an important role in increasing breast mass and cell differentiation. A group of peptides, including angiotensin II, gonadotropin-releasing hormone (GnRH), and vasopressin, stimulate the release of prolactin. The mammary ducts and alveoli mature and proliferate as prolactin levels steadily rise from the normal nonpregnancy level of 10 to 20 ng/mL to a peak of 200 to 400 ng/mL at term (Tyson et al., 1972).

Progesterone and estrogen levels abruptly drop after a woman gives birth. In turn, the anterior pituitary gland, no longer inhibited by these two hormones, releases pulses of prolactin 7 to 20 times in 24 hours and greater amounts during sleep; thus, for accurate measurement of prolactin, samples should be taken in close intervals around the clock (Madden et al., 1978). Episodic peaks are superimposed on a stable ongoing level of secretion. Because human placental lactogen (HPL) competes with prolactin for binding to breast receptors, the decline of the HPL level after delivery of the placenta also promotes prolactin action. Figure 3-9 describes the rise and fall of hormones during pregnancy and lactation.

Following lactogenesis II, when milk secretion shifts from endocrine to autocrine control, prolactin secretion continues to be controlled by the

---

Figure 3-9 Hormone Levels During Pregnancy and Lactation.

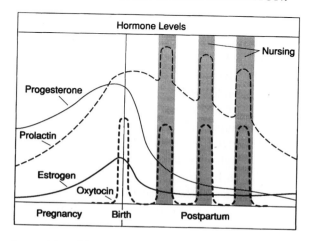

Source: Adapted from Love, 1990.

hypothalamus. This control is largely inhibitory; that is, whenever the pathway between the hypothalamus and the pituitary is disrupted, prolactin levels rise. During galactopoiesis, the hypothalamus is dependent upon removal of milk for lactation to continue. When the nipple is stimulated and milk is removed from the breast, the hypothalamus inhibits the release of dopamine, a prolactin-inhibiting factor; this drop in dopamine stimulates the release of prolactin and promotes milk production (Chao, 1987).

Plasma prolactin levels increase the most in the immediate postpartum period but rise and fall in proportion to the frequency, intensity, and duration of nipple stimulation. Prolactin concentration in blood doubles in response to suckling and peaks approximately 45 minutes after the beginning of a breastfeeding session (Noel et al., 1974). If lidocaine is applied to the nipples to deaden sensation, the prolactin level does not increase (Neville, 2001).

Prolactin levels remain elevated throughout the first 6 months postpartum in women who breastfeed at regular intervals. At 6 months postpartum, serum prolactin can still more than double in response to suckling (Battin et al., 1985). If a mother does not breastfeed, prolactin levels usually reach nonpregnant levels by 7 days postpartum (Tyson et al., 1972).

During lactation, maternal prolactin levels are described as follows:

- They follow a circadian rhythm; levels during the night (sleep) are higher than during the day.
- They decline slowly over the course of lactation (Battin et al., 1985; Cox et al., 1996) but remain elevated for as long as the mother breastfeeds, even if she breastfeeds for years (Stallings et al., 1996).
- They rise with suckling: The more feedings, the higher the level of serum prolactin. More than 8 breastfeedings per 24 hours prevents decline of the concentration of prolactin before the next breastfeeding (Cox et al., 1996; Tay et al., 1996).
- They are not necessarily proportional to milk yield, especially after lactation becomes

established (Hill et al., 1999; Ueda et al., 1994), although feeding two babies simultaneously doubles the prolactin surge (Tyson et al., 1972).
- They delay the return of ovulation by inhibiting the ovarian response to follicle-stimulating hormone, and prolactin levels are higher in amenorrheic women than in cycling women during the first year' postpartum (Battin et al., 1985; Stallings et al., 1996).
- They are not related to the degree of postpartum breast engorgement (West, 1979).
- They drop with cigarette smoking (Baron et al., 1986) and rise with beer drinking (Mennella & Beauchamp, 1993).
- They rise with anxiety and psychological stress (Hill et al., 1999) even though feeding at the breast and the milk-ejection reflex are calming (because of oxytocin release).
- Depressed mothers have lower serum prolactin levels (Groer, 2005a).

Normal prolactin levels in nonpregnant or nonlactating women are 20 ng/mL or less. In lactating women, mean baseline prolactin levels are 90 ng/mL at 10 days postpartum; afterward, these levels slowly decline but remained elevated at 180 days postpartum (44.3 ng/mL). Women who remain amenorrheic have higher baseline prolactin levels (approximately 110.0 ng/mL) as compared to women who menstruate prior to 180 days (approximately 70.1 ng/mL) (Battin et al., 1985). Figure 3-10 provides an overview of prolactin serum levels during pregnancy and breastfeeding.

Prolactin is also present in breastmilk. The release of prolactin into intra-alveolar secretions of the breast plays a role in establishing and maintaining lactation. Milk prolactin concentration is lower than its concentration in blood plasma and is highest in early transitional milk (approximately 43 ng/mL) and foremilk rather than hindmilk (Cox et al., 1996). This early transmission of prolactin in the aqueous foremilk is thought influence intestinal fluid and electrolyte exchange in the newborn (Yuen, 1988). Milk prolactin levels are about the same between the left and right breasts and are highest in the morning (Cregan et al., 2002). Breastmilk prolactin

Figure 3-10 FLUCTUATION OF HUMAN PLACENTAL LACTOGEN AND PROLACTIN SERUM LEVELS IN PREGNANCY AND LACTATION.

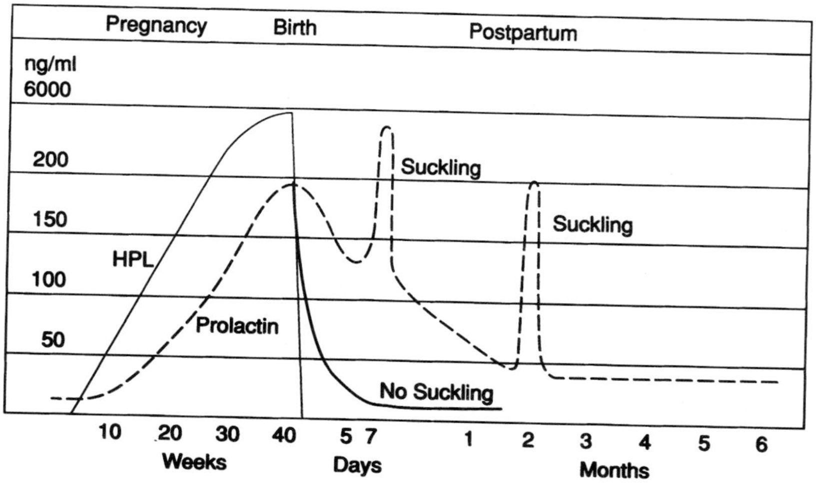

Source: Data from Battin D et al. Effect of suckling on serum prolactin, lutenizing hormone, follicle-stimulating hormone, and estradiol during prolonged lactation. *Obstet. Gynecol.* 1985;65:785–788; Tyson JE et al. Studies of prolactin in human pregnancy. *Am J Obstet Gynecol.* 1972;113:14–20; Speroff L, Glass RH, Kase NG. Clinical gynecology, endocrinology and infertility. 4th ed. Baltimore, MD: Williams & Wilkins; 1989:283.

steadily declines, but remains detectable in mature milk (approximately 11 ng/mL) until weaning up to 40 weeks postpartum (Yuen, 1988).

De Carvalho et al. (1983) postulated that frequent feeding in early lactation stimulates a faster increase in milk output because suckling stimulates the development of receptors to prolactin in the mammary gland. According to this theory, the number of receptors per cell increases in early lactation and remains constant thereafter (Hinds & Tyndale-Biscoe, 1982; Sernia & Tyndale-Biscoe, 1979).

Some understanding of the impact of early breastfeeding on prolactin receptors is provided by Zuppa et al. (1988). In their study, although serum prolactin levels were slightly lower in multiparous mothers as compared with primiparous mothers in the first 4 postpartum days, the volume of milk obtained by the infants of the multiparous mothers was significantly higher. The researchers concluded that multiparous women had a greater number of mammary gland receptors for prolactin. The implication is

that the controlling factor in breastmilk output is the number of prolactin receptors, rather than the amount of prolactin in serum. More receptors may result in more than adequate milk production, even in the presence of lower prolactin levels. This finding helps to explain why infants of multiparous mothers begin gaining weight somewhat faster than do those of primiparous mothers.

Cortisol

Cortisol, one of the main glucocorticoids in the body, acts synergistically on the mammary system in the presence of prolactin (Neville & Berga, 1983). The final differentiation of the alveolar epithelial cell in a mature milk cell takes place because prolactin is present, but only after prior exposure to cortisol and insulin. Glucocorticoids are hormones secreted by the adrenal glands that help to regulate water transport across the cell membranes during lactation. A high cortisol level is associated with a delay in lactogenesis (Chen et al., 1998).

Thyroid-Stimulating Hormone

Thyroid-stimulating hormone (TSH) promotes mammary growth and lactation through a permissive rather than a regulatory role. Dawood et al. (1981) established that a marked and significant increase in plasma thyroid-stimulating hormone level occurs on the third to fifth postpartum days.

Prolactin-Inhibiting Factor

Prolactin-inhibiting factor (PIF) is a hypothalamic substance, either dopamine itself or mediated by dopamine. It stimulates dopamine releases and, therefore, inhibits prolactin secretions (dopamine agonist). Bromocriptine, a drug that suppresses lactation, is an example of a dopamine agonist. Dopamine antagonists have the opposite effect. Nipple stimulation and milk removal suppresses PIF and dopamine, causing prolactin levels to rise and the breast to produce milk. Drugs such as domperidone, metoclopramide, phenothiazines, and reserpine derivatives increase breastmilk production because they inhibit PIF (Asztalos et al., 2012; Bohnet & Kato, 1985; Donovan & Buchanon, 2012).

Oxytocin

In response to suckling, release of the posterior pituitary hormone oxytocin causes the milk-ejection reflex (MER) or letdown, a contraction of the myoepithelial cells surrounding the alveoli necessary for the removal of milk from the breast. Oxytocin is released in pulsatile waves and is carried though the bloodstream to the breast, where it interacts with receptors on myoepithelial cells, causing contraction and forcing milk from the alveoli into the ducts where it becomes available to the newborn through the nipple openings. Many women feel pressure and a tingling, warm sensation during milk ejection, and a significant increase in milk-duct diameter can be observed via ultrasound imaging when the milk ejection is sensed. After lactation becomes established, many women will experience multiple milk ejections during a feed. In a study of 45 Australian mothers, 88% were able to sense the initial milk ejection; however, none sensed subsequent milk ejections (Ramsay Mitoulas, et al., 2005).

Oxytocin plays a major role in the continuance of lactation. During suckling or breast stimulation, this hormone is released in discrete pulses. Oxytocin blood levels rise within 1 minute on stimulation, and they return to baseline levels within 6 minutes after the cessation of nipple stimulation. This rise and fall of oxytocin levels continues at each feeding throughout the lactation course, even when the mother breastfeeds for an extended period (Leake et al., 1983). The posterior pituitary contains a surprisingly large store of oxytocin (3000–9000 mU) as compared with the amount required to elicit the ejection reflex (50–100 mU) (Lincoln & Paisley, 1982).

Oxytocin has another important function—to contract the mother's uterus. Uterine contractions help to control postpartum bleeding and aid in uterine involution. The uterus not only contracts during breastfeeding, but also continues to contract rhythmically for as long as 20 minutes after the feeding. These cramps may be painful during the first few days postpartum. After involution is complete, however, these rhythmical pulsations may be a source of pleasure to the mother. Oxytocin also has peripheral effects—notably, dilation of peripheral vascular beds and increased blood flow without increased systemic arterial pressure. As a result, breastfeeding is accompanied by increased skin temperature not unlike that of a menopausal hot flash (Marshall et al., 1992). New mothers often report an increase in thirst while breastfeeding, which appears to be closely related to the increase in plasma oxytocin (James et al., 1995). Women who have had emergency cesarean births (Nissen et al., 1996) or are under stress (Ueda et al., 1994) have significantly fewer oxytocin pulses during breastfeeding. Breast massage raises the maternal plasma oxytocin level (Yokoyama et al., 1994).

Through oxytocin mediation, these afferent pathways become so well established that letdown can occur even when the mother merely thinks of her baby. Many anecdotal reports describe spontaneous lactation in mothers who have weaned. Milk synthesis is a complex interplay of the hypothalamic–pituitary–gonadal axis (Figure 3-11),

Figure 3-11 (A) RELEASE AND EFFECT OF PROLACTIN ON MILK EJECTION.
(B) RELEASE AND EFFECT OF OXYTOCIN.

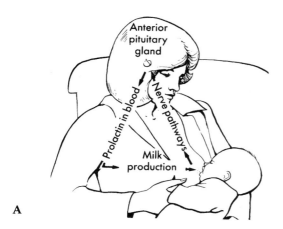

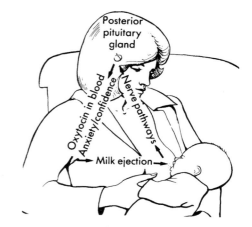

A

B

which is susceptible to emotional upheaval and can potentially inhibit the letdown reflex.

The calmness while breastfeeding that mothers report is partly governed by oxytocin. Oxytocin infusion in rats produces sedation, lower blood pressure, and lower levels of corticosteroids (Uvnas-Moberg, 1997). Groer and Davis (2002) make the case that breastfeeding women have a diminished response to stressors and to pain. Perceived stress is significantly lower in breastfeeding mothers compared to formula-feeding mothers (Groer, 2005b). When exposed to stress, lactating women have been found to have lower levels of ACTH, cortisol, glucose, and norepinephrine compared to nonlactating women (Altemus et al., 1996).

Johnstone and Amico (1986) measured the influence of supplemental feedings on oxytocin and prolactin peaks. They discovered that mothers who were exclusively breastfeeding had higher oxytocin levels over time than women who were giving their babies replacement feedings. The exclusively breastfeeding women's oxytocin levels not only remained higher but also tended to climb over time, so that their oxytocin levels were higher at 15 to 24 weeks postpartum than they were at earlier periods (2–4 weeks and 5–14 weeks postpartum). In sharp contrast, the oxytocin levels of the mothers who were

supplementing their babies with formula-feeding were lower at all times examined, and no rise in oxytocin peaks was noted over time. In both groups of women, prolactin levels tended to decline over time. Among mothers who were not supplementing, however, prolactin levels were consistently higher at all times examined. These data suggest that over time prolactin levels can be expected to fall, whereas oxytocin levels will continue to climb. However, when a mother supplements her child with formula-feedings, prolactin levels decline markedly and fall even further over time, and oxytocin levels remain depressed and do not climb.

Milk Production

With the closure of the tight junctions between the cells of the alveoli (see Figure 3-8) and through the mediation of the hypothalamus, the alveolar cells respond with milk secretion at the base of the alveolar cell, where small droplets form and migrate through the cell membrane and into the alveolar ducts for storage (see Figure 3-7). The rate of milk synthesis after each breastfeeding episode varies, ranging from 17 mL/hr to 33 mL/hr in one study (Arthur et al., 1989). Milk synthesis is related to the degree of breast fullness. For example, a woman who does not breastfeed her baby for 6 hours will have a lower rate of milk synthesis than if she had breastfed every 90 minutes (Cregan & Hartmann, 1999).

The highly vascularized secretory cells extract water, lactose, amino acids, fats, vitamins, minerals, and numerous other substances from the mother's blood, converting them into milk for her infant. Stores of adipose tissue laid down during pregnancy are drawn upon to provide a substrate for milk synthesis. When the milk "comes in" or rapidly increases in volume, creating breast fullness 3 to 4 days after birth, closure of the junctional complexes between the mammary alveolar cells prevents direct access of extracellular space to the lumen of the mammary alveoli (Neville, 2001). In turn, sodium, chloride, and lactose concentrations are altered. Mothers then begin to feel a tightening in their breasts as the myoepithelial cells contract to expel the milk (see Color Plate 3). This physiologic response is known as the milk-ejection reflex formerly called "letdown."

Autocrine Versus Endocrine

It is at this point that lactation shifts from endocrine control (hormone driven) to autocrine control (milk removal driven) (Prentice et al., 1989). It follows, then, that the amount of colostrum secreted by non-breastfeeding women during the first few days postpartum is similar to that of breastfeeding women; however, this pattern reverses abruptly after the first few days. Thus breastfeeding is not a major factor for the initiation of lactation but it is essential for the continuation of lactation (Kulski & Hartmann, 1981). From a clinical standpoint, the onset of copious milk secretion after birth or the milk "coming in" will happen whether the baby is being put to the breast or not, as it is hormonally driven.

Feedback Inhibitor of Lactation

An autocrine feedback mechanism, the feedback inhibitor of lactation (FIL) appears to locally control milk synthesis. The specific mechanism by which FIL works to inhibit breastmilk synthesis is not clear, but it appears to involve a compound within the milk, not the distension of the breast that slows the build-up of milk. It is thought that this mechanism of local control of milk synthesis must comprise a relationship between the filling and emptying cycle of the alveoli. More detailed information on how this mechanism works would be useful to clinicians in treating oversupply or undersupply problems (Cregan & Hartmann, 1999).

Galactopoiesis

Galactopoiesis is the maintenance of the established milk production (Table 3-1). The breast is not a passive container of milk, but rather an organ of active production that is infant rather than hormone driven. The removal of milk from the breasts facilitates continued milk production; conversely, lack of adequate milk removal or stasis tends to limit breastmilk synthesis in the breasts. It is the quantity and quality of infant suckling or milk removal that governs breastmilk synthesis. Milk production reflects the infant's appetite rather than the woman's ability to produce milk, which in fact can be several-fold higher than the infant's ability to remove milk (Daly & Hartmann, 1995). As long as milk is removed regularly from the breast, the alveolar cells will continue to secrete milk almost indefinitely.

This phenomenon—that is, the supply–demand response—is a feedback control mechanism that regulates the production of milk to match the intake of the infant. A common adage that expresses this response is "The more the mother breastfeeds, the more milk there will be" (La Leche League International, 1997). Because lactation is an energy-intensive process, it makes teleological sense that there should be safeguards against wasteful overproduction as well as mechanisms to ensure a prompt response to the infant's need.

A case of a new mother who became pregnant 3 months after having a pituitary resection supports the concept of autocrine control (de Coopman, 1993). After delivering a healthy infant, this mother had sufficient milk to completely sustain her baby by breastfeeding without supplementation. This unusual situation was attributable to the pituitary abscess that caused milk production to continue through her pregnancy after she weaned her first child; thus her milk yield postpartum was based on milk removal as much as on hormonal stimulation.

Galactorrhea

Galactorrhea is the spontaneous secretion of milk from the breast under nonphysiological circumstances. Small amounts of milk or serous fluid are commonly expressed for weeks, months, or years from women who have previously been pregnant or lactating. Many anecdotal reports of spontaneous lactation present an intriguing enigma. Thyrotoxicosis, certain drugs (reserpine, methyldopa, phenothiazines, antipsychotics), and the use of intrauterine devices containing copper (Horn & Scott, 1969) can trigger abnormal milk secretion.

Surprisingly, only 30% of women with galactorrhea have higher-than-normal prolactin levels (Frantz et al., 1972); these women are otherwise healthy and have no history of menstrual irregularity or infertility but may be overly sensitive to normal circulating prolactin levels (Friesen & Cowden, 1989). In other women, galactorrhea is a symptom of a larger problem of hyperprolactinemia; in addition to a spontaneous milk secretion, these women may complain of amenorrhea, difficulty in becoming pregnant, and lack of libido. Any woman with persistent galactorrhea should be referred to a physician for a thorough physical examination and biochemical assessment.

Clinical Implications: Mother

Breast Assessment

Prenatal assessment of the breast and nipples is important to recognizing risk factors for successful lactogenesis. Physicians, nurse–midwives, nurses, and lactation consultants practicing as primary caregivers are the ideal people to perform a prenatal breast assessment.

Ideal for teaching as well as for data gathering, physical assessment of the breast and nipples includes both inspection and palpation. While one is assessing the breasts, the following observations and questions are relevant.

Inspection

Size, symmetry, and shape of the breasts proper have minimal effect on lactation. The assessment provides the opportunity to reassure the woman with small breasts that she will be able to breastfeed and have a sufficient supply of milk. Asymmetry of breast size is usually normal, but marked asymmetry may be an indication of insufficient glandular tissue (IGT)/primary hypoplasia in a small minority of women (see Color Plate 27). Hypoplasia (lack of breast tissue) signified by a wide space between breasts (intramammary space), a short breast that has a dog-eared appearance (high inframammary fold), and thin, tubular breasts are anatomic "red flags" associated with insufficient lactation (Huggins et al., 2000; Neifert et al., 1985, 1990). When mothers with possible hypoplasia (underdeveloped breasts) are identified, their newborn babies should be monitored closely for adequate milk intake. Inadequate glandular tissue might prevent the mother from exclusively breastfeeding her baby; however, she can continue to enjoy the breastfeeding relationship if she provides the baby with additional nutrition while feeding from the breast.

For the woman with large breasts, discussing the importance of a well-fitted bra and locations where such a bra may be obtained is helpful. Holding and feeding her infant will not be the same for the large-breasted woman as for mothers with average-size breasts. Instead of simply holding the breast, the mother with large breasts may need to lift her breast and hold or push part of the breast back to permit her infant to grasp the nipple and maintain an adequate airway. Using semi-reclining positions for feeding to lift the breast away from the postpartum belly and bringing the baby down to where the nipple naturally falls, rather than lifting the heavy breast, can be helpful alternatives. During prenatal discussions, the mother may talk about some of her deeper feelings about having large breasts and her decision to breastfeed (also see the *Breast-Related Problems* chapter).

The skin of the breast should be inspected for any deviations. Skin turgor and elasticity can be assessed by gently pinching the skin, although the effect of elasticity on lactation is questionable:

women who have been pregnant before have more elastic skin because it has been stretched from a previous pregnancy; women pregnant for the first time have firmer tissue.

A lateral incision in the vicinity of the cutaneous branch of the fourth intercostal nerve made during breast augmentation or reduction surgery may mean severed innervation of the nipple and areola (Farina et al., 1980). Surgery on the breast, especially if it involves an incision at the areolar margin, is likely to interfere to some degree with milk production. However, even having undergone such surgery, most mothers still can breastfeed. Breast-reduction surgery, because of the greater likelihood of the removal of nipple tissue (Hurst, 1996), is more likely than augmentation surgery to negatively influence later lactation performance (Neifert et al., 1990). Scar tissue from injury should be evaluated for its effect on skin elasticity and the degree to which nerve sensitivity may have been affected (also see the *Breast-Related Problems* chapter).

Note should also be taken of any skin thickening and dimpling of the breast or nipple tissue. Although rare in a woman of childbearing age, such a change could be an early sign of a tumor and should be promptly referred to a physician for evaluation.

The breast assessment is the time for the nurse or lactation consultant to ask questions: "Have your breasts grown during pregnancy?" "Have you had any tenderness and soreness?" An increase in breast size, swelling, and tenderness usually indicates adequately functioning breast tissue responsive to hormonal changes.

Next, the nipple should be carefully inspected. (For the purpose of this discussion, *nipple* will refer to the areola as well as the nipple shaft and pores.) If the nipples appear small, explain that the size of a woman's nipples is of secondary importance to their functional ability. Likewise, any nipple structural abnormality such as inversion should be assessed only in terms of its function.

The look of the breast does not dictate its ability to function. A case in point may be women who have sustained significant scarring from burns (see Color Plate 25). Second- and third-degree burns rarely extend so deeply into the parenchyma that

they destroy the glandular tissue of the breast, even when the burns have occurred in adulthood. Significant scarring of the dermis and epidermis, however, may result in (1) reduced maternal sensation when the infant suckles; (2) minimal tissue elasticity, requiring the mother to alter the baby's position at the breast; and (3) reduced milk ejection if a nipple has been surgically reconstructed. Nevertheless, scar tissue on the breast or nipple does not, by itself, preclude breastfeeding.

Palpation

After a thorough washing of the hands, the nurse or lactation consultant should assess the nipple by compressing or palpating the areola between the forefinger and the thumb just behind the base of the nipple (the pinch test). This action simulates the compression that occurs when the infant is at the breast. Because of possible nipple adhesions within the underlying connective tissue, a nipple that initially appears everted may retract inwardly on stimulation. Conversely, a nipple that appears flattened or inverted may, on palpation, evert; therefore, differentiation must be made between structure and function in assessing the nipples.

The classification of nipple function in Table 3-3 is suggested as standard terminology. It must be emphasized that although many primigravidas have nipples that tend to retract during pregnancy, most evert easily by the end of pregnancy and do not interfere with breastfeeding. Thus nipple assessment should be performed periodically through the pregnancy to track changes and to inform the mother how her body is preparing to feed her baby.

Classification of Nipple Function

When the nipple is compressed using the pinch test, it responds in one of the ways identified in Figure 3-12. This response may reflect degree of function.

Flat or retracted nipples may be treatable during pregnancy. Dysfunction may be present in one nipple while the other is perfectly normal, or it may be present in both nipples. Retraction or inversion can prevent the infant from effectively removing milk

Table 3-3 CLASSIFICATION OF NIPPLE FUNCTION

Protraction	Nipple moves forward; considered a normal functional response. No special interventions are needed.
Retraction	Instead of protracting, the nipple moves inward.
Minimal	An infant with a strong suck exerts sufficient pressure to pull the nipple forward. A weak or premature infant may have difficulties at first.
Moderate to severe	Nipple retracts to a level even with or behind the surrounding areola. Intervention is helpful to stretch the nipple outward and improve protractility.
Inversion	On visual inspection, all or part of the nipple is drawn inward within the folds of the areola.
Simple	The nipple moves outward to protraction with manual pressure or when cold (pseudoinversion).
Complete	The nipple does not respond to manual pressure because adhesions bind the nipple inward; very rarely there is congenital absence of the nipple.

from milk ducts that lie beneath the areola. Retraction or simple inversion identified in early pregnancy, however, does not necessarily foretell later difficulty. The infant forms a teat not only from the nipple but also from the surrounding breast tissue. When inversion is noted early in pregnancy, time is on the mother's side. As pregnancy progresses, hormonal changes increase the size and protractility of the nipples. The mother also has time to use interventions that help prevent subsequent feeding problems (also see the *Breast-Related Problems* chapter).

Concepts to Practice

Encouraging early and frequent breastfeeding is a simple, low-cost recommendation for breastfeeding initiation. If the infant is able to suckle effectively at the breast soon after birth, there is a direct relationship between the frequency and strength of suckling and subsequent availability of breastmilk. There appears to be an early "window of opportunity" for the infant's suckling to stimulate prolactin receptors (discussed earlier in this chapter), which in turn enhances milk production. A basic knowledge of anatomy and physiology is put to valuable use when the lactation consultant or nurse translates basic concepts into easily understandable teaching materials. If a client realizes a stressful environment

may temporarily inhibit her milk ejection, she may take action to reduce stressful situations over which she has control. If a woman understands that the reason she needs less covering when she breastfeeds is that she literally has "hot flashes" during feedings, she will take measures to "keep cool." Examples of the application of basic biologic principles of maternal lactation are legion and form the basis of many of the chapters that follow in this text.

Newborn Oral Development

Infants perform a series of complex oral movements to obtain sufficient nutriment from their mother's breast to meet daily nutritional requirements and to support rapid growth, especially during the first few months of life. The act of suckling entails far more than simply obtaining food. The infant's earliest autonomous functions are focused about his mouth and pharynx area. The infant's mouth is the cockpit of his awareness and is the principal site of interaction with his environment.

In the embryo, facial and pharyngeal regions develop from neural-crest cells at about the time of neural-tube closure. Further development occurs due to tissue differentiation from the endoderm, which later forms the digestive tract. During gestation, the fetus is able to swallow amniotic fluid as

Figure 3-12 (A) PROTRACTING NORMAL NIPPLE. (B) MODERATE TO SEVERE RETRACTION. (C) INVERTED-APPEARING NIPPLE THAT, WHEN COMPRESSED USING A PINCH TEST, WILL EITHER INVERT FARTHER INWARD OR WILL PROTRACT FORWARD. (D) TRUE INVERSION; NIPPLE INVERTS FURTHER.

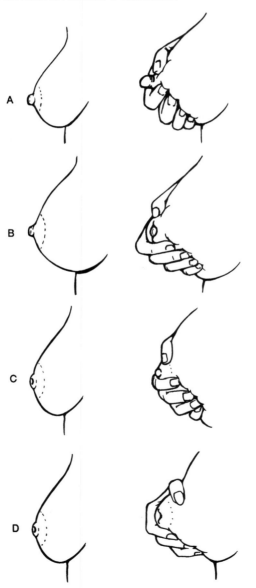

early as 11 weeks (Miller, 1982) and has a suck reflex at 24 weeks (Herbst, 1981). Older studies reported that the rooting response and the link between sucking and swallowing was not established until 32 weeks (Amiel-Tison, 1967) and not well coordinated until 37 weeks (Bu'Lock et al., 1990). However, in a study of Swedish preterm infants (Nyqvist et al., 1999), efficient rooting, areolar grasp, and latching-on at the breast were observed at 28 weeks—much earlier than previously thought.

At birth, the infant's mouth is vertically short in comparison with that of the adult. There is so little room that when the newborn's mouth is closed, the tongue is in lateral contact with the gums and with the roof of the mouth, helping to broaden and lower the palate. Other proportional differences in size and shape distinguish the infant and the adult skull (Figures 3-13 and 3-14). Notably, the infant's lower jaw (mandible) is small and somewhat receded.

The Palate

Whereas the adult's hard palate is deeply arched and situated on a higher plane relative to the base of

Figure 3-13 MIDSAGITTAL SECTION OF CRANIAL AND ORAL ANATOMY OF AN ADULT WHILE SWALLOWING.

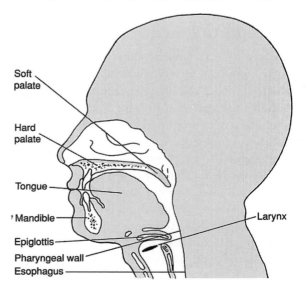

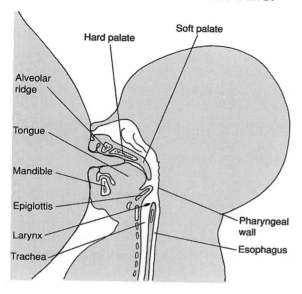

Figure 3-14 MIDSAGITTAL SECTION OF CRANIAL AND ORAL ANATOMY OF AN INFANT WHILE SWALLOWING.

the skull, the infant's hard palate is short, wide, and only slightly arched at birth. Corrugated transverse folds (rugae) on the hard palate assist the newborn in holding the breast during sucking. While the hard palate works with the tongue to compress the nipple and maintain its position, the soft palate, a muscular flap, seals to the back of the tongue during sucking and elevates to seal off the nasal cavity during swallowing (Wolf & Glass, 1992).

The hard palate is shaped by tongue movements. A high, narrow palate might signal tongue-tie or low muscle tone. Another potentially troublesome palate shape is the "bubble" palate. Described by Marmet and Shell (1984) as a concavity in the hard palate, it can cause sore, abraded nipples if the nipple is pulled into the bubble rather than staying elongated to near the juncture of the hard and soft palates (Jacobs et al., 2007). To bring the position of the tongue forward, the mother lies in a supine (on back) position with pillows to support her, with the baby placed on the chest to breastfeed (Snyder, 1997). Photographs of prone positions can be found in the *Supporting Sucking Skills in Breastfeeding Infants*

chapter by Catherine Watson Genna (Marmet & Shell, 2013).

The Tongue and Lips

Because the infant's tongue fills the small oral cavity, his tongue movements are well supported by contact with other oral structures. Taste buds on the tongue (mostly on the tongue tip) are present at birth, and the newborn sucks faster in response to sweet tastes.

The entire surface of the tongue is within the oral cavity. Elad and colleagues (2014) demonstrated that the anterior tongue moves as a 'stiff body' along with the jaw, while the posterior tongue undulates in a peristaltic wave. Downward displacement of the tongue and jaw creates subatmospheric pressure, which allows milk to flow from the breast (Elad et al., 2014, Geddes et al., 2008), where milk is under positive pressure due to the milk-ejection reflex. The peristaltic movements are likely most important in swallowing, as they provide positive pressure to move the bolus to the pharynx. Three-dimensional ultrasound has revealed that peristaltic tongue movements are visible only in a true mid-sagittal view (Burton et al., 2013) and that a slightly off-center view makes the tongue movements appear to be up and down only.

Once the baby's tongue tip grasps the breast and draws it into the mouth, the tongue grooves around the newly formed teat to hold it in place in the infant's mouth. The lips then seal to the areola. The infant's lips are well adapted to assist the tongue in creating an airtight closure around the breast. The lips are partially everted so that the oral mucosa presents slightly externally; they have tiny swellings on the inner surface (eminences of the pars villosa) that facilitate holding the breast and areola in place.

The Epiglottis

The infant's epiglottis lies just below the soft palate, unlike the adult's (as seen in Figure 3-14). This arrangement reduces the risk of aspiration by directing milk laterally rather than straight down. The epiglottis protects the airway during the swallow by tilting over the airway to direct milk around the infant's trachea and into the esophagus, closing off the pathway to the lungs when the infant swallows.

The Larynx

Relative to an adult larynx, the infant larynx is much higher in the oral cavity and occupies a larger space. It is short and funnel-shaped. As fluid passes through the mouth, the larynx elevates and moves under the base of the tongue so that fluid can move easily into the pharynx. Because the larynx is high and elevated during swallowing, it depends much less on the action of the epiglottis and on closure of the vocal folds to protect the airway. The shape of the pharynx gradually changes as the child grows. At birth, the pharynx curves very gradually downward to join the oral cavity. This curvature challenges speech production, as does the need to develop central nervous system control for speech articulation. By puberty, the posterior walls of the nasal and oral segments join almost at a right angle.

The Cheeks

The infant has pads of fat on both cheeks to assist with suckling. Each pad is a circumscribed layer of fat enclosed within its own capsule of fibrous connective tissue. It lies between the buccinator and masseter muscles. The buccal fat pads provide stability for tongue grooving during sucking and provide structural integrity to the cheeks during sucking. When babies suck their own tongues, the degree of negative pressure collapses the cheeks, creating a characteristic dimpling. Collapsing of the cheeks is more likely in a premature baby who lacks the layer of fat (including that in the cheeks) that gives full-term infants their characteristic plump facial appearance.

The largest increments in craniofacial growth occur during the first 4 years of life. During the first year after birth, the lower jaw grows downward, creating a larger intraoral space. Active breastfeeding encourages facial and temporo mandibular development and strengthens the jaw muscles. The tongue also gradually descends. By the time the child reaches 4 or 5 years of age, the tongue is attached directly to the epiglottis of the larynx. The frenulum is a fold of mucous membrane midline on the undersurface of the tongue that provides traction on the orifices of the salivary glands during tongue movements, promoting salivation. If the frenulum is too short to allow freedom of tongue movement or is placed too far forward to permit tongue extension upward or forward, it can interfere with an infant's ability to suck (Notestine, 1990).

The shape and softness of the human breast are beneficial to shaping the infant's hard palate into a round U-shaped configuration because the breast broadens and flattens in response to the infant's tongue movements. Compared with the V shape associated with bottle-fed children, the broad and wide palate of a breastfed child is physiologically ideal because it expands the choanal airway and aligns teeth properly (Palmer, 1998).

Sucking

Sucking behavior develops early in gestation. Fetuses display a suck reflex by 24 weeks' gestation. By 28 weeks, preterm babies can coordinate the suck/swallow/breathe cycle at the breast; by 32 weeks, they can suck in repeated bursts of more than 10 sucks and in maximum sucking bursts of more than 30 sucks (Nyqvist et al., 1999).

The precise way in which infants use their oral and facial muscles to efficiently take in nourishment from their mothers' breasts is vital information for health professionals, because some breastfeeding infants have initial difficulty getting on the breast, and a few continue to have sucking dysfunction. In a study of spontaneous feeding behavior, infants placed in a prone position between their mothers' breasts after an unmedicated delivery began licking, sucking, and rooting movements after about 15 minutes, began hand-to-mouth movements after about 34 minutes, and spontaneously began to suck after 55 minutes. Licking movements both preceded and followed the rooting reflex in alert infants (Widstrom et al., 1987), as did hand-to-mouth and hand-to-breast movements (Widstrom et al., 2011). Infants exposed to labor medications, including epidural analgesia, require twice the length of uninterrupted skin-to-skin contact after birth to find and attach to the breast and suckle (up to 2 hours). There are long-lasting consequences for breastfeeding and the maternal–infant relationship if continuous skin-to-skin contact is interrupted in those first 2 hours after birth and especially before the first breastfeeding (Bystrova et al., 2009). For more information on the effect of birth interventions on breastfeeding, see *The Impact of Birthing Practices on Breastfeeding* by Linda Smith and Mary Kroeger (2010).

The first research report in which the development of sucking was followed during the first 4 hours post birth was conducted by Gene Cranston Anderson at the University of Illinois Medical Center in Chicago (Anderson et al., 1982). This study was conducted because of the controversy about the most appropriate time to begin feeding newborns. At the time of Anderson's study in the early 1970s, common practice called for hospital-born infants to be separated from their mothers, isolated, and fasted, often for as long as 12 hours. Anderson measured sucking pressures using a "suckometer" to show that in the first few hours after birth, neonates had a strong sucking ability and should be fed.

In fact, sucking might be strongest in neonates soon after delivery. When sucking ability was measured using the Neonatal Oral Motor Assessment Scale (NOMAS), an instrument to digitally assess oral motor behavior and sucking ability, younger newborns had a stronger suck than did older newborns (MacMullen & Kulski, 2000).

The position of the neonate's tongue is critical to the feeding. After the rooting stimulus, the infant opens the mouth wide (gape response), keeping the tongue at the bottom of the mouth. This tongue position enables the infant to "catch" the mother's breast to draw the nipple area into the mouth. An infant places the tongue in the palate when crying, which might be a security reflex, to prevent obstruction of the trachea during the inspiration phase. Consequently forcing a crying baby to the breast might cause the infant to place the tongue in his or her palate, a defensive response that inhibits sucking and disturbs the rooting-tongue reflex system (Widstrom & Thingstrom-Paulsson, 1993).

In the literature, *sucking* and *suckling* are often are used interchangeably to refer to suckling. In this text, we also use these terms interchangeably, although some individuals feel strongly about the distinction (Montagu, 1979):

> The baby is said to "suck" at its mother's nipple. The baby knows better than to do anything so foolish, for were he to "suck" the nipple all he would, for the most part, succeed in achieving would be to produce a partial vacuum in his mouth and fail to develop the ability to suckle properly. A baby sucks at the nozzle on the top of a bottle, but at the mother's breast a baby suckles.

Does the infant suckle or suck at the breast? Now that we have discovered that the mechanism by which babies extract milk from the breast differs considerably from the method that they use on a bottle teat, we urge that separate words are needed to differentiate the two acts. The word *suckle* seems ideal for breastfeeding, and it has come to be used in this sense in modern American breastfeeding literature. However, this term still retains its original meaning in the breastfeeding literature of many of the British Commonwealth countries. The Oxford English Dictionary (1961) defines the two words thus:

> Suck: (1) the action or an act of sucking milk from the breast; the milk or other fluid sucked at one time; (2) to apply the lips to a teat, breast, the mother, nurse, or dam, for the purpose of extracting milk from, with the mouth.

> Suckle: (1) To give suck to; to nurse (a child) at the breast; (2) to cause to take milk from the breast or udder; to put to suck.

Babies suck and swallow at a frequency of about once per second or more slowly when breastmilk is actively flowing. This rate is similar to that of other primates. If the milk flow lessens or stops, the infant will increase this rate to about two suckles per second (Wolff, 1968). In other words, when the milk flow increases, the rate of suckling decreases. Conversely, when milk flow is low, the rate of suckling is higher. Non-nutritive sucking (on a pacifier or finger, or before milk flow) has a stable rhythm determined by the brain stem's central pattern generator (Barlow & Estep, 2006). Healthy breastfeeding infants are able to adjust their sucking rate on a continuum to adjust to milk flow. In addition to yielding milk and calories, sucking facilitates feelings of calm, reduces heart rate and metabolic rate, and elevates both the baby's and mother's pain threshold (Blass, 1994; Gray et al., 2002; Groer & Davis, 2002).

Non-nutritive sucking has important implications for infant development, especially under special circumstances such as prematurity. Non-nutritive sucking in premature infants increases peristalsis, enhances secretion of digestive fluids, and decreases crying in these infants (Measel & Anderson, 1979). Kangaroo mother care and non-nutritive sucking at the breast are developmentally appropriate ways of providing non-nutritive sucking. "Emptying" the breast is usually unnecessary: preterm infants will not transfer milk until they are able to safely coordinate swallowing. Swallowing small boluses helps preterm infants transition to full feeding more rapidly (Lau & Smith, 2012).

Suckling at the breast has been examined in great detail. With the advent of ultrasonography and other technologies, it is now possible to accurately quantify suckling patterns, replacing earlier descriptions that only inferred what actually occurred. When infants feed from both breasts, milk transfer from the second breast decreases by 58% as compared with the first breast, even though there are no significant changes in suckling pressure (Prieto et al., 1996). Jacobs et al. (2007), Marmet and Shell (1984), Woolridge (1986, 2011), McBride and Danner (1987), and Smith et al. (1985) described infant suckling mechanics at the breast. The following description of functional suckling is based on the work of these investigators. Figure 3-15 illustrates the complete suck cycle.

1. The nipple and its surrounding areola and underlying breast tissue are drawn deeply into the infant's mouth; the infant's tongue, lips, and cheeks then form a seal. The infant's lips are flanged outward around the mother's breast and are minimally involved.

2. The tip of the infant's tongue is maintained over the lower gum while the anterior tongue grooves around the areola of the breast.

3. During the feeding, the mother's highly elastic nipple elongates (two to three times its resting length) into a teat by suction created

Figure 3-15 COMPLETE SUCK CYCLE. THE BABY IS SHOWN IN MEDIAN SECTION. THE BABY EXHIBITS GOOD FEEDING TECHNIQUE: THE NIPPLE IS DRAWN WELL INTO THE MOUTH, EXTENDING BACK TO THE JUNCTION OF THE HARD AND SOFT PALATE (THE LACTIFEROUS SINUSES ARE DEPICTED WITHIN THE TEAT, ALTHOUGH THESE CANNOT BE VISUALIZED ON SCANS).

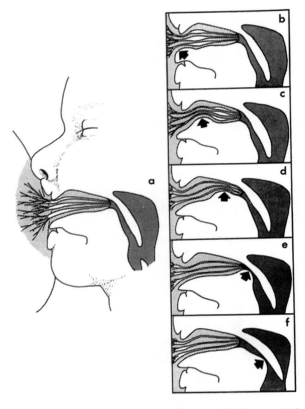

Source: Used with permission from Woolridge MW. The "anatomy" of infant sucking. *Midwifery.* 1986;2:164–167.

within the baby's mouth. The nipple extends back near the junction between the hard and soft palates (Jacobs et al., 2007). At its base, the nipple is held between the upper gum and tongue that covers the lower gum. The mother's nipple and areolar tissue undergo extensive changes during feeding.

4. The tongue muscles press upward in a wave beginning at the tongue tip and moving back (peristalsis). The soft palate is pressed to the back of the tongue, creating a sealed oral cavity around the teat. The jaw simultaneously elevates, compressing the maternal areola against the infant's alveolar ridge. The masseter is the jaw muscle that is most active during suckling; it raises the jaw and causes it to protrude preparing for compression on the breast (Gomes et al., 2006).

5. A new wave of compression begins, and the mandible moves downward, dragging the mid- and posterior tongue with it and increasing the amount of space in the sealed oral cavity, thereby reducing intraoral pressure. Milk flows from the area of high pressure (the breast, under influence of the milk-ejection reflex) to the area of low pressure (the infant's mouth). Milk is delivered into the central groove of the tongue.

6. The jaw elevates and a new wave of peristalsis begins, pushing the milk back along the tongue. If there is sufficient milk to trigger a swallow, the infant's vocal folds close, the epiglottis tilts over the airway, the larynx is drawn upward under the base of the tongue, and finally the soft palate elevates to seal the back of the nose. The pharyngeal muscles contract, making the pharynx shorter. Finally, the tongue pushes the milk backward into the pharynx under positive pressure. Once milk has safely passed by the airway and entered the esophagus, the soft palate returns to its resting position against the back of the tongue and the airway reopens.

7. The infant lowers the jaw, and a new cycle begins. A rhythm is created by this sequence of vertical jaw movements superimposed on the peristaltic movements of the tongue, which results in depression and elevation of the posterior tongue while the anterior tongue maintains the seal on the breast.

The differences between bottle-feeding and breastfeeding are summarized in Table 3-4. Generally, breastfeeding infants suckle more times per day and maintain a higher level of oxygen pressure (tcPO$_2$) and skin temperature (Mathew, 1988; Meier & Anderson, 1987) than do bottle-feeding infants. The differences between bottle-feeding and breast-feeding premature infants are even greater (Chen et al., 2000; Meier & Pugh, 1985).

Breathing, Suckling, and Pacing

In a normal, coordinated, nutritive suckling cycle, breathing appears to continue throughout the sucking cycle; however, at the onset of the swallow, as the bulk of the bolus enters the pharynx, airflow is momentarily interrupted and then immediately restored. Deglutition (swallowing) apnea lasts about 0.5 second. In a perfectly coordinated cycle of suckling, swallowing, and breathing, breathing movements appear to be related in a 1:1:1 sequence. The rate of suckling is high for the first 1 or 2 minutes until the milk-ejection reflex occurs, then slows down as milk flow increases. This sequence reoccurs with each milk ejection during a feeding. As the feeding progresses, suckling bursts become shorter with more frequent and longer respiratory pauses, reflecting infant fatigue and the need to restore oxygen levels.

Suckling patterns change as the infant develops. At first suckling is a reflexive action; however, the infant quickly learns through experimental opportunities, sensory inputs, and neurological maturation so that feeding and swallowing change from a reflex to a volitional process and the pattern of breathing–swallowing coordination changes (Bronwen et al., 2007). This evolution is important to keep in mind and to share with parents when working with a baby with feeding problems—things probably will improve as the baby grows and practices breastfeeding.

Although suckling, swallowing, and breathing are generally well coordinated during a feeding, mild cyanosis is a relatively common event, especially in neonates. The neonate almost always recovers spontaneously and often continues to suckle and swallow despite cyanosis. The infant's oxygen saturation normally declines during a feeding. Mean levels drop from 96% (during feeding) to 93% (post feeding) in breastfed infants and from 95%

Table 3-4 COMPARISONS BETWEEN BREASTFEEDING AND BOTTLE-FEEDING IN FULL-TERM INFANTS

Breastfeeding	Bottle-feeding	References
More frequent suckling/min	Less frequent suckling/min	Drewett & Woolridge, 1979; Mathew, 1988; Wolff, 1968
Nutritive: 1 suckle/second		
Non-nutritive: 2 suckles/second		
Breathing patterns	Breathing patterns	Mathew, 1988
Shortening of expiration	Prolonged expiration	
Prolonging of inspiration	Shortening of inspiration	
Oxygen saturation < 90%	Oxygen saturation < 90%	Mathew, 1988
2 of 10 infants	5 of 10 infants	
Bradycardia	Bradycardia	Hammerman & Kaplan, 1995; Mathew, 1988
0 of 10 infants	2 of 10 infants	
Extended opening of mouth to grasp mother's nipple	Less extension to grasp rubber teat	Marmet & Shell, 1984
Infant's lips flanged outward, relaxed and resting against the breast to make a seal	Lips closer together and pursed to maintain contact with rubber teat	McBride & Danner, 1987
Extensive mandibular (jaw) action	Minimal mandibular action	Palmer, 1998
Tongue grooved around nipple; remains under nipple throughout feeding; moves in peristaltic, rolling action from front to back	Tongue upward and thrust forward against end of teat, "piston-like," to control milk flow	Marmet & Shell, 1984; Weber et al., 1986; Woolridge, 1986
Silent, except for soft swallow sounds, and (in older infants), cooing or "singing"	High-pitched squeak at end of intake of air prior to new suck	
Duration of feeding varies from short (few minutes) to long (30 minutes or longer)	Duration of feeding is usually 5–10 minutes	Ardran et al., 1958
Includes nutritive and non-nutritive suckling throughout the feeding but less distinct differences	Involves nearly exclusively nutritive suckling	Ardran et al., 1958; Hornell, 1999; Woolridge, 1986
Swallowing occurs nonrandomly between breaths and does not interfere with breathing	Swallowing patterns are different according to type of bottle/nipple	Goldfield, 2006

(during feeding) to 92% (post feeding) in bottle-fed infants (Hammerman & Kaplan, 1995). When term babies were given bottle-feedings with breastmilk, formula, and distilled water, the infants receiving breastmilk were found to have better coordination between swallowing and breathing, which helps prevent subclinical aspiration (Mizuno et al., 2002).

Unless hypoxic, the newborn is usually a nose breather, owing in part to the positioning of the soft palate and to the lack of space in the mouth through which air can travel. Although it is true that babies have ventilatory problems when the nasal passages are occluded, an infant is capable of breathing through the mouth when necessary (Rodenstein et al., 1985). Fatigue is common when beginning to nipple feed, especially with low-birth-weight babies. Observe the infant's cues to identify the need for a rest. Pacing the feeding includes removing the nipple (or removing milk from the nipple) at the first sign of disorganized feedings and/or swallowing to allow the infant a breathing break to recover and rest. Supportive positioning (side-lying) can also help the infant coordinate swallowing and breathing during bottle-feeding. For breastfeeding, prone positioning on a reclined mother and pressure on the breast to occlude some ducts during rapid milk flow are effective pacing techniques. More information on pacing feedings of children with neurologic disorders is provided in later chapters of this text.

Feeding and swallowing are sensitive indicators of the child's neurologic function. Birth injury, congenital defects, or other situations of neurologic dysfunction interfere with normal suckling. It may be necessary to bottle-feed infants with any of these conditions until breastfeeding can be initiated. Therefore a basic review of neural control of sucking

and swallowing, from either a bottle or breast, is in order. Coordination of more than 20 pairs of muscles and 5 cranial nerves is required just for swallowing! The cranial nerves involved include the trigeminal (V), facial (VII), glossopharyngeal (IX), vagus (X), and hypoglossal (XII) (Figure 3-16).

An example of the neural complexity and overlap is described by Wolf and Glass (1992). A breast-feeding infant who has sucking disorganization should be further evaluated neurologically to help understand the specific reason for the feeding dysfunction.

Wolf and Glass (1992) describe bottle-feeding sucking patterns in Figure 3-17:

- Normal sucking coordination of sucking, swallowing, and breathing in Figure 3-17a

Figure 3-16 OVERLAPPING FUNCTION OF CRANIAL NERVES IN SUCK–SWALLOW–BREATHE.

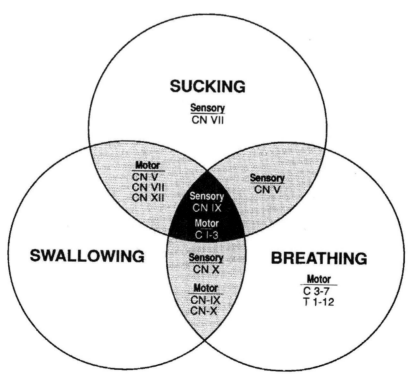

Source: Reproduced from Wolf LS, Glass RP. Feeding and swallowing disorders in infancy: assessment and management. Used with permission of Hammill Institute on Disabilities.

Figure 3-17 NORMAL COORDINATION OF SUCKING, SWALLOWING, AND BREATHING COMPARED TO ABNORMAL PATTERNS. EACH TRIANGLE REPRESENTS A SWALLOW.

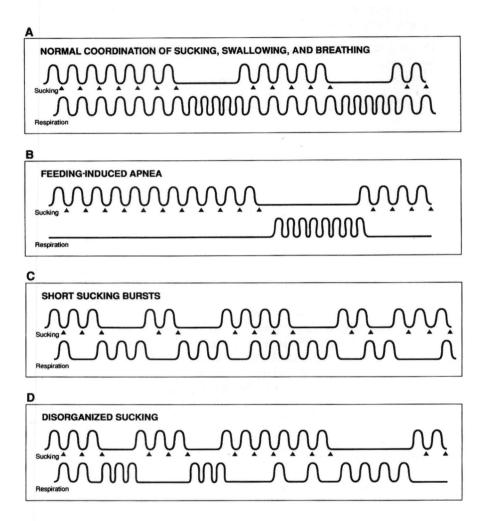

Source: Reproduced from Wolf LS, Glass RP. Feeding and swallowing disorders in infancy: assessment and management. Used with permission of Hammill Institute on Disabilities.

is organized into a series of sucking bursts and pauses.

- In feeding-induced apnea (Figure 3-17b), the infant is unable to pace himself and has lengthy sucking bursts without breathing at appropriate intervals. Sucking may cease, with the infant then compensating for the

previous lack of breathing with rapid panting breaths. This can lead to fatigue or poor coordination of swallowing, reflected by sputtering and coughing and putting the infant at risk for aspiration.

- In short sucking bursts (Figure 3-17c), the infant takes only one to five sucks and swallows before pausing. This pattern is seen in infants with low aerobic capacity, such as preterm infants or those with respiratory or cardiac instability. It can be a functional pattern if the infant is not rushed and is allowed to feed frequently. Careful monitoring of milk transfer is advised in infants with short sucking bursts, as well as medical evaluation.

- Very disorganized sucking (Figure 3-17d) may reflect general disorganization because of a neurologic deficit, respiratory problems, or a too-fast nipple-flow rate.

Frequency of Feedings

How often does the exclusively breastfed infant feed? Hornell et al. (1999) recorded the daily number of feedings of 506 Swedish infants for the first 6 months after births. In Sweden, breastfeeding is the norm. Each mother in this study had previously breastfed at least one infant for at least 4 months, and all mothers considered that they breastfed on demand.

During the first 6 months of life, the median frequency of feeds was eight feeds per 24 hours. This finding is consistent with the data published by Howie et al. (1981) and Quandt (1986), but different from the studies published by Butte et al. (1985) and de Carvalho et al. (1982), who noted a decline in feeding frequency during the first months. It also differs from a study of La Leche League mothers, who showed an average daily number of 15 feedings (Cable & Rothenberger, 1984).

In the Hornell et al. (1999) study, the median frequency of daytime feeds of exclusively breastfed infants was slightly less than 6 during the first 26 weeks of life. The median number of night feeds declined from 2.2 at 2 weeks to 1.3 at 12 weeks, after which it increased to 1.8 at 20 weeks (Figure 3-18). The frequency and duration of daily feedings varied widely among mothers. For example, at 2 weeks, the frequency of feeds during the day ranged from 2.9 to 10.8 and night feeds from 1.0 to 5.1. Daytime sucking duration ranged from 20 minutes to more than 4 hours and nighttime duration from 0 to 2 hours, 8 minutes. Increased

Figure 3-18 NUMBER OF BREASTFEEDS DURING (A) DAYTIME, (B) NIGHTTIME, AND (C) 24 HOURS AT DIFFERENT AGES. MEDIAN, 25TH, AND 75TH PERCENTILES AND RANGE.

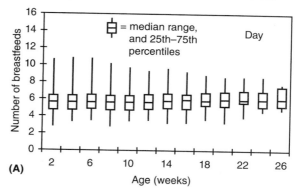

(A)

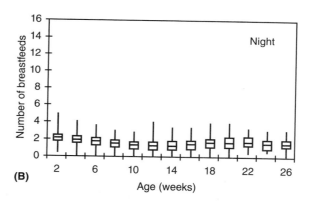

(B)

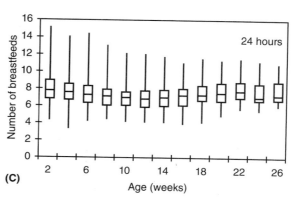

(C)

Source: Used with permission from Hornell A et al. Breastfeeding patterns in exclusively breastfed infants: a longitudinal prospective study in Uppsala, Sweden. *Acta Paediatr*. 1999;88:203–211.

feeding frequencies or so-called appetite or growth spurts were not observed in this study.

Australian mothers were found to breastfeed in similar patterns. Specifically, infants exclusively breastfed an average of 11 times in 24 hours (range 6–18) (Kent et al., 2005).

The neonate's ability to suckle effectively at the breast takes time and practice. For the first few feedings, even in full-term infants, suckling is usually disorganized. Drugs given to the mother during childbirth can also inhibit early suckling. Usually, after several attempts, the infant latches onto the breast and begins to suckle vigorously and effectively. These first feedings are critical because they imprint a suckling pattern that tends to be repeated in subsequent feedings. A healthy infant unaffected by labor or birth analgesia or anesthesia should be allowed to demonstrate hunger before being offered the breast. Practicing lactation consultants are fully aware that it is difficult, if not impossible, to "make" a baby breastfeed when he is in a deep sleep. Forcing the infant to the breast might abolish the rooting reflex and disturb placement of the tongue (Widstrom & Thingstrom-Paulsson, 1993).

Consistent breastfeeding assessment and identification of early problems so that they can be resolved before they worsen is essential. Several breastfeeding assessment tools have been developed. The more popular breastfeeding assessment tools are discussed in the *Infant Assessment* chapter. The PIBBs breastfeeding tool, developed for assessing preterm infants, can be found as an appendix to the *Use of Human Milk and Breastfeeding in the Neonatal Intensive Care Unit* chapter.

SUMMARY

Knowledge of maternal breast anatomy and the physiology of lactation are necessary antecedents to clinical practice. The fundamental biological principles of lactation discussed in this chapter are used, albeit not always consciously, in almost every clinical situation in which lactation is involved. Knowledge of the structure and function of the normal breast and of infant suckling are necessary for assessment; knowing what is normal must precede recognizing the abnormal and recommending actions designed to support an optimal breastfeeding experience. Enabling the natural physiological mechanisms to function optimally is more likely to lead to an uncomplicated breastfeeding experience; conversely, interference with these mechanisms can result in difficulty with breastfeeding for mother and infant. For example, restrictive policies on breastfeeding of preterm babies are commonly based on bottle-feeding studies, not on knowledge about the early development of infants' capacity for suckling at the breast (Chen et al., 2000; Nyqvist, 2013; Nyqvist et al., 1999).

At the same time, anatomy and physiology are the building blocks in a larger picture of the breastfeeding and lactation experience. Most women are physiologically equipped to produce sufficient milk for their infant or infants—yet the most commonly cited problem in breastfeeding worldwide is the mother's perception that she has insufficient milk (Hill & Humenick, 1989). Social and cultural influences play a major role in the mother's perceptions of her ability to nourish her infant from her breasts. Succeeding chapters build on the anatomy and physiology of lactation and address the clinical implications as well as its social and cultural aspects.

KEY CONCEPTS

- Early milk removal helps calibrate milk production. Initiating breastfeeding in the first 2 hours after birth increases milk production, as does increasing the number of early feedings on day 2 and 3. If milk is not removed by day 3 postpartum, mammary involution begins.
- Three factors are necessary for lactation: (1) oxytocin release from the posterior pituitary; (2) removal of breastmilk by the infant, hand, or pump; and (3) prolactin release from the anterior pituitary, which stimulates lactogenesis and initiates milk secretion.
- Lactogenesis (secretory activation) can be delayed in cases of extensive maternal–infant separation, late initiation of milk removal, and maternal metabolic derangements.

- The short-term rate of milk synthesis is considerably higher when most of the available milk has been removed from the breast. Frequent breast emptying stimulates the development of more lactocytes (milk-making cells) and up-regulates hormone receptors on existing cells.

- Frequency of breastfeedings varies widely; however, exclusively breastfed term infants (living in a country where breastfeeding is the norm) feed a median of 8 times per day (6 times during the day, and twice during the night).

- Mammary ducts do not widen into sinuses behind the nipple as previously thought, but the ducts are distensible and expand as they fill with milk during the milk-ejection process.

- Suspensory ligaments of the breast are called Cooper's ligaments.

- Each breast of an adult woman weighs, on average 150 to 200 g. The breast doubles in weight to 400 to 500 g (approximately 1 pound) during lactation.

- Nerves that supply the breast are from the second to the sixth intercostal nerves. The fourth intercostal nerve, which penetrates the left breast at the 4–5 o'clock position and the right breast at the 7–8 o'clock position, supplies the greatest amount of sensation to the nipple and areola.

- If the lowermost nerve branch of the fourth intercostal nerve is severed, the mother loses sensation to the nipple and areola.

- Breast asymmetry is common; the left breast is often larger than the right.

- Marked asymmetry and breast hypoplasia may indicate problems with milk production.

- Areola and nipple color vary according to complexion: lighter (pink to tan) in fairer women and darker in women with more melanin (brown to black).

- Supernumerary nipples (accessory nipple), which occur in 1% to 5% of the population, form at any point along the milk line from the axilla to the groin.

- Poor nipple protractility occurs in 10% to 35% of women during their first pregnancy.

- Nipple inversion is found in about 3% of women, and it is bilateral in 87% of these women. Only 4% of inverted nipples are tethered.

- Prolactin influences nipple growth; increase in breast volume attributable to areolar growth is related to serum placental lactogen; the ductal system proliferates and differentiates under the influence of estrogen; and progesterone promotes enlargement of the lobes, lobules, and alveoli.

- Lactogenesis, stage I (secretory differentiation) occurs in mid- to late pregnancy when breast size increases as epithelial cells of the alveoli differentiate into secretory cells for milk production.

- Lactogenesis II (secretory activation, days 2 to 8 postpartum) is the onset of copious milk secretion after birth when milk volume increases rapidly and then abruptly levels off.

- Before lactogenesis II, large gaps exist between the alveolar epithelial cells. These gaps close as the activating lactocytes grow and contact each other through adhesion structures called desmosomes, which close the intercellular spaces. These tight junctions allow better control of the ion content of mature milk. Once the tight junctions form, transfer of most drugs into milk decreases. During mastitis, gap junctions reopen as lactocytes shrink and milk production in the affected breast declines.

- Maternal conditions that can delay or impair lactogenesis include primiparity, cesarean birth, type 1 diabetes, labor analgesia and fluid balance, obesity, polycystic ovary syndrome, gestational ovarian theca lutein cysts, placental retention, Sheehan's syndrome, severe stress, isolated prolactin (PRL) deficiency, and breast surgery.

- The developmental cycle of the mammary gland includes four phases: (1) mammogenesis, (2) lactogenesis, (3) galactopoiesis, and (4) involution.

- After delivery, progesterone levels drop and prolactin levels rise; both of these hormones act synergistically with cortisol, thyroid-stimulating hormone, insulin, and oxytocin to establish and maintain lactation.

- Following lactogenesis II (secretory activation), milk production shifts from endocrine to autocrine control. When the nipple is stimulated and milk removed from the breast, the hypothalamus inhibits dopamine, which in turn stimulates the release of prolactin, which then catalyzes milk production.

- The basic unit of the breast is the alveolus, which is surrounded by a contractile unit of myoepithelial cells responsible for ejecting milk into the ductules. Each ductule merges into a larger duct. The ducts are lined with epithelium and highly vascular connective tissue.

- Milk is secreted into the alveolar lumina, where it is stored until the posterior pituitary hormone oxytocin causes the milk-ejection reflex or letdown, a contraction of the myoepithelial cells surrounding the alveoli.

- Oxytocin plays a major role in lactation. Blood levels of this hormone rise within 1 minute of suckling, remain elevated during the feeding, and return to baseline levels within 6 minutes. Oxytocin in the blood also stimulates prolactin release from the pituitary.

- Oxytocin contracts the mother's uterus, which helps to control postpartum bleeding and aids in uterine involution.

- The supply–demand response is a feedback control mechanism that regulates the production of milk to match the intake of the infant.

- Galactorrhea is the unexpected spontaneous secretion of milk from the breast. It is often due to excessive prolactin levels from a pituitary adenoma or use of dopamine-suppressing medications.

- Milk production is controlled by a shifting balance of endocrine and autocrine factors throughout the course of lactation.

- If the frenulum—a fold of mucous membrane midline on the undersurface of the baby's tongue—is too short or is too far forward, it can interfere with an infant's ability to suckle.

- The sucking reflex is present at 24 weeks' gestation. By 28 weeks, preterm babies can coordinate the suck/swallow/breathe cycle; by 32 weeks, they can suck in repeated bursts.

- Forcing a crying baby to the breast evokes a defensive response (tongue to palate) that inhibits latch and sucking and disturbs the rooting-tongue reflex system.

- Nutritive sucking occurs during rapid milk flow and usually proceeds at a rate of one suck per second; non-nutritive sucking is a faster sucking rate that occurs when milk flow is slow or absent.

- Breastfeeding infants feed more times per day and maintain a higher level of oxygen pressure (tcPO2) and skin temperature compared with bottle-fed infants.

- Suck training, an emerging area of lactation practice, involves oral stimulation and manipulation to treat feeding problems in infants.

REFERENCES

Alexander JM, Grant AM, Campbell MJ. Randomized controlled trial of breast shells and Hoffman's exercises for inverted and non-protractile nipples. *Br Med J*. 1992;304:1030–1032.

Altemus J, Deuster PA, Galliven E, et al. Suppression hypothalamic–pituitary–adrenal axis responses to stress in lactating women. *J Clin Endocr Metab*. 1996;80:2954–2959.

Amiel-Tison C. Neurological evaluation of the maturity of newborn infant. *Arch Dis Child*. 1967;43:89.

Anderson AM. Disruption of lactogenesis by retained placental fragments. *J Hum Lact*. 2001;17:142–144.

Anderson GC, McBride MR, Dahm J, et al. Development of sucking in term infants from birth to four hours post-birth. *Res Nurs Health*. 1982;5:21–27.

Ardran GM, Kemp MB, Lind J. A cineradiographic study of breast feeding. *Br J Radiol*. 1958;31:156–162.

Arthur PG, Jones TJ, Spruce J, Hartmann PE. Measuring short-term rates of milk synthesis in breast-feeding mothers. *Q J Exp Physiol*. 1989;74:419–428.

Asztalos EV, Campbell-Yeo M, daSilva OP, et al. Enhancing breast milk production with Domperidone in mothers of preterm neonates (EMPOWER trial). *BMC Pregnancy Childbirth*. 2012;12:87. doi: 10.1186/1471-2393-12-87.

Barlow SM, Estep M. Central pattern generation and the motor infrastructure for suck, respiration, and speech. *J Commun Disord*. 2006;39:366–380.

Baron JA, Bulbrook RD, Wang DY, Kwa HG. Cigarette smoking and prolactin in women. *Br Med J.* 1986;293:482.

Battin D, Marrs RP, Fleiss PM, Mishell DR Jr. Effect of suckling on serum prolactin, luteinizing hormone, follicle-stimulating hormone, and estradiol during prolonged lactation. *Obstet Gynecol.* 1985;65:785–788.

Berman MA, Davis GD. Lactation from axillary breast tissue in the absence of a supernumerary nipple: a case report. *J Reprod Med.* 1994;39:657–659.

Betzold CM, Hoover KL, Snyder CL. Delayed lactogenesis II: a comparison of four cases. *J Midwifery Womens Health.* 2004;49:132–137.

Blaikeley J, Clarke S, Mackeith R, Ogden KM. Breastfeeding: factors affecting success. *J Obstet Gynaecol Br Emp.* 1953;60:657–669.

Blass EM. Behavioral and physiological consequences of suckling in rat and human newborns. *Acta Paediatr Suppl.* 1994;397:71–76.

Bohnet HG, Kato K. Prolactin secretion during pregnancy and puerperium: response to metoclopramide and interactions with placental hormones. *Obstet Gynecol.* 1985;65:789–792.

Bronwen KN, Huckabee ML, Jones RD, Frampton CM. The first year of human life: coordinating respiration and nutritive swallowing. *Dysphagia.* 2007;23:37–43.

Bu'Lock F, Woolridge MW, Baum JD. Development of coordination of sucking, swallowing and breathing: ultrasound study of term and preterm infants. *Dev Med Child Neurol.* 1990;32:669–778.

Burton P, Deng J, McDonald D, Fewtrell MS. Real-time 3D ultrasound imaging of infant tongue movements during breast-feeding. *Early Hum Dev.* 2013;89:635–641. doi: 10.1016/j.earlhumdev.2013.04.009.

Butte NF, Wills C, Jean CA, et al. Feeding patterns of exclusively breast-fed infants during the first four months of life. *Early Hum Dev.* 1985;12:291–300.

Bystrova K, Ivanova V, Edhborg M, et al. Early contact versus separation: effects on mother-infant interaction one year later. *Birth.* 2009;36:97–109.

Cable TA, Rothenberger LA. Breast-feeding behavioral patterns among La Leche League mothers: a descriptive survey. *Pediatrics.* 1984;73:830.

Chantry CJ, Nommsen-Rivers LA, Peerson JM, et al. Excess weight loss in first-born breastfed newborns relates to maternal intrapartum fluid balance. *Peds.* 2011;127:171–179.

Chao S. The effect of lactation on ovulation and fertility. *Clin Perinatol.* 1987;14:39–49.

Chapman DJ, Perez-Escamilla R. Identification of risk factors for delayed onset of lactation. *J Am Diet Assoc.*1999;99:450–455.

Chapman DJ, Perez-Escamilla R. Maternal perception of the onset of lactation is a valid, public health indicator of lactogenesis stage II. *J of Nutr.* 2000;130:2972–2980.

Chen CH, Wang TM, Chang HM, Chi CS. The effect of breast- and bottle-feeding on oxygen saturation and body temperature in preterm infants. *J Hum Lact.* 2000;16:21–27.

Chen DC, Nommsen-Rivers L, Dewey KG, Lonnerdal B. Stress during labor and delivery and early lactation performance. *Am J Clin Nutr.* 1998;68:335–344.

Clemente CD. *Anatomy: a regional atlas of the human body.* Philadelphia, PA: Lea & Febiger; 1978.

Cooper AP. *Anatomy of the breast.* London: Longman, Orme, Green, Browne and Longmans; 1840.

Courtiss EH, Goldwyn RM. Breast sensation before and after plastic surgery. *Plast Reconstr Surg.* 1976;58:1–12.

Cox DB, Owens RA, Hartmann PE. Blood and milk prolactin and the rate of milk synthesis in women. *Exp Physiol.* 1996;81:1007–1020.

Cregan M, Hartmann PE. Computerized breast measurement from conception to weaning: clinical implications. *J Hum Lact.* 1999;15:89–95.

Cregan MD, Mitoulas LR, Hartmann PE. Milk prolactin, feed volume, and duration between feeds in women breast-feeding their full-term infants over a 24-hour period. *Exp Physiol.* 2002;87:207–214.

Daly SEJ, Hartmann PE. Infant demand and milk supply. Part 1: infant demand and milk production in lactating women. *J Hum Lact.* 1995;11:21–23.

Dawood MY, Khan-Dawood FS, Wahi RS, Fuchs F. Oxytocin release and plasma anterior pituitary and gonadal hormones in women during lactation. *J Clin Endocrinol Metab.* 1981;52:678–683.

Dawson EK. A histological study of the normal mamma in relation to tumour growth: 1. Early development to maturity. *Edinb Med J.* 1934;41:653–682.

de Carvalho M, Robertson S, Merkatz R, Klaus M. Milk intake and frequency of feeding in breast-fed infants. *Early Hum Dev.* 1982;7:155–163.

de Carvalho M, Robertson S, Friedman A, Klaus M. Effect of frequent breast-feeding on early milk production and infant weight gain. *Pediatrics.*1983;72:307–311.

de Coopman J. Breastfeeding after pituitary resection: support for a theory of autocrine control of milk supply? *J Hum Lact.* 1993;9:35–40.

Dewey KG, Nommsen-Rivers LA, Heinig J, Cohen RJ. Risk factors for suboptimal infant breastfeeding behavior, delayed onset of lactation, and excess neonatal weight loss. *Peds.* 2003;112:607–619.

Dökmetaş HS, Kilicli F, Korkmaz S, Yonem O. Characteristic features of 20 patients with Sheehan's syndrome. *Gynecol Endocrinol.* 2006 May;22(5):279–283.

Donovan TJ, Buchanan K. Medications for increasing milk supply in mothers expressing breastmilk for their preterm hospitalised infants. *Cochrane Database Syst Rev.* 2012 Mar 14;3:CD005544. doi: 10.1002/14651858.CD005544.pub2.

Doucet S, Soussignan R, Sagot P, Schaal B. An overlooked aspect of the human breast: areolar glands in relation with breastfeeding pattern, neonatal weight gain, and the dynamics of lactation. *Early Hum Dev.* 2012

Feb;88(2):119–28. doi: 10.1016/j.earlhumdev
.2011.07.020.

Drewett RF, Woolridge M. Sucking patterns of human babies on the breast. *Early Hum Dev*. 1979;315:315–321.

Elad D, Kozlovsky P, Blum O, et al., Biomechanics of milk extraction during breastfeeding. *PNAS*, 111(14): 5230–5235, 2014 doi:10.1073/pnas.1319798111.

Farina MA, Newby BG, Alani HM. Innervation to the nipple–areola complex. *Plast Reconstr Surg*. 1980;66: 497–501.

Frantz A, Kleinberg DL, Noel G. Studies on prolactin in man. *Recent Prog Horm Res*. 1972;28:527–534.

Friesen HG, Cowden EA. Lactation and galactorrhea. In: DeGroot LJ, ed. *Endocrinology in pregnancy*. Philadelphia, PA: Saunders; 1989:2074–2086.

Geddes DT. Inside the lactating breast: the latest anatomy research. *J Midwifery Women's Health*. 2007;52:556–563.

Geddes DT, Kent JC, Mitoulas LB, et al. Tongue movement and intra-oral vacuum in breastfed infants. *Early Hum Dev*. 2008;84(7):471–477.

Goldfield EC, Richardson MJ, Lee KG, Margetts S. Coordination of sucking, swallowing, and breathing and oxygen saturation during early infant breast-feeding and bottle-feeding. *Ped Res*. 2006;60:450–455.

Gomes CF, Trezza EM, Murade EC, Padovani CR. Surface electromyography of facial muscles during natural and artificial feeding of infant. *J Pediatr*. 2006;82:103–109.

Grajeda R, Perez-Escamilla R. Stress during labor and delivery is associated with delayed onset of lactation among urban Guatemalan women. *J Nutr*. 2002;132: 3055–3060.

Gray L, Miller LW, Philipp BL, Blass EM. Breastfeeding is analgesic in healthy newborns. *Pediatrics*. 2002;109: 590–593.

Groer M. Differences between exclusive breastfeeding, formula-feeders and controls: a study of stress, mood, and endocrine variables. *Biol Res Nurs*. 2005a;7:106.

Groer M. Neuroendocrine and immune relationships in postpartum fatigue. *Am J Matern Child Nurs*. 2005b;30:133–138.

Groer M, Davis MW. Postpartum stress: current concepts and the possible protective role of breastfeeding. *JOGN Nursing*. 2002;31:411–417.

Grossl NA. Supernumerary tissue: historical perspectives and clinical features. *South Med J*. 2000;93:29–32.

Gusterson BA, Stein T. Human breast development. *Semin Cell Dev Biol*. 2012 Jul;23(5):567–73. doi: 10.1016/ j.semcdb.2012.03.013. Epub 2012 Mar 16.

Hale TW. *Medications and mother's milk: a Manual of lactational pharmacology*, 14th ed. Amarillo, TX: Hale Publishing; 2010.

Hammerman C, Kaplan M. Oxygen saturation during and after feeding in healthy term infants. *Biol Neonate*. 1995;67:94–99.

Hartmann P, Cregan M. Lactogenesis and the effects of insulin-dependent diabetes mellitus and prematurity. *J Nutr*. 2001;131:3016S–20S.

Hartmann PE, Sherriff JL, Kent JC. Maternal nutrition and milk synthesis. *Proc Nutr Soc*. 1995;54:379–389.

Herbst JJ. Development of suck and swallowing. In: Lebenthal E, ed. *Textbook of gastroenterology and nutrition in infancy*, Vol. 1. New York, NY: Plenum; 1981: 97–107.

Hildebrandt HM. Maternal perception of lactogenesis time: a clinical report. *J Hum Lact*. 1999;15:317–323.

Hill PD, Chatterton RT, Aldag AC. Serum prolactin in breastfeeding: state of the science. *Biol Res Nurs*. 1999;1:65–75.

Hill PD, Humenick SS. Insufficient milk supply. *Image*. 1989;21:145–148.

Hinds LA, Tyndale-Biscoe CH. Prolactin in the marsupial *Macropus engenii* during the estrous cycle, pregnancy, and lactation. *Biol Reprod*. 1982;26:391–398.

Hoover K, Barbalinardo L, Pia Platia M. Delayed lactogenesis 2 secondary to gestational ovarian theca lutein cysts in two normal singleton pregnancies. *J Hum Lact*. 2002;18:264–268.

Horn HW, Scott JM. IUD insertion and galactorrhea. *Fertil Steril*. 1969;20:400–404.

Hornell A, Aarts C, Kylberg E, et al. Breastfeeding patterns in exclusively breastfed infants: a longitudinal prospective study in Uppsala, Sweden. *Acta Paediatr*. 1999;88: 203–211.

Howie PW, McNeilly AS, Houston MJ, et al. Effect of supplementary food on suckling patterns and ovarian activity during lactation. *Br Med J*. 1981;283:757–759.

Huggins K, Petok E, Mireles O. Markers of lactation insufficiency: a study of 34 mothers. In: Auerbach K, ed. *Current issues in clinical lactation*. Sudbury, MA: Jones and Bartlett; 2000:25–35.

Humenick SS, Hill PD, Thompson J, Hart AM. Breast-milk sodium as a predictor of breastfeeding patterns. *Can J Nurs Res*. 1998;30:67–81.

Hurst N. Lactation after augmentation mammoplasty. *Obstet Gynecol*. 1996;87:30–34.

Hytten FE. Clinical and chemical studies in lactation: IX. Breastfeeding in hospital. *Br Med J*. 1954;18: 1447–1452.

Hytten FE, Baird D. The development of the nipple in pregnancy. *Lancet*. June 7, 1958;1:1201–1204.

Iwama S, Welt CK, Romero CJ, et al. Isolated prolactin deficiency associated with serum autoantibodies against prolactin-secreting cells. *J Clin Endocrinol Metab*. 2013 Oct;98(10):3920-5. doi: 10.1210/jc.2013–2411.

Jacobs LA, Dickinson JE, Hart PD, et al. Normal nipple position in term infants measured on breastfeeding ultrasound. *J Hum Lact*. 2007;23:52–59.

James RJA, Irons DW, Holmes C, et al. Thirst induced by a suckling episode during breast feeding and its relation with plasma vasopressin, oxytocin and osmoregulation. *Clin Endocrinol*. 1995;43:277–282.

Johnstone JM, Amico JA. A prospective longitudinal study of the release of oxytocin and prolactin in response to infant suckling in long-term lactation. *J Clin Endocrinol Metab*. 1986;62:653.

Kent JC, Mitoulas LR, Cregan MD, et al. Volume and frequency of breastfeeding and fat content of breast milk throughout the day. *Pediatrics*. 2005;117: e387–e395.

Kopans DB. *Breast imaging*. Philadelphia, PA: Lippincott; 1989:20.

Kulski JK, Hartmann PE. Changes in human milk composition during the initiation of lactation. *Aust J Exp Biol Med Sci*. 1981;59:101–114.

La Leche League International. *The womanly art of breastfeeding*, 6th ed. Schaumberg, IL: La Leche League; 1997.

Lau C, Smith EO. Interventions to improve the oral feeding performance of preterm infants. *Acta Paediatr*. 2012; 101:e269–e274.

Leake R, Waters CB, Rubin RT, et al. Oxytocin and prolactin responses in long-term breast-feeding. *Obstet Gynecol*. 1983;62:565–568.

Lincoln DW, Paisley AC. Neuroendocrine control of milk ejection. *J Reprod Fertil*. 1982;65:571–586.

Love S. *Dr. Susan Love's breast book*. Boston, MA: Addison-Wesley; 1990:34.

MacMullen NJ, Kulski LA. Factors related to suckling ability in healthy newborns. *JOGN Nursing*. 2000;29: 390–396.

MacPherson EE, Montagna W. The mammary glands of rhesus monkeys. *J Invest Derm*. 1974;63:17–18.

Madden JD, Boyar RM, MacDonald PC, Porter JC. Analysis of secretory patterns of prolactin and gonadotropins during twenty-four hours in a lactating woman before and after resumption of menses. *Am J Obstet Gynecol*. 1978;132:436–441.

Marasco L, Marmet C, Shell E. Polycystic ovary syndrome: a connection to insufficient milk supply? *J Hum Lact*. 2000;16:143–148.

Marmet C, Shell E. Training neonates to suck correctly. *MCN*. 1984;9:401–407.

Marmet C, Shell E. Therapeutic positioning for breastfeeding. In: Genna CW, ed. *Supporting sucking skills in breastfeeding infants*. Sudbury, MA: Jones and Bartlett; 2013: 305–325.

Marshall WM, Cumming DC, Fitzsimmons GW. Hot flushes during breast feeding? *Fertil Steril*. 1992;57:1349–1350.

Mathew OP. Regulation of breathing patterns during feeding. In: Mathew OP, Sant Ambrogio G, eds. *Respiratory function of the upper airway*. New York, NY: Marcel Dekker; 1988:535–560.

McBride MC, Danner SC. Sucking disorders in neurologically impaired infants: assessment and facilitation of breast-feeding. *Clin Perinatol*. 1987;14:109–130.

Measel CP, Anderson GC. Nonnutritive suckling during tube feedings: effect on clinical course in premature infants. *JOGN Nursing*. 1979;8:265–272.

Meier P, Anderson GC. Responses of small preterm infants to bottle- and breast-feeding. *MCN*. 1987;12: 97–105.

Meier P, Pugh EJ. Breastfeeding behavior in small preterm infants. *MCN*. 1985;10:396–401.

Mennella JA, Beauchamp GK. Beer, breastfeeding, and folklore. *Dev Psychobiol*. 1993;26:459–466.

Miller AJ. Deglutition. *Physiol Rev*. 1982;62:129–183.

Mizuno K, Ueda A, Takeuchi T. Effects of different fluids on the relationship between swallowing and breathing during nutritive sucking in neonates. *Bio Neonate*. 2002;81:45–50.

Montagna W, MacPherson EE. Some neglected aspects of the anatomy of the breasts. *J Invest Derm*. 1974;63:10–16.

Montagu A. Breastfeeding and its relation to morphological, behavioral, and psychocultural development. In: Rapheal D, ed. *Breastfeeding and food policy in a hungry world*. New York, NY: Academic; 1979:189–193.

Morton JA. The clinical usefulness of breast milk sodium in the assessment of lactogenesis. *Pediatrics*. 1994;93: 802–806.

Neifert M, DeMarzo S, Seacat J, et al. The influence of breast surgery, breast appearance, and pregnancy-induced breast changes on lactation sufficiency as measured by infant weight gain. *Birth*. 1990 Mar;17(1):31–38.

Neifert MR, McDonough SL, Neville MC. Failure of lactogenesis associated with placental retention. *Am J Obstet Gynecol*. 1981;140:477–478.

Neifert MR, Seacat JM, Jobe WE. Lactation failure due to insufficient glandular development of the breast. *Pediatrics*. 1985 Nov;76(5):823–828.

Neubauer SH, Ferris AM, Chase CG, et al. Delayed lactogenesis in women with insulin-dependent diabetes mellitus. *Am J Clin Nutr*. 1993;58:54–60.

Neville, MC. Anatomy and physiology of lactation. In: Schanler RJ, ed. Breastfeeding 2001, Part 1: The evidence for breastfeeding. *Pediatr Clin North Am*. 2001;48:13–34.

Neville MC, Berga SE. Cellular and molecular aspects of the hormonal control of mammary function. In: Neville MC, Neifert MR, eds. *Lactation: physiology, nutrition, and breast-feeding*. New York, NY: Plenum; 1983: 141–177.

Nissen E, Uvnäs-Moberg K, Svensson K, et al. Different patterns of oxytocin, prolactin but not cortisol release during breast-feeding in women delivered by cesarean section or by the vaginal route. *Early Hum Dev*. 1996; 45:103–108.

Noel GL, Suh HK, Frantz AG. Prolactin release during nursing and breast stimulation in postpartum and non-postpartum subjects. *J Clin Endocrinol Metab*. 1974;38: 413–423.

Nommsen-Rivers LA, Chantry CJ, Peerson JM, et al. Delayed onset of lactogenesis among first-time mothers is related to maternal obesity and factors associated with ineffective breastfeeding. *Am J Clin Nutr*. 2010;92: 574–584.

Notestine GE. The importance of the identification of ankyloglossia (short lingual frenulum) as a cause of breastfeeding problems. *J Hum Lact*. 1990;6:113–115.

Nyqvist KH. Lack of knowledge persists about early breast-feeding competence in preterm infants. *J Hum Lact.* 2013;29:296–299.

Nyqvist K, Sjoden PO, Ewald U. The development of preterm infants' breastfeeding behavior. *Early Hum Dev.* 1999;55:247–264.

Oliveira AM, Cunha CC, Phenha-Silva N, et al. Interference of the blood glucose control in the transition between phases I and II of lactogenesis in patients with type 1 diabetes mellitus. *Braz Arch of Endocrinology Metabolism.* 2008;52:473–481.

Oxford English dictionary, Vol. 10. Oxford, England: Clarendon Press, 1961.

Palmer B. The influence of breastfeeding on the development of the oral cavity: a commentary. *J Hum Lact.* 1998;14:93–99.

Park HS, Yoon CH, Kim HJ. The prevalence of congenital inverted nipple. *Aesthetic Plast Surg.* 1999;23:1446.

Prentice A, Addey CVP, Wilde CJ. Evidence for local feedback control of human milk secretion. *Biochem Soc Trans.* 1989;17:489–492.

Prieto CR, Cardenas H, Salvatierra AM, et al. Sucking pressure and its relationship to milk transfer during breastfeeding in humans. *J Reprod Fertil.* 1996;108:69–74.

Quandt SA. Patterns of variation in breast-feeding behaviors. *Soc Sci Med.* 1986;23:445–453.

Ramsay DT, Kent JC, Hartmann RA, Hartmann PE. Anatomy of the lactating human breast redefined with ultrasound imaging. *J Anat.* 2005;206:525–534.

Ramsay DT, Mitoulas LR, Kent JC, et al. The use of ultrasound to characterize milk ejection in women using an electric breast pump. *J Hum Lact.* 2005;21:421–428.

Rasmussen KM, Hilson JA, Kjolhede CL. Obesity may impair lactogenesis 2. *J Nutr.* 2001;131:3009S–3011S.

Rasmussen KM, Kjolhede CL. Prepregnant overweight and obesity diminish the prolactin response to suckling in the first week postpartum. *Peds.* 2004;113:465–471.

Riordan J, Gross A, Angeron J, et al. The effect of labor pain relief on neonatal suckling and breastfeeding duration. *J Hum Lact.* 2000;16:7–12.

Rodenstein DO, Perlmutter N, Stanescu DC. Infants are not obligatory nose breathers. *Am Rev Respir Dis.* 1985;131:343–347.

Russo J, Russo IH. Development of the human mammary gland. In: Neville MD, Daniel CW, eds. *The mammary gland: development, regulation, and function.* New York, NY: Plenum; 1987:67–93.

Russo J, Russo IH. Development of the human breast. *Maturitas.* 2004 Sep 24;49(1):2–15.

Sakalidis VS, Williams TM, Hepworth AR, et al. A comparison of early sucking dynamics during breastfeeding after cesarean section and vaginal birth. *Breastfeed Med.* 2013;8:79–85.

Salazar H, Tobon H. Morphologic changes of the mammary gland during development, pregnancy, and lactation.

In: Josimovich J, ed. *Lactogenic hormones, fetal nutrition and lactation.* New York, NY: Academic Press; 1974:1–18.

Schaal B, Doucet S, Sagot P, et al. Human breast areolae as scent organs: morphological data and possible involvement in maternal–neonatal coadaptation. *Dev Psychobiol.* 2006;48(2):100–110.

Sernia C, Tyndale-Biscoe CH. Prolactin receptors in the mammary gland, corpus luteum and other tissues of the Tammar wallaby, *Macropus engenii. J Endocrinol.* 1979; 26:391–398.

Sert M, Tetiker T, Kirim S, Kocak M. Clinical report of 28 patients with Sheehan's syndrome. *Endocr J.* 2003;50(3):297–301.

Smith DM. Montgomery's areolar tubercle: a light microscopic study. *Arch Pathol Lab Med.* 1982;106:60–63.

Smith L, Kroeger M. *The impact of birthing practices on breast-feeding,* 2nd edition. Sudbury MA: Jones & Bartlett; 2010.

Smith WL, Erenberg A, Nowak A, Franken EA Jr. Physiology of sucking in the normal term infant using real-time ultrasound. *Radiology.* 1985;156:379–381.

Snyder JB. Bubble palate and failure-to-thrive: a case report. *J Hum Lact.* 1997;13:139–143.

Sozmen M. Effects of early suckling of cesarean-born babies on lactation. *Biol Neonate.* 1992;62:67–68.

Speroff L, Glass RH, Kase NG. *Clinical gynecology, endocrinology and infertility,* 4th ed. Baltimore, MD: Williams & Wilkins; 1989:283.

Stallings JF, Worthman CM, Panter-Brick C, Coates RJ. Prolactin response to suckling and maintenance of postpartum amenorrhea among intensively breastfeeding Nepali women. *Endocrinol Res.* 1996;22:1–28.

Sternlicht MD, Kouros-Mehr H, Lu P, Werb Z. Hormonal and local control of mammary branching morphogenesis. *Differentiation.* 2006;74:365–381.

Tay CCK, Glasier AF, McNeil AS. Twenty-four hour patterns of prolactin secretion during lactation and the relationship to suckling and the resumption of fertility in breast-feeding women. *Hum Reprod.* 1996;11:950–955.

Telles NC, ed. *Atlas of breast ultrasound.* Philadelphia, PA: Department of Radiology and Department of Pathology, Thomas Jefferson University Medical College and Hospital; 1980:121.

Thibaudeau S, Sinno H, Williams B. The effects of breast reduction on successful breastfeeding: a systematic review. *Journal of Plastic, Reconstructive & Aesthetic Surgery.* 2010;63:1688–1693e.

Tyson JE, Hwang P, Guyda H, Friesen HG. Studies of prolactin in human pregnancy. *Am J Obstet Gynecol.* 1972;113:14–20.

Ueda T, Yokoyama Y, Irahara M, et al. Influence of psychological stress on suckling-induced pulsatile oxytocin release. *Obstet Gynecol.* 1994;84:259–262.

Uvnas-Moberg K. Oxytocin linked antistress effects: the relaxation and growth response. *Acta Physiol Scand Supp.* 1997;640:38–42.

Vanky E, Isaksen H, Moen MH, Carlsen SM. Breastfeeding in polycystic ovary syndrome. *Acta Obstet Gynecol Scand.* 2008;87:531–535. doi: 10.1080/00016340802007676.

Vorherr H. Development of the female breast. In: Vorherr H, ed. *The breast.* New York, NY: Academic; 1974: 1–18.

Waller H. The early failure of breastfeeding. *Arch Dis Child.* 1946;21:1–12.

Watson CJ. Involution: apoptosis and tissue remodeling that convert the mammary gland from milk factory to quiescent organ. *Breast Cancer Res.* 2006;8(2):203.

Weber F, Woolridge MW, Baum JD. An ultrasonographic study of the organization of sucking and swallowing by newborn infants. *Dev Med Child Neurol.* 1986;28: 19–24.

West CP. Hormonal profiles in lactating and non-lactating women immediately after delivery and their relationship to breast engorgement. *Am J Obstet Gynecol.* 1979; 86:501–506.

Widstrom AM, Lilja G, Aaltomaa-Michalias P, et al. Newborn behaviour to locate the breast when skin-to-skin: a possible method for enabling early self-regulation. *Acta Paediatr.* 2011;100:79–85.

Widstrom AM, Ransjö-Arvidson AB, Christensson K, et al. Gastric suction in healthy newborn infants: effects on circulation and developing feeding behaviour. *Acta Paediatr Scand.* 1987;76:566–572.

Widstrom AM, Thingstrom-Paulsson J. The position of the tongue during rooting reflexes elicited in newborn infants before the first suckle. *Acta Paediatr.* 1993;82: 281–283.

Wilson-Clay B, Hoover K. *The breastfeeding atlas,* 5th ed. Manchaca, TX: LactNews Press; 2013.

Wolf LS, Glass RP. *Feeding and swallowing disorders in infancy: assessment and management.* San Antonio, TX: Therapy Skill Builders; 1992:9–10, 133–137.

Wolff PH. The serial organization of sucking in the young infant. *Pediatrics.* 1968;42:943–956.

Woolridge MW. The "anatomy" of infant sucking. *Midwifery.* 1986;2:164–171.

Woolridge M. The mechanisms of breastfeeding revised—new insights into how babies feed provided by fresh ultrasound studies of breastfeeding. *Evidence-Based Child Health,* 2011;6(suppl 1):46–46.

Yokoyama Y, Ueda T, Irahara M, Aono T. Releases of oxytocin and prolactin during breast massage and suckling in puerperal women. *Eur J Obstet Gynecol Reprod Biol.* 1994;53:17–20.

Yuen BH. Prolactin in human milk: the influence of nursing and duration of postpartum lactation. *Am J Obstet Gynecol.* 1988;158:583–586.

Ziemer M. Nipple skin changes and pain during the first week of lactation. *JOGN Nursing.* 1993;22:247–256.

Zuppa AA, Tornesello A, Papacci P, et al. Relationship between maternal parity, basal prolactin levels and neonatal breast milk intake. *Biol Neonate.* 1988;53:144–147.

Appendix 3-A

Suck Training for Breastfeeding

Suck training, or digital sucking exercises, is an emerging area of lactation practice for treating feeding problems related to immature and/or abnormal suckling in infants. Sucking problems may be the result of a lack of normal development such as in low-birth-weight infants and/or an early sign of neurologic impairment. Suck training can be as simple as placing one's finger in the neonate's mouth to orally stimulate a baby who is "slow" to latch on to the breast—a practice trial whereby the infant learns how to grasp the mother's nipple. Parents unintentionally perform suck training when they place their "pinky" finger in their baby's mouth while holding him in their crossed arms.

We also might consider finger-feeding, described elsewhere in this text, to be a form of suck training. For example, until the baby matures sufficiently, mothers of preterm infants might first breastfeed and then finger-feed the remainder of the breastmilk or formula. Essentially, suck training is a method of oral stimulation and manipulation to teach the baby how to effectively suckle a bottle nipple or a breast; it is an umbrella term for any therapy used to correct an infant suckling problem.

Most problems can be avoided or corrected by facilitating an effective latch onto the breast. However, for a multitude of reasons described elsewhere in this text, some babies have suckling problems even when the baby has a good latch (Marmet & Shell, 1984).

Practitioners in this area usually are speech and language therapists, occupational therapists, or other specialists with a background in neurodevelopmental training (NDT) who understand the anatomy and physiology of the breast and the infant's oral structures. These specialists were trained to help bottle-feed babies; however, a few have subspecialized in breastfeeding sucking problems. If specialists are not available to assist breastfeeding mothers, lactation consultants can fill this role, educating themselves to do so by attending continuing education courses, through self-study, and in clinical practice.

A form of suck training is used in the neonatal intensive care unit (NICU) to improve suckling ability of low-birth-weight babies. For example, when introducing the first oral feedings to a low-birth-weight baby, the nurse or lactation consultant places a finger in the baby's mouth and slowly introduces one or two drips of expressed breastmilk or formula to see how the baby reacts, to observe the baby's ability to swallow, and to assess for tongue thrusting and gagging.

The pressure to discharge the baby (including the low-birth-weight baby) early because of reimbursement issues and insurance requirements has generated great interest in suck training. Suck training, if effective, hastens discharge to home, but there are very few studies that substantiate that when infants receive suck training, they are discharged earlier.

Research on suck training techniques to test their effectiveness is sparse and mostly limited to bottle-feeding, but findings do indicate that suck training is beneficial. Gaebler and Hanzlik (1996) demonstrated that preterm infants receiving perioral and intraoral stimulation just before bottle-feedings scored better on the standardized feeding assessment scale NOMAS (see the *Infant Assessment* chapter), had greater weight gain, and experienced fewer days of hospitalization. Fucile et al. (2002) reaffirmed that preterm infants who received oral stimulation were able to feed significantly earlier. Until studies on suck training of breastfed infants are done, this knowledge gap is being filled by clinical experience and opinion of experts.

Some practitioners find suck training techniques helpful; others think they are invasive and controlling and should never be used. The literature on the care of premature infants who required intubation documents that the irritation of the infant's oral cavity can cause the baby to avoid having anything further put into the mouth, including the breast. For those clinicians determined to forge ahead, we emphasize the need for gentleness and close following of infant signals: if the baby does not like your finger in its mouth, take it out!

Therapists use a variety of suck training techniques to improve feedings at the breast. There are probably as many techniques as there are babies with suckling problems. While no standard protocols for suck training for breastfeeding could be found at the time of this writing other than the Marmet and Shell Basic Suck-Training Technique, several techniques for treating specific sucking dysfunctions exist. Most have evolved from bottle-feeding protocols and then were adapted to breastfeeding. They usually involve oral stimulation in which the baby's mouth, tongue, gums, and palate are massaged and manipulated, as well as positioning and cheek and chin support.

Basic Suck-Training Technique

The most well-known suck training technique for breastfeeding infants was developed by Chele Marmet and Ellen Shell and published in *Maternal Child Nursing* in 1984. This article has become a classic treatise on suck training in the lactation field. Marmet and Shell developed the Basic Suck-Training Technique and the Alternate Suck-Training Technique as a result of working with numerous mothers and babies who came to their lactation clinic seeking help with getting their infants to effectively latch and suckle. The basic concept underlying their technique is that properly filling the baby's mouth with a finger will teach the baby the correct depth of latch on the breast. This action brings the baby's tongue forward so that the tongue tip covers the alveolar ridge and rests on the lower lip as it troughs and cups (Figure 3-19).

Technique

1. Stroke the baby's cheek toward the lips.
2. Brush the baby's lips until they relax.
3. Using the pad of the finger, massage the outside of the lower gums, the top of the lower gums, the outside of the upper gums, and the top of the upper gums.
4. Insert the finger into the baby's mouth nail down, pad up. Gently slide the finger to the juncture of the hard and soft palates (S spot). Women typically use their first finger and men their small "pinky" finger. Only light pressure is needed. Most babies love to suckle and will quickly draw the finger back to the S spot, the place to where the nipple usually extends.
5. Press down and forward with the fingernail portion of the finger as the baby suckles. Alternate rubbing the baby's hard palate with downward and forward pressure. Give praise and encouragement to the baby for the correct motion.

If the baby holds his posterior tongue in a humped position, periodically press down on the humped area with the nail side of the finger for a few seconds and then return to light pressure to the S spot. The tongue may relax after repeating this exercise several times.

Figure 3A-1 BASIC SUCK-TRAINING TECHNIQUE.

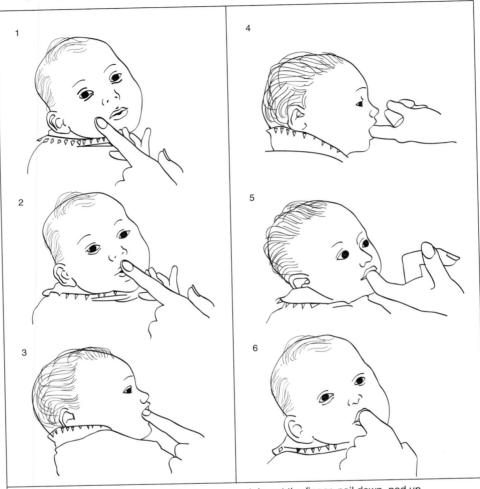

1. Stroke the baby's cheek toward the lips.

2. Brush the lips.

3. Massage the outside of the lower gums, the top of the lower gums, the outside of the upper gums, and the top of the upper gums.

4. Insert the finger, nail down, pad up.

5. Gently start rubbing the hard palate and progress to the soft palate to initiate sucking. As the baby sucks, gently press down and forward with the fingernail portion of the finger. Alternate rubbing the baby's hard palate with downward and forward pressure. Give verbal praise and encouragement to the baby for correct motion.

6. Alternate method. Insert finger, nail side toward the roof of the mouth. Position the pad of the finger at the place where the baby's tongue begins to slant downward toward the pharynx. Use the finger to pull the tongue forward. An eyedropper can be used instead of a finger or in addition to a finger when the baby needs a food reward for behavior modification to occur. The baby is rewarded with expressed breast milk or formula as the tongue is placed into the correct position with the dropper.

Source: Adapted from Marmet C, Shell E. Training neonates to suck correctly. *MCN*. 1984;9:401–407.

La Leche League Technique

Other versions of basic suck training have appeared in the literature since Marmet and Shell's work. La Leche League leaders adopted an oral motor technique that patterns the front-to-back peristaltic movements of the tongue (Mohrbacher, 2010, pp. 806–807).

Technique

1. Touch the infant's cheek with a finger, moving toward the lips. Then brush the lips a few times with a clean index finger to encourage the infant to open its mouth.
2. Massage the outside of the infant's gum with the index finger, beginning each stroke at the middle of the baby's upper or lower gum and moving toward either side.
3. Use the tip of the index finger to press down firmly on the top of the tip of the baby's tongue and count slowly to three before releasing the pressure.
4. Release the pressure while keeping the finger in the infant's mouth, and move back slightly on his tongue, pressing again to a count of three.
5. Move back on the tongue one or two more times.
6. If the baby gags, bring the finger forward.
7. Repeat the "tongue walk" three or four times before each breastfeeding.

Sensorial Oral Stimulation in Infants with Suck Feeding Disabilities

The Sensorial Oral Stimulation technique is a feeding program for high-risk infants meant to avoid hospital complications associated with oral gastric feeding, intubation, and so on.

Technique

1. Explore the rooting reflex by making light contact over the lips and cheeks with five fingertips.
2. Use circular massage on the upper lip and anterior gum side for 5 minutes.
3. Continue massage toward the lateral gum side and inside the cheek for 3 minutes.
4. Apply tactile stimulus to the lower lip with little pressure.
5. Place pressure on the suckling point (located in the central area of the hard palate behind the upper gum).

A blind study (Rendon-Macias et al., 1999) was done to determine the clinical and physiological changes in suck feeding after sensorial oral stimulation in 14 infants. Five of these infants received mother's milk and were described as being breastfed, but it was not clear to what extent the babies fed directly from the mother versus received the milk by other means. The results showed increased milk intake and significant improvement in suckling using this technique.

Suck-Training Methods for Specific Dysfunctions

The following techniques were described by Catherine Watson Genna (2013) as being specifically useful for certain problems.

Tongue Tip Elevation

If the tongue tip elevates during latch attempts, the tongue becomes a physical barrier to the mother's nipple entering the infant's oral cavity. The tongue can be humped or bunched. The tongue may be retracted in addition to being elevated.

1. Calm the baby.
2. Tickle the tongue tip down with a finger just before attachment.
3. Use finger-feeding to teach the infant that milk should be on top of the tongue (Genna, 2013, p. 32).

Tongue Humping (Posterior Elevation)

When the tongue is humped, it blocks the oral cavity. To use this technique, massage the posterior tongue in a circular motion with exaggeration of the outward movement or finger-feed with counter-pressure on the humped area of the tongue (Genna, 2013, p. 33).

Tongue Retracted

This dysfunction occurs when the retracted tongue is held posteriorly in the mouth with the tongue tip well behind the alveolar ridges. Tongue retraction impedes the ability of the infant to grasp the breast and draw the nipple into his mouth, as tongue contact with the breast is the salient stimulus for latch. If the infant manages to latch, a retracted tongue position reduces the ability of the tongue to keep the breast in place and produce suction. The bite reflex is stimulated by contact between the breast and the infant's lower gum without the tongue interposed.

To reduce tongue retraction, massage the anterior tongue with a fingertip until it extends over the lower gum. If the infant is unable to maintain the tongue in a forward position, finger-feeding for one or more feedings while massaging the tongue forward may help (Genna, 2013, p. 33). Assess the infant with significant tongue retraction or humping for tongue-tie.

Suck-Training Method for Infants with Neurologic Dysfunction

Neurologically impaired infants have immature, damaged, or abnormally developed nervous systems that may cause abnormalities of suckling and swallowing. Suckling abnormalities usually present as absence of the suckling response, weakness or incoordination of suckling and swallowing, or some combination of these problems. McBride and Danner (1987) studied the effect of suck training for depressed suckling in a neurologically impaired infant and recommended the following technique.

Technique

1. Place the infant's head and body in a flexed position.

2. Gently stroke or press on the infant's cheeks to encourage suckling.
3. Gently move a finger or another long, soft object in all directions in the infant's mouth, touching the tongue and buccal (cheek) mucosa. Press the finger pad gently onto the hard palate and the fingertip onto the soft palate.
4. If this does not elicit a suck, encircle the infant's mouth with the fingertip several times. Repeat the sequence after tapping with the fingertips using gentle and even pressure around the mouth.
5. Vibrating the laryngopharyngeal musculature with the fingertips beginning under the chin and along either side of the larynx to the sternal notch may be helpful.

Additional exercises for neurologically impaired infants can be found in *The Ill Child: Breastfeeding Implications* chapter.

INTERNET RESOURCES

Craniosacral Therapy Association of North America: http://www.craniosacraltherapy.org
Neuro-Development Treatment Association: http://www.ndta.org

REFERENCES

Fucile S, Gisel EG, Lau C. Oral stimulation accelerates the transition from tube to oral feeding in preterm infants. *J Pediatr.* 2002;141:230–236.

Gaebler CP, Hanzlik JR. The effects of a prefeeding stimulation program on preterm infant. *Am J Occup Ther.* 1996;50:184–192.

Genna CW. *Supporting sucking skills in breastfeeding infants*, 2nd ed. Burlington, MA: Jones and Bartlett; 2013:32–33.

Marmet C, Shell E. Training neonates to suck correctly. *MCN.* 1984;9:401–407.

McBride M, Danner S. Sucking disorders in neurologically impaired infants. *Clin Perinatol.* 1987;14:109–130.

Mohrbacher N. *Breastfeeding answers made simple.* Amarillo, TX: Hale; 2010.

Rendon-Macias ME, Perez LA, Mosco-Peralta MR, et al. Assessment of sensorial oral stimulation in infants with suck feeding disabilities. *Indian J Pediatr.* 1999;66:319–329.

Chapter 4

The Biological Specificity of Breastmilk

Jan Riordan

Considered similar to the placental blood of intrauterine life, human milk resembles unstructured living tissue, such as blood, and is capable of transporting nutrients, affecting biochemical systems, enhancing immunity, and destroying pathogens (Eidelman et al., 2012). With the use of sophisticated laboratory techniques, many scientific investigators have substantiated the life-sustaining properties of breastmilk. Organs themselves provide evidence of the profound influence of breastfeeding. For example, the thymus plays a role in the development of the immune system by providing the environment for T-cell differentiation and maturation. At age 4 months, the thymus is about twice as large in exclusively breastfed infants as in infants fed only infant formula. This difference in size persists until the child is at least 10 months old (Hasselbalch et al., 1999). Although thymus size can be influenced by many factors, it would not be unreasonable to envision a variety of hypothetical mechanisms whereby breastfeeding might influence thymic size (Prentice & Collinson, 2000).

Breastmilk, like all other animal milks, is species specific. It has been adapted throughout human existence to meet nutritional and anti-infective requirements of the human infant to ensure optimal growth, development, and survival. The evolutionary origins of milk appear to be found in the secretions of primitive apocrine-like glands. As the secretory fluid and the glands that produced it became more complex, the volumes produced became greater (Oftedal, 2012). Milk composition changes depending on the infant's gender or whether conditions are good or bad. At birth, the baby's immune system is small but complete. It expands in response to the child's exposure to newly acquired bacteria but takes time before the infant develops full capacity to defend itself (Larsson, 2004). National and international health organizations consistently recommend that mothers breastfeed for the entire first year of life and thereafter as long as it is beneficial to the mother and infant (U.S. Department of Health and Human Services [DHHS], 2010).

Because an infant's birth weight normally requires about 4 to 6 months to double, the nutritional needs of the human baby must be substantially different from those of other mammals whose birth weight doubles much more rapidly. In addition, breastmilk enhances brain development: breastfed children may be more intelligent than children not breastfed. A meta-analysis of 11 studies in which confounding variables were adjusted showed an average 3.2-point higher cognitive development score among breastfed infants. This advantage was seen early on and continued through childhood (Anderson et al., 1999). Deoni et al.'s (2013) examination of the relationship between breastfeeding duration and white matter in the brain revealed those children who breastfed longer had increased white matter development. Positive relationships between white matter microstructure and breastfeeding duration were exhibited in several brain regions.

This chapter breaks down the general properties of human milk into specific components and describes for each component species-specific "biochemical messages" that contribute to the well-being of the baby and mother. The chapter also explores the concept that these "messages" can be nutritional programming, triggering an early stimulus or insult during a critical or sensitive period with long-term effects on health and disease (Lucas, 1998; Nommsen-Rivers, 2003). Knowledge of biological constructs of lactation is critical to the clinician because it forms the rationale for effective practice in the clinical setting.

Milk Synthesis and Maturational Changes

Major components of human milk (protein, fat, lactose) are synthesized and secreted by the mammary secretory epithelial cells. Cregan and Hartmann (1999) labeled these cells "lactocytes." During pregnancy, these cells further develop under the influence of prolactin. Four of the five pathways necessary for milk secretion are synchronized in the alveolar cell of the mammary gland. In the fifth milk-secretion pathway, the passage of components is between epithelial cells, rather than through them, forming the paracellular pathway (Neville et al., 2001).

Factors that influence milk composition include stage of lactation, gestational age of the infant, stage (beginning or end) of the feeding, frequency of the baby's demand for milk, and degree of fullness or emptiness of the breasts. As discussed in the *Anatomy and Physiology of Lactation* chapter, lactogenesis occurs in two stages. Stage I refers to the development, during late pregnancy, of the mammary gland's capacity to synthesize milk. Stage II, traditionally based on postpartum day, refers to the onset of copious milk secretion or the time at which the mother feels her milk "coming in."

Arthur, Smith, and Hartmann (1989) and Humenick (1987) proposed two different biological markers as objective measures to define stages of breastmilk maturation. On the one hand, Arthur, Smith, and Hartmann hold that in the first stage of lactogenesis, average concentrations of lactose, citrate, and glucose are low. A sudden and rapid increase in concentrations of these components between 24 to 48 hours after birth heralds the transition from stage I to stage II lactogenesis. Stage II lactogenesis markers (lactose, citrate, and total nitrogen) take an additional 24 hours to attain the same concentrations in women who have insulin-dependent diabetes compared with women who do not (Hartmann & Cregan, 2001). On the other hand, Humenick et al. (1994) consider the breakdown of an emulsion dependent on the ratio of sterols plus phospholipids to fat content of milk (Maturation Index of Colostrum and Milk [MICAM]) as the biological marker for breastmilk maturation (Figure 4-1).

Both of these methods appear to be valid in that they were positively related to greater milk yield (Casey et al., 1985; Saint et al., 1984), infant weight gain, and lower transcutaneous bilirubinometer readings (Humenick, 1987). Studies also show that breastmilk maturation during lactogenesis proceeds more rapidly in some mothers than in others and is not consistent with the coming in of the milk. Neville et al., (2001) believed that the terms "colostrum" and "transitional milk" used to describe breastmilk during the early postpartum period do not define clear-cut changes in milk composition and are not a useful distinction. Instead, Neville suggested, they should be viewed as part of a continuum of events where changes in breastmilk occur rapidly during the first few days after birth and are followed by

Figure 4-1 MILK TYPE BY DAY.

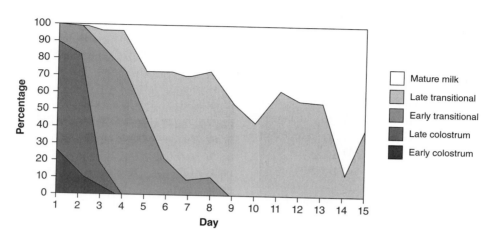

Source: Used with permission from Humenick SS. The clinical significance of breastmilk maturation rates. *Birth*. 1987;14:174–179.

slow changes. The time at which mothers report that their milk comes in is highly variable and ranges from 38 to 98 hours after birth, with an average of 50 to 59 hours (Arthur, Jones, et al., 1989; Hildebrandt, 1999; Kulski & Hartmann, 1981).

Compared with mature milk, colostrum is richer in protein and minerals and lower in carbohydrates, fat, and some vitamins. This high concentration of total protein and total ash (minerals) and whey in colostrum and early milk gradually changes to reflect the infant's needs over the first 2 to 3 weeks as lactation becomes established. The total dose of such key components as immunoglobulins, which the infant receives from breastmilk, remains relatively constant throughout lactation, regardless of the amount of breastmilk provided by the mother. This happens because concentrations decrease as total volume increases while lactation is established; at weaning, concentration increases as total volume decreases.

At birth the neonate's intestine is sterile, but it is rapidly colonized thereafter. Breastfed infants have an intestinal ecosystem that contains a high concentration of bifidobacteria and lactobacilli. Following birth, breastmilk delivers beneficial bacteria from the mother's gut to her baby's digestive system.

Energy, Volume, and Growth

Human milk is rich in nutrient proteins, nonprotein nitrogen compounds, lipids, oligosaccharides, vitamins, and certain minerals. In addition, it contains hormones, enzymes, growth factors, and many types of protective agents. Human milk contains about 10% solids for energy and growth; the rest is water, which is vital for maintaining hydration. The pH of early colostrum is 7.45; it falls to a low of 7.0 during the second week of lactation. Thereafter, the pH of milk remains at 7.0 and then rises gradually to 7.4 by 10 months postpartum. The significance of these changes is not known (Morriss et al., 1986). Infants can digest breastmilk much more rapidly than formula. The average gastric half-emptying time for breastmilk is substantially less (48 minutes) than for infant formula (78 minutes) (Cavell, 1981).

Healthy infants, even preterm infants, who consume enough breastmilk to meet their energy needs receive enough fluid to satisfy their requirements even in hot and dry environments (Almroth & Bidinger, 1990; Ashraf et al., 1993; Brown, Black, et al., 1986; Cohen et al., 2000; Sachdev et al., 1991). Exclusive and prolonged breastfeeding in healthy infants enhances infant growth during the first 3 months of life and does not affect the normal growth pattern during the first year (Kramer et al., 2002, 2003; Kramer & Kakuma, 2004; Wells et al., 2012).

Caloric Density

The caloric content or energy density of human milk is generally considered to be 65 kcal/dL, although published values differ. Garza et al. (1983) reported 57.7 kcal/dL, Lepage et al. (1984) reported 66.6 kcal/dL, and Lemons et al. (1982) reported 72.2 kcal/dL. Mitoulas and colleagues (2002) analyzed milk samples over the first 12 months and found milk energy content varied from 59.7 to 67.1 kcal/dL. Using breastmilk as the "gold standard," the American Academy of Pediatrics (Eidelman et al., 2012) recommended a calorie content of 67 kcal/dL for commercial formulas.

Nature abhors waste, and breastmilk is efficiently utilized. During their first 4 months, exclusively breastfed infants attain adequate growth with nutrient intakes substantially less than the current dietary recommendation (Butte et al., 1990). The energy requirements of breastfed infants are approximately 20% less than recommended levels (Butte et al., 2000; Stuff & Nichols, 1989). Breastmilk of women who have been lactating for more than 1 year has significantly increased fat and energy compared with breastmilk of women who have been lactating for shorter periods (Mandel et al., 2005). Caloric intake does not increase after solid foods are added to the baby's diet, strongly suggesting that the calorie value of breastmilk feeds is sufficient for the infants' needs. Kilocalories of breastmilk ingested per kilogram of body weight for exclusively breastfed babies decrease significantly during the first few months of life (Table 4-1).

The energy intakes of breastfed and formula-fed infants differ significantly because their energy expenditure differs greatly. Total daily energy expenditure, minimal rates of energy expenditure, metabolic rates during sleep, rectal temperature, and heart rates are all lower in breastfed infants. Total

Table 4-1 KILOCALORIES OF BREASTMILK INGESTED PER KILOGRAM ACCORDING TO INFANT AGE

Time Post Birth	kcal per kg
14 days	128
3rd month	70–75
5th month	62.5

Data from: Garza, Stuff, & Butte, 1986; Wood et al., 1988

body water and fat-free mass is smaller, and body fat is higher in breastfed infants at 4 months of age (Butte et al., 1995). By 8 months, breastfed infants have consumed about 30,000 kcal less than bottle-fed infants (Butte et al., 1990). Hindmilk may have two to three times the concentration of milk fat found in foremilk (Ballard & Morrow, 2013).

Although this difference in energy intake should result in about a 2.7-kg mean difference of weight, such is not the case. To explain this discrepancy, Garza, Stuff, and Butte (1986) suggested that (1) differences in intake in the general population are not as great as those found in the babies studied; (2) energy expenditure differs substantially between breastfed and bottle-fed infants; or (3) composition of newly acquired tissue differs between these two groups. One possibility is that the energy density of milk taken by a 4-month-old is higher on the average than that taken by the same baby 3 months earlier. The 4-month-old baby's suckle is more active, leading to a higher intake that more than compensates for the volumes needed, because breastmilk is used more completely and with less waste than is artificial milk. Figure 4-2 depicts the differences in energy density among expressed breastmilk, preterm milk, foremilk, and hindmilk.

Milk Volume

The volume of milk must provide sufficient caloric energy to permit normal growth and development. Small amounts of colostrum—averaging about 37 mL (range, 7–123 mL)—are yielded in the first 24 hours postpartum (Hartmann, 1987; Hartmann

Figure 4-2 MEAN PROTEIN CONTENT
(A) AND ENERGY DENSITY (B) OF
FULL-TERM DONOR AND PRETERM
MILK AND FULL-TERM FORE- AND
HINDMILK DURING THE FIRST 6 MO.
OF LACTATION. VERTICAL LINES
SHOW STANDARD ERRORS OF MEANS.

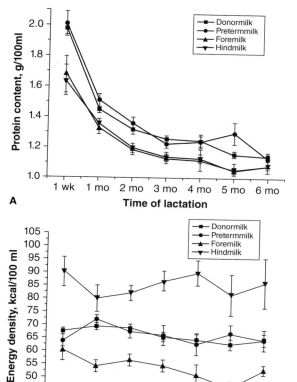

A

B

Source: Used with permission from Saarela AT, Kokkonen J,
Koivisto M. Macronutrient and energy contents of human milk
fractions during the first six months of lactation. *Acta Paediatricia.*
2005,94:1176–1181.

& Prosser, 1984); the infant ingests approximately
7 to 14 mL at each feeding (Houston et al., 1983).
This milk yield gradually increases for the first
36 hours, but then is followed by a dramatic increase

during the next 49 to 96 hours. By day 5, volume
is about 500 mL/day; it increases more slowly to
about 800 mL/day at month 6 of full breastfeeding,
with a range between 550 mL and 1150 mL (Cox et
al., 1996; Cregan et al., 2002; Daly, Owens, et al.,
1993; Neville et al., 1988). On average, a baby
takes only 67% of the available breastmilk. These
researcher-identified volumes are similar to others established by test-weighing the infant (using
prefeeding and postfeeding infant weighing). The
volume of milk taken by thriving breastfed infants
varies little from 1 to 4 months. By 1 month, intake
averages 750 to 800 mL per day. Breastmilk intake
slowly declines as other foods are added to the
baby's diet.

Even if a mother feels that she had insufficient
milk to feed her first baby, health professionals
should reassure women that it is well worth trying a second time. Multiparous mothers produce
more breastmilk (about 140 mL) at 1 week than
women giving birth for the first time (Ingram et al.,
2001). Breastmilk of adolescent mothers is not different from breastmilk of adult women, although
adolescents in one study breastfed fewer times per
day (Motil, Sheng, et al., 1997).

It is well established that breastmilk production
and intake are related to infant demand. Infants
have the capacity to self-regulate their own milk
intake. This important concept of lactation has been
extensively studied. Australian researchers measured the short-term rates of milk synthesis using
a computerized system in which a camera relays
video images to a computer that produces a model
of the chest by active triangulation (Daly et al.,
1993). Newer research using ultrasound imaging to
re-investigate the anatomy of the lactating breast,
milk production measured by 24 hour test weights,
and storage capacity as measured through creamatocrit determination of breast fullness offer further
evidence that infant appetite determines milk production (Ramsay et al., 2005). Their findings and
practical applications are summarized in Box 4-1
(Cregan & Hartmann, 1999; Daly & Hartmann,
1995a, 1995b; Ramsay et al., 2005).

BOX 4-1 APPLICATION OF PHYSIOLOGICAL PRINCIPLES

Principle from Physiological Research	Application in Practice
The breast does balance supply to meet the infant's demand for breastmilk.	Watch the baby for hunger cues.
The breast can rapidly change its rate of milk synthesis from one feed to the next.	Encourage the mother when she thinks she has "run out of milk."
The breasts have the capacity to synthesize more milk than the infant usually requires.	As above.
The left and right breasts rarely produce the same amount of milk. Data on 24-hour milk production of individual breasts confirm that one breast is usually more productive than the other.	Mothers often refer to having one "good" breast, or state that the baby prefers one breast to the other.
There is no correlation between milk production and the amount of glandular tissue, the number of ducts or the mean diameter of the milk ducts, nor is there a correlation between the amount of glandular tissue and the storage capacity in the breast. Therefore, milk production is controlled by infant appetite.	Mothers should feed baby based on cues that demonstrate appetite/hunger.
There is no relationship between total milk storage capacity and total 24-hour milk production.	Women with smaller breasts can produce as much milk as women with larger breasts but they must breastfeed more often.
The greater the degree of emptying at a breastfeed, the greater the rate of milk synthesis after that feed.	Advise the mother to avoid fast "switching" from one breast to another and to try to empty one breast as much as possible.
The length of time between feeds (up to 6 hours) does not appear to decrease milk synthesis.	Feeding interval can be flexible once lactation is established.

Breastfeeding Patterns and Milk Production

Within the first feeding, babies show a wide variation in the amount, variations, and patterns of amount of milk they take (Khan et al., 2013). The infant may feed from one breast only, feed from both breasts within 30 minutes, or have a cluster of breastfeeds (feed again from the first breast within 30 minutes of feeding on the second breast), among other patterns. It is uncommon for the left and right breasts to produce the same amount of breastmilk at any one feeding. If there is a difference, the right breast is usually more productive (Cox et al., 1996).

Differences in Milk Volume Between Breasts

As noted previously, milk output is more often greater from the right breast versus the left breast (Cox et al., 1996; Daly, Owens, et al., 1993; Engstrom et al., 2007; Kent et al., 1999; Ramsay et al., 2005), even though right-handed mothers instinctively use the right hand to position the baby and breast, thereby making it easier to feed from the left breast. In addition, in all cultures there is a preference of mothers to hold their babies in their left arm, thus facilitating feeding at the left breast (Engstrom et al., 2007). A likely explanation for the difference in left-side versus right-side milk production is that the right breast receives more blood flow than the left breast (Aljazaf, 2004).

Daly, Owens, et al. (1993) were able to determine the rate of synthesis of human milk. Figure 4-3A shows the volume of milk produced by one woman who had a storage capacity of 111 mL for her right breast and a capacity of 81 mL for her left breast. As shown in the figure, the maximum amount of milk that the mother appeared to be able to store was about 20% of her infant's 24-hour milk intake. From her breast volume changes over time, it appears that her infant met its demand for milk by breastfeeding frequently. Conversely, Figure 4-3B depicts the milk production of another woman who produced similar volumes of milk but with larger storage

Figure 4-3 (**A**) THE RIGHT AND LEFT BREAST VOLUME CHANGES OF ONE SUBJECT OVER A PERIOD OF 24 HOURS.

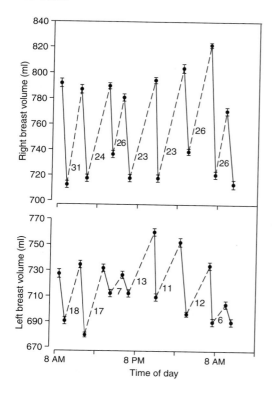

Figure 4-3 (**B**) BREAST VOLUME CHANGES. THE RIGHT AND LEFT BREAST VOLUME CHANGES OF ONE SUBJECT OVER A PERIOD OF 28 HOURS. EACH POINT REPRESENTS THE MEAN PLUS OR MINUS THE STANDARD ERROR OF THE MEAN OF REPLICATE BREAST-VOLUME MEASUREMENT. LINES LINK PREFEEDING AND POSTFEEDING MEAN BREAST VOLUMES. DASHED LINES LINK POSTFEEDING MEAN BREAST VOLUME OF A BREASTFEEDING TO THE PREFEEDING MEAN BREAST VOLUME OF THE NEXT BREAST; THEIR SLOPES THUS INDICATES RATE OF MILK SYNTHESIS BETWEEN THE TWO BREASTFEEDINGS. RATE OF MILK SYNTHESIS ALSO IS GIVEN BY THE NUMBER OF (IN MILLILITERS PER HOUR) ACCOMPANYING EACH DASHED LINE.

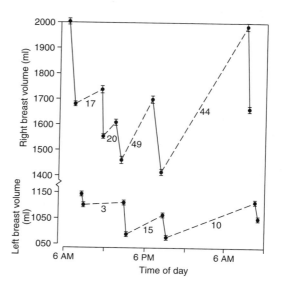

Source: Used with permission from Daly SE, Owens RA, Hartmann PE. The short-term synthesis and infant-regulated removal of milk in lactating women. *Exp Physiol.* 1993;78:209–220.

capacities for her breasts (right breast, 600 mL; left breast, 180 mL), allowing her to store nearly 90% of her infant's 24-hour milk intake. Further, there was no relationship between total milk storage capacity and 24-hour milk production. Thus we can conclude that *breast size does not restrict a woman's ability to provide milk for her infant.* By comparison, mothers with a greater storage capacity do have more flexibility with patterns of breastfeeding.

There appear to be wide differences among women in terms of their rate of milk synthesis, which among some women can be double or triple the rate of other women (Arthur et al., 1989; Daly et al., 1992). Milk volume between breasts also differs; left and right breasts rarely produce the same volume of milk (Kent et al., 2006), demonstrating that the rate of milk synthesis within one breast is independent of the rate of milk synthesis in the other breast (Cox et al., 1996; Daly, Owens, et al., 1993).

The amount of milk available in the breast is not necessarily an important determinant of the amount removed by the infant at feedings. Infant intake of breastmilk also varies widely. For example, at 5 months, infant intake of breastmilk can range from 200 mL/day for partial breastfeeding to 3500 mL/day if a wet nurse is used (Neville & Oliva-Rasbach, 1987). These differences appear to be culturally based. Australian women, for example, have been reported to make more breastmilk than do U.S. women. The average daily yield of well-nourished Australian mothers during the first 6 months of lactation was found to be in excess of 1100 mL in one study (Hartmann, 1987) and to range from 535 mL to 1078 mL in another study (Daly, Owens, et al., 1993).

Khan et al. (2013) measured breastmilk intake over a 24-hour period in a study of 15 women. They found no difference between mean (standard deviation [SD]) 24-hour milk intake of babies from the left breast (400 [128] g) and right breast (402 [104] g), and no difference for single feeds from the left breast (64 [16] g) and right breast (62 [18] g). Furthermore, there was no difference between the left and right breasts in terms of the time between feeds during a 24-hour period.

A healthy, breastfeeding, full-term neonate breastfeeds an average of 4.3 times during the first 24 hours of life (range, 0–11) and 7.4 times during the next 24 hours (range, 1–22) (Yamauchi & Yamanouchi, 1990), and an overall median of 8 times per day after the first several days post birth (see Hornell et al., 1999). Breastmilk intake shows little or no correlation with maternal factors, such as weight-for-height, weight gain, nursing frequency, maternal age, and parity (Dewey & Lönnerdal, 1983). Although birth weight is not a strong predictor of milk intake throughout lactation, infant weight at 1 month is. Thus lactation performance during the first 4 weeks postpartum is a strong predictor of milk output during the subsequent period of full lactation (Neville & Oliva-Rasbach, 1987).

Infant Growth

Normal human growth is greatest during infancy. The infant gains about 10 g/kg/day (about 5 to 7 oz/week) until about 4 weeks post birth; at that point, the gain drops to 1 g/kg/day (about 3 oz/week) by the end of the first year of life.

Some growth differences between breastfed and formula-fed infants have been noted. Infants breastfed exclusively have the same or somewhat greater weight gain in the first 3 to 4 months than do bottle-fed or mixed-fed infants (Fawzi et al., 1997; Juex et al., 1983; Motil, Sheng, et al., 1997). After this time, bottle-fed or mixed-fed infants clearly weigh more. The greatest differences are evident between 6 and 20 months of age, when breastfed infants weight less than corresponding bottle-fed or mixed-fed infants (Dewey et al., 1993, 1995; Yoneyama et al., 1994). Increases in length and head circumference growth remain the same for both groups. Length is a reliable indicator for evaluating infant growth, and the absence of any significant difference in length between breastfed and formula-fed infants suggests that formula-fed infants are overfed. Small for gestational age infants who are breastfed show faster postnatal growth and are more likely to have significant catch-up growth than those who are fed a standard term infant formula (Lucas et al., 1997).

In 2006, the World Health Organization (WHO) released updated global growth standards derived from the Multicenter Growth Reference Study (MGRS). All of the planning, methodology, and results are posted on WHO's website (World Health Child Growth Standards, http://www.who .int/childgrowth/en/). The new standards were developed from a large and detailed prospective study of infant growth and developmental milestones among *optimally breastfed* infants in Brazil, Ghana, India, Norway, Oman, and the United States ($N \approx 8000$ between 1997 and 2003). These standards have been adopted by industrial and non-industrial countries representing approximately 75% of the world's population younger than 5 years (de Onis et al., 2012). Grummer-Strawn, Reinold, & Krebs, (2010) advocated that these growth curves should be used to monitor all infants, regardless of feeding method. (See the *Low Intake in the Breastfed Infant: Maternal and Infant Considerations* chapter for additional detail on use of the growth curves.)

Color

Breastmilk comes in several colors. Normally, it is white or yellowish. It can be green if the mother is eating an unusual amount of green vegetables or taking a medication such as nifedipine, or it can be yellow from eating yellow vegetables such as carrots. The "rusty pipe syndrome," in which the milk is tinged with pink or red, reflects old ductal bleeding. A variety of colors of breastmilk are shown in color photos in *The Breastfeeding Atlas* (Wilson-Clay & Hoover, 2013).

Nutritional Values

Around the world, breastmilk composition is remarkably stable, varying only within a relatively narrow range. The nutritional status of the mother does not appear to affect milk volume unless the mother is malnourished (Brown et al., 1986; Forman et al., 1990).

Constituents of colostrum and breastmilk and their amounts are shown in Appendix 4-A at the end of this chapter. Figure 4-4 presents a profile of lactose protein and lipid concentrations in human

milk for the first 30 days of lactation. Yet, because breastfeeding is an interactive process, the infant helps to determine composition of the feed. During

Figure 4-4 LACTOSE PROTEIN AND TOTAL LIPID CONCENTRATION IN HUMAN MILK.

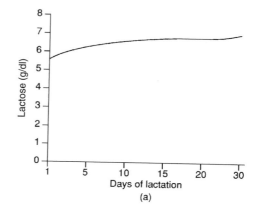

(a)

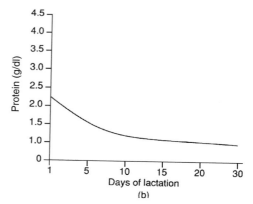

(b)

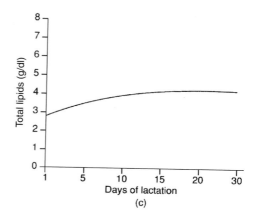

(c)

weaning (involution phase), for example, the concentrations of sodium and protein in breastmilk progressively increase and the milk becomes saltier; in contrast, concentrations of potassium, glucose, and lactose gradually decrease (Prosser et al., 1984).

Fat

The fat of human milk, which provides about half of the milk's calories, is its most variable component. Fat varies from one mother to another, and from early to late lactation. The total fat content of human milk ranges from 22 to 62 g/L and is independent of breastfeeding frequency (Kent et al., 2006). Hindmilk contains at least twice the amount of fat compared to foremilk (Saarela et al., 2005) (see again Figure 4-2). The energy density of preterm mother's milk is much greater than that of full-term mother's milk, owing to a 30% higher fat concentration (Atkinson et al., 1980). Triglycerides—the main constituent (98–99%) of milk fat—are readily broken down to free fatty acids and glycerol by the enzyme lipase, which is found not only in an infant's intestine but also in the breastmilk itself.

Analysis of fat content at four time periods showed that this content was higher during the day and lower at night—a finding consistent with previous reports. The average fat content in breastmilk was not associated with intervals between feeds, the number of breastfeeds during the day, the volume during the feed, and the 24-hour milk intake from each feed duration The average 24-hour intake of fat was 34.8 (8.4) g/liter and was not related to the duration of the feed or the frequency of breastfeeds (Khan et al., 2013). Infants get the same amount of energy from their mother's milk throughout the day regardless of their feeding behavior—that is, fats provide about half of the baby's energy intake.

The lipid fraction of human milk provides essential fatty acids. The main concern about fatty acid intake is its effect on brain growth. The rate of brain growth is greatest in the last trimester of pregnancy and continues throughout the first year of life. Tissues of breastfed and formula-fed infants have distinctly different plasma fatty acid compositions. Breastmilk contains a wide range of long-chain polyunsaturated fatty acids (LC-PUFAs), which represent 88% of milk fat and are the most variable element in milk (Jensen, 1999). Interestingly, levels of fatty acids are low in lactating women, which indicates that transfer to breastmilk occurs at the expense of the maternal stores (Koletzko & Rodriquez-Palmero, 1999).

DHA and AA

LC-PUFAs include docosahexaenoic acid (DHA) and arachidonic acid (AA), which are associated with higher visual acuity and cognitive ability of the child. Together, DHA and AA account for approximately 20% of the fatty acid content of the brain and are involved in early neurodevelopment by promoting healthy neurological growth, repair, and myelination (Guesnet & Alessandri, 2011). An analysis of studies of human-milk feedings, DHA-supplemented, and unsupplemented formula documented advantages of DHA for visual acuity (SanGiovanni et al., 2000). Other studies, however, show that DHA supplementation of the pregnant or breastfeeding woman has no impact on either infant development or visual function (Malcolm et al., 2003). AA content in human milk is stable and does not vary widely throughout the world. The content of DHA, in contrast, varies according to diet; therefore an increased supply of DHA may not always be beneficial. In the case of coastal populations with high intakes of fish, for example, few or no effects will be noted because infants already receive breastmilk with high DHA levels (Brenna et al., 2007).

Another reason that not all breastfed infants have higher cognitive development and intelligence is that there are two forms of a gene known as *RADS2*. In infants who carry the C form of this gene, breastfeeding raises intelligence by producing an enzyme that helps convert fatty acids in breastmilk into components that spur neurons to sprout connections, a factor that may enhance intelligence, memory, and creativity. The 10% of infants who do not carry the C form of the gene lack this enzyme; therefore they derive no cognitive benefit from breastmilk (Caspi et al., 2007).

An essential fatty acid that enhances the developing human visual system, DHA is found in extremely high levels in the photoreceptors and the visual cortex and may ameliorate neurovisual developmental disorders such as the retinopathy of prematurity (Hylander et al., 2001). Breastfed infants accumulate DHA in the cortex, whereas formula-fed infants merely maintain the same amount of DHA that is present at birth. As a result, breastfed infants have higher levels of DHA than an age-matched group of formula-fed infants (Baur et al., 2000).

The prevailing consensus is that children who were breasted have higher scores on IQ tests and cognitive function than do children who were formula-fed. These findings are complemented by brain imaging studies in adolescents showing increases in total white matter, sub-gray gray matter, and cortical thickness in those who were breastfed, as well as a relationship between duration of breastfeeding and IQ (Hallowell & Spatz, 2012; Issac et al., 2012; Kafouri et al., 2013).

Breastfed infants have a higher proportion of acetic acid in the short-chain fatty acid spectra than do formula-fed infants; this factor, along with the monoglycerides generated by milk lipases, acts to protect them against envelope viruses, bacteria, and fungi (Garza et al., 1987; Siigur et al., 1993). The paler color, softer consistency, and milder odor of breastmilk stools, as compared with formula stools, are due in part to a higher concentration of fatty acid soaps (Quinlan et al., 1995). Fatty acid composition also differs between mothers whose babies develop atopic manifestation during the first year of life and those whose babies remain healthy. Specifically, the lower levels of α-linolenic acid and n-3 long-chain polyunsaturated fatty acid in the mature milk of atopic mothers, especially in those with atopic babies, suggest that low levels of this fatty acid could be associated with the development of atopy in the infants (Duchen et al., 1999).

Although maternal dietary fat intake does not affect the total amount of fat in a mother's milk, the types of fat in the diet do influence the composition of fatty acids in milk. For example, black mothers in South Africa who consume a traditional maize diet have higher levels of monounsaturated fatty acid in their milk than do their urban counterparts who eat more animal fats (van der Westhuyzen et al., 1988). If the mother eats a high-carbohydrate, energy-replete diet, the proportion of triglycerides of medium-chain fatty acid increases (Garza et al., 1987).

The effects of breastfeeding can depend on the formerly breastfed individual's age. A prime example of this effect is seen with cholesterol. Because cholesterol levels (10–20 mg/dL) in human milk are considerably higher than those in formulas derived from bovine milk (Wagner & Stockhausen, 1988), one would expect cholesterol levels in adulthood to be higher in breastfed individuals. The reverse, however, is true. Exposure to cholesterol in breastmilk may have long-term benefits for cardiovascular health. Coronary artery disease in persons up to 20 years of age is less frequent in individuals who were breastfed (Bergstrom et al., 1995). Serum total cholesterol and low-density lipoprotein (LDL) levels (1) tend to be higher among breastfed infants compared to nonbreastfed infants, (2) are not different by infant-feeding group by 18 months of age (Demmers et al., 2005) and during childhood, and (3) tend to be lower among adults who were breastfed rather than artificially fed as infants (Owen et al., 2002). In addition to higher cholesterol concentration, adults who were bottle-fed demonstrate higher plasma glucose concentrations and impaired glucose tolerance (Ravelli et al., 2000).

Fat content of milk changes throughout a breastfeeding and, generally speaking, increases more steeply as more milk is taken. This content varies according to the degree to which the breast is emptied at that breastfeeding, with fat content increasing markedly after most of the milk in the breast has been taken (Daly, Owens, et al., 1993). The longer the time interval between two breastfeedings, the less likely the infant is to empty the breast and, therefore, the lower the fat concentration will be in the subsequent feeding. Although the work of Daly, Owens, et al. (1993) indicated that the pattern of feedings dictates the infant's fat intake, this is not necessarily the case. Woolridge et al (1990) studied mothers who fed in two patterns—either feeding at one breast or feeding at two breasts during the same session. The infants were able to regulate their fat intake and to achieve stable fat intakes despite the disparate patterns of feedings. These findings support the call for flexible "baby-led" feedings.

Lactose

Lactose, a disaccharide, accounts for most of the carbohydrates in human milk, although small quantities of oligosaccharides, galactose, and fructose are also present. Although lactose concentration is relatively constant (7.0 g/dL) in mature milk, it is affected by maternal diet: the more frequent the feeds, the higher the concentration of lactose.

Lactose enhances calcium absorption and metabolizes readily to galactose and glucose, which supply energy to the rapidly growing brain of the infant. Some oligosaccharides promote the growth of *Lactobacillus bifidus*, thereby increasing intestinal acidity and stemming the growth of pathogens (Dai et al., 2000).

The enzyme lactase is necessary to convert lactose into simple sugars that can be easily assimilated by the infant. This enzyme is present in the infant's intestinal mucosa from birth. Congenital or primary lactase deficiency is exceedingly rare (Montgomery et al., 1991). Lactose intolerance, however, is common in many mammals as they grow older and is the result of diminishing activity of intestinal lactase after weaning. In humans, lactose intolerance is more prevalent in adults of Asian and African heritage.

Probiotic and Prebiotic Bacteria

Probiotic bacteria are live microorganisms that can be a health benefit. For example, some probiotic bacteria that have *Lactobacillus* strains act by competing with other bacteria for nutrients, thereby reducing the numbers of potentially pathogenic microbes. Certain *Lactobacillus* strains may ameliorate the symptoms of rotavirus infections (Larsson, 2004). Lactobacilli colonize breastfed babies' oral cavities more frequently than those who are formula-fed. The dominant *Lactobacillus* is *L. gasseri* (Romani Vestman et al., 2013).

Protein

Protein content of mature human milk from well-nourished mothers is about 0.8 to 0.9 g of protein per deciliter. The average 24-hour total protein intake is 10.9 g and is independent of the duration of duration and interval between feeds (Khan et al., 2013). Some of the protein in human milk is probably not nutritionally available to the infant; it serves immunological purposes instead. The high quality of protein in human milk and its precisely balanced quantity meet the energy needs of infants (Gaull, 1985; Raiha, 1985). As seen in Figure 4-2, the protein content in breastmilk decreases rapidly during the first several months postpartum (Saarela et al., 2005).

Human milk contains casein and whey protein. Levels change as lactation progresses to meet the nutritional needs of the infant. The casein concentration is lower in early lactation, but then increases rapidly. Whey proteins are at their highest concentration in early lactation, but then gradually fall. These changes result in a whey/casein ratio of about 90:10 in early lactation, 60:40 in mature milk, and 50:50 in late lactation (Kunz & Lönnerdal, 1992). Whey proteins are acidified in the stomach, forming soft, flocculent curds. These materials are quickly digested, supplying a continuous flow of nutrients to the baby. By contrast, caseins (the primary protein in untreated bovine milk) form a tough, less digestible curd that requires high expenditure of energy for an incomplete digestive process.

Whey protein is composed of five major components: (1) α-lactalbumin, (2) serum albumin, (3) lactoferrin, (4) immunoglobulins, and (5) lysozyme. The latter three elements play important roles in immunological defense. The lactoferrin concentration in milk is higher in iron-deficient women as compared with well-nourished mothers; therefore, milk lactoferrin may also help protect the infant against iron deficiency (Raiha, 1985). A large number of other proteins (enzymes, growth modulators, and hormones) are present in low concentrations.

Nonprotein Nitrogen

Milk proteins are synthesized from amino acids derived from the bloodstream. Nonprotein nitrogen contains a number of free amino acids, including glutamic acid, glycine, alanine, valine, leucine, aspartic acid, serine, threonine, proline, and taurine. When amino acids exist singly or in free form, they are known as free amino acids. Of these, leucine, valine, and threonine are essential amino acids; they must be consumed in the diet because the body does not manufacture them.

The percentage of protein in human colostrum is greater than that in mature breastmilk. This high level is due to the fact that in colostrum, lactose and water have not yet flooded the milk production system; it also reflects the presence of additional amino acids and antibody-rich proteins, especially secretory IgA and lactoferrin. All 10 essential amino acids are present in colostrum and account for approximately 45% of its total nitrogen content.

Nucleotides

Nucleotides are low-molecular-weight compounds with a nitrogenous base. Necessary for energy metabolism, enzymatic reactions, and growth and maturation of the developing gastrointestinal tract, they also play several roles in immune function, including enhancing lymphocytic proliferation, stimulating immunoglobulin production in lymphocytes, and increasing natural killer-cell activity. Infant formula manufacturers seek to emulate the many nucleotides of breastmilk in their formulas (Cosgrove, 1998; Leach et al., 1995).

The importance to the baby of available nitrogen cannot be overstated. Atkinson, Anderson, and Bryan (1980) have shown that the concentration of nitrogen in the milk of women who deliver preterm infants is 20% greater than that in the milk of women delivering at term. The higher levels of available protein and fat in preterm mother's milk underscore the importance of using the milk of the preterm infant's mother rather than pooled milk from women in other stages of lactation (Table 4-2). Donated milk (not preterm milk), however, can be modified with components from other human milk to make a preterm human milk formula with none of the dangers of commercial bovine-based preterm formulas.

Vitamins and Micronutrients

The amounts of vitamins and micronutrients in human milk vary from one mother to another because of diet and genetic differences. However, it is generally true that human milk will satisfy the micronutrient requirements of a full-term healthy infant and, therefore, can be taken as the primary yardstick of dietary recommendations, or reference values. Generally, as lactation progresses, the level of water-soluble vitamins in breastmilk increases, and the level of fat-soluble vitamins declines. The levels of fat-soluble vitamins (A, D, K, E) in human milk are minimally influenced by recent maternal diet, as these vitamins can be drawn from storage in the body.

Table 4-2 COMPOSITION OF TERM AND PRETERM MILK DURING THE FIRST MONTH OF LACTATION

	3–5 Days		8–11 Days		15–18 Days		26–29 Days	
Nutrients	Full Term	Preterm	Full Term	Preterm	Full Term	Preterm	Full Term	Preterm
Energy (kcal/dl)	48	58	59	71	62	71	62	70
Lipid (gm/dl)	1.85	3.00	2.9	4.14	3.06	4.33	3.05	4.09
Protein (gm/dl)	1.87	2.10	1.7	1.86	1.52	1.71	1.29	1.41
Lactose (gm/dl)	5.14	5.04	5.98	5.55	6.00	5.63	6.51	5.97

Data from Anderson CH. Human milk feeding. *Pediatr Clin No Amer*. 1985;32:335–352.

Vitamin A

Human milk is a good source of vitamin A (200 IU/dL), which is present mainly as retinol (40–53 ng/dL). Required for vision and maintenance of epithelial structures, vitamin A reaches its highest levels in breastmilk in the first week after birth and then gradually declines. Deficiency of vitamin A is a serious health problem for young children in many developing countries, leading to blindness through damage to the corneal epithelium (xerophthalmia) and to increased morbidity from infectious diseases. The prolongation of even partial breastfeeding provides an important source of vitamin A to children in developing countries (Bates & Prentice, 1994).

Vitamin D

Human milk contains very little fat-soluble vitamin D; consequently, breastfed infants can develop rickets, although such an event is uncommon. The risk of rickets is greatest for dark-skinned children living in inner-city areas, children whose clothing deters skin exposure to the sun, and children of mothers eating vegetarian diets that exclude meat, fish, and dairy products. However, the child who is adequately exposed to the sun (and thus to radiation-formed precursors of vitamin D) and whose mother consumes adequate nutrients may not need routine vitamin D supplements (Greer & Marshall, 1989). Vitamin D may constitute an exception to the general rule that breastmilk micronutrient levels are protected from the effect of maternal deficiency. Wagner and colleagues (2008, 2012) contend that we should no longer see vitamin D as a "vitamin" important in childhood but rather view it as a complex prehormone and potent mediator of the immune system tied to inflammatory or long-latency diseases.

Evidence points to a vitamin D dose of 400 IU/day as adequate (Wagner et al., 2008) to achieve serum 25(OH)D concentration greater than 11 ng/mL in nearly all infants, although high-risk populations may need more. In the United States, the American Academy of Pediatrics recommends that all breastfed infants be supplemented with 400 IU of vitamin D per day from birth (Wagner, Greer, & AAP, 2008).

Vitamin E

Human colostrum is particularly rich in vitamin E (tocopherol). Milk of mothers with preterm and term infants have similar levels of vitamin E (3 IU/100 kcal) and carotenoid levels, which are higher than those in bovine milk (Ostrea et al., 1986) and in formula (Sommerburg et al., 2000). A deficiency of vitamin E in infancy can result in hemolytic anemia, especially in the premature infant. Because it is an antioxidant, vitamin E protects cell membranes in the retina and lungs against oxidant-induced injury. The requirement for vitamin E increases with intake of polyunsaturated fatty acids in breastmilk. Mothers who eat foods high in polyunsaturated fats and "fast foods" add to oxidant stress (Guthrie et al., 1977). Newer research confirms that human milk is a source of antioxidative vitamins and that their concentrations decrease throughout the period of lactation, while their total antioxidative properties increase, suggesting an additional system of antioxidants in human milk. Furthermore, the phase of lactation does not affect the degree of human milk's lipid oxidative damage.

Vitamin K

Vitamin K, which is required for the synthesis of blood-clotting factors, is present in human milk in small amounts. A few days after birth, a baby normally produces vitamin K in sufficient quantities by enteric bacteria. However, neonates are susceptible to vitamin K deficiency until ingestion of copious amounts of breastmilk can promote gastrointestinal bacterial colonization, which enhances their low levels of vitamin K. Vitamin K supplements taken by the mother will increase breastmilk levels and infant plasma levels of the vitamin (Greer, 1999).

Insufficient vitamin K in neonates can lead to vitamin K–responsive hemorrhagic disease. To prevent hemorrhage and to raise prothrombin levels, 1 mg vitamin K is routinely given intramuscularly postpartum. Alternatively, a 1 mg oral dose of vitamin K administered at birth, at 1 to 2 weeks, and at 4 to 6 weeks is absorbed in the intestinal tract in amounts sufficient to prevent bleeding, and the infant is spared the pain of an injection and the risk of nerve damage that is always present with any intramuscular injection. Formula-fed infants need not receive vitamin K routinely because formula (other than soy) contains vitamin K (Medves, 2002).

Water-soluble vitamins—ascorbic acid, nicotinic acid, B_{12}, riboflavin, and B_6—are readily influenced by the maternal diet. If maternal supplements are present, the vitamin levels in the milk increase and then plateau. Although supplementation may be beneficial for undernourished women, it is not necessary if the mother is well nourished and eating a diet that contain foods close to their natural state.

Vitamin B_{12}

Vitamin B_{12} is needed for early development of the baby's central nervous system. A mother eating a vegan diet (i.e., without meat or dairy products) may produce milk deficient in vitamin B_{12}. A deficiency of B vitamin folate during pregnancy is associated with neural tube defects. In the United States, the March of Dimes campaign to educate women on the importance of taking folic acid supplements during preconception and pregnancy has reduced neural tube deformities.

Unlike other micronutrients, folate (which is bound to a folate-binding protein) remains at the same level throughout all stages of lactation. Maternal stores of folate diminish slightly from 3 to 6 months to maintain milk folate levels (Mackey & Picciano, 1999).

Vitamin B_6

High pharmacological doses of vitamin B_6 have been reported to suppress prolactin and, therefore, lactation. However, low nutritionally relevant doses have no effect on plasma prolactin or on breastmilk volume. A dose as high as 4.0 mg of vitamin B_6 taken as part of a vitamin B complex supplement is considered safe for both the lactating mother and the infant (Andon et al., 1985).

Minerals

The total mineral content in human milk is fairly constant. Except for magnesium, minerals tend to reach their highest concentration in human milk in the first few days after birth and then decrease

slightly in a consistent pattern throughout lactation, with little diurnal variation or variation within feedings. Maternal age, parity, and diet, even when the mother takes supplements, usually have minimal influence on mineral concentrations in milk, probably because of their regulation from maternal body stores (Butte et al., 1987; Casey et al., 1989).

Sodium

Breastmilk sodium is elevated in early colostrum but falls dramatically by the third day postpartum and subsequently declines at a slower rate for 6 months. Elevated levels of sodium in human milk occur during weaning, in women with mastitis, and during the first months of gestation. A high concentration of sodium has also been found in the milk of mothers whose infants develop malnutrition, dehydration, and hypernatremia. Persistent high levels may be a marker for impaired lactation (Morton, 1994).

Zinc

Zinc is actively transported into the mammary gland. Zinc levels rise to a peak on the second day postpartum and then decline for the duration of lactation (Casey et al., 1989). Zinc is eight times as abundant in human colostrum as in mature milk. Requirements for this mineral are relatively high in the very young infant, but decrease with increasing age of the infant (Krachler et al., 1998; Krebs & Hambidge, 1986). For fully breastfed infants, a combination of high absorption and efficient conservation of intestinal endogenous zinc suffice to retain enough zinc to meet the demands of infant growth in the face of modest intake (Abrams et al., 1996; Krebs et al., 1996). Zinc supplements, when taken by women with normal zinc levels, do not affect the infant's growth, morbidity, or motor development (Heinig et al., 2006).

Zinc dramatically improves acrodermatitis enteropathica, a rare but serious congenital metabolic disorder that manifests itself in part as severe dermatitis (Evans & Johnson, 1980). While infants with this disorder continue to receive human milk, they have no symptoms. The high bioavailability of zinc in human milk is brought about by a low-molecular-weight zinc-binding ligand that facilitates zinc absorption. Abnormally low zinc levels in breastmilk are rare but can sometimes occur in mothers of infants with low birth weight or if there is an inherited genetic condition (Chowanadisai et al., 2006). A slowing growth rate and persistent perioral or perianal rash (with or without diarrhea) in infants fed solely breastmilk may be due to zinc depletion (Atkinson et al., 1989). These infants should continue to breastfeed but may require zinc supplementation.

Maternal diet does not affect breastmilk zinc levels. In the rare case where a woman has low concentrations of breastmilk zinc, she is likely to have delivered her infant prematurely (Lönnerdal, 2000).

Iron

Although human milk contains only a small amount of iron (0.5–1.0 mg/L), breastfed babies are rarely iron deficient. They maintain their iron status at the same level as that of formula-fed infants receiving iron supplements for up to 9 months (Duncan et al., 1985; Salmenpera et al., 1986; Siimes et al., 1984). Breastfed infants are sustained by sufficient iron stores laid down in utero and by the high lactose and vitamin C levels in human milk, which facilitate iron absorption. Iron in human milk is absorbed five times as well as a similar amount from cow milk.

For the first few months of life, healthy, full-term infants draw on the extensive iron reserves that are generally present in their bodies at birth. Normally, an infant's hemoglobin level is high (16–22 g/dL) at birth and decreases rapidly as physiological adjustment is made to extrauterine life. At 4 months of age, normal hemoglobin ranges between 10.2 and 15 g/dL. Iron is well absorbed by older infants and such absorption is not affected by mineral intake from solid foods in the diet or by vegetarianism (Abrams et al., 1996; Dorea, 2000; Lönnerdal, 2000). Breastmilk iron is affected by the mother's iron intake only when the mother is severely anemic, but not in those women with mild to moderate anemia (Kumar et al., 2008).

Unless the infant is anemic, iron supplementation is not usually needed and may, in fact, be detrimental to the breastfeeding baby during the first 6 months after birth. Excess iron tends to saturate lactoferrin, thereby diminishing its anti-infective properties. The authors of a randomized double-blind controlled trial concluded that routine iron supplementation of Swedish and Honduran breastfed infants with normal hemoglobin presented a greater risk of diarrhea (Dewey et al., 2002).

Calcium

Like iron, calcium appears in only small quantities in human milk (20–34 mg/dL), yet babies absorb 67% of the calcium in human milk as compared to only 25% of that in cow milk. Neonatal hypocalcemia and tetany are more commonly seen in the formula-fed infant, because cow milk has a much higher concentration of phosphorus (its calcium/phosphorus ratio is 1.2:1.0 versus the ratio of 2:1 seen in human milk), which leads to decreased absorption and increased excretion of calcium. Calcium and phosphorus supplements are sometimes given to breastfed infants with low birth weight, who should be monitored for hypercalcemia (calcium > 11 mg/dL) (Steichen et al., 1987).

Magnesium

Magnesium is present in low levels in breastmilk and decreases in mature milk over the course of 3 to 6 months (Picciano, 2001). Women who have been treated with magnesium sulfate for preeclampsia have high milk magnesium concentrations for the first day postpartum. After that time, levels return to normal (Lönnerdal, 2000).

Other Minerals

Copper levels are highest on the first few days postpartum, decrease for about 5 to 6 months, and then tend to remain stable. The mother's serum levels have no influence on milk concentration (Dorea, 2000). Selenium concentrations are usually higher in human milk than in formula (Kumpulainen et al., 1987; Smith et al., 1982). Minute amounts of aluminum, iodine, chromium, and fluorine are also found in breastmilk.

Formula-fed infants ingest as much as 80 times more manganese than do breastfed infants. Because manganese enters the neonatal brain at a much higher rate than in the adult brain, neonates are at risk of neurotoxicity from excess manganese. High manganese levels in infant formula have been identified as being possibly related to neurocognitive deficits (Tran et al., 2002).

Very little is known about the mechanisms or control of the secretion of trace elements into human milk.

Preterm Milk

The milk of a woman who delivers a preterm infant is different from that of a woman who delivers at term, probably to meet the special needs of the low-birth-weight neonate. Compared with term breastmilk, preterm breastmilk has higher levels of energy, lipids, protein, nitrogen, fatty acids, some vitamins, and minerals (see again Table 4-2). In addition, preterm breastmilk has higher levels of immune factors, including cells, immunoglobulins, and anti-inflammatory elements than term breastmilk. The *Breastfeeding the Preterm Infant* chapter discusses preterm breastmilk in more detail.

Anti-infective Properties

Breastmilk offers the newborn protection against disease and can reduce the risk of death for infants. When researchers compared Centers for Disease Control and Prevention (CDC) records of children who died between 28 days and 1 year, children who were breastfed had 20% lower risk of dying between 28 days and 1 year than children who were not breastfed. The longer the breastfeeding, the lower the risk for illness (Chen & Rogan, 2004).

Only in the last few decades have investigators begun to identify the specific anti-infective components of human milk that make it a peerless substance for feeding the human infant. Breastmilk has been viewed from ancient times as living tissue, and rightly so. This "white blood" contains enzymes, immunoglobulins, and leukocytes in abundance. These components, one frequently enhancing the

efficacy of another, account for most of the unique anti-infective properties of human milk. In some cultures, fresh breastmilk is used as eye drops to treat conjunctivitis; elsewhere, it is common practice to apply breastmilk on the skin to heal cracked nipples. Breastmilk provides several tiers of defense against diseases of infants, including a top tier of secretory antibodies against specific pathogens, followed by a tier of fatty acids and lactoferrin that provide broad-spectrum protection, followed by glycoconjugates and oligosaccharides, each protecting against one or more specific pathogens (Newburg et al., 1998). Table 4-3 lists the major components of human milk and their functions.

Recent innovations to infant formula have included probiotics as a way of making the flora of formula-fed babies more like that of the breastfed baby. Probiotics are viable nonpathogenic bacteria, so-called healthy bacteria that colonize the intestine and modify the intestinal microflora to contain less pathogenic bacteria than are present in formula-fed infants. Prebiotics are nondigestible food components that stimulate the growth of bifidobacteria. Oligosaccharides, which are prebiotic soluble fibers, play an important role in postnatal development of intestinal flora but have not been found in infant formulas until recently. Infant formulas containing probiotics and prebiotics are new on the market, leading formula companies to compete against one another to advertise and sell these products.

Human milk can be called a "symbiotic," referring to a mixture of probiotics and prebiotics that is beneficial to the infant by improving the survival and implantation of live dietary microorganisms in the gastrointestinal tract. Breastmilk provides a continuous source of microbes to the infant's gastrointestinal tract during the first few weeks after birth. Bacteria commonly isolated include staphylococci, streptococci, micrococci, lactobacilli, and enterococci. Although we tend to think of these bacteria as producing disease, some are natural microbes; once in the gastrointestinal tract, such bacteria stimulate the neonate's immune system to grow, thereby helping to protect the infant against infectious diseases (Martin et al., 2005). Microbes that colonize the neonate's gastrointestinal tract

Table 4-3 MAJOR COMPONENTS OF HUMAN MILK AND THEIR FUNCTIONS

Cells	Function
Phagocytes (macrophages)	Engulf and absorb pathogens; release IgA; polymorphonuclear and mononuclear.
Lymphocytes	T cells and B cells; essential for cell-mediated immunity; antiviral activity; memory T cells give long-term protection.
Anti-inflammatory Factors	
Prostaglandins PGE1, PGE2	Cytoprotective
Cytokines/chemokines	Immunodulating agents that bind to specific cellular receptors, activate the immune system, promote mammary growth, and move lymphocytes into breastmilk and across neonatal bowel wall. TGF-β is the dominating cytokine in colostrum.
Growth factors	Promote gut maturation, epithelial cell growth. EGF is a type of cytokine.
Enzymes	
Amylase	Facilitates infant digestion of polysaccharides.
Lipase	Hydrolizes fat in infant intestine; bacteriocidal activity.
Growth Factors/Hormones	
Human growth factors	Polypeptides that stimulate proliferation of intestinal mucosa and epithelium; strengthens mucosal barrier to antigens.
Cortisol, insulin, thyroxine cholecystokinin (CCK)	Promotes maturation of the neonate's intestine and intestinal host-defense process. Thyroxin protects against hypothyroidism; CCK enhances digestion.
Prolactin	Enhances development of B and T lymphocytes.
Lipids (Fat)	Major source of calories.
Long-chain polyunsaturated fatty acids (LC-PUFA)	DHA and AA associated with higher visual acuity and cognitive ability; breastmilk content dependent on maternal diet.
Free fatty acids (FFA)	Anti-infective effects.
Triglycerides	Largest source of calories for infant; broken down to free fatty acids and glycerol by lipase; types of fat depend on maternal diet.
Lactose	Carbohydrate, major energy source; breaks down into galactose and glucose; enhances absorption of Ca, Mg, and Mn.
Oligosaccharides	Microbial and viral ligands.
Glycoconjugates	Microbial and viral ligands.
Minerals	Regulates normal body functions; minimal influence by maternal diet.
Protein	
Whey	Contains lactoferrin, lysozyme, and immunoglobulins, alpha-lactalbumin.
Immunoglobulins (SIgA, IgM, IgG)	Immunity response to specific antigens in environment. SIgA pathways to mammary gland called GALT and BALT.
Lactoferrin	Antibacterial especially against *E. coli*; iron carrier.

Table 4-3 MAJOR COMPONENTS OF HUMAN MILK AND THEIR FUNCTIONS (CONTINUED)

Cells	Function
Lysozyme	Bacteriocidal and anti-inflammatory; activity progressively increases starting 6 months after delivery.
Taurine	Abundant amino acid; associated with early brain maturation and retinal development.
Casein	Inhibits microbial adhesion to mucosal membranes.
Vitamins A, C, E	Anti-inflammatory action; scavenges oxygen radicals.
Water	Constitutes 87.5% of human milk volume; provides adequate hydration to infant.

during and after birth are safest if they come from the mother because she can provide a defense against them. These microbes, especially those in the gastrointestinal tract, serve as a stimulus for the growth and development of the infant's immune system (Larsson, 2004).

Studies continue to reaffirm the significance of breastmilk in preventing infections (Dewey et al., 1995; Frank et al., 1982; Kovar et al., 1984; Kramer et al., 2001; Pullan et al., 1980; Rosenberg, 1989; Victora et al., 1987). These studies have been joined by additional new research showing reductions in otitis media, respiratory tract infections, bronchiolitis, atopic disease, gasteroenteritis, and sudden infant death syndrome (SIDS) in breastfed infants. Specifically, evidence of protection following exclusive breastfeeding is seen in otitis, respiratory disease, gastroenteritis, atopic disease, SIDS, and cognitive development (Eidelman et al., 2012; Ip et al., 2007). The evidence is strongest for bacterial infections, gastroenteritis, and necrotizing enterocolitis but is less convincing for respiratory infections (Kramer et al., 2001).

Gastroenteritis and Diarrheal Disease

Wherever infant morbidity and mortality are high, breastfeeding conclusively helps to prevent infantile diarrhea and gastrointestinal infections (Almroth & Latham, 1982; Brown et al., 1989; Clavano, 1982; Duffy et al., 1986; Espinoza et al., 1997;

Grantham-McGregor & Back, 1972; Habicht et al., 1988; Jason et al., 1984; Koopman et al., 1985; Kovar et al., 1984; Mitra & Rabbani, 1995; Perera et al., 1999; Ravelomanana et al., 1995; Ruuska, 1992). Breastfeeding minimizes diarrhea both by providing protective factors and by reducing exposure to other foods or water that may contain enteropathogens (Van Derslice et al., 1994). As antibiotic resistance becomes a global problem, discoveries about the protective effects of breastfeeding become even more important (Hakansson et al., 2000).

Such protection is dose dependent, however. In a review of field studies conducted to identify the effect of breastfeeding on childhood diarrhea in Bangladesh, children who were partially breastfed had a greater risk of diarrhea than had those who were exclusively breastfed (Glass & Stoll, 1989). Although breastmilk's protective effect is most easily demonstrated in areas of poverty and malnutrition, evidence of this protection can be seen worldwide. In China, Chen, Yu, and Li (1988) showed that compared with breastfed infants, artificially fed infants are more likely to be admitted to the hospital for gastroenteritis and other conditions. In the Cebu region of the Philippines, giving water, teas, and other liquids to breastfed babies doubled or tripled the likelihood of diarrhea (Popkin et al., 1990). Young Nicaraguan children who develop rotavirus infections very early in life are partially protected by specific IgA antibodies in their mothers' milk. Rotavirus in stool samples of such children was found to be correlated significantly with the concentration of antirotavirus IgA antibodies in colostrum (Espinoza et al., 1997). Canadian infants exclusively breastfed for the first 2 months had significantly fewer episodes of diarrhea than did infants bottle-fed from birth (Chandra, 1979). Breastfed children in Burma required less oral rehydration solution compared to those who were not breastfed during the early acute phase of diarrhea and recovered from diarrhea more quickly (Khin-Maung-U et al., 1985).

A major methodological problem in breastfeeding research on disease is the dose-response effect—the greater the amount of breastmilk the infant receives, the greater the protection against disease; protection improves with the duration of breastfeeding. A lack of a clear consistent definition of breastfeeding is a flaw in many breastfeeding studies given the fact that there is a wide variation in feeding practices and that mothers often erroneously report supplements given to the infant (Aarts et al., 2000; Zaman et al., 2002). Moreover, it is neither feasible nor ethical to randomly assign mother–infant dyads to breastfeeding or formula-feeding groups.

Kramer et al. (2001) got around this problem by looking at infant outcomes of hospitals and clinics in Belarus that introduced breastfeeding-friendly hospital initiatives and comparing them with outcomes of hospitals and clinics that continued their traditional practices. Their results indicated that infants at the intervention site were more likely to breastfeed to any degree at 12 months and were more likely to be exclusively breastfeeding at 3 and 6 months. The risk of gastrointestinal infections and atopic eczema were significantly lower in the intervention group, but a significant reduction in respiratory tract infection was not observed. A follow-up study (years 2002–2005) involving the children who were in the breastfeeding promotion intervention modeled on the Baby-Friendly Hospital Initiative scored higher means on the Wechsler Intelligence Test (Kramer et al., 2008).

Epidemiological evidence indicates that human milk continues to confer protection even with supplementation. Indeed, partial breastfeeding is better than no breastfeeding at all. This protection is specific to pathogens in the mother's and infant's environment. Moreover, the infant receives protection against the pathogens it is most likely to encounter. Table 4-4 summarizes the ameliorating and protective effects of human milk. This table assumes that breastfeeding is the norm and that artificial feeding is a deviation from the norm that brings about hazards to infant health.

Two infant health problems exacerbated by lack of breastfeeding—respiratory illness and otitis media—are discussed next. Other disease-related issues are discussed throughout this text. The impact of exclusive breastfeeding on the economy is stunning. If 90% of U.S. families would comply with medical recommendations to breastfeed exclusively for 6 months after birth, the United States would save $1.3 billion per year and prevent 911 infant deaths (Bartick & Reinhold, 2010). If babies are not breastfed for a year or more, the added costs to the healthcare system for four illnesses would total more than $1 billion (Riordan, 1997).

Respiratory Illness

Studies of the protective effects of breastfeeding against respiratory tract infections are conflicting and complex because of errors in parents' reports and other conditions not related to feeding. Several studies suggest that breastfeeding helps to prevent respiratory illnesses (Abdulmoneim & Al-Gamdi, 2001; Cushing et al., 1998; Lopez-Alarcon et al., 1997), whereas others indicate that this practice provides little protection (Dewey et al., 1995; Kramer et al., 2001). There is, however, strong evidence that breastmilk protects against respiratory syncytial virus (RSV) infection (Bell et al., 1988; Downham et al., 1976; Duffy et al., 1986; Holberg et al., 1991; Naficy et al., 1999; Newburg et al., 1998; Rahman et al., 1987). Downham et al. (1976) compared 115 infants hospitalized with RSV who were younger than 12 months with 162 control infants. Only 7% of the hospitalized infants were breastfed, compared with 27.5% of the control infants—a statistically significant difference. In the case of pneumonia caused by *Streptococcus*, researchers

Table 4-4 AMELIORATION OF DISEASE IN INFANTS AND CHILDREN BY HUMAN MILK

Disease in Child	Ameliorating Properties of Human Milk
Acrodermatitis enteropathica	More efficient zinc absorption (Evans & Johnson, 1980).
Appendicitis	Anti-inflammatory properties (Pisacane et al., 1995b).
Asthma	Introduction of milk other than human milk prior to four months is a risk factor for asthma at age 6 years (Dell & To, 2001; Oddy, 2000). Risk of asthma reduced 4% with each additional month of exclusive breastfeeding (Oddy et al., 2004). Breastfeeding provides protection against asthma in children with family history of atopy (Gdalevich et al., 2001), especially if the child is exposed to tobacco smoke (Chulada et al., 2003).
Atherosclerosis	Having been breastfed is inversely associated with carotid intima-media thickness, carotid plaque, and femoral plaque (Martin et al., 2005).
Bacterial infections, neonatal sepsis	Leukocytes, lactoferrin, immune properties (Ashraf et al., 1993; Fallot, Boyd & Oski, 1980; Leventhal et al., 1986).
Cardiovascular disease	Dietary cholesterol in infancy elevates plasma total cholesterol levels through direct mechanisms that persists only until weaning (Demmers et al., 2005). High adult erythrocyte sedimentation rate, a moderate risk factor for coronary heart disease among those bottle-fed compared to those breastfed (Gunnarsdottir et al., 2007).
Celiac disease	Longer duration and greater exclusivity of breastfeeding associated with later diagnosis. Protects against development of villous atrophy in intestinal mucosa. Later introduction of gluten in breastfeeders (Ascher et al., 1997; Auricchio, 1983; Bouguerra et al., 1998; Greco et al., 1988; Ivarsson et al., 2000; Kelly et al., 1989; Logan, 1990).
Childhood cancer (lymphoma, leukemia, neuroblastoma)	Modulates and strengthens defenses against carcinogenic insult by enhancing long-term development of infant immune system (Davis, 1998). Cancer cells undergo apoptosis (destruction) in human milk (Bener, Denic, & Galadari, 2001; Daniels et al., 2002; Davis, Savitz, & Graubard, 1988; Franke, Custer, & Tanaka, 1998; Gimeno & de Suza, 1997; Hakansson et al., 1995; Kwan et al., 2004; Martin et al., 2005; Mathur et al., 1993; Shu et al., 1995; Smulevich et al., 1999; Svanborg et al., 2003); Swartzbaum et al., 1991).
Colitis	Less exposure to cow's milk proteins (Anveden-Hertzberg, 1996; Jenkins et al., 1984; Rigas et al., 1993).
Crohn's disease	Uncertain (Bergstrand & Hellers, 1983; Koletzko et al., 1989; Rigas et al., 1993).
Diabetes, type 1 (IDDM)	Lack of antigenic peptides helps protect against autoimmune disease. Lessens risk 2–26%. Short duration of breastfeeding associated with induction of beta-cell autoantibodies (Borch-Johnson et al., 1984; Gimeno & de Suza, 1997; Kostraba et al., 1993; Mayer et al., 1988; Perez-Bravolt et al., 1996; Rosenbauer, Herzig, & Giani, 2008; Verge et al., 1994; Virtanen et al., 1992; Wahlberg, Vaarala, & Ludvigsson, 2006; Wasmuth & Kolb, 2000; and many more articles).
Dental caries	Less occurrence of dental caries (Erickson, 1999).

(continues)

Table 4-4 AMELIORATION OF DISEASE IN INFANTS AND CHILDREN BY HUMAN MILK (CONTINUED)

Disease in Child	Ameliorating Properties of Human Milk
Gastrointestinal infection/diarrheal disease	Humoral and cellular anti-infectious factors (Dewey et al., 1995; Espinoza et al., 1997; Howie et al., 1990; Long et al., 1999; Sadeharju et al., 2007). Numerous other studies discussed throughout this text.
Gastroesophageal reflux	More rapid gastric emptying; lower esophageal pH (Heacock et al., 1992).
Hypertrophic pyloric stenosis	Uncertain; breastfeeding may prevent pyloric spasm and edema (Habbick, Kahnna, & To, 1989).
Hypertension	Children breastfed until at least 6 months have lower systolic blood pressure than those breastfed for a shorter duration (Lawlor, 2004).
Inguinal hernia	Hormones in breastmilk might stimulate neonatal testicular function to close inguinal canal and promote descent of testes. One-fourth incidence (Pisacane et al., 1995a).
Juvenile rheumatoid arthritis	Anti-inflammatory properties protect against autoimmune disease (Mason et al., 1995).
Liver disease	Protease inhibitors (including antitrypsin) protect children with alpha-antitrypsin deficiency (Udall et al., 1985).
Malocclusion	Physiological suckling patterns (Labbok & Hendershot, 1987).
Multiple sclerosis	Protects against autoimmune disease (Pisacane et al., 1994).
Necrotizing enterocolitis	Immunological factors, macrophages, osmolarity of human milk, high levels of platelet-activating acetyl-hydrolase; suppression of (IL)-8 (Akisu et al., 1998; Lucas & Cole, 1990; Minekawa et al., 2004).
Otitis media	Antibody, T- and B-cell protection; lack of irritation from cow's milk; upright feeding position (Aniansson et al., 1994; Duncan et al., 1993; Sassen, Brand, & Grote, 1994).
Oral development	Fewer malocclusions and reduced need for orthodontic intervention because breastfed children have well-rounded, U-shaped dental arch. Fewer problems with snoring and sleep apnea in later life (Palmer, 1998).
Respiratory syncytial virus	IgA, IgG antibody transmitted to breastmilk and infant through gut-associated or bronchus-associated lymphoid tissue (GALT & BALT). Lactadherin, a glycoprotein, binds to rotavirus and inhibits activity (Bell, 1988; Duffy et al., 1986; Holberg et al., 1991; Naficy et al., 1999; Newburg, et al., 1998; Rahman et al., 1987).
Lower respiratory tract disease	Meta-analysis of 33 studies on healthy infants in developed nations. Severe respiratory tract illnesses with hospitalization were tripled for infants who were not breastfed compared with those who were exclusively breastfed for 4 months (Bachrach, Schwarz, & Bachrach, 2003).
Retinopathy of prematurity	Antioxidants (inositol, vitamin E, beta-carotene) and DHA may protect against the development of retinopathy of prematurity (Hylander et al., 2001).
Sudden infant death syndrome	Uncertain; possibly anti-infectious, antiallergic (Ford et al., 1993; Gilbert et al., 1995; Kum-Nji, 2001).
Urinary tract infections	Antibacterial properties (sIgA) bind to bacteria and prevent them from reaching the urinary tract. Protection is greatest in girls (Marild et al., 2004; Pisacane et al., 1990).

discovered a novel folding variant of α-lactalbumin that is a naturally occurring antibacterial compound in breastmilk (Hakansson et al., 2000).

As with gastroenteritis, the preventive effect of breastmilk can be seen on a global scope. When Chen, Yu, and Li (1988) looked for an association between type of feeding and hospitalization of infants in Shanghai, they found that artificial feeding was associated with more frequent hospitalizations for respiratory infections during the first 18 months of life. About one-fourth of hospitalizations of U.K. infants with lower respiratory tract infection could have been prevented if those infants had been exclusively breastfed (Quigley et al., 2007). In Brazil, babies who were not breastfed were 17 times more likely than those who were exclusively breastfed to be admitted to the hospital for pneumonia (Cesar et al., 1999). Similar protection has been established for *Haemophilus influenzae* bacteremia and meningitis (Cochi et al., 1986; Istre et al., 1985; Takala et al., 1989).

Otitis Media

Breastfeeding protects against ear infections (otitis media) for reasons that are not completely clear. However, immunological factors, the feeding position, and lack of irritation from bovine-based formula may explain this phenomenon. Saarinen et al. (1982) followed healthy term infants for 3 years. Prior to 6 months of age, no infant had otitis during the period of exclusive breastfeeding, whereas 10% of the babies who were given any cow milk did. These significant differences persisted up to 3 years of age. Other studies (Aniansson et al., 1994; Dewey et al., 1995) support an inverse relationship between ear infections and breastfeeding.

Controversies and Claims

In contrast to global evidence that breastfeeding helps to protect infants against health problems, Bauchner, Levanthal, and Shapiro (1986) and Leventhal et al. (1986) challenged the claim that breastfeeding protects infants in developed countries, citing lack of control for potentially confounding factors, such as low birth weight, parental smoking, crowding, sanitation, and other characteristics of socioeconomic status. Howie et al. (1990) settled this controversy by examining the effect of breastfeeding on childhood illness in Scotland in a study using an adequate sample that met the methodological criteria set by Bauchner et al. (1986). Howie concluded that breastfeeding during the first 13 weeks of life confers protection against gastrointestinal illness beyond the period of breastfeeding itself.

A few years later, Fuchs, Victor, and Martines (1996) questioned this long-term protection for diarrhea. They found that children who had stopped breastfeeding in the previous 2 months were vulnerable to developing dehydrating diarrhea. Certain supplemental foods, such as herbal teas, prolonged diarrheal disease in Mexican children (Long et al., 1999).

In a prospective multicenter study on the effect of breastmilk in preventing necrotizing enterocolitis in premature infants, Lucas and Cole (1990) found that the disease was 6 to 10 times more common in exclusively formula-fed babies than in exclusively breastfed babies. This held true even though the human milk received was often pooled and not derived from the baby's mother. These findings support the contention that breastfeeding is more than a lifestyle choice; it has profound implications for the health of the child.

Parents sometimes ask how long breastmilk's protective effects last. Table 4-5 presents research on the length of breastfeeding and expected protection.

Chronic Disease Protection

The protection offered by breastmilk against illness extends beyond infancy to childhood and adulthood. Breastfeeding contributes to prevention of celiac disease, diabetes, multiple sclerosis, sudden infant death syndrome, childhood cancer, and many other health problems that are discussed throughout this text. The longer the duration of breastfeeding and the more complete exclusivity of breastmilk, the greater its protective effect.

Table 4-5 Minimum Length of Breastfeeding for Protection Against Infectious Diseases

Health Problem	Minimum Length of Breastfeeding	Length of Protection	Source
Gastroenteritis/diarrheal disease	13 weeks	7 years	Howie, 1990
Otitis media	4 months	3 years	Duncan et al., 1993
Respiratory infections	15 weeks	7 years	Wilson et al., 1998
Wheezing bronchitis	—	6–7 years	Burr et al., 1993; Porro et al., 1993
Haemophilus influenzae, type b	—	10 years	Silfverdal et al., 1997
Hodgkin's disease	6 months	Not specified	Davis, 1998

Childhood Cancer

Does a mother's milk modulate the interaction between the developing infant immune system and infectious agents that protects an infant against carcinogenic insults? The evidence on this point is conflicting. When Davis (1998) reviewed nine case-control studies on the association between infant feeding and childhood cancer, she confirmed that children who are never breastfed or are breastfed for a short term have a higher risk of developing Hodgkin's disease than those who are breastfed for at least 6 months. It is possible that a type of human α-lactalbumin found in breastmilk lessens the risk of childhood cancer. This α-lactalbumin, a protein–lipid complex called HAMLET, induces apoptosis-like death in tumor cells but leaves fully differentiated cells unaffected (Hakansson et al., 1995; Svanborg et al., 2003).

A meta-analysis (Martin et al., 2005) concluded that breastfeeding reduces the risk of childhood acute lymphoblastic leukemia (ALL) and acute myeloblastic leukemia (AML); however, the public health importance of this finding may be small. Increasing breastfeeding from 50% to 100% of all infants would prevent at most 5% of cases of childhood acute leukemia or lymphoma. In another meta-analysis, Kwan et al. (2004) found that long-term breastfeeding was linked to a 24% lower risk of ALL. Breastfeeding for 6 months or less appeared

to reduce ALL risk by 12%. The next year, this same researcher concluded that there was no evidence that breastfeeding affects the occurrence of childhood ALL (Kwan et al., 2005). Evidence showing that breastfeeding is protective against childhood cancer is inconsistent.

Allergies and Atopic Disease

The incidence of food-induced allergic disease in children has been estimated to range between 0.3% and 7.5% (Metcalfe, 1984). Heredity is a significant predictor of allergic disease, even when the mother is on a milk-free diet during late pregnancy and lactation (Lovegrove et al., 1994). Sixty percent of all those who will develop atopic eczema do so within the first year of life, and 90% do so within the first 5 years. Before 6 to 9 months of age, the infant intestinal mucosa is permeable to proteins; moreover, secretory immunoglobulin A (IgA), which will later "paint" the mucosa and bind sensitizing proteins to itself, is not yet functioning effectively. After following 150 infants from birth to 17 years of age, Saarinen and Kajosaari (1995) concluded that breastfeeding is prophylactic against allergies—including eczema, food allergy, and respiratory allergy—throughout childhood and adolescence.

Cow milk is the most common single allergen affecting infants. Several proteins in cow milk are known to act as allergens, including lactoglobulin, casein, bovine serum albumin, and lactalbumin. Modern heat treatment of formula has reduced—but certainly not eliminated—the allergic potential of these proteins. The problem is probably exacerbated by the sizable dose of allergens in formula and by the large volume of formula ingested. At 2 to 4 months of age, for example, infants consume their body weight in milk each week. This is the equivalent of nearly 7 quarts per day for an adult—truly a macrodose!

Vomiting, diarrhea, colic, and occult bleeding are symptoms of allergy. This condition also affects the respiratory tract (runny nose, cough, asthma) and the skin (dermatitis, urticaria). Because its symptoms are varied and nonspecific, the diagnosis of allergy is often mistaken or missed.

At birth, the immunoglobulin E (IgE) system is defective in the potentially allergic infant, and problems arise if this system is activated by allergens. When the introduction of foreign proteins is delayed for 4 to 6 months, the baby's own IgA system is permitted to become more fully functional; thus allergic responses may be minimized or entirely avoided. Exclusive consumption of breastmilk facilitates the early maturation of the intestinal barrier and provides a passive barrier to potentially antigenic molecules until the baby's own natural barriers develop.

Chemokines such as interleukin 8 (IL-8) are present in higher concentrations in the breastmilk of allergic women who also have significantly more interleukin 4 (IL4) in their milk; the latter chemokine is needed for the production of IgE. High levels of neonatal blood IgE are thought to predict later development of atopic symptoms. When the relationship between fecal IgE levels (a reliable indicator of serum IgE levels) was compared in infants 1 month old, formula-fed babies showed a higher incidence of high fecal IgE levels than did breastfed infants (Sasi et al., 1994).

A few breastfed infants develop atopic eczema. Of those who do, the culprit is often foods ingested by the mother—especially cow milk. Cow milk antigen can be detected in breastmilk

(Axelsson et al., 1986; Cavagni et al., 1988; Odze et al., 1995; Paganelli et al., 1986). Early and occasional exposure to cow milk protein sensitizes neonates so that even minute amounts of bovine milk protein in human milk may later act as booster doses that elicit allergic reactions (Host et al., 1988). Prolonged breastfeeding exclusively or combined with infrequent exposure to small amounts of cow milk during the first 8 weeks induces the development of IgE-mediated cow milk allergy (Saarinen et al., 2000). By almost completely excluding milk, other dairy products, eggs, fish, beef, and peanuts from mothers' diets throughout pregnancy and lactation, Chandra et al. (1986) documented a significant reduction in the incidence and severity of atopic eczema among breastfed infants of these mothers at high risk for allergy.

The "hygiene hypothesis" maintains that early exposure to microbes helps prevent allergies in children. As Larsson (2004) explains it, normal bacteria in the gut are important for the maturation of the immune system so that it learns to react against microbes rather than its own tissue. The infant who is exposed early to microbes develops an immunological tolerance to food, pollen, mites, and other structures instead of reacting against them, causing allergic reactions. Thus having pets such as cats or dogs and ingestion or inhalation of endotoxin-containing material appears to help prevent allergies (Larsson, 2004).

Although an enormous number of epidemiological studies have been published on breastfeeding and risk of atopic disease in children, their results remain inconsistent. The reasons for the different outcomes are probably related to flaws in study design such as absence of control of family history (Pohlabeln et al., 2010). When the infant is identified as breastfed, does that mean that the baby received no other nutriments? If so, for how long was breastfeeding continued? After conducting a meta-analysis of 22 original research reports on infant feeding and atopic disease, Kramer (1988) decided that errors in the research methods used to investigate these issues have often led to conflicting results and seriously flawed study designs.

Asthma

Outcomes of epidemiological and clinical studies on asthma and breastfeeding are inconsistent, and the longstanding question of whether breastfeeding prevents or reduces the incidence of asthma has been controversial. To help settle this question, Gdalevich, Mimouni, and Mimouni (2001) conducted a meta-analysis of research on the effect of breastfeeding on bronchial asthma. They found 41 studies that showed a protective effect, 5 studies that had no association, and 2 studies that had a positive association. Twelve of these studies were prospective and met the standards for study methodology as determined by Kramer (1988). Meta-analysis of these 12 studies showed that exclusive breastfeeding during the first months after birth is associated with lower asthma rates during childhood (odds ratio [OR], 0.70; 95% confidence interval [CI], 0.60 to 0.81). Oddy (2000, 2004) has carefully researched the effect of breastfeeding on asthma in children in Western Australia. He has found an association with less exclusive breastfeeding and asthma.

Finally, in regard to breastfeeding's protective effect against chronic disease, Palmer (1998) makes a convincing case that artificial feedings alter normal early oral cavity development so much that it can cause later problems such as snoring, sleep apnea, and malocclusion. For the mother herself, breastfeeding promotes health because it helps to prevent breast and ovarian cancer (see the *Women's Health and Breastfeeding* chapter).

The Immune System

The notion of a separate immune system as an integral part of a body capable of fighting disease at all of the body's surfaces is relatively new, having emerged in the mid-1900s. Although it had long appeared that breastfeeding enhances immunity, a cause–effect relationship was not acknowledged as a scientific fact until more was known about the existence of an immune system outside of the bloodstream (Koerber, 2006). Because the human immune system is not fully developed at birth,

infants are particularly vulnerable to infections and gastrointestinal illnesses. Breastmilk stimulates and supplements the infant's developing immune system.

The body's overall immune system is known as the systemic immune system. Another immune system, the secretory immune system, involves surfaces of the body (such as the breast) and acts locally. Lymphocytes in the secretory immune system differ from other lymphocytes. Sensitized to antigens found in the gastrointestinal or the respiratory tracts, these lymphocytes travel through mucosal lymphoid tissues (e.g., breasts, salivary glands, bronchi, intestines, and genitourinary tract), where they secrete antibodies.

Most antigens to which a mother has been exposed sensitize lymphocytes migrating to the breast. There they secrete immunoglobulins into the milk—hence, the term "secretory IgA" (sIgA). These components are described later in this chapter where immunoglobulins are discussed. Lawrence and Pane (2007) have presented an extensive review of the immunology of human milk.

Active Versus Passive Immunity

Immunity occurs both actively and passively. Maternal antibodies passed to the fetus through the placenta before birth represent an example of passive immunity. Passive immunological protection is only temporary, as the infant's immune system has not itself responded.

Breastfeeding can also confer long-term protection by stimulating an active immune response. Active immunity is a specific immunity whereby the immune system formulates a long-term memory of exposure to a certain antigen. Later exposure to the same antigen will produce an immune response. Poliovirus or rubella immunization or any attenuated virus immunization of the mother provides active immunity to the infant, as the virus will likely appear in her milk, thereby immunizing the infant. Reports indicate that enhanced vaccine responses are observed in breastfed infants compared with those not breastfeeding. After being vaccinated for measles–mumps–rubella (MMR), only breastfed children demonstrated increased production of interferon-gamma (Pabst et al., 1997). Another example of active immunity is the breastfed infant's immune response to cytomegalovirus in human milk.

Cells

Human milk contains two main types of white blood cells (leukocytes): phagocytes and lymphocytes (Figures 4-5 and 4-6). Although phagocytes (mostly macrophages) are the most abundant (90%) of the white blood cells, the lymphocyte population (10%) has significant protective effects in the recipient infant. The concentration of these cells and the predominant cell type vary with the duration of lactation. After birth, the number of these cells is higher than at any other time; their number declines progressively thereafter.

Phagocytes

Macrophages, a type of leukocyte, are the dominant phagocyte in human milk. They engulf and absorb pathogens. Macrophages release IgA, although they probably do not synthesize it. Macrophages are both polymorphonuclear (PMN) and mononuclear. Because PMN cell numbers increase dramatically during inflammation of the breast, they may function to protect the mammary tissue per se rather than to impart protection to the newborn (Buescher & Pickering, 1986). Macrophages also produce complement, lactoferrin, and lysozyme (discussed later in this chapter).

Neutrophils are yet another phagocytic leukocyte. Short lived but effective, they are the first white blood cells to arrive at an inflamed site, such as when mastitis occurs.

Lymphocytes

Lymphocytes are also leukocytes; they include T cells, B cells, and assorted T-cell subsets. Lymphocytes account for approximately 4% of the total leukocytes in early lactation; about 83% of the lymphocytes are T cells that appear to transfer

Figure 4-5 WHILE CELLS OF THE BLOOD.

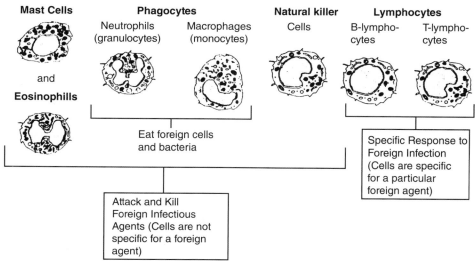

Source: Fan H, Conner R, Villareal L. *The biology of AIDS.* Boston, MA: Jones and Bartlett; 1989:28.

Figure 4-6 MICROSCOPE VIEW OF LIVING CELLS IN HUMAN MILK. THE 4000 CELLS PER CENTIMETER OF HUMAN MILK CONSIST MAINLY OF MACROPHAGES AND T-CELL AND B-CELL LYMPHOCYTES. MACROPHAGES SECRETE LYZOZYME, WHICH HELP DESTROY THE CELL WALLS OF BACTERIA.

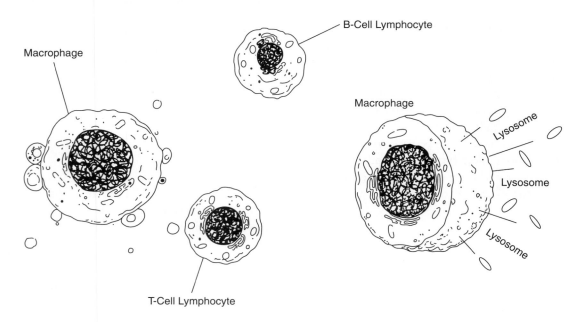

through human milk to infants (Wirt et al., 1992). The various ways in which lymphocytes recognize and help to destroy antigens are collectively called cell-mediated immunity. Such immunity is important in the destruction of viruses, because the cells within which viruses live shield them from the action of antibodies. Formula-fed and breastfed infants possess different types of lymphocyte subsets (Hawkes & Gibson, 2001).

A population of white blood cells that decreases rapidly in the first week after birth and continues to decline steadily, T cells are a special and separate immune component that can be activated into memory T cells (Wirt et al., 1992). These memory cells are the key to active immunity. Antibodies persist for only a few weeks before breaking down; however, memory cells can live for years, providing long-lasting protection. It is not clear whether T cells are activated in human milk or whether some

specific homing of activated and memory T lymphocytes to the breast occurs.

B cells have functional capabilities similar to those of T cells. They mature into plasma-like cells that travel to epithelial tissues in the breast and release antibodies (Bellig, 1995; Newman, 1995) that reflect exposure to pathogens encountered in their environment. For example, milk from mothers living in Nigeria and exposed to malaria was compared with milk from a control population of mothers living in Washington, DC. The Nigerian mothers carried a high IgA level of antimalaria antibodies compared with the Washington mothers (Kassim et al., 2000).

Stem Cells

Australian Mark Cregan (Cregan et al., 2007), a molecular biologist who studies the complex cellular components of human milk, was the first to

Figure 4-7 MAMMARY STEM CELLS ISOLATED FROM HUMAN BREASTMILK.

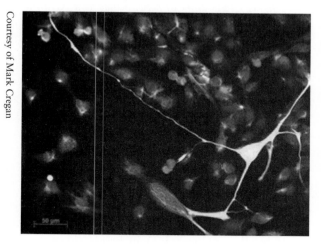

Courtesy of Mark Cregan

This is an exciting development because it opens up the possibility of a nonfetal—and, therefore, less controversial—source of stem cells for regenerative medicine in conditions such as diabetes, Parkinson's disease, and spinal injuries. This readily available and noninvasive source of multiple lineages of mammary stem cells could be used to treat a multitude of health problems.

Cregan's finding of stem cells indicates that breastmilk does much more than provide for the baby›s nutritional needs. Just as immune cells transferred through breastmilk have been shown to survive in the digestive tract of infants, so further research may well demonstrate that stem cells guide the baby's development and disease resistance ex utero as a new mother's mammary glands take over from the placenta.

The stem cell content of human milk ranges between 10,000 and 13 million cells/mL; therefore infants ingest thousands to millions of viable stem cells with every breastfeeding. The amount varies widely between studies and also between women from a single study. Colostrum and early-lactation milk often contain more cells than mature breastmilk. The presence of stem cells in human milk shows the ability of breastmilk cells to expand in culture and for colony types.

Breast stem cells are alive when consumed by the baby, which suggests they might have benefits beyond what is currently known. More study of this issue may revolutionize the fields of lactation and physiology and open new avenues for understanding the importance of breastfeeding from a biosystem perspective rather than as simply a source of food.

discover stem cells in breastmilk. Cregan's research team cultured cells from breastmilk and found some of them contained the protein nestin, which acts as a marker that allows for the identification and isolation of stem cells. Embryonic stem cells were previously known to exist in amniotic fluid and in the umbilical cord, but the breastmilk discovery marked the first time these cells had been found in an adult (Figure 4-7).

Since Cregan's discovery, embryonic stem cells, which account for approximately 2% of all cells in human breastmilk, have been harvested in large quantities. Mammary stem cells exist in a quiescent state but become activated during pregnancy and lactation as they undergo a controlled program of proliferation, differential action, and apoptosis (death) stimulated by hormones.

In 2012, researcher Foteini Hassiotou published a paper in the journal *Stem Cells* demonstrating that breastmilk stem cells can turn into cells that represent all three embryonic germ layers: endoderm, mesoderm, and ectoderm. These basic cells have the potential to differentiate into specialized cells such as pancreatic cells that produce their own insulin.

Antibodies and Immunoglobulins

Antibodies are immunoglobulins that recognize and act on a particular antigen. Immunoglobulins are proteins produced by plasma cells in response to an immunogen. There are five types of immunoglobulins: IgG, IgA, IgM, IgE, and IgD. Both IgA and IgE play critical roles in the biological specificity of human milk for the recipient infant.

Secretory IgA (sIgA) is the major immuno-globulin in human secretions. sIgA provides the initial bolus that supplements immunoglobulins transferred earlier across the placenta to the fetus. It is the immunoglobulin most frequently noted in medical literature as having immense immuno-logical value to the neonate. The concentration of sIgA, which is both synthesized and stored in the breast, may reach up to 5 mg/mL in colostrum; it then decreases to 1 mg/mL in mature milk. Inter-leukin-6 in human milk may be partly responsible for the genesis of IgA- and IgM-producing cells in the mammary gland (Rudloff et al., 1993). As the mother yields more milk, the infant receives more sIgA, so that the total dose of sIgA the baby receives throughout lactation is constant or even increases (depending on the milk intake). Mothers of infants with a systemic infection and poor suckling have higher IgA levels in their breastmilk (Feist et al., 2000), and low-income women have nearly three times the milk sIgA of high-income women (Groer et al., 2004).

Synthesis of sIgA via the secretory immune sys-tem utilizes an elegant lymphocyte traffic pathway called gut-associated lymphoid tissue (GALT) or bronchus-associated lymphoid tissue (BALT). This pathway leads to the development of lymphoid cells in the mammary gland, which produce IgA antibodies after exposure to specific microbial or environmental antigens on the intestinal or the respiratory mucosa (Goldman et al., 1983; Oka-moto & Ogra, 1989). The migration of immuno-logical responsiveness from both BALT and GALT to the mammary glands supports the unique con-cept of a common mucosal immune system.

Because the infant's own IgA is deficient and increases only slowly during the first several months after birth, sIgA in human milk provides important passive immunological protection to the digestive tract of newborn infants. sIgA protects the new-born's entire intestinal tract. It is only minimally absorbed from the intestine because it is bound to the human milk fat globule membrane, travels through the newborn's entire intestinal tract, and is found unaltered in the newborn feces (Schroten et al., 1999).

A number of IgA antibodies in human milk appear to act upon viruses or bacteria that cause respiratory and gastrointestinal tract infections. These infecting agents include *Escherichia coli*, *Vib-rio cholerae*, *Clostridium difficile*, *Salmonella*, *Giardia lamblia*, *Entamoeba histolytica*, *Campylobacter*, rota-virus, and poliovirus (Pickering & Kohl, 1986; Ruiz-Palacios et al., 1990). As stated earlier, immu-nizing breastfeeding women with poliovirus or rubella creates IgA antibodies in milk that specifi-cally target these agents. IgA4 may also play a role in host defense of mucosal surfaces; in some women, IgA4 is produced locally in the mammary gland (Keller et al., 1988).

In addition to IgA, other Ig classes, including IgD, may be involved in local immunity of the breast. Several investigators (Litwin et al., 1990; Steel & Leslie, 1985) have demonstrated high lev-els of locally produced IgD in breast tissues and breastmilk. Another immune messenger, sCD14, has been found in significant quantities in breast-milk (25,100 ng/mL) versus formula (0.6 ng/mL). sCD14 plays an important role in enabling intesti-nal epithelial cells to prevent gastrointestinal gram-negative infections and stimulating the newborn immune system (Blais et al., 2006).

As shown in Figure 4-8, clear biological rhythms of protective factors predictably rise and fall as lac-tation progresses. The reasons for waxing and wan-ing of various anti-infective components are not always clear but are assumed to be adapted to the needs of the infant.

Nonantibody Antibacterial Protection

Nonantibody factors in human milk make up an elegant and intricate system that protects the infant against bacterial infection. These factors include lactoferrin, the bifidus factor, lactoperoxidase, and oligosaccharides.

Lactoferrin

Lactoferrin, a potent bacteriostatic iron-binding protein, is abundant in human milk (1–6 mg/mL) and is also present in bovine milk. Its concentration

Figure 4-8 A LONGITUDINAL STUDY OF SELECTED RESISTANCE FACTORS IN HUMAN MILK. (A) TOTAL (.) AND SECRETORY (.) IgA. (B) LYSOZYME. (C) LACTOFERRIN. (D) MACROPHAGES-NEUTROPHILS (._.) AND LYMPHOCYTES (._.).

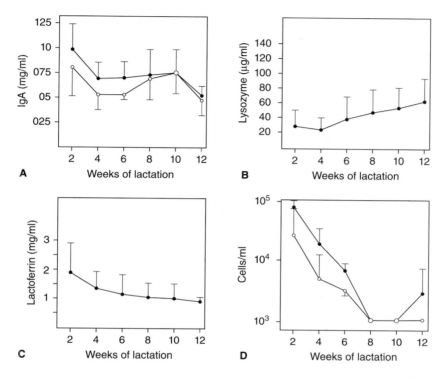

Adapted from Goldman AS, Garza C, Nichols BL, Goldblum RM. Immunologic factors in human milk during the first year of lactation. *J Pediatr.* 1982;100:563–567.

declines sevenfold as lactation progresses. Lactoferrin is present in higher proportions relative to total protein in preterm milk (de Ferrer et al., 2000). After pasteurization at 62.5°C for 30 minutes, only 39% of the original lactoferrin remains in the milk. Lactoferrin inhibits adhesion *of E. coli* to cells and helps prevent diarrheal disease (de Araujo & Giugliano, 2001). In the presence of IgA antibody and bicarbonate, it readily absorbs enteric iron, thereby preventing pathogenic organisms, particularly *E. coli* and *Candida albicans* (Borgnolo et al., 1996; Kirkpatrick et al., 1971), from obtaining the iron needed for their survival. Because exogenous iron may well interfere with the protective effects of lactoferrin, the benefits and drawbacks of giving iron supplements to the healthy breastfed infant

must be carefully weighed. Lactoferrin also has been shown to be an essential growth factor for human B and T lymphocytes (Hashizume et al., 1983) to inhibit fungal growth and a key modulator of inflammatory disorders such as cancer, allergy, and arthritis (Legrand et al., 2008).

The Bifidus Factor

The intestinal flora of breastfed infants is dominated by gram-positive lactobacilli, especially *Lactobacillus bifidus*. This bifidus factor in human milk, first recognized by Gyorgy (1953), promotes the growth of these beneficial bacteria. The buffering capacities of breastmilk (bifidus factor), together with the low protein and phosphate levels, contribute to the low pH (5–6) of stools. This acid environment, which is present even in the first days of life of the breast-feeding infant (Rubaltelli et al., 1998), discourages replication of enteropathogens such as *Shigella*, *Salmonella*, and some *E. coli* strains. This protection does not appear to be complete, however. Although breastmilk inhibits bacterial–cellular adhesion to intestinal epithelial cells (a sign of the beginning of the infectious process), it does not prevent loss of the epithelial barrier (Kohler et al., 2002). Whether the breastfed infants in the study demonstrating this point were fed other liquids and foods was not addressed.

Lactoperoxidase

Although levels of the enzyme lactoperoxidase are low in neonates, substantial amounts are present in the newborn's saliva. It is thought that IgA in milk enhances the ability of lactoperoxidase to kill streptococci.

Oligosaccharides

Oligosaccharides (carbohydrates composed of a few monosaccharides) in human milk help to block antigens from adhering to the epithelium of the gastrointestinal tract. This blocking mechanism prevents the attachment of *Pneumococcus*, which is particularly adhesive (Goldman et al., 1986). There are approximately 130 different oligosaccharides in human milk. Breastmilk contains many times the amount of oligosaccharides that is found in bovine milk or formula. Although a few formula companies have begun adding a limited number of simple oligosaccharides to infant formula, the oligosaccharides found in human milk can be thought of as 130 reasons to breastfeed (McVeagh & Miller, 1997). Because of their complexity, synthetic oligosaccharides with structures identical to human milk oligosaccharides are not yet available; instead non-milk-derived oligosaccharides are being used in formula and other foods.

Cytokines and Chemokines

Cytokines are protein signals secreted by lymphocytes, monocytes, macrophages, and other cells. Pro-inflammatory cytokines are responsible for the body responses of swelling, tenderness, and fever. Chemokines are pro-inflammatory cytokines that signal the immune system to bring in more phagocytic cells to an infected or inflamed site (Larsson, 2004). They are also called immunomodulators, in recognition of the fact that they operate in networks and orchestrate activation of the immune system (Goldman et al., 1996), probably by moving lymphocytes into breastmilk and across the neonatal bowel wall (Michie et al., 1998).

Several different cytokines and chemokines have been discovered in human milk recently, and the list is growing rapidly (Garofalo & Goldman, 1998). In addition to activating the immune system to protect the infant against infection (Wallace et al., 1997), these biologically active molecules appear to play a role in growth and differentiation of the mammary gland (Goldman et al., 1996). Groer and Shelton (2009) measured cytokines and stress levels in breastfeeding and formula-feeding women. Exercise was associated with elevated pro-inflammatory cytokines in breastmilk (Groer & Shelton, 2009); however, formula-feeding women had decreased levels of cytokines, suggesting that breastfeeding was more protective against stress. Much has yet to be learned about cytokines.

Anti-inflammatory and Immunomodulating Components

Many host defense agents in human milk have more than one function. Secretory IgA, lactoferrin, and lysozyme are examples. Human milk, which is rich in anti-inflammatory agents, supplies key protection during the vulnerable period of infancy. Major biochemical pathways of inflammations are either absent or poorly represented in breastmilk. Garofalo and Goldman (1999) identified several anti-inflammatory factors in breastmilk, such as antioxidants (vitamins A, C, and E, and enzymes), alpha$_1$-antitrypsin, cortisol, epidermal growth factor, IgA, lysozyme, prostaglandins, and cytokines. The anti-inflammatory effects of these components have not yet been directly demonstrated in the nursing infant, but they are thought to modulate cytokine responses to infection and facilitate defense mechanisms while minimizing tissue damage (Kelleher & Lönnerdal, 2001).

Goldman et al. (1996) suggest that the immunomodulating properties of human milk have a long-term influence on the development of the immune system and explain why the long-term risk for many diseases is lessened by breastfeeding. An immunomodulator changes the function of another defense agent, thereby altering the quality or magnitude of the immune response. Fibronectin in human milk is an example of an immunomodulator that acts by augmenting the clearance of bacteria and intravascular debris. Interferon-alpha is not found in human milk, yet breastfed infants with respiratory syncytial virus infection have higher blood levels of this element than nonbreastfed infants. Cytokines are also thought to immunomodulate the immune system. For example, interleukin-18, which is activated by macrophages, is present in higher concentrations in colostrum compared with early milk and mature milk. Interleukin-10 increases the development of IgA antibody production, so it plays an important role in host defense of neonates (Takahata et al., 2001). Other anti-inflammatory properties of human milk such as sIgA are more indirect.

Bioactive Components

Hamosh (2001) designates a special group of substances in human milk as bioactive components. These substances promote growth and development of the newborn by special activities that continue after the infant ingests breastmilk. Many are not available to the infant in commercial infant formula. Research on bioactive components is a growing area of investigation. These bioactive components may play a significant role in child health.

Enzymes

Mammalian milk contains a large number of enzymes, some of which appear to have a beneficial effect on the development of the newborn. The enzyme content of human milk and that of bovine milk differ substantially (Hamosh, 1996). For example, lysozyme activity is several thousand times greater in human milk than in bovine milk. The alkaline pH of the human infant's stomach has a limited effect on the antitrypsin activity of breastmilk, thereby protecting children with alpha-antitrypsin deficiency against severe liver disease and early death (Udall et al., 1985). Most mammal milks contain many enzymes that appear to be species specific because of their varying level of activity in different species. The enzymes discussed next either serve a digestive function in the infant or may be important to neonatal development.

Lysozyme

Lysozyme, a major component of human milk whey fraction, produces both bacteriocidal and anti-inflammatory action. It acts with peroxide and ascorbate to destroy *E. coli* and some *Salmonella* strains (Pickering & Kohl, 1986). Lysozyme is much more abundant in human milk (400 µg/mL) than in bovine milk. Rather than slowly declining as lactation progresses, however, lysozyme activity increases progressively, beginning about 6 months after delivery (Goldman et al., 1982; Prentice et al., 1984). Lysozyme differs from other protective factors in this respect because babies begin receiving solid foods around 6 months, and high levels of lysozyme may be a teleological, practical safeguard against the greater risk from pathogens and diarrheal disease that the infant experiences at this time.

Lipase

For human infants to digest fat, adequate lipase activity and bile salt levels must be present. The bile salt–stimulated lipase and lipoprotein lipase present in human milk compensate for immature pancreatic function and for the absence of amylase in neonates, especially in the premature infant. When human milk is frozen or refrigerated (Hamosh et al., 1997), lipase is not affected; however, heating severely reduces lipase activity. Several protozoa—*G. lamblia*, *E. histolytica*, and *Trichomonas vaginalis*—have been shown in vitro to be killed rapidly by exposure to salt-stimulated lipase, which is found only in the milk of humans and mountain gorillas (Blackberg et al., 1980).

Amylase

Amylase is necessary for the digestion of starch. Although amylase is synthesized and stored in the pancreas of the newborn, it is 6 months before this enzyme is released into the duodenum. Human milk contains about 10 to 60 times as much alpha-amylase as does normal human serum, thus providing an alternative source of this starch-digestive substance. No alpha-amylase is present in bovine, goat, or swine milk, suggesting that this enzyme appeared late in the evolutionary continuum. Breastfed infants have fewer problems digesting solid foods than do formula-fed infants, even if these foods are introduced early, because of the alpha-amylase provided by breastmilk. Amylase is stable when refrigerated; that is, it demonstrates 95–100% activity after 24 hours storage at 15–25°C (Hamosh et al., 1997).

Leptin

Leptin, a hormone that regulates appetite, food intake, and energy metabolism, is present in breastmilk but not in formula. Leptin is produced mainly by the adipose tissue and its level varies significantly between people. Leptin concentrations in breastmilk decrease with time during lactation and show significant relationships with other maternal hormones. For example, Miralles et al. (2006) demonstrated that leptin in breastmilk may regulate body weight during infancy. The higher the milk leptin concentration, the lower the infant's BMI—indicating that milk leptin could explain, at least partially, the greater risk of obesity in formula-fed infants compared with breastfed infants (Savino, Sorrenti, et al., 2012).

Growth Factors and Hormones

Human milk contains growth-promoting components also known as growth factors or growth modulators. Like the components that produce the anti-infective properties of breastmilk, these substances are more pronounced in colostrum than in mature milk. Neither their biological significance nor their method of action is clear as yet, but it appears that they have a greater synergistic effect when combined with each other. The source of growth factors is epithelial and stromal cells and macrophages in the breast. These factors exert growth-promoting and protective effects on the neonatal gastrointestinal tract that cannot be provided by commercial formula (Kobata et al., 2008). Different growth factors may have overlapping functions, both stimulating cell growth and indirectly affecting the infant's defense mechanisms against disease (Morriss et al., 1986).

Epidermal Growth Factor

Epidermal growth factor (EGF), a type of cytokine, is a major growth-promoting agent in breastmilk that stimulates proliferation of intestinal mucosa and epithelium and strengthens the mucosal barrier to antigens (Carpenter, 1980; Petschow, Carter, & Hutton, 1993). A polypeptide that contains 53 amino acids, EGF has its highest concentration in human milk after delivery; its level decreases rapidly thereafter (Matsuoka & Idota, 1995). There is no diurnal variation or variation between preterm and term milk. EGF is also present in plasma, saliva, and amniotic fluid, but human milk contains a higher concentration. This growth factor may also be involved in the development of LDL receptors and in cholesterol metabolism.

Human Milk Growth Factors I, II, and III

Three polypeptides—called human milk growth factors (HMGF) I, II, and III—have been isolated (Shing & Klagsburn, 1984). HMGF III stimulates DNA synthesis and cellular proliferation, suggesting that it is an epidermal growth factor. In vivo studies (Heird et al., 1984; Widdowson et al., 1996) on growth factors in animal milk have shown striking increases in the mass of intestinal mucosa. Growth factors in human milk influence the growth of target tissues in the breastfed infant by provoking an endogenous hormonal response that is different from that provoked by formula—a possible stimulus of nutritional programming.

Insulin-Like Growth Factor

An insulin-like growth factor (IGF-I) in human milk is thought to have a growth-promoting role. The concentration of this factor in colostrum is about 30 times that in human serum, significantly higher than the concentration in cow milk, and very low to almost absent in formula (Shehadeh et al., 2001). These high levels (4.1 nmol/L) decrease rapidly (to 1.3 nmol/L) as colostrum gives way to transitional milk (Read et al., 1984) but do not decline further. In fact, Corps et al. (1988) found that the concentration of an insulin-like growth factor in human milk increased (to 2.5 nmol/L) by the sixth week postpartum.

Thyroxine and Thyrotropin-Releasing Hormone

Thyroxine is present in human milk in small quantities but is not found in commercial formulas. Its concentration in colostrum is low, increases by the first week postpartum, and gradually declines thereafter. It has been suggested that thyroxine may stimulate the maturation of the infant's intestine (Morriss, 1985).

Although the thyroxine level is significantly higher in breastfed children than in formula-fed children at 1 and 2 months of age (Rovet, 1990), it is unclear whether breastfeeding protects breastfed infants against clinical evidence of congenital hypothyroidism (Latarte et al., 1980; Rovet, 1990). Some infants receive sufficient thyroxine in their mother's milk to compensate for hypothyroidism; thus the symptoms of this imbalance may be masked for several months. Although this does not appear to be true for all infants, the results of thyroid studies after the first week of life should be interpreted with caution in breastfed infants and should include measurements of both thyroxine and thyroid-stimulating hormone (TSH) concentrations.

Cortisol

Cortisol is present in relatively high concentrations in colostrum, but its level declines rapidly by the second day postpartum and remains low thereafter. Its role in infant physiology is not clear. Three theories have been presented concerning the function of cortisol in infants. The first is that it may control the transport of fluids and salts in an infant's gastrointestinal tract (Kulski & Hartmann, 1981).

A second theory suggests that it may play a role in the growth of an infant's pancreas (Morrisset & Jolicoeur, 1980). Finally, cortisol may serve as a hormone released during chronic stress. A mother's higher level of satisfaction with breastfeeding is associated with lower levels of cortisol in her milk. The amount of cortisol in milk is inversely related to sIgA, suggesting that cortisol may suppress the function of immunoglobulin-producing cells in milk (Groer et al., 1994).

Cholecystokinin

Cholecystokinin (CCK) is a gastrointestinal hormone that enhances digestion, sedation, and a feeling of satiation and well-being. During suckling, vagal stimulation causes CCK release in both mother and infant, producing a sleepy feeling. The infant's CCK level peaks twice after suckling. The first peak occurs immediately after the feeding, and then the level peaks again 30 to 60 minutes later. The first CCK rise is probably induced by suckling; the second by the presence of milk in the gastrointestinal tract (Marchini & Linden, 1992; Uvnas-Moberg et al., 1993).

Beta-Endorphins

Beta-endorphin concentrations are higher in the colostrum of women who delivered (1) prematurely, (2) vaginally, and (3) without epidural analgesia. It is hypothesized that elevated beta-endorphin concentrations in colostrum may contribute to postnatal fetal adaptation to overcoming birth stress of natural labor and delivery, while simultaneously enhancing the postnatal development of several related biological functions of the growing newborn (Zanardo et al., 2001).

Prostaglandins

Prostaglandins, a special group of lipids, are present in most mammal cells and tissues and affect almost every biological system. Formed by numerous body tissues, prostaglandins affect many physiological functions, including local circulation, gastric and mucous secretion, electrolyte balance, zinc absorption, and release of brush border enzymes. The protective activity of milk lipids is thought to be due to the presence of two prostaglandins, PGE_2 and PGF_{2a}, present both in colostrum and in mature milk. Concentrations there are about 100 times as great as their levels in adult plasma (Lucas & Mitchell, 1980). PGE_2, in particular, is thought to exert a cytoprotective action (protection against inflammation and necrosis) on the gastric mucosa by promoting the accumulation of phospholipids in the neonatal stomach (Reid et al., 1980). The full extent of the beneficial effects of prostaglandins in human milk awaits future scientific investigation.

Taurine

Taurine, which is not found in bovine milk, is the second most abundant amino acid in human milk (Raiha, 1985). This unusual amino acid, which may function as a neurotransmitter, plays an important role in early brain maturation (Gaull, 1985). Before 1983, taurine was thought to act only in the conjugation of bile acids. Infants who do not receive taurine in their diet conjugate bile acids with glycine, which less effectively assists in absorbing dietary fats. Although deleterious effects of low taurine levels are not known in humans, deficiencies have caused retinal problems in cats and monkeys (Jensen et al., 1988). Taurine was added to most commercial formulas when formula-fed infants were found to have plasma taurine levels only half as high as those of breastfed infants.

Implications for Clinical Practice

Human milk is a species-specific fluid of diverse composition that includes both nutrient and non-nutrient substances, all of which protect the infant. Although the significance to young infants of these components is well known, the influence of their nutritional programming on the subsequent health of infants is a relatively new field.

An understanding of the biological components of human and bovine milks and of manufactured formulas is essential for the healthcare specialist who is providing lactation assistance. When prenatal discussion with the parents and prenatal classes include information about the immunological protection available from breastmilk but absent from formula, parents can then make an informed choice of infant feeding method.

This chapter objectively describes human milk components—but what about mothers' views of their breastmilk? Bottorff and Morse (1990) revealed that mothers clearly recognize the difference between colostrum and mature breastmilk. Because of the relative thickness of colostrum, some mothers believe it is the "strongest" milk, significant for its "rich" supply of antibodies rather than for its nutritional properties. Breastmilk was frequently described by using fat-related terms (e.g., lean, creamy, rich) and evaluated by drawing comparisons to cow milk and infant formula, as if some similarities should exist between the two.

Knowledge of lactation physiology and breastmilk components provides us direction for lactation practice and advice to mothers. For example, the high fat content (and thus calories) in hindmilk—the milk that appears when the breast is nearly empty—implies caution in routinely recommending "switch" nursing (repeatedly switching feedings from breast to breast during a breastfeeding) (Woolridge & Fisher, 1988). In fact, infants whose requirements may fluctuate with time are amazingly adept at self-regulating their nutrient intake (Woolridge et al., 1990). Thus we can encourage women to be flexible about breastfeedings and to be led by their infant's cues that tell the mother when to continue and when to stop a feeding.

Given the differences between the growth patterns of breastfed infants and infants fed human-milk substitutes, practitioners need to evaluate infant growth using standardized growth charts based on breastfed infants. Otherwise, breastfeeding mothers might be told that their babies are gaining too slowly and that their milk production must be insufficient, when their babies are actually healthy in all respects. (See the *Low Intake in the Breastfed Infant: Maternal and Infant Considerations* chapter on slow weight gain for a more detailed discussion of this issue.)

The drop in infant CCK levels 10 minutes after a feeding implies that a "window" exists within which the infant can be awakened to feed from the second breast or to reattach to the first side for additional fat-rich milk. To wait 30 minutes after the feeding before laying the baby down takes advantage of the second CCK peak to help the infant stay asleep.

The studies cited in this chapter support giving fresh, rather than heat-treated or frozen, human milk whenever possible. Some living cells are killed by both of these treatments. Pasteurization significantly decreases concentrations of IgM, IgA, IgG, and lysozymes (Koenig et al., 2005). Also, due to the action of the bile salt–stimulated lipase, fat in fresh human milk is absorbed more completely than that in pasteurized milk. Mixing mother's milk with formula is acceptable. This approach is particularly important for premature infants, who lack digestive enzymes, as mixing fresh human milk with formula improves fat absorption. Ideally, preterm infants will be receiving high volumes of their own mother's milk or mother's milk enriched with human milk components, both of which sustain excellent growth without the risks associated with bovine milk.

During the assessment phase of working with a breastfeeding family, the practitioner needs to ask if there is a family history of allergies. If so, the mother should be encouraged to breastfeed for a minimum of 12 months and to delay feeding the infant solid foods until the baby shows signs of readiness for this transition. Because of the risk of sensitization to allergenic proteins, particularly in babies who have a family history of allergies, even occasional formula supplements can trigger an allergic reaction and should be avoided as long as possible. In addition to preventing allergies, infant malabsorption problems, such as celiac disease, are lessened when the baby is breastfed and solid foods are delayed. Solid foods are usually started around 6 months of age as a baby's intestinal enzymes mature and become increasingly capable of digesting complex proteins and starches. After 6 months, babies can eat whatever they like and in any order they want.

In the maternal diet, dairy products are particularly potential allergens to the breastfeeding baby. If the mother notices that a particular food seems to cause an allergic response in her infant, she needs to consider eliminating it from her diet. A case report (Wilson et al., 1990) describes rectal bleeding in a 4-day-old infant who was exclusively breastfed: her mother was drinking four to five glasses of cow milk per day. Although this case is extreme and rare, it demonstrates the potential for problems when a breastfeeding mother drinks large quantities of cow milk. Discussion of diet and appropriate substitution should be part of the care provided the mother by the healthcare worker offering lactation consultation and support.

SUMMARY

The nutritional components of human milk, combined with its immune and antiallergic properties, make it the ideal foundation for optimal infant health. The immunological and allergy protection conferred by breastmilk are obvious, but it is more difficult to substantiate the protection offered by breastfeeding against inflammatory and immunologically determined disorders that emerge later in life. There appears to be a threshold level for passive immunity conferred by breastmilk that is related to the amount of breastmilk a baby receives—a dose-response effect exists such that exclusively breastfed infants benefit far more than infants who receive minimum amounts of breastmilk (Raisler et al., 1999). Geddes and Prescott (2013) remind us of the dramatic rise in chronic noncommunicable diseases that has resulted in far more than 60% of global deaths. What role has breastfeeding (or lack thereof) played in the increased incidence of obesity, heart disease, cancer, allergies. and other immune diseases? All of these conditions can be prevented.

Allowed to breastfeed at will in response to their own needs, infants generally obtain milk in amounts that satisfy their energy needs and maintain normal growth. Practical experience clearly supports the benefits of breastfeeding. In recent years, scientific data from all parts of the world confirm what the practitioner has long observed.

It is ironic that many of the complex properties of human milk described in this chapter have been identified through research funded by formula companies, which stand to make large sums of money if they can develop products that can accurately claim a close resemblance to human milk.

KEY CONCEPTS

- Human milk—the gold standard for infant nutriment—has between 57 to 65 kcal of energy per deciliter.
- Breastfed infants ingest less volume than formula-fed infants because human milk is more energy efficient.
- Babies do not usually remove all the milk available in the breast during a single feeding; instead, they usually take about two-thirds of available breastmilk in the breast.
- Small amounts of colostrum are produced in the first day or two after delivery, followed by rapid increases to about 500 mL at five days postpartum.
- Babies take 11 breastfeeds per day on average, but this frequency ranges from 6 to 18 feeds per day.
- Differences in milk output from the right and left breasts are common.
- Milk storage capacity differs among women. Women with larger breasts have a greater milk storage capacity and may breastfeed less often; women with small breasts may need to breastfeed more often. Otherwise, breast size does not affect the ability to breastfeed.
- Milk synthesis and volume differ between breasts.
- The nutritional status of a lactating mother has a minimal effect on milk volume unless she is malnourished.
- Multiparous women produce more breastmilk than primiparous women; mothers produce significantly more breastmilk with their second baby.
- Breastfed infants grow at about the same rate as those not breastfed for the first 3 to 4 months.

- Fat in human milk varies according to the degree to which the breast is emptied. High volume is associated with low milk fat content; accordingly, fat content progressively increases during a single feeding.
- Breastfeeding should occur early and frequently; the longer the interval between feedings, the lower the fat content.
- The type of fat the mother eats affects the type of fatty acids present in her milk.
- Primary or congenital lactose deficiency or intolerance in infants is rare or nonexistent.
- Lactose in human milk supplies quick energy to the infant's rapidly growing brain.
- Human milk contains two main proteins: casein and whey. Casein is tough and less digestible curd; whey is soft and flocculent, and is digested rapidly.
- The amount of protein in colostrum is greater than that in mature milk because of the immune factors (IgA, lactoferrin) present in colostrum.
- Preterm mother's milk contains high levels of protein and fat compared with nonpreterm milk; thus using the milk of the preterm infant's own mother is preferred.
- Generally speaking, human milk contains sufficient amounts of vitamins and minerals to meet the needs of full-term infants. Exceptions are premature infants and vitamin D supplementation for dark-skinned babies living in northern climates.
- Mineral content in human milk is fairly constant, tending to be highest right after birth and decreasing slightly throughout lactation.
- Healthy infants who consume enough breastmilk to meet their energy needs receive enough fluid to satisfy their requirements even in hot and dry environments.
- In the first 1 to 2 days after birth, the infant ingests small amounts, approximately 7 to 14 mL, of colostrum at each feeding. Milk yield gradually increases for the first 36 hours, then rapidly increases. By day 5, volume is about 500 mL/day; it reaches 800 mL/

day (range, 550 to 1150) during months 1 to 6 of full breastfeeding.

- Immunity occurs actively and passively. Colostrum is densely packed with antibodies and immunoglobulins.
- Human milk contains two types of white cells: phagocytes and lymphocytes. Phagocytes (1) engulf and absorb pathogens and (2) release IgA. Lymphocytes (83% are T cells) protect an infant by destroying the cell walls of viruses in a process called cell-mediated immunity.
- Antibodies are immunoglobulins that act against specific antigens or pathogens. Secretory IgA is the major immunoglobulin. Total sIgA remains relatively constant throughout lactation.
- sIgA passes from the mother's mucosa (intestinal, respiratory) to the mammary gland/breastmilk through lymphocyte traffic pathways (GALT and BALT).
- Immunity has a dose-response effect—the more breastmilk the infant ingests, the greater the immunity.

REFERENCES

Aarts E, Kylberg A, Hornell A, et al. How exclusive is breastfeeding? A comparison of data since birth with current status data. *Int J Epidemiol.* 2000;29:1041–1046.

Abrams SA, Wen H, Stuff JE. Absorption of calcium, zinc, and iron from breast milk by five- to seven-month-old infants. *Pediatr Res.* 1996;39:384–390.

Abdulmoneim I, Al-Gamdi SA. Relationship between breastfeeding duration and acute respiratory infections in infant. *Saudi Med J.* 2001;22:347–350.

Akisu M, Kultursay N, Ozkayin N, et al. Platelet-activating factor levels in term and pre-term milk. *Biol Neonate.* 1998;74:289–283.

Aljazaf KMNH. *Ultrasound imaging in the analysis of the blood supply and blood flow in the human lactating breast* [Dissertation]. Medical Imaging Science, Curtin University of Technology, Perth, Australia, 2004.

Almroth S, Bidinger PD. No need for water supplementation for exclusively breast-fed infants under hot and arid conditions. *Trans Roy Soc Trop Med Hyg.* 1990;84:602–604.

Almroth SG, Latham MC. Breast feeding practices in rural Jamaica. *J Trop Pediatr.* 1982;28:103–109.

Anderson CH. Human milk feeding. *Pediatr Clin North Am.* 1985;32:335–352.

Anderson JW, Johnstone BM, Remley DT. Breastfeeding and cognitive development: a meta-analysis. *Am J Clin Nutr.* 1999;70:25–35.

Andon MB, Howard MP, Moser PB, Reynolds RD. Nutritionally relevant supplementation of vitamin B$_6$ in lactating women: effect on plasma prolactin. *Pediatrics.* 1985;76:769–773.

Aniansson G, Alm B, Andersson B, et al. A prospective cohort study on breast-feeding and otitis media in Swedish infants. *Pediatr Infect Dis J.* 1994;13:183–188.

Anveden-Hertzberg L. Proctocolitis in exclusively breast-fed infants. *Eur J Pediatr.* 1996;155:464–467.

Arthur PG, Jones TJ, Spruce J, Hartmann PE. Measuring short-term rates of milk synthesis in breast-feeding mothers. *Q J Exp Physiology.* 1989;47:419–428.

Arthur PG, Smith M, Hartmann PE. Milk lactose, citrate, and glucose as markers of lactogenesis in normal and diabetic women. *J Pediatr Gastroenterol Nutr.* 1989;9:488–496.

Ascher H, Krantz I, Rydberg L, et al. Influence of infant feeding and gluten intake on celiac disease. *Arch Dis Child.* 1997;76:113.

Ashraf RN, Jalil F, Aperia A, Lindblad BS. Additional water is not needed for healthy breast-fed babies in a hot climate. *Acta Paediatr Scan.* 1993;82:1007–1011.

Atkinson SA, Anderson G, Bryan MH. Human milk: comparison of the nitrogen composition of milk from mothers of premature infants. *Am J Clin Nutr.* 1980;33:811–815.

Atkinson SA, Whelan D, Whyte RK, Lönnerdal B. Abnormal zinc content in human milk: risk for development of nutritional zinc deficiency in infants. *Am J Dis Child.* 1989;143:608–611.

Auricchio S, Follow D, de Ritis G, et al. Does breast feeding protect against the development of clinical symptoms of celiac disease in children? *J Pediatr Gastroenterol Nutr.* 1983;2:428–433.

Axelsson I, Jakobsson I, Lindberg T, Benediktsson B. Bovine beta-lactoglobulin in the human milk. *Acta Pediatr Scand.* 1986;75:702.

Bachrach VR, Schwarz E, Bachrach LR. Breastfeeding and the risk of hospitalization for respiratory disease in infancy: a meta-analysis. *Arch Pediatr Adolesc Med.* 2003;157:237–243.

Ballard O, Morrow AL. Human milk composition: nutrients and bioactive factors. *Pediatr Clin North Am.* 60;2013:49–74.

Bartick M, Reinhold A. The burden of suboptimal breastfeeding in the United States: a pediatric cost analysis. *Peds.* 2010; 125(5):e1048–1056.

Bates CJ, Prentice A. Breast milk as a source of vitamins, essential minerals and trace elements. *Pharmacol Ther.* 1994;62:193–220.

Bauchner J, Levanthal JM, Shapiro ED. Studies of breastfeeding and infections: how good is the evidence? *JAMA.* 1986;256:887–892.

Baur LA, O'Connor J, Pan DA, et al. Relationships between the fatty acid composition of muscle and erythrocyte membrane phospholipid in young children and the effect of type of infant feeding. *Lipids.* 2000;35:77–82.

Bell LM, Clark HF, Offit PA, et al. Rotavirus serotype-specific neutralizing activity in human milk. *Am J Dis Child.* 1988;142:275–278.

Bellig LL. Immunization and the prevention of childhood diseases. *J Obstet Gynecol Neonatal Nurs.* 1995;24:469–477.

Bener A, Denic S, Galadari S. Longer breast-feeding and protection against childhood leukaemia and lymphomas. *European J Cancer.* 2001;37:234–238.

Bergstrand O, Hellers G. Breast-feeding during infancy in patients who develop Crohn's disease. *Scand J Gastroenterol.* 1983;18:903–906.

Bergstrom O, Hernell O, Persson LA, Vessby B. Serum lipid values in adolescents are related to family history, infant feeding, and physical growth. *Atherosclerosis.* 1995;17:1–13.

Blackberg LD, Hernell O, Olivecrona T, et al. The bile salt–stimulated lipase in human milk is an evolutionary newcomer derived from a non-milk protein. *FEBS Lett.* 1980;112:151.

Blais DR, Harrold J, Altosaar I. Killing the messenger in the nick of time: persistence of breastmilk sCD14 in the neonatal gastrointestinal tract. *Pediatr Res.* 2006;59:371–376.

Borch-Johnson K, Joner G, Mandrup-Poulsen T, et al. Relation between breast-feeding and incidence rates of insulin-dependent diabetes mellitus. *Lancet.* 1984;2:1083–1086.

Borgnolo G, Barbone F, Scornavacca G, et al. A case-control study of *Salmonella* gastrointestinal infection in Italian children. *Acta Paediatr.* 1996;85:804–808.

Bottorff JL, Morse JM. Mother's perceptions of breast milk. *JOGN Nursing.* 1990;19:518–527.

Bouguerra F, Haijem S, Guilloud-Bataille M, et al. Effect of breastfeeding relative to the age at onset of celiac disease. *Arch Pediatr.* 1998;5:621.

Brenna JT, Varamini B, Jensen RG, et al. Docosahexaenoic and arachidonic acid concentrations in human breastmilk worldwide. *Am J Clin Nutr.* 2007;85:1457–1464.

Brown KH, Akhtar NA, Robertson AD, Ahmed MG. Lactational capacity of marginally nourished mothers: relationships between maternal nutritional status and quantity and proximate composition of milk. *Pediatrics.* 1986;78:909–919.

Brown KH, Black RE, Lopez de Romaña G, Creed de Kanashiro H. Infant-feeding practices and their relationship with diarrheal and other diseases in Huascar (Lima), Peru. *Pediatrics.* 1989;83:31–40.

Brown KH, Creed de Kanashiro H, del Aguila R, et al. Milk consumption and hydration status of exclusively breast-fed infants in a warm climate. *J Pediatr.* 1986;108:677–680.

Buescher ES, Pickering LK. Polymorphonuclear leukocytes in human colostrum and milk. In: Howell RR, Morriss FH, Pickering LK, eds. *Human milk in infant nutrition and health.* Springfield, IL: Thomas; 1986:160–173.

Burr ML, Limb ES, Maguire, MJ, et al. Infant feeding, wheezing, and allergy: a prospective study. *Arch Dis Child.* 1993;68:724–728.

Butte NF, Garza C, Smith EO, et al. Macro- and trace-mineral intakes of exclusively breast-fed infants. *Am J Clin Nutr.* 1987;45:42–47.

Butte NF, Smith EO, Garza C. Energy utilization of breast-fed and formula-fed infants. *Am J Clin Nutr.* 1990;51:350–358.

Butte NF, Wong WW, Fiorotto M, et al. Influence of early feeding mode on body composition of infants. *Biol Neonate.* 1995;67:414–424.

Butte NF, Wong WW, Hopkinson JM, et al. Energy requirements derived from total energy expenditure and energy deposition during the first 2 years of life. *Am J Clin Nutr.* 2000;72:1558–1569.

Carpenter G. Epidermal growth factor is a major growth-promoting agent in human milk. *Science.* 1980;210:198–199.

Casey CE, Hambidge KM, Neville MC. Studies in human lactation: zinc, copper, manganese and chromium in human milk in the first month of lactation. *Am J Clin Nutr.* 1985;41:1193–1200.

Casey CE, Neville MC, Hambidge KM. Studies in human lactation: secretion of zinc, copper, and manganese in human milk. *Am J Clin Nutr.* 1989;49:773–785.

Caspi A, Williams B, Kim-Cohen J. Moderation of breast-feeding effect on the IQ by genetic variation in fatty acid metabolism. *Proc Natl Acad Sci USA.* 2007;104(47):188860–188865.

Cavagni G, Paganelli R, Caffarelli C, et al. Passage of food antigens into circulation of breast-fed infants with atopic dermatitis. *Ann Allergy.* 1988;61:361–365.

Cavell B. Gastric emptying in infants fed human or infant formula. *Acta Paediatr Scand.* 1981;70:639–641.

Cesar JA, Victoria CG, Barros FC. Impact of breastfeeding on admission for pneumonia during postneonatal period in Brazil: nested case-control study. *Br Med J.* 1999;318:1316–1320.

Chandra RK. Prospective studies of the effect of breast-feeding on incidence of infection and allergy. *Acta Paediatr Scand.* 1979;68:691–694.

Chandra RK, Puri S, Suraiya C, Cheema PS. Influence of maternal food antigen avoidance during pregnancy and lactation on incidence of atopic eczema in infants. *Clin Allergy.* 1986;16:563–569.

Chen A, Rogan WJ. Breastfeeding and the risk of post neonatal death in the United States. *Pediatrics.* 2004;113:435–439.

Chen Y, Yu S, Li W. Artificial feeding and hospitalization in the first 18 months of life. *Pediatrics.* 1988;81:58–62.

Chowanadisai W, Lönnerdal B, Kelleher SL. Identification of a mutation in SLC30A2 (ZnT-2) in women with low milk zinc concentration that results in transient neonatal zinc deficiency. *J Biol Chem.* 2006;281:39699–39707.

Chulada PC, Arbes SJ, Dunson D, Z. Breast-feeding and the prevalence of asthma and wheeze in children: analyses from the third national health and nutrition examination survey, 1988–1994. *J Allergy Clin Immunol.* 2003;111:328–336.

Clavano NR. Mode of feeding and its effect on infant mortality and morbidity. *J Trop Pediatr.* 1982;28:287–293.

Cochi SL, Fleming DW, Hightower AW, et al. Primary invasive *Haemophilus influenzae* type b disease: a population-based assessment of risk factors. *J Pediatr.* 1986;108:87–96.

Cohen RJ, Brown KH, Rivera LL, Dewey KG. Exclusively breastfed, low birth weight term infants do not need supplemental water. *Acta Paediatr.* 2000;89:550–552.

Corps AN, Brown KD, Rees LH, Carr J, Prosser CG. The insulin-like growth factor I content in human milk increases between early and full lactation. *J Clin Endocrinol Metab.* 1988;67:25–29.

Cosgrove M. Perinatal and infant nutrition: nucleotides. *Nutrition.* 1998;14:748.

Cox DB, Owens RA, Hartmann PE. Blood and milk prolactin and the rate of milk synthesis in women. *Exp Physiol.* 1996;81:1007–1020.

Cregan MD, Fan Y, Appelbee A, et al. Identification of nestin-positive putative mammary stem cells in human breastmilk. *Cell Tissue Res.* 2007;329:129–136.

Cregan MD, Hartmann PE. Computerized breast measurement from conception to weaning: clinical implications. *J Hum Lact.* 1999;15:89–95.

Cregan MD, Mitoulas LR, Hartmann PE. Milk prolactin, feed volume, and duration between feeds in women breastfeeding their full-term infants over a 24-hour period. *Exp Physiol.* 2002;87:207–214.

Cushing AH, Samet JM, Lambert WE, et al. Breastfeeding reduces the risk of respiratory illness in infants. *Am J Epidemiol.* 1998; 147:863–870.

Dai D, Nanthkumar NN, Newburg DS, Walker WA. Role of oligosaccharides and glycoconjugates in intestinal host defense. *J Pediatr Gastroenterol Nutr.* 2000;30(suppl):23.

Daly SE, Di Rosso A, Owens RA, Hartmann PE. Degree of breast emptying explains changes in the fat content, but not fatty acid composition of human milk. *Exp Physiol.* 1993;78:741–755.

Daly SE, Hartmann PE. Infant demand and milk supply. Part 1: infant demand and milk production in lactating women. *J Hum Lact.* 1995a;11:21–26.

Daly SE, Hartmann PE. Infant demand and milk supply. Part 2: the short-term control of milk synthesis in lactating women. *J Hum Lact.* 1995b;11:27–36.

Daly SE, Kent JC, Huynh DQ, et al. The determination of short-term breast volume changes and the rate of

synthesis of human milk using computerized breast measurement. *Exp Physiol.* 1992;77:79–87.

Daly SE, Owens RA, Hartmann PE. The short-term synthesis and infant-regulated removal of milk in lactating women. *Exp Physiol.* 1993;78:209–220.

Daniels JL, Olshan AF, Pollock BH, et al. Breast-feeding and neuroblastoma, USA and Canada. *Cancer Causes Control.* 2002;13:401–405.

Davis MK. Review of the evidence for an association between infant feeding and childhood cancer. *Int J Cancer.* 1998;S11:29–33.

Davis MK, Savitz DA, Graubard B. Infant feeding and childhood cancer. *Lancet.* 1988;2(8607):365–368.

de Araujo AN, Giugliano LG. Lactoferrin and free secretory component of human milk inhibits the adhesion of enteropathic *Escherichia coli* to HeLa cells. *BMC Microbiol.* 2001;1:25.

de Ferrer PA, Baroni A, Sambucetti ME, et al. Lactoferrin levels in term and preterm milk. *J Am College Nutr.* 2000;19:370–373.

Dell S, To T. Breastfeeding and asthma in young children: findings from a population-based study. *Arch Pediatr Adolesc Med.* 2001;155:1261–1265.

Demmers TA, Jones PJ, Wang Y, et al. Effects of early cholesterol intake on cholesterol biosynthesis and plasma lipids among infants until 28 months of age. *Pediatrics.* 2005;115:1594–1601.

Deoni S, Dean DC, Pityatinsky I, O'Muircheartaigh J. Breastfeeding and early white matter development: a cross-sectional study. *NeuroImage.* 2013;82:77–86.

de Onis M, Onyango A, Borghi E, et al. Worldwide implementation of the WHO child growth standards. *Public Health Nutr.* 2012;15(9):1603–1610.

Dewey KG, Domellöf M, Cohen RJ, et al. Iron supplementation affects growth and morbidity of breast-fed infants: results of a randomized trial in Sweden and Honduras. *J Nutr.* 2002;132:3249–3255.

Dewey KG, Heinig J, Nommsen-Rivers LA. Differences in morbidity between breast-fed and formula-fed infants. *J Pediatr.* 1995;126:697–702.

Dewey KG, Heinig MJ, Nommsen LA, et al. Breast-fed infants are leaner than formula-fed infants at 1 year of age: the DARLING study. *Am J Clin Nutr.* 1993;57:140–145.

Dewey KG, Lönnerdal B. Milk and nutrient intake of breast-fed infants from 1 to 6 months: relation to growth and fatness. *J Pediatr Gastroenterol Nutr.* 1983; 2:497–506.

Dewey KG, Peerson JM, Brown KH, et al. Growth of breast-fed infants deviates from current reference data: a pooled analysis of US, Canadian, and European data sets. *Pediatrics.* 1995; 96:495–503.

Dorea JG. Iron and copper in human milk. *Nutrition.* 2000;16:209–220.

Downham MA, Scott R, Sims DG, et al. Breast-feeding protects against respiratory syncytial virus infection. *Br Med J.* 1976;2:274–276.

Duchen K, Yu G, Björkstén B. Polyunsaturated fatty acids in breast milk in relation to atopy in the mother and her child. *Int Arch Allergy Immunol.* 1999;118:321–323.

Duffy LC, Byers TE, Riepenhoff-Talty M, et al. The effects of infant feeding on rotavirus-induced gastroenteritis: a prospective study. *Am J Public Health.* 1986;76:259–263.

Duncan B, Schifman RB, Corrigan JJ Jr, Schaefer C. Iron and the exclusively breast-fed infant from birth to six months. *J Pediatr Gastroenterol Nutr.* 1985;4:412–425.

Duncan J, Ey J, Holberg CJ, et al. Exclusive breast-feeding for at least 4 months protects against otitis media. *Pediatrics.* 1993;91:867–872.

Eidelman AI, Schanler RJ, American Academy of Pediatrics, Section on Breastfeeding Executive Committee. Breastfeeding and the use of human milk. *Pediatrics.* 2012:129:e827–e841.

Engstrom JL, Meier PP, Jegier B et al. Comparison of milk output from the right and left breasts during simultaneous pumping in mothers of very low birth weight infants. *Breastfeed Med.* 2007;2:83–91.

Erickson PR, Mazhari E. Investigation of the role of human breast milk in caries development. *Pediatr Dent.* 1999;21:86–90.

Espinoza E, Paniagua M, Hallander H, et al. Rotavirus infections in young Nicaraguan children. *Pediatr Infect Dis.* 1997;16:564–571.

Evans GS, Johnson PE. Characterization and quantitation of a zinc-binding ligand and human milk. *Pediatr Res.* 1980;14:876–880.

Fallot MB, Boyd JL, Oak FA. Breast-feeding reduces incidence of hospital admissions for infections in infants. *Pediatrics.* 1980;65:1121–1124.

Fawzi WW, Forman MR, Levy A, et al. Maternal anthropometry and infant feeding practices in Israel in relation to growth in infancy: the North African Infant Feeding Study. *Am J Clin Nutr.* 1997;65:1731–1737.

Feist N, Berger D, Speer CP. Anti-endotoxin antibodies in human milk: correlation with infection of the newborn. *Acta Paediatr.* 2000;89:1087–1092.

Ford RPK, Taylor BJ, Mitchell EA, et al. Breastfeeding and the risk of sudden infant death syndrome. *Int J Epidemiol.* 1993;22:885–890.

Forman MR, Guptill KS, Chang DN, et al. Undernutrition among Bedouin Arab infants: the Bedouin Infant Feeding Study. *Am J Clin Nutr.* 1990;51:339–343.

Frank AL, Taber LH, Glezen WP, et al. Breast-feeding and respiratory virus infection. *Pediatrics.* 1982;70:239–245.

Franke AA, Custer LJ, Tanaka Y. Isoflavones in human breast milk and other biological fluids. *Am J Clin Nutr.* 1998;68(suppl):1466S–1473S.

Fuchs SC, Victor CG, Martines J. Case-control study of risk of dehydrating diarrhoea in infants in vulnerable period after full weaning. *Br Med J.* 1996;313:391–394.

Garofalo RP, Goldman AS. Cytokines, chemokines, and colony-stimulating factors in human milk. *Biol Neonate.* 1998;74:134–142.

Garofalo RP, Goldman AS. Expression of functional immunomodulating and anti-inflammatory factors in human milk. *Clin Perinatol.* 1999;26:361.

Garza C, Johnson CA, Smith EO, Nichols BL. Changes in the nutrient composition of human milk during gradual weaning. *Am J Clin Nutr.* 1983;37:61–65.

Garza C, Schanler RJ, Butte NF, Motil KJ. Special properties of human milk. *Clin Perinatol.* 1987;14:11–31.

Garza C, Stuff J, Butte N. Growth of the breast-fed infant. In: Goldman AS, Atkinson SA, Hanson LA, eds. *Human lactation: the effects of human milk on the recipient infant.* New York, NY: Plenum; 1986:109–121.

Gaull GE. Significance of growth modulators in human milk. *Pediatrics.* 1985;75(suppl):142–145.

Gdalevich M, Mimouni D, Mimouni M. Breast-feeding and the risk of bronchial asthma in childhood: a systematic review with meta-analysis of prospective studies. *J Pediatr.* 2001;139:261–266.

Geddes DT. Prescott SL. Developmental origins of health and disease: the role of human milk in preventing disease in the 21st century. *J Hum Lact.* 2013;29(2):123–127.

Gilbert RE, Wigfield RE, Fleming PJ, et al. Bottle-feeding and the sudden infant death syndrome. *BMJ.* 1995; 310:88–90.

Gimeno SGA, de Suza JMP. IDDM and milk consumption. *Diabetes Care.* 1997;20:1256–1260.

Glass RI, Stoll BJ. The protective effect of human milk against diarrhea: a review of studies from Bangladesh. *Acta Paediatr Scand.* 1989;351(suppl):131–136.

Goldman AS, Garza C, Nichols BL, Goldblum RM. Immunologic factors in human milk during the first year of lactation. *J Pediatr.* 1982;100:563–567.

Goldman AS, Goldblum RM, Garza C, Nichols BL, Smith EO. Immunologic components in human milk during gradual weaning. *Acta Paediatr Scand.* 1983;72:133–134.

Goldman AS, Thorpe LW, Goldblum RM, Hanson LA. Anti-inflammatory properties of human milk. *Acta Paediatr Scand.* 1986;75:689–695.

Goldman AS, Thorpe LW, Goldblum RM, Hanson LA. Cytokines in human milk: properties and potential effects upon the mammary gland and the neonate. *J Mammary Gland Biol Neoplasia.* 1996;1:251–258.

Grantham-McGregor SM, Back EH. Breast feeding in Kingston, Jamaica. *Arch Dis Child.* 1972;45:404–409.

Greco L, Auricchio S, Mayer M, Grimaldi M. Case control study on nutritional risk factors in celiac disease. *J Pediar Gastroenterol Nutr.* 1983;7:395–399.

Greer FR. Vitamin K status of lactating mothers and their infants. *Acta Paediatr.* 1999;88(suppl):95.

Greer FR, Marshall S. Bone mineral content, serum vitamin D metabolite concentrations and ultraviolet B light exposure in infants fed human milk with and without vitamin D$_2$ supplements. *J Pediatr.* 1989;114:204–212.

Groer M, Davis M, Steele K. Associations between human milk sIgA and maternal immune, infections, endocrine, and stress variables. *J Hum Lact.* 2004;20:153–158.

Groer MW, Humenick S, Hill P. Characterizations and psychoneuroimmunologic implications of secretory immunoglobulin A and cortisol in preterm and term breast milk. *J Perinat Neonatal Nurs.* 1994;7:42–51.

Groer MW, Shelton, MM Exercise is associated with elevated proinflammatory cytokines in human milk. *JOGNN.* 2009;36:35–41.

Grummer-Strawn LM, Reinold C, Krebs NF. Use of World Health Organization and CDC growth charts for children aged 0–59 months in the United States. *MMWR Recomm Rep.* 2010;59(RR-9):1–15. Available at: http://www.cdc.gov/mmwr/preview/mmwrhtml/rr5909a1.htm.

Guesnet P, Alessandri JM. Docosahexaenoic acid (DHA) and the developing central nervous system (CNS) e implications for dietary recommendations. *Biochimie.* 2011;93: 7–12.

Gunnarsdottir I, Aspelund T, Birgidsdottir BE, et al. Infant feeding patterns and midlife erythrocyte sedimentation rate. *Acta Paediatrica.* 2007;96:852–856.

Guthrie HA, Picciano MF, Sheehe D. Fatty acid patterns of human milk. *J Pediatr.* 1977;90:39–41.

Gyorgy P. A hitherto unrecognized biochemical difference between human milk and cow's milk. *Pediatrics.* 1953;11:98–104.

Habbick BF, Kahnna C, To T. Infantile hypertropic pyloric stenosis: a study of feeding practices and other possible causes. *Can Med Assoc J.* 1989;140:401–404.

Habicht JP, DaVanso J, Butz WP. Mother's milk and sewage: their interactive effects on infant mortality. *Pediatrics.* 1988;81:456–460.

Hakansson A, Svensson M, Mossberg A-K, et al. A folding variant of α-lactalbumin with bactericidal activity against *Streptococcus pneumoniae. Molec Microbiol.* 2000;35:589–600.

Hakansson A, Zhivotovsky B, Orrenius S, et al. Apoptosis induced by a human protein. *Proc Natl Acad Sci.* 1995;92:8064.

Hallowell SG, Spatz DL. The relationship of brain development and breastfeeding in the late-preterm infant. *J Pediatr Nurs.* 2012;27(2):154–162. doi: 10.1016/j.pedn.2010.12.018. Epub March 2, 2011.

Hamosh M. Human milk: digestion in the neonate. *Clin Perinatol.* 1996;23:191.

Hamosh M. Bioactive factors in human milk. *Ped Clin North Am.* 2001;48:69–86.

Hamosh M, Henderson TR, Ellis LA, et al. Digestive enzymes in human milk: stability at suboptimal storage temperatures. *J Pediatr Gastroenterol Nutr.* 1997;24:38–43.

Hartmann PE. Lactation and reproduction in Western Australian women. *J Reprod Med.* 1987;32:543–557.

Hartmann PE, Cregan M. Lactogenesis and the effects of insulin-dependent diabetes mellitus and prematurity. *J Nutrition.* 2001;131:3016S–3020S.

Hartmann PE, Prosser CG. Physiological basis of longitudinal changes in human milk yield and composition. *Fed Proc.* 1984;43:2448–2453.

Hashizume S, Kuroda K, Murakami H. Identification of lactoferrin as an essential growth factor for human lymphocytic cell lines in serum-free medium. *Biochem Biophys Acta.* 1983;763:377.

Hasselbalch H, Engelmann MD, Ersboll AK, et al. Breastfeeding influences thymic size in late infancy. *Eur J Pediatr.* 1999;158:964–967.

Hassiotou F1, Beltran A, Chetwynd E, et al. Breastmilk is a novel source of stem cells with multilineage differentiation potential. Stem Cells. 2012 Oct;30(10):2164–74. doi: 10.1002/stem.1188.

Hawkes JS, Gibson RA. Lymphocyte subpopulations in breast-fed and formula-fed infants at six months of age. *Adv Exp Med Biol.* 2001;501:497–504.

Heacock H, Jeffrey HE, Baker JL, Page M. Influence of breast versus formula milk on physiological gastroesophageal reflux in healthy, newborn infants. *J Pediatr Gastroenterol.* 1992;14:41–46.

Heinig J, Brown KH, Lönnerdal B, Dewey KG. Zinc supplementation does not affect growth, morbidity, or motor development of US term breastfed infants at 4–10 mo of age. *Am J Clin Nutr.* 2006;84:594–601.

Heird WC, Schward SM, Hansen IH. Colostrum-induced enteric mucosal growth in beagle puppies. *Pediatr Res.* 1984;18:512.

Hildebrandt HM. Maternal perception of lactogenesis time: a clinical report. *J Hum Lact.* 1999;15:317–323.

Holberg CJ, Wright AL, Martinez FD, et al. Risk factors for respiratory syncytial virus-associated lower respiratory illnesses in the first year of life. *Am J Epidemiol.* 1991;133:1135–1151.

Hornell A, Aarts C, Kylberg E, et al. Breastfeeding patterns in exclusively breastfed infants: a longitudinal prospective study in Uppsala, Sweden. *Acta Paediatr.* 1999;88:203–211.

Host A, Husby S, Osterballe O. A prospective study of cow's milk allergy in exclusively breast-fed infants. *Acta Paediatr Scand.* 1988;77:663–670.

Houston MJ, Howie PW, McNeilly AS. Factors affecting the duration of breast feeding: 1. Measurement of breast milk intake in the first week of life. *Early Hum Dev.* 1983;8:49–54.

Howie PW, Forsyth JS, Ogston SA, et al. Protective effect of breast feeding against infection. *Br Med J.* 1990;300:11–16.

Humenick SS. The clinical significance of breastmilk maturation rates. *Birth.* 1987;14:174–179.

Humenick SS, Mederios D, Wreschner TB, et al. The Maturation Index of Colostrum and Milk (MICAM): a measurement of breast milk maturation. *J Nurs Measurement.* 1994;2:16–86.

Hylander MA, Strobino DM, Pezzullo JC, Dhanireddy R. Association of human milk feedings with a reduction in retinopathy of prematurity among very low birth weight infants. *J Perinatology.* 2001;21:356–362.

Ingram JC, Woolridge MS, Greenwood RJ. Breastfeeding: it is worth trying with the second baby. *Lancet.* 2001;358:986–987.

Ip S, Chung M, Raman G. *Breastfeeding and maternal and infant health outcomes in developed countries.* Evidence Report/Technology Assessment No. 153 (Prepared by Tufts-New England Medical Center Evidence-Based Practice Center, under Contract No. 290-02-0022). AHRQ Publication No. 07-E007. Rockville, MD: Agency for Healthcare Research and Quality; 2007. Available at: http://citeseerx.ist.psu.edu/viewdoc/download?doi=10.1.1.182.8429&rep=rep1&type=pdf.

Issac C, Sivakumar A, Kumar C. Lead levels in breast milk, blood plasma and intelligence quotient: a health hazard for women and infants. *Bull Environ Contam Toxicol.* 2012;88:145–149. doi: 10.1007/s00128-011-0475-9.

Istre GR, Conner JS, Broome CV, et al. Risk factors for primary *Haemophilus influenzae* disease: increased risk from day care attendance and school-aged household members. *J Pediatr.* 1985;106:190–195.

Ivarsson A et al. Epidemic of celiac disease in Swedish children. *Acta Pediatr.* 2000;89:165.

Jason JM, Niebury P, Marks JS. Mortality and infectious disease associated with infant-feeding practices in developing countries. *Pediatrics.* 1984;74(suppl):702–727.

Jenkins HR, Pincott JR, Soothill JF, et al. Food allergy: the major cause of infantile colitis. *Arch Dis Child.* 1984;59:326–329.

Jensen RG. Lipids in human milk. *Lipids.* 1999;34:1243.

Jensen RG, Ferris AM, Lammi-Keefe CJ, Henderson RA. Human milk as a carrier of messages to the nursing infant. Nutr Today. 1988;23:20–25.

Juex G, Díaz S, Casado ME, et al. Growth pattern of selected urban Chilean infants during exclusive breast feeding. *Am J Clin Nutr.* 1983;38:462–468.

Kafouri S, Kramer M, Leonard G, et al. Breastfeeding and brain structure in adolescence. *Int J Epidemiol.* 2013;42(1):150–159. doi: 10.1093/ije/dys172.

Kassim OO, Ako-Anai KA, Torimiro SE, et al. Inhibitory factors in breast milk, maternal and infant sera against in vitro growth of *Plasmodium falciparum* malaria parasite. *J Trop Pediatr.* 2000;46:92–96.

Kelleher SL, Lönnerdal B. Immunological activities associated with milk. *Adv Nutr Res.* 2001;10:39–65.

Keller MA, Gendreau-Reid L, Heiner DC, et al. IgAG$_4$ in human colostrum and human milk: continued local production or selective transport form serum. *Acta Paediatr Scand.* 1988;77:24–29.

Kelly DW, Phillips AD, Elliot EJ, et al. Rise and fall of coeliac disease 1960–1985. *Arch Dis Child.* 1989;64:1157–1160.

Kent JC, Mitoulas LR, Cregan MD, et al. Volume and frequency of breastfeedings and fat content of breast-milk throughout the day. *Pediatrics.* 2006;117:387–395.

Kent JC, Mitoulas L, Cox DB, et al. Breast volume and milk production during extended lactation in women. *Exp Physiol.* 1999;82:435–447.

Khan S, Hepworth AR, Prime DK, et al. Variation in fat, lactose, and protein composition in breast milk over 24 hours: association with infant feeding patterns. *J Hum Lact.* 2013;29:81–89.

Khin-Maung-UJ, Nyunt-Nyunt-Wai, Myo-Khin, et al. Effect of clinical outcome of breastfeeding during acute diarrhea. *Br Med J.* 1985;290:587–589.

Kirkpatrick CH, Green I, Rich RR, Schade AL, et al. Inhibition of growth of *Candida albicans* by iron-unsaturated lactoferrin: relation to host defense mechanisms in chronic mucocutaneous candidiasis. *J Infect Dis.* 1971;124:539.

Kobata R, Tsukahara H, Ohshima Y, et al. High levels of growth factors in human breast milk. *Early Hum Dev.* 2008;84:67–9.

Koenig A, de Albuquerque Diniz EM, Barbosa SF, Vaz FA. Immunologic factors in human milk: the effects of gestational age and pasteurization. *J Hum Lact.* 2005;21(4):439–443.

Koerber A. From folklore to fact: the rhetorical history of breastfeeding immunity, 1950–1997. *J Med Humanity.* 2006;27:151–166.

Kohler H, Donarski S, Stocks B, et al. Antibacterial characteristics in the feces of breast-fed and formula-fed infants during the first year of life. *J Pediatr Gastroenterol Nutr.* 2002;34:188–193.

Koletzko B, Rodriquez-Palmero M. Polyunsaturated fatty acids in human milk and their role in early human development. *J Mammary Gland Biol Neoplasia.* 1999; 4:269.

Koletzko S, Sherman P, Corey M, et al. Role of infant feeding practices in development of Crohn's disease in childhood. *Br Med J.* 1989;298:1617–1618.

Koopman JS, Turkish VJ, Monto AS. Infant formulas and gastrointestinal illness. *Am J Public Health.* 1985;75:477–480.

Kostraba JN, Cruickshanks KJ, Lawler-Heavner J, et al. Early exposure to cow's milk and solid foods in infancy, genetic predisposition and risk of IDDM. *Diabetes.* 1993;42:288–295.

Kovar MG, Serdula MK, Marks JS, Fraser DW. Review of the epidemiologic evidence for an association between infant feeding and infant health. *Pediatrics.* 1984; 74(suppl):615–638.

Krachler M, Rossipal SE, Irgolic KJ. Changes in the concentrations of trace elements in human milk during lactation. *J Trace Elements Biol.* 1998;12:159–176.

Kramer MS. Infant feeding, infection, and public health. *Pediatrics.* 1988;81:164–166.

Kramer MS, Aboud F, Mironova E, et al. Breastfeeding and child cognitive development: new evidence from a large randomized trial. *Arch Gen Psychiatry.* 2008;65:578–584.

Kramer MS, Guo T, Platt RW, et al. Infant growth and health outcomes associated with 3 compared with 6 mo of exclusive breastfeeding. *Am J Clin Nutr.* 2003;78(2):291–295.

Kramer MS, Kakuma R. The optimal duration of exclusive breastfeeding: a systematic review. *Adv Exp Med Biol.* 2004;554:63–77.

Kramer MS, Chalmers B, Hodnett ED, et al. Promotion of Breastfeeding Intervention Trial (PROBIT): a randomized trial in the Republic of Belarus. *JAMA.* 2001;285:413–420.

Kramer MS, Guo T, Platt RW, et al. Breastfeeding and infant growth: biology or bias? *Pediatrics.* 2002;110:343–347.

Krebs NF, Hambidge KM. Zinc requirements and zinc intakes of breast-fed infants. *Am J Clin Nutr.* 1986;43:288–292.

Krebs NF, Reidinger CJ, Miller LV, Hambidge KM. Zinc homeostasis in breast-fed infant. *Pediatr Res.* 1996;39:661–665.

Kulski JK, Hartmann PE. Changes in the concentration of cortisol in milk during different stages of human lactation. *Aust J Exp Biol Med Sci.* 1981;59:769–778.

Kum-Nji P, Mangrem CL, Wells PJ. Reducing the incidence of sudden infant death syndrome in the delta region of Mississippi: a three-pronged approach. *South Med J.* 2001;94:704–710.

Kumar A, Rai AK, Basu S, et al. Cord blood and breast milk iron status in maternal anemia. *Pediatrics.* 2008;121:e673–e677.

Kumpulainen J, Salmenperä L, Siimes MA, et al. Formula feeding results in lower selenium status than breastfeeding or selenium-supplemented formula feeding: a longitudinal study. *Am J Clin Nutr.* 1987;45:49–53.

Kunz C, Lönnerdal B. Re-evaluation of the whey protein/casein ratio of human milk. *Acta Paediatr.* 1992;81:107–112.

Kwan ML, Buffler PA, Abrams B, Kiley VA. Breastfeeding and the risk of childhood leukemia: a meta-analysis. *Public Health Rep.* 2004;119:521–535.

Kwan ML, Buffler PA, Wiemels JL, et al. Breastfeeding patterns and risk of childhood acute lymphoblastic leukaemia. *Br J Cancer.* 2005;93:379–384.

Labbok M, Hendershot GE. Does breast-feeding protect against malocclusion? An analysis of the 1981 Child Health Supplement to the National Health Interview survey. *Am J Priv Med.* 1987;3:227–232.

Larsson LA. *Immunobiology of human milk.* Amarillo, TX: Pharmasoft; 2004:32.

Latarte J, Guyda H, Dussault JH, Glorieux J. Lack of protective effect of breast-feeding in congenital hypothyroidism: report of 12 cases. *Pediatrics.* 1980;65:703–705.

Lawlor DA, Najman JM, Sterne J, et al. Associations of parental, birth, and early life characteristics with systolic blood pressure at 5 years of age. *Circulation.* 2004;110:2417–2423.

Lawrence RM, Pane CA. Human breast milk: current concepts of immunology and infectious diseases. *Curr Probl Pediatr Adolesc Health Care.* 2007;37:7–36.

Leach JL, Baxter JH, Molitor BE, et al. Total potentially available nucleotides of human milk by stage of lactation. *Am J Clin Nutr.* 1995;61:1224–1230.

Legrand D, Pierce A Elass E, et al. Lactoferrin structure and functions. Adv Exp Med Biol. 2008;606:163-94.

Lemons JA, Moye L, Hall D, Simmons M. Differences in the composition of preterm and term human milk during early lactation. *Pediatr Res.* 1982;16:113–117.

Lepage G, Collet S, Bouglé D, et al. The composition of preterm milk in relation to the degree of prematurity. *Am J Clin Nutr.* 1984;40:1042–1049.

Leventhal JM, Shapiro ED, Aten CB, et al. Does breastfeeding protect against infection in infants less than 3 months of age? *Pediatrics.* 1986;78:896–903.

Litwin SD, Zehr BD, Insel RA. Selective concentration of IgD class-specific antibodies in human milk. *Clin Exp Immunol.* 1990;80:262–267.

Logan RF. Coeliac disease. *Lancet.* 1990 Sep 8;336(8715):633.

Long K, Vasquez-Garibay E, Mathewson J, et al. The impact of infant feeding patterns on infection and diarrheal disease due to entero-toxigenic *Escherichia coli. Salud Publica Mex.* 1999;41:263–270.

Lönnerdal B. Regulation of mineral and trace elements in human milk: exogenous and endogenous factors. *Nutr Review.* 2000;58:223–229.

Lopez-Alarcon M, Villalpando S, Fajardo A. Breast-feeding lowers the frequency and duration of acute respiratory infection and diarrhea in infants under six months of age. *J Nutr.* 1997;127:436–443.

Lovegrove JA, Hampton SM, Morgan JB. The immunological and long-term atopic outcome of infants born to women following a milk-free diet during late pregnancy and lactation: a pilot study. *Br J Nutr.* 1994;71:223–238.

Lucas A. Programming by early nutrition: an experimental approach. *J Nutr.* 1998;128:401S–406S.

Lucas A, Cole TJ. Breast milk and neonatal necrotizing enterocolitis. *Lancet.* 1990;336:1519–1523.

Lucas A, Fewtrell MS, Davies PS, et al. Breastfeeding and catch-up growth in infants born small for gestational age. *Acta Paediatr.* 1997;86:564–569.

Lucas A, Mitchell MD. Prostaglandins in human milk. *Arch Dis Child.* 1980;55:950.

Mackey AD, Picciano MF. Maternal folate status during extended lactation and the effect of supplemental folic acid. *Am J Clin Nutr.* 1999;69:285.

Malcolm CA, McCulloch DL, Montgomery C, et al. Maternal docosahexaenoic acid supplementation during pregnancy and visual evoked potential development in term infants: a double blind, prospective, randomised trial. *Arch Dis Child.* 2003;88:F383.

Mandel D, Lubetzky R, Dollberg S, et al. Fat and energy contents of expressed human breast milk in prolonged lactation. *Pediatrics.* 2005;116:e432–e435.

Marchini G, Linden A. Cholecystokinin, a satiety signal in newborn infants? *J Dev Physiol.* 1992;17:215–219.

Marild S, Hansson S, Jodal U, et al. Protective effect of breast-feeding against urinary tract infection. *Acta Paediatr.* 2004;93:164–167.

Mason T, Rabinovich CE, Fredrickson DD, et al. Breast feeding and the development of juvenile rheumatoid arthritis. *J Rheumatol.* 1995;22:1166–1170.

Martin RM, Gunnell D, Owen CG, Smith GD. Breast-feeding and childhood cancer: a systematic review with meta-analysis. *Int. J Cancer.* 2005;117:1020–1031.

Martin R, Olivares M, Marín ML, et al. Probiotic potential of 3 lactobacilli strains isolated from breast milk. *J Hum Lact.* 2005;21:8–17.

Mathur GP, Gupta, N, Mathur S, et al. Breastfeeding and childhood cancer. *Indian Pediatr.* 1993;30:651–657.

Matsuoka Y, Idota T. The concentration of epidermal growth factor in Japanese mother's milk. *J Nutr Sci Vitaminol.* 1995;41:24–51.

Mayer EJ, Hamman RF, Gay EC, et al. Reduced risk of IDDM among breast-fed children. *Diabetes.* 1988;37:1625–1632.

McVeagh P, Miller JB. Human milk oligosaccharides: only the breast. *J Paediatr Child Health.* 1997;33:281–286.

Medves JM. Three infant care interventions: reconsidering the evidence. *JOGNN.* 2002;31:563–569.

Metcalfe DD. Food hypersensitivity. *J Allergy Clin Immunol.* 1984;73:749–762.

Michie, Tantscher E, Schall T, Rot A. Physiological secretion of chemokines in human breast milk. *Eur Cytokine Netw.* 1998;9:123–129.

Minekawa R, Takeda T, Sakata M, et al. Human breast milk suppresses the transcriptional regulation of IL-1(beta)-induced NF-(kappa)B signaling in human intestinal cells. *Am J Physiol.* 2004;287:C1404–C1411.

Miralles O, Sánchez J, Palou A, Picó C. A physiological role of breast milk leptin in body weight control in developing infants. *Obesity.* 2006;14:1371–1377.

Mitoulas LR, Kent JC, Cox DB, et al. Variation in fat, lactose and protein in human milk over 24 h and throughout the first year of lactation. *Br J Nutr.* 2002;88:29–37.

Mitra AK, Rabbani F. The importance of breastfeeding in minimizing mortality and morbidity from diarrhoeal diseases: the Bangladesh perspective. *J Diarrhoeal Dis Res.* 1995;13:1–7.

Montgomery RK, Büller HA, Rings EH, Grand RJ. Lactose intolerance and the genetic regulation of intestinal lactose-phlorizin hydrotase. *Fed Am Soc Exp Biol J.* 1991;5:2824–2832.

Morriss FH. Method for investigating the presence and physiologic role of growth factors in milk. In: Jensen RG, Neville MC, eds. *Human lactation: milk components and methodologies.* New York, NY: Plenum; 1985:193–200.

Morriss FH, Brewer ED, Spedale SB, et al. Relationship of human milk pH during course of lactation to concentrations of citrate and fatty acids. *Pediatrics.* 1986;78:458–464.

Morrisset J, Jolicoeur L. Effect of hydrocortisone on pancreatic growth in rats. *Am J Physiol.* 1980;239:295.

Morton JA. The clinical usefulness of breast milk sodium in the assessment of lactogenesis. *Pediatrics.* 1994;93:802–806.

Motil KJ, Krtz B, Thotathuchery M. Lactation performance of adolescent mothers show preliminary differences from that of adult women. *J Adolescent Med.* 1997;20:442–449.

Motil KJ, Sheng HP, Montandon CM, Wong WW. Human milk protein does not limit growth of breast-fed infants. *J Pediatr Gastroenterol Nutr.* 1997;24:10–17.

Naficy AB, Abu-Elyazeed R, Holmes JL, et al. Epidemiology of rotavirus diarrhea in Egyptian children and implications for disease control. *Am J Epidemiol.* 1999;150:770–777.

Neville MC, Keller R, Seacat J, et al. Studies in human lactation: milk volumes in lactating women during the onset of lactation and full lactation. *Am J Clin Nutr.* 1988;48:1375–1386.

Neville MC., Morton J, Umemora S. Lactogenesis: Transition from pregnancy to lactation. *Ped Clin North Am.* 2001;48:35–52.

Neville MC, Oliva-Rasbach J. Is maternal milk production limiting for infant growth during the first year of life in breast-fed infants? In: Goldman AS, Atkinson SA, Hanson LA, eds. *Human lactation,* Vol. 3. New York, NY: Plenum; 1987:123–133.

Newburg DS, Peterson JA, Ruiz-Palacios GM, et al. Role of human-milk lactadherin in protection against symptomatic rotavirus infection. *Lancet.* 1998;351:1160.

Newman J. How breast milk protects newborns. *Sci Am.* December 1995:76–79.

Nommsen-Rivers L. The long-term effects of early nutrition: the role of breastfeeding on cholesterol levels. *J Hum Lact.* 2003;19:103–104.

Oddy WH. Breastfeeding and asthma in children: findings from a West Australian study. *Breastfeed Rev.* 2000;8:5–11.

Oddy WH, Sherriff JL, de Klerk NH, et al. The relation of breastfeeding and body mass index to asthma and atopy in children: a prospective cohort study to age 6 years. *Am J Public Health.* 2004;94:1531–1537.

Odze RD, Wershil BK, Leichtner AM, Antonioli DA. Allergic colitis in infants. *J Pediatr.* 1995;126:163–170.

Oftedal OT. The evolution of milk secretion and its ancient origins. *Animal.* 2012;6(3):355–368.

Okamoto Y, Ogra P. Antiviral factors in human milk: implications in respiratory syncytial virus infection. *Acta Paediatr Scand.* 1989;351(suppl):137–143.

Ostrea EM, Balun JE, Winkler R, Porter T. Influence of breast-feeding on the restoration of the low serum concentration of vitamin E and beta-carotene in the newborn infant. *Am J Obstet Gynecol.* 1986;154:1014–1017.

Owen CD, Whincup PH, Odoki K, et al. Infant feeding and blood cholesterol: a study in adolescents and a systematic review. *Pediatrics.* 2002;110:597–608.

Pabst HE, Spady DW, Pilarski LM, et al. Differential modulation of the immune response to breast- or formula-feeding of infants. *Acta Paediatr.* 1997;86:1291–1297.

Paganelli R, Cavagni G, Pallone F. The role of antigenic absorption and circulating immune complexes in food allergy. *Ann Allergy.* 1986;57:330–336.

Palmer B. The influence of breastfeeding on the development of the oral cavity: a commentary. *J Hum Lact.* 1998;14:93–99.

Perera BJ, Ganesan S, Jayarasa J, Ranaweera S. The impact of breastfeeding practices on respiratory and diarrhoeal disease in infants: a study from Sri Lanka. *J Trop Pediatr.* 1999;45:115–118.

Perez-Bravolt F, Carrasco E, Guiterrez-Lopez MD, et al. Genetic predisposition and environmental factors leading to the development of insulin-dependent diabetes mellitus in Chilean children. *J Mol Med.* 1996;74:105–109.

Petschow B, Carter DL, Hutton GD. Influence of orally administered epidermal growth factor on normal and damaged intestinal mucosa in rats. *J Pediatr Gastroenterol Nutr.* 1993;17:49–57.

Picciano MF. Nutrient composition of human milk. *Ped Clin North Am.* 2001;48:53-67.

Pickering LK, Kohl S. Human milk humoral immunity and infant defense mechanisms. In: Howell RR, Morriss FH, Pickering LK, eds. *Human milk in infant nutrition and health.* Springfield, IL: Thomas; 1986:123–140.

Pisacane A, Graziano L, Mazzarella G, et al. Breast feeding and urinary tract infection. *Lancet.* 1990;336:50.

Pisacane A, Impagliazzo N, Russo M, et al. Breast feeding and multiple sclerosis. *Br Med J.* 1994;308:1411–1412.

Pisacane A, de Luca U, Vaccaro F, et al. Breast-feeding and inguinal hernia. *J Pediatr.* 1995a;127:109–111.

Pisacane A, de Luca U, Impagliazzo N, et al. Breast feeding and acute appendicitis. *BMJ.* 1995b;310:836–837.

Pohlabeln H, Nuhlenbruch K, Jacobs S, et al. Frequency of allergic diseases in 2-year old children in relationship to prenatal history of allergy and breastfeeding. *J Investig Allergol Clin Immunol.* 2010;20(3):195–200.

Porro E, Indinnimeo L, Anotognoni G, et al. Early wheezing and breast feeding. *Asthma.* 1993;30:23–28.

Popkin BM, Adair L, Akin JS, et al. Breast-feeding and diarrheal morbidity. *Pediatrics.* 1990;86:874–882.

Prentice AM, Collinson AC. Does breastfeeding increase thymus size? *Acta Paediatr.* 2000;89:8–10.

Prentice AM, Prentice AM, **Cole TJ**, et al. Breast-milk antimicrobial factors of rural Gambian mothers. I. Influence of stage of lactation and maternal plane of nutrition. *Acta Paediatr Scand.* 1984;73:796–812.

Prosser CG, Saint L, Hartmann PE. Mammary gland function during gradual weaning and early gestation in women. *Aust J Exp Biol Med Sci.* 1984; 62:215–228.

Pullan CR, Toms GL, Martin AJ, et al. Breast-feeding and respiratory syncytial virus infection. *Br Med J.* 1980;281(6247):1034–1036.

Quigley MA, Kelly YJ, Sacker A. Breastfeeding and hospitalization for diarrheal and respiratory infection in the United Kingdom Millennium Cohort Study. *Pediatrics.* 2007;119:e837–e842.

Quinlan PT, Lockton S, Irwin J, Lucas AL. The relationship between stool hardness and stool composition in breast- and formula-fed infants. *J Pediatr Gastroenterol Nutr.* 1995;20: 81–90.

Rahman MM, Yamauchi M, Hanada N, et al. Local production of rotavirus specific IgA in breast tissue and transfer to neonates. *Arch Dis Child.* 1987;62:401–405.

Raiha NCR. Nutritional proteins in milk and the protein requirement of normal infants. *Pediatrics.* 1985;75 (suppl):136–141.

Raisler J, Alexander C, Campo P. Breastfeeding and infant illness: a dose-response relationship? *Am J Public Health.* 1999;89:25–30.

Ramsay DT, Kent JC, Hartmann RA, Hartmann PE. Anatomy of the lactating human breast redefined with ultrasound imaging. *J Anat.* 2005;206:525–534.

Ravelli A, van der Meulen JH, Osmond C, et al. Infant feeding and adult glucose tolerance, lipid profile, blood pressure, and obesity. *Arch Dis Child.* 2000;82:248–252.

Ravelomanana N, Razafindrakoto O, Rakotoarimanana DR, et al. Risk factors for fatal diarrhoea among dehydrated malnourished children in a Madagascar hospital. *Eur J Clin Nutr.* 1995;49:91–97.

Read L, Upton FM, Francis GL, et al. Changes in the growth-promoting activity of human milk during lactation. *Pediatr Res.* 1984;18:133–138.

Reid B, Smith H, Friedman Z. Prostaglandins in human milk. *Pediatrics.* 1980;66:870–872.

Rigas A, Rigas B, Glassman M, et al. Breast-feeding and maternal smoking in the etiology of Crohn's disease and ulcerative colitis in childhood. *Ann Epidemiol.* 1993;3:387–392.

Riordan JM. The cost of not breastfeeding: a commentary. *J Hum Lact.* 1997;13(2):93–97.

Romani Vestman N, Timby N, Holgerson P, et al. Characterization and in vitro properties of oral lactobacilli in breastfed infants. *BMC Microbiology.* 2013; 13:193.

Rosenbauer J, Herzig P, Giani G. Early infant feeding and risk of type 1 diabetes mellitus—a nationwide population-based case-control study in pre-school children. *Diabetes Metab Res Rev.* 2008;24:211–222.

Rosenberg M. Breast-feeding and infant mortality in Norway 1860–1930. *J Biosoc Sci.* 1989;21:335–348.

Rovet JF. Does breast-feeding protect the hypothyroid infant whose condition is diagnosed by newborn screening? *Am J Dis Child.* 1990;144:319–323.

Rubaltelli FR, Biadaioli R, Pecile P, Nicoletti P. Intestinal flora in breast- and bottle-fed infants. *J Perinat Med.* 1998;26:186–191.

Rudloff EH, Schmalstieg FC Jr, Palkowetz KH, et al. Interleukin-6 in human milk. *J Reprod Immunol.* 1993;23:13–20.

Ruiz-Palacios GM, Calva JJ, Pickering LK, et al. Protection of breast-fed infants against *Campylobacter* diarrhea by antibodies in human milk. *J Pediatr.* 1990;116:707–713.

Ruuska R. Occurrence of acute diarrhea in atopic and non-atopic infant: the role of prolonged breast-feeding. *J Pediatr Gastroenterol Nutr.* 1992;14:27–33.

Saarela AT, Kokkonen J, Koivisto M. Macronutrient and energy contents of human milk fractions during the first six months of lactation. *Acta Paediatrica.* 2005;94:1176–1181.

Saarinen UM. Prolonged breast feeding as prophylaxis for recurrent otitis media. *Acta Paediatr Scand.* 1982;71:567–571.

Saarinen KM, Juntunen-Backman K, Järvenpää AL, et al. Breast-feeding and the development of cow's milk protein allergy. *Adv Exp Med Biol.* 2000;478:121–130.

Saarinen UM, Kajosaari M. Breastfeeding as prophylaxis against atopic disease: prospective follow-up study until 17 years old. *Lancet.* 1995;346:1065–1069.

Sachdev HP, Krishna J, Puri RK, et al. Water supplementation in exclusively breastfed infants during summer in the tropics. *Lancet.* 1991;337(8747):929–933.

Saint L, Smith M, Hartmann PE. The yield and nutrient content of colostrum and milk of women giving birth to 1 month postpartum. *Br J Nutr.* 1984;52:87–95.

Salmenpera L, Perheentupa J, Siimes MA. Folate nutrition is optimal in exclusively breast-fed infants but inadequate in some of their mothers and in formula-fed infants. *J Pediatr Gastroenterol Nutr.* 1986;5:283–289.

SanGiovanni JP, Parra-Cabrera S, Colditz GA, et al. Meta-analysis of dietary essential acuity in healthy preterm infants. *Pediatrics.* 2000;105:1292–1298.

Sasai K, Furukawa S, Kaneko K, et al. Fecal IgE in infants at 1 month of age as indicator of atopic disease. *Allergy.* 1994;49:791–794.

Sassen ML, Brand R, Grote JJ. Breast-feeding and acute otitis media. *Amer J Otolaryngol.* 1994;15:351–357.

Savino F, Sorrenti M, Risistin and leptin in breastmilk and infants in early life. *Early Hum Dev.* 2012:888:779–782.

Schroten H, Bosch M, Nobis-Bosch R, et al. Secretory immunoglobulin A is a component of the human milk fat globule membrane. *Pediatr Res.* 1999;45:82–86.

Shehadeh N, Gelertner L, Blazer S, et al. Importance of insulin content in infant diet: suggestion for a new infant formula. *Acta Paediatr.* 2001;90:93–95.

Shing YW, Klagsburn M. Human and bovine milk contain different sets of growth factors. *Endocrinology.* 1984;115:273.

Shu XO, Clemens J, Zheng, et al. Infant breastfeeding and the risk of childhood lymphoma and leukaemia. *Int J Epidemiol.* 1995;24:27–34.

Siigur U, Ormission A, Tamm A. Faecal short-chain fatty acids in breast-fed and bottle-fed infants. *Acta Paediatr.* 1993;82:536–538.

Siimes MA, Salmenperä L, Perheentupa J. Exclusive breast-feeding for nine months: risk of iron deficiency. *J Pediatr.* 1984;104:196–199.

Silfverdal SA, Bodin L, Hugosson S, et al. Protective effect of breastfeeding on invasive Haemophilus influenzae infection: a case-control study in Swedish preschool children. *Int J Epidemiol.* 1997 Apr;26(2):443–450.

Smith AM, Picciano MF, Milner JA. Selenium intakes and status of human milk and formula fed infants. *Am J Clin Nutr.* 1982;35:521.

Smulevich, VB, Solionova LG, Belyakova, SV. Parental occupation and other factors and cancer risk in children: 1. Study methodology and non-occupational factors. *Int J Cancer.* 1999;83:712.

Sommerburg O, Meissner K, Nelle M, et al. Carotenoid supply in breast-fed and formula-fed neonates. *Eur J Pediatr.* 2000;159:86–90.

Steel MG, Leslie GA. Immunoglobulin D in rat serum, saliva and milk. *Immunology.* 1985;55:571–577.

Steichen JJ, Krug-Wispe SK, Tsang RC. Breastfeeding the low birth weight preterm infant. *Clin Perinatol.* 1987;14:131–171.

Stuff JE, Nichols GL. Nutrient intake and growth performance of older infants fed human milk. *J Pediatr.* 1989;115:959–968.

Svanborg C, Agerstam H, Aronson A, et al. HAMLET fills tumor cells by an apoptosis-like mechanism—cellular, molecular, and therapeutic aspects. *Adv Cancer Res.* 2003;8:1–29.

Swartzbaum JA, George SL, Pratt CB, Davis B. An exploratory study of environmental and medical factors potentially related to childhood cancer. *Med Pediatr Oncol.* 1991;19:115–121.

Takahata Y, Takada H, Nomura A, et al. Interleukin-18 in human milk. *Pediatr Res.* 2001;50:268–272.

Takala AK, Eskola J, Palmgren J, et al. Risk factors of invasive *Haemophilus influenzae* type b disease among children in Finland. *J Pediatr.* 1989;115:694–701.

Tran TT, Chowanadisai W, Lönnerdal B, et al. Effects of neonatal dietary manganese exposure on brain dopamine levels and neurocognitive functions. *Neurotoxicology.* 2002;145:1–7.

Udall JN, Dixon M, Newman AP, et al. Liver disease in α_1-antitrypsin deficiency. *JAMA.* 1985;253:2679–2682.

U.S. Department of Health and Human Services (DHHS). *Healthy people 2020.* Washington, DC: DHHS; 2010. Available at: http://www.healthypeople.gov/2020/topicsobjectives2020/objectiveslist.aspx?topicId=26.

Uvnas-Moberg K, Marchini G, Windberg J. Plasma cholecystokinin concentrations after breastfeeding in healthy 4 day old infants. *Arch Dis Child.* 1993;68:46–48.

Van Derslice J, Popkin B, Briscoe J. Drinking-water quality, sanitation, and breast-feeding: their interactive effects on infant health. *Bull WHO.* 1994;72:589–601.

van der Westhuyzen, Chetty M, Atkinson PM. Fatty acid composition of human milk from South African black mother consuming a traditional maize diet. *Eur J Clin Nutr.* 1988;42:213–220.

Verge CF, Howard NJ, Irwig L, et al. Environmental factors in childhood IDDM: a population-based case-control study. *Diabetes Care.* 1994;17:1381.

Victora CG, Smith PG, Vaughan JP, et al. Evidence for protection by breastfeeding against infant deaths from infectious diseases in Brazil. *Lancet.* 1987;2:319–321.

Virtanen SM, Rasanen L, Aro A, et al. Childhood diabetes in Finland Study Group: feeding in infancy and the risk of type 1 diabetes mellitus in Finnish children. *Diabet Med.* 1992;9:815.

Wagner CL, Greer FR, American Academy of Pediatrics Section on Breastfeeding. Committee on Nutrition. Prevention of rickets and vitamin D deficiency in infants, children and adolescents. *Pediatrics.* 2008;122:1142–1152.

Wagner CL, Taylor TS, Holis BW. Does vitamin D make the world go round? *Breastfeed Med.* 2008;3:239–250.

Wagner C, Taylor SN, Johnson DD, HollisBW. The role of vitamin D in pregnancy and lactation: emerging concepts. *Women's Health.* 2012;8(3):323–340.

Wagner V, Stockhausen JG. The effect of feeding human milk and adapted milk formulae on serum lipid and lipoprotein levels in young infants. *Eur J Pediatr.* 1988;147:292–295.

Wahlberg J, Vaarala O, Ludvigsson J. Dietary risk factors of the emergence of type 1 diabetes-related autoantibodies in 2 1/2 year-old Swedish children. *Br J Nutr.* 2006;95:603–608.

Wallace JM, Ferguson SJ, Loane P, et al. Cytokines in human milk. *Br J Biomed Sci.* 1997;54:85–87.

Wasmuth HE, Kolb H. Cow's milk and immune-mediated diabetes. *Proc Nutr Soc.* 2000;59:573–579.

Wells JC, Jonsdottir OH, Hibberd PL, et al. Randomized controlled trial of 4 compared with 6 mo of exclusive breastfeeding in Iceland: differences in breast-milk intake by stable-isotope probe. *Am J Clin Nutr.* 2012;96(1):73–79. doi: 10.3945/ajcn.111.030403.

Widdowson EM, Colombo VE, Artavanis CA. Changes in the organs of pigs in response to feeding for the first 24 hours after birth: II. The digestive tract. *Biol Neonate.* 1996;28:272.

Wilson AC, Forsyth JS, Greene SA, et al. Relation of infant diet to childhood health: seven year follow up of cohort of children in Dundee infant feeding study. *BMJ.* 1998;316:21–25.

Wilson JV, Self TW, Hamburger R. Severe cow's milk-induced colitis in an exclusively breast-fed neonate. *Clin Pediatr.* 1990;29:77–80.

Wilson-Clay B, Hoover K. *The breastfeeding atlas,* 5th ed. Manchaca, TX: LactNews Press; 2013.

Wirt DP, Adkins LT, Palkowetz KH, et al. Activated and memory T lymphocytes in human milk. *Cytometry.* 1992;13:282–290.

Woolridge MW, Fisher C. Colic, "overfeeding," and symptoms of lactose malabsorption in the breast-fed baby: a possible artifact of feed management? *Lancet.* 1988;2:382–384.

Woolridge MW, Ingram JC, Baum JD. Do changes in pattern of breast usage alter the baby's nutrient intake? *Lancet.* 1990;336:395–397.

Yamauchi Y, Yamanouchi I. Breast-feeding frequency during the first 24 hours after birth in full-term neonates. *Pediatrics.* 1990;86:171–175.

Yoneyama K, Nagata H, Asano H. Growth of Japanese breast-fed and bottle-fed infants from birth to 20 months. *Ann Hum Biol.* 1994;21:597–608.

Zaman K, Sack DA, Chakraborty J, et al. Children's fluid intake during diarrhoea: a comparison of questionnaire responses with data from observations. *Acta Paediatr.* 2002;91:376–382.

Zanardo V, Nicolussi S, Carlo G, et al. Beta endorphin concentrations in human milk. *J Pediatr Gastroenterol Nutr.* 2001;33:160–164.

Composition of Human Colostrum and Mature Breastmilk

Constituent (per 100 mL)	Colostrum 1–5 days	Mature Milk > 30 days	Constituent (per 100 mL)	Colostrum 1–5 days	Mature Milk > 30 days
Energy, kcal	58	70	*Vitamins (Water Soluble)*		
Lactose, g	5.3	7.3	Thiamine, µg	15	16
Total nitrogen, mg	360	171	Riboflavin, µg	25	35
Protein nitrogen, mg	313	129	Niacin, µg	75	200
Nonprotein nitrogen, mg	47	42	Folic acid, µg	—	5.2
Total protein, g	2.3	0.9	Vitamin B_6, µg	12	28
Casein, mg	140	187	Vitamin B_{12}, ng	200	26
α-lactalbumin, mg	218	161	Vitamin C, mg	4.4	4.0
Lactoferrin, mg	330	167	*Minerals and Trace Elements*		
IgA, mg	364	142	Calcium, mg	23	28
Urea, mg	10	30	Sodium, mg	48	15
Creatine, mg	—	3.3	Potassium, mg	74	58
Total fat, g	2.9	4.2	Iron, µg	45	40
Cholesterol, mg	27	16	Zinc, µg	540	166
Vitamins (Fat Soluble)					
Vitamin A, µg	89	47			
Beta-carotene, µg	112	23			
Vitamin D, µg	—	0.04			
Vitamin E, µg	1280	315			
Vitamin K, µg	0.2	0.21			

Source: Used with permission from Casey CE, Hambidge KM. Nutritional aspects of human lactation. In: Neville MC, Neifert MR, eds. *Lactation: physiology, nutrition and breastfeeding.* New York: Plenum; 1983:203–204.

Hilary Rowe
Teresa E. Baker
Thomas W. Hale

Chapter 5

Drug Therapy and Breastfeeding

Introduction

Over the past 5 years, more mothers have been attempting to breastfeed and to continue to breastfeed exclusively due to the national and international campaigns to educate the public about the numerous health and economic benefits of this practice (Centers for Disease Control and Prevention [CDC], 2013). The CDC's 2012 breastfeeding report card data support this hypothesis, as 74.6% of women in America breastfed in the early postpartum period and 47.2% continued breastfeeding at 6 months (16% exclusively, up from 11% in 2007). Human milk provides the infant's first and best choice for protection against infectious disease during the first year of life. Not only is it perfectly suited for the infant's gastrointestinal (GI) tract, but its numerous growth factors enhance growth and maturation of a relatively permeable GI tract. Key benefits to the infant include perfect nutrition, enhanced neurocognitive development, stronger immune function, and significant reductions in infectious disease, such as upper respiratory infections, otitis media, sudden infant death syndrome, and necrotizing enterocolitis (Cochi et al., 1986; Ford et al., 1993; Goldman, 1993; Goldman et al., 1994; Piscane et al., 1992).

Even though the initiation rates of breastfeeding are on the rise, as noted earlier, the number of women who do not exclusively breastfeed or discontinue breastfeeding before 6 months is still too high (CDC, 2013). There are numerous reasons for this high discontinuation rate, including common misconceptions about medications in breastmilk. Surveys in Western countries indicate that 90% to 99% of women who breastfeed will receive at least one medication during the first week postpartum (Bennett, 1996). While it is not known for sure how many women discontinue breastfeeding due to concerns associated with using various medications, at least one Scandinavian study suggests that among mothers who discontinue breastfeeding prematurely, the use of medications is a major reason (Matheson, 1985).

Healthcare professionals often advise women to discontinue breastfeeding because they are unsure about the suitability of the medication in breastmilk for infants, and often their concerns are reinforced if they consult a medication product monograph to aid in their clinical decision making. Many manufacturers' prescribing inserts discourage breastfeeding to avoid risks of litigation. Some even suggest that no data are available, even when dozens of published works clearly show the safety of their product. However, sometimes the safety of a product for a breastfeeding child is not absolutely clear. This is particularly true of new medications, which never have breastfeeding data when they are first launched.

Certain pharmacokinetic parameters can be used to help distinguish between safe and unsafe medications. Certainly the most useful data available are studies already present in the literature that disclose the amount of drug that enters milk, but, as noted previously, this information is not available for new medications. Therefore, the healthcare practitioner must sometimes use available kinetic tools to evaluate the overall risk to the infant.

The following review is designed to aid readers in their evaluation of medications in breastfeeding mothers and to provide our current insight into this field. Lactation consultants and other healthcare providers can use the following pharmacokinetic information, the most up-to-date literature, and the lactation risk categories (e.g., safer, probably safe) to evaluate the mother's need for drug therapy and determine the true risk to her infant from the medication (Hale, 2012).

The Alveolar Subunit

The parenchyma of the breast consists of approximately 8–12 ductal regions that ultimately drain toward the nipple (Figure 5-1). Ducts migrate through the mammary fat during pregnancy as progestin, estrogen, and placental lactogen levels rise. The forming ducts canalize themselves through the fat pad during the first and second trimesters of pregnancy, ultimately ending in extensive lobulo-alveolar clusters, which are lined by the alveolar epithelium that actually creates milk (Neville et al., 1998).

The alveolar unit is lined with specialized epithelial cells called lactocytes. The entire alveolar unit is thoroughly perfused with capillaries and lymphatics and is innervated with small nerves. Closely juxtapositioned to the basal membrane of the alveolus are numerous capillaries that serve as the primary source of immunoglobulins, fats, and many other components (including drugs) needed for the production of human milk (Figure 5-2). During pregnancy, the size and number of alveolar complexes increase significantly due to the high level of maternal

Figure 5-1 STRUCTURE OF THE ALVEOLAR SUBUNIT WITH BLOOD SUPPLY AND OTHER STRUCTURES.

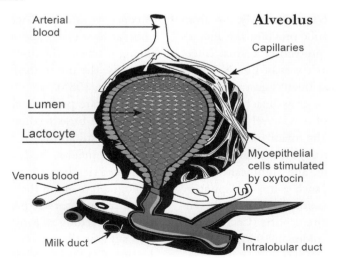

Source: Adapted from Hale TW, Hartmann PE. Textbook of Human Lactation. Amarillo: Hale Publishing; 2007

Figure 5-2 TRANSPORT OF DRUGS AND OTHER SUBSTANCES THROUGH THE ALVEOLAR EPITHELIAL CELL.

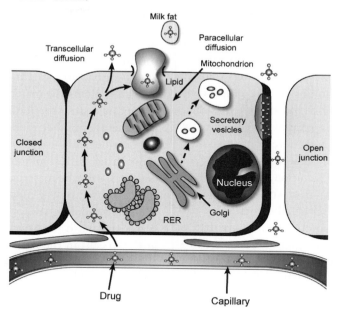

Source: Adapted from Hale TW, Hartmann PE. Textbook of Human Lactation. Amarillo: Hale Publishing; 2007

estrogen, progesterone, placental lactogen, prolactin, and oxytocin, all of which act directly on the mammary gland to bring about developmental changes (Neville, McFadden, & Forsyth, 2002). At this stage, milk production is largely suppressed by the high levels of progestins. With delivery of the placenta, however, progestins and estrogens rapidly disappear from the plasma of the mother, and the lactocytes begin a rapid change from a quiescent state to a fully active secretory state (secretory lactogenesis).

During the early stages of lactation (colostral phase), when the lactocytes are small in size and the intercellular spaces are large, maternal substances, including drugs, lymphocytes, immunoglobulins, proteins, and other plasma substances, can easily transfer into human milk via these large intercellular gaps. Over time, with the drop in progestins, the lactocytes grow in size and subsequently narrow the intercellular gaps, eventually closing most of them.

As can be seen from the transition from colostrum to mature milk, changes in breastmilk occur due to rapid growth of the lactocytes, ending in closure of the tight junctions between the cells. At 36 hours following delivery, a major change in the components of milk occurs, which is complete by 5 days postpartum. With closure of the intercellular spaces, the transfer of maternal medications and other maternal proteins into the mother's milk is greatly reduced.

Drug Transfer into Human Milk

Drugs transfer into human milk largely as a function of their physicochemical characteristics, which include their molecular weight, lipid solubility, protein binding, and pK_a (Atkinson & Begg, 1990; Hale et al., 2007). Maternal factors that affect the rate of drug transfer include the relative oral absorption of the medication and the plasma levels of the medication. Of these many factors, the following are the most influential:

- Maternal plasma levels of the drug
- Molecular weight of the medication
- Oral bioavailability of the medication in mother and infant
- Protein binding of the medication

Passive Diffusion of Drugs into Milk

The transfer of drugs into human milk is usually facilitated by passive diffusion down a concentration gradient formed by the non-ionized, free drug on each side of the semipermeable membrane (Miller, Banerjee, & Stowe, 1967). Normally, drugs transfer from areas of high concentration to areas of low concentration (passive diffusion). As described earlier, the overall rate and degree of transfer may be initially affected by the stage of alveolar development and the junctional condition of the lactocytes.

In the first 2–3 days of lactation, which are characterized by the production of small volumes of colostrum, the alveolar epithelial structure of the breast is quite open and porous. Thus many maternal proteins, lipids, immunoglobulins, and medications easily transfer into the milk compartment. Often drug levels in milk reach equilibrium with the plasma compartment (milk/plasma ratio = 1). As the lactocytes begin to swell after several days, the intercellular junctions close. This subsequently leads to dramatically lower levels of drugs in the milk compartment after the first week postpartum. While the transfer of medications or any substance into milk may be higher during the initial stages of early lactation, the absolute amount of colostrum delivered is often quite low (50–60 mL/day on days 1 and 2), so the clinical dose of medication delivered to the infant during this time is actually very low.

Milk and maternal plasma should be viewed as distinct and separate compartments. For most drugs, their transfer in and out of the milk compartment is accomplished by passive diffusion. While some active transport systems exist for immunoglobulins, electrolytes, and particularly iodides, facilitated transport systems are rather limited. Indeed, fewer than 10 drugs appear to be selectively transported into human milk. Transport systems for medications may be indicated by drugs that have high milk/plasma ratios, although many drugs are ion trapped in milk due to the lower pH of milk and the higher pK_a of the medication (as discussed in the next subsection). Regardless, in the case of higher milk/plasma ratios, it is apparent that either the drug is ion trapped in the milk or it is pumped into milk at higher levels (e.g., iodides).

Drugs enter and exit the milk compartment largely as a function of their physiochemistry. The retrograde diffusion of drugs from the milk back into the plasma is well documented and is probably controlled by the same kinetic factors as influence drugs' entry into breastmilk (Schadewinkel-Scherkl et al., 1993). As the maternal plasma level of medication increases, so does the transfer into milk. Then, as the mother metabolizes or eliminates the medication and her plasma levels begin to drop, most drugs diffuse out of the milk compartment and back into the maternal plasma compartment to be eliminated by the mother (Figure 5-3). Following this reasoning, it is obvious that the diffusional forces that push medications into milk are highest at C_{max} (peak) in the mother and lowest during the trough period when the mother is eliminating the medication. Thus, with drugs having a shorter half-life, one can avoid higher exposure to the medications by avoiding breastfeeding when the maternal plasma levels are highest, instead breastfeeding when the maternal levels are much lower. While this timing mechanism works to curtail transfer of some drugs, however, it will not work for medications with long half-lives, as the time period between C_{max} and trough is prolonged in this case.

Ion Trapping

Because the pH of milk is slightly more acidic than that of plasma (milk pH = 7.2; plasma pH = 7.4), certain weak bases ($pK_a > 8$) may become more polarized and, therefore, fail to diffuse backward into the plasma once in milk. As a consequence, they become "trapped" in milk (ion trapping) and may produce higher milk/plasma ratios (Rasmussen, 1971). Ion trapping probably occurs with medications such as the barbiturates and ranitidine, among many others. Conversely, a weak acid is often trapped in the plasma compartment, where it is more polar and enters milk relatively poorly due to its polarized state. In such a case, it is unable to transfer through the lactocyte bilayer lipid membranes due to its high state of polarity.

Figure 5-3 COMPARTMENT REPRESENTATION OF DRUG TRANSFER FROM PLASMA TO THE MILK COMPARTMENT.

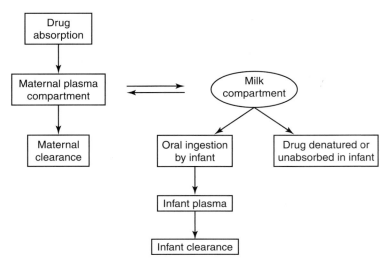

Molecular Weight

With closure of the intercellular gaps, most medications that transfer into breastmilk enter via the "transcellular" pathway. To do so, they must enter the basal membrane of the lactocyte, diffuse gently through the cell, and exit via the luminal surface. The smaller the molecular weight of the medication (300 daltons or less), the greater the rate of diffusion across the bilayer lipid membranes. As the molecular weight of the medication exceeds 500–800 daltons, it becomes increasingly difficult to diffuse through the bilayer membranes and enter milk. Thus medications whose molecular weights exceed 1000 daltons seldom enter the milk compartment in clinically relevant amounts. Medications such as heparin, insulin, interferon, and other high-molecular-weight drugs simply do not pass into milk in clinically relevant amounts (Kumar, Hale, & Mock, 2000). In contrast, a medication such as lithium, which has no protein binding and low molecular weight, transfers into milk readily (Sykes, Quarrie, & Alexander, 1976). Many of the psychotropic drugs, such as the amphetamines, have low molecular weights and are highly lipid soluble, which accounts for their rapid entry into

the central nervous system as well as their higher milk/plasma ratios in human milk.

Lipophilicity

Although plasma contains lipids, the concentration is relatively low compared to the 5–15% triglycerides found in human milk. As such, some medications that are lipid soluble may immerse themselves in the lipid fraction of milk and transfer to the infant. We actually know very little about the diffusion into and out of the lipid fraction of milk, but it appears that by selectively extracting the lipid fraction in milk, certain drugs accumulate in higher concentrations. Some medications during their transfer through the lactocyte dissolve themselves in the lipid droplets and are subsequently dumped into the alveolar lumen. Others may pass completely through the cell and subsequently transfer into the lipid droplets within the milk itself. For highly lipid-soluble drugs, such as many neuroleptic drugs (e.g., diazepam, chlorpromazine), a vast majority of the drug is found in the lipid fraction (Syversen & Ratkje, 1985).

While scientifically interesting, the clinical utility of this information is relatively small. The most important feature of lipid solubility is that the more lipid soluble the medication, the more likely it will transfer into human milk. A more practical feature of this relationship is that most central nervous system (CNS)–active drugs are both low in molecular weight and very lipid soluble—two kinetic parameters that permit them to transfer through the blood–brain barrier as well as into human milk. Hence, greater concern for the infant should be taken with CNS-active drugs.

Milk/Plasma Ratio

The ratio of the concentration of drug in the milk to that in the plasma is known as the milk/plasma ratio (M/P). The M/P ratio is quite useful in determining the relative transfer of medication into milk, but there are significant difficulties in accurately measuring it. Because of differences in the rate of drug transfer, changes in plasma and milk concentrations of medications do not always follow one another, and the time at which the samples are drawn becomes incredibly important. For example, the M/P ratio may be 1.14 at zero time and 0.31 at 3 hours following administration (Hale et al., 2002). As a result, the M/P ratio actually reflects the differential rate of entry of drug into plasma and milk and will often change from hour to hour (Sykes et al., 1976). Most importantly, the M/P ratio is of limited clinical use in assessing the likelihood that a clinically relevant dose will be transferred to the infant during breastfeeding. Even with some drugs that have high M/P ratios (e.g., ranitidine), the absolute dose transferred to the infant is still subclinical. Ultimately, it is the concentration of drug in the milk (relative infant dose) and the volume of milk ingested that determine the clinical dose transferred to the infant. For this reason, low M/P ratios suggest that very little drug enters the milk. Conversely, high M/P ratios may or may not indicate high levels in milk because the key factor is the maternal plasma level of medication.

Maternal Plasma Levels

Ultimately, one of the most important kinetic factors determining drug transfer to the infant is the maternal plasma level of the drug. Plasma concentrations of drugs vary according to the dose administered, the half-life of the medication, the volume of distribution, the oral bioavailability, and the proclivity for protein binding. Drugs vary enormously in potency, with some requiring only microgram doses whereas others require huge doses (grams). Because of the enormous difference in potency, plasma levels of various drugs can vary from nanograms per milliliter to milligrams per milliliter. In general, as the molar concentration of a drug in solution increases, the equilibrium gradient also increases to force the drug into other compartments. Thus, the more drug present, the higher the forces pushing it into the milk compartment. For this reason alone, the degree and rate of transfer of a drug into milk generally correlate with the plasma concentration curve. As the concentration in the plasma peaks (C_{max}), it is quite common that milk levels peak as well. While this is certainly not always true, such as with metformin, the majority of drugs exhibit this feature. Thus it is important to understand that if a drug is not absorbed in the mother or is rapidly depleted from her plasma compartment to other compartments (rapid redistribution), the transfer to her milk compartment will be quite low. Drugs with brief half-lives will be eliminated so quickly that they seldom pose a major risk to the infant, unless the infant is feeding at C_{max}.

Bioavailability

The bioavailability of a medication generally refers to the amount of drug that reaches the systemic circulation after administration. Depending on the route of administration (oral, intravenous [IV], intramuscular [IM], subcutaneous [SC], topical), medications may ultimately pass into the systemic circulation prior to reaching their intended site of action or the milk compartment. Fortunately, many medications are unstable in the gastric milieu or are incompletely absorbed by infants. Most, but not all, topical medications are poorly absorbed transcutaneously, so they seldom attain significant plasma levels. When drugs are administered orally, the liver sequesters or metabolizes many medications, preventing their entry into the plasma compartment. Thus the poor bioavailability of many products reduces the exposure level in breastfed infants.

Because infants receive drugs via the mother's milk, oral bioavailability is of major importance in evaluating potential risks to the infant. The absolute dose of a medication received via milk must be decreased by the percent oral bioavailability. Obviously, drugs with poor bioavailability are ideal for breastfeeding mothers, as their absorption in the infant is likely poor. Examples of medications with poor oral bioavailability include low-molecular-weight heparins, proton pump inhibitors (e.g., omeprazole), and vancomycin. In some instances, however, the active medication may become concentrated in the GI tract of the infant, causing problems. Diarrhea and thrush are common complications following the use of various antibiotics, for example.

Drug Metabolites

Ordinarily, the primary function of drug metabolism is to make the drug more soluble so that the kidneys will excrete it. However, in many situations, the parent drug (prodrug) is actually metabolized to the active drug. This is true of valacyclovir, codeine, hydroxyzine, fluoxetine, and many other medications. Some of these metabolites actually have much longer half-lives than the parent drug—for example, norfluoxetine (from Prozac), normeperidine (from Demerol), and cetirizine (from Atarax, hydroxyzine). Thus, in some cases, the metabolite and the parent drug both must be evaluated for their levels in milk and side effects. In the case of meperidine, it is the metabolite (normeperidine) that is believed to account for some of the toxicities of this drug.

Calculating Infant Exposure

Perhaps the most important clinical parameter is to calculate the actual dose (D_{inf}) received by the infant. To do so, you must know the actual concentration of medication in the milk and the volume of milk transferred. While this information is not always available, many drugs do have published studies providing the peak (C_{max}) concentrations or the average (C_{av}) concentrations for the drug. In many previous studies, C_{max} was the most commonly reported value.

Unfortunately, this measure frequently overestimates the amount of drug actually delivered to the infant. More recent studies now calculate the area under the curve (AUC) value for the medication. This methodology accurately estimates the average daily intake by the infant and is much more accurate than the C_{max} estimates.

The volume of milk ingested is highly variable and depends on the age of the infant and the extent to which the infant is exclusively breastfed. Many clinicians use a 150 cc/kg/day value to estimate the amount of milk ingested by the infant. The following formula estimates the clinical dose to the infant:

$$D_{inf} = \text{Drug concentration in milk}$$
$$(\text{at } C_{max} \text{ or } C_{av}) \times \text{Volume of milk ingested}$$

However, the most useful and accurate measure of exposure is to calculate the relative infant dose (RID):

$$\text{Relative infant dose} = D_{inf}(\text{mg/kg/day}) / \text{Maternal dose (mg/kg/day)}$$

This value, which is generally expressed as a percentage of the mother's dose, provides a standardized method of relating the infant's dose to the maternal dose. In full-term infants, Bennett (1996) recommends that a relative infant dose of more than 10% should be the theoretical "level of concern" for most medications. Nevertheless, the 10% level of concern is relative, and each situation should be individually evaluated according to the overall toxicity of the medication. In premature infants, this "level of concern" may need to be lowered appropriately, depending on the medication. In this regard, it should always be remembered that many neonates may have been exposed in utero to drugs taken by their mothers and that in utero exposure may be an order of magnitude greater than that received via breastmilk. Thus infants exposed in utero to methadone go through significant withdrawal upon delivery, even when breastfeeding.

Unique Infant Factors

A good clinical exam of the infant is mandatory to evaluate the relative risk of the medication to the infant.

All infants should be categorized as low, moderate, or high risk for the medication of interest. Low-risk infants are generally older infants (6–18 months), who can metabolize and handle drugs relatively efficiently. Mothers in the terminal stage of lactation (more than 1 year after giving birth) often produce relatively smaller quantities of milk. Thus the absolute clinical dose transferred is often low to nil. Moderate-risk infants are those younger than 6 months who suffer from various metabolic problems, such as complications of delivery, apnea, GI anomalies, or other metabolic problems. High-risk infants include premature infants, newborns, unstable infants, and infants with poor renal output.

Fewer than 1% of all therapeutic agents used today have recommended dosing guidelines for the newborn or premature infant. The infant's GI tract is undergoing dynamic changes early in the postnatal period. During the first week of life, a state of relative achlorhydria exists; the pH continues to decrease slowly toward adult values in the next 2 years. Medications that are weak acids may have reduced absorption (phenobarbital) in infants, and drugs that are weak bases may have enhanced absorption. Because the infant's exposure occurs via the oral route, the oral bioavailability of the medication is of paramount importance. Drugs with high first-pass clearance (e.g., morphine) are rapidly cleared from the portal circulation and sequestered in the liver, even in infants. Drugs with poor stability in the gut (e.g., aminoglycosides, domperidone, heparin, proton pump inhibitors) are rapidly degraded in the stomach or intestine and remain unabsorbed. Poor biliary function subsequently leads to poor lipid absorption and relative steatorrhea in newborn or premature infants. Therefore, lipid-soluble drugs, even if present in milk, would have poorer oral bioavailability in the infant. Gastric emptying time is much prolonged in premature infants and in some cases may alter the absorption kinetics altogether. The values for total body water are higher than in adults, protein binding is decreased in neonates, and the oxidative and conjugative capacity of the liver is greatly reduced in neonates (Besunder, Reed, & Blumer, 1988). Interestingly, while the metabolic capacity of the liver is reduced at first, it increases rapidly and actually approximates adult capacity by 9–12 months (Morselli, Franco-Morselli, & Bossi, 1980).

Ultimately, the evaluation of the safety of drugs in breastmilk depends on at least four major factors: the amount of medication present in milk, the oral bioavailability of the medication, the inherent toxicity of the drug, and the ability of the infant to clear the medication. Table 5-1 lists medications with particularly high risk levels that should be avoided or used with caution in breastfeeding mothers. While we know milk levels for many hundreds of drugs and their approximate bioavailability, the ability of the infant to clear the medication is highly variable and still requires individual evaluation by the clinician. Begg (2000) estimated infant clearance to be 5%, 10%, 33%, 50%, 66%, and 100% of adult maternal levels at 24–28, 28–34, 34–40, 40–44, 44–68, and more than 68 weeks postconceptual age, respectively.

Maternal Factors

The plasma compartment is the only source of medication for the milk compartment. If drugs are not absorbed by the mother and do not produce significant plasma levels, then they pose no risk to an infant. Medications that are not orally bioavailable in the mother (e.g., oral vancomycin, magnesium hydroxide, magnesium sulfate) do not normally attain significant plasma levels and, therefore, are not likely to be hazardous to a breastfed infant. This group also includes most—but not all—topical preparations. Many topical steroids, antibiotics, and retinoids used over minimal surface areas are not well absorbed through the skin and are virtually undetectable in the plasma compartment. One-time injections of local anesthetics (such as for dental procedures) provide so little drug that plasma levels are minuscule. Hence, the acute use of many medications is not usually problematic, as the overall dose transferred to the infant is small over time.

The amount of milk the mother produces is very important as well. Milk production on the first and second days postpartum is so small that the overall dose of medication transferred is usually insignificant. Mothers who are 1–2 years postpartum also generally have a significantly reduced milk supply,

Table 5-1 DRUGS TO GENERALLY AVOID OR USE WITH CAUTION IN BREASTFEEDING MOTHERS

Drug	Clinical Significance	Lactation Risk Category (Hale, 2012)
ACE inhibitors	Use caution in premature infants; compatible thereafter. Preferred ACEIs are captopril and enalapril (Devlin & Fleiss, 1981).	Safer
Acebutolol	Potential hypotension in infants (Boutroy et al., 1986).	Probably safe
Alcohol	May reduce milk production significantly (Mennella & Beauchamp, 1991).	Probably safe
Amiodarone	Avoid long-term use. Brief use okay. High risk of accumulation due to long half-life and high volume of distribution; cardiovascular risks are high; thyroid suppression is significant (McKenna et al., 1983; Plomp et al., 1992).	Possibly hazardous acute/hazardous chronic
Amphetamines	Potentially high milk levels; stimulation of infant (Steiner et al., 1984).	Probably safe
Anticancer agents	Cytotoxicity, immune suppression.	Hazardous
Aspirin	81 mg dose probably okay; avoid higher doses. Wait 2 hours postdose to avoid (Putter et al., 1974).	Probably safe
Caffeine	Milk levels small, but neonatal half-life long. Symptoms include jitteriness and stimulation (Ryu, 1985).	Safer
Chloramphenicol	Blood dyscrasia and aplastic anemia are possible in mother, but not reported as a result of breastfeeding (Havelka et al., 1968).	Possibly hazardous
Cocaine	Potential high milk levels; intoxication, stimulation of infant (Winecker et al., 2001).	Hazardous
Doxepin	Dangerous sedation and respiratory arrest reported (Matheson et al., 1985).	Hazardous
Iodine	High levels in milk. May inhibit thyroid function in neonate (Saenz, 2000).	Possibly hazardous
Lithium	Levels high in milk; risk high to infant unless monitored closely (Sykes et al., 1976).	Probably safe with close observation
Marijuana	May suppress prolactin and/or milk supply. Infant will be drug-screen positive for long periods (Astley & Little, 1990).	Hazardous
Meperidine	Neonatal sedation reported, neurobehavioral delay in neonates (Wittels et al., 1990).	Probably safe
Methotrexate and immuno-suppressants	Levels in milk are apparently low, with a relative infant dose of approximately 0.12% (Johns et al., 1972). Potential for a range of symptoms associated with suppression of the immune system. Methotrexate may concentrate in neonatal GI cells (Fountain et al., 1953).	Probably safe
Ribavirin	No reported milk levels, but following chronic use may lead to hemolytic anemia; caution is recommended (Schering Corporation, 2001).	Possibly hazardous
Sulfonamides	Avoid early postnatally. They displace bilirubin from its binding site. Hyperbilirubinemia possible. Do not use in G6PD deficiency (Rasmussen, 1958).	Probably safe
Tetracycline (chronic)	Brief use okay (< 3 weeks); chronic use not recommended (Morganti et al., 1968; Shetty, 2002).	Safer (short term) Hazardous (chronic use)

and their infants are much older. Thus the clinical dose transferred in late-stage lactation is often reduced as well. As a consequence, the risk of a medication in a mother with an 18-month-old infant is relatively small unless the drug is extraordinarily toxic (radioactive or anticancer drugs).

Minimizing the Risk

The following factors may profoundly reduce infant exposure to medications and the risk for adverse effects:

- Avoid feeding the infant or pump and discard the mothers' milk at C_{max}. Because milk levels are invariably a function of maternal plasma levels, avoiding breastfeeding at the peak concentration (C_{max}) will always reduce infant exposure to higher drug levels in milk. While useful for shorter half-life medications, this advice is of questionable use with medications having a long half-life, and its feasibility in real life is questionable.
- Temporarily withhold breastfeeding for brief exposures. If the mother can store sufficient milk for a brief exposure to medication (e.g., radiocontrast test), then the risk to the infant is eliminated. Milk produced during the exposure can be pumped and discarded.
- Choose medications that have minimal levels in milk, and when possible choose the medication in a class of drugs with the smallest relative infant dose. However, all medications should be evaluated for their efficacy in the specific syndrome. Sometimes, there are no better alternatives.

- Choose medications that are commonly used in pediatric patients and are considered safe.
- Choose medications with high protein binding (e.g., warfarin), because tissue and milk levels will be lower.
- Choose medications with poor penetration into the CNS, as they usually produce lower milk levels.
- Choose medications with higher molecular weights (e.g., heparin), as this factor greatly reduces transfer into milk.

Effect of Medications on Milk Production

Drugs That May Inhibit Milk Production

Some medications are well known to affect the rate of milk production. Because infant weight gain and development are directly associated with milk production, even modest changes in milk supply can produce major growth complications for the infant. Drugs that may potentially inhibit milk production include ergot alkaloids (bromocriptine, cabergoline, ergotamine), estrogens, progestogens, pseudoephedrine, and, to a minor degree, alcohol (Aljazaf et al., 2003; Mennella & Beauchamp, 1991; Sweezy, 1992; Treffers, 1999). Box 5-1 lists drugs that are known to negatively affect milk production.

Estrogens have a long but poorly documented history of suppressing milk (Booker & Pahl, 1967; Booker, Pahl, & Forbes, 1970; Gambrell, 1970). It has been hypothesized that oral contraceptives

---

BOX 5-1 DRUGS THAT MAY REDUCE MILK PRODUCTION

- Bromocriptine
- Cabergoline
- Ergotamine
- Estrogens
- Progestins
- Ethanol
- Pseudoephedrine

may interfere with the natural decrease in progesterone levels after delivery, which is the trigger for lactogenesis II to occur; therefore, if hormones are initiated too early, this therapy may decrease milk production (Kennedy, Short, & Tully, 1997). In a study from 1983 that included 330 women who used nonhormonal contraceptives (NHC), combined oral contraceptives (COCs), and copper intrauterine devices (Cu IUDs) starting on day 30 postpartum, researchers found more infants were weaned from breastmilk at 6 and 8 months in the COC group (16.3% COC, 9% NHC, and 4.7% Cu IUD at 6 months) (Croxatto et al., 1983). However, by the end of 1 year, an equivalent number of women (approximately 40%) in each of the three groups were no longer breastfeeding. Although infants of the COC-using mothers were within the normal range for their weight, they did have significantly smaller weight gains at 6 and 12 months when compared to infants of NHC-using mothers.

A double-blind randomized trial published in 2012 compared the effect of initiating progestin-only contraceptives (0.35 mg norethindrone) to COCs (0.035 mg ethinyl estradiol + 1 mg norethindrone) at 2 weeks postpartum (Espey et al., 2012). The researchers found there was no difference in continuation of breastfeeding between the two groups at 8 weeks (64.1% combined pills versus 63.5% progestin-only contraceptives) or 6 months. In both groups, women were more likely to stop breastfeeding if they supplemented their infants with formula or had concerns about inadequate milk supply. Although this study did not find a difference between the two hormonal contraceptives and the changes in milk production, there was no comparison of rates of breastfeeding discontinuation with a placebo group, and only the mother's perception of changes in milk volume—not actual volumes—was analyzed.

The progestin-only implants and intrauterine devices that are used for contraception contain levonorgestrel. Several studies have demonstrated that levonorgestrel has limited, if any, effect on milk volume; moreover, because its concentrations are lowest in the plasma of IUD users, it is thought that the IUD is the contraceptive option least likely to affect milk production (Shaaban, Salem, & Abdullah, 1985).

Among 120 women who used progestin implants, there were no reported changes in breastfeeding at 5–6 weeks postpartum (Shaaban, 1991). In a study of 163 and 157 women who used levonorgestrel IUDs and copper IUDs, respectively, no changes in breastfeeding, infant growth, and infant development were noted over 12 months in either group (Shaamash et al., 2005). Although the levonorgestrel IUD data suggest minimal to no effect on breastmilk supply, some caution is recommended, as the authors have received numerous reports of milk suppression following insertion of this product.

Due to the conflicting data, when hormonal contraception is necessary, low-dose progesterone-only oral contraceptives should be used or, if combined oral contraceptives are required, a product with a low estrogen level should be recommended. The most sensitive time for suppression is in the early postpartum period, before the mother's milk supply is established; therefore, waiting as long as possible (minimum 4 weeks) prior to use is advised (Queenan, 2012). All mothers who take hormonal contraception should be forewarned of possible effects on milk production and should be counseled to observe any changes in breastfeeding.

Some members of the ergot family are well known to suppress prolactin levels. Bromocriptine has been used in the past to reduce engorgement and inhibit milk production, although it was associated with numerous cases of cardiac dysrhythmias, stroke, intracranial bleeding, cerebral edema, convulsions, and myocardial infarction (Dutt, Wong, & Spurway, 1998; Iffy et al., 1998; Pop et al., 1998). A newer analog, cabergoline, has proved much safer and is now recommended for both hyperprolactinemia and inhibition of lactation (Ferrari, Piscitelli, & Crosignani, 1995; Webster et al., 1992). Doses of 1 mg cabergoline administered in the early postpartum period will completely inhibit lactation. For established lactation, 0.25 mg twice daily for 2 days has been found to completely inhibit lactation (Caballero-Gordo et al., 1991; "Single Dose Cabergoline," 1991). In cases where mothers have received cabergoline inappropriately, immediate pumping and breastfeeding will probably return their milk supply to normal.

Recent suggestions propose that the nasal decongestant pseudoephedrine may suppress milk production (Aljazaf et al., 2003). More studies are still needed to confirm this relationship, but mothers should be cautious about using pseudoephedrine, particularly if they are in late-stage lactation (more than 8 months) or have poor milk supply.

Drugs That May Stimulate Milk Production

The pituitary hormone prolactin is one of the major controllers of milk production. It is well known that while prolactin levels must be elevated for milk production to occur, higher levels of prolactin do not necessarily increase production (Chatterton et al., 2000). In essence, you have to have enough prolactin to maintain milk synthesis, but overwhelmingly high levels do not make more milk. Thus prolactin levels and milk production are not necessarily related. Initially, prenatal prolactin levels are quite high (200 ng/mL or higher), but then drop significantly over the next 6 months, to slightly elevated levels in the 70 ng/mL range. Mothers whose prolactin levels fall to the nonpregnant, nonlactating range of less than 20 ng/mL may suffer from poor milk synthesis.

In some mothers, particularly those with premature infants, prolactin levels may not be sufficient to support adequate lactation. In these patients, medications that inhibit dopamine receptors in the hypothalamus (e.g., metoclopramide, domperidone) may or may not stimulate milk production. Prolactin release from the pituitary is inhibited by dopamine from the hypothalamus. Consequently, any drug that inhibits dopamine will ultimately increase prolactin release.

Dopamine antagonists, such as domperidone, metoclopramide, risperidone, and the phenothiazine neuroleptics, are well known to stimulate milk production in some patients. The two most commonly used dopamine antagonists are metoclopramide (Reglan) and domperidone (Motilium) (Budd et al.,

1993; Ehrenkranz & Ackerman, 1986; Hofmeyr & Van Iddekinge, 1983; Hofmeyr, Van Iddekinge, & Blott, 1985; Kauppila, Kivinen, & Ylikorkala, 1981; Kauppila et al., 1983; Petraglia et al., 1985). Metoclopramide is the most commonly used agent, and in some cases, profoundly stimulates milk production as much as 100%. Unfortunately, it may induce significant depression if therapy is continued for more than a month. The prolactin-stimulating effect of metoclopramide is dose related, with doses of 10–15 mg three times daily required for efficacy. The amount transferred into milk is small, ranging from 28 to 157 μg/L in the early puerperium, which is far less than the clinical dose administered directly to infants (800 μg/kg/day) (Kauppila et al., 1981). The most significant side effects of metoclopramide are extrapyramidal symptoms, gastric cramping, and (in some cases) major depression.

Domperidone is apparently better tolerated because it does not penetrate the blood–brain barrier; thus no or few CNS side effects occur. However, this medication is not available in the United States other than via compounding pharmacies; in 2004, the U.S. Food and Drug Administration (FDA) issued a warning to mothers about using this unapproved medication for increasing milk production, because several published reports and case studies indicate that domperidone is associated with cardiac arrhythmias, cardiac arrest, and sudden death in patients receiving its intravenous form. Domperidone continues to be used in many other countries, however. One study of this agent suggested that it can produce a mean milk volume increase of 44.5% over 7 days (da Silvia et al., 2001). Reported levels of domperidone in milk were only 1.2 ng/mL.

Dopamine antagonists clearly do not always stimulate milk production in patients with elevated prolactin levels or in those patients with inadequate breast tissue. Nevertheless, in many mothers with premature infants, these drugs may be quite efficacious. Because a mother's milk supply is dependent on an "elevated" prolactin level, the precipitous withdrawal of these agents may result in a significant loss of milk supply. A slow withdrawal is generally recommended over several weeks to a month to prevent loss of milk supply. The dopamine antagonists are often used inappropriately to stimulate milk production in mothers with moderate to low milk production. Before these agents are employed, mothers should be advised to breastfeed more often, pump after breastfeeding, and reduce the intervals between breastfeeding. In those cases where maternal prolactin levels are already elevated, the dopamine antagonists often fail to work at all. Thus measuring baseline prolactin levels just before breastfeeding or approximately 3 hours after breastfeeding will provide an accurate estimate of the mother's trough or baseline prolactin levels; these should be somewhere above 50–70 ng/mL.

The stimulation of milk production by use of herbal medications is extraordinarily common therapy today. However, good supporting data suggesting that these agents stimulate milk production are minimal to nil. Fenugreek is the most commonly used herbal for this purpose. In an abstract describing 10 women who were exclusively breast pumping, a comparison of their milk production diaries was made 1 week prior to fenugreek use and 1 week after they ingested three capsules three times daily; the average milk production during the fenugreek week increased significantly from 207 mL/day (range 57–1057 mL) to 464 mL/day (range 63–1140 mL) (Swafford & Berens, 2000). However, a more recent abstract from 2011 produced data from 26 mothers of premature infants who took fenugreek 1725 mg three times a day for 3 weeks and found there was no effect on either prolactin levels or volume of breastmilk (Reeder, Legrand, & O'Conner-Von, 2011). Although no major adverse effects were reported in these abstracts, herbal products are not controlled by the FDA, so the quality and consistency of the products available in the United States are likely to vary and may put the mother or infant at risk of unknown adverse effects. Fenugreek is not recommended to improve breastmilk production at this time.

Review of Selected Drug Classes

Analgesics

Analgesics are the most commonly used medications in breastfeeding mothers. While nonsteroidal anti-inflammatory drugs (NSAIDs) are the most frequently used agents for this purpose, opioids, such as morphine, fentanyl, and hydrocodone, are most commonly given during the early postpartum period for pain relief. Selected analgesics are reviewed in Table 5-2.

NSAIDs

Of the various NSAID family members, ibuprofen and ketorolac are perhaps ideal agents, with low relative infant doses (less than 0.6%). Naproxen is suitable for short-term use (a few days), but bleeding, hemorrhage, and acute anemia have been reported with its use in a 7-day-old infant (Figalgo, 1989). Data from our laboratories on the newer cyclooxygenase 2 (COX2) inhibitors, such as celecoxib, suggest that their milk levels are quite low, much less than 66 µg/L (Hale, McDonald, & Boger, 2004).

Aspirin, due to its causal association with Reye's syndrome, is not generally recommended in breastfeeding mothers. However, given the very short half-life (31 minutes) of aspirin, the transfer of aspirin itself into milk is probably low to nil. The relative infant dose varies enormously and is reported to range from 0.04% to as high as 10% of the maternal dose (Bailey et al., 1982). Nevertheless, the amount of aspirin in milk is usually low, and it could be used in low maternal doses (82 mg/day) to inhibit platelet function. We do not know if the incidence of Reye's syndrome is dose related with aspirin. Would a single 82 mg/day dose increase the risk of Reye's syndrome? We do not know, but the possibility appears to be extraordinarily remote. Most cases of Reye's syndrome occur in children 10–13 years old who are exposed to therapeutic doses of aspirin during a viral illness; the syndrome

Table 5-2 Relative Infant Dose and Clinical Significance of Selected Analgesic Agents

Drug	Relative Infant Dose (%)	Clinical Significance	Lactation Risk Category (Hale, 2012)
Ibuprofen	0.65 (Weibert et al., 1982)	None detected in infants; no adverse effects reported.	Safest
Ketorolac	0.2 (Wischnik et al., 1989)	Milk levels are very low; no untoward effects reported.	Safer
Naproxen	3.3 (Jamali & Stevens, 1983)	Long half-life; may accumulate in infant. Bleeding, anemia, vomiting, and drowsiness have been reported in breastfed infants (Figalgo, 1989). Short-term use is acceptable; avoid chronic use.	Probably safe Possibly/hazardous (chronic)
Indomethacin	1 (Lebedevs et al., 1991)	Milk levels low; plasma levels low to undetectable in infants; use with caution as there has been one report of seizure in a breastfed infant at 7 days of age (Eeg-Olofsson et al., 1978).	Probably safe
Morphine	9.1 (Feilberg et al., 1989)	Poor oral bioavailability; milk levels generally low; considered safe; observe for sedation.	Probably safe
Hydromorphone	0.7 (Edwards et al., 2003)	Potent semisynthetic narcotic, lowest relative infant dose of the opioid medications.	Probably safe
Oxycodone	8 (Marx et al., 1986)	Use of doses greater than 40 mg/day should be avoided, as adverse effects such as CNS depression in the infant appear to be dose related (Lam et al., 2012).	Probably safe
Codeine	8.1 (Findlay et al., 1981)	There have been case reports of respiratory depression in infants. Caution is advised due to variable CYP 2D6 metabolism (Koren et al., 2006).	Probably safe
Fentanyl	3 (Leuschen et al., 1990)	Milk levels low; no untoward effects from exposure to milk.	Safer

is rarely reported in infants. Lastly, acetylsalicylic acid is rapidly deacetylated to it metabolite, salicylic acid. At 2 hours in adults, aspirin is largely undetectable. We do not think that salicylic acid is associated with Reye's syndrome, so a brief wait of 2 hours after administering aspirin to breastfeed would probably reduce the risk of Reye's syndrome in a breastfed infant.

Methadone

Methadone is widely used in the treatment of opiate addiction and is commonly used in pregnant patients. Methadone levels in milk depend on the dose, but generally range from 2.8% to 5.6% of the maternal dose (Begg et al., 2001; Wojnar-Horton et al., 1997). Because of these low levels in milk, neonatal abstinence syndrome may occur in a high percentage of breastfed newborns whose mothers took methadone during pregnancy (Ostrea, Chavez, & Strauss, 1976; Strauss et al., 1974). In a study by McCarthy and Posey (2000), methadone concentrations in milk ranged from 27 to 260 µg/L in patients receiving 25–180 mg/day. Assuming milk intake of 475 mL/day, the average infant would receive only 50 µg/day or 0.97% of the maternal dose in these studies.

Morphine and Congeners

The data on morphine are unfortunately somewhat inconsistent. Older studies suggested the amount of morphine in milk was minimal to undetectable. In a study of epidural morphine, the concentration in milk following two 4 mg epidural doses was only 82 µg/L (Wittels, Scott, & Sinatra, 1990). Other studies suggest higher levels (10–100 µg/L) were present (Robieux et al., 1990). Given its poor oral bioavailability (less than 25%) and minimal milk levels, morphine does not appear to be significantly hazardous to most breastfeeding infants, as long as the maternal doses remain low to moderate and the infant is stable. Nevertheless, all infants should be closely monitored for respiratory distress, sedation, or poor feeding.

Although some cases of neonatal sedation and apnea have been reported with codeine, the majority of infants are unaffected. While the codeine studies are poor, they suggest that milk levels are low after 48 hours of exposure to 12 doses of 60 mg codeine; the estimated dose of codeine in 2000 mL of milk was only 0.7 mg, or 0.1% of the maternal dose. A recent fatal overdose in one infant with codeine use has suggested clinicians should reevaluate the use of this medication during lactation (Koren, Cairns et al., 2006). Due to the unpredictability of the mother's metabolism of codeine and risk of her rapidly metabolizing the codeine to morphine, it has been suggested that codeine be avoided in breastfeeding (Koren, Cairns et al., 2006). Apparently, hydrocodone is not subject to genetic variations in its metabolism, so it is probably a better choice than codeine in most mothers.

Meperidine

The use of meperidine in the perinatal period is increasingly controversial, as many studies have identified harm to the infant whereas others advocate that short-term use has little risk (Al-Tamimi et al., 2011; Brackbill et al., 1974a). Although the use of meperidine in obstetrics was once common, it has fallen into disfavor as more and more cases of sedation and poor breastfeeding have been reported in newborn infants. Meperidine administered to mothers has been found to produce neonatal respiratory depression, decreased Apgar scores, lower oxygen saturation, respiratory acidosis, and abnormal neurobehavioral scores (Brackbill et al., 1974a, 1974b; Hodgkinson et al., 1978, 1979). Meperidine is metabolized to normeperidine, which is both active and has a half-life of approximately 62–73 hours in newborns. Because of this prolonged half-life, neonatal depression after exposure to meperidine may be profound and prolonged (Brackbill et al., 1974b). Small but significant amounts of meperidine and normeperidine are secreted into human milk and have been found to produce changes in neurocognitive function in some infants (Quinn et al., 1986; Wittels et al., 1997).

Fentanyl

The transfer of fentanyl into human milk is low. In women receiving doses varying from 50 to 400 µg intravenously during labor, the amount found in milk was exceedingly low, generally below the limit of detection (less than 0.05µg/L) (Leuschen et al., 1990).

Antibiotics and Antifungals

Aside from analgesics, the most commonly used class of medications in breastfeeding mothers are the antibiotics. Virtually all of the penicillins and cephalosporins have been studied and are known to produce only trace levels in milk; however, some changes in intestinal flora are to be expected (Table 5-3) (Blanco et al., 1983; Bourget, Quinquis-Desmaris, & Fernandez, 1993; Kafetzis et al., 1980, 1981; Matsuda, 1984; Shyu et al., 1992; Yoshioka et al., 1979).

The transfer of the older tetracyclines into human milk is very low (Morganti et al., 1968). When these medicines are mixed with calcium salts, their bioavailability is significantly reduced, and it is

Table 5-3 RELATIVE INFANT DOSE AND CLINICAL SIGNIFICANCE OF ANTIBIOTICS

Drug	Relative Infant Dose (%)	Clinical Significance	Lactation Risk Category (Hale, 2012)
Amoxicillin	1 (Kafetzis et al., 1981)	The penicillins have minimal transfer into human milk. They have been used for years in breastfeeding and have not had any serious adverse events reported in infants (Benyamini et al., 2005). Observe for changes in intestinal flora.	Safest
Ampicillin	0.3 (Matsuda, 1984)		Safest
Ampicillin + sulbactam	0.5 (Foulds et al., 1985)		Safest
Gentamicin	2.1 (Celiloglu et al., 1994)	Gentamicin produced measurable blood levels (0.41 µg/mL) in 5 of 10 infants when women were given gentamicin 80 mg IM q8h (Celiloglu et al., 1994). The expected intake for an infant was negligible at 307 µg/day (Celiloglu et al., 1994). Observe for changes in intestinal flora.	Safer
Tobramycin	0–2.6 (Festini et al., 2006; Uwaydah et al., 1975)		Probably safe
Cefazolin	0.8 (Yoshioka et al., 1979)	The cephalosporins are also suitable in lactation, as they have low relative infant doses and no major adverse effects in infants have been reported after years of use. Observe for changes in intestinal flora.	Safest
Cephalexin	0.5 (Ilett et al., 2006)		Safest
Cefuroxime	0.6 (Takase & Uchida, 1979)		Safer
Ceftriaxone	4.1 (Bourget et al., 1993)		Safest
Cefotaxime	0.3 (Kafetzis et al., 1980)		Safer
Ceftazidime	0.9 (Blanco et al., 1983)		Safest
Cefepime	0.3 (Sanders, 1993)		Safer
Meropenem	0.18 (Sauberan et al., 2012)	There is one published case report demonstrating minimal transfer into human milk (Sauberan et al., 2012). Observe for changes in intestinal flora.	Probably safe
Erythromycin	1.4 (Knowles, 1972)	Hypertonic pyloric stenosis has been reported in one case with erythromycin (Stang, 1986). Observe for changes in intestinal flora.	Safest
Clarithromycin	2.1 (Sedlmayr et al., 1993)		Safest
Azithromycin	5.9 (Kelsey et al., 1994)		Safer
Clindamycin	1.6 (Smith & Morgan, 1975)	Pseudomembranous colitis (bloody stools) has been reported in one infant (Mann, 1980). Observe for changes in intestinal flora.	Safer

unlikely the infant would absorb the small levels present in milk. However, doxycycline absorption is delayed, not blocked, and over time its absorption may be significant. Short-term administration of these compounds for as long as 3 weeks is permissible. Long-term use, such as for acne, is not recommended in breastfeeding mothers due to the possibility of dental staining in the infant and reduced growth rate in the epiphyseal growth plates (Shetty, 2002).

The use of fluoroquinolones is somewhat controversial in breastfeeding mothers, as these antibiotics are contraindicated in the pediatric population (Ghaffar et al., 2003). Fluoroquinolones have caused arthrotoxicity (cartilage blisters, fissures, and erosions) in animal studies using beagle dogs 13–16 weeks of age and have also caused reversible musculoskeletal adverse effects in adults; none of these changes, however, has been found in the pediatric population (Ghaffar et al., 2003; von Keutz et al., 2004). Due to the low dose received via milk and limited reports of arthropathy in the pediatric population, fluoroquinolones are thought to be suitable for use in lactating women. Pseudomembranous colitis has been reported in one infant who was exposed to ciprofloxacin in breastmilk; however, this adverse effect can occur with any antibiotic (Harmon, Burkhart, & Applebaum, 1992).

Studies of the new fluoroquinolones suggest that ofloxacin (and its derivatives) probably lead to the lowest concentrations in milk (Giamarellou et al., 1989). Ciprofloxacin concentrations in human milk vary over a wide range, but are generally quite low (2.1–2.6%) (Cover & Mueller, 1990; Gardner, Gabbe, & Harter, 1992; Giamarellou et al., 1989). Ciprofloxacin was approved in 2001 for use in breastfeeding mothers by the American Academy of Pediatrics (AAP, 2001). Ciprofloxacin ophthalmic products are poorly absorbed and the dose used in these formulations is low, so these products may be used in breastfeeding mothers.

Metronidazole is a commonly used antimicrobial in pediatric patients. Older studies in rodents suggesting that metronidazole may be mutagenic have never been duplicated in humans (Schwebke, 1995). Following an oral dose of 400 mg three times daily, the maximum concentration in milk averaged 15.5 mg/L (Passmore et al., 1988). Relative infant doses reported are moderate, approximating 10% to 13% of the maternal dose. Thus far, no untoward effects have been reported in breastfed infants other than a metallic taste imparted to the milk. High maternal doses (oral), such as 2 g for treatment of trichomoniasis, may potentially produce high milk levels. In these patients, a brief interruption of breastfeeding is recommended for 12–24 hours (Erickson, Oppenheim, & Smith, 1981).

Following the use of intravenous metronidazole, milk levels of the antibiotic have not been reported; however, the IV route is also considered suitable in lactation. In addition, intravaginal and topical applications do not produce significant plasma levels and do not require changes in breastfeeding recommendations.

The macrolide antibiotics are considered to be compatible with breastfeeding, as their milk levels are quite low. Following a dose of 2 g erythromycin daily, milk levels varied from 1.6 to 3.2 mg/L of milk (Knowles, 1972). When clarithromycin 250 mg twice daily was given to 12 breastfeeding mothers, the relative infant dose was estimated to be 2.1% (Sedlmayr et al., 1993). Azithromycin transfer to milk is minimal and produces a clinical dose of approximately 0.4 mg/kg/day (Kelsey et al., 1994). Erythromycin may not be a good choice in early postnatal mothers, however, as it is known to increase the risk of hypertrophic pyloric stenosis, even in breastfed infants (Sorenson et al., 2003).

Sulfonamides displace bilirubin from its albumin binding site, so they should not be used in newborns. However, they can be used later, generally after 22 days of life in most infants, when bilirubin levels drop to baseline. Sulfisoxazole milk levels are low, and only 1% of the maternal dose is transferred to the infant (Kauffman, O'Brien, & Gilford, 1980). Only minimal transfer of trimethoprim, which is commonly used in sulfonamide products, occurs.

There are numerous other antibiotics in common use, and the reader is referred to other sources for a complete compilation of these drugs (Hale, 2012; Hale & Hartman, 2007).

The use of antifungals in breastfeeding mothers is popular due to suggestions of topical and intraductal candidiasis associated with lactation. However, recent evidence suggests that *Candida albicans* may not be present in the ductal system of breastfeeding women at all, and some sources have suggested that this pain may be instead associated with *Staphylococcus aureus* infections (Hale et al., 2009; Livingston & Stringer, 1999). While it is clear that *C. albicans* may reside on the nipple as a result of contact with the infant's saliva (at least 80% of infants have oral *Candida* by 3 weeks of age), the simple presence of *Candida* on the nipple does not infer it is infectious. The transfer of fluconazole has been studied and is reported to be about 16% of the maternal dose (Force, 1995). This is still considerably less than the clinical dose commonly used in neonates.

Box 5-2 Suitability of Commonly Used Vaccines in Lactation

- Measles, mumps, rubella (MMR): Generally considered safe
- Diphtheria, pertussis, tetanus (dPT): Generally considered safe
- Hepatitis A: Considered safe
- Hepatitis B: Considered safe
- Influenza intranasal (FluMist): Probably safe, but injectable formulation preferred
- Influenza injectable: Generally considered safe
- Varicella: Generally considered safe
- Human papillomavirus (HPV, Gardasil): Generally considered safe

Source: Data from: Hale TW. Medications and Mothers' Milk. Amarillo, TX: Hale; 2012.

While there is some risk of elevated liver enzymes, no such cases have been reported following exposure to fluconazole in breastmilk. Antifungals such as nystatin, clotrimazole, and miconazole are often used topically to treat candidiasis and are considered safe as long as minimal amounts are applied to limit oral absorption by the infant.

Vaccines

During lactation, women may need to update their vaccinations, receive the yearly flu vaccine, or get vaccines they have never previously received prior to travel. Although most vaccines are compatible with breastfeeding, the practitioner should check each vaccine prior to administration, as some vaccines do pose significant risk to the infant when exposed via breastmilk (Box 5-2) (Hale, 2012).

One vaccine with known risk in lactation is the yellow fever vaccine (a live, attenuated vaccine). There have been two case reports, one from Canada and one from Brazil, where breastfed infants younger than 3 weeks of age developed confirmed cases of encephalitis after the vaccine was given to their mothers (Couto et al., 2010; Kuhn et al., 2011). This vaccine is not recommended for use during lactation; however, if its administration is necessary, then the mother should be advised to avoid breastfeeding for about 2 weeks after vaccination (80–100% of persons develop neutralizing antibodies by 10 days after receiving the vaccine and 99% by 28 days) (Staples & Fischer, 2010).

The oral polio vaccine is also associated with a potential risk and is not recommended in breastfeeding mothers with infants younger than the age of 6 weeks, as this vaccine contains three live, attenuated polio viruses (Adcock & Greene, 1971). This vaccine is not known to have any adverse effects when infants are exposed via breastmilk, but some concern has arisen that the effectiveness of the vaccine may be altered when given to the infant directly. If a breastfeeding mother requires the polio vaccine, then the inactivated polio vaccine may be used and the infant can still be immunized without the concern that the vaccine's efficacy could be altered. Most other vaccines have been cleared for maternal use by the CDC.

Antihypertensives

Antihypertensive agents are commonly used early postnatally and sometimes much longer in breastfeeding mothers, but as a family, they require a higher degree of caution. Several beta blockers (e.g., atenolol, acebutolol) have been reported to produce dangerous cyanosis, bradycardia, and hypotension in some breastfed infants (Boutroy et al., 1986). Infants should be closely monitored for these symptoms following therapy. Certain beta blockers are safer than others, and the careful selection of an appropriate medication is highly recommended.

Angiotensin-converting enzyme inhibitors (ACEIs) are becoming popular therapies in numerous health conditions including hypertension, hypertensive urgency, heart failure, myocardial infarction, diabetes, and kidney disease. The two ACEIs with the most breastfeeding data are captopril and enalapril. In a study of 12 women who took captopril 100 mg three times a day, the estimated relative infant dose was 0.002% (Devlin & Fleiss, 1981). In a study where 5 mothers were given a 20 mg dose of enalapril, the average maximum milk concentrations of enalapril and its active metabolite enalaprilat were 1.74 μg/L and 1.72 μg/L, respectively; the relative infant dose was estimated to be about 0.175% (Redman, Kelly, & Cooper, 1990). Although there are many ACEIs on the market, along with another class of medications that are similar to ACEIs called angiotensin receptor blockers (ARBs), captopril and enalapril are preferred due to the lack of safety data for these other medications.

Among the calcium-channel blockers, nifedipine and verapamil are known to have low levels in breastmilk. Nifedipine is commonly used to treat pregnancy-induced hypertension and hypertension early in the postpartum period. While the amount in milk varies depending on the study, the clinical dose received by the infant is generally less than 8 μg/kg/day (Penny & Lewis, 1989). Four other studies of verapamil transfer into milk have reported relative infant doses of 0.1%, 0.2%, 0.3%, and 1.0%—all of which are subclinical levels (Andersen, 1983; Anderson et al., 1987; Inoue et al., 1984; Miller et al., 1986).

Other antihypertensives, such as hydralazine and methyldopa, are commonly used in pregnant patients. Studies suggest that their breastmilk levels are quite low and do not produce clinical changes in breastfed infants (Jones & Cummings, 1978; Liedholm et al., 1982; White, Andreoli, & Cohn, 1985).

Antiplatelet and Anticoagulant Therapy

Women may require the use of antiplatelet and anticoagulant therapy during lactation for the prevention and treatment of numerous cardiac and thromboembolic diseases. The use of low-dose acetylsalicylic acid (81 mg) is compatible with breastfeeding; older studies of acetylsalicylic acid used 1 g orally and found a suitable relative infant dose of 9.4% (Putter, Satravaha, & Stockhausen, 1974). Although the risk of using 81–325 mg aspirin daily is probably quite low, little is known about the dose in breastmilk and the risk of Reye's syndrome in the infant (Bailey et al., 1982).

In one of the larger warfarin studies, which included 13 mothers, there were no breastmilk samples with detectable levels of this medication, and no one reported adverse events in their breastfed infant (Orme et al., 1977). Warfarin is compatible with breastfeeding because it is highly protein bound, undetectable in breastmilk, and has no reported adverse events after years of experience in lactation.

Heparin, including low-molecular-weight heparins (LMWHs), is considered compatible with breastfeeding and is commonly used post-cesarean section for prophylaxis of deep vein thrombosis and pulmonary embolism (McEvoy, 1992). Heparin has a high molecular weight (12,000–15,000 daltons) and consequently is unlikely to enter breastmilk or be absorbed orally (McEvoy, 1992). Dalteparin, a LMWH, has been studied in 15 patients approximately 6 days post-cesarean section. Its levels in breastmilk were found to be very low, less than 0.005–0.037 IU/mL (Richter et al., 2001). Oral absorption of dalteparin and other LMWHs is also unlikely (Richter et al., 2001).

Unfortunately, no human data on clopidogrel in breastmilk have been published to date (Sanofi-Aventis Canada, 2012). Because its metabolite covalently bonds with platelet receptors with a long half-life of 11 days, this drug is not preferred for use in breastfeeding women. Due to clopidogrel's irreversible inhibition of platelet aggregation, the infant's platelet function could be inhibited for a long period of time if any drug reached the infant via breastmilk. Clopidogrel has a reasonable molecular weight of 420 daltons, it is not significantly protein bound, and its oral bioavailability is 50%. This drug has the potential to enter breastmilk and would not be the drug of choice in breastfeeding mother; however, if required, it would not be contraindicated.

Psychotherapeutic Agents

Sedatives and Hypnotics

The most commonly used sedative medications for anxiety and sleep are the benzodiazepines. Most of the benzodiazepine anxiolytics have been thoroughly studied in breastfeeding mothers. Levels of diazepam, lorazepam, and midazolam have been reported and are quite low (Table 5-4) (Matheson, Lunde, & Bredesen, 1990; Summerfield & Nielsen, 1985; Wesson et al., 1985; Whitelaw, Cummings, & McFadyen, 1981). A recent study examined adverse event rates in infants exposed to benzodiazepines via breastmilk (Kelly et al., 2012). Among the 124 women participating, only 1.6% (2 of 124) of the infants (2–24 months old) had CNS depression. There was no correlation between infant sedation and maternal benzodiazepine dose or duration of breastfeeding; however, in the two mothers who reported sedation, it was noted that they were taking a mean of 3.5 medications, versus 1.7 medications for the other mothers, that could

Table 5-4 RELATIVE INFANT DOSE AND CLINICAL SIGNIFICANCE OF PSYCHOTROPIC DRUGS

Antidepressant	Relative Infant Dose (%)	Comments	Lactation Risk Category (Hale, 2012)
Citalopram	3.6 (Rampono et al., 2000)	Majority of infants have few adverse effects; however, there have been two cases of excessive somnolence, decreased feeding, and weight loss with citalopram (Frannsen, 2006; Schmidt et al., 2000). Fluoxetine has caused colic, fussiness, and crying (Lester et al., 1993; Taddio et al., 1996).	Safer
Escitalopram	5.3 (Rampono et al., 2006)		Safer
Fluvoxamine	1.6 (Hagg et al., 2000)		Safer
Fluoxetine	5–9 (Lester et al., 1993; Taddio et al., 1996)		Safer
Sertraline	0.54 (Stowe et al., 2003)		Safer
Paroxetine	1.4 (Ohman et al., 1999)		Safer
Venlafaxine	8.1 (Newport et al., 2009)	No adverse events have been reported in the literature.	Probably safe
Desvenlafaxine	6.8 (Rampono et al., 2011)		Probably safe
Duloxetine	0.1 (Lobo et al., 2008)		Probably safe
Olanzapine	1.6 (Croke et al., 2002)	No adverse events have been reported in the literature.	Probably safe
Quetiapine	0.09 (Rampono et al., 2007)		Safer
Risperidone	4.3 (Hill et al., 2000)		Probably safe
Valproic acid (VPA)	1.4–1.7 (von Unruh et al., 1984)	One case report of a breastfed 3-month-old who developed thrombocytopenia, petechiae, a minor hematoma, and anemia 6 weeks after his mother's dose doubled. This reaction may have been due to a viral illness (Stahl et al., 1997). There are numerous controversies about long-term neurodevelopment; until more data are available, caution is advised (Meador et al., 2010).	Probably safe

Table 5-4 RELATIVE INFANT DOSE AND CLINICAL SIGNIFICANCE OF
PSYCHOTROPIC DRUGS (CONTINUED)

Carbamazepine	5.9 (Shimoyama et al., 2000)	Levels in milk low; there is one report of elevated liver function tests in a 9-day-old infant (Shimoyama et al., 2000).	Safer
Lithium	30.1 (Moretti et al., 2003)	RID is variable so lithium should be used only if found to be most suitable mood stabilizer for the mother, and the infant is full term and healthy. Monitoring serum creatinine, BUN, and thyroid function in the infant is recommended (Moretti et al., 2003; Viguera et al., 2007).	Probably safe with close observation
Lamotrigine	9.2 (Newport et al., 2008)	Reports of significant plasma levels have occurred; none high enough to produce side effects. It may be helpful to monitor infant's plasma levels (Newport et al., 2008; Ohman et al., 2000).	Probably safe
Topiramate	24.5 (Ohman et al., 2002)	Levels in infants are 10–20% of mothers; no adverse effects have been reported (Ohman et al., 2002).	Probably safe

also cause CNS depression. The three benzodiazepines most commonly taken by mothers in this study were lorazepam (52%), clonazepam (18%), and midazolam (15%). Therefore, if benzodiazepine use is needed during lactation, administering a medication with a shorter half-life and limiting concomitant use of other sedating drugs are recommended.

The intermittent use of diazepam, midazolam, or lorazepam has not been associated with significant sedation in breastfed infants. In a prospective study of 42 women ingesting sedatives while breastfeeding, there were only three reports of slight sedation in their infants (Ito et al., 1993). Lorazepam has a shorter half-life than diazepam (12 hours) and when administered as premedication in 3.5 mg oral doses, milk concentrations are only 8–9 µg/L, which is far too low to be clinically relevant (Summerfield & Nielson, 1985). Other studies have suggested high levels (23–82 µg/L) of this medication are found

in breastmilk, but do not produce neurobehavioral effects in breastfed infants (McBride et al., 1979).

In a mother who received oral alprazolam 0.5 mg two to three times daily during pregnancy, a neonatal withdrawal syndrome was reported in the breastfed infant the first week postpartum (Anderson & McGuire, 1989). These data suggest that the amount of alprazolam in breastmilk is insufficient to prevent a withdrawal syndrome following prenatal exposure. Further, in another case of infant exposure solely via breastmilk, the mother took alprazolam (dosage unspecified) for 9 months while breastfeeding and withdrew herself from the medication over a 3-week period (Anderson & McGuire, 1989). In this case, the mother reported withdrawal symptoms in the infant, including irritability, crying, and sleep disturbances. Thus short-term use of certain benzodiazepines (i.e., diazepam, midazolam, or lorazepam) over a week or two is unlikely to produce problems, but long-term daily exposure could be problematic.

Antidepressants

Recent data from 17 American states indicate that postpartum depression affects 12% to 20% of women. These estimates suggest that rates have either risen or patients are reporting their symptoms more openly, as previously documented rates were much lower—between 10% and 15% (Brett, 2008; O'Hara et al., 1990). In the past, the use of antidepressants in breastfeeding mothers was discouraged. However, recent information suggests that depression itself has major negative implications for infants and that it may interfere with optimal parenting, producing significant neurobehavioral delays in infants (Lee & Gotlib, 1991; Sinclair & Murray, 1998; Zekoski, O'Hara, & Wills, 1987). Many women presenting with depressive symptoms may not require pharmacotherapy. Early postpartum sleep deprivation and stress are clearly normal, and general support may be all that is required. Nevertheless, in some patients with severe depression, therapy is clearly indicated. For these reasons, it is important that major depression in breastfeeding women be closely monitored and, if necessary, treated.

In the past, the older tricyclic antidepressants were the mainstay of depressive therapy. While they have been thoroughly studied in breastfeeding mothers and are generally considered safe, their poor side-effect profile generally precludes their use (Bader & Newman, 1980; Brixen-Rasmussen, Halgrener, & Jorgensen, 1982). Weight gain, sedation, and anticholinergic symptoms such as dry mouth, blurred vision, and constipation are major drawbacks to their use as antidepressants. However, these agents still have a prominent use in prevention of migraine headaches and in chronic pain syndromes. When used for these conditions, lower doses at bedtime suffice and tend to reduce the untoward effects associated with this family. Thus they are still commonly used for pain and migraine prevention.

With the introduction of the selective serotonin reuptake inhibitors (SSRIs), the use of antidepressants has increased enormously. In general, the SSRIs are well tolerated and highly effective, and an increasing number of studies show that they are quite safe in breastfeeding mothers. Clinical studies of sertraline (Zoloft) and paroxetine (Paxil) clearly suggest that transfer of these agents into milk is quite minimal, and virtually no side effects have been reported in numerous breastfed infants (Altshuler et al., 1995; Kristensen et al., 1998; Stowe et al., 1997, 2000). Withdrawal in newborns (characterized by poor adaptation, jitteriness, irritability, and other signs and symptoms) has been reported from in utero exposure with sertraline, paroxetine, and other SSRIs (Chambers et al., 1996; Sanz et al., 2005; Stiskal et al., 2001).

At least three case reports of colic, prolonged crying, vomiting, tremulousness, and other symptoms have been reported following the use of fluoxetine (Prozac) in breastfeeding women, although these numbers are probably quite small compared to the thousands of infants who have breastfed without side effects (Hale, Shum, & Grossberg, 2001; Lester et al., 1993; Spencer & Escondido, 1993). In addition, there is some question as to whether these symptoms arose due to withdrawal from fluoxetine, rather than from serotonergic overload.

Citalopram is an SSRI antidepressant similar in effect to fluoxetine and sertraline, although more selective for the receptor site. In an excellent study of seven women receiving an average of 0.41 mg/kg/day of this medication, the average peak level (C_{max}) was 154 µg/L for citalopram and 50 µg/L for demethylcitalopram (Rampono et al., 2000). However, average milk concentrations (AUC) were lower, averaging 97 µg/L for citalopram and 36 µg/L for demethylcitalopram during the dosing interval. Low concentrations of citalopram (2–2.3 µg/L) were detected in only three of the seven infants' plasma. The authors estimate the daily intake to be approximately 3.7% of the maternal dose. Although no infant adverse effects were reported in this study, citalopram has been associated with two reported cases of infant sedation (Frannsen et al., 2006; Schmidt, Olesen, & Jensen, 2000). In the first case, the infant's sedation may have been caused by in utero exposure and subsequent withdrawal from the antidepressant in the first few weeks of life (Frannsen et al., 2006). In the second case, the changes in the infant's sleep were reversed when the maternal dose was decreased (Schmidt et al., 2000).

The active metabolite of citalopram, escitalopram (Lexapro), has recently been studied. In a case report of a mother taking escitalopram (5 mg/day) while breastfeeding her newborn at 1 week of age, the reported milk level was 24.9 ng/mL (Castberg & Spigset, 2006). The infant daily dose was 3.74 µg/kg. At 7.5 weeks of age, the mother was taking 10 mg/day and the milk concentration level was 76.1 ng/mL; the infant daily dose was 11.4 µg/kg. There were no adverse events reported in the infant. Another study of eight breastfeeding women taking an average of 10 mg/day showed the total relative infant dose of escitalopram and its metabolite to be 5.3% of the mothers' dose (Rampono et al., 2006). The drug and its metabolite were undetectable in most of the infants tested. No adverse events in the infants were reported.

The mixed serotonin and norepinephrine reuptake inhibitors (SNRIs)—venlafaxine, desvenlafaxine, and duloxetine—are all considered compatible with breastfeeding. Venlafaxine has now been studied in 20 breastfeeding women (Ilett et al., 1998, 2002; Newport et al., 2009). In the 20 infants, the relative infant doses from the three studies ranged from 6.8% to 8.1% for this medication's active metabolite (*o*-desmethylvenlafaxine). Moreover, no adverse effects were noted in their infants despite milk concentrations of up to 8.2 mg/kg/day. Another report has suggested the infants born of mothers consuming venlafaxine may be at higher risk for a more severe withdrawal and that these symptoms may actually be reduced by breastfeeding (Koren, Moretti, & Kapur, 2006).

Bupropion (Wellbutrin, Zyban) is an antidepressant that can also be used as a tobacco cessation therapy. In a study that enrolled 10 breastfeeding mothers who took bupropion 150 mg SR (sustained release) daily for 3 days and then 300 mg SR daily for 4 more days, the relative infant dose was estimated on day 7 to be 0.14% (Haas et al., 2004). There has been one case report of a 6-month-old infant who experienced seizures on day 4 of exposure to bupropion via breastmilk (Chaudron, 2004). The mother discontinued taking the medication and no further seizure activity occurred in the infant. The author has also received three case reports suggesting that bupropion may reduce milk supply. Close monitoring of infant weight gain and the mother's milk supply is suggested.

Antimanic Preparations

The treatment of bipolar syndrome in breastfeeding mothers is somewhat controversial. Lithium, valproate, and carbamazepine have relatively well-established efficacy in acute mania. However, due to the significant toxicity of lithium, some caution is recommended. Lithium is both small in molecular weight and unbound in the plasma compartment. As such, it produces relatively high levels in human milk and some reported toxicity (Llewellyn, Stowe, & Strader, 1998; Sykes et al., 1976; Tunnessen & Hertz, 1972). Research data suggest that lithium plasma levels in breastfed infants are moderate, approximately 30% to 40% of the maternal level (Fries, 1970; Sykes et al., 1976). However, lithium plasma levels can change dramatically depending on the individual's state of hydration, particularly in the infant with dehydration, and careful monitoring of plasma lithium levels in both mother and infant is strongly recommended. Because lithium affects thyroid function, thyroid function tests should be routinely ordered as well.

Newer studies of valproic acid suggest that this medication is quite efficacious in treating acute mania. It has a more rapid onset of action, and two placebo-controlled studies have reported clinically significant superiority of divalproex over placebo (Bowden et al., 1994; Pope et al., 1991). The transfer of valproic acid into milk is generally considered quite low. In a study of six women receiving 9.5–31 mg/kg/day valproic acid, milk levels averaged 1.4 mg/L while maternal serum levels averaged 45.1 mg/L (Nau et al., 1981). The average milk/serum ratio was 0.027. Most authors agree that the amount of valproic acid transferred to the infant via milk is low. However, recent information suggests that exposure of the fetus to valproic acid significantly increases the risk of autism spectrum and other mental disorders in the offspring (Christensen et al., 2013). This increased risk presumably could persist during lactation as well. Thus the use of valproic acid in breastfeeding mothers should be avoided if other suitable treatments are available. In addition, the infant should be closely monitored for liver and platelet changes.

Lamotrigine (Lamictal) is now approved for the treatment of mania. In numerous studies in breastfeeding mothers, relative infant doses varied according to maternal dose; with doses of 200-400 mg/day, the RID ranged from 7.6% to 13% (Ohman, Vitols, & Tomson, 2000; Page-Sharp et al., 2006; Rambeck et al., 1997; Tomson, Ohman, & Vitols, 1997).

Antipsychotics

The published literature on the transfer of antipsychotics into breastmilk is growing. However, older data seem to suggest that the phenothiazines and thioxanthenes transfer into milk in rather limited amounts.

In a number of small studies, the relative infant dose of chlorpromazine from breastmilk ranged from 0.25% to 0.14% after single doses of 1200 mg and 40 mg, respectively (Blacker, 1962; Ohkubo, Shimoyama, & Sugawara, 1992; Wiles, Orr, & Kolakowska, 1978). In general, normal neurobehavioral development has been reported in infants exposed to chlorpromazine via breastmilk, although drowsiness and lethargy was reported in one infant who ingested milk containing 92 µg/L of chlorpromazine (Ayd, 1973; Wiles et al., 1978). However, in another study, three infants exposed to both chlorpromazine and haloperidol via breastmilk showed developmental delays, and an infant exposed only to chlorpromazine was unaffected (Yoshida et al., 1998). However, chlorpromazine and other phenothiazines have been associated with neonatal apnea and sudden infant death syndrome; thus they are poor choices for use in breastfeeding mothers (Boutroy, 1994; Pollard & Rylance, 1994). For these reasons, the older phenothiazines and thiozanthines should probably be avoided in breastfeeding women.

Haloperidol transfers into breastmilk in moderately low concentrations, and reported relative infant doses range from 0.2% to 11.2% (Ohkubo et al., 1992; Stewart, Karas, & Springer, 1980; Sugawara, Shimoyama, & Ohkubo, 1999; Whalley, Blain, & Prime, 1981). While adverse effects have been minimal in at least two cases, in at least three other cases following exposure to both haloperidol and chlorpromazine via milk, neurobehavioral developmental milestones were not met (Whalley et al., 1981; Yoshida et al., 1998).

The newer atypical antipsychotics may be the best choice of therapy for breastfeeding mothers. These agents include olanzapine, risperidone, quetiapine, and aripiprazole.

Olanzapine transfer into milk has been studied in a total of 14 cases. Relative infant doses ranged from 0.9% to 1.6% following maternal doses of 2.5–20 mg daily (Ambresin et al., 2004; Croke et al., 2002; Gardiner et al., 2003; Kirchheiner, Berghöfer, & Bolk-Weischedel, 2000). In 7 of the infants, olanzapine was undetectable in the serum.

The transfer of quetiapine into human milk has been studied in a total of eight cases. The relative infant dose ranged from 0.09% to 0.27% (Lee et al., 2004; Misri et al., 2006; Rampono et al., 2007). In none of the reported cases were side effects noted in the breastfed infant.

The transfer of risperidone into human milk is also low and has been described in five women and four mother–baby pairs. Risperidone levels are reportedly quite low, with an estimated relative infant dose of 4.3% (Hill et al., 2000). The metabolite was detected in infant plasma in one case, and the concentrations of both risperidone and its metabolite were below the analytical limit of detection in another case. No adverse effects were detected in the four exposed infants studied (Aichhorn, Stuppaeck, & Whitworth, 2005; Ilett et al., 2004; Ratnayake & Libretto, 2002).

Aripiprazole is a newer second-generation antipsychotic; this medication has also been found to have minimal levels in breastmilk. In one mother who took aripiprazole 18 mg once daily throughout pregnancy and then during lactation, 38.7 µg/L was measured in her breastmilk 6 days postpartum (Watanabe et al., 2011). In a second case report, a mother was taking aripiprazole 15 mg/day and her breastmilk levels of the drug were found to be considerably lower—13 µg/L on day 15 and 14 µg/L on day 16 (Schlotterbeck et al., 2007).

Corticosteroids

The corticosteroids, in general, apparently do not transfer well into human milk. Following moderately high doses of prednisone (80 mg), the clinical dose transferred via breastmilk is only 10 µg/kg, which is approximately 10% of the body's endogenous production (Ost et al., 1985). Prednisone and prednisolone transfer into milk has been found to be limited, even with larger doses (Berlin, 1979). Even following chronic doses of methylprednisolone (6–8 mg/day), no untoward side effects were noted in the infants (Coulam et al., 1982).

Steroids used via inhalation, such as fluticasone or budesonide, pose no problem for a breastfeeding mother or infant. Maternal plasma levels are low, and milk levels should be lower still, although no studies in breastfeeding mothers have been published to date. These drugs were designed to have potent local effects, but minimal to nil oral absorption. Hence, milk levels will likely be minimal.

In the case of high intravenous doses (1–2 g prednisone), such as for multiple sclerosis or acute immune reactions, plasma levels of these steroids fall rapidly due to redistribution. A brief interruption of up to 12 hours should suffice to limit infants' exposure via breastmilk (Hale & Ilett, 2002).

With most lower-potency topical steroids, the transcutaneous absorption is generally minimal. However, following the use of high-potency topical steroids over a large body surface, significant plasma levels may be measured. In these instances, a risk-versus-benefit assessment may be required concerning breastfeeding, particularly because these agents are extremely potent. In essence, the recommendation is to use low- to moderate-potency topical steroids if possible.

Thyroid and Antithyroid Medications

The primary objective of treating patients with thyroid supplements is to increase their plasma thyroxine levels into the euthyroid range. Hence, it should be obvious that once accomplished, supplementation with thyroxine is no different than breastfeeding in a normal euthyroid mother. Regardless, the amount of thyroxine transferred into human milk is invariably low (Mizuta et al., 1983; Oberkotter, 1983). There are no contraindications to breastfeeding and using thyroid supplements as long as normal thyroxine levels in the maternal plasma are maintained.

In hyperthyroid states, both propylthiouracil (PTU) and methimazole have been thoroughly studied. PTU levels in breastmilk are at least 10-fold lower than the maternal plasma level. Following a dose of 400 mg, the average amount of PTU transferred over 4 hours was found to be only 99 µg (Kampmann et al., 1980). Using radiolabeled PTU, only 0.08% of the maternal dose was transferred into milk over 24 hours (Low, Lang, & Alexander, 1979). To date, no changes in infants' thyroid function have been reported.

Carbimazole is metabolized to the active metabolite, methimazole. Its levels depend on the maternal dose, but appear too low to produce a clinical effect in the breastfeeding infant. In one study of a patient receiving 2.5 mg methimazole every 12 hours, the dose to the infant was calculated as 16–39 µg/day (Tegler & Lindstrom, 1980). This was equivalent to 7% to 16% of the maternal dose. In a study of 35 lactating women receiving 5–20 mg/day of methimazole, no changes in the infant thyroid function were noted in any infant, even those whose mothers received higher doses (Azizi, 1996).

Further, in a study of 11 women who were treated with a methimazole derivative, carbimazole (5–15 mg daily, equal to 3.3–10 mg methimazole), all 11 infants had normal thyroid function following maternal treatments (Lamberg et al., 1984). In a large study of more than 139 thyrotoxic lactating mothers and their infants, even at methimazole doses of 20 mg/day, no changes in infant thyroid-stimulating hormone (TSH), T_4, or T_3 levels were noted in more than 12 months of study (Azizi et al., 2000).

Drugs of Abuse

Certain drugs of abuse are of major concern to a breastfeeding infant, and mothers need to be advised that the risk of the drug is simply too high to continue to breastfeed their infant. The risk-versus-benefit determination in women who have a history of drug abuse and who want to breastfeed is enormously difficult. Each healthcare provider must evaluate the relative risk that the mother will return to the use of these various medications. While with some of these drugs the overall risk posed by the medication may be lower, some drugs of abuse are detrimental to breastfeeding infants. In these cases, the risk assessment is extremely important. Mothers who appear unlikely to adhere to a drug-free environment while breastfeeding should probably be advised to feed their infants with formula.

Because most drugs of abuse are psychotropics, they readily pass into the brain and, in most instances, the breastmilk compartment as well. The most dangerous compounds are the hallucinogens, such as LSD and phencyclidine. Mothers who are drug-screen positive for these substances should be strongly warned that these agents are the most dangerous of this group and pose significant hazards to their infants. Amphetamines and methylphenidate also pass into milk, but the levels may not be high enough to pose a major hazard to most infants, although this is as yet unclear. Milk/plasma ratios with the amphetamines range from 3 to 7 (Steiner et al., 1984). Interestingly, cocaine levels in milk have never been reported, but based on this stimulant's kinetics we can be certain that cocaine readily enters milk.

The effect of marijuana in breastfeeding mothers is rather unclear. To date, neurobehavioral effects on infants have not been reported, even in heavy smokers (Perez-Reyes & Wall, 1982). Marijuana passes rapidly out of the plasma compartment and enters adipose tissue (stored for weeks to months). Because of this rapid redistribution, milk levels are apparently low.

Analysis of breastmilk in a chronic heavy user of marijuana revealed an eightfold accumulation of this drug in breastmilk compared to plasma, although the dose received was insufficient to produce significant side effects in the infant. Studies have shown significant absorption and metabolism in infants, although long-term sequelae are conflicting. In one study of 27 women who smoked marijuana routinely during breastfeeding, no differences were noted in growth, mental, and motor development outcomes (Tennes et al., 1985).

Another study suggested that marijuana use should be strongly discouraged, as significant changes in the endocannabinoid system, which regulates mood, cognition, reward, and goal-directed behavior, were found to occur after fetal exposure (Astley & Little, 1990). Marijuana in breastmilk was shown to

be associated with a slight decrease in infant motor development at 1 year of age, especially when used during the first month of lactation; interestingly, no detectable effect on infant mental development was observed at 1 year of age. However, because this study included marijuana use during the first trimester of pregnancy, it is difficult to determine the effects of the drug from lactation alone.

The ingestion of heroin in breastfeeding mothers has not been well studied. Heroin is almost instantly deacetylated to its metabolite, morphine. While morphine is considered a good choice as an analgesic for breastfed infants, the major problem with heroin ingestion is the enormous dose sometimes used. Hence, levels of the metabolite (morphine) in milk could be potentially quite large and, therefore, hazardous to the infant.

Mothers should be advised that all of these psychotropic drugs of abuse readily enter milk and that their infants may be at high risk of sedation, apnea, or death if the dose is high enough. Further, all mothers should be advised that regardless of the clinical effect on the infant, their infants will be drug-screen positive for many days, and perhaps weeks, following their use. Suggested pumping and discarding periods are suggested in Table 5-5.

Table 5-5 SUGGESTED DURATION FOR INTERRUPTED BREASTFEEDING FOLLOWING USE OF DRUGS OF ABUSE

Drug	Interrupt Feeding
Cocaine, crack	24 hours
Amphetamines, Ecstasy, MDMA	24–36 hours
Barbiturates	48 hours
Phencyclidine, PCP	1–2 weeks
LSD	48 hours
Ethanol	1 hour per drink, or until sober
Heroin, morphine	24 hours
Marijuana	24 hours

Radioactive Agents

Radioisotopes

The use and transfer of radiolabeled substances are of major importance to breastfeeding mothers. Commonly used as diagnostic tools, the majority of these radioactive compounds have rather brief half-lives and do not pose a major problem for breastfeeding mothers. They can simply pump and discard their milk for 12–24 hours and continue to breastfeed. However, with the use of iodine-131, gallium-67, or thallium-201, longer pumping periods may be necessary and may preclude breastfeeding altogether.

A thorough summary of the most current literature concerning radioisotope transmission into human milk is available (Hale, 2012). Mothers who are required to take these medications are urged to follow the guidelines set forth by various texts (Hale, 2012).

The most dangerous radioisotope is iodine-131. It is concentrated in human milk (approximately 16- to 23-fold), may potentially destroy the infant's thyroid, and could ultimately increase the risk of thyroid carcinoma in the infant exposed to this isotope via milk. The Nuclear Regulatory Commission (NRC) recommends discontinuing breastfeeding altogether. Because the level of radioactive iodine in breast tissue is so high, women who require high doses of I-131 should probably discontinue breastfeeding for several weeks prior to use to avoid high radiation doses to their breast tissues.

Radiocontrast Agents

Radiocontrast agents or radio-opaque agents are used to enhance visualization of various tissue compartments. Two types are used: one group of agents contains high concentrations of iodine, and the other group contains the gadolinium ion. The iodinated groups are used for computed axial tomography (CAT) scans, while the gadolinium products are used for magnetic resonance imaging (MRI) scans.

In general, we recommend against the use of iodine-containing products in breastfeeding mothers. In the case of the radiocontrast agents, however, the iodine molecule is covalently bound to the structure and is only minimally released. Thus, following the use of radiocontrast agents, the amount of free iodine is minimal, and these products are not considered a risk to breastfed infants. In addition, the plasma half-life of these agents is quite short—less than 1 hour for most—and the oral bioavailability is virtually nil. Therefore, the risk that breastfeeding infants will absorb clinically relevant amounts is low.

Table 5-6 provides the pharmacokinetic data and published milk levels on some radiocontrast agents. While most of the package inserts for these products suggest a 24-hour pumping and discarding of milk, this step is obviously not necessary. The American College of Radiology (ACR) has published a guideline on this subject and suggests that radiocontrast agents are not contraindicated in breastfeeding mothers (ACR Committee on Drugs and Contrast Media, 2001).

In MRI scans, gadolinium-containing compounds are used. Milk levels of gadopentetate are reported to be very low (Rofsky, Weinreb, & Litt, 1993). In the Rofsky et al. study, only 0.23% of the maternal dose was excreted over 24 hours of exposure. Further, the oral bioavailability of the gadolinium products is about 0.8%.

SUMMARY

The data supporting the health benefits of breastfeeding are now significant, and this practice is strongly supported by numerous national academies and healthcare organizations. Far too often, however, mothers are given inaccurate information and advised to discontinue breastfeeding so that they can be treated with a medication. In most cases, drugs are quite safe for breastfeeding mothers to consume, and the healthcare practitioner is advised to seek accurate advice prior to disturbing the provision of the most wonderful source of nutrition and health care an infant will ever receive.

It is true that all medications transfer into human milk. However, the vast majority do so in levels that are incredibly low, are almost always subclinical,

Table 5-6 RADIOCONTRAST AGENTS AND THEIR REPORTED MILK CONCENTRATIONS

Drug	Dose	Milk (C_{max})	Clinical Significance	Bioavailability	Lactation Risk Category (Hale, 2012)
Gadopentetate	6.5 g	3.09 µmol/L (Rofsky et al., 1993)	Only 0.023% of maternal dose; total dose = 0.013 µmol/24 hours; safe.	0.8%	Safer
Iohexol	0.755 g/kg	35 mg/L (Nielsen et al., 1987)	Mean milk level was only 11.4 mg/L; virtually unabsorbed; safe.	< 0.1%	Safer
Iopanoic acid	2.77 g	20.8 mg/ 19–29 hours (Holmdahl, 1956)	Only 0.08% of maternal dose; virtually unabsorbed; safe.	Nil	Safer
Metrizamide	5.06 g	32.9 mg/L (Ilett et al., 1981)	Only 0.02% of maternal dose recovered over 44.3 hours; poor oral absorption; safe.	0.4%	Safer
Metrizoate	580 mg	14 mg/L (Nielsen et al., 1987)	Mean milk level 11.4 mg/24 hours; only 0.3% of maternal dose; safe.	Nil	Safer

and pose no real risk for most infants. Nevertheless, all infants should be evaluated for risk prior to their mothers taking medications, and those infants deemed at high risk should be exposed to only medications that carry a minimal risk associated with their use. In reality, we do have a rather extensive database on drugs and their transfer into human milk.

By understanding the various mechanisms of transfer and those medications that pose the greatest risks, the clinician can usually develop strategies that can provide for the safe use of medications in mothers who breastfeed their infants. Such strategies involve using a safer medication or breastfeeding when the medication is low in the maternal plasma supply or, as a last resort, pumping and discarding the milk while the mother is treated.

Physicians and patients are advised to carefully choose those medications with lower relative infant doses and limited side-effect profiles. This might not always be possible, however, and each physician and mother must, as a team, determine the best choice for the individual case. Almost always, with the proper choice of medication, the mother can continue to breastfeed while undergoing drug therapy.

KEY CONCEPTS

- Avoid using medications when not absolutely necessary. This includes most herbal drugs.
- Choose drugs with shorter half-lives over those with longer half-lives.
- Choose drugs with less toxicity and those commonly used in infants.
- Choose drugs with poorer bioavailability to reduce oral absorption in infants.
- Choose drugs for which published milk studies are available.
- Evaluate the infant's medications. See if there are drug interactions.
- Evaluate the age, stability, and condition of the infant to determine whether the infant can handle exposure to the medication.
- Preterm or unstable neonates may be more susceptible to adverse effects of medications because their clearance mechanisms have not matured.
- Understand that drugs that enter the CNS will also likely enter breastmilk. An increased level of concern is recommended with such medications.
- Always advise the mother to watch for changes in milk production with various drugs. Mothers forewarned are more observant of subtle changes.
- Most drugs can be safely used in breastfeeding mothers, after a risk-versus-benefit assessment has been done and the mother has been counseled about side effects to watch for in the infant and when to report them to a healthcare professional.
- Only a very few medications are unsafe under any circumstances.
- A relative infant dose of less than 10% is generally considered compatible with breastfeeding.

REFERENCES

ACR Committee on Drugs and Contrast Media. Administration of contrast medium to breastfeeding mothers. *Am Coll Radiol.* 2001;57(10):13.

Adcock E, Greene H. Poliovirus antibodies in breast-fed infants. *Lancet.* 1971;2(7725):662–663.

Aichhorn W, Stuppaeck C, Whitworth AB. Risperidone and breast-feeding. *J Psychopharmacol.* 2005;19(2):211–213.

Aljazaf K, Hale TW, Ilett KF, et al. Pseudoephedrine: effects on milk production in women and estimation of infant exposure via breastmilk. *Br J Clin Pharmacol.* 2003;56(1):18–24.

Al-Tamimi YIK, Paech MJ, O'Halloran SJ, Hartmann PE. Estimation of infant dose and exposure to pethidine and norpethidine via breast milk following patient-controlled epidural pethidine for analgesia post caesarean delivery. *Int J Obstet Anesth.* 2011;20:128–134.

Altshuler LL, Burt VK, McMullen M, Hendrick V. Breast-feeding and sertraline: a 24-hour analysis. *J Clin Psychiatry.* 1995;56(6):243–245.

Ambresin G, Berney P, Schulz P, Bryois C. Olanzapine excretion into breast milk: a case report. *J Clin Psychopharmacol.* 2004;24(1):93–95.

American Academy of Pediatrics (AAP). Transfer of drugs and other chemicals into human milk. *Pediatrics.* 2001;108(3):776–789.

Andersen HJ. Excretion of verapamil in human milk. *Eur J Clin Pharmacol.* 1983;25(2):279–280.

Anderson P, Bondesson U, Mattiasson I, Johansson BW. Verapamil and norverapamil in plasma and breast milk during breast feeding. *Eur J Clin Pharmacol.* 1987;31(5):625–627.

Anderson PO, McGuire GG. Neonatal alprazolam withdrawal: possible effects of breast feeding. *DICP.* 1989;23 (7–8):614.

Astley SJ, Little RE. Maternal marijuana use during lactation and infant development at one year. *Neurotoxicol Teratol.* 1990;12(2):161–168.

Atkinson HC, Begg EJ. Prediction of drug distribution into human milk from physicochemical characteristics. *Clin Pharmacokinet.* 1990;18(2):151–167.

Ayd F Jr. Excretion of psychotropic drugs in human breast milk. *Int Drug Ther News Bull.* 1973;8(9,10):33–40.

Azizi F. Effect of methimazole treatment of maternal thyrotoxicosis on thyroid function in breast-feeding infants. *J Pediatr.* 1996;128(6):855–858.

Azizi F, Khoshniat M, Bahrainian M, Hedayati M. Thyroid function and intellectual development of infants nursed by mothers taking methimazole. *J Clin Endocrinol Metab.* 2000; 85(9):3233–3238.

Bader TF, Newman K. Amitriptyline in human breast milk and the nursing infant's serum. *Am J Psychiatry.* 1980;137(7):855–856.

Bailey DN, Weibert RT, Naylor AJ, Shaw RF. A study of salicylate and caffeine excretion in the breast milk of two nursing mothers. *J Anal Toxicol.* 1982;6(2):64–68.

Begg EJ. *Clinical pharmacology essentials: the principles behind the prescribing process.* Auckland, New Zealand: Adis International; 2000.

Begg EJ, Malpas TJ, Hackett LP, Ilett KF. Distribution of *R*- and *S*-methadone into human milk at steady state during ingestion of medium to high doses. *Br J Clin Pharmacol.* 2001;52(6):681–685.

Bennett PN. Use of the monographs on drugs. In: *Drugs and human lactation.* Amsterdam, Netherlands: Elsevier; 1996:67–74.

Benyamini L, Merlob P, Stahl B, et al. The safety of amoxicillin/clavulanic acid and cefuroxime during lactation. *Ther Drug Monit.* 2005;27:499–502.

Berlin CM. Excretion of prednisone and prednisolone in human milk. *Pharmacologist.* 1979;21:264.

Besunder JB, Reed MD, Blumer JL. Principles of drug biodisposition in the neonate: a critical evaluation of the pharmacokinetic–pharmacodynamic interface (Part II) [Review]. *Clin Pharmacokinet.* 1988;14(5): 261–286.

Blacker KH. Mothers milk and chlorpromazine. *Am J Psychiatry.* 1962;114:178–179.

Blanco JD, Jorgensen JH, Castaneda YS, Crawford SA. Ceftazidime levels in human breast milk. *Antimicrob Agents Chemother.* 1983;23(3):479–480.

Booker DE, Pahl IR. Control of postpartum breast engorgement with oral contraceptives. *Am J Obstet Gynecol.* 1967;98(8):1099–1101.

Booker DE, Pahl IR, Forbes DA. Control of postpartum breast engorgement with oral contraceptives. II. *Am J Obstet Gynecol.* 1970;108(2):240–242.

Bourget P, Quinquis-Desmaris V, Fernandez H. Ceftriaxone distribution and protein binding between maternal blood and milk postpartum. *Ann Pharmacother.* 1993;27(3):294–297.

Boutroy MJ. Drug-induced apnea. *Biol Neonate.* 1994;65 (3–4):252–257.

Boutroy MJ, Bianchetti G, Dubruc C, Vert P, Morselli PL. To nurse when receiving acebutolol: is it dangerous for the neonate? *Eur J Clin Pharmacol.* 1986;30(6):737–739.

Bowden CL, Brugger AM, Swann AC, et al. Efficacy of divalproex vs lithium and placebo in the treatment of mania. The Depakote Mania Study Group. *JAMA.* 1994;271(12):918–924.

Brackbill Y, Kane J, Manniello RL, Abramson D. Obstetric meperidine usage and assessment of neonatal status. *Anesthesiology.* 1974a;40(2):116–120.

Brackbill Y, Kane J, Manniello RL, Abramson D. Obstetric premedication and infant outcome. *Am J Obstet Gynecol.* 1974b;118(3):377–384.

Brett K. Prevalence of self-reported postpartum depressive symptoms—17 states, 2004–2005. *Morb Mortal Wkly Rep.* 2008;57(14):361–366.

Brixen-Rasmussen L, Halgrener J, Jorgensen A. Amitriptyline and nortriptyline excretion in human breast milk. *Psychopharmacology (Berl).* 1982;76(1):94–95.

Budd SC, Erdman SH, Long DM, et al. Improved lactation with metoclopramide: a case report. *Clin Pediatr (Phila).* 1993;32(1):53–57.

Caballero-Gordo A, Lopez-Nazareno N, Calderay M, et al. Oral cabergoline: single-dose inhibition of puerperal lactation. *J Reprod Med.* 1991;36(10):717–721.

Castberg I, Spigset O. Excretion of escitalopram in breast milk. *J Clin Psychopharmacol.* 2006;26(5):536–538.

Celiloglu M, Celiker S, Guven H, et al. Gentamicin excretion and uptake from breast milk by nursing infants. *Obstet Gynecol.* 1994;84(2):263–265.

Centers for Disease Control and Prevention (CDC). Breastfeeding report card—United States 2012. January 27, 2013. Available at: http://www.cdc.gov/breastfeeding/pdf/2012BreastfeedingReportCard.pdf.

Chambers CD, Johnson KA, Dick LM, et al. Birth outcomes in pregnant women taking fluoxetine [Comments]. *N Engl J Med.* 1996;335(14):1010–1015.

Chatterton RT, Hill PD, Aldag JC, et al. Relation of plasma oxytocin and prolactin concentrations to milk production in mothers of preterm infants: influence of stress. *J Clin Endocrinol Metab.* 2000;85(10):3661–3668.

Chaudron LH. Bupropion and breastfeeding: a case of possible infant seizure. *J Clin Psychiatry.* 2004;65(6):881–882.

Christensen J, Gronborg TK, Sorensen MJ et al. Prenatal valproate exposure and risk of autism spectrum disorders and childhood autism. *JAMA.* 2013;309(16):1696–1703.

Cochi SL, Grønborg TK, Sørensen MJ, et al. Primary invasive *Haemophilus influenzae* type b disease: a population-based assessment of risk factors. *J Pediatr.* 1986;108(6):887–896.

Coulam CB, Moyer TP, Jiang NS, Zincke H. Breastfeeding after renal transplantation. *Transplant Proc.* 1982;14(3):605–609.

Couto AM, Schermann MT, Mohrdieck R, Suzuki A. Transmission of yellow fever vaccine virus through breast-feeding—Brazil, 2009. *Morb Mortal Wkly Rep.* 2010;59(5):130–132.

Cover DL, Mueller BA. Ciprofloxacin penetration into human breast milk: a case report [Comments]. *DICP.* 1990;24(7–8):703–704.

Croke S, Buist A, Hackett LP, et al. Olanzapine excretion in human breast milk: estimation of infant exposure. *Int J Neuropsychopharmacol.* 2002;5(3):243–247.

Croxatto HB, Diaz S, Peralta O, et al. Fertility regulation in nursing women: IV. Long-term influence of a low-dose combined oral contraceptive initiated at day 30 postpartum upon lactation and infant growth. *Contraception.* 1983;27(1):13–25.

da Silva OP, Knoppert DC, Angelini MM, Forret PA. Effect of domperidone on milk production in mothers of premature newborns: a randomized, double-blind, placebo-controlled trial. *CMAJ.* 2001;164(1): 17–21.

Devlin RG, Fleiss PM. Captopril in human blood and breast milk. *J Clin Pharmacol.* 1981;21(2):110–113.

Dutt S, Wong F, Spurway JH. Fatal myocardial infarction associated with bromocriptine for postpartum lactation suppression. *Aust N Z J Obstet Gynaecol.* 1998;38(1):116–117.

Edwards JE, Rudy AC, Wermeling DP, et al. Persistence of amethopterin in normal mouse tissues. *Proc Soc Exp Biol Med.* 1953;83(2):369–373.

Edwards JE, Rudy AC, Wermeling DP, et al. Hydromorphone transfer into breast milk after intranasal administration. Pharmacotherapy. 2003 Feb;23(2):153-8. PMID: 12587803 [PubMed - indexed for MEDLINE]

Eeg-Olofsson O, Malmros I, Elwin CE, Steen B. Convulsions in a breast-fed infant after maternal indomethacin [Letter]. *Lancet.* 1978;2(8082):215.

Ehrenkranz RA, Ackerman BA. Metoclopramide effect on faltering milk production by mothers of premature infants. *Pediatrics.* 1986;78(4):614–620.

Erickson SH, Oppenheim GL, Smith GH. Metronidazole in breast milk. *Obstet Gynecol.* 1981;57(1):48–50.

Espey E, Ogburn T, Leeman L, et al. Effect of progestin compared with combined oral contraceptive pills on lactation. *Obstet Gynecol.* 2012;119(1):5–13.

Feilberg VL, Rosenborg D, Broen CC, Mogensen JV. Excretion of morphine in human breast milk. *Acta Anaesthesiol Scand.* 1989;33(5):426–428.

Ferrari C, Piscitelli G, Crosignani PG. Cabergoline: a new drug for the treatment of hyperprolactinaemia. *Hum Reprod.* 1995;10(7):1647–1652.

Festini F, Ciuti R, Taccetti G, et al. Breast-feeding in a woman with cystic fibrosis undergoing antibiotic intravenous treatment. *J Matern Fetal Neonatal Med.* 2006;19(6):375–376.

Figalgo I. Anemia aguda, rectaorragia y hematuria asociadas a la ingestion de naproxen. *Anales Espanoles de Pediatrica.* 1989;30:317–319.

Findlay JW, DeAngelis RL, Kearney MF, et al. Analgesic drugs in breast milk and plasma. *Clin Pharmacol Ther.* 1981;29(5):625–633.

Force RW. Fluconazole concentrations in breast milk. *Pediatr Infect Dis J.* 1995;14(3):235–236.

Ford RP, Taylor BJ, Mitchell EA, et al. Breastfeeding and the risk of sudden infant death syndrome. *Int J Epidemiol.* 1993;22(5):885–890.

Foulds G, Miller RD, Knirsch AK, Thrupp LD. Sulbactam kinetics and excretion into breast milk in postpartum women. *Clin Pharmacol Ther.* 1985;38(6):692–696.

Fountain JR, Hutchison DJ, Waring GB, Burchenal JH. Persistence of amethopterin in normal mouse tissues. *Proc Soc Exp Biol Med.* 1953;83(2):369–373.

Frannsen EJMV, Ettaher F, Valerio PG, et al. Citalopram serum and milk levels in mother and infant during lactation. *Ther Drug Monit.* 2006;28(1):2–4.

Fries H. Lithium in pregnancy. *Lancet.* 1970;1(7658):1233.

Gambrell RDJ. Immediate postpartum oral contraception. *Obstet Gynecol.* 1970;36(1):101–106.

Gardiner SJ, Kristensen JH, Begg EJ, et al. Transfer of olanzapine into breast milk, calculation of infant drug dose, and effect on breast-fed infants. *Am J Psychiatry.* 2003;160(8):1428–1431.

Gardner DK, Gabbe SG, Harter C. Simultaneous concentrations of ciprofloxacin in breast milk and in serum in mother and breast-fed infant. *Clin Pharm.* 1992;11(4):352–354.

Ghaffar F, McCracken GH, Hooper DC, Rubinstein E. *Quinolones in pediatrics: quinolone antimicrobial agents.* Washington, DC: ASM Press; 2003:343–354.

Giamarellou H, Kolokythas E, Petrikkos G, et al. Pharmacokinetics of three newer quinolones in pregnant and lactating women. *Am J Med.* 1989;87(5A):49S–51S.

Goldman AS. The immune system of human milk: antimicrobial, antiinflammatory and immunomodulating properties. *Pediatr Infect Dis J.* 1993;12(8):664–671.

Goldman AS, Chheda S, Keeney SE, et al. Immunologic protection of the premature newborn by human milk. *Semin Perinatol.* 1994;18(6):495–501.

Haas JS, Kaplan CP, Barenboim D, et al. Bupropion in breast milk: an exposure assessment for potential treatment to prevent post-partum tobacco use. *Tobacco Control.* 2004;13(1):52–56.

Hagg S, Granberg K, Carleborg L. Excretion of fluvoxamine into breast milk. *Br J Clin Pharmacol.* 2000;49(3):286–288.

Hale TW. *Medications and mothers' milk.* Amarillo, TX: Hale; 2012.

Hale TW, Bateman TL, Finkelman MA, Berens PD. The absence of *Candida albicans* in milk samples of women with clinical symptoms of ductal candidiasis. *Breastfeed Med.* 2009;4(2):57–61.

Hale TW, Hartman PE. *Textbook of human lactation.* Amarillo, TX: Hale; 2007.

Hale TW, Ilett KF. *Drug therapy and breastfeeding: from theory to clinical practice.* London, UK: Parthenon Press; 2002.

Hale TW, Kristensen JH, Hackett LP, et al. Transfer of metformin into human milk. *Diabetologia.* 2002;45(11):1509–1514.

Hale TW, Kristensen JH, Ilett KF. The transfer of medications into human milk. In: Hale TW, Hartmann PE, eds. *Textbook of human lactation.* Amarillo, TX: Hale; 2007:465–478.

Hale TW, McDonald R, Boger J. Transfer of celecoxib into human milk. *J Hum Lact.* 2004;20(4):397–403.

Hale TW, Shum S, Grossberg M. Fluoxetine toxicity in a breastfed infant. *Clin Pediatr (Phila).* 2001;40(12):681–684.

Harmon T, Burkhart G, Applebaum H. Perforated pseudomembranous colitis in the breast-fed infant. *J Pediatr Surg.* 1992;27(6):744–746.

Havelka J, Hejzlar M, Popov V, et al. Excretion of chloramphenicol in human milk. *Chemotherapy.* 1968;13(4):204–211.

Hill RC, McIvor RJ, Wojnar-Horton RE, et al. Risperidone distribution and excretion into human milk:

case report and estimated infant exposure during breast-feeding [Letter]. *J Clin Psychopharmacol.* 2000;20(2):285–286.

Hodgkinson R, Bhatt M, Grewal G, Marx GF. Neonatal neurobehavior in the first 48 hours of life: effect of the administration of meperidine with and without naloxone in the mother. *Pediatrics.* 1978;62(3):294–298.

Hodgkinson R, Huff RW, Hayashi RH, Husain FJ. Double-blind comparison of maternal analgesia and neonatal neurobehaviour following intravenous butorphanol and meperidine. *J Int Med Res.* 1979;7(3):224–230.

Hofmeyr GJ, Van Iddekinge B. Domperidone and lactation [Letter]. *Lancet.* 1983;1(8325):647.

Hofmeyr GJ, Van Iddekinge B, Blott JA. Domperidone: secretion in breast milk and effect on puerperal prolactin levels. *Br J Obstet Gynaecol.* 1985;92(2):141–144.

Holmdahl KH. Cholecystography during lactation. *Acta Radiol.* 1956;45(4):305–307.

Iffy L, O'Donnell J, Correia J, Hopp L. Severe cardiac dysrhythmia in patients using bromocriptine postpartum. *Am J Ther.* 1998;5(2):111–115.

Ilett KF, Hackett LP, Ingle B, Bretz PJ. Transfer of probenecid and cephalexin into breast milk. *Ann Pharmacother.* 2006;40(5):986–989.

Ilett KF, Hackett LP, Dusci LJ, et al. Distribution and excretion of venlafaxine and *O*-desmethylvenlafaxine in human milk. *Br J Clin Pharmacol.* 1998;45(5):459–462.

Ilett KF, Hackett LP, Kristensen JH, et al. Transfer of risperidone and 9-hydroxyrisperidone into human milk. *Ann Pharmacother.* 2004;38(2):273–276.

Ilett KF, Hackett LP, Paterson JW, McCormick CC. Excretion of metrizamide in milk [Letter]. *Br J Radiol.* 1981;54(642):537–538.

Ilett KF, Kristenson JH, Hackett LP, et al. Distribution of venlafaxine and its *O*-desmethyl metabolite in human milk and their effects in breastfed infants. *Br J Clin Pharmacol.* 2002;53(1):17–22.

Inoue H, Unno N, Ou MC, et al. Level of verapamil in human milk [Letter]. *Eur J Clin Pharmacol.* 1984;26(5):657–658.

Ito S, Unno N, Ou MC, Iwama Y, Sugimoto T. Prospective follow-up of adverse reactions in breast-fed infants exposed to maternal medication. *Am J Obstet Gynecol.* 1993;168(5):1393–1399.

Jamali F, Stevens DR. Naproxen excretion in milk and its uptake by the infant. *Drug Intell Clin Pharm.* 1983;17:910–911.

Johns DG, Rutherford LD, Leighton PC, Vogel CL. Secretion of methotrexate into human milk. *Am J Obstet Gynecol.* 1972;112(7):978–980.

Jones HM, Cummings AJ. A study of the transfer of alpha-methyldopa to the human foetus and newborn infant. *Br J Clin Pharmacol.* 1978;6(5):432–434.

Kafetzis DA, Lazarides CV, Siafas CA, et al. Transfer of cefotaxime in human milk and from mother to foetus. *J Antimicrob Chemother.* 1980;6(suppl A):135–141.

Kafetzis DA, Siafas CA, Georgakopoulos PA, Papadatos CJ. Passage of cephalosporins and amoxicillin into the breast milk. *Acta Paediatr Scand.* 1981;70(3):285–288.

Kampmann JP, Johansen K, Hansen JM, Helweg J. Propylthiouracil in human milk: revision of a dogma. *Lancet.* 1980;1(8171):736–737.

Kauffman RE, O'Brien C, Gilford P. Sulfisoxazole secretion into human milk. *J Pediatr.* 1980;97(5):839–841.

Kauppila A, Arvela P, Koivisto M, et al. Metoclopramide and breast feeding: transfer into milk and the newborn. *Eur J Clin Pharmacol.* 1983;25(6):819–823.

Kauppila A, Kivinen S, Ylikorkala O. A dose response relation between improved lactation and metoclopramide. *Lancet.* 1981;1(8231):1175–1177.

Kelly LE, Poon S, Madadi P, Koren G. Neonatal benzodiazepines exposure during breastfeeding. *J Pediatrics.* 2012; 16:448–451.

Kelsey JJ, Moser LR, Jennings JC, Munger MA. Presence of azithromycin breast milk concentrations: a case report. *Am J Obstet Gynecol.* 1994;170(5 Pt 1):1375–1376.

Kennedy KI, Short RV, Tully MR. Premature introduction of progestin-only contraceptive methods during lactation. *Contraception.* 1997;55(6):347–350.

Kirchheiner J, Berghöfer A, Bolk-Weischedel D. Healthy outcome under olanzapine treatment in a pregnant woman. *Pharmacopsychiatry.* 2000;33:78–80.

Knowles JA. Drugs in milk. *Pediatr Currents.* 1972;21: 28–32.

Koren G, Cairns J, Chitayat D, et al. Pharmacogenetics of morphine poisoning in a breastfed neonate of a codeine-prescribed mother. *Lancet.* 2006;368(9536):704.

Koren G, Moretti M, Kapur B. Can venlafaxine in breast milk attenuate the norepinephrine and serotonin reuptake neonatal withdrawal syndrome? *J Obstet Gynaecol Can.* 2006;28(4):299–302.

Kristensen JH, Ilett KF, Dusci LJ, et al. Distribution and excretion of sertraline and *N*-desmethylsertraline in human milk. *Br J Clin Pharmacol.* 1998;45(5):453–457.

Kuhn ST-ML, MacDonald J, Webster P, Law B. Case report: probable transmission of vaccine strain of yellow fever virus to an infant via breast milk. *CMAJ.* 2011;183(4):E243–E245.

Kumar AR, Hale TW, Mock RE. Transfer of interferon alfa into human breast milk. *J Hum Lact.* 2000;16(3):226–228.

Lam J, Kelly L, Ciszkowski C, et al. Central nervous system depression of neonates breastfed by mothers receiving oxycodone for postpartum analgesia. *J Pediatr.* 2012;160:33–37.

Lamberg BA, Ikonen E, Osterlund K, et al. Antithyroid treatment of maternal hyperthyroidism during lactation. *Clin Endocrinol (Oxf).* 1984;21(1):81–87.

Lebedevs TH, Wojnar-Horton RE, Yapp P, et al. Excretion of indomethacin in breast milk. *Br J Clin Pharmacol.* 1991;32(6):751–754.

Lee A, Giesbrecht E, Dunn E, Ito S. Excretion of quetiapine in breast milk. *Am J Psychiatry.* 2004;161(9):1715–1716.

Lee CM, Gotlib IH. Adjustment of children of depressed mothers: a 10-month follow-up. *J Abnorm Psychol.* 1991;100(4):473–477.

Lester BM, Cucca J, Andreozzi L, et al. Possible association between fluoxetine hydrochloride and colic in an infant. *J Am Acad Child Adolesc Psychiatry.* 1993;32(6):1253–1255.

Leuschen MP, Wolf LJ, Rayburn WF. Fentanyl excretion in breast milk [Letter]. *Clin Pharm.* 1990;9(5):336–337.

Liedholm H, Wåhlin-Boll E, Hanson A, et al. Transplacental passage and breast milk concentrations of hydralazine. *Eur J Clin Pharmacol.* 1982;21(5):417–419.

Livingston V, Stringer J. The treatment of *Staphylococcus aureus* infected sore nipples: a randomized comparative study. *J Hum Lact.* 1999;15(3):241–246.

Llewellyn A, Stowe ZN, Strader JRJ. The use of lithium and management of women with bipolar disorder during pregnancy and lactation. *J Clin Psychiatry.* 1998;59(suppl 6):57–64; discussion 6557–6564.

Lobo ED, Loghin C, Knadler MP, et al. Pharmacokinetics of duloxetine in breast milk and plasma of healthy postpartum women. *Clin Pharmacokinet.* 2008;47(2):103–109.

Low LC, Lang J, Alexander WD. Excretion of carbimazole and propylthiouracil in breast milk [Letter]. *Lancet.* 1979;2(8150):1011.

Mann CF. Clindamycin and breast-feeding. *Pediatrics.* 1980;66(6):1030–1031.

Marx CM, Pucin F, Carlson JD, et.al. Oxycodone excretion in human milk in the puerperium. *Drug Intell Clin.* 1986;20:474.

Matheson I. Drugs taken by mothers in the puerperium. *Br Med J (Clin Res Ed).* 1985;290(6481):1588–1589.

Matheson I, Lunde PK, Bredesen JE. Midazolam and nitrazepam in the maternity ward: milk concentrations and clinical effects. *Br J Clin Pharmacol.* 1990;30(6):787–793.

Matheson I, Pande H, Alertsen AR. Respiratory depression caused by *N*-desmethyldoxepin in breast milk. *Lancet.* 1985;2(8464):1124.

Matsuda S. Transfer of antibiotics into maternal milk. *Biol Res Pregnancy Perinatol.* 1984;5(2):57–60.

McBride RJ, Dundee JW, Moore J, et al. A study of the plasma concentrations of lorazepam in mother and neonate. *Br J Anaesth.* 1979;51(10):971–978.

McCarthy JJ, Posey BL. Methadone levels in human milk. *J Hum Lact.* 2000;16(2):115–120.

McEvoy GE, ed. *AFHS drug information 1992.* Bethesda, MD: American Society of Health-System Pharmacists; 1992.

McKenna WJ, Harris L, Rowland E, et al. Amiodarone therapy during pregnancy. *Am J Cardiol.* 1983;51(7):1231–1233.

Meador KJ, Baker GA, Browning N, et al. Effects of breast-feeding in children of women taking antiepileptic drugs. *Neurology.* 2010;75(22):1954–1960. Pubmed Central PMCID: PMC3014323.

Mennella JA, Beauchamp GK. The transfer of alcohol to human milk: effects on flavor and the infant's behavior [Comments]. *N Engl J Med.* 1991;325(14):981–985.

Miller GE, Banerjee NC, Stowe CM Jr. Diffusion of certain weak organic acids and bases across the bovine mammary gland membrane after systemic administration. *J Pharmacol Exp Ther.* 1967;157(1):245–253.

Miller MR, Withers R, Bhamra R, Holt DW. Verapamil and breast-feeding. *Eur J Clin Pharmacol.* 1986;30(1):125–126.

Misri S, Corral M, Wardrop AA, Kendrick K. Quetiapine augmentation in lactation: a series of case reports. *J Clin Psychopharmacol.* 2006;26(5):508–511.

Mizuta H, Amino N, Ichihara K, et al. Thyroid hormones in human milk and their influence on thyroid function of breast-fed babies. *Pediatr Res.* 1983;17(6):468–471.

Moretti ME, Koren G, Verjee Z, Ito S. Monitoring lithium in breast milk: an individualized approach for breast-feeding mothers. *Ther Drug Monit.* 2003;25(3):364–366.

Morganti G, Ceccarelli G, Ciaffi G. [Comparative concentrations of a tetracycline antibiotic in serum and maternal milk]. *Antibiotica.* 1968;6(3):216–223.

Morselli PL, Franco-Morselli R, Bossi L. Clinical pharmacokinetics in newborns and infants: age-related differences and therapeutic implications. *Clin Pharmacokinet.* 1980;5(6):485–527.

Nau H, Rating D, Koch S, Häuser I, Helge H. Valproic acid and its metabolites: placental transfer, neonatal pharmacokinetics, transfer via mother's milk and clinical status in neonates of epileptic mothers. *J Pharmacol Exp Ther.* 1981;219(3):768–777.

Neville MC, McFadden TB, Forsyth I. Hormonal regulation of mammary differentiation and milk secretion. *J Mammary Gland Biol Neoplasia.* 2002;7(1):49–66.

Neville MC, Medina D, Monks J, Hovey RC. The mammary fat pad. *J Mammary Gland Biol Neoplasia.* 1998;3(2):109–116.

Newport DJ, Pennell PB, Calamaras MR, et al. Lamotrigine in breast milk and nursing infants: determination of exposure. *Pediatrics.* 2008;122(1):e223–e231.

Newport DJ, Ritchie JC, Knight BT, et al. Venlafaxine in human breast milk and nursing infant plasma: determination of exposure. *J Clin Psychiatry.* 2009;70(9):1304–1310.

Nielsen ST, Matheson I, Rasmussen JN, et al. Excretion of iohexol and metrizoate in human breast milk. *Acta Radiol.* 1987;28(5):523–526.

Oberkotter LV. Thyroid function and human breast milk [Letter]. *Am J Dis Child.* 1983;137(11):1131.

O'Hara MW, Zekoski EM, Philipps LH, Wright EJ. Controlled prospective study of postpartum mood disorders: comparison of childbearing and nonchildbearing women. *J Abnorm Psychol.* 1990;99(1):3–15.

Ohkubo T, Shimoyama R, Sugawara K. Measurement of haloperidol in human breast milk by high-performance liquid chromatography. *J Pharm Sci.* 1992;81(9): 947–949.

Ohman I, Vitols S, Luef G, et al. Topiramate kinetics during delivery, lactation, and in the neonate: preliminary observations. *Epilepsia.* 2002;43(10):1157–1160.

Ohman I, Vitols S, Tomson T. Lamotrigine in pregnancy: pharmacokinetics during delivery, in the neonate, and during lactation. *Epilepsia.* 2000;41(6):709–713.

Ohman R, Hagg S, Carleborg L, Spigset O. Excretion of paroxetine into breast milk. *J Clin Psychiatry.* 1999;60(8):519–523.

Orme ML, Lewis PJ, De Swiet M, et al. May mothers given warfarin breast-feed their infants? *Br Med J.* 1977;1(6076):1564–1565.

Ost L, Wettrell G, Björkhem I, Rane A. Prednisolone excretion in human milk. *J Pediatr.* 1985;106(6):1008–1011.

Ostrea EM, Chavez CJ, Strauss ME. A study of factors that influence the severity of neonatal narcotic withdrawal. *J Pediat.* 1976;88(4 Pt. 1):642–645.

Page-Sharp M, Kristensen JH, Hackett LP, et al. Transfer of lamotrigine into breast milk. *Ann Pharmacother.* 2006;40(7–8):1470–1471.

Passmore CM, McElnay JC, Rainey EA, D'Arcy PF. Metronidazole excretion in human milk and its effect on the suckling neonate. *Br J Clin Pharmacol.* 1988;26(1):45–51.

Penny WJ, Lewis MJ. Nifedipine is excreted in human milk. *Eur J Clin Pharmacol.* 1989;36(4):427–428.

Perez-Reyes M, Wall ME. Presence of delta9-tetrahydrocannabinol in human milk [Letter]. *N Engl J Med.* 1982;307(13):819–820.

Petraglia F, De Leo V, Sardelli S, et al. Domperidone in defective and insufficient lactation. *Eur J Obstet Gynecol Reprod Biol.* 1985;19(5):281–287.

Pisacane A, Graziano L, Mazzarella G, et al. Breast-feeding and urinary tract infection. *J Pediatr.* 1992;120(1):87–89.

Plomp TA, Vulsma T, de Vijlder JJ. Use of amiodarone during pregnancy. *Eur J Obstet Gynecol Reprod Biol.* 1992;43(3):201–207.

Pollard AJ, Rylance G. Inappropriate prescribing of promethazine in infants [Letter]. *Arch Dis Child.* 1994;70(4):357.

Pop C, Metz D, Matei M, et al. Postpartum myocardial infarction induced by Parlodel. *Arch Mal Coeur Vaiss.* 1998;91(9):1171–1174.

Pope HG Jr, McElroy SL, Keck PE Jr, Hudson JI. Valproate in the treatment of acute mania: a placebo-controlled study. *Arch Gen Psychiatry.* 1991;48(1):62–68.

Putter J, Satravaha P, Stockhausen H. [Quantitative analysis of the main metabolites of acetylsalicylic acid: comparative analysis in the blood and milk of lactating women (authors' translation)]. *Z Geburtshilfe Perinatol.* 1974;178(2):135–138.

Queenan J. Exploring contraceptive options for breastfeeding mothers. *Obstet Gynecol.* 2012;119(1):1–2.

Quinn PG, Kuhnert BR, Kaine CJ, Syracuse CD. Measurement of meperidine and normeperidine in human breast milk by selected ion monitoring. *Biomed Environ Mass Spectrom.* 1986;13(3):133–135.

Rambeck B, Kurlemann G, Stodieck SR, May TW, Jürgens U. Concentrations of lamotrigine in a mother on lamotrigine treatment and her newborn child. *Eur J Clin Pharmacol.* 1997;51(6):481–484.

Rampono J, Hackett LP, Kristensen JH, et al. Transfer of escitalopram and its metabolite demethylescitalopram into breastmilk. *Br J Clin Pharmacol.* 2006;62(3):316–322.

Rampono J, Kristensen JH, Hackett LP, et al. Citalopram and demethylcitalopram in human milk: distribution, excretion and effects in breast fed infants. *Br J Clin Pharmacol.* 2000; 50(10):263–268.

Rampono J, Kristensen JH, Ilett KF, et al. Quetiapine and breastfeeding. *Ann Pharmacother.* 2007;41(4):711–714.

Rampono J, Teoh S, Hackett LP, et al. Estimation of desvenlafaxine transfer into milk and infant exposure during its use in lactating women withpostnatal depression. *Arch Womens Ment Health.* 2011;14(1):49–53.

Rasmussen F. Mammary excretion of sulphonamides. *Acta Pharmacol Toxicol.* 1958;15:138–148.

Rasmussen F. *Excretion of drugs by milk.* In: Brodie BB, Gillette JR, Ackerman HS eds. *Concepts in biochemical pharmacology. Part 1.* New York, NY: Springer-Verlag; 1971:390–402.

Ratnayake T, Libretto SE. No complications with risperidone treatment before and throughout pregnancy and during the nursing period. *J Clin Psychiatry.* 2002;63(1): 76–77.

Redman CW, Kelly JG, Cooper WD. The excretion of enalapril and enalaprilat in human breast milk. *Eur J Clin Pharmacol.* 1990;38(1):99.

Reeder C, Legrand A, O'Conner-Von S. The effect of fenugreek on milk production and prolactin levels in mothers of premature infants [Abstract]. *J Hum Lact.* 2011;27:74.

Richter C, Sitzmann J, Lang P, et al. Excretion of low molecular weight heparin in human milk. *Br J Clin Pharmacol.* 2001;52(6):708–710.

Robieux I, Koren G, Vandenbergh H, Schneiderman J. Morphine excretion in breast milk and resultant exposure of a nursing infant. *J Toxicol Clin Toxicol.* 1990;28(3):365–370.

Rofsky NM, Weinreb JC, Litt AW. Quantitative analysis of gadopentetate dimeglumine excreted in breast milk. *J Magn Reson Imaging.* 1993;3(1):131–132.

Ryu JE. Caffeine in human milk and in serum of breast-fed infants. *Dev Pharmacol Ther.* 1985;8(6):329–337.

Saenz RB. Iodine-131 elimination from breast milk: a case report. *J Hum Lact.* 2000;16(1):44–46.

Sanders CC. Cefepime: the next generation? *Clin Infect Dis.* 1993;17(3):369–379.

Sanofi-Aventis Canada Inc. *Pharmaceutical manufacturer prescribing information: clopidogrel.* 2012.

Sanz EJ, De-las-Cuevas C, Kiuru A, et al. Selective serotonin reuptake inhibitors in pregnant women and neonatal withdrawal syndrome: a database analysis. *Lancet.* 2005;365(9458):482–487.

Sauberan J, Bradley J, Blumer J, Stellwagen L. Transmission of meropenem in breast milk. *Pediatr Infect Dis J.* 2012;31:832–834. Pubmed Central PMCID: 22544050.

Schadewinkel-Scherkl AM, Rasmussen F, Merck CC, et al. Active transport of benzylpenicillin across the blood–milk barrier. *Pharmacol Toxicol.* 1993;73(1):14–19.

Schering Corporation. Rebetol (ribavirin) product information. 2001. Available at: http://archives.who.int/eml/expcom/expcom15/applications/newmed/ribaravin/APP_REBETOL.pdf.

Schlotterbeck PLD, Kircher T, Hiemke C, Grunder G. Aripiprazole in human milk. *Int J Neuropsychopharmacol.* 2007;10(3):433.

Schmidt K, Olesen OV, Jensen PN. Citalopram and breast-feeding: serum concentration and side effects in the infant. *Biol Psychiatry.* 2000;47(2):164–165.

Schwebke JR. Metronidazole: utilization in the obstetric and gynecologic patient. *Sex Transm Dis.* 1995;22(6):370–376.

Sedlmayr T, Peters F, Raasch W, Kees F. [Clarithromycin, a new macrolide antibiotic: effectiveness in puerperal infections and pharmacokinetics in breast milk]. *Geburtshilfe Frauenheilkd.* 1993;53(7):488–491.

Shaaban MM. Contraception with progestogens and progesterone during lactation. *J Steroid Biochem Mol Biol.* 1991;40(4–6):705–710.

Shaaban MM, Salem HT, Abdullah KA. Influence of levonorgestrel contraceptive implants, Norplant, initiated early postpartum upon lactation and infant growth. *Contraception.* 1985;32(6):623–635.

Shaamash AH, Sayed GH, Hussien MM, Shaaban MM. A comparative study of the levonorgestrel-releasing intrauterine system Mirena® versus the Copper T380A intrauterine device during lactation: breast-feeding performance, infant growth and infant development. *Contraception.* 2005;72(5):346–351.

Shetty AK. Tetracyclines in pediatrics revisited. *Clin Pediatr.* 2002;41:203–209.

Shimoyama R, Ohkubo T, Sugawara K. Monitoring of carbamazepine and carbamazepine 10,11-epoxide in breast milk and plasma by high-performance liquid chromatography. *Ann Clin Biochem.* 2000;37(Pt 2):210–215.

Shyu WC, Shah VR, Campbell DA, et al. Excretion of cefprozil into human breast milk. *Antimicrob Agents Chemother.* 1992;36(5):938–941.

Sinclair D, Murray L. Effects of postnatal depression on children's adjustment to school: teacher's reports. *Br J Psychiatry.* 1998;172:58–63.

Single dose cabergoline versus bromocriptine in inhibition of puerperal lactation: randomised, double blind, multi-centre study. European Multicentre Study Group for Cabergoline in Lactation Inhibition [see comments]. *Br Med J.* 1991;302(6789):1367–1371.

Smith JA, Morgan JR. Clindamycin in human breastmilk. *Can Med Assoc J.* 1975;112:806.

Sorensen HT, Skriver MV, Pedersen L, et al. Risk of infantile hypertrophic pyloric stenosis after maternal postnatal use of macrolides. *Scand J Infect Dis.* 2003;35(2):104–106.

Spencer MJ, Escondido CA. Fluoxetine hydrochloride (Prozac) toxicity in a neonate. *Pediatrics.* 1993;92(5):721–722.

Stahl MM, Neiderud J, Vinge E. Thrombocytopenic purpura and anemia in a breast-fed infant whose mother was treated with valproic acid. *J Pediatr.* 1997;130:1001–1003.

Stang H. Pyloric stenosis associated with erythromycin ingested through breastmilk. *Minn Med.* 1986;69(11):669–670, 682.

Staples JEGM, Fischer M. Yellow fever vaccine: recommendations of the Advisory Committee on Immunization Practices (ACIP). *MMWR Recomm Rep.* 2010;59(RR-7):1–27.

Steiner E, Villén T, Hallberg M, Rane A. Amphetamine secretion in breast milk. *Eur J Clin Pharmacol.* 1984;27(1):123–124.

Stewart RB, Karas B, Springer PK. Haloperidol excretion in human milk. *Am J Psychiatry.* 1980;137(7):849–850.

Stiskal JA, Kulin N, Koren G, et al. Neonatal paroxetine withdrawal syndrome. *Arch Dis Child Fetal Neonatal Ed.* 2001;84(2):F134–F135.

Stowe ZN, Cohen LS, Hostetter A, et al. Paroxetine in human breast milk and nursing infants. *Am J Psychiatry.* 2000;157(2):185–189.

Stowe ZN, Hostetter AL, Owens MJ, et al. The pharmacokinetics of sertraline excretion into human breast milk: determinants of infant serum concentrations. *J Clin Psychiatry.* 2003;64(1):73–80.

Stowe ZN, Owens MJ, Landry JC, et al. Sertraline and desmethylsertraline in human breast milk and nursing infants [Comments]. *Am J Psychiatry.* 1997;154(9):1255–1260.

Strauss ME, Andresko M, Stryker JC, et al. Methadone maintenance during pregnancy: pregnancy, birth, and neonate characteristics. *Am J Obstet Gynecol.* 1974;120(7):895–900.

Sugawara K, Shimoyama R, Ohkubo T. Determinations of psychotropic drugs and antiepileptic drugs by high-performance liquid chromatography and its monitoring in human breast milk. *Hirosaki Med J.* 1999;51(suppl):S81–S86.

Summerfield RJ, Nielsen MS. Excretion of lorazepam into breast milk [Letter]. *Br J Anaesth.* 1985;57(10):1042–1043.

Swafford S, Berens P. Effect of fenugreek on breast milk production. *BM News and Views.* September 11–13, 2000;6(3). Annual meeting abstracts.

Sweezy SR. Contraception for the postpartum woman. *NAACOGS Clin Issue Perinat Womens Health Nurs.* 1992;3(2):209–226.

Sykes PA, Quarrie J, Alexander FW. Lithium carbonate and breast-feeding. *Br Med J.* 1976;2(6047):1299.

Syversen GB, Ratkje SK. Drug distribution within human milk phases. *J Pharm Sci.* 1985;74(10):1071–1074.

Taddio A, Ito S, Koren G. Excretion of fluoxetine and its metabolite, norfluoxetine, in human breast milk. *J Clin Pharmacol.* 1996;36(1):42–47.

Takase Z SH, Uchida M. Fundamental and clinical studies of cefuroxime in the field of obstetrics and gynecology. *Chemother (Tokyo).* 1979;27(suppl 6):600–602.

Tegler L, Lindstrom B. Antithyroid drugs in milk. *Lancet.* 1980;2(8194):591.

Tennes K, Avitable N, Blackard C, et al. Marijuana: prenatal and postnatal exposure in the human. *NIDA Res Monogr.* 1985; 59:48–60.

Tomson T, Ohman I, Vitols S. Lamotrigine in pregnancy and lactation: a case report. *Epilepsia.* 1997;38(9):1039–1041.

Treffers PE. [Breastfeeding and contraception]. *Ned Tijdschr Geneeskd.* 1999;143(38):1900–1904.

Tunnessen WWJ, Hertz CG. Toxic effects of lithium in newborn infants: a commentary. *J Pediatr.* 1972; 81(4):804–807.

U.S. Food and Drug Administration (FDA). FDA talk paper: FDA warns against women using unapproved drug, domperidone, to increase milk production. 2004. Available at: http://www.fda.gov/Drugs/DrugSafety/InformationbyDrugClass/ucm173886.htm. Accessed January 27, 2013.

Uwaydah M, Bibi S, Salman S. Therapeutic efficacy of tobramycin: a clinical and laboratory evaluation. *J Antimicrob Chemother.* 1975;1(4):429–437.

Viguera AC, Newport DJ, Ritchie J, et al. Lithium in breast milk and nursing infants: clinical implications. *Am J Psychiatry.* 2007;164(2):342–345.

von Keutz E, Ruhl-Fehlert C, Drommer W, Rosenbruch M. Effects of ciprofloxacin on joint cartilage in immature dogs immediately after dosing and after a 5-month treatment-free period. *Arch Toxicol.* 2004;78:418–424.

von Unruh GE, Froescher W, Hoffmann F, Niesen M. Valproic acid in breast milk: how much is really there? *Ther Drug Monit.* 1984;6(3):272–276.

Watanabe NKM, Sugibayashi R, Nakamura T, et al. Perinatal use of aripiprazole: a case report. *J Clin Psychopharmacol.* 2011;31(3):377–379.

Webster J, Piscitelli G, Polli A, et al. Dose-dependent suppression of serum prolactin by cabergoline in hyperprolactinaemia: a placebo controlled, double blind, multicentre study. European Multicentre Cabergoline Dose-finding Study Group. *Clin Endocrinol (Oxf).* 1992;37(6):534–541.

Weibert RT, Townsend RJ, Kaiser DG, Naylor AJ. Lack of ibuprofen secretion into human milk. *Clin Pharmacol.* 1982;1(5):457–458.

Wesson DR, Camber S, Harkey M, Smith DE. Diazepam and desmethyldiazepam in breast milk. *J Psychoactive Drugs.* 1985;17(1):55–56.

Whalley LJ, Blain PG, Prime JK. Haloperidol secreted in breast milk. *Br Med J (Clin Res Ed).* 1981;282(6278):1746–1747.

White WB, Andreoli JW, Cohn RD. Alpha-methyldopa disposition in mothers with hypertension and in their breast-fed infants. *Clin Pharmacol Ther.* 1985;37(4):387–390.

Whitelaw AG, Cummings AJ, McFadyen IR. Effect of maternal lorazepam on the neonate. *Br Med J (Clin Res Ed).* 1981;282(6270):1106–1108.

Wiles DH, Orr MW, Kolakowska T. Chlorpromazine levels in plasma and milk of nursing mothers. *Br J Clin Pharmacol.* 1978;5(3):272–273.

Winecker RE, Goldberger BA, Tebbett IR, et al. Detection of cocaine and its metabolites in breast milk. *J Forensic Sci.* 2001;46(5):1221–1223.

Wischnik A, Manth SM, Lloyd J, et al. The excretion of ketorolac tromethamine into breast milk after multiple oral dosing. *Eur J Clin Pharmacol.* 1989;36(5):521–524.

Wittels B, Glosten B, Faure EA, et al. Postcesarean analgesia with both epidural morphine and intravenous patient-controlled analgesia: neurobehavioral outcomes among nursing neonates. *Anesth Analg.* 1997;85(3):600–606.

Wittels B, Scott DT, Sinatra RS. Exogenous opioids in human breast milk and acute neonatal neurobehavior: a preliminary study. *Anesthesiology.* 1990;73(5):864–869.

Wojnar-Horton RE, Kristensen JH, Yapp P, et al. Methadone distribution and excretion into breast milk of clients in a methadone maintenance programme. *Br J Clin Pharmacol.* 1997;44(6):543–547.

Yoshida K, Smith B, Craggs M, Kumar R. Neuroleptic drugs in breast-milk: a study of pharmacokinetics and of possible adverse effects in breast-fed infants. *Psychol Med.* 1998;28(1):81–91.

Yoshioka H, Cho K, Takimoto M, et al. Transfer of cefazolin into human milk. *J Pediatr.* 1979;94(1):151–152.

Zekoski EM, O'Hara MW, Wills KE. The effects of maternal mood on mother–infant interaction. *J Abnorm Child Psychol.* 1987;15(3):361–378.

Viral Infections and Breastfeeding

E. Stephen Buescher

Introduction

Mother-to-child transmission (MTCT) of a viral infectious agent can occur during pregnancy, at birth, and/or during the postpartum period. Transmission during pregnancy usually results from transplacental passage of the infectious agent. Transmission at birth occurs via contact with an infected birth canal or contact with infectious maternal body fluid (e.g., blood). Transmission during the postpartum period results from either the close proximity of the mother to the infant (e.g., contact or respiratory spread) or infant ingestion of infected maternal fluids (e.g., breastmilk, blood). Thus concerns about viral infectious disease transmission to the infant in the postpartum period are pertinent to both infections acquired by the mother but not transmitted via her milk and infections that are potentially transmitted in breastmilk. The following questions are addressed in this chapter:

1. Which viruses are found in the milk of infected or seropositive women?
2. What are the risks for transmission of these viruses by breastfeeding?
3. What outcomes do infections with these viruses lead to in children?
4. Do maternal breastmilk protective factors limit transmission of specific viruses or reduce the severity of a given viral infection in the infant?
5. Are effective treatments available for the mother or the infant?

Unfortunately, the completeness of the answers to these questions varies. Some answers are quite extensive, well understood, and supported with excellent science and clinical experience. Others are incomplete or based on one or two anecdotal cases, are purely epidemiologic observations, or are based on laboratory rather than clinical observations. This chapter addresses these questions, although we recognize that there are no simple answers to the complex puzzle of viral transmission from mother to infant.

Human milk is a "human infant support system" that provides the nursing infant with protection, information, and nutrition. However, because human milk is capable of transmitting infectious agents, it may also represent a potential threat to the nursing infant. The "protection against infection" widely acknowledged to result from breastfeeding is mediated by both classical and novel immunologic mechanisms of milk that protect against a surprisingly broad array of pathogens and infectious conditions. However, this "protection" is typically incomplete—that is, it decreases but does not eliminate the possibility of infectious illness. This is an important realization when discussing the "pros and cons" and "benefits versus risks" of breastfeeding, because these considerations change from one infectious agent to the next.

Human Immunodeficiency Virus

Background

Human immunodeficiency virus (HIV) is classified as a retrovirus, a name that implies that its genetic material, RNA, must be "retrograde converted" or "reverse transcribed" to DNA to infect a cell. HIV can be detected in human milk both as a "provirus" (the DNA form of HIV that is integrated into a cell's genetic material) and as free virus (the mature, infectious RNA form of the virus) (Lewis et al., 1998; Ruff et al., 1994). HIV is estimated to infect approximately 0.8% of the current world population between 15 and 49 years old, and approximately 0.6% of adults in North America (range 0.1–4% of adults by region worldwide) (Kaiser Foundation, 2012). The World Health Organization's (WHO) *2011 Global HIV/AIDS Response Progress Report* states that at the end of 2010 there were 34.0 million persons living with HIV/AIDS. Worldwide, an estimated 390,000 children younger than 15 years of age became HIV infected in 2011.

Risks for Transmission

HIV infection is spread by exchange of infected blood or by mucous membrane contact with infected blood and body fluids. In adults, IV drug use and sexual activity are the most common activities associated with acquisition. In infants and small children, either perinatal or breastmilk MTCT of HIV accounts for most infections. In the United States, the estimated number of perinatal HIV infections peaked in 1991, but has since declined primarily due to interventions instituted since that time (discussed later in this section). The current rate of perinatal HIV transmission in the United States is 1.4% (Read et al., 2012), compared to rates of 25–30% before the interventions were started.

Outcomes of HIV Infection

Infection with HIV, when left untreated, results in destruction of T-cell immunity that allows recurrent, severe, and ultimately life-threatening opportunistic infections to manifest as acquired immunodeficiency syndrome (AIDS). Progression from infection to AIDS occurs over years in adults; by comparison, in perinatally infected infants, AIDS usually presents before the first birthday.

Interventions/Treatments

The interventions that have so markedly decreased perinatal HIV infections in the United States include routine HIV screening of pregnant women, use of antiretroviral therapy (ART) for control and prevention of maternal infection, and avoidance of breastfeeding. Since the last edition of this text was published, ongoing research has more closely examined breastfeeding and prevention of MTCT transmission.

Breastfeeding by HIV-positive mothers is associated with HIV transmission. However, the risk of acquisition is modified by details of how breastfeeding occurs. Exclusive breastfeeding lowers the early (first 6 weeks of lactation) risk of breastmilk HIV transmission, but research shows that the risk of transmission persists as long as breastfeeding continues (Coovadia et al., 2007). The same study showed that replacement feedings (no breastmilk) had about the same risk of HIV acquisition by 6 months of age as did exclusive breastfeeding, and that mixed feedings (human milk plus other feeding types) had the highest rates of early HIV transmission. However, because infants on mixed feedings transitioned to full replacement feedings quickly, their period of risk for HIV acquisition was short (no risk after about 3 weeks) compared to the exclusively breastfed infants, who were at risk throughout the entire time they breastfed. In this study, noting that the sizes of these groups were *not* comparable, the infants with a brief, high HIV transmission risk (mixed feeding) and those with a prolonged, low HIV transmission risk (exclusive breastfeeding) were associated with about the same probability of HIV-free survival at 6 months (approximately 75%). Perhaps the most striking observation from this study, however, was that infant mortality at 3 months of age was nearly 2.5 times higher in those infants who received replacement feeds (no breastmilk) compared to the exclusively breastfed infants—reiterating the importance of breastfeeding as a means to prevent infant mortality in the developing world. Thus breastfeeding by the HIV-positive mother who does not have access to alternative foods that are "acceptable, feasible, affordable, sustainable, and safe" remains a tradeoff of one risk versus another. This likely explains why studies of prevention of MTCT of HIV have shifted away from manipulating feedings to emphasize maternal ART and infant prophylaxis (Bulterys, Ellington, & Kourtis, 2010) so that breastfeeding by the HIV-infected mother will carry less risk of HIV acquisition by the infant.

Approximately 80% of U.S. HIV-infected women are of childbearing age. Routine HIV testing and counseling for all pregnant women, and ART for those who are HIV positive, is now the standard of care in the United States. Both the Centers for Disease Control and Prevention (CDC) and the World Health Organization continue to recommend avoidance of breastfeeding and use of replacement feedings by HIV-infected women when such feedings are "acceptable, feasible, affordable, sustainable, and safe." In developed countries, these requirements are easily met and breastfeeding by HIV-infected women has virtually ceased, with concomitant elimination of MTCT of HIV via breastfeeding. In underdeveloped countries, when alternative feedings cannot meet the "acceptable, feasible, affordable, sustainable, and safe" criteria, the HIV-infected mother has little choice but to breastfeed. If she must, the recommendation is for breastfeeding to be exclusive, and for as short a duration as feasible. The WHO recommendation is that once feedings are no longer exclusively breastmilk and supplements are given, HIV-infected women should avoid breastfeeding completely.

In developed/"resource-rich" countries, availability of ART is good and its use readily controls HIV infection, decreasing the likelihood of disease complications, including MTCT of HIV. In the underdeveloped world, ART is only now becoming generally available, and its use is slowly broadening from only the *symptomatic* HIV-infected population to include the asymptomatic (but potentially infectious) HIV-infected population. The childbearing/breastfeeding mother in these countries is typically a member of the latter group. Based on the successes achieved with ART to control HIV infection in the developed world, emerging opinion is that similar approaches, if they can be implemented, are likely to control HIV infection in less developed countries (Becquet et al., 2009). The impediments to achieving this goal, however, are great, including societal expectations, access to care and cost of medications.

Nonetheless, the WHO (2010) now recommends that "mothers known to be HIV-infected should be provided with lifelong antiretroviral therapy or antiretroviral prophylaxis interventions to reduce HIV transmission through breastfeeding." It is likely this approach will become the mainstay for prevention of MTCT of HIV in the future. Thus ongoing study of other and better approaches to prevention of breastfeeding-related MTCT of HIV has been pursued, with the recognition that maternal/infant ART/prophylaxis may be the best approach for the future.

Maternal/Infant Antiretroviral Treatment/Prophylaxis

Prior to 1994, the perinatal rate of MTCT of HIV was 25–30% in the United States. Protocol 076—the use of zidovudine (AZT) treatment of mothers during pregnancy, labor, and delivery, and AZT prophylaxis of the newborn postpartum—decreased peripartum MTCT of HIV to less than 2%. In underdeveloped countries where the 076 protocol approach has not been feasible, use of a simpler approach has been investigated: administration of a single oral dose of an inexpensive, slowly metabolized antiretroviral agent (nevirapine) to the mother during labor and to the infant after birth.

In the initial study, this approach decreased peripartum MTCT of HIV by approximately 47% (McCarthy, 1999). This observation led to a series of subsequent studies examining neviripine with and without other ART agents as perinatal prophylaxis, with the unanticipated observation that single-dose neviripine in the mother resulted in subsequent development of neviripine-resistant HIV in approximately15% of women (Cunningham et al., 2002). Resistance could also develop in neviripine-exposed infants if their peripartum prophylaxis failed (Palumbo et al., 2010).

Because neviripine was found to persist in the blood of women who received a single oral dose for as long as 3 weeks, and because most HIV transmission via breastmilk occurs early following delivery, it was of interest to see if neviripine treatment of the mother postpartum could alter MTCT of HIV infection via breastfeeding. In two words, it does. Compared to an AZT regimen, single-dose neviripine treatment of HIV-infected mothers during labor resulted in a 41% decrease in the relative risk of the infant acquiring HIV infection over the first 18 months of life (Jackson et al., 2003). Because of the drug resistance seen with single-dose "monotherapy" neviripine treatments, other ART agents in combination with neviripine are actively being examined for both prevention of breastfeeding transmission of HIV in parts of Africa and in south and southeast Asia, and for long-term suppression of maternal HIV disease (see the summary by Lala & Merchant, 2012).

General guidelines for avoiding perinatal transmission of HIV include the following:

- Screening for HIV. Knowing a mother's HIV status is critical for preventing transmission.
- Prenatal ART to decrease the mother's HIV viral load and reduce the risk of perinatal transmission.
- Continued maternal ART postpartum to suppress the mother's HIV viral load, improve her health, and minimize breastmilk viral load.
- Use of "replacement feedings" (formula-feeding) by HIV-infected mothers where acceptable, feasible, affordable, sustainable, and safe

alternatives are available. (The U.S. Department of Health and Human Services states that HIV-infected women should neither breastfeed nor provide their breastmilk for the nutrition of their own or other infants.)

- When breastfeeding cannot be avoided, antiretroviral prophylaxis of the breastfeeding infant throughout the breastfeeding period, continued for 1–2 weeks after complete weaning.
- Exclusive breastfeeding of the infant if safe alternative supplements are not available. Where safe replacement feedings are not feasible, promotion of exclusive breastfeeding reduces risk of HIV-1 transmission to the baby. If replacement infant feedings are used, the risk of HIV transmission is exchanged for the risk of diarrhea and pneumonia when fuel to boil water (for replacement feeding preparation, sterilization, or bottles), nutritional additives, and equipment are not available (Savage & Lhotska, 2000).
- After the cessation of exclusive breastfeeding, complete avoidance of breastfeeding by HIV-infected women.
- Pregnancy deferral. HIV-infected women who are not receiving ART should defer pregnancy and begin ART. In countries where cesarean section delivery is available, surgical delivery decreases infant exposure to maternal blood and body fluids, thereby reducing risk of MTCT of HIV.
- Avoidance of artificial rupture of membranes and insertion of scalp electrodes in the case of vaginal birth.
- Avoidance of practices that increase the risk of HIV exposure. HIV-negative mothers who are breastfeeding should avoid high-risk practices for HIV acquisition (e.g., drug abuse or a sexual partner who is bisexual or has engaged in practices linked to HIV transmission). Primary infection with HIV is associated with high blood viral loads, and high blood viral loads increase the risk of HIV transmission by breastfeeding.

- Maintenance of breast health. In HIV-infected women, breast conditions such as mastitis, breast abscess, and nipple fissure may increase the risk of HIV transmission through breastfeeding—the latter two likely because of blood contamination of the milk (Lunney et al., 2010).

Healthcare Practitioners

Practitioners who work with human milk or with breastfeeding women need to be concerned about their own protection. The CDC recommends "standard precautions" be used when handling blood and/or body fluids of all patients regardless of their infection status. "Standard precautions" apply to blood and other body fluids that contain visible blood (e.g., semen, vaginal secretions, or milk), but they *do not obligatorily apply* to human milk unless it contains visible blood (Occupational Safety and Health Administration [OSHA] Standard 1910.1030) and occupational exposure to human milk has not been implicated in the transmission of HIV. Nevertheless, it may be reasonable and prudent for the healthcare worker who comes in frequent contact with human milk (e.g., via breast pump cleaning, working in human milk banking) to wear gloves. Gloves are not needed when touching the breasts (e.g., in breast assessment). If the mother has an open wound on her breast, use of gloves is indicated for the protection of both the mother and the care provider. Staff routinely wear gloves during delivery and for newborn care. Vigorous hand washing by the care provider—both before and after any physical contact with a patient or with any body fluid—is standard practice for infection control and should be performed consistently to prevent transmission of *any* infection to the mother, the child, and the healthcare worker.

There are currently insufficient data to guarantee that pasteurization of breastmilk will eliminate the risk of HIV transmission. Multiple different approaches for "decreasing" or "preventing" MTCT of HIV by treatment of breastmilk have been proposed and examined, and many have shown the ability to decrease virus content in milk, but none has been demonstrated to "eliminate" risk of transmission. The American Board of Pediatrics states that "these methodologies are unlikely to eliminate HIV from milk completely," and it does not support their use because of cost, cultural acceptability, and potential effects on other protective activities in human milk (Read & Committee on Pediatric AIDS, 2003).

Counseling

If nothing else, the last 10 years have clearly demonstrated the scientific, therapeutic, cultural, geographic, and practical complexity of MTCT of HIV infection. WHO technical guidelines have previously emphasized that all HIV-infected mothers should receive feeding counseling that includes general information about the risks and benefits of various infant feeding options, and specific guidance in selecting the option most likely to be suitable for their situation (Coutsoudis, 2000). Having moved into the era of ART that effectively suppresses HIV infection, we now have the perspective that exclusive breastfeeding is one of several tools available to decrease (but not eliminate) the risk of MTCT of HIV. Because no epidemic in human history has ever been controlled by treatment approaches, HIV infection both as an individual health problem and as a public health problem is better avoided than treated. Zero risk of acquisition is the public health objective, and exclusive breastfeeding decreases but does not eliminate the risk of HIV for the breastfed infant. In the underdeveloped world, exclusive breastfeeding may be an imperfect but practically acceptable "best option" considering the various cultural, therapeutic, and practical realities. In the developed world, exclusive breastfeeding is not a "zero-risk" approach. For the present, the "zero-risk" approach for MTCT of HIV involves avoidance of human milk feeding. Perhaps in the future, with ongoing research, an approach that allows breastfeeding by the HIV-infected mother with negligible or no risk of HIV transmission to her infant will be found. Until that time, optimal prevention of acquisition, modified by practical realities, remains the worldwide goal of efforts to control

MTCT of HIV. Along the same lines, prevention can be facilitated at even earlier phases by ensuring understanding of the modes of and risk factors for transmission of HIV. The great majority of HIV infections in women occur as sexually transmitted infections (STIs), and as for many other STIs, barrier precautions/safe sex approaches mitigate these risks. Teaching women "safe sex" approaches is, therefore, appropriate as a complementary approach to prevention of MTCT of HIV infection.

HIV-infected women come from all walks of life. Whatever the direct cause of their illness, their lives can be shattered by the knowledge that they are HIV infected. Few illnesses are associated with such stigmatization and social isolation. Although HIV-infected women desperately need help from family, friends, and other support groups, they may be isolated from these supports because HIV is a "secret" disease. Their counseling needs are necessarily complex, because these women must make difficult decisions while trying to cope with the implications of HIV for themselves and their families. In areas where antiretroviral drugs are available, the importance of adherence to the drug therapy is an essential topic.

Herpes Simplex Virus

The condition referred to as herpes, caused by the herpes simplex virus (HSV), is a common infection of humans. HSV-1 is a DNA virus that manifests "latency," meaning that after the initial infection, the viral DNA is incorporated into cellular DNA (usually in nerve cells) in a "latent" state, and this "latent" virus has the capacity to leave latency and cause clinical illness repeatedly at subsequent times in the host's life. No matter at what age it is acquired, HSV is a recurrent infection whose usual manifestation consists of painful fluid-filled vesicles at the site of initial inoculation. HSV recurrences are due to the latent virus becoming reactivated, not to new infections.

Different forms of illnesses are seen in different age groups. In adults, the most common forms of disease are mouth/lip "fever blisters" and "genital herpes," a sexually transmitted disease. The former is typically caused by HSV type 1 (HSV-1), the

latter by HSV-2. In children, the most common form of infection is "primary" (i.e., first infection) herpetic gingivo-stomatitis: an ulcerating infection of the lips, mouth, and pharynx (extension to other body sites without direct contact with infected saliva is unusual). Herpetic gingivo-stomatitis is usually self-limited, and recurrences typically arise in the mouth or on the lips as "canker sores" or "fever blisters." In both adults and children, herpes encephalitis (brain infection) can occur but is, thankfully, uncommon. In newborn and young infants, three forms of herpes simplex disease occur: herpes encephalitis (approximately 25% of cases), disseminated herpes infection (40% of cases), and skin/eye/mucous membrane herpes (45% of cases). Disseminated herpes infection and herpes encephalitis are typically severe illnesses with high morbidity and mortality. Skin/eye/mucous membrane disease tends to be limited to those areas that give it its name and has low morbidity and mortality compared to disseminated disease and encephalitis.

Although infant HSV disease can be acquired from contact with an active skin, lip, or mouth lesion, the usual mode of acquisition is via delivery through a birth canal with active herpes infection. Birth through *recurrent* genital HSV infection is associated with a less than 5% risk of the infant developing clinical herpetic infection. Birth through a *primary* genital herpes infection is linked to a 50% rate of developing clinical infection. Development of clinical illness typically occurs 7–20 days after delivery, but is observed earlier if a larger HSV exposure occurs or primary maternal infection is present at the time the infant is delivered. Despite the high incidence of genital herpes in the general population, the incidence of neonatal herpes is low, ranging from 1/2000 to 1/10,000 births (Brown, 1995).

Vaginal delivery is safe in most women with a history of recurrent genital herpes unless active lesions are present at term. Cesarean section should be performed within 6 hours of rupture of membranes if active lesions are present. Cesarean delivery is not recommended when a woman with a history of recurrent infection does not have obvious lesions or clinical symptoms of the infection at the time of delivery.

Outcomes

In infants beyond the neonatal period, children, and adults, HSV infection is usually localized and self-limited, even without treatment. Recurrences throughout life are to be expected. In immunocompromised hosts, including the neonatal infant, HSV infection can have high morbidity and mortality, depending on the extent of spread, whether the central nervous system is involved, and how rapidly treatment is initiated.

HSV and Breastfeeding

It is doubtful that this infection is transmitted through human milk. A single report describes detection of HSV DNA in human breastmilk (Kotronias & Kapranos, 1999), and one report proposes transmission to a newborn via breastmilk (Dunkle, Schmidt, & O'Connor, 1979). Transmission during breastfeeding is more likely due to occur from direct contact with a herpetic lesion on the breast.

One report of HSV transmission from mouth to breast involved a nursing toddler who transmitted HSV to the mother through breastfeeding (Sealander & Kerr, 1989). The child had lesions on the inner aspect of the lower lip, and the mother developed painful blisters on her nipples. Both the child's oral lesions and the mother's nipple lesions were positive for HSV-1. Breastfeeding was suspended for a week and the mother was treated with oral acyclovir for 5 days with improvement, after which she resumed breastfeeding. The authors commented that when a young child develops oral HSV lesions, inquiry regarding whether the mother is breastfeeding the child should be made so the risks can be evaluated and interventions can be begun.

A second report described a mother who developed an areolar lesion postpartum and continued to breastfeed (Sullivan-Bolyai et al., 1983). After an uneventful nursery course, the infant was discharged home on day 2 of life. The infant developed vesicles in the mouth and chin on day 4, and HSV-1 was isolated from these lesions on day 6 and from the mother's breast lesion on day 7. The infant died on day 11. This case illustrates the seriousness of

perinatally acquired HSV for the infant and points out the need to prevent direct infant contact with any lesion suggestive of HSV (because the vesicle fluid in an HSV lesion is rich in infectious virus).

Breast lesions are seldom the first clinical evidence of herpes in the family (Sullivan-Bolyai et al., 1983). A primary herpetic infection may occur in another family member who then passes it on to the infant (e.g., the father during sexual activity with the mother, or a sibling/grandparent who kisses their little brother/sister or "grandbaby"). Therefore, transmission may occur on a mother-to-infant, infant-to-mother, or other-family-member-to-infant basis, with the infant then passing the virus on to the mother during feedings.

Breastmilk Protective Factors

No factors in human milk are known to be protective against HSV.

Counseling

HSV is an emotionally difficult and anxiety-provoking topic because the infection in an infant is most often acquired from the genital tract of the mother. Feelings of guilt and concerns regarding disclosure of intimate details and/or conjugal fidelity can all arise in the setting of neonatal HSV infection, because invariably the questions "Where did it come from?" and "How did I get it?" are asked, and there is often a perceived need to blame someone. The best approach in these situations is emphasize the present/future rather than the past and the need of the infant for their parents' support.

Treatment/Interventions

Women with herpetic lesions on their breast should refrain from feeding from the involved breast; active lesions should be covered (American Academy of Pediatrics [AAP], 2012c) to prevent contact by the suckling infant. In the absence of breast lesions, the infant of a mother with HSV-1 or HSV-2 infection (assuming the infant is well) may breastfeed and "room-in" with the mother. Scrupulous hand washing, gowning, and covering of any lesions must be practiced to prevent possible transmission of the virus to the infant. The mother need not wear latex/nitrile gloves while breastfeeding.

Treatment of maternal HSV infection, depending on its severity, is usually directed at symptomatic relief and prevention of spread. Three antiviral treatments are approved for HSV infection: acyclovir (Zovirax), valacyclovir, and famciclovir. Aggressive and early use of intravenous acyclovir is the usual management of severe infection in the mother and any infection in the infant. Oral or topical acyclovir may be used for less severe episodes in the mother. Routine administration of acyclovir to pregnant women with a history of recurrent HSV infection is not recommended (Cline, Bailey-Dorton, & Cayelli, 2000). Two over-the-counter antiviral creams, Abreva and Viroxyn, are now available for symptomatic treatment of cold sores and fever blisters. The effectiveness of these medications for prevention of HSV shedding is not known. Cleaning herpetic lesions with povidone-iodine (Betadine) solution is rational and may prevent a secondary bacterial infection, and application of Burrow's solution (aluminum acetate) may give symptomatic relief of some of the discomfort.

Varicella-Zoster Virus (Chickenpox/Varicella/Zoster/Shingles)

Varicella-zoster virus (VZV) is another member of the herpesvirus family and is the cause of two main illnesses, chickenpox and zoster (shingles). Infection is lifelong, with the virus persisting in nerve cells of the host in a latent state. Chickenpox is a childhood rash illness and represents the primary VZV infection. It is remarkably contagious: individuals who develop chickenpox are contagious 48 hours *before* appearance of the rash and remain so until the rash is fully crusted. Active childhood immunization against chickenpox began in 1995 in the United States, resulting in dramatic declines in this infection's incidence.

Most adults have immunity to varicella-zoster virus because of either previous infection or immunization; therefore, the question of whether mothers with chickenpox can breastfeed is infrequent. Individuals without immunity to chickenpox who are exposed to it are potentially infectious from day 10 through day 21 *following* exposure. The skin lesions of chickenpox classically begin on the neck or trunk and spread to the face, scalp, mucous membranes, and extremities. They first appear as small, spherical vesicles of clear fluid on an erythematous base ("a dewdrop on a rose petal"), which then develop into flattened vesicles containing progressively more cloudy fluid. The fluid in the vesicles is highly contagious. The vesicles appear in crops, and "crust" over a period of 2–5 days. A live, attenuated virus vaccine is given in two doses (at 12–15 months and 4–6 years of age) and the same vaccine, administered in a larger dose, is now used for prevention of shingles in individuals 60 years and older. The CDC recommends vaccination against chickenpox for all *susceptible* healthcare workers.

Transmission of VZV

Because chickenpox can be acquired by susceptible individuals of any age, a woman may develop this infection while she is breastfeeding. In such a case, she should continue to breastfeed. Because of the window of contagiousness for chickenpox, the infant will already be exposed to the infection *before* the mother is recognized to have chickenpox skin lesions. Infants typically tolerate chickenpox well, although they tend to have more skin lesions than older children.

Outcomes of Infection

Intrauterine infection with VZV (congenital varicella) can occur if the mother develops chickenpox while she is pregnant. The timing of the disease during pregnancy is important for several reasons. "Congenital varicella syndrome" is a severe manifestation of intrauterine infection that occurs when VZV is contracted in the first half of pregnancy. Limb hypoplasia, neurologic and ocular abnormalities, and characteristic cicatricial skin scarring, often in a dermatomal pattern (Gnann, 2012), are seen in the infant at birth. Fortunately, this form of congenital infection is rare (1–6/100,000 births).

Third-trimester varicella in the mother can also results in infection of the fetus, but this is usually well tolerated: these infants are at higher risk for developing zoster during infancy.

The mother who develops chickenpox in the peripartum period (between 5 days prepartum to 2 days postpartum) presents a special medical problem. Neonates in this situation have as much as a 50% risk of developing varicella that has a mortality approaching 30%, presumably due to lack of transplacentally transferred anti-VZV antibodies. Treatment of the newborn infant at birth with high-titer varicella immune globulin decreases the mortality of this condition. Even if the mother received varicella immune globulin during her pregnancy, the infant still requires treatment.

Breastmilk Protective Factors

No protective factors against VZV have been proven to be present in human milk.

Treatments and Interventions

Spread of varicella-zoster virus occurs by both respiratory and contact routes; thus a woman with varicella admitted to the hospital for delivery requires both airborne and contact precautions (gowns, gloves, and masks) for infection control. After delivery, the mother and baby should be isolated from other mothers and infants, but need not be isolated from each other. Breastfeeding should be encouraged (Heuchan & Isaacs, 2001). If appropriate, mother and infant should be discharged promptly to minimize risk to other hospitalized individuals, but this approach must be individualized. The mother should pump/express her breastmilk if the baby is temporarily housed elsewhere. The baby should be protected from direct contact with the mother's skin lesions until they are fully crusted. Development of maternal zoster during pregnancy has not been associated with intrauterine VZV infection (presumably due to preexisting maternal anti-VZV antibody).

Non-immune healthcare workers who have been exposed to chickenpox should not have contact with non-immune patients/mothers/babies from day 10 to day 21 following their exposure. Non-immune, nonpregnant, VZV-exposed healthcare workers should be vaccinated against VZV.

Cytomegalovirus

Cytomegalovirus (CMV) is a member of the herpesvirus family and is probably the most common congenital infection worldwide. Infection is lifelong, with the virus persisting in a latent state in multiple cell types of the host. The prevalence of antibodies against CMV in adults varies from approximately 50% (in developed countries) to 90% (in developing countries), suggesting that infection with CMV often occurs at an early age. The prevalence of CMV antibody in young children is highest in developing countries and in countries in which communal child care and breastfeeding are common.

Risks for Transmission

CMV can commonly be found in many body fluids (human milk, the genital tract, urine, and pharyngeal secretions) and is transmitted by contact with any of these fluids. Breastfeeding transmission of CMV occurs in 60% to 70% of mother–infant pairs, depending on how long breastfeeding continues and the content of CMV in the milk.

Outcomes

In full-term infants, MTCT by breastfeeding is nearly always asymptomatic, so breastfeeding by a CMV-infected mother is appropriate (Plosa et al., 2012). The greatest risks from CMV infection arise with the fetus (usually in a woman who has her primary CMV infection during pregnancy; Damato, 2002) and the preterm infant who acquires the infection from breastmilk (Luck & Sharland, 2009). In primary CMV infection during pregnancy, approximately half of the fetuses are infected by CMV (Nelson & Demmler, 1997), and about 10% of these congenitally infected newborns will show symptoms at birth (hepatitis, neutropenia, thrombocytopenia, sepsis-like syndrome) that lead to recognition of their syndrome at that time. Of these symptomatic infants, 40% to 60% will go on to develop auditory, cognitive, or motor impairment. Of the 90% of infants who are asymptomatic at birth, 10% to 15% will develop sensorineural deafness during childhood (Pass, 2010). Premature infants who acquire CMV infection are more likely to manifest symptoms of infection than are term infants (Maschmann et al., 2001). These symptoms may include sepsis syndrome, pneumonia, necrotizing enterocolitis, hepatitis, thrombocytopenia, or neutropenia, all of which predictably prolong the NICU course of these infants. Whether CMV-positive breastmilk should be given to extremely premature infants is a topic of ongoing discussion (Plosa et al., 2012).

Breastmilk Protective Factors

No protective factors against CMV have been proven to be present in the milk of CMV-naïve mothers.

Counseling

It is clear that CMV infection can be transmitted via breastfeeding, and that in the small, premature infant, severe illness can result from breastmilk MTCT of CMV. Although this risk of severe illness cannot be accurately estimated, it is likely small—but it is real. In weighing the risks versus benefits of breastmilk transmission of CMV, most would say that in the small, young, unstable, and highly vulnerable premature infant in the NICU, the risk likely exceeds the benefit. CMV-negative donor breastmilk or banked breastmilk may be safer options in such cases. In the older, "feeder and grower" premature infant, the risk-to-benefit ratio may be more permissive for breastmilk feeding, but this is best determined on a case-by-case basis.

Management/Interventions

Pasteurization of milk inactivates CMV; freezing milk at −20°C (−4°F) decreases viral titers but does not reliably eliminate CMV. Because milk banks pasteurize their donor milks before storage and distribution, they are expected to be free of infectious CMV.

CMV infection is not usually treated, except in immunocompromised individuals and congenitally infected infants. At present, four agents are FDA approved for CMV treatment: ganciclovir, valganciclovir, foscarnet, and cidifovir. Unfortunately, their clinical application is limited by their toxicities, poor oral absorption, and potential for development of drug resistance by CMV with prolonged use.

Rubella

Rubella virus is the cause of a once-prevalent childhood rash illness called rubella, "German measles," or "3-day measles." Although it caused a self-limited, usually mild illness in children, it was well known that if a pregnant woman acquired infection, there was significant risk of congenital infection causing severe birth defects of the eye, heart, and brain. This severe outcome from intrauterine infection was largely responsible for development of an effective vaccine that is now routinely given to children (the measles/mumps/rubella {MMR} vaccine) and has nearly eliminated rubella in developed countries.

Risks for Transmission

Because of its known teratogenicity, it might be easy to assume that rubella virus transmitted in human milk would likewise be dangerous to the infant. Based on studies of postpartum rubella vaccine recipients, rubella virus can be passed via maternal milk lymphocytes to the infant, and infants may transiently develop blood antibodies against the vaccine virus (indicating infection). The infant exposed to the rubella vaccine virus in this manner does not develop illness (Losonsky et al., 1982). The applicability of these observations to wild-type rubella infections is uncertain but support the premise that rubella virus can be transmitted via breastmilk and cause infection in the infant (Klein, Byrne, & Cooper, 1980). Whether infection with wild-type virus would remain asymptomatic is not known.

Outcomes of Infection

In infants and children, rubella is also called the "3-day measles," owing to its short duration and associated rash. The accompanying fever is usually mild and swollen glands are common. In pregnant women, fetal outcomes can be poor.

Breastmilk Protective Factors

No protective factors against rubella have been proven to be present in milk from rubella-naïve mothers.

Treatments/Interventions

The American Academy of Pediatrics (2012b) recommends that "women with rubella or women who have been immunized recently with live-attenuated rubella virus vaccine may continue to breastfeed."

Hepatitis B

Hepatitis B virus (HBV) causes infection of the liver that has the potential to produce systemic manifestations (depending on the severity and chronicity of the infection). In children and adults, acute infection may be asymptomatic or manifest as any severity of illness from mild "flu-like" symptoms to rapidly progressive liver failure. Acute infection can either resolve completely or become a chronic, lifelong infection. The latter is associated with development of hepatocellular carcinoma after three to four decades.

Risks for Transmission

HBV is transmitted by contact with infected blood or body secretions. Thus transmission of infection via contact with an infected individual's blood or during sexual intercourse is a possibility. An estimated 3% to 13% of neonatal HBV infections result from intrauterine infection prior to labor (Guo et al., 2010). The remaining large majority of perinatally acquired infections result from HBV acquisition from blood/body fluid contact preceding or during the birthing process. This fact explains why immunoprophylaxis and vaccination against HBV are performed immediately after birth.

Hepatitis B virus antigens and DNA are commonly present in the milk of mothers with both acute and chronic hepatitis B infection, and because hepatitis B is the "blood-and body fluid–transmitted" hepatitis, these breastmilk specimens should transmit infection. However, epidemiologic studies of infants of hepatitis B–infected mothers indicate no difference in rates of infection when breastfed and nonbreastfed infants are compared if the infants received appropriate peripartum passive and active immunization against hepatitis B (Shi et al., 2011). The explanation for this paradox is incomplete, but some propose that blood exposure—for example, at birth or in blood-contaminated breastmilk—is the real risk for hepatitis B infection, rather than the potential exposure from routine breastfeeding.

Breastmilk Protective Factors

No protective factors against hepatitis B have been proven to be present in milk from hepatitis B–naïve mothers.

Outcomes of Infection

The large majority of perinatally acquired HBV infections are asymptomatic. Approximately 90% of perinatal infections become chronic HBV infections, with the accordant risks of late hepatocellular carcinoma development.

Treatments/Interventions

Screening mothers for their HBV status prepartum is a standard of care in the United States. Testing of a woman's HBV status can be confusing, however, because different test results have different clinical implications. The most important tests for determining infection status and infectious risk are the following:

- Hepatitis B surface antigen (HBsAg): This is the material covering the surface of the hepatitis B virion and, if positive, indicates either the presence of intact virus in the blood or partial virus particles. If HBsAg is positive, the individual can transmit HBV with his or her body fluids.
- Hepatitis B e antigen (HBeAg): This is a component of the infectious virus particle, and its presence in the blood indicates active production of infectious virions. If HBeAg is positive, the risk of transmission from blood or body fluid contact is extreme and HBV can be transmitted with even tiny blood/body fluid exposures.

- Hepatitis B DNA (HB-DNA): If this test is positive, it suggests the presence of HBV virions in the blood.

The following tests are the most important ones for determining immunity:

- Antibody to HBsAg (anti-HBsAg): If this test is positive, the patient has either been vaccinated or is convalescent from distant acute HBV infection.
- Antibody to hepatitis B core antigen (anti-HBcAg): If this test is positive, the patient may be (1) convalescent from distant acute HBV infection or (2) in the process of responding to HBV infection (and is potentially infectious).

Because interpretation of hepatitis B tests may be complicated, specialty consultation is common to determine the implications of test results.

All infants born to HBsAg-positive mothers (who have been exposed to maternal blood, amniotic fluid, and vaginal secretions during delivery) should receive hepatitis B immunoglobulin (HBIg) and their first dose of HBV vaccine within 12 hours after birth. These infants may breastfeed. For infants with birth weights greater than 2000 g, a second dose of vaccine is given at age 1–2 months and a third dose at age 6 months. For infants with birth weights less than 2000 g, the initial dose of vaccine should be given within 12 hours of birth and followed with three doses of HBV vaccine given at 1, 2–3, and 7 months of age. This four-dose series is used in small infants because responses to the standard three-dose series in this weight group may be less than adequate. Infants of HBsAg-positive mothers should be tested for both HBsAg and anti-HBsAg after completion of the vaccine series to determine if prevention of infection has been successful (AAP, 2012a).

It is considered safe for a mother infected with hepatitis B to breastfeed her infant. Should a mother develop nipple injury/fissuring that causes obvious blood contamination of her milk, it may be prudent to refrain from feeding from the affected breast until the obvious bleeding ceases.

Treatment of hepatitis B infection is currently reserved for adults with chronic infections and is largely investigational. Agents used include interferon-α, lamivudine, and tenofovir, as well as other investigational drugs.

Hepatitis B vaccination is recommended for all infants as part of the routine childhood immunization schedule.

Hepatitis C

Hepatitis C virus (HCV) is the agent formerly called "non-A, non-B hepatitis." Adult infection is acquired from contact with blood from a HCV-infected individual (e.g., via blood or blood product transfusion, intravenous drug use), and is associated with development of chronic hepatitis in 70% to 80% of infected adults. Sexual transmission has been proposed as a mechanism of spread, but is difficult to demonstrate except in HIV-infected individuals. In childhood, HCV infection is mainly acquired through vertical transmission. The perinatal MTCT rate is approximately 6%, and relates to the presence and intensity of maternal viremia (i.e., the presence of virus RNA in the blood) and high viral load at delivery (Tajiri et al., 2001).

Risks for Transmission

Despite detection of HCV RNA (i.e., presumably infectious virus) in some breastmilk samples, there is no strong evidence that breastfeeding confers risk of HCV infection (Polywka et al., 1999; Tajiri et al., 2001), and no definite case of mother-to-infant transmission via breastmilk has been reported. The overall rate of MTCT of HCV among breastfed infants is not different from that seen among formula-fed infants, indicating no additional risk from breastfeeding.

Outcomes of Infection

After acquiring HCV infection, 20% to 30% of individuals spontaneously clear their infection. The 70% to 80% of patients who develop chronic infection experience long-term insidious progression that produces liver cirrhosis (chronic HCV infection is the most common reason that liver transplantation is performed in the United States), liver failure, and/or hepatocellular carcinoma.

Breastmilk Protective Factors

No protective factors against HCV infection have been proven to be present in human milk.

Treatment/Management

HCV-infected women should be allowed to breastfeed (Lin et al., 1995). Because HCV transmission relates to blood contact, it has been proposed that cracks or fissuring of the nipples from breastfeeding might pose a risk for HCV transmission (Buckhold, 2000; Roberts & Yeung, 2002). This consideration is hypothetical, but it may be reasonable and prudent to avoid breastfeeding during obvious situations of blood contamination of the milk because HCV has a high rate of converting to chronic infection, and chronic infection, in turn, is associated with high rates of development of cirrhosis and liver failure.

Treatment of HCV infection is largely investigational, and utilizes agents such as ribavirin and pegylated interferon-α.

Human T-Cell Lymphotropic Viruses

Human T-cell lymphotrophic viruses 1 and 2 (HTLV-1 and HTLV-2) are closely related viruses that are members of the delta retrovirus family. HTLV-1 is endemic in southwestern and northern Japan, Africa, Australia, Alaska, South America, and the Caribbean. HTLV-2 occurs in select Amerindian and Central African populations and IV-drug users. HTLV-1 infection is linked with adult T-cell leukemia and lymphoma, myelopathy/tropical spastic paraparesis, and uveitis. HTLV-2 infection is associated with milder forms of myelopathy/tropical spastic paraparesis, arthritis, bronchitis, and pneumonia. Both viruses are rare in the United States.

Risks for Transmission

The risk of MTCT of HTLV-1 via breastfeeding is 15% to 25% (compared to 3% without breastfeeding) (Ribeiro et al., 2011). The risk for HTLV-2 MTCT is thought to be similar. The duration of breastfeeding appears to be an important risk factor for transmission of HTLV-1. In the largest summary study to date, the HTLV-1 acquisition rates for infants breastfed for less than 6 months versus more than 6 months were 7.4% versus 20.3%, respectively; the rate for bottle-fed infants over the same period was lower (2.5%), reiterating the importance of any breastfeeding in HTLV-1 transmission.

Outcomes of Infection

Data on the frequency of development of T-cell leukemia/lymphoma or myelopathy/tropical spastic paraparesis following HTLV-1 or HTLV-2 infection are not available.

Breastmilk Protective Factors

No protective factors against HTLV-2 or HTLV-2 infection have been proven to be present in the milk of HTLV-1– or HTLV-2–naïve mothers.

Treatment/Interventions

Avoidance of breastfeeding by HTLV-1–positive mothers continues to be recommended in Japan. HTLV-2–positive mothers are also recommended to avoid breastfeeding (Hino, 2011). Freezing and thawing breastmilk eliminates HTLV-1 infectivity (Ando et al., 2004).

West Nile Virus

West Nile fever, a condition caused by West Nile virus (WNV), was an exclusively Asian/European/African disease until its introduction into the northeastern United States in 1999. Since that time, WNV has spread across North America as a mosquito-borne virus whose reservoir in nature is birds. Since its arrival in North America, modes of transmission for WNV other than mosquito bite have been documented, including via blood transfusion and probably via both intrauterine and breastmilk MTCT.

Risks for Transmission

Transmission through breastfeeding appears to be rare (Hinckley, O'Leary, & Hayes, 2007) and current recommendations are that women with WNV infection may continue to breastfeed (AAP, 2012d).

Outcomes of Infection

WNV infection can be asymptomatic (approximately 80% of cases), can cause a mild febrile illness called West Nile fever (20%), or can cause West Nile encephalitis (less than 1%) (Rossi, Ross, & Evans, 2010).

Breastmilk Protective Factors

No protective factors against WNV infection have been proven to be present in milk from WNV-naïve mothers.

Treatment/Management

There are no treatments for West Nile virus infection. Prevention of infection is via use of insect repellents to reduce exposure to mosquitos.

Implications for Practice

Except for HIV and HTLV-1, viral infection in the mother rarely requires avoidance of breastfeeding of the term infant. From a practical standpoint, the infant has often already been exposed to the virus infecting the mother by the time her illness is recognized. For the hospitalized mother–infant dyad, if the mother is well enough to care for her infant and the infant does not require special hospital care, it is reasonable to have the mother and infant stay in the same room.

For the breastfeeding mother with a viral disease, isolation precautions should be used while she is hospitalized to prevent exposure of other mothers, infants, or healthcare workers. This is usually achieved via scrupulous hand hygiene and gowning/masking (if indicated) to prevent possible cross-contamination. The effectiveness of alcohol-based agents for hand hygiene varies depending on the virus and the active ingredients in the rub (Iwasawa et al., 2012). For example, these agents have poor effectiveness against rhinoviruses (Savolainen-Kopra et al., 2012), but good choices against influenza viruses (Grayson et al., 2009). In contrast, hand washing appears to be predictably effective (Grayson et al., 2009). While the hand-rub solutions are more convenient than hand washing in many situations, hand washing is always required if the hands are visibly contaminated, to remove foreign materials. No data indicate that "antiseptic" soaps are superior to non-antiseptic soaps for preventing infection or transmission of infection. The mother does not need to wear rubber gloves while breastfeeding her infant; for hospital staff, the most effective way to prevent the spread of viral infections among neonates, parents, and fellow staff is to maintain appropriate infection control precautions (gloves, gowns, and masks as appropriate).

We should be cognizant that a new mother is already under stress. Giving her the information that she has a viral infection (irrespective of the mechanism of transmission) may cause her to feel pain, anger, and guilt. These feelings may be compounded by fear that breastfeeding her infant may cause harm. Encouraging the mother to express her fears, answering her questions, and then supporting her desires is a vital contribution that the nurse or lactation consultant can make to her care and well-being.

Acknowledgments

Jan Riordan, a founding editor and author of this text, was the original author of this chapter. For this fifth edition, as the new solo author, I have made a number of changes in organization and updated the evidence, but the content honors Dr. Riordan's initial and ongoing work in this important text.

SUMMARY

Beginning at about the 28th week of gestation, the fetus receives passive immunity from the mother as transplacentally passed IgG antibody. The term infant is, therefore, born with the "immunologic repertoire" of the mother. This "passive immunity" from the mother is protective for 3–6 months following birth, with small amounts of maternal antibody remaining in the infant's circulation for as long as 12–15 months. During breastfeeding, the infant absorbs negligible amounts of antibody from the mother's milk, although the milk antibody very likely performs antibody functions within the intestinal lumen, providing protection against intestinal infections and toxins. In addition, other non-nutritional milk components such as the oligosaccharides provide a second level of protection against intestinal infections and toxins.

Significant concern for MTCT of viral infection through breastmilk applies to HIV and HTLV-1/2 and, in specific situations, to varicella, CMV, HSV, and hepatitis B and C. For most other viral infections, it is appropriate for breastfeeding to continue. The potential for HIV transmission by human milk is clear, and in the future, studies of antiretroviral therapy in the breastfeeding mother suggest ART for the mother and breastfeeding infant may ultimately be the best approach to preventing transmission in underdeveloped countries.

KEY CONCEPTS

- HIV-infected women should not breastfeed where safe, affordable infant food alternatives are available. It is well established that HIV can be transmitted from mother to infant through breastfeeding. Where HIV-infected women have no other option but to breastfeed, exclusive breastfeeding for as short a period as possible should be promoted. HIV-infected pregnant women should receive feeding counseling that includes general information about the risks and benefits of infant feeding options, and specific guidance in selecting the option most suitable for their particular situation.

- For the healthcare worker, breastmilk is considered a human body fluid, and has the potential to transmit disease when it has obvious contamination from blood. Wearing gloves to prevent contact with breastmilk is a reasonable and prudent precaution.

- If a mother has an open wound on her breast, wearing personal protective equipment (gloves at minimum) is warranted, just as it is with wounds at any other site (Siegel et al., 2007). In the absence of breast lesions, the newborn of a mother with HSV-1 may breastfeed if the baby is well and be with the mother in her room; however, scrupulous hand washing, gowning, and covering of any lesions must be practiced to prevent possible transmission to the infant.

- Women with herpetic lesions on their breasts should refrain from breastfeeding until the lesion has crusted.

- If a mother develops chickenpox within 5 days before delivery or within 48 hours after birth, her infant is a candidate for varicella-zoster immune globulin treatment. In addition, the mother should delay breastfeeding until her chickenpox lesions have crusted, in the interim using a breast pump to maintain her milk supply. Infection control precautions for healthcare workers using gowns, gloves, and masks are indicated. Following birth, the mother and baby should be isolated from others and discharged as soon as possible. The baby should be protected from direct contact with the mother's skin lesions. If the infant develops chickenpox lesions after birth, the child can be isolated with the mother, and breastfeeding may occur uninterrupted.

- Cytomegalovirus, a prevalent infection, can be found in human milk, genital tract secretions, urine, and pharyngeal secretions. It is transmitted by any close contact. Transmission through breastmilk is documented, but in term infants, serious illnesses and clinical symptoms do not result from this transmission. In premature and very-low-birth-weight infants, there is concern that serious illness and clinical symptoms might occur due to breastmilk transmission. The major risk of CMV infection is transmission to the fetus by a woman who has a primary infection during pregnancy.

- The rubella vaccine virus can be passed via maternal milk lymphocytes to the infant, suggesting that the wild-type rubella virus might do the same. Infants who acquire rubella vaccine virus in this way transiently show serum antibody responses and do not develop illness, but whether asymptomatic infection would also be the case for infants acquiring wild-type rubella virus via breastmilk is not known.

- Infants born to a HBsAg-positive mother have already been exposed to maternal blood during delivery and may breastfeed. The infant should receive hepatitis B immune globulin (HBIg) and hepatitis B vaccine within 12 hours of birth.. These infants should subsequently be followed up with screening for HBsAg to determine whether their postnatal prophylaxis was effective.

- There is no direct evidence that breastfeeding confers risk for MTCT of hepatitis C virus.

- Women who are HTLV-1 or HTLV-2 seropositive are advised not to breastfeed. In children who must be breastfed for socioeconomic reasons, longer breastfeeding confers a higher risk of transmission. Children of infected mothers who do not acquire the infection still acquire passive maternal antibodies that disappear by 9 months of age.

- Mothers with West Nile virus can breastfeed.

Internet Resources

Position papers on HIV/AIDs and breastfeeding: http://global-breastfeeding.org

HIV/AIDS Surveillance Report. Statistics, teaching tools, PowerPoint presentations: http://www.cdc.gov/hiv/stats.htm

World Health Organization. Guidelines for antiretroviral drugs for treating pregnant women and preventing HIV infection in infants: http://www.who.int/hiv/pub/guidelines/en/

World Health Organization: http://www.who.int/hiv/pub/me/monitoring_framework/en/

References

American Academy of Pediatrics (AAP). Hepatitis B. In: *2012 red book: report of the Committee on Infectious Diseases* (29th ed.). Elk Grove Village, IL: Author; 2012a:369–390.

American Academy of Pediatrics (AAP). Rubella. In: *2012 red book: report of the Committee on Infectious Diseases* (29th ed.). Elk Grove Village, IL: Author; 2012b:629–634.

American Academy of Pediatrics (AAP). Transmission of infectious agents via human milk. In: *2012 red book: report of the Committee on Infectious Diseases* (29th ed.). Elk Grove Village, IL: Author; 2012c:128–132.

American Academy of Pediatrics. West Nile virus. In: *2012 red book: report of the Committee on Infectious Diseases* (29th ed.). Elk Grove Village, IL: Author; 2012d:792–795.

Ando Y, Ekuni Y, Matsumoto Y, et al. Long-term serological outcome of infants who received frozen-thawed milk from human T-lymphotropic virus type-I positive mothers. *J Obstet Gynaecol Res.* 2004;30(6):436–438.

Becquet R, Ekouevi DK, Arrive E, et al. Universal antiretroviral therapy for pregnant and breast-feeding HIV-1–infected women: towards the elimination of mother-to-child transmission of HIV-1 in resource-limited settings. *Clin Infect Dis.* 2009;49:1936–1945.

Brown ZA. Preventing transmission of herpes simplex to newborns. *Contemp Nurse Pract.* September–October 1995:29–35.

Buckhold KM. Who's afraid of hepatitis C? *Am J Nurs.* 2000;100:26–31.

Bulterys M, Ellington S, Kourtis AP. HIV-1 and breastfeeding: biology of transmission and advances in prevention. *Clin Perinatol.* 2010;37:807–824.

Cline MK, Bailey-Dorton C, Cayelli M. Update in maternity care: maternal infections diagnosis and management. *Primary Care.* 2000;27:13–33.

Coovadia HM, Rollins NC, Bland RM, et al. Mother-to-child transmission of HIV-1 infection during exclusive breastfeeding in the first 6 months of life: an intervention cohort study. *Lancet.* 2007;369:1107–1116.

Coutsoudis A. Promotion of exclusive breastfeeding in the face of the HIV pandemic [Commentary]. *Lancet.* 2000;356:1620–1621.

Cunningham CK, Chaix M-L, Rekacewicz C, et al. Development of resistance mutations in women receiving standard antiretroviral therapy who received intrapartum nevirapine to prevent perinatal human immunodeficiency virus type 1 transmission: a substudy of Pediatric AIDS Clinical Trials Group Protocol 316. *J Infect Dis.* 2002;186:181–188.

Damato EG. Cytomegalovirus infection: perinatal complications. *JOGN Nurs.* 2002;31:86–92.

Dunkle LM, Schmidt R, O'Connor DM. Neonatal herpes simplex infection possibly acquired via maternal breast milk. *Pediatrics.* 1979;63:250–251.

Gnann JW. Varicella-zoster virus: prevention through vaccination. *Clin Obstet Gynecol.* 2012;55:560–570.

Grayson ML, Melvani S, Druce J, et al. Efficacy of soap and water and alcohol-based hand-rub preparations against live H1N1 influenza virus on the hands of human volunteers. *Clin Infect Dis.* 2009;48:285–291.

Guo Y, Liu J, Meng L, et al. Survey of HBsAg-positive pregnant women and their infants regarding measures to prevent maternal–infantile transmission. *BMC Infect Dis.* 2010;10:26–30.

Heuchan A, Isaacs D. The management of varicella-zoster virus exposure and infection in pregnancy and the newborn period. *Med J Aust.* 2001;174(6):288–292.

Hinckley AF, O'Leary DR, Hayes EB. Transmission of West Nile virus through human breast milk seems to be rare. *Pediatrics.* 2007;119:e666.

Hino S. Establishment of the milk-borne transmission as a key factor for the peculiar endemicity of human T-lymphotropic virus type 1 (HTLV-1): the ATL Prevention Program Nagasaki. *Proc Jpn Acad Ser B.* 2011;87:152–166.

Iwasawa A, Niwano Y, Kohno M, Ayaki M. Virucidal activity of alcohol-based hand rub disinfectants. *Biocontrol Sci.* 2012;17:45–49.

Jackson B, Musoke P, Fleming T, et al. Intrapartum and neonatal single-dose nevirapine compared with zidovudine for prevention of mother-to-child transmission of HIV-1 in Kampala, Uganda: 18-month follow-up of the HIVNET 012. *Lancet.* 2003;362:859–868.

Kaiser Foundation. HIV/AIDS fact sheet. December 2012. Available at: http://kaiserfamilyfoundation.files.wordpress.com/2013/01/3030-17.pdf.

Klein EB, Byrne T, Cooper LZ. Neonatal rubella in a breast-fed infant after postpartum maternal infection. *J Pediatr.* 1980;97:774–775.

Kotronias D, Kapranos N. Detection of herpes simplex virus DNA in maternal breast milk by in situ hybridization with tyramide signal amplification. *In Vivo.* 1999;13(6):463–466.

Lala MM, Merchant RH. Prevention on parent to child transmission of HIV: what is new? *Indian J Pediatr.* 2012;1491–1500.

Lewis P, Nduati R, Kreiss JK, et al. Cell-free human immunodeficiency virus type 1 in breast milk. *J Infect Dis.* 1998 Jan;177(1):34–39.

Lin HH, Kao JH, Hsu HY, et al. Absence of infection in breast-fed infants born to hepatitis C virus–infected mothers. *J Pediatr.* 1995;126:589–591.

Losonsky GA, Fishaut JM, Strussenberg J, et al. Effect of immunization against rubella on lactation products: I. Development and characterization of specific

immunologic reactivity in breast milk. *J Infect Dis.* 1982;145:661–666.

Luck S, Sharland M. Postnatal cytomegalovirus: innocent bystander or hidden problem? *Arch Dis Child Fetal Neonatal Ed.* 2009;94:F58–F64.

Lunney KM, Iliff P, Mutasa K, et al. Associations between breast milk viral load, mastitis, exclusive breastfeeding, and postnatal transmission of HIV. *Clin Infect Dis.* 2010;50:762–769.

Maschmann J, Hamprecht K, Dietz K, et al. Cytomegalovirus infection of extremely low-birth weight infants via breast milk. *Clin Infect Dis.* 2001;33:1998–2003.

McCarthy M. Low-cost drug cuts perinatal HIV-transmission rate. *Lancet.* 1999;354(9175):309.

Nelson CT, Demmler GJ. Cytomegalovirus infection in the pregnant mother, fetus, and newborn infant. *Clin Perinatol.* 1997;24:151–160.

Occupational Safety and Health Administration (OSHA). OSHA Standard 1910.1030. Available at: http://www.osha.gov/pls/oshaweb/owadisp.show_document?p_table=STANDARDS&p_id=10051#1910.1030%28b%29.

Palumbo P, Lindsey JC, Hughes MD, et al. Antiretroviral treatment for children with peripartum nevirapine exposure. *N Engl J Med.* 2010;363:1510–1520.

Pass RF. Congenital cytomegalovirus infection: screening and treatment. *J Pediatr.* 2010;157:179–180.

Plosa EJ, Esbenshade JC, Fuller MP, Weitkamp JH. Cytomegalovirus infection. *Pediatr Rev.* 2012;33:156–164.

Polywka S, Schröter M, Feucht HH, Zöllner B, Laufs R. Low risk of vertical transmission of hepatitis C virus by breast milk. *Clin Infect Dis.* 1999;29:1327–1329.

Read JS, Cohen RA, Hance LF, et al. Missed opportunities for prevention of mother-to-child transmission of HIV-1 in the NISDI Perinatal and LILAC cohorts. *Int J Gynecol Obstet.* 2012;119:70–75.

Read JS, Committee on Pediatric AIDS. Human milk, breastfeeding, and transmission of human immunodeficiency virus type 1 in the United States. *Pediatrics.* 2003;112:1196.

Ribeiro MA, Martins ML, Teixeira C, et al. Blocking vertical transmission of human T cell lymphotropic virus type 1 and 2 through breastfeeding interruption. *Pediatr Infect Dis J.* 2011;31:1139–1143.

Roberts EA, Yeung L. Maternal–infant transmission of hepatitis C virus infection. *Hepatology.* 2002;36(5 suppl 1):S106–S113.

Rossi SL, Ross TM, Evans JD. West Nile virus. *Clin Lab Med.* 2010;30(1):47–65.

Ruff AJ, Coberly J, Halsey NA, et al. Prevalence of HIV-1 DNA and p24 antigen in breast milk and correlation with maternal factors. *J Acquir Immune Defic Syndr.* 1994;7(1):68–73.

Savage F, Lhotska L. Recommendations on feeding infants of HIV positive mothers. *Adv Exp Med Biol.* 2000;478:225–230.

Savolainen-Kopra C, Korpela T, Simonen-Tikka M-L, et al. Single treatment with ethanol hand rub is ineffective against human rhinovirus: hand washing with soap and water removes the virus efficiently. *J Med Virol.* 2012;84:543–547.

Sealander JY, Kerr CP. Herpes simplex of the nipple: infant-to-mother transmission. *Am Family Pract.* 1989;39:111–113.

Shi Z, Yang Y, Wang H, et al. Breastfeeding of newborns by mothers carrying hepatitis B virus: a meta-analysis and systematic review. *Arch Pediatr Adolesc Med.* 2011;165(9):837–846.

Siegel JD, Rhinehart E, Jackson M, et al. Guideline for isolation precautions: preventing transmission of infectious agents in healthcare settings. 2007. Available at: http://www.cdc.gov/ncidod/dhqp/pdf/isolation2007.pdf.

Sullivan-Bolyai JS, Fife KH, Jacobs RF, et al. Disseminated neonatal herpes simplex virus type 1 from a maternal breast lesion. *Pediatrics.* 1983;71:455–457.

Tajiri H, Miyoshi Y, Funada S, et al. Prospective study of mother-to-infant transmission of hepatitis C virus. *Pediatr Infect Dis J.* 2001;20:10–14.

World Health Organization (WHO). Guidelines on infant feeding and HIV 2010: principles and recommendations for infant feeding in the context of HIV and a summary of evidence. 2010. Available at: http://whqlibdoc.who.int/publications/2010/9789241599535_eng.pdf.

World Health Organization (WHO). 2011 global HIV/AIDS response progress report. 2011. Available at: http://www.who.int/hiv/pub/progress_report2011/en/.

Section Three

Prenatal, Perinatal, and Postnatal Periods

CHAPTER 7   Perinatal and Intrapartum Care

CHAPTER 8   Postpartum Care

CHAPTER 9   Breast-Related Problems

CHAPTER 10   Low Intake in the Breastfed Infant: Maternal and Infant Considerations

CHAPTER 11   Jaundice and the Breastfed Baby

CHAPTER 12   Breast Pumps and Other Technologies

CHAPTER 13   Breastfeeding the Preterm Infant

CHAPTER 14   Donor Milk Banking

A caring approach, knowledge, and clinical skills merge in lactation consultant services during pregnancy, the intrapartum, and the immediate postpartum. Problems that are most likely to be of concern in the early days of breastfeeding relate to method of birth, breast engorgement, sore nipples, and other problems that resolve quickly. Most infants are born at or close to term and are healthy and thrive with only breastmilk. A few grow poorly when breastfed. Does this problem derive from the mother, the baby, or the hospital? How can the problem be resolved without compromising the breastfeeding relationship? Those infants who are born early or at risk represent a small percentage of the total, yet they require extra caregiving by their mothers and the specialized technologies and caretaking available in neonatal intensive care units. Donor milk banks represent a means of obtaining human milk for the occasional situation where it is needed to achieve exclusive breastfeeding. More and more hospitals keep human milk in their freezers for use when a baby needs supplements to his or her own mother's milk.

Chapter 7

Perinatal and Intrapartum Care

Kay Hoover

Helping women breastfeed is rewarding. With a basic understanding of the anatomy and physiology of the breast, infant behavior, infant suckling, and the nutritional and immunological properties of breastmilk, the healthcare worker can contribute greatly to a woman's breastfeeding experience. Being prepared to offer practical assistance supported by relevant research findings will meet the urgent needs of mothers with little or no breastfeeding experience. The provider must also be able to assist new mothers who, despite previous breastfeeding experience, are still anxious.

Mothering and breastfeeding are learned behaviors, and a mother's best "teacher" is her own baby. Lactation is a part of the reproductive cycle and is automatic. Milk production begins during pregnancy and increases in volume after birth. However, it is the baby's need, expressed through the behavior of breastfeeding, that determines how much milk is made and how long milk continues to be produced. The baby breastfeeds within the caregiving environment that the mother provides, and everything that a woman has learned in her lifetime contributes to her ability to accept the role of a breastfeeding mother. When reaffirmed as a person and supported in her early efforts to breastfeed, a mother will have most of what she needs to assume her new role and relish the unique joys it will provide her.

Breastfeeding Preparation

The best preparation for breastfeeding is for the woman to learn as much as possible before she embarks on her own childbearing adventure. Learning about breastfeeding can be accomplished in any number of ways. The prospective or new mother can attend sessions held by a community-based breastfeeding group, such as La Leche League, Breastfeeding USA, Nursing Mothers, or the Australian Breastfeeding Association. Each of these groups conducts regularly scheduled meetings to provide education and support for breastfeeding women. The woman may also choose to take a prenatal breastfeeding class. Classes may be offered by healthcare facilities, such as hospitals or prenatal care providers' offices, independent lactation consultants, and public health or nutrition programs, such as the Special Supplemental Nutrition Program for Women, Infants, and Children (WIC) in the United States. Moreover, the woman may have been raised in a breastfeeding community and have friends and family who have breastfed and have learned what she needs to know to get started without going to classes or groups.

In addition to attending breastfeeding groups or classes, mothers can prepare by reading books, by watching DVDs about breastfeeding, and by talking to women who have breastfed. Discussing breastfeeding with women who have had positive experiences is a good way to learn. The experienced breastfeeding mother acts as a mentor to the less knowledgeable woman. She can respond to the new mother's concerns and feelings and advise her on aspects of breastfeeding that are more difficult to address in written form or in a less personal setting.

Doulas and Childbirth Educators

Doulas are educated to provide support for women throughout labor and delivery (Trainor, 2002). During labor, continuous support by a trained doula reduces the need for analgesics, shortens the length of labor, decreases cesarean deliveries, and improves breastfeeding outcomes (Campbell et al., 2006; Montgomery & Hale, 2012). Doulas and childbirth educators encourage breastfeeding and integrate breastfeeding information into their prenatal teaching.

Prenatal Nipple Changes

Production of colostrum starts during pregnancy. In some women, colostrum spontaneously leaks in late pregnancy or during sexual intercourse due to oxytocin release. During pregnancy, the nipples become more elastic and enlarge, which may explain why some women characterize their nipples as "flat" or "inverted" at the beginning of pregnancy but not at the end. How the nipple looks when the baby is not suckling bears little resemblance to its appearance in the baby's mouth, and it is not necessary for the nipple to be everted when not in the baby's mouth. If the nipples appear functional and are not inverted, the best preparation is to do nothing.

Early Feedings

Skin-to-Skin Care Stabilizes the Newborn

Skin-to-skin care was originally used with premature infants, as seen in Figure 7-1. Today, it is also recommended for parents of full-term babies. A plethora of research and books published over the past 30 years uniformly support skin-to-skin care. Box 7-1 summarizes the risks of *not* using skin-to-skin care during the perinatal period. Therefore, following birth, the baby should be dried and placed skin-to-skin on the mother's chest (Figure 7-2). At this

Figure 7-1 SKIN-TO-SKIN, OR KANGAROO, CARE.

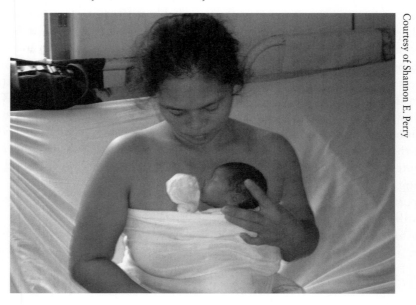

Courtesy of Shannon E. Perry

Figure 7-2 NEWBORN PLACED ON MOTHER'S CHEST.

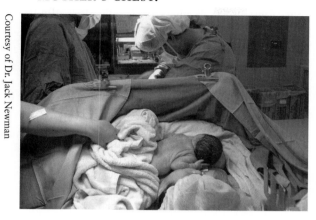

time, the mother and father have their first bonding experience with their new baby, which is almost always very emotional. If the perineum needs to be repaired, it can be done while the baby has skin-to-skin contact. It is important for babies to be placed skin-to-skin immediately at birth and to remain there during the first transition hours after birth.

"Skin-to-skin" means the mother and baby are in a chest-to-chest position. The baby's arm should not be between them. The baby's shoulders should be touching the mother's chest. The baby's head should be turned to the side so the nose is not blocked, and there should be lots of space between the baby's chest and the baby's chin to keep the airway open—in other words, the head should be in extension (Andres et al., 2011; Gnigler et al., 2013).

Takahashi et al. (2011) compared infants placed skin-to-skin by 5 minutes after birth to babies placed skin-to-skin after 5 minutes, as well as those spending less than 60 minutes to those spending more than 60 minutes in skin-to-skin care. The earlier skin-to-skin contact and the longer skin-to-skin contact group had better cardiopulmonary stability and reduced infant stress. For most babies, there is no need to weigh the baby right away. However, some hospitals have policies that require a weight measurement to ascertain if the baby needs to have blood sugars checked frequently. If that is the case, dry the baby off while waiting at least 30 to 60 seconds with the infant maintained at or below the level of the placenta before clamping the cord (American College of Obstetrics and Gynecology

---

BOX 7-1 RISKS OF *NOT* USING SKIN-TO-SKIN CARE DURING THE PERINATAL PERIOD

- Unstable temperatures in the baby (Bergman et al., 2004; Fransson et al., 2005; Walters et al., 2007)
- Shorter duration of exclusive breastfeeding (Vaidya et al., 2005)
- More maternal stress and less satisfaction with breastfeeding (Anderson et al., 2004)
- Stress of separation as demonstrated by higher vasoconstriction in the periphery and more crying
- Less desire by the mother to hold her infant (Anderson et al., 2004)
- Less ability of the baby to smell the natural scent of his mother's milk (Marlier & Schaal, 2005), resulting in less milk ingestion in preterm babies and a longer hospital stay (Raimbault et al., 2007)
- Greater pain and more crying during painful procedures such as heel-lancing and blood collection (Johnston et al., 2003; Marin Gabriel et al., 2013)
- More maternal depressive symptoms and physiological stress in the first postpartum month when mothers did not hold their babies skin-to-skin for several hours each day (Bigelow et al., 2012)

[ACOG], 2012). In preterm babies, one study found higher initial glucose levels (Mercer et al., 2003). Do a quick weight check, and then place the baby skin-to-skin with the mother. Put several thicknesses of a warmed blanket over the baby and the mother, and then put a hat on the baby's head. No matter how the baby is going to be fed, or whether the baby was born by cesarean section or vaginally, all newborns transition to their extra-uterine life better when they are in skin-to-skin care with their mothers.

The recommendations from the American Academy of Pediatrics (AAP) and the American College of Obstetricians and Gynecologists (ACOG, 2012) and the AAP's neonatal resuscitation guidelines (2010) say that if the baby is breathing, has good color, and has good muscle tone, then immediately at birth the baby should be dried off and placed skin-to-skin on the mother and covered with several thicknesses of warm blankets. While the baby is in skin-to-skin contact, the baby goes through nine stages—birth cry, relaxation, awakening, activity, crawling, resting, familiarization, suckling, and sleeping (Widström et al., 2011).

Skin-to-skin care accelerates the baby's adaptation to extrauterine life, reduces crying, and increases the baby's blood glucose and temperature. Mother–infant body contact is as effective as supplemental heat in maintaining the healthy newborn's temperature (Bergman et al., 2004; Christensson et al., 1998; Fransson et al., 2005; Johanson et al., 1992; Walters et al., 2007). With twins, each breast will independently maintain the proper temperature for each baby (Ludington-Hoe et al., 2006). Skin-to-skin contact also colonizes the baby with the mother's harmless bacteria, thereby protecting the infant from pathogenic bacteria.

Skin-to-Skin Care Promotes Breastfeeding

Ideally, the first breastfeeding will take place in the first hour after birth. When healthy infants are placed skin-to-skin on the mother's abdomen and chest shortly after birth, they are alert, and they can crawl, stimulated by the mother's touch, across her abdomen to reach her breast. The baby's hands massage the mother's breast. Each time the baby touches the breast, oxytocin is released, causing nipple erection (Matthiesen et al., 2001). The baby smells, mouths, and licks the mother's nipple and finally attaches to the breast and feeds. See the appendix at the end of this chapter for a listing of research and scholarly papers regarding the newborn's reactions to the smell of mother's milk and/or secretions from Montgomery's glands on the breast areola. Leaving the amniotic fluid on the baby's hands helps the baby find the breast (Varendi et al., 1996).

Neonates who are kept in skin-to-skin contact with their mothers immediately after birth are more likely to suckle effectively than those who are separated. In general, full-term infants demonstrate a well-organized sequence of suckling behaviors, including bringing the hand to the mouth, rooting, and suckling within the first hour after birth (Widström et al., 1990). The placenta is normally expelled soon after birth, often before the infant latches on for the first time. Walters et al. (2007) noticed that having the baby skin-to-skin did not increase nurses' workload, and in the unusual case of an episiotomy repair, the discomfort seemed to be minimized for the mother. The baby should remain in skin-to-skin contact at least until the first breastfeeding is complete.

Early (in the first hour after birth) and frequent breastfeeding are encouraged for optimal functioning of both the infant and the mother for the following reasons:

- Suckling stimulates uterine contractions, aids in the expulsion of the placenta, and helps to control maternal blood loss.
- Mothers will breastfeed for a longer duration (Ekström et al., 2003; Lawson & Tulloch, 1995; Lothian, 1995; Mizuno et al., 2004; Wright et al., 1996).
- The infant's suckling reflex is usually intense after birth. Gratification of this reflex "imprints" this biobehavior to facilitate learning to suckle (Anderson et al., 1982).
- The infant promptly receives the immunological components of the colostrum.

- The infant's digestive peristalsis is stimulated, thereby promoting elimination of the byproducts of hemoglobin breakdown. Jaundice is more likely to occur when feeding and peristalsis are delayed (see the *Jaundice and the Breastfed Baby* chapter).

- Breast engorgement is minimized by the early and frequent removal of milk from the breast (Moon & Humenick, 1989).

- Lactation is accelerated, more milk is produced, and early and frequent intake of breastmilk lessens infant weight loss after birth (Chen et al., 1998; de Carvalho et al., 1982).

- Frequent removal of milk keeps the breast as empty as possible and stimulates the synthesis of breastmilk (Cregan & Hartmann, 1999).

- Attachment and bonding are enhanced at a time when both the mother and the infant are in a heightened state of readiness.

- When babies are placed skin-to-skin immediately at birth and remain there for 2 hours following birth, the duration of exclusive breastfeeding at 48 hours and 6 weeks are significantly higher than when babies are separated from their mothers at birth (Thukral et al., 2012).

- When the baby feeds within the first hour, the parents as well as the professional caregivers relax because the baby is fed.

With the mother on her back and slightly reclined between 30 and 40 degrees, the baby should breastfeed in the delivery room/birthing suite. The ambience and homey comforts of a birthing suite encourage early breastfeeding. The father can share the enjoyment of these first moments together and can help position the mother and infant comfortably in the birthing bed.

Newborns usually lick or nuzzle the nipple at first. Given ample opportunity, the baby is able to crawl to the mother's breast, self-attach, and suckle strongly within an hour (Righard, 1995; Righard & Alade, 1990). Those babies who have been affected by a long labor or a difficult birth may suckle only

minimally at this time, but they should have an opportunity to lick or nuzzle the nipple. Mothers whose infants have come in contact with their nipple–areolar complex typically choose to keep their babies with them for more time during the hospital stay (Widström et al., 1990). Explaining to the mother that "nuzzling" is normal behavior will help her to see this activity as a positive response rather than as disinterest in actual breastfeeding. For newborns, the volatile compounds originating in the areolar secretions or the milk reduce crying, stimulate eye opening, and release mouthing movements (Doucet et al., 2007).

In one study (Gomez et al., 1998), infants were eight times more likely to breastfeed spontaneously if they spent more than 50 minutes skin-to-skin with their mothers immediately after birth; thus the amount of time spent in skin-to-skin contact might be a critical component in breastfeeding success. The more time the baby spent skin-to-skin, the more likely the baby was to exclusively breastfeed during the hospital stay (Gomez et al., 1998). Bramson and colleagues (2010) summarized their study findings as follows: "We determined that the longer a mother experiences early skin-to-skin contact during the first three hours following birth, the more likely that she will breastfeed exclusively during the maternity hospitalization" (p. 134).

Mothers who held their infants skin-to-skin indicated a strong preference for the same type of postdelivery care in the future (86%), whereas only 30% of mothers who held their infants swaddled indicated that they would most certainly prefer this type of care in the future. Infants held skin-to-skin were more than twice as likely to breastfeed successfully during their first postbirth feeding than those who were held swaddled in blankets (Carfoot et al., 2005).

On rare occasions, the first breastfeeding takes place after the mother and her newborn are transferred from the delivery area to their room. Wherever it may be, if the mother is awake and oriented, it is best that she put her baby to breast as soon as possible (see Figures 7-3 and 7-4).

Figure 7-3 LACTATION CONSULTANT ASSISTING MOTHER AT EYE LEVEL DURING FIRST BREASTFEEDING.

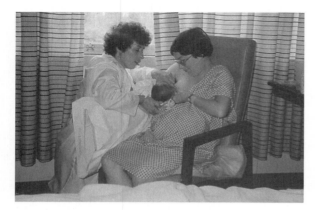

Figure 7-4 BABY PUT TO BREAST RIGHT AFTER DELIVERY.

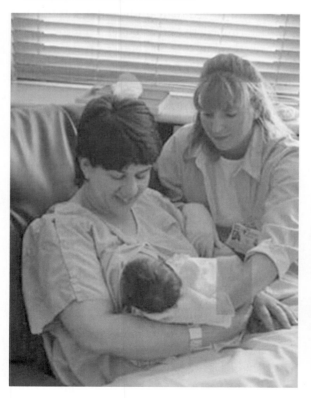

Skin-to-Skin Contact After Cesarean Birth

The neonatologist can evaluate the baby when the baby is on the mother's chest (Barbero et al., 2013). In the twenty-first century, more and more research and quality improvement projects have identified ways that hospitals can institute skin-to-skin after cesarean births (Gouchon et al., 2010; Hung & Berg, 2011; Nolan & Lawrence, 2009; Smith et al., 2008). Anecdotal evidence indicates that parents are very appreciative of the opportunity following the surgical birth (see Figure 7-5).

Epidurals and Other Birth Practices

Some neonates will take longer to learn how to latch onto the breast and feed effectively than others. Interventions during labor, birth, and the post-birth care influence the baby's feeding skills. Most women in the United States and many who live in South American and European countries have epidurals during labor; indeed, in certain places, more than 90% of women receive such care, and the trend is toward more use of epidurals. Epidurals are popular with women; some call it "the best thing since sliced bread." These women are unaware that such

Figure 7-5 NEWBORN SKIN-TO-SKIN AFTER CESAREAN SECTION.

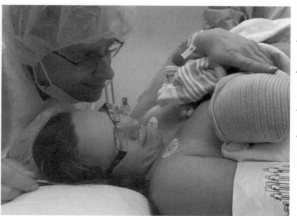

Courtesy of Kay Hoover, MEd, IBCLC

analgesia can delay and diminish neonatal suckling and be associated with shorter breastfeeding duration (Beilin et al., 2005; Crowell et al., 1994; Jordan et al., 2005; Ransjö-Arvidson et al., 2001; Riordan et al., 2000; Sepkoski et al., 1992; Smith, 2010; Torvaldsen et al., 2006), especially if the amount of analgesia administered is high. Fortunately, anesthetists have been using less analgesia in recent years.

Epidurals can have a "domino" effect—usually labor slows down after placement of the epidural—necessitating one intervention after another. For example, the body temperature of the mother and the baby may be elevated with epidurals (Lieberman et al., 1997; Ransjö-Arvidson et al., 2001; Viscomi, 2000), resulting in separation and septic workup to determine if an infection is present. Other research on the effect of epidurals on breastfeeding has concluded that epidural use does not lead to breastfeeding problems or poor infant neurobehavior (Chang & Heaman, 2005). These more recent studies reflect the use of smaller analgesic dosages for epidurals. Women who have a vacuum extraction during birth may abandon breastfeeding early (Hall et al., 2002), possibly due in part to a long, drawn-out, and stressful labor and infant injury. If the birth was by cesarean delivery, it takes longer for the mother's milk to increase in volume.

About one-third of women report their childbirth experiences to be traumatic. In such cases, as Beck and Watson (2008) found from their phenomenological research, the mothers either breastfed because they wanted to do something right after "failing at childbirth" or decided not to breastfeed because they needed to protect themselves from another trauma. If their negative childbirth experiences led them down the path to breastfeed, it was to prove to themselves that they could be good mothers, to atone for themselves to their infants, or to mentally heal themselves and their babies. For women whose negative childbirth experiences impeded breastfeeding, breastfeeding felt like one more way to be violated. These women wanted to reclaim some power for themselves. Some women had flashbacks to the trauma they experienced during childbirth when they breastfed; others felt a disturbing detachment from their babies. This phenomenological study helps us to understand how stressful births can result in abandonment of breastfeeding.

Suctioning

Another disruption to early breastfeeding is routine suctioning of the infant's mouth and nose after birth. The suction tends to cause the infant to have nasal edema and "stuffiness." Because the baby's airway is somewhat obstructed, the baby does not feed well until the swelling subsides. Oral suctioning can lead to breastfeeding difficulties because the baby's mouth or throat may be sore (Widström et al., 1987). In a randomized controlled pilot study, newborns receiving bulb suctioning showed a statistically significant lower heart rate during the first 20 minutes after birth (Waltman et al., 2004). One pediatrician observed rough suctioning with a bulb syringe that resulted in perforation in the soft palate (Soppas, personal communication, June 2003). The 2012 *Guidelines for Perinatal Care* from the AAP and the ACOG (p. 270) state, "When the newborn is vigorous . . . there is no evidence that nasopharyngeal suctioning is necessary."

Postbirth Care of the Newborn

The Academy of Breastfeeding Medicine Protocol #5 (Holmes et al., 2013) as well as the breastfeeding policy statement from the AAP (Eidelman & Schanler, 2012) and *Guidelines for Perinatal Care* (AAP & ACOG, 2012) recommend that hospitals "discontinue disruptive policies that interfere with early skin-to-skin contact" (Eidelman & Schanler, 2012, p. e-834). In addition, under Table 5, "Recommendations on Breastfeeding Management for Healthy Term Infants," the policy recommends:

- "Direct skin-to-skin contact with mothers immediately after delivery until the first feeding is accomplished and encouraged throughout the postpartum period
- Delay in routine procedures (weighing, measuring, bathing, blood tests, vaccines, and eye prophylaxis) until after the first feeding is completed

- Delay in administration of intramuscular vitamin K until after the first feeding is completed but within six hours of birth" (p. e-835)

There have been two interesting studies on delaying the neonate' first bath. One suggested that waiting to bathe the baby may reduce infections (Akinbi et al., 2004). The other study showed that waiting for 12 hours or more before the first bath increased in-hospital breastfeeding rates (Preer et al., 2013).

Hearing Screening

Hearing tests can be done while the baby is held skin-to-skin with one of the parents. Delaying the hearing exam until after 48 hours for cesarean-born babies and for at least the first 24 hours for vaginal-birth babies will increase the likelihood that the baby will pass the test, thus reducing maternal anxiety. In addition, delaying the screening will decrease interruptions of early breastfeeding (Smolkin et al., 2012).

Normal Newborn Sleep and Eating Patterns

Newborns spend 64% of their time sleeping (Sadeh et al., 1996). When skin-to-skin care is practiced and the mother and baby stay together throughout the hospital stay, the breastfeeding neonate exhibits a sleep pattern similar to that indicated in Table 7-1. The initial alertness for the first 2 hours after birth and the eagerness of the baby to breastfeed are followed by deeper sleep for several hours and then increased wakefulness and interest in breastfeeding. During this period of increased wakefulness, the baby will feed frequently, alternating between relatively short periods of light sleep and quiet wakefulness (Williams & Mueller, 1989). Mothers may interpret these "cluster feedings" as indicators that the baby is not getting any milk or is getting an insufficient amount. However, they actually constitute a series of mini-feedings, snacks, or courses in a larger banquet that is part of a single breastfeeding episode. A cluster of mini-feedings

Table 7-1 FIRST-DAY SLEEP PATTERNS OF NEONATES

Infant State	Time Period
Alert	Birth–2 hours
Light and deep sleep	2–20+ hours
Increasing wakefulness*	20–24 hours

*Often includes a cluster of 5 to 10 feeding episodes over 2 to 3 hours followed by deep sleep of 4 to 5 hours.

by the baby is usually followed by a period of deep sleep, during which time the mother should be encouraged to sleep.

A positive, satisfying birthing experience gets breastfeeding off to a good start, and parents often recall this experience in great detail many years later. The caregiver's unhurried, nurturing approach helps to establish rapport with the mother. It is important to explain to the first-time mother that breastfeeding is not as automatic for her as the suckling and rooting reflexes are for her baby. Yet the experience is new to the baby, too, and the first few times at breast offer opportunities for each partner to learn from the other. Early breastfeeding is optimized in the following ways:

- Wash your hands thoroughly. An alcohol-based hand rub may be used *in addition* to hand washing. Gloves (nonlatex) are worn as appropriate. Artificial fingernails should not be worn (Hedderwick et al., 2000; Winslow & Jacobson, 2000). Wearing these nails encourages growth of pathogens, and their sharp edges can hurt the mother and baby.
- Arrange for privacy. Concentrating on learning a new skill is easier when it is private. Ask visitors to leave as appropriate. Sometimes mothers are too polite to ask visitors to leave so that they can feed the baby (and/or rest!), and it is up to the nurse or lactation consultant to make this request. Shut the door of the mother's room or pull the curtains around her bed if she wishes. Privacy door hangers are helpful in reducing interruptions for breastfeeding families (Albert & Heinrichs-Breen, 2011).

- Help the mother to find the most comfortable position and ensure that several pillows are available. Full frontal contact of the baby's body with the mother's chest is a natural position and often works well for breastfeeding. Help the mother place the baby on her chest and recline back, with her body totally supported. The baby should be snuggled securely in the mother's arms and facing toward her. This permits the mother to easily maintain eye contact with her baby. Be sure there is no pressure on the back of the baby's head. The baby's head should be free so he can move it in the event that his nostrils become blocked.

- Many hours after the birth, women who have had a cesarean birth may prefer to sit in the hospital bed; others find it more comfortable to breastfeed while sitting in a comfortable chair with low arms. To provide support, arrange pillows on the woman's lap, behind her back, and under her arms. If the mother is in bed, raise the back of the bed for additional support or put the bed in a semi-Fowler's position. The mother who must remain flat may lie on her back or side with pillows at her back and between her knees. If wearing a hospital gown, open the snaps on the shoulders to pull down and expose the breast as needed.

- Work with the mother at her eye level. If she is in a chair or bed, pull up a chair; if the bed is electronically operated, raise the bed to bring her to your eye level. When an individual is engaging in a new activity, anyone standing higher may provoke anxiety in the learner (see again Figure 7-3). Standing at the baby's feet seems to be the best angle when assisting with breastfeeding. Suggest that the mother support her breast with her hand if needed. Advise her to keep her thumb and fingers well behind the areola in a C-hold—a position in which the hand is shaped into a *C* (Figure 7-6).

- Help the mother to position her baby so that his nose is at the level of the mother's nipple. Ask the mother to bring the baby's chin in contact with her breast. When the

Figure 7-6 THE C-HOLD.

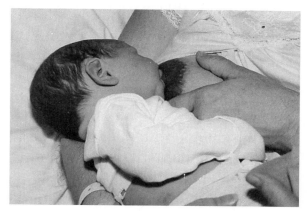

infant opens his mouth wide (rooting reflex) in response to this stimulus, he can self-attach or the mother can bring his shoulders to her breast in one quick movement of her hand or forearm, aiming the nipple toward the soft palate. By placing your hand behind the mother's hand or arm, you can assist her in bringing the baby in close when the baby opens with a wide gape to maximize the amount of breast tissue he grasps.

- Once latched, the baby's lips should be flanged outward and his nose slightly away from the surface of the breast so that he can breathe easily (Figure 7-7). If the mother is concerned about the baby's ability to breathe, ask her to bring the baby's hips in close to her body, or lift her breast slightly so she can easily maintain the infant's airway. Keep in mind that the baby has not breastfed before, and the suckle–swallow–breathe pattern is a relatively complex series of actions that requires learning and practice.

- Explain that an infant should be allowed to breastfeed as long and as often as he wants to stimulate and maintain the milk production. In some cases, the neonate will take only one breast before falling asleep, but most babies will take both breasts. As long as each breast is offered frequently, single-breast feedings of whatever duration the baby wishes are an appropriate option (Woolridge et al., 1990).

Figure 7-7 LATCH-ON. (A) MOUTH GAPED OPEN. (B) GRASPING BREAST.

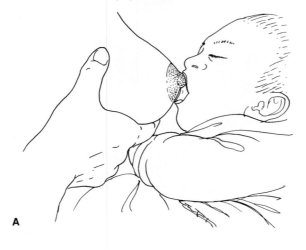

A

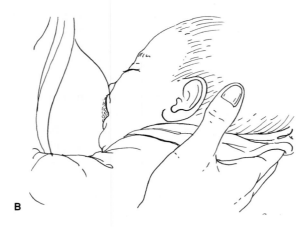

B

"Take turns with the breast you start on" and "Allow the baby to finish the first breast and come off on his or her own before offering the other breast" are easy suggestions. Four researchers have concluded that the baby should be the one to determine the length of the feeding.

◄ "It is suggested that the duration of a breast feed should be determined by the infant's response and not by an arbitrary time schedule" (Howie et al., 1981, p. 71).

◄ "... the infant should be permitted to self-regulate feeding, that is to be allowed to control the feeding process. This means that mothers must learn to trust their infants to exercise control and healthcare professionals must find ways to empower mothers to exercise such trust" (Woolridge & Baum, 1991, p. 118).

◄ "It seems reasonable that a baby should be allowed to finish the first breast and, if still hungry, be offered the second breast. The baby's appetite is the deciding factor" (Righard et al., 1993, p. 182).

◄ "Breastfed infants should be encouraged to feed on demand, day and night, rather than conform to an average that may not be appropriate for the mother–infant dyad" (Kent et al., 2006, p. e-387).

• Teach "baby watching." The recommendation is, "Watch the baby, not the clock." Feed the baby at the *earliest* sign of hunger. Crying is a *late* sign of hunger. A crying baby cannot latch on; the baby needs time to be consoled and to "settle down" emotionally and physiologically before he will become interested in feeding again. With crying, both the infant's blood pressure and intracranial pressure rise causing oxygen-depleted blood to flow back into the systemic circulation rather than into the lungs (Anderson, 1989). Box 7-2 describes the stages of the baby readying to feed.

• Suggest that the mother feed until she notes cues from the infant suggesting satiety (suckling activity ceases, baby falls asleep and lets go of the breast himself). The length of the feeding is up to the baby. If the baby lets go of the breast within 2 to 5 minutes, suggest to the mother that she burp the baby and return the baby to the same breast. Once the baby has fallen asleep and has come off the breast on his own, she can offer the other breast when the baby gives feeding cues again. Toward the end of the feeding, the mother will probably become relaxed to the point of sleepiness—a delightful side effect of oxytocin secretion (Mulford, 1990).

BOX 7-2 CUES IN BABY WATCHING	
Baby Cue	**Stage of Readiness to Feed**
Wiggling, moving arms or legs	Early
Rooting, fingers to mouth	Early
Fussing, squeaky noises	Mid
Restless, crying intermittently	Mid
Full cry, aversive screaming pitch, color turns red	Late

Data from Anderson, 1989.

Early feedings are a critical time for learning new information, especially for the first-time mother, who usually asks many questions. For example, noisy breathing during feedings indicating a "stuffy" nose may worry some mothers who are concerned that the baby is having trouble getting enough oxygen. If the baby is feeding well, nasal stuffiness is usually not a problem and will resolve on its own. Neonates are obligate nose breathers. In a few instances, a newborn's nares are congested to the point where the baby refuses to breastfeed because he cannot breathe and feed at the same time. In this case, saline drops or a hydrocortisone solution in the nose will help alleviate the problem. Mothers also worry if the baby gets the hiccups, another normal baby behavior.

If breastfeeding is painful after the first 30 seconds, the mother should be taught how to break the infant's suction on the breast by placing her finger in the corner of his mouth between his gums so she can take him off and start over again. If the mother and baby are having problems with latching, the mother can compress her breast to assist the baby in taking more breast tissue into his mouth.

Pain Medications

A common question asked of lactation specialists in the perinatal period concerns the use of pain medications for nursing mother. Acetaminophen and ibuprofen are commonly used for pain control postpartum. Both are safe and effective.

Meperidine should not be used, as it can cause cyanosis, respiratory depression, risk of apnea, and somnolence, and it reduces the frequency of breastfeeding in infants. (See the *Drug Therapy and Breastfeeding* chapter.) Morphine or fentanyl is preferred to meperidine for patient-controlled IV analgesia after a cesarean birth (Montgomery & Hale, 2012).

While oxycodone is a popular pain medication post cesarean births, it is not usually recommended for use in breastfeeding mothers because of its higher risk of sedation and dependence in the mother. While it has a relative infant dose of 1.5% to 3.5% of the mother's dose, higher doses have been noted to lead to higher levels in breastmilk. In one study, while milk levels as high as 168 ng/mL were detected, the limited milk volume reduced the overall dose to the infant. In this study, only 1 out of 50 infants exposed to maternal milk had detectable plasma levels. At particularly high doses, breastfed infants may receive more than 10% of a therapeutic infant dose, which poses only minimal risk to the infant because of the low volume of breastmilk ingested in the first few days after delivery (Seaton et al., 2007).

Hydrocodone, the most commonly used opiate analgesic in the United States, is associated with a relative infant dose of only 2.4% to 3.7%. At low to moderate doses, it appears to have few complications in breastfed infants. However, severe constipation in mothers is a common clinical complaint.

Feeding Positions

There are many ways to hold a baby while breast-feeding. The commonly taught positions are the laid-back (Colson et al., 2008) (Figure 7-8), the cradle (Figure 7-9), the cross-cradle (across-the-lap; Figure 7-10A), the football (or clutch or under-the-arm; Figure 7-10B), and the side-lying (Figure 7-11) positions. Although there is nothing magical about a particular position, with help in the hospital the mother can be encouraged to try a few different positions to find out what is most comfortable for her and her infant (Table 7-2). Mothers who had vaginal deliveries have reported less fatigue if they breastfeed in the side-lying position rather than the sitting position (Milligan et al., 1996).

Latch-On and Positioning Techniques

Methods for teaching new mothers how to latch the baby onto the breast are considered fundamental in lactation clinical practice. When problems arise, achieving optimal latch and positioning is often the first and often the only treatment needed to fix most breastfeeding problems.

Different methods list techniques for achieving a "correct," "proper," or "good" latch and/or positioning. Some include the exact alignment that the baby's head must be with his body during a feeding. One recommends that the baby's chin be buried in the breast, his nose not touching the breast (Newman & Pitman, 2006). Rebecca Glover's video,

Figure 7-8 LAID-BACK POSITION.

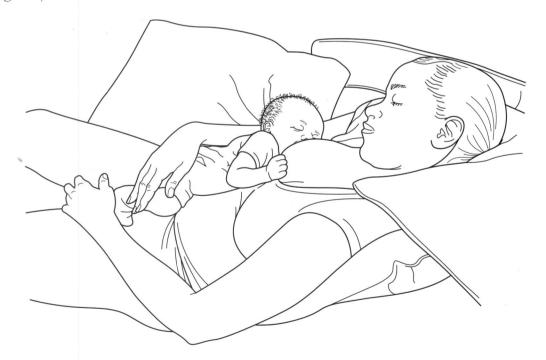

Figure 7-9 MADONNA (CRADLE) POSITION. (A) FRONT VIEW. (B) SIDE VIEW.

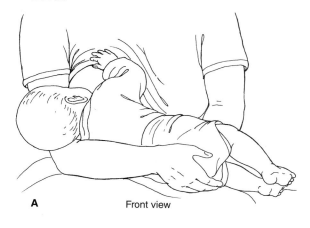

A Front view

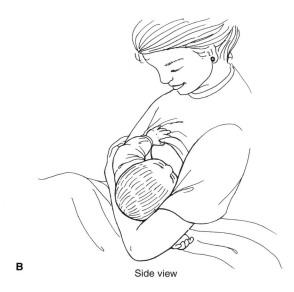

B Side view

Figure 7-10 (A) CROSS-CRADLE OR MODIFIED CLUTCH HOLD. (B) FOOTBALL OR CLUTCH HOLD.

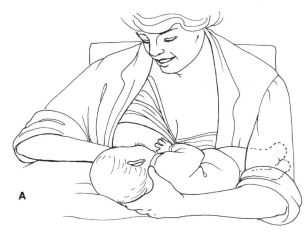

A

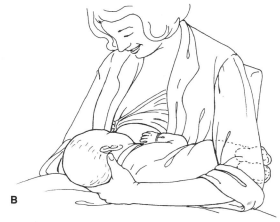

B

Follow Me Mum, emphasizes the use of one finger to tilt the nipple toward the baby's nose. Suzanne Colson and colleagues (2008) recommend the "postnatal lie" with full frontal contact of the baby with the mother. Christina Smillie and Kittie Frantz's video, *Baby-Led Breastfeeding*, recommends that the baby be angled across the mother's body and allowed to self-attach. Chele Marmet and Ellen Shell describe more than 20 types of therapeutic positioning at the breast in *Supporting Sucking Skills in Breastfeeding Infants* (Genna, 2013).

An example of another technique is teaching the mother the mechanics of breastfeeding using the sandwich analogy:

> Using the sandwich as a model, the breast must be first shaped into an oval and then approached from below starting with the nose near the sandwich stuffing. The head tips back slightly and the mandible comes up and forward to fix itself well back on the sandwich. The upper lip is the last part to land on the sandwich, and it is then possible to take a large and satisfying bite. (Wiessinger, 1998)

The many methods for latching the baby onto the breast reflect a growing interest in clinical

Figure 7-11 SIDE-LYING POSITION.

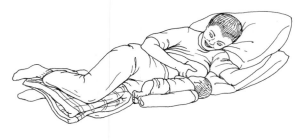

techniques to help breastfeeding women by placing the baby on the breast a certain way. These techniques are useful because they emphasize to the mother (and father) that getting off to the right start by getting the baby to take the breast a certain way will optimize breastfeeding. Basically the mother needs to find a position and latch-on technique that works for her and her baby.

The Infant Who Has Not Latched On

Occasionally, an otherwise healthy newborn will not latch onto his mother's breast, even after several attempts. Most nurses and lactation consultants have witnessed the frustrating situation in which a distraught mother repeatedly tries to breastfeed her neonate, only to have the baby fall into a deep sleep. This is a great time to teach the mother how to hand-express drops of milk directly onto the baby's lips.

The appropriate action in this situation is to keep the baby skin-to-skin with his mother and teach her to watch for cues that the baby has cycled through the period of deep sleep and is beginning to awaken. Movement of head, arms, and legs; mouthing; and grimacing are all early cues that the baby is slowly awakening. This is the time to be alert to his interest in latching. Teaching parents these baby cues is

Table 7-2 POSITIVE AND NEGATIVE ELEMENTS OF INFANT FEEDING POSITIONS

Positioning	Positive Elements	Negative Elements
Laid-back	Babies are abdominal feeders. Allows for self-attachment. Provides good support for the baby and relaxation for the mother.	May not work for some women with extremely large breasts. Not enough photos and drawings of this position, so mothers are not familiar with it.
Cradle	"Classic" position. Most frequently pictured and most often used.	Baby's head tends to wobble around on the mother's arm. Mother has minimal control over baby's head.
Football or clutch	Provides control of baby's head. Good for low-birth-weight, preterm, or late-preterm babies with minimum head control. Avoids incision of cesarean birth. Best position to be able to see the baby's mouth.	Some teaching and coaching required on how to position baby. Baby's bottom needs to be against the back of mother's chair so his head can extend back and there is room between his chin and chest.
Cross-cradle	Provides good head control. Along with football hold, allows for ease with bringing the baby to the breast.	Least familiar to caregivers. Some mothers are not comfortable holding their babies in this manner.
Side-lying	Minimizes fatigue (Milligan et al., 1996). Enables mother to rest more completely than is possible if she is sitting up.	Not always taught in hospital. Mothers may fear smothering baby in this position. Difficult for the mother to see to assist the infant with attachment.

a valuable element in early postpartum care. Poor latch-on in this very early time is common (Dewey et al., 2003) and is not oral aversion or a breastfeeding "strike" discussed in other sections of this text. The baby's lack of interest may be due to labor- or birth-related issues, or to the infant's neurological immaturity. Forcing the baby on the breast before the baby is ready to wake and show active interest may result in an aversive reaction (Widström & Thingström-Paulsson, 1993).

In the unusual event of an infant who cannot attach to the breast after several attempts, a visual evaluation of the infant's mouth is appropriate. The roof of the mouth should be wide and gently domed. The tongue should be long enough to extend over the lower gum. The baby's response to a feather-light stroking of the center of the lower lip should be noted. In most cases, the alert infant will open his mouth wide and the tongue will come forward in response to such stimulation, as if seeking its source. The infant's frenulum (the small tissue tag under the tongue) should be evaluated during suckling. If the frenulum appears tight, a visual examination should be performed to determine whether the frenulum prevents the tongue from elevating or extending sufficiently to produce the wavelike motion necessary for effective suckling (Burton et al., 2013).

Most hospital protocols call for supplementation with the mother's expressed milk to be started if the baby has not latched on by *12 hours postpartum*; a few hospitals use *24 hours* as the cutoff time. The sooner the mother starts providing her milk for her baby, the faster the milk increases in volume.

The inability of the baby to latch onto the breast during the hospital stay does not bode well for breastfeeding. Mercer et al. (2010) found five situations that remained highly significant for predicting discontinuation of breastfeeding by 7 to 10 days postpartum:

- Young maternal age
- No previous breastfeeding experience
- Latching difficulty/sore nipples
- Long stretches of time between breastfeeding sessions
- Use of two or more bottles during the hospital stay

Babies with attachment problems need extra attention and their mothers need additional support.

Digital Examination

Occasionally, a digital examination may be appropriate. The healthcare provider must use a clean, gloved finger with a short nail. A finger (pad side up, nail side down) is slid into the baby's mouth with the baby's permission. The tongue should groove around the finger. When the pad of the fingertip lightly touches the back of the hard palate, the baby usually initiates a suck response that includes massaging by the tongue on the underside of the finger from knuckle to the fingertip.

In a healthy newborn, the strength of the oral negative pressure is such that the examiner will feel as if the nail bed is being pulled deeper into the baby's mouth. The nature of the suckling action should be rhythmic, although some neonates quickly realize that the finger does not reward suckling and so cease doing so after several attempts. Because the finger is not a breast, with its soft areolar and nipple tissue, suckling at the breast should be the first experience for the infant. Thereafter, a finger assessment may be attempted, although it is not necessary in most cases and should be used judiciously.

Even if the baby is found to have an anatomic variation, it may not interfere with effective suckling. However, infants with a cleft palate, a high palatal arch, or a short tongue may require interventions provided by a therapist knowledgeable in treating these oral problems before the baby can breastfeed effectively.

Most maternal and infant problems resolve with time. The full-term infant is born with additional extracellular fluid (shed in the first few days after birth) that sustains him for a short time. Urine output usually exceeds fluid intake for the first 3 to 4 days after birth (Wight, 2003). However, after 24 hours without receiving fluid nutriment, the neonate is at risk for dehydration. Figure 7-12 presents a flowchart that can be used as an algorithm indicating appropriate actions for early feedings or lack of feedings. Box 7-3 contains guidelines for intervention when the infant does not latch onto the breast by 12 to 24 hours after birth.

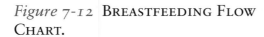

Figure 7-12 Breastfeeding Flow Chart.

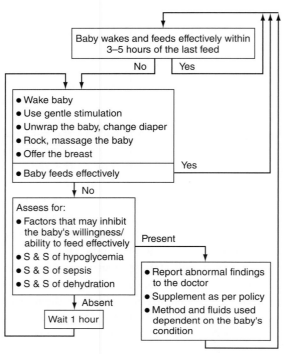

Source: Reprinted with permission from Glover J. Supplementation of breastfeeding newborns: a flowchart for decision-making. *J Hum Lact* 1995;11:127–31.

Plan for the Baby Who Has Not Latched On

The most important concern when a baby is not latching is to feed the baby. One easy technique is to teach the mother how to hand-express her milk onto a spoon, and then feed her baby the drops of colostrum from the spoon. Often when staff members hear "feed the baby," they picture a bottle in the baby's mouth. If a baby is not latching, giving a bottle can lead to the discontinuation of breastfeeding (Howard et al., 2003). Supplementing in the first 24 hours can be done using a spoon or a feeding syringe with drops of colostrum or, once the volume of milk has increased to 10 mL or more, with finger-feeding or cup-feeding.

Women produce a relatively small amount of milk during the first few days postpartum (Casey et al., 1986; Santoro et al., 2010). These small amounts of colostrum give the baby an opportunity to practice the suck–swallow–breathe pattern. The baby should have lots of practice time before the milk increases in volume. Table 7-3 lists expected breastmilk intake for the neonate's first 4 days after birth. After 1 week, the baby should be taking a full volume of milk. Multiply the baby's birth weight in pounds times 2.5, and the result will equal the number of

---

Box 7-3 Guidelines for the Infant Who Does Not Latch-On (According to Hours Postpartum)

0–24 Hours

- For full-term healthy baby, no supplement is necessary providing that the baby has periods of awake and quiet, and vital signs and blood sugar are within normal limits.
- Attempt to breastfeed during quiet, alert times or at least every 3 hours.
- Teach hand expression to provide drops of milk for the baby at least every 3 hours.
- Have parents hold baby skin-to-skin.
- Encourage a quiet environment.
- If not latched-on by 18–24 hours, provide electric pump and instruct in use, breast massage, and hand expression. Pump and/or hand express at least 8 times in 24 hours.

24–48 Hours

- In hospital (every 3 hours) attempt to breastfeed.
- If unsuccessful after 10 minutes, feed baby with expressed breastmilk + water to equal 5 to 15 cc.

Use formula if no breastmilk available.

- Apply nipple shield if the baby is too weak to latch or mother has flat or inverted nipple(s).
- Continue to pump.
- After discharge attempt to breastfeed every 3 hours.

If unsuccessful after 10 minutes, feed baby expressed breastmilk to equal 5 to 15 cc.

- Use alternative feeding methods as appropriate: finger feed, spoon, cup, slow flow nipple.
- Continue skin-to-skin contact and quiet environment.
- Continue to pump at least 8 times/24 hours.

48–72 Hours

- Attempt to breastfeed baby every 2–3 hours.
- If unsuccessful, feed baby with expressed breastmilk = 15 to 30 cc or expressed breastmilk + formula to equal 15 to 30 cc. Use formula if no breastmilk available.
- Consider nipple shield if the baby is too weak to latch or mother has flat or inverted nipple(s).
- Use alternative feeding method: cups, finger feed, slow flow nipple.
- Continue skin-to-skin contact and quiet environment.
- Continue to pump at least 8 times/24 hours.

72–96 Hours

Continue same as above, increasing volumes to 30 to 60 cc.

Table 7-3 AVERAGE INTAKE BY HEALTHY NEWBORNS

Age	mL per Feeding
First 24 hours	2–10
24 to 48 hours	5–15
48 to 72 hours	15–30
72 to 96 hours	30–60

Data from Wight NE, Cordes R. Academy of Breastfeeding Medicine Clinical Protocol #3: Hospital guidelines for the use of supplementary feedings in the healthy term breastfed neonate. *Breastfeeding Medicine*. 2009;4(3):175–182.

ounces the baby needs in 24 hours when the baby is a week old (160 mL/kg/day) . Once the baby has regained birth weight, use the baby's current weight to calculate the volume needed during the early weeks (10 weeks). After several months the volume per weight goes down (see energy requirements in the *Biological Specificity of Breastmilk* chapter).

This equation works for the first 2 to 3 months when weight gain is the fastest it will ever be. After that, a baby needs less in proportion to his weight (Heinig et al., 1993). Between 1 month and 6 months after birth, babies take in about the same amount of milk daily (Kent et al., 2013; Neville & Oliva-Rasbach, 1987). Neville and Oliva-Rasbach (1987) found a 24 mL per month increase in the volume of intake between 1 and 6 months of age—that is, a difference of only 4 ounces between 1 and 6 months.

Establishing the Milk Supply

When a baby is not latching onto the breast, the mother needs to establish her milk supply through alternative means. Combining hand expression and use of an electric pump has been shown to produce more milk than pumping alone (Morton et al., 2009). Before the mother in this situation leaves the hospital, a multiple-user, hospital-grade electric breast pump with a double-pump kit should be made available to her. She should pump both her breasts at the same time for about 10 to 15 minutes, 8 to 10 times in 24 hours. While she is pumping, she can massage her breasts. The postpartum nurses can show the mother how to hold both pump kits to her breasts with one arm, so she has a hand free to massage her breasts while pumping. The hospital should provide a form for her to keep a record of the milk expressed each time.

When a baby has not latched on yet, it is important for the mother and baby to remain skin-to-skin for as many hours each day as possible (Meyer & Anderson, 1999). Skin-to-skin contact will help the baby learn to breastfeed (Svensson et al., 2013). Part of the discharge teaching by the postpartum nurse and/or lactation consultant needs to include the importance of continuing skin-to-skin holding until the baby has learned to breastfeed well.

It is important for the mother to remove as much milk as she possibly can. Thus, once her milk supply increases in amount (usually on the third day postpartum), she needs to pump until the milk drips or sprays subside, stop pumping, massage her breasts, and begin pumping again. Repeat the process two times. She should be able to complete the pumping process within 30 minutes.

Mother's Nipples and Breast Problems

When a baby is having difficulty latching, it is usually a baby problem, but the mother's nipples may be a contributing factor. On occasion, the woman's nipples may be too big for the newborn to accommodate all of her nipple and enough of the breast tissue to extract milk. In such a case, the mother will need to bring in the milk supply herself, feed her milk to her baby, and wait for the baby to grow into her nipple size.

If the mother's nipple is flat, is inverted, or retracts when the baby compresses the breast with his gums, it is difficult for the baby to attach. Many babies figure out how to make their mother's breasts work for them, but other babies need some help.

Teaching the mother to compress and shape her breast tissue for the baby to feel in his mouth when the nipple retracts may be just enough of a signal for the baby to continue suckling. Other techniques that have been tried, but not formally researched, include the following:

- Pull back on the breast tissue so the nipples will protrude.
- Express some milk to soften the breast for the baby if the woman is engorged.
- Reverse-pressure softening also pushes fluids back into the breast, softening the areola to help make latch easier (Cotterman, 2004; Miller & Riordan, 2004).
- Breast shells worn between feedings might help push areolar puffiness back into the breast (see the section on breast edema later in this chapter) so the baby can latch.
- Pump the breasts just before the feed to pull out the nipples.
- Use a nipple shield (must pump or express after feedings, monitor diaper output, and weigh the baby twice weekly).

There is some evidence related to use of "nipple-expanding" devices to pull out flat or inverted nipples, such as commercial expanders (e.g., Evert It, Niplette, Supple Cups, Latch Assist). For example, in a pilot study by Bouchet-Horwitz (2011), two pregnant women with inverted nipples that did not appear functional had very good results using Supple Cups the last 3 weeks of their pregnancies and the first 2 postpartum weeks. Chanprapaph et al. (2013) published the results of their randomized study of pregnant women with short nipples. They found that women using breast cups during pregnancy for 8 hours during the day increased the length of short nipples and enhanced the exclusive breastfeeding rate at 12 weeks compared to a group of women who did not use the breast cups.

Large-breasted women sometimes find breastfeeding challenging simply because they have difficulty dealing with their large breasts and the newborn at the same time. Finding a surface for the baby to be secure and to support the breast can be the answer for these women. Once the baby and the breast are well supported, the mother can use both hands to hold the end of her breast for her baby. Care should be taken to position the baby so the weight of the breast is not resting on the baby's chest.

Women are creative in finding a position that will work for them. Positions women with large breasts have used successfully to find a way to support both the breast and the baby include the following:

- Sitting in a chair next to her hospital bed with the bed elevated to the level of her breast. The baby and her breast are supported by the bed.
- In the hospital, possibly sitting up to the meal tray table to support both.
- Using a side-lying position with a bed or the floor supporting the baby and her breast.
- Using a pillow for breastfeeding twins that is big enough to support both.
- Using the dining room table at home to support the baby and the breast.

Baby Problems That May Cause Difficulty with Latch-On

To latch on successfully, the baby needs an intact palate, a tongue that can cup and extend over the lower lip, lips that flange and seal, and a mouth that does not hurt. If the baby is having any problems along these lines, he may not be able to attach well to the breast to breastfeed.

The baby needs to be able to breathe while feeding at the breast. A baby with laryngomalacia (floppy laryngeal structures pulled into the airway upon inspiration with audible stridor) or tracheomalacia (softening of the cartilaginous ring surrounding the trachea with stridor upon expiration) will need careful positioning to be able to breastfeed. A side-lying position with the baby's head in extreme extension may work well for these babies. In time, the baby will grow bigger and the lack of muscle tone will not affect breathing. Reassure the family that the baby will outgrow the problem by about 1 year. Also explain that feedings will take longer, because the baby will need to pause frequently to catch his breath more often (Genna, 2013).

The baby who is in pain resulting from birth trauma or surgical intervention may be temporarily unable to respond to internal hunger cues or external stimuli. A fractured clavicle, sore head, cranial suture out of line, hematoma, forceps marks, vacuum extraction trauma, and circumcision may all contribute to an apparent disinterest in feeding for several hours. Feeding the baby with drops of the mother's milk from a spoon is a good way to get colostrum into the baby during the first 48 hours.

Sometimes a baby will refuse one breast. This could be due to pain on one side of the body such as from a broken clavicle, an injury on one side of his head, torticollis, or a painful shoulder. A few women have related stories of their children who were blind in one eye who resisted breastfeeding when the seeing-eye was blocked. One woman reported the same response from her baby who was deaf in one ear and did not like to feed lying on the side that blocked his "hearing" ear.

Some babies exhibit an exaggerated gag reflex. They may act as if they are backing away from the breast. Practicing sucking on the mother's clean finger and gradually moving the fingertip to the junction of the hard and soft palates may be an effective way to help these babies. If the baby has a tendency to hold his tongue in the wrong place, several strategies may be used to assist the baby. If the baby is sucking the roof of his mouth, the baby may be working at stabilizing his jaw. By providing chin support, the baby may be able to lower his tongue. If the baby holds his tongue behind the lower gum, the parents can play an imitation game with the baby and stick their tongues out at him. Babies tend to imitate their parents. Also, gently tapping a finger on the baby's lips should elicit interest on the baby's part to stick out his tongue in search of the finger.

When a baby is having difficulty latching, keep an eye, ear, and nose out for potential stimuli that could be obnoxious to the baby. The smell of perfume, soaps, body lotions, room deodorizers, and so on may disturb him. Loud noises, such as barking dogs or a mother yelling at older children, can scare the newborn. If anything is touching the baby's cheeks, such as his undershirt, a baby blanket, or the mother's fingers, the baby may turn toward them and ultimately away from the breast. Removing anything that could be in the way will help the baby. The most disturbing stimulus of all is pressure on the back of the baby's head. The baby becomes very worried that his nose will become blocked. Suggest that the mother support the baby's shoulders and hold the baby's ears with her index finger and thumb. The web between the finger and thumb make a "collar" for the baby. In this way the baby knows he has control of his head and can lift his head back to free his airway if needed.

Previous negative experiences may cause aversion to the breast. If the baby's head has been pushed into the breast, the baby may start to cry when offered the breast. If the negative experience persists, the baby is likely to shut down when offered the breast. The parents may describe the baby as "falling asleep" every time they attempt to breastfeed. When the baby has breast aversion, feeding the baby another way is important (see the *Low Intake in the Breastfed Infant: Maternal and Infant Considerations* chapter). Have the mother hold the baby skin-to-skin on her chest at nonfeeding times. Gradually move the baby, over the course of several days, to the breastfeeding position. Once the baby can be placed in the mother's arms in a breastfeeding position without the aversive behavior, the baby can be offered the breast after having been fed half of his milk for that feeding. Attempts to latch should be kept to a short time. These attempts should stop before the baby or mother gets upset. Babies who are hypertonic or hypotonic may need the additional help of a curled or flexed position for breastfeeding.

Late-Preterm Infants

The average length of gestation in the United States is 39 weeks, not 40 weeks, largely because of the increase in births between 34 and 36 completed weeks of gestation. Births between 34 completed weeks and less than 37 completed weeks are called *late-preterm infants*, and babies born at 37 0/7 to 38 6/7 weeks are called *early term infants* (ACOG, 2013). In 2012, late-preterm babies accounted for 8.1% of all U.S. births (Hamilton et al., 2013). In the past, these late-preterm babies were placed in a special nursery; now, however, they are placed on the regular postpartum unit with their mothers. This practice is good for establishing breastfeeding, but as lactation consultants working in the postpartum area will testify, most late-preterm infants require considerable time and effort before they are able to breastfeed effectively.

Mothers of late-preterm babies are more likely to have a medical problem such as hypertension, antepartum hemorrhage, diabetes, prolonged rupture of membranes, or cesarean delivery that may affect breastfeeding (Shapiro-Mendoza et al., 2008).

Characteristics of the late-preterm infant may include the following (see Color Plate 40):

- Neurologic disorganization and poor behavioral state control. These infants can go from a highly alert state to deep sleep rapidly, and the environment should be kept quiet to avoid overstimulation.
- Poor muscle tone or floppiness that requires careful positioning and extra support during feedings.
- Poor temperature control because of less body fat.
- Tendency to demonstrate thermal and metabolic stress in response to unnecessary suction or excessive handling (Wight, 2003).
- An uncoordinated suckle–swallow–breathe pattern. The baby may have a weak suck, or a small mouth in relation to the mother's nipple size.
- More susceptible to infections.
- Unstable respirations.
- Greater risk for hypothermia, hypoglycemia, excessive weight loss, and dehydration.
- Slow to gain weight and may have failure to thrive.
- More susceptible to high bilirubin, longer to excrete bilirubin, and perhaps more prone to kernicterus.
- More likely to have apnea events.
- Rehospitalization (Edmonson et al.,1997; Soskolne et al., 1996).
- Breastfeeding failure.
- Excessive sleepiness.

Many of these characteristics are related to the immaturity of the brain. More than one-third of the brain volume develops in the last 6 to 8 weeks of gestation. The white matter volume in the brain increases fivefold in those last weeks, with development including maturation of the neuronal and synaptic connections (Hallowell & Spatz, 2012).

The incidence of sudden infant death syndrome is 1.37 per 1000 births in late-preterm babies versus 0.67 per 1000 births in full-term babies (Hunt, 2006). In short, the immaturity of the late-preterm baby leads to more vulnerability.

During breastfeeding, the late-preterm baby will need good shoulder girdle support for head control. The baby should be placed facing the mother, with the baby's arms separated and hugging the breast, and the baby's hips should be well supported. Figure 7-13 shows a 36-week-old premature baby at breast. The usual pattern of these infants is to grasp the breast and suckle for a short time and then stop to rest (pacing the feed). Once a bolus of milk is in the baby's mouth and he drops his tongue to swallow, he may not have the maturity to bring his tongue into position to initiate the next suckle. The inability of these babies to maintain sustained periods of at least 10 suck–swallow–breathe cycles before a pause limits milk transfer and puts them at risk for high bilirubin levels, hypoglycemia, dehydration, and insufficient weight gain. Interventions for these infants must be individualized; however, skin-to-skin holding, keeping them warm, allowing uninterrupted periods of rest between feedings, and limiting stimulation are all important for optimizing the baby's ability to feed well when awake.

Three basic principles apply to breastfeeding the late-preterm baby (Wight, 2003):

- Feed the baby the mother's pumped milk.
- Establish and maintain the mother's milk supply.

Figure 7-13 **A 36-Week-Old Premature Baby at Breast.**

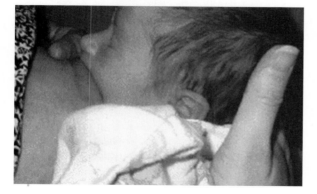

- Provide support while she waits for her baby to mature.

Many of these babies do not feed well until they are close to term age, at which time they begin to waken for feedings voluntarily. Until the late-preterm baby reaches a full-term age, the mother will need to pump after each breastfeeding to establish her milk production. This expressed milk can be given to the baby if the baby cannot obtain enough milk by breastfeeding. The baby's intake can be determined by measuring prefeeding and postfeeding weights on an electronic scale that is accurate to 2 g. Durable medical equipment companies should carry such equipment for families to rent. Because this small baby is learning to breastfeed, an alternative feeding method that does not involve sucking, such as cup or spoon, are options to consider. Nipple shields work well for these babies if they are having trouble maintaining the latch and the mother has a good milk supply.

The mother–baby dyad will need extra care in such cases. Follow-up phone calls and early return for weight checks is mandatory. Mothers of 34 to 37 weeks' gestation babies who have breastfed a full-term baby previously need just as much help as first-time breastfeeders. These women will remember a vigorous baby who knows how to feed effectively, but their past experience does not prepare them for a sleepy baby who gives little feedback. With late-preterm babies, it may be wise to keep mother and baby in the hospital an additional day or two.

Late-preterm infants treated as full-term infants pose a special situation. They fall between the cracks—they are not considered preterm infants unless they have medical problems, but they do not behave exactly like full-term infants. These vulnerable infants have the same risks for complications as infants born prematurely (Simpson & Creehan, 2008). The unborn baby gains about 0.5 lb per week, so babies born at 34 weeks may be 1.5 lb smaller than those born at 37 weeks.

Feeding Methods

Cup-Feeding

Babies can be fed by cup from birth, and many low-birth-weight infants are cup-fed around the world until they are mature enough to exclusively breast-feed (Gupta et al., 1999). Many maternity units in the United Kingdom and elsewhere give supplements by cup so as not to use bottles.

The oro-motor skills used in sipping and lapping from a cup differ from those used while suckling at the breast or at the bottle because there is no object in the baby's mouth (Mizuno & Kani, 2005). Despite these differences, cup-feeding low-birth-weight infants was found to be at least as safe as bottle-feeding, with no differences in physiological stability, choking, spitting, apnea, and bradycardia during feeds for both feeding methods (Malhotra et al., 1999; Marinelli et al., 2001; Mizuno & Kani, 2005). In a controlled trial (Howard et al., 2003), 700 healthy term infants were randomized to early or late introduction to a pacifier and within each group to cup or bottle for any supplement. The authors concluded that administration time, amounts ingested, and physiologic stability did not differ with cup- and bottle-feeding.

In another study, infants took less volume and required more time to feed when they were learning to cup-feed than when learning to bottle-feed (Dowling et al., 2002). Freer (1999) found that a drop in oxygen saturation can occur in the preterm infant while cup-feeding. Other drawbacks include milk spillage and the fact that the baby is deprived of sucking. In two very early cup-feeding studies (Davis et al., 1948; Freeden, 1948), full-term babies cup-fed efficiently, taking milk faster by cup than by bottle or breast. In the 1940s, newborns were in the hospital for 10 days. Given more time, they became very proficient at cup-feeding.

The following are appropriate times to cup-feed:

- When baby is unable to latch onto the breast for whatever reason
- When the mother is not present on the neonatal unit
- When parents and staff wish to avoid the infant developing a preference for bottle nipples
- When breastfeeding is not possible for any reason

The following are *not* appropriate times to cup-feed:

- When the infant has been recently extubated with possible damage to the vocal cords
- When the infant has a poor gag reflex
- When the infant is extremely lethargic
- When the infant has neurological deficits
- With a preterm baby with an unstable respiratory condition

For cup-feeding, a small cup with a rounded edge is preferred. In India, a special cuplike device called a *paladai* is used for feeding premature babies in some neonatal intensive care units. The nurses in these units prefer the *paladai* to a regular cup (Malhotra et al., 1999). Medicine cups that hold small quantities are readily available in hospitals. Check the rim to be sure it is soft and rounded. Medicine cups can be used for early feedings when volume will rarely exceed an ounce. Commercial feeding cups for newborns are also available.

How to Cup-Feed

The following recommendations for how to cup-feed can be given to help the mother:

- Hold the baby in an upright sitting position that is comfortable for both mother and the infant (see Figure 7-14).
- Secure the baby's arms and hands to prevent him from knocking the cup.
- Place a cloth diaper under the baby's chin to catch spillage (weigh before and after feeding). Bring the cup to a position resting on

Figure 7-14 **Baby Cup-Feeding.**

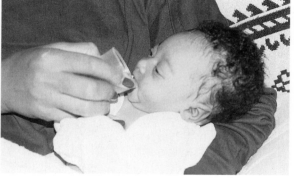

Courtesy of Kay Hoover, MEd, IBCLC

his lower lip, with the rim at the corners of his mouth. Avoid putting pressure on the lower lip.

- Tip the cup slightly to allow the fluid to come in complete contact with the upper lip. Do *not* pour the milk into the baby's mouth.
- Let baby "pace" the feeding by watching his cues. Keep cup in position while the baby pauses.

Cup-feeding can be difficult for parents to learn. Teaching them this technique should include a "return demonstration" to make certain they are doing it safely (Hedberg-Nyqvist, 1999; Wilson-Clay & Hoover, 2013). As long as the caregiver does not attempt to pour too much milk into the baby's mouth, the risk of aspiration is minimal and the feeding can be accomplished quickly (Lang et al., 1994; Thorley, 1997). Some infants will "fight" the cup and refuse to drink milk from it. Each infant must be treated individually.

Finger-Feeding

Finger-feeding with a feeding tube is an alternative feeding method for neonates (Figure 7-15). It is used by some lactation consultants when the baby is too sleepy to breastfeed, if the baby does not latch on well for any reason, if the mother and baby are separated, or if the baby cannot bottle-feed. Proponents of finger-feeding believe that it facilitates proper use of the oral muscles, allows the baby to feel the fingertip at the junction of the hard and soft palates, promotes optimal coordination of the suck–swallow–breathe pattern, and allows the baby to pace the feeding (Hazelbaker, 1997). Critics

Figure 7-15 FINGER-FEEDING. THE TECHNIQUE IS USED TO FEED AN INFANT BREASTMILK AND AVOID ARTIFICIAL NIPPLES WHEN THE INFANT IS NOT LATCHING ONTO THE BREAST.

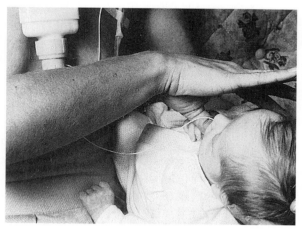

Courtesy of Pat Bull

claim that the technique is invasive and addictive. Instructions for finger-feeding a neonate are presented in Box 7-4.

Nipple Shields

Nipple shields have a controversial history, largely due to the bad reputation of the old type of shields that were made of rubber or latex. Babies of mothers using these old types of shields were unable to ingest sufficient breastmilk, often resulting in slow weight gain and failure to thrive. As a result,

---

BOX 7-4 FINGER-FEEDING A NEONATE

- Ensure that your hands are clean and the nail on the finger or thumb you use is cut short before you begin. Wearing a latex-free glove or finger cott is preferable when the baby is finger-fed by someone other than the mother or father.
- Prop the baby, making sure his head is stable and slightly tilted back.
- If using a feeding-tube device (#5 French, 15 in. long), the tube can be held close to the end of the finger.

(continues)

Box 7-4 (*CONTINUED*)

- Connect the feeding tube with a syringe or feeding bottle with expressed breastmilk or, if necessary, formula, depending on the situation. If using a bottle, the feeding tube can be inserted through a cut made in the rubber nipple. If using a syringe, choose the size most appropriate for the circumstances (usually 10 to 30 cc).
- Select a large digit, since the breast fills the baby's mouth.
- Stroke the baby's lips gently until the baby opens his mouth. Slide your finger or allow the baby to suck the finger in with the nail bed resting on his tongue and the pad side up. The tip of the finger needs to extend to the juncture of the hard and soft palates. The tube can be taped to the pad side of the parent's finger. In most instances, the baby will begin sucking as soon as he feels the finger pad on the hard palate.
- Push milk from the syringe into the baby's mouth ONLY if the baby is sucking.
- If the baby is sucking effectively, the person who is finger-feeding the baby will feel a pulling sensation along the nail bed with each exertion of negative pressure (suckle), as if the nail is being pulled deeper into the baby's mouth.
- Monitor color and vital signs, especially if the baby is low birth weight or has poor muscle tone or oral structural deficits.
- Record the amount of human milk (or formula) that the baby takes.
- Show the mother (and the father) how to finger-feed.

---

nipple shields came to be viewed as interfering with breastfeeding, rather than assisting the new mother in breastfeeding. The newer ultrathin silicone nipple shields are especially helpful for a mother with flat or inverted nipples, for preterm or late-preterm babies who have trouble latching and maintaining suction, or for babies who have developed a preference for a bottle nipple and thus refuse the breast.

When a woman first uses a silicone nipple shield, she needs to use a multiuser electric pump (like the ones used in the hospitals) and pump her milk four to six times a day after breastfeeding to establish a milk supply. The baby needs to be weighed twice a week and diapers monitored for adequate stools and wetness. Once the baby is gaining well (about an ounce a day), the mother can gradually wean herself off pumping as long as the baby continues to gain appropriately.

In many cases, the short-term use of a nipple shield will preserve the breastfeeding relationship while the baby learns to breastfeed (Meier et al., 2000; Nicholson, 1993; Wilson-Clay, 1996). A La Leche League mother movingly described how

a silicone nipple shield "saved her breastfeeding relationship" with her baby (Clemmit, 2003).

Placing a feeding tube (attached to a syringe with the mother's milk supplement) inside of the nipple shield during a feed may help (Figure 7-16). This technique offers several benefits for the baby:

- An immediate reward for latching on and suckling
- An opportunity to stimulate the breast and remove breastmilk
- Control over the amount and flow of supplement ingested
- Nutriment (calories and fluids)

To apply a silicone nipple shield, wet the shield with a thin layer of water inside the nipple shield brim, then flip up the brim of the shield (like that of a sombrero), and turn one-third of the teat of the shield in on itself. Center the shield directly over the nipple, and gently pat down the brim (Wilson-Clay, 2003). The silicone will reshape itself and pull the nipple partway into the shield teat, thus helping the weak baby to draw the nipple into the

Figure 7-16 FEEDING TUBE DEVICE UNDER A SILICONE NIPPLE SHIELD. (A) FEEDING TUBE DEVICE PLACED UNDER NIPPLE SHIELD. BABY WOULD NEED TO BE ABLE TO SUCK WELL IN ORDER TO PULL THE MILK OUT OF THE BOTTLE AND THROUGH THE TUBING. THIS IS A GOOD TECHNIQUE TO KEEP THE BABY FEEDING AT THE BREAST UNTIL HE CAN LATCH ON TO THE BREAST AND GET OUT ENOUGH MILK DIRECTLY. IT COULD ALSO BE USED FOR A BABY WHO HAS BECOME ACCUSTOMED TO A BOTTLE NIPPLE. (B) BABY RECEIVES SUPPLEMENTATION FROM FEEDING TUBE AND BREASTFEEDS AT THE SAME TIME. AS SOON AS BABY ATTACHES, MILK CAN BE SQUEEZED INTO THE NIPPLE SHIELD TO GIVE THE BABY AN IMMEDIATE REWARD FOR ANY ATTEMPTS MADE AT THE BREAST. USE WITH BABY WHO HAS GOTTEN USED TO BOTTLE-FEEDING, HAS A WEAK SUCKLE, OR HAS DIFFICULTY LATCHING ONTO THE BREAST.

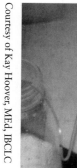

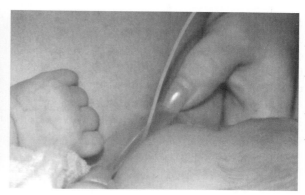

shield. For additional discussion on nipple shields, see the *Breast Pumps and Other Technologies* chapter.

Hypoglycemia

Newborns experience a decrease in blood glucose for the first 2 hours after birth as they adapt to the extra-uterine environment, but then regain blood glucose over the next several days (Eidelman, 2001). This transient hypoglycemia in the immediate postpartum period occurs in almost all mammalian species (Wight & Marinelli, 2006), and is an adaptive phenomenon as the newborn changes from the fetal state of continuous transplacental glucose feeding to that of intermittent feeding after birth. This dynamic process is self-limiting and is usually not pathologic.

Hypoglycemia is partially a matter of definition. Whether a baby is considered to have a low blood glucose level depends on the laboratory values used

as criteria for hypoglycemia and the reliability of the methods used to measure blood glucose. Before deciding what is abnormal, one must first establish what is normal. What are normal blood sugar levels for newborns? Hypoglycemia protocols vary widely according to region, and routine glucose testing after birth is common even though it is not recommended by the Academy of Breastfeeding Medicine and other physician organizations. On the whole, breastfed infants have lower blood sugar levels (58 mg/dL) than formula-fed infants (72 mg/dL), according to a study conducted by Hawdon et al. (1992). In the same study, blood sugar levels were correlated with the intervals between the feeds—the more frequent the feeding, the higher the glucose concentration.

While there are still no universally accepted "cutoff" glucose levels for hypoglycemia, several guidelines have been recommended. Alkalay and colleagues (2006) conducted a population meta-analysis and recommended low thresholds for blood glucose based on hours after birth (Table 7-4). These hypoglycemia guidelines were incorporated into the ABM *Guidelines for Glucose Monitoring and Treatment of Hypoglycemia in Breastfed Neonates* (Wight & Marinelli, 2006). In addition, the ABM guidelines include information on general management recommendations around feeding and screening for hypoglycemia in the breastfed newborn, as well as specific management of documented hypoglycemia (available at http://www.bfmed.org/Media/Files/Protocols/hypoglycemia.pdf). On the basis of research findings from a large sample of well, full-term infants, Heck and Erenberg (1987) recommend that hypoglycemia in full-term infants be defined as a serum glucose concentration of less than 30 mg/dL on the first day after birth or less than 40 mg/dL on the second day after birth. Srinivasan et al. (1986) recommended similar levels. If the higher level of 40 mg/dL were used for the first day postpartum, 20.6% of well, full-term infants would be considered hypoglycemic and would receive unnecessary supplements (Sexson, 1984). Brand et al. (2005) evaluated the effects of transient hypoglycemia on the first day after birth in 75 healthy, term, large-for-gestational-age infants in terms of their later neurodevelopment. There were no significant differences between children with normal glycemic levels and hypoglycemia defined as such at 4-year follow-up using standardized development scales.

Severe neonatal hypoglycemia leads to potential brain damage and can result in serious sequelae such as seizures. Prolonged hypoglycemia can be avoided by close clinical observation of vulnerable infants while avoiding excessive invasive management (Moore & Perlman, 1999). Clinical symptoms that indicate possible hypoglycemia in neonates include the following:

- Jitteriness
- Exaggerated reflexes
- High-pitched cry
- Seizures
- Lethargy
- Rapid breathing
- Hypothermia
- Poor suck and refusal to feed

Hypoglycemia is of particular concern in conjunction with certain health conditions: the infant of a mother with diabetes, a postmature neonate, or an infant who is small for gestational age. The infant of a mother with diabetes is most apt to experience hypoglycemia shortly after birth, because he continues to produce a high level of insulin, which depletes the blood glucose within hours after birth. The degree of infant hypoglycemia usually reflects the success achieved in controlling the mother's blood glucose during her pregnancy. Hypoglycemia may be avoided in these babies if they are kept warm skin-to-skin and allowed unrestricted access to the breast. If they become symptomatic, they require 10% to 15% glucose intravenously until they stabilize. As long as they are neurologically stable, they should continue to breastfeed as they work toward discontinuing the IV glucose.

Postmature infants also need early, frequent breastfeedings to normalize their glucose levels. Lethargy and poor feeding in these babies may contribute to hypoglycemia; thus any interest shown in feeding should be followed by immediate, unrestricted access to the breast for as often and as long as the baby wishes. Most postmature neonates, after a first breastfeeding, show increased interest in

Table 7-4 RECOMMENDED LOW THRESHOLD: PLASMA GLUCOSE LEVEL (PGL)

Hour After Birth	5th Percentile PGL (mg/dL)
1–2 (lowest point)	28 (1.6 mmol/L)*
3–47	40 (2.2 mmol/L)
48–72	48 (2.7 mmol/L)

* To convert mmol/L of glucose to mg/dL, multiply by 18.
To convert mg/dL of glucose to mmol/L, divide by 18 or multiply by 0.055.
Data from Alkalay AL Sarnat HB, Flores-Sarnat L, et al. Population meta-analysis of low plasma glucose thresholds in full-term normal newborns. *Am J Perinatol.* 2006;23(2):115–119.

subsequent breastfeeding, thus reducing the risk of continued hypoglycemia.

The newborn who is small for his gestational age is also at risk for hypoglycemia. A prompt first breastfeeding, followed by very frequent breastfeeding sessions thereafter, is usually sufficient to bring the baby's blood glucose level to normal. In some cases, continued poor feeding may require a supplement. In such a case, it is recommended to start with the mother's own milk. If no milk can be obtained with hand expression and there is no banked human milk, then formula may have to be used. This practice need not be repeated once the baby is breastfeeding well.

In summary, the following conditions are associated with low blood sugar:

- Small-for-gestational-age infants
- Postmature infants
- Discordant twin (smaller)
- Large-for-gestational-age infants: greater than 90th percentile of weight
- Infants of diabetic mothers
- Low-birth-weight infants: less than 2500 g
- Postasphyxia, cold stress, sepsis, and other stresses

Intrapartum management plays a role in the neonate's glucose level. Use of hypertonic glucose infusions during labor can lead to elevation in maternal blood glucose, which in turn can result in fetal hyperglycemia and hyperinsulinemia and eventually neonatal hypoglycemia.

The blood level is first measured at the bedside using glucose testing strips. These strips are cheap and practical, but their results may vary significantly from the true blood glucose level. Studies comparing different reagent strips have estimated that as many as 20% of truly normal glycemic infants are falsely labeled as hypoglycemic when such measurements are used, leading to unnecessary lab tests and treatments. Ho et al. (2004) compared five glucometer devices and found that *none* were satisfactory as the sole measuring device. Measuring blood glucose concentrations in asymptomatic babies in the first 2 postnatal hours is unnecessary and can cause parents to become anxious and worried for no reason. It also interferes with establishing breastfeeding and can result in serious disruption of the initiation and duration of breastfeeding (Haninger & Farley, 2001).

Placing the baby skin-to-skin with his mother helps stabilize his blood sugar. Christensson et al. (1998) reported average blood glucose of 57.6 mg/dL in a skin-to-skin group of infants and 46.6 mg/dL in a group of neonates cared for away from their mothers. Walters et al. (2007) reported an average glucose level of 65 mg/dL at 60 minutes post birth.

If the neonate has low blood sugar and is unable to suckle or feedings are not tolerated, begin IV therapy. If glucose remains low despite feedings, IV glucose should be started and the IV rate adjusted by monitoring changes in blood glucose. Infants with symptoms of hypoglycemia should have more aggressive therapy.

Cesarean Birth

In 2012, the cesarean birth rate in the United States was 32.8%. The U.S. rates from 2010 through 2012 remained steady (Hamilton et al., 2013). Many European and South American countries have similar and even higher rates of surgical births.

The impact of cesarean delivery on breastfeeding has been extensively studied. Although its effects are difficult to disentangle from other interventions, generally breastfeeding rates and duration among mothers who deliver by cesarean birth are about the same as those among mothers who have vaginal births. The mother's commitment to breastfeeding plays a substantial role despite unexpected birth outcomes. A greater commitment to breastfeeding, regardless of the manner of birth, results in longer duration of breastfeeding (Janke, 1988).

Cesarean births are associated with delayed lactogenesis and a delay in initiating breastfeeding (Chen et al., 1998; Dewey et al., 2003; Evans et al., 2003; Grajeda & Perez-Escamilla, 2002; Leung et al., 2002; Rowe-Murray & Fisher, 2002). Recovery from major surgery takes more time, is more painful and stressful, and represents additional risks compared to an uneventful vaginal birth, which explains why breastfeeding occurs later. One-third of the women delivered by cesarean birth believed that their ability to breastfeed was affected negatively to a large or very large extent by postoperative pain (Karlstrom et al., 2007).

Women's reactions to having a cesarean birth vary. Although some women may interpret an unexpected cesarean birth as a reflection of their adequacy as a mother, these births are so frequent now that parents tend to view them as a normal or alternative mode of delivery. Childbirth educators and others have effectively conveyed the messages that cesarean birth does not have to be a threat and that women can be awake to experience the event and the baby's father can be present at the birth (Gouchon et al., 2010; Hung & Berg, 2011; Nolan & Lawrence, 2009; Smith et al., 2008). The baby can be placed skin-to-skin with mother (or father) in the operating room during the surgery. This is a good time to point out to the parents that the baby calms once placed skin-to-skin with either mother or father. Of course, the baby needs to be monitored while skin-to-skin (Andres et al., 2011; Jarrell et al., 2009; Pejovic & Herlenius, 2013). The baby can be transported on the mother's chest from the operating room to the recovery area. The baby may breastfeed whenever ready.

In working with a mother who has experienced a cesarean birth, the nurse needs to assess the mother's degree of physical comfort and awareness. If she is not fully conscious, the baby will need to be carefully watched (Dageville et al., 2008). While the mother is on her back, the baby can be placed prone on top of her. Relieve discomfort with pain medicine. Once the mother is awake and able to sit up, assist the mother in positioning the baby so there is no pressure near her abdominal incision. A clutch/football hold (see again Figure 7-10B) will avoid the sensitive incision area. As the pain of her incision decreases, the mother can be instructed and assisted in the use of positions other than the football hold. By the second or third day postpartum, the side-lying position is generally comfortable, especially if the mother is adequately supported with pillows at her back and beneath her abdomen.

The baby born by cesarean section may be lethargic, particularly if the birth followed a long labor. If so, encourage skin-to-skin care and teach the mother hand expression to feed drops of breastmilk to the baby.

Breast Engorgement

Breast engorgement is a major issue in the early postpartum period as the breasts, under the influence of hormonal shifts, increase milk production rapidly from 36 to 96 hours postpartum. Although the gradual buildup of fluid in the breasts following parturition is a welcome sign of breastmilk, breast engorgement is a common problem in the early days after birth and a common reason for early weaning. Because women leave the hospital before their breasts become full or engorged, this situation is usually handled at home or in a postdischarge visit at a clinic or medical office.

For most women, engorgement reaches its height from 3 to 5 days after birth and slowly recedes; for some women, however, it may last as long as 2 weeks (Humenick et al., 1994). During normal engorgement, the mother's breast tissue usually remains compressible, thus enabling the infant to attach comfortably and efficiently, without risk of trauma to the breast or nipple tissue. Extreme breast fullness rarely lasts more than 24 hours, during which time breastfeeding can continue without discomfort. The mother with breast fullness should be encouraged to view this state as a transitory indication of milk production that will begin to regulate to meet the baby's needs as the infant breastfeeds.

Multiparous women are more likely to report more intense engorgement than primiparous women, and distinct patterns of breast engorgement can be identified (Humenick et al., 1994). Severe breast engorgement—a pathologic condition, and often the consequence of mismanagement—is painful. It can be caused by any situation that allows milk stasis to occur. There are several situations that lead to uncomfortable engorgement:

- Supplements (Wright et al., 1996)
- Delayed initiation of feedings at the breast
- Infrequent feedings
- Time-limited feedings

- Removing the baby from the first breast to ensure feeding from both breasts at every feeding (Lawson & Tulloch, 1995)
- Breast implants

Sometimes the tissue around the nipple and areola becomes so taut that the infant is unable to grasp the nipple. When the baby is unable to latch onto the breast, the mother's discomfort mounts, and her breast and nipple tissue may be so tight that even leaking cannot occur. Under such conditions, further trauma to the tissue is apt to occur when a vigorous baby attempts unsuccessfully to grasp and draw the breast into his mouth.

Research on engorgement is unique in that the condition slowly and inevitably resolves itself no matter which treatment is used; thus, in studies of this phenomenon, a group of mothers (preferably randomized) receiving the treatment must be compared simultaneously with a group who do not receive the treatment. Mangesi and Dowswell (2010) analyzed eight randomized control trials involving 744 women receiving treatments for breast engorgement in an attempt to discover which treatments were effective. They concluded that acupuncture, cabbage leaves, cold gel packs, pharmacological treatments, and ultrasound treatments were all ineffective.

The mother should be encouraged to offer the breast frequently to avoid painful engorgement. During the first 2 weeks of life, the average number of minutes a baby spends breastfeeding in 24 hours is about 2.7 hours (de Carvalho et al., 1982). If the baby is being offered the breast fewer than eight times in 24 hours, and for less than an average of 20 minutes per feeding, it may not be enough. If the mother is unable to increase the number of feedings, she may obtain relief with the judicious use of hand expression or a breast pump. A fever of unknown origin in a mother during the first week postpartum may be another sign of breast engorgement. Occasionally, fever from engorgement can be 101°F or higher.

Breast Edema

Women who receive excessive intravenous fluids throughout labor may develop edema of their breast. This edema differs from the normal physiologic engorgement that precedes lactogenesis. The mother's breasts can be as "hard as rocks" and the nipples distended. As a result, the neonate may be unable to latch onto her breasts until the edema has subsided. Breast edema can be treated with areolar compression, a method to reduce nipple/areola edema manually by using gentle positive pressure (Miller & Riordan, 2004).

- Ask the mother to wash her hands thoroughly. Her nails should be short and preferably unpolished, with no artificial nails.
- Instruct her to apply firm but gentle pressure with the index finger and thumb on either side of the areola behind the nipple. Have her hold it there until the edema can be felt to be giving way. Suggest she remove her fingers to see if there are finger impressions remaining in the tissue. If there are, then areolar edema is present.
- Ask her to apply pressure again slightly behind the softened spot and hold the pressure until the area under her fingers softens. Applying steady inward pressure toward the chest wall for 60 seconds or longer, concentrating on the areola where it joins the base of the nipple, and moving the fingers behind the softened area to the firm tissue and applying pressure again should bring about the desired softening. If her fingernails are short, the mother can press with the curved fingertips of both hands simultaneously, with the nail nearly touching the sides of the nipple. The goal is to create a ring of small "dimples" or pits on the areola at the base of the nipple. (If performed by the healthcare provider, the flat part of two thumbs or two fingers can also be used. This will require another 60 seconds of pressure in opposite quadrants to soften the same general area.)
- Rotating the finger pressure, continue displacing the edema into the breast tissue until the areola is soft and the nipple is pliable. Plan on the procedure taking anywhere from a few minutes to 30 minutes to move the edema out enough to latch the infant onto the breast. The length of time will depend on the severity of the edema.

- The effects of areolar compression, also called reverse pressure softening (Cotterman, 2004), are fourfold: (1) it moves excess interstitial fluid inward in the direction of natural lymphatic drainage; (2) it relieves overdistension of the milk ducts and reduces latch discomfort; (3) it enables the infant to draw the breast deeply into his mouth so that milk can be removed; and (4) it stimulates the nerves supplying the nipple and areolar complex, thus triggering the milk-ejection reflex (Cotterman, 2004).
- Areolar compression should be done *before* pumping the breast. Pumping the breast first before areolar compression can cause further accumulation of edema in the areola, especially when maximum settings on the pump are used. The negative pressure of a pump tends to draw excess interstitial fluid *toward* the areola and nipple instead of moving it *away* from the area, thus worsening the problem. Once edema is displaced, the nipple will stretch outward, making latching easier.

Hand Expression

Although many women in the United States think first of using a breast pump to obtain milk, expressing milk by hand is a skill that has been used by many women for millennia. The mother's own hands offer several advantages over breast pumps:

- They cost her nothing.
- They may trigger a more effective milk-ejection reflex.
- They are always available.
- They compress the breast for milk removal.

After the mother has practiced this skill, she may find that she can obtain more milk more quickly than women who use an electric device for the same purpose. Techniques vary across cultures and are most effective when the breasts are compressed well behind the nipple (Figure 7-17). Every postpartum nurse and every lactation consultant should be able to instruct a mother in hand expression. Pushing back toward the chest wall with her fingers and then rolling the fingers together is recommended rather than sliding the fingers down the breast, to avoid inadvertently bruising or abrading the skin. The mother should be cautioned that she might have greater difficulty with expression if she is attempting to relieve engorgement or if her breasts are very tender. If breast massage and breast warming (Yigit et al., 2012) are practiced with each expression, encourage the mother to avoid creating a ritual that becomes so time consuming that it interferes with the process. This is particularly relevant if the mother is expressing her milk at work or some other site where she has only a limited time in which to accomplish it. An experienced mother who can demonstrate the technique to the novice can often provide the most effective teaching. If she has given birth to a preterm baby, expressing milk in the first hour after birth will increase the amount of milk the mother is able to express during the whole first week postpartum, according to a pilot study conducted by Parker et al. (2012).

Clinical Implications

Assessment is a critical first step in working with a mother who has a newborn. For example, if the baby is sleepy and is breastfeeding infrequently, the hospital caregiver can do the following:

- Encourage and facilitate the mother to hold her baby skin-to-skin.
- Teach her how to hand-express her milk and feed the baby the drops of milk with a spoon or feeding syringe. Small amounts of milk will usually awaken the baby.
- Encourage the mother to take every opportunity when the baby is awake to offer the breast.
- Suggest that the mother let the baby stay on the first breast until he has let go on his own before offering the second breast.
- Provide specific suggestions regarding home visitation and follow-up with a lactation consultant in private practice and a community-based breastfeeding mothers' group. If the mother experienced difficulty in breastfeeding with an earlier baby, the caregiver may need to reassure the concerned or anxious mother that a similar situation need not recur, or if it does recur, explain what to do about it.

Figure 7-17 HAND EXPRESSION. (A) WASH HANDS AND ANY COLLECTION EQUIPMENT TO BE USED. SIT COMFORTABLY, AND PLACE THE COLLECTION CUP UNDER THE BREAST. APPLY WARM, MOIST TOWEL TO ENHANCE MILK FLOW. MASSAGE BREASTS AND NIPPLES TO STIMULATE MILK EJECTION REFLEX. USE GENTLE PRESSURE USING A CIRCULAR MOTION, MOVING AROUND THE BREAST. (B) SQUEEZE THE BREAST GENTLY, ROLLING THE HANDS FORWARD FROM THE CHEST TOWARD THE NIPPLE. (C) PLACE THUMB AND FOREFINGERS APPROXIMATELY 2 TO 3 CM (1 TO 1 1/2 INCHES) BEHIND THE NIPPLE AND PRESS INTO THE BREAST. (D) PRESS INWARD TOWARD THE CHEST WALL SQUEEZING GENTLY WITH A SLIGHT ROLLING ACTION TOWARD THE NIPPLE. RELEASE PRESSURE AND REPEAT AS NEEDED TO OBTAIN MILK. IF PAIN RESULTS, SOMETHING IS WRONG AND THE MOTHER SHOULD BE OBSERVED IN ORDER TO IDENTIFY WHAT MAY BE CAUSING THE MOTHER DISCOMFORT. (E) CHANGE POSITION OF THE FINGERS AROUND THE AREOLA TO EXPRESS MILK FROM AS MANY DUCTS AS POSSIBLE. WITHIN 3 TO 5 MINUTES, THE MILK FLOW MAY SLOW; THIS IS A SIGNAL TO EXPRESS MILK FROM THE OTHER BREAST. BOTH SIDES MAY BE EXPRESSED AS OFTEN AS THE MOTHER WISHES IN A GIVEN SESSION OR UNTIL SHE TIRES. PARTICULARLY IN THE BEGINNING, THE MOTHER SHOULD EXPECT TO SPEND 20 TO 30 MINUTES EXPRESSING MILK. AS SHE BECOMES MORE ADEPT AT IT, THE TIME WILL DECREASE EVEN AS THE AMOUNT OF MILK OBTAINED INCREASES.

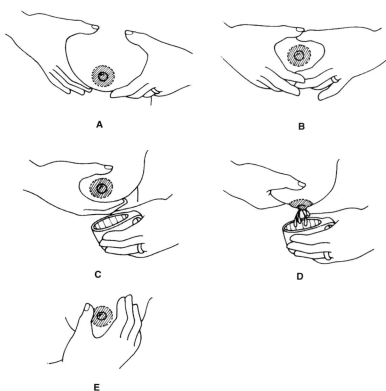

Breastfeeding Assessment

The infant's first few times breastfeeding should be assessed early in the neonatal period. Such assessment enables the healthcare worker to determine how well the infant roots, latches on, and suckles. Minor adjustments of maternal position or infant position can be made without interrupting or interfering with the mother and infant as they begin to learn how to breastfeed together. Several assessment tools specific to feedings at the breast are available, as described in the *Infant Assessment* chapter.

Assessment tools are useful for evaluating infant suckling over several feedings to show mothers that their babies are learning with each feeding and are becoming more efficient at obtaining milk. They can also be used to alert the caregiver to specific "red flags." If the mother–baby dyad is not feeding effectively, they may need special attention to prevent a problem with dehydration and weight loss. Breastfeeding assessment tools remind the mother that what her baby does is both complex and predictable and that her baby needs lots of opportunities to practice, just as she needs many opportunities to learn how to hold and position him for optimal breastfeeding. Of the commonly used breastfeeding indicators, audible swallowing best predicts the actual intake of breastmilk after 96 hours post birth (Riordan et al., 2005). Certain perinatal events predict the mother will stop breastfeeding by 7 to 10 days postpartum (Hall et al., 2002; Mercer et al., 2010), so mothers who experience these events need extra help (see Table 7-5).

Weight Loss

Infants are routinely weighed in the hospital. Exclusively breastfed neonates lose more weight than those completely or partially formula-fed, according to a study of 773 Canadian infants (Box 7-5; Martens & Romphf, 2007). If the parents are not aware that neonatal weight loss is normal in the first few days after birth, they should be reassured that their baby will begin to gain weight in a few days.

Table 7-5 RISKS FACTORS PREDICTING LIKELIHOOD FOR BREASTFEEDING CESSATION BY 7 TO 10 DAYS POSTPARTUM

History	In Hospital
Young maternal age	Latch difficulties
Previous unsuccessful breastfeeding experience	Long intervals between breastfeeding sessions
Pregnancy-induced hypertension	Two or more supplemental bottles

Data from Mercer AM, Teasley SL, Hopkinson J, et al. Evaluation of a breastfeeding assessment score in a diverse population. *J Hum Lact.* 2010;26(1):42–48.

Basic Feeding Techniques

The following basic feeding techniques can be reviewed with the parents before discharge:

- Feed the baby frequently (8 or more feedings in a 24-hour period). Using a visual aid such as the size of the baby's fist to demonstrate the size of the newborn's stomach is an excellent way to illustrate why the neonate needs frequent feedings: his stomach is simply too small to hold large quantities at a time! Additionally, the curds formed by human milk are digested quickly. By comparison, artificial baby milk forms large curds that take longer to digest than human milk. Thus the formula-fed infant feeds fewer times.
- Start the feedings on alternate breasts. Offer (and keep the baby on) the first breast until he has completed that side. If he wants more, offer the second breast for as long as the baby wants. Some babies will be satiated with one breast; others prefer two, and still others may have marathon feedings in which they move from one breast to the other several times! Avoid watching the clock. The best timer of the feeding is the baby.

> **BOX 7-5 PERCENTAGE OF INFANT WEIGHT LOSS AT HOSPITAL DISCHARGE ACCORDING TO TYPE OF FEEDING**
>
> | Exclusively breastfed | 5.49 |
> |---|---|
> | Partially breastfed | 5.52 |
> | Completely formula-fed | 2.43 |
>
> Data from Martens & Romphf, 2007.

- Avoid the use of pacifiers for the first 3 to 4 weeks, until breastfeeding is well established (Eidelman & Schanler, 2012).

Ways to Reassure Parents That the Baby Is Consuming Enough Milk

Identify various ways in which the mother can recognize that her infant is getting sufficient milk. These include the following:

- Listening for and identifying the infant's swallows
- The baby waking on his own for at least 8 feedings in 24 hours
- Stool color change from black to yellow on average by 6 days after birth (Nommsen-Rivers et al., 2008)

Keeping feeding records "may be a valuable tool in self-regulating breastfeeding and promoting a longer duration of full breastfeeding" (Pollard, 2011). Ultimately the baby's weight proves the baby's intake.

Signs That Intervention Is Needed

Slow infant weight gain is addressed in depth in the *Low Intake in the Breastfed Infant: Maternal and Infant Considerations* chapter. Briefly, the following signs indicate a need for healthcare intervention:

- Scant, concentrated urine; brick dust urine (from urate crystals) after day 2; or no urine at all
- Infrequent stools (fewer than four per day after day 3)
- Stools that have not turned yellow by day 6

- Lethargy (baby not waking by himself to feed at least eight times in 24 hours)
- Extreme fretfulness (never contented after any feeding)
- No swallowing heard during feedings after 96 hours
- Mother experiencing nipple soreness that is more intense if it existed earlier, or that suddenly develops if it was previously absent
- Mother's breasts are clinically engorged and very painful, making it difficult or impossible for the baby to breastfeed
- Baby not latching onto the breast

Discharge Planning

Over the past 30 years, the average length of the birth hospital stay in the United States has declined significantly. The average length of stay for all births in non-federal hospitals in the U.S. in 2009–2010 was 2.6 days (National Center for Health Statistics, 2013). Mandated by law in 1996, mothers and infants return home 48 hours after a vaginal birth and 96 hours after a cesarean birth (Centers for Medicare and Medicaid Services, n.d.). Early discharge from the hospital—a fact of life for most new mothers and their neonates—has had a major impact on postpartum care. It is the responsibility of the hospital caregiver to highlight critical points that parents need to pay attention to when they are newly home with their baby. Foremost among these concerns is seeing to it that the baby feeds often and effectively.

Early discharge does not appear to negatively affect breastfeeding; in fact, some studies indicate that mothers who leave the hospital early breastfeed longer (Edmonson et al., 1997; Lee et al., 1995; Margolis & Schwartz, 2000). At the same time, early discharge may negatively influence the mother's feeling of competence in her mothering, particularly if she is unprepared or unsure of how to care for her newborn. Contact with mother-to-mother organizations can help the mother to place her experiences in the context of other women's comments about their breastfeeding course. In addition, more home health visits are provided instead of longer hospitalization. Pediatricians and other physicians, cognizant of the postdischarge void in medical coverage, are routinely scheduling appointments with the family of a breastfed baby within 48 to 72 hours after discharge as recommended by the American Academy of Pediatrics.

The goals of discharge planning are twofold: to prevent common problems and to provide emotional support (Page-Goertz, 1989). With such a brief time in the hospital, the mother needs a caregiver who imparts as much basic information as possible without overwhelming her. She also needs reinforcement of her self-confidence in her role as a new mother. These two goals are mutually reinforcing: as the caregiver instructs the mother in the prevention of problems, this provider is in a position to simultaneously enhance the new mother's self-esteem and self-confidence; in short, the mother is able to "take control" of her experience (Hall & Carty, 1993). The mother's perceptions of her infant not only reflect how she and the baby will interact, but can also influence how long she breastfeeds. Guidelines for discharge teaching about breastfeeding are available from both the American Academy of Pediatrics and the Academy of Breastfeeding Medicine (Eidelman & Schanler, 2012; Evans, 2007).

Written Instructions with Referral Information for Community Support

At discharge, the parents need clear, simply written materials that provide step-by-step information and are individualized as much as possible. Materials with drawings or photographs of positioning, hand expression of milk, and other techniques are helpful. The hospital caregiver should establish a definite plan for follow-up: making a phone call to the mother at a specific time postdischarge or providing her with phone numbers for the hospital "warmline" and for lactation consultants or La Leche League leaders in the area. If the baby has breastfeeding problems, it is appropriate at discharge to refer the family to the hospital outpatient breastfeeding services, home health, nurse casemanager, follow-up at a breastfeeding clinic, or a lactation consultant in the community.

In many countries other than the United States, midwives and home health visitors routinely visit new mothers. The optimal time for a follow-up visit or telephone call is no later than 2 to 4 days after discharge from the hospital. This is an especially crucial period because enough time has passed to make an accurate evaluation of the mother's milk supply and the infant's intake. All pediatric care providers should assure assessment of breastfeeding babies soon after discharge as recommended by the American Academy of Pediatrics (Eidelman & Schanler, 2012; Evans, 2007).

Commercial Formula Advertisement

Distribution of commercial marketing bags to maternity patients at hospital discharge should stop, as such practices reduce exclusive breastfeeding. Supplying her with containers of formula can undermine the mother's confidence and plant doubts about her ability to breastfeed, especially for the immigrant mother (see the *Cultural Context of Breastfeeding* chapter). Past systematic reviews comparing breastfeeding rates and duration among new mothers who received marketing discharge packs and those who received no packs or nonmarketing packs have shown that exclusive breastfeeding was reduced at all time points in the presence of commercial hospital discharge packs, but mixed feeding (nonexclusive breastfeeding) was not affected (Snowden et al., 2000). Two recent studies validated past studies showing marketing bags distributed by hospitals reduced exclusive breast-feeding (Feldman-Winter, Grossman, et al., 2012; Sadacharan et al., 2014). Sadacharan et al. (2011) reported that an increased proportion of U.S. hospitals have discontinued marketing for the formula industry. In fact, all birthing facilities in Rhode Island and Massachusetts no longer distribute marketing bags to maternity patients.

Discharge packs may not exert as large an influence on breastfeeding duration as some other determinants, but many of the other more powerful influences—such as education, race, income, marital status, and return to work—are not as readily amenable to change (Howard & Howard, 1997). In addition, the marketing bags contain powdered formula. The Centers for Disease Control and Prevention (CDC) recommends avoiding powdered formula for newborns, preterm babies, and any at-risk babies because powdered formula is not sterile. An article in *Pediatrics* clearly stated that "the exclusive use of breast milk or ready to feed formula for infants less than two months old should be encouraged" (Jason, 2012, p. 1). Hospitals set themselves up for liability by distributing powdered infant formula.

The Baby-Friendly Hospital Initiative

The Baby-Friendly Hospital Initiative is a global strategy to increase support for breastfeeding. As of October 2013, 169 hospitals and birth centers in the United States had achieved the designation. In addition, more than 600 hospitals and birth centers are on the pathway to become designated as Baby-Friendly, and many more are interested in starting the process. There are approximately 3000 birthing hospitals and centers in the United States. With about one-third of the birthing facilities working in the direction of adopting the evidence-based practices that support breastfeeding, the United States is well on the way to implementing the global recommendations. All 60 birthing hospitals in New Zealand already practice the 10 steps of the Baby-Friendly Hospital Initiative.

The Kaiser Permanente health system in California has asked all 29 of its hospitals to become Baby-Friendly and adopt the practices that have been shown through research to support breastfeeding. The state of California is working on legislation requiring all birthing hospitals to support breastfeeding by putting into place the evidence-based practices that support breastfeeding by 2025.

A quick overview of the 10 steps to supporting breastfeeding in hospitals is provided here:

1. Write a breastfeeding policy that includes all the evidence-based practices to support successful breastfeeding and that is reviewed annually by the hospital breastfeeding committee, and have a system in place to ensure these practices are being followed.
2. Educate healthcare practitioners and new staff members so they can fulfill the breastfeeding policy.
3. Educate parents and family members prenatally about breastfeeding.
4. Provide skin-to-skin care of the newborn at birth, keep mothers and babies together, allow time for the baby to breastfeed, delay procedures until the baby has finished the first breastfeeding, and perform routine procedures while the baby is skin-to-skin with the mother.
   These procedures include the following:
   - Apgar evaluation
   - Listening to the baby's heartbeat
   - Baby's footprints
   - Placing ID bands on the baby
   - Eye ointment
   - Taking temperature
   - Drawing blood
   - Monitoring the mother—temperature, blood pressure, and other vital signs
5. If the mother and baby need to be separated, teach the mother how to bring in her milk supply and maintain it until her baby can breastfeed effectively.
6. Assess the breastfeeding sessions and teach mothers how the baby shows an interest in feeding and signs of satiety.

7. Do not use pacifiers and bottle nipples until the baby is 3 to 4 weeks old, so the baby learns breastfeeding well.

8. Keep the baby in the family's postpartum room 24 hours a day. Provide for the care of the mother and the baby in the family's postpartum room.

9. Give breastfeeding babies no food or drink other than breastmilk. Keep track of breastfeeding exclusivity rates at hospital discharge.

10. Establish safeguards in the community for follow-up once families leave the hospital so that breastfeeding will be supported after discharge.

All birthing facilities can follow evidence-based practices to support breastfeeding. The Academy of Breastfeeding Medicine, the American Academy of Pediatrics, the International Lactation Consultant Association, as well as several U.S. state health departments provide model breastfeeding policies that birthing facilities may use (AAP, 2009; Feldman-Winter et al., 2012; Philipp, 2010).

ACKNOWLEDGMENT

Jan Riordan is the original author of this chapter. Her many years of experience working with mothers and babies and her career as a nurse, nurse educator, and researcher shaped the chapter. After hearing my presentation "When Babies Do Not Latch," Linda Smith suggested that I ask Jan about including the information in her book. When I approached Jan, she graciously suggested that it be added to her chapter, *Perinatal and Intrapartum Care*. Thus, I am now an author of this chapter.

Jan has been an inspiration to all professional lactation consultants. A quick pubmed.gov search revealed more than 20 articles written by Jan, starting with *JOGNN* articles in 1980. Her areas of interest include medications in breastmilk, sore nipples, mastitis, breast edema, conducting research, and labor medications and their effect on infants' sucking abilities. Her later career has focused on indicators of effective breastfeeding and estimates of milk intake. She was the first to publish on the cost of not

breastfeeding. Her online breastfeeding education course, which increased the number of lactation consultants, was the first of its kind. I appreciate collaborating with Jan, a true breastfeeding pioneer, on this chapter.

SUMMARY

Consumer advocacy, the expectations of parents, childbirth and breastfeeding education, early hospital discharge, frequent cesarean births, and new technologies all affect birthing and early breastfeeding. No longer do we view the mother and her infant as separate entities; rather, we care for them as a natural, single unit. Many hospitals boast a family-centered birthing unit or labor-delivery room providing postpartum care where the mother and infant are cared for together in one room. Birthing rooms today look much like a bedroom, with a comfortable reclining chair for the mother's support person and hookups for medical equipment that are concealed behind wall prints and other decorations. A major benefit of this kind of mother and baby care is that families receive more comprehensive, coordinated care, which facilitates breastfeeding.

At the same time that we are seeing improvements in mother and baby care, the use of medical interventions, particularly epidural analgesia, has skyrocketed. Two opposing forces appear to be battling each other for control of childbirth: on one side are childbirth education, midwifery, doula services, and free-standing birthing centers; on the other side are hospitals with routine epidural injections, high rates of cesarean births, and other technologies that medicalize the intrapartum experience.

New mothers need reassurance that they can enjoy an uncomplicated breastfeeding experience and that common concerns can be easily managed. Families need to learn about breastfeeding during pregnancy. There is rarely enough time during the hospital stay for the family to receive as much education about breastfeeding as they need to ensure an enjoyable breastfeeding experience. The few days in the hospital provide the baby with the opportunity to practice breastfeeding before the mother's milk increases in volume. During this time, the mother should be spending time falling in love with her baby and learning to read her baby's feeding cues.

Government and insurance companies are becoming more aware of the cost savings associated with breastfeeding. Insurance companies are required to provide breastfeeding support, and breastfeeding sustains the baby's health. Breastfeeding is being promoted as the feeding of choice. Public awareness about breastfeeding has grown. Breastfeeding is socially responsible.

KEY CONCEPTS

- The best preparation for breastfeeding is to learn as much as possible about mothering before the birth of the baby and find a breastfeeding support system.

- Nipple preparation during pregnancy is not necessary.

- If there are no complications, the first breastfeeding should take place during the first hour after the infant's birth.

- After the infant has been dried, he can be placed skin-to-skin on the mother's body to help the baby transition to extrauterine life.

- Neonates are initially alert for about 2 hours after birth; this period is followed by deep sleep until 20 hours, and then increased wakefulness and interest in frequent breastfeeding.

- Privacy, comfortable positioning, and optimal latch-on are all basic skills necessary to assist mothers and neonates in early breastfeeding.

- When a baby is not latching onto the breast, it is important to encourage skin-to-skin holding, feed the baby mother's milk, establish the mother's milk supply, and find hands-on help to correct any problematic situations.

- If cup-feeding is done carefully, it can be as safe as bottle-feeding.

- During the first 2 days after birth, infants who are bottle-fed often consume too much milk.

- New parents should watch the baby, not the clock, to determine when the baby is ready to feed. Feed the baby at the *earliest* sign of hunger. Crying is a *late* sign of hunger.

- Late-preterm infants (born between 34 and 37 weeks' gestation) need special help and careful, frequent follow-up, as these babies tend to breastfeed poorly at first. Once they reach full-term age, they breastfeed well.

- Short-term use of a silicone nipple shield (followed by pumping) in certain situations (nipple inversion, low-birth-weight infants) can preserve the breastfeeding relationship while waiting for the baby to mature.

- The generally accepted criterion for hypoglycemia in full-term infants is serum glucose concentration of less than 30 mg/dL in the first 24 hours after birth or less than 40 mg/dL after the first 24 hours. Early skin-to-skin care, frequent breastfeeding, close clinical observation, and reducing stress for the baby (e.g., delaying the bath for many hours, doing painful procedures while the baby is skin-to-skin and breastfeeding, delayed cord clamping, and not separating mother and baby) reduce the risk of low blood sugar.

- Generally speaking, women who deliver by cesarean birth breastfeed as frequently and for as long as those who have vaginal births. Special concerns related to breastfeeding post cesarean delivery are pain control, comfortable positioning, and early initiation of breastfeeding.

- Normal breast engorgement starts at 3 to 5 days after birth and then slowly recedes over the first 2 weeks postpartum.

- During normal engorgement, the mother's breast tissue usually remains compressible, thus enabling the infant to suckle comfortably and efficiently. Early and frequent breastfeeding minimizes severe engorgement.

- The full-term infant is born with additional extracellular fluid that sustains him for a short time. Urine output usually exceeds fluid intake for the first 3 to 4 days after birth.

- Excessive intravenous fluids during labor can lead to postpartum breast edema. The technique of areolar compression can help reshape the breast and nipple area so that the neonate is able to latch onto the breast.

- Hand expression is a time-honored skill that costs nothing, is easy to learn, and is always available.

- Early discharge does not appear to affect breastfeeding, if there is adequate postpartum care and support. If follow-up care is not provided, costly readmissions to the hospital may result.

- The goal of discharge planning is to prevent common problems and to provide emotional support to the new parents. With such a brief time in the hospital, the mother needs a caregiver who imparts as much basic information as possible without overwhelming her and is able to answer her questions with research-based information.

- At hospital discharge 2 to 3 days postpartum, the average weight loss of exclusively breastfed neonates is about twice that of formula-fed neonates.

- Basic and priority discharge teaching includes teaching the mother how to recognize her baby's feeding cues, how to latch her baby onto the breast, how to know the baby is getting enough milk, who to call for help with breastfeeding, and how to hand-express her milk.

- Providing marketing bags with formula reduces the length of exclusive breastfeeding; however, the availability of these products does not exert as large an influence on breastfeeding duration as some other determinants.

- When birthing facilities follow the *Ten Steps to Successful Breastfeeding*, the initiation, duration, and exclusivity of breastfeeding are improved.

Internet Resources

Academy of Breastfeeding Medicine—clinical protocols: http://www.bfmed.org

Video of newborn crawling to mother's breast: http://www.breastcrawl.org

Video of doctor teaching hand expression: http://newborns.stanford.edu/Breastfeeding/HandExpression.html

Hospital brochure about skin-to-skin care immediately after birth: http://lomalindahealth.org/common/pdf/PSN%20Skin%20to%20Skin%20Care%20Brochure%2007.pdf

Singing rap song about postbirth care: http://www.youtube.com/watch?v=N9KptD3t110&feature=youtu.be

Cesarean birth with baby going skin-to-skin with mother: http://www.youtube.com/watch?v=m5RIcaK98Yg

Skin-to-skin and kangaroo care information—DrBarbCNM.com http://www.skintoskincontact.com/susan-ludington.aspx

References

Akinbi HT, Narendran V, Pass AK, et al. Host defense proteins in vernix caseosa and amniotic fluid. *Am J Obstet Gynecol*. 2004;191(6):2090–2096.

Albert J, Heinrichs-Breen J. An evaluation of a breastfeeding privacy sign to prevent interruptions and promote successful breastfeeding. *J Obstet Gynecol Neonatal Nurs*. 2011;40(3):274–280.

Alkalay AL, Sarnat HB, Flores-Sarnat L, et al. Population meta-analysis of low plasma glucose thresholds in full-term normal newborns. *Am J Perinatol*. 2006;23(2):115–119.

American Academy of Pediatrics (AAP). Sample hospital breastfeeding policy for newborns. American Academy of Pediatrics Section on Breastfeeding. 2009. Available at: http://www2.aap.org/breastfeeding/curriculum/documents/pdf/Hospital%20Breastfeeding%20Policy_FINAL.pdf. Accessed January 20, 2014.

American Academy of Pediatrics (AAP). Special report—neonatal resuscitation: 2010 American Heart Association guidelines for cardiopulmonary resuscitation and emergency cardiovascular care. *Pediatrics*. 2010;126(5):e1400–e1413.

American Academy of Pediatrics (AAP), American College of Obstetrics and Gynecology (ACOG). *Guidelines for perinatal care*, 7th ed. Elk Grove Village, IL: AAP; 2012.

American College of Obstetrics and Gynecology (ACOG), Committee on Obstetric Practice. *Timing of umbilical cord clamping after birth*. Committee Opinion Number 543. December 2012. Available at: https://www.acog

.org/Resources_And_Publications/Committee _Opinions/Committee_on_Obstetric_Practice /Timing_of_Umbilical_Cord_Clamping_After_Birth. Accessed April 23, 2014.

American College of Obstetrics and Gynecology (ACOG), Committee on Obstetric Practice, Society for Maternal–Fetal Medicine. Committee Opinion Number 560. Medically indicated late-preterm and early-term deliveries 2013. Available at: http://www .acog.org/~/media/Committee%20Opinions /Committee%20on%20Obstetric%20Practice/co560 .pdf?dmc=1&ts=20130411T0359492289. Accessed April 22, 2014.

Anderson GC. Risk in mother–infant separation postbirth. *Image: J Nurs Schol.* 1989;21(4):196–199.

Anderson GC, Chiu S-h, Morrison B, et al. Skin-to-skin care for breastfeeding difficulties postbirth. In: Field T, ed. *Touch and massage in early child development.* New Brunswick, NJ: Johnson & Johnson; 2004:116–136.

Anderson GC, McBride MR, Dahm J, et al. Development of sucking in term infants from birth to four hours postbirth. *Res Nurs Health.* 1982;5(1):21–27.

Andres V, Garcia P, Rimet Y, et al. Apparent life-threatening events in presumably healthy newborns during early skin-to-skin contact. *Pediatrics.* 2011;127(4):e1073–e1076.

Barbero P, Madamangalam AS, Shields A. Skin to skin after cesarean birth. *J Hum Lact.* 2013;29(4):446–448.

Beck CT, Watson S. Impact of birth trauma on breastfeeding: a tale of two pathways. *Nurs Res.* 2008;57(4):228–236.

Beilin Y, Bodian CA, Weiser J, et al. Effect of labor epidural analgesia with and without fentanyl on infant breast-feeding: a prospective, randomized, double-blind study. *Anesthesiology.* 2005;103(6): 1211–1217.

Bergman NJ, Linley LL, Fawcus SR. Randomized controlled trial of skin-to-skin contact from birth versus conventional incubator for physiological stabilization in 1200- to 2199-gram newborns. *Acta Paediatr.* 2004;93(6):779–785.

Bigelow A, Power M, MacLellan-Peters J, et al. Effect of mother/infant skin-to-skin contact on postpartum depressive symptoms and maternal physiological stress. *JOGNN.* 2012;41(3):369–382.

Bouchet-Horwitz J. The use of Supple Cups for flat, retracting, and inverted nipples. *Clin Lact.* 2011;2(3): 30–33.

Bramson L, Lee JW, Moore E, et al. Effect of early skin-to-skin mother–infant contact during the first 3 hours following birth on exclusive breastfeeding during the maternity hospital stay. *J Hum Lact.* 2010;26(2):130–137.

Brand PL, Molenaar NL, Kaaijk C, et al. Neurodevelopmental outcome of hypoglycaemia in healthy, large for gestational age, term newborns. *Arch Dis Child.* 2005;90(1):78–81.

Burton P, Deng J, McDonald D, et al. Real-time 3D ultrasound imaging of infant tongue movements during breastfeeding. *Early Hum Dev.* 2013;89(9): 635–641.

Campbell D, Scott KD, Klaus MH, et al. Female relatives or friends trained as labor doulas: outcomes at 6 to 8 weeks postpartum. *Birth.* 2006;34(3):220–227.

Carfoot S, Williamson P, Dickson R. A randomised controlled trial in the north of England examining the effects of skin-to-skin care on breastfeeding. *Midwifery.* 2005;21(1):71–79.

Casey CE, Neifert MR, Seacat JM, Neville MC. Nutrient intake by breastfed infants during the first five days after birth. *Am J Dis Child.* 1986;140(9):933–936.

Centers for Medicare and Medicaid Services. Newborns' and Mothers' Health Protection Act (NMHPA) n.d. Available at: http://www.cms.gov/CCIIO/Programs-and-Initiatives/Other-Insurance-Protections/nmhpa _factsheet.html. Accessed April 22, 2014.

Chang ZM, Heaman MI. Epidural analgesia during labor and delivery: effects on the initiation and continuation of effective breastfeeding. *J Hum Lact.* 2005;21(3): 305–314.

Chanprapaph P, Luttarapakul J, Siribaribuck S, et al. Outcome of non-protractile nipple correction with breast cups in pregnant women: a randomized controlled trial. *Breastfeed Med.* 2013;8(4):408–412.

Chen DC, Nommsen-Rivers L, Dewey KG, Lonnerdal B. Stress during labor and delivery and early lactation performance. *Am J Clin Nutr.* 1998;68(2):334–344.

Christensson K, Bhat GJ, Amadi BC, et al. Randomised study of skin-to-skin versus incubator care for rewarming low-risk hypothermic neonates. *Lancet.* 1998;352(9134):1115.

Clemmit S. Nipple shield perspective. *New Beginnings.* 2003;20(2):58–59.

Colson SD, Meek JH, Hawdon JM. Optimal positions for the release of primitive neonatal reflexes stimulating breastfeeding. *Early Hum Dev.* 2008;84(7):441–449.

Cotterman K. Reverse pressure softening: a simple tool for easier latching during engorgement. *J Hum Lact.* 2004;20(2):227–237.

Cregan M, Hartmann PE. Computerized breast measurement from conception to weaning: clinical implications. *J Hum Lact.* 1999;15(2):89–96.

Crowell MK, Hill PD, Humenick SS. Relationship between obstetric analgesia and time of effective breastfeeding. *J Nurse Midwifery.* 1994;39(3):150–156.

Dageville C, Pignol J, De Smet S. Very early neonatal apparent life-threatening events and sudden unexpected deaths: incidence and risk factors. *Act Paediatr.* 2008;97(7):866–869.

Davis HV, Sears RR, Miller HC, Brodbeck AJ. Effects of cup, bottle and breastfeeding on oral activities of newborn infants. *Pediatrics.* 1948;2:549–558.

de Carvalho M, Robertson S, Merkatz R, et al. Milk intake and frequency of feeding in breastfed infants. *Early Hum Dev.* 1982;7(2):155–163.

Dewey KG, Nommsen-Rivers LA, Heinig MJ, et al. Risk factors for suboptimal infant breastfeeding behavior, delayed onset of lactation, and excess neonatal weight loss. *Pediatrics.* 2003;112(3):607–619.

Doucet S, Soussignan R, Sagot P, Schaal B. The "smellscape" of mother's breast: effects of odor masking and selective unmasking on neonatal arousal, oral, and visual responses. *Dev Psychobiol.* 2007;49(2):129–138.

Dowling DA, Meier PP, DiFiore J, et al. Cup-feeding for preterm infants: mechanics and safety. *J Hum Lact.* 2002;18(1):13–20.

Edelstein S, Sharlin J. *Life cycle nutrition: an evidence-based approach.* Sudbury, MA: Jones and Bartlett; 2010:167.

Edmonson MB, Stoddard JJ, Owen LM. Hospital readmission with feeding-related problems after early postpartum discharge of normal newborns. *JAMA.* 1997;278(4):299–303.

Eidelman A. Hypoglycemia and the breastfed neonate. *Pediatr Clin North Am.* 2001;48(2):377–387.

Eidelman AI, Schanler RJ. Breastfeeding and the use of human milk. *Pediatrics.* 2012;129(3):e827–e841.

Ekström A, Widström AM, Nissen E. Duration of breast-feeding in Swedish primiparous and multiparous women. *J Hum Lact.* 2003;19(2):172–178.

Evans A. Academy of Breastfeeding Medicine Clinical Protocol #2: guidelines for hospital discharge of the breastfeeding term newborn and mother: "the going home protocol." *Breastfeed Med.* 2007;2(3):158–165.

Evans KC, Evans RG, Royal R, et al. Effect of caesarean section on breast milk transfer to the normal term newborn over the first week of life. *Arch Dis Child Fetal Neonatal Ed.* 2003;88(5):F380–F382.

Feldman-Winter L, Grossman X, Palaniappan A, et al. Removal of industry-sponsored formula sample packs from the hospital: does it make a difference? *J Hum Lact.* 2012;28(3):380–388.

Feldman-Winter L, Procaccini D, Merewood A. A model infant feeding policy for Baby-Friendly designation in the USA. *J Hum Lact.* 2012;28(3):304–311.

Fransson AL, Karlsson H, Nilsson K. Temperature variation in newborn babies: importance of physical contact with the mother. *Arch Dis Child Neonatal Ed.* 2005;90(6):F500–F504.

Freeden RC. Cup-feeding of newborn infants. *Pediatrics.* 1948;2:544–548.

Freer Y. A comparison of breast and cup-feeding in preterm infants: effect on physiological parameters. *J Neonatal Nurs.* 1999;5:15–21.

Genna CW, ed. *Supporting sucking skills in breastfeeding infants,* 2nd ed. Burlington, MA: Jones & Bartlett Learning; 2013.

Glover J. Supplementation of breastfeeding newborns: a flowchart for decision-making. *J Hum Lact.* 1995;11(2):127–131.

Glover R. *Follow me mum: the key to successful breastfeeding* [DVD]. 2005.

Gnigler M, Ralser E, Karall D, et al. Early sudden unexpected death in infancy (ESUDI): three case reports and review of the literature. *Acta Paediatr.* 2013;102:e235–e238.

Gomez P, Baiges Nogues MT, Batiste Fernandez MT, et al. Kangaroo method in delivery room for full-term babies. *Anales Espanoles de Pediatria.* 1998;48(6):631–633.

Gouchon S, Gregori D, Picotto A, el al. Skin-to-skin contact after cesarean delivery: an experimental study. *Nurs Res.* 2010;59(2):78–84.

Grajeda R, Perez-Escamilla R. Stress during labor and delivery is associated with delayed onset of lactation among urban Guatemalan women. *J Nutr.* 2002;132(10):3055–3060.

Gupta A, Khanna K, Chattree S. Cup-feeding: an alternative to bottle feeding in a neonatal intensive unit. *J Trop Pediatr.* 1999;45(2):108–110.

Hall RT, Mercer AM, Teasley SL, et al. A breastfeeding assessment score to evaluate the risk for cessation of breastfeeding by 7 to 10 days of age. *J Pediatr.* 2002;141(5):659–664.

Hall WA, Carty EM. Managing the early discharge experience: taking control. *J Adv Nurs.* 1993;18(4):574–582.

Hallowell SG, Spatz DL. The relationship of brain development and breastfeeding in the late-preterm infant. *J Pediatr Nurs.* 2012;27(2):154–162.

Hamilton BE, Martin JA, Ventura SJ. Births: preliminary data for 2012. *National Vital Statistics Reports.* 2013;62(3):1–33.

Haninger NC, Farley CL. Screening for hypoglycemia in healthy term neonates: effects on breastfeeding. *J Midwifery Women's Health.* 2001;46(5):292–301.

Hawdon JM, Ward-Platt MP, Aynsley-Green A. Patterns of metabolic adaptation for preterm and term infants in the first neonatal week. *Arch Dis Child.* 1992;67(4):357–365.

Hazelbaker AK. In defense of finger-feeding. *Medela Rental Round-up.* 1997;14(2):10–11.

Heck LJ, Erenberg A. Serum glucose levels in term neonates during the first 48 hours of life. *J Pediatr.* 1987;110(1):119–122.

Hedberg-Nyqvist K. A cup feeding protocol for neonates: evaluation of nurses' and parents' use of two cups. *J Neonatal Nurs.* 1999;5:31–35.

Hedderwick SA, McNeil SA, Lyons MJ, et al. Pathogenic organisms associated with artificial fingernails worn by healthcare workers. *Infect Control Hosp Epidemiol.* 2000;21(8):505–509.

Heinig MJ, Nommsen LA, Peerson JM, et al. Energy and protein intakes of breastfed and formula-fed infants during the first year of life and their association with growth velocity: the DARLING study. *Am J Clin Nutr.* 1993;58(1):152–161.

Ho HT, Yeung WK, Young BW. Evaluation of "point of care" devices in the measurement of low blood glucose in neonatal practice. *Arch Dis Child Fetal Neonatal Ed.* 2004;89(4):F356–F359.

Holmes AV, McLeod AY, Bunik M. Academy of Breastfeeding Medicine Protocol #5: peripartum breastfeeding management for the healthy mother and infant at term. *Breastfeed Med.* 2013;8(6):469–473.

Howard C, Howard F. Discharge packs: how much do they matter? *Birth.* 1997;24(2):98–101.

Howard C, Howard FM, Lanphear B, et al. Randomized clinical trial of pacifier use and bottle-feeding or cupfeeding and their effect on breastfeeding. *Pediatrics.* 2003;111(3):511–518.

Howie PW, Houston MJ, Cook A, et al. How long should a breast feed last? *Early Hum Dev.* 1981;5(1):71–77.

Humenick SS, Hill PD, Anderson MA. Breast engorgement: patterns and selected outcomes. *J Hum Lact.* 1994;10(2):87–93.

Hung KJ, Berg O. Early skin-to-skin after cesarean to improve breastfeeding. *MCN.* 2011;36(5):318–324.

Hunt CE. Ontogeny of autonomic regulation in late preterm infants born at 34–37 weeks postmenstrual age. *Semin Perinatol.* 2006;30(2):73–76.

Janke JR. Breastfeeding duration following cesarean and vaginal births. *J Nurs Midwifery.* 1988;33(4):159–164.

Jarrell JR, Ludington-Hoe SM, Aboaelfettah A. Kangaroo care with twins: a case study in which one infant did not respond as expected. *Neonatal Network.* 2009;28(3):157–163.

Jason J. Prevention of invasive *Cronobacter* infections in young infants fed powdered infant formulas. *Pediatrics.* 2012;130(5):1–9.

Johanson RB, Spencer SA, Rolfe P, et al. Effect of post-delivery care on neonatal body temperature. *Acta Paediatr.* 1992;81(11):859–862.

Johnston CC, Stevens B, Pinelli J, et al. Kangaroo care is effective in diminishing pain response in preterm neonates. *Arch Pediatr Adolesc Med.* 2003;157(1):1084–1088.

Jordan S, Emery S, Bradshaw C, et al. The impact of intrapartum analgesia on infant feeding. *BJOG.* 2005;112(7):927–934.

Karlstrom A, Engstrom-Olofsson R, Norbergh KG, et al. Postoperative pain after cesarean birth affects breastfeeding and infant care. *JOGNN.* 2007;36(5):430–440.

Kent JC, Hepworth AR, Sherriff JL, et al. Longitudinal changes in breastfeeding patterns from 1 to 6 months of lactation. *Breastfeed Med.* 2013;8(4):401–407.

Kent J, Mitoulas LR, Cregan MD, et al. Volume and frequency of breastfeedings and fat content of breast milk throughout the day. *Pediatrics.* 2006;117(3):e387–e395.

Lang S, Lawrence CJ, Orme RL. Cup-feeding: an alternative method of infant feeding. *Arch Dis Child.* 1994;71(4):365–369.

Lawson T, Tulloch MI. Breastfeeding duration: prenatal intentions and postnatal practices. *J Adv Nurs.* 1995;22(5):841–849.

Lee KS, Perlman M, Ballantyne M, et al. Association between duration of neonatal hospital stay and readmission rate. *J Pediatr.* 1995;127(5):758–766.

Leung GM, Lam TH, Ho LM. Breast-feeding and its relation to smoking and mode of delivery. *Obstet Gynecol.* 2002;99(5 pt 1):785–794.

Lieberman E, Lang JM, Frigoletto F Jr, et al. Epidural analgesia, intrapartum fever, and neonatal sepsis evaluation. *Pediatrics.* 1997;99(3):415–419.

Lothian JA. It takes two to breastfeed: the baby's role in successful breastfeeding. *J Nurs Midwifery.* 1995;40(4):328–334.

Ludington-Hoe S, Lewis T, Morgan K, et al. Breast and infant temperatures with twins during shared kangaroo care. *JOGNN.* 2006;35(2):223–231.

Malhotra N, Vishwambaran L, Sundaram KR, et al. A controlled trial of alternative methods of oral feeding in neonates. *Early Hum Dev.* 1999;54(1):29–38.

Mangesi L, Dowswell T. Treatments for breast engorgement during lactation. *Cochrane Database Syst Rev.* 2010;8(9):CD006946.

Margolis L, Schwartz JB. The relationship between the timing of maternal postpartum hospital discharge and breastfeeding. *J Hum Lact.* 2000;16(2):121–128.

Marin Gabriel MA, Del Rey Hurtado de Mendoza B, Jimenez Figueroa L, et al. Analgesia with breastfeeding in addition to skin-to-skin contact during heel prick. *Arch Dis Child Fetal Neonatal Ed.* 2013;98(6):F499–F503.

Marinelli K, Burke GS, Dodd VL. A comparison of the safety of cupfeedings and bottlefeedings in premature infants whose mothers intend to breastfeed. *J Perinatol.* 2001;21(6):350–355.

Marlier L, Schaal B. Human newborns prefer human milk: conspecific milk odor is attractive without postnatal exposure. *Child Dev.* 2005;76(1):155–168.

Martens P, Romphf L. Factors associated with newborn in-hospital weight loss: comparisons by feeding method, demographics, and birthing procedures. *J Hum Lact.* 2007;23(2):233–241.

Matthiesen AS, Ransjö-Arvidson AB, Nissen E, Uvnas-Moberg K. Postpartum maternal oxytocin release by newborns: effects of infant hand massage and sucking. *Birth.* 2001;28(1):13–19.

Meier PP, Brown LP, Hurst NM, et al. Nipple shields for preterm infants: effect on milk transfer and duration of breastfeeding. *J Hum Lact.* 2000;16(2):106–114.

Mercer AM, Teasley SL, Hopkinson J, et al. Evaluation of a breastfeeding assessment score in a diverse population. *J Hum Lact.* 2010;26(1):42–48.

Mercer JS, McGrath MM, Hensman A, et al. Immediate and delayed cord clamping in infants born between 24 and 32 weeks: a pilot randomized controlled trial. *J Perinatol.* 2003;23(6):466–472.

Meyer K, Anderson GC. Using skin-to-skin (kangaroo) care in a clinical setting with full-term infants having breastfeeding difficulties. *MCN.* 1999;24(4):190–192.

Miller V, Riordan J. Treating postpartum breast edema with areolar compression. *J Hum Lact.* 2004;20(2):223–226.

Milligan RA, Flenniken PM, Pugh LC. Positioning intervention to minimize fatigue in breastfeeding women. *Appl Nurs Res.* 1996;9(2):67–70.

Mizuno K, Kani K. Sipping/lapping is a safe alternative feeding method to suckling for preterm infants. *Acta Paediatr.* 2005;94(5):574–580.

Mizuno K, Mizuno N, Shinohara T, et al. Mother–infant skin-to-skin contact after delivery results in early recognition of own mother's milk odour. *Acta Paediatr.* 2004;93(12):1640–1645.

Montgomery A, Hale TW. Academy of Breastfeeding Medicine. ABM Clinical Protocol #15: analgesia and anesthesia for the breastfeeding mother. *Breastfeed Med.* 2012;7(6):547–553.

Moon JL, Humenick SS. Breast engorgement: contributing variables and variables amenable to nursing intervention. *JOGNN.* 1989;18(4):309–315.

Moore AM, Perlman M. Symptomatic hypoglycemia in otherwise healthy, breastfed, term newborns. *Pediatrics.* 1999;103(4 pt 1):837–839.

Morton J, Hall JY, Wong RJ, et al. Combining hand techniques with electric pumping increases milk production in mothers of preterm infants. *J Perinatol.* 2009;29(11):757–764.

Mulford C. Subtle signs and symptoms of the milk ejection reflex. *J Hum Lact.* 1990;6(4):177–178.

National Center for Health Statistics. *Health, United States, 2012: with special feature on emergency care.* Hyattsville, MD. 2013. Available at: http://www.cdc.gov/nchs/data/hus/hus12.pdf#097. Accessed April 23, 2014.

Neville M, Oliva-Rasbach J. Is maternal milk production limiting for infant growth during the first year of life in breast-fed infants? In Goldman A, Atkinson S, Hanson L, eds. *Human lactation 3.* New York: Plenum Press; 1987:123–133.

Newman J, Pitman T. *The latch.* Amarillo, TX: Hale; 2006.

Nicholson WL. The use of nipple shields by breastfeeding women. *Aust Coll Midwives J.* 1993;6(2):18–24.

Nolan A, Lawrence C. A pilot study of a nursing intervention protocol to minimize maternal–infant separation after cesarean birth. *JOGNN.* 2009;38(4):430–442.

Nommsen-Rivers LA, Heinig MJ, Cohen RJ, et al. Newborn wet and soiled diaper counts and timing of onset of lactation as indicators of breastfeeding inadequacy. *J Hum Lact.* 2008;24(1):27–33.

Page-Goertz S. Discharge planning for the breastfeeding dyad. *Pediatr Nurs.* 1989;15(5):543–544.

Parker LA, Sullivan S, Krueger C, et al. Effect of early breast milk expression on milk volume among mother of very low birth weight infants. *J Perinatol.* 2012;32(3):205–208.

Pejovic NJ, Herlenius E. Unexpected collapse of healthy newborn infants: risk factors, supervision and hypothermia treatment. *Acta Paediatr.* 2013;102(7):680–688.

Philipp BL. Academy of Breastfeeding Medicine Clinical Protocol #7: model breastfeeding policy. *Breastfeed Med.* 2010;5(4):173–177.

Pollard DL. Impact of a feeding log on breastfeeding duration and exclusivity. *Matern Child Health J.* 2011;15(3):395–400.

Preer G, Pisegna JM, Cook JT, et al. Delaying the bath and in-hospital breastfeeding rates. *Breastfeed Med.* 2013;8(6):485–490.

Puri P, Hollwarth M. *Pediatric surgery, diagnosis and management.* New York: Springer; 2009:76.

Raimbault C, Saliba E, Porter RH. The effect of the odour of mother's milk on breastfeeding behaviours of premature neonates. *Acta Paediatr.* 2007;96(3):368–371.

Ransjö-Arvidson AB, Matthiesen AS, Lilja G, et al. Maternal analgesia during labor disturbs newborn behavior: effects on breastfeeding, temperature and crying. *Birth.* 2001;28(1):5–12.

Righard L. How do newborns find their mother's breast? *Birth.* 1995;22(3):174–175.

Righard L, Alade MO. Effect of delivery room routines on success of first breastfeed. *Lancet.* 1990;336(8723):1105–1107.

Righard L, Flodmark CE, Lothe L, et al. Breastfeeding patterns: comparing the effects on infant behavior and maternal satisfaction of using one or two breasts. *Birth.* 1993;20(4):182–185.

Riordan J, Gill-Hopple K, Angeron J. Indicators of effective breastfeeding and estimates of breast milk intake. *J Hum Lact.* 2005;21(4):406–412.

Riordan J, Gross A, Angeron J, et al. The effect of labor pain relief medication on neonatal suckling and breastfeeding duration. *J Hum Lact.* 2000;16(1):7–12.

Rowe-Murray HJ, Fisher JR. Baby Friendly Hospital practices: cesarean section is a persistent barrier to early initiation of breastfeeding. *Birth.* 2002;29(2):124–131.

Sadacharan R, Grossman X, Matlak S, Merewood A. Hospital discharge bags and breastfeeding at 6 months: data from the Infant Feeding Practices Study II. *J Hum Lact.* 2014;30(1):73–79. doi: 10.1177/0890334413513653.

Sadacharan R, Grossman X, Sanchez E, Merewood A. Trends in US hospital distribution of industry-sponsored infant formula sample packs. *Pediatrics.* 2011;128(4):702–705. doi: 10.1542/peds.2011-0983.

Sadeh A, Dark I, Vohr B. Newborns' sleep–wake patterns: the role of maternal, delivery, and infant factors. *Early Hum Dev.* 1996;44(2):113–126.

Santoro W Jr, Martinez FE, Ricco RG, et al. Colostrum ingested during the first day of life by exclusively breastfed healthy newborn infants. *J Pediatr.* 2010;156(1):29–32.

Seaton S, Reeves M, McLean S. Oxycodone as a component of multimodal analgesia for lactating mothers after caesarean section: relationships between maternal plasma, breastmilk and neonatal plasma levels. *Aust NZJ Obstet Gynaecol.* 2007;47(3):181–185.

Sepkoski CM, Lester BM, Ostheimer GW, et al. The effects of maternal epidural anesthesia on neonatal behavior during the first month. *Dev Med Child Neurol.* 1992;34(12):1072–1080.

Sexson WR. Incidence of neonatal hypoglycemia: a matter of definition. *J Pediatr.* 1984;105(1):149–150.

Shapiro-Mendoza CK, Tomashek KM, Kotelchuck M, et al. Effect of late-preterm birth and maternal medical conditions on newborn morbidity risk. *Pediatrics.* 2008;121(2):e223–e232.

Simpson KR, Creehan PA. *Perinatal nursing*, 3rd ed. Philadelphia: Lippincott Williams & Wilkins, AWHONN; 2008:636.

Smillie CM. *Baby-led breastfeeding: the mother–baby dance* [DVD]. Geddes Productions, 2007.

Smith J, Plaat F, Fisk NM. The natural caesarean: a woman-centered technique. *BJOG.* 2008;115:1037–1042.

Smith L. *Impact of birthing practices on breastfeeding*, 2nd ed. Sudbury, MA: Jones and Bartlett; 2010.

Smolkin T, Mick O, Dabbah M, et al. Birth by cesarean delivery and failure on first otoacoustic emissions hearing test. *Pediatrics.* 2012;130(1):e95–e100.

Snowden HM, Renfrew MJ, Woolridge MW. Commercial hospital discharge packs for breastfeeding women (Cochrane review). In: *The Cochrane library.* Oxford, UK: 2000; Issue 2.

Soskolne EI, Schumacher R, Fyock C, et al. The effect of early discharge and other factors on readmission rates of newborns. *Arch Pediatr Adolesc Med.* 1996;150(4):373–379.

Srinivasan G, Pildes RS, Cattamanchi G, et al. Plasma glucose values in normal neonates: a new look. *J Pediatr.* 1986;109(1):114–117.

Svensson KE, Velandia MI, Matthiesen A-ST, et al. Effects of mother–infant skin-to-skin contact on severe latch-on problems in older infants: a randomized trial. *Int Breastfeed J.* 2013;8(1):1.

Takahashi Y, Tamakoshi K, Matsushima M, et al. Comparison of salivary cortisol, heart rate, and oxygen saturation between early skin-to-skin contact with different initiation and duration times in healthy, full-term infants. *Early Hum Dev.* 2011;87(3):151–157.

Thorley V. Cup-feeding: problems caused by incorrect use. *J Hum Lact.* 1997;13(1):54–55.

Thukral A, Sankar MJ, Agarwal R. Early skin-to-skin contact and breastfeeding behavior in term neonates: a randomized controlled trial. *Neonatology.* 2012;102(2):114–119.

Torvaldsen S, Roberts CL, Simpson JM, et al. Intrapartum epidural analgesia and breastfeeding: a prospective cohort study. *Int Breastfeed J.* 2006;1:24.

Trainor C. Valuing labor support. *AWHONN Lifelines.* 2002;6:387–389.

Vaidya K, Sharma A, Dhungel S. Effect of early mother–baby close contact over the duration of exclusive breastfeeding. *Nepal Med Coll J.* 2005;7(2):138–140.

Varendi H, Porter RH, Winberg I. Attractiveness of amniotic fluid odor: evidence of prenatal olfactory learning? *Acta Pediatr.* 1996; 85(10):1223–1227.

Viscomi CM. Maternal fever, neonatal sepsis evaluation and epidural labor analgesia. *Reg Anesth Pain Med.* 2000;25(5):549–553.

Walters MW, Boggs KM, Ludington-Hoe S, et al. Kangaroo care at birth of full term infants: a pilot study. *Am J Maternal Child Nurs.* 2007;32(6):375–381.

Waltman PA, Brewer JM, Rogers BP, et al. Building evidence for practice: a pilot study of newborn bulb suctioning at birth. *J Midwifery Women's Health.* 2004;49(1):32–38.

Widström AM, Lilja G, Aaltomaa-Michalias P, et al. Newborn behaviour to locate the breast when skin-to-skin: a possible method for enabling early self-regulation. *Acta Paediatr.* 2011;100(1):79–85.

Widström AM, Ransjö-Arvidson AB, Christensson K, et al. Gastric suction in healthy newborn infants: effects on circulation and developing feeding behaviors. *Acta Paediatr Scand.* 1987;76(4):566–572.

Widström AM, Thingström-Paulsson J. The position of the tongue during rooting reflexes elicited in newborn infant before the first suckle. *Acta Paediatr.* 1993;82(3):281–283.

Widström AM, Wahlberg V, Matthiesen AS, et al. Short-term effects of early suckling and touch of the nipple on maternal behavior. *Early Hum Dev.* 1990;21(3):153–163.

Wiessinger D. A breastfeeding teaching tool using a sandwich analogy for latch-on. *J Hum Lact.* 1998;14(1):51–56.

Wight N. Breastfeeding the borderline (near-term) preterm infant. *Pediatr Ann.* 2003;32(5):329–337.

Wight NE, Marinelli KA. Academy of Breastfeeding Medicine Clinical Protocol #1: guidelines for glucose monitoring and treatment of hypoglycemia in breastfed neonates. *Breastfeed Med.* 2006;1(3):178–184.

Williams J, Mueller S. A message to the nurse from the baby. *J Hum Lact.* 1989;5(1):19.

Wilson-Clay B. Clinical use of silicone nipple shields. *J Hum Lact.* 1996;12(4):279–285.

Wilson-Clay B. Nipple shields in clinical practice: a review [Editorial]. *Breastfeed Abstr.* 2003;22(2):11–12.

Wilson-Clay B, Hoover K. *The breastfeeding atlas*, 5th ed. Austin, TX: LactNews Press; 2013.

Winslow EH, Jacobson AF. Can a fashion statement harm the patient? Long and artificial nails may cause nosocomial infections. *Am J Nurs.* 2000;100(9):63–65.

Woolridge MW, Baum JD. Infant appetite control and the regulation of breast milk supply. *Children's Hospital Quarterly.* 1991;3(2):113–199.

Woolridge MW, Ingram JC, Baum JD. Do changes in pattern of breast usage alter the baby's nutrient intake? *Lancet.* 1990;336(8712):395–397.

Wright A, Rice S, Wells S. Changing hospital practices to increase the duration of breastfeeding. *Pediatrics.* 1996;97(5):669–675.

Yigit F, Cigdem Z, Temizsoy E, et al. Does warming the breasts affect the amount of breastmilk production? *Breastfeed Med.* 2012;7(6):487–488.

Research and Scholarly Papers on the Newborn's Reactions to the Smell of Mother's Milk or Secretions from the Montgomery Glands on the Areola

Delaunay-El Allam M, Soussignan R, Patris B, et al. Long-lasting memory for an odor acquired at the mother's breast. *Dev Sci.* 2010;13(6):849–863.

Doucet S, Soussignan R, Sagot P, Schaal B. The "smellscape" of mother's breast: effects of odor masking and selective unmasking on neonatal arousal, oral, and visual responses. *Dev Psychobiol.* 2007;49(2):129–138.

Doucet S, Soussignan R, Sagot P, Schaal B. The secretion of areolar (Montgomery's) glands from lactating women elicits selective, unconditional responses in neonates. *PLoS One.* 2009;4(10):e7579.

Marlier L, Schaal B. Human newborns prefer human milk: conspecific milk odor is attractive without postnatal exposure. *Child Dev.* 2005;76(1):155–168.

Mizuno K, Mizuno N, Shinohara T, et al. Mother–infant skin-to-skin contact after delivery results in early recognition of own mother's milk odour. *Act Paediatr.* 2004;93(12):1640–1645.

Nishitani S, Miyamura T, Tagawa M, et al. The calming effect of a maternal breast milk odor on the human newborn infant. *Neurosci Res.* 2009;63(1):66–71.

Raimbault C, Saliba E, Porter RH. The effect of the odour of mother's milk on breastfeeding behaviour of premature neonates. *Acta Paediatr.* 2007;96(3):368–371.

Rodriguez NA, Meier PP, Groer MW, et al. Oropharyngeal administration of colostrum to extremely low birth weight infants: theoretical perspectives. *J Perinatol.* 2009;29(1):1–7.

Schaal B, Doucet S, Sagot P, et al. Human breast areolae as scent organs: morphological data and possible involvement in maternal–neonatal coadaptation. *Dev Psychobiol.* 2006;48:100–110.

Sullivan RM, Toubas P. Clinical usefulness of maternal odor in newborns: soothing and feeding preparatory responses. *Biol Neonate.* 1998;74(6):402–408.

Varendi H, Christensson K, Porter RH, Winberg J. Soothing effect of amniotic fluid smell in newborn infants. *Early Hum Dev.* 1998;51:47–55.

Varendi H, Porter RH. Breast odour as the only maternal stimulus elicits crawling towards the odour source. *Acta Paediatr.* 2001;90(4):372–375.

Varendi H, Porter RH, Winberg I. Attractiveness of amniotic fluid odor: evidence of prenatal olfactory learning? *Acta Paediatr.* 1996;85(10):1223–1227.

Varendi H, Porter RH, Winberg I. Natural odour preferences of newborn infants change over time. *Acta Paediatr.* 1997;86(9):985–990.

Yildiz A, Arikan D, Gözüm S, et al. The effect of the odor of breast milk on the time needed for transition from gavage to total oral feeding in preterm infants. *J Nurs Schol.* 2011;43(3):265–273.

Postpartum Care

Linda J. Smith

This chapter follows the mother–infant dyad after birth in the early postpartum period. It first addresses normal behavior and physiology, and then covers common problems during the "fourth trimester" for the mother, the baby, and the family.

As of early 2013, the majority (77%) of U.S. mothers initiated breastfeeding (Centers for Disease Control and Prevention [CDC], 2013a). Of infants born in 2010, 49% were breastfeeding at 6 months, and 16% continued breastfeeding at 1 year. These rates are the highest reported to date. Unfortunately, 60% of mothers who intended to exclusively breastfeed their children were not meeting their own breastfeeding goals (Odom et al., 2013). An astounding 92% of mothers reported problems in the first week after birth, with difficulty with the infant feeding at the breast leading the list, followed by breast pain and milk quantity (Wagner et al., 2013). Breastfeeding problems peaked on day 3, and remained significant at day 7. Clearly, there is a need for more robust, prevalent, and skilled support in the early days and weeks following childbirth.

Immediate Postbirth Events

Normally, the mother–baby dyad will be assured immediate and uninterrupted skin-to-skin contact immediately after birth for at least 1 hour or until after the first successful breastfeed (World Health Organization [WHO] & United Nations Childrens Fund [UNICEF], 2009). The mother and baby are kept warm, and the baby remains in continuous skin-to-skin contact with the mother's chest or abdomen during this period (Dumas et al., 2013). Within 5–70 minutes, the baby is able to use his inborn capabilities to move through nine specific behaviors to crawl, wiggle, or scoot his way to one breast or the other, latch on comfortably, and receive a bolus of colostrum due to the powerful oxytocin responses following birth (Widstrom et al., 2011). Simultaneously, the mother's and baby's central nervous systems are flooded with hormones and pleasurable, familiar experiences including those related to smell, hearing, touch, and warmth. The mother's body is the baby's natural habitat, which provides all basic biological needs and determines behavior. The newborn both initiates and maintains breastfeeding; the mother responds with caring and maintains breastfeeding while continuing to transition into her new role as a mother (Dumas et al., 2013).

First Weeks: Principles and Expectations

The early weeks of the mother–baby dyad's new relationship are characterized by symbiotic functions and rhythmicity. Sleeping rhythms of mother and baby are congruent when they are in close physical contact, but can be profoundly different (and disruptive) when mother and baby are not in close physical contact (McKenna et al., 2007). Mothers need rest to recover physically and emotionally from even relatively uncomplicated births; babies need rest, food, and comfort to continue developing all body systems. Both need nourishing food frequently to build tissue and strength, and both respond profoundly to multiple sensory messages of the other. Shared sleep is inextricably connected with and significantly supportive of breastfeeding (Huang et al., 2013; McKenna et al., 1997), yet bedsharing has been the subject of much controversy. This practice is addressed later in this chapter.

The key principles during this period are (1) feed the baby, (2) protect the mother's milk production, and (3) keep the mother and baby together. Time is generally on your side, and virtually all problems can be resolved.

Feeding, Sleeping, and Behavior Patterns of the Neonate

Newborns' sleep cycles are approximately 60–90 minutes long (Bergman, 2013; Jenni et al., 2006), with no particular pattern of day–night differentiation (circadian rhythms) emerging for several months. Babies *begin* consolidating multiple sleep cycles into longer sleep stretches (Parmelee et al., 1964) and gravitate toward more sleep during dark (nighttime hours) only in the *second* 6 months of life (Coons & Guilleminault, 1982, 1984). Sleep is intrinsically interrelated with breastfeeding, especially in the first half-year of the baby's life (Galbally et al., 2013). Newborns nurse approximately hourly (Bergman, 2013) and virtually every time they wake up, day and night, for many months (Kent et al., 2006).

The baby's gastric and metabolic functions closely parallel his developing circadian sleep cycle and the mother's lactation synthesis patterns. A baby's stomach empties of human milk in about 60–90 minutes. The capacity of a baby's stomach at birth is about 20 mL (Bergman, 2013). The average volume of a single letdown reflex is about 35–40 mL (Ramsay et al., 2005). From days 2 through 6, babies have 5–10 daily breastfeeding sessions, with milk intake increasing rapidly to between 395 and 868 mL (Kent, 2007). During the first 6 months

of life, babies take an average volume of milk of 750–800 mL per day (Kent et al., 2006). Surprisingly, this intake does not substantially change during the first 12 months. Given the baby's stomach capacity, the negative consequences of overfeeding (gastric distension, discomfort, vomiting/spitting, reflux), the rapid gastric emptying time of human milk, and the total daily calories needed for growth, we can expect that a baby will breastfeed many times per day and night. After all, the baby will double his weight in about 4 months, and needs frequent feeds to accomplish this important developmental stage.

Kent et al. (2006) published an analysis of 24-hour feeding patterns of healthy, exclusively breastfeeding babies aged 1–6 months. Thirteen percent of the babies always took both breasts at a feed, 30% never took both breasts (i.e., they fed from only one breast per feed), and most alternated between one and both breasts. Feeds ranged from 6 to 18 per day, and on average, the babies took 11 feeds per day, with between-feed intervals varying between 50 minutes to 6 hours. A large feed did not predict a long interval before the next feed; conversely, a small feed did not predict a short interval before the next meal. Baby-initiated feeds are the biologically driven norm. Either the mother or the baby may terminate a specific feed; if the baby signals again, restarting a feed is appropriate. Mother-directed (scheduled) feeding was a concept that developed in the late 1800s and flourished during the formula-feeding era, but it failed to consider the interrelated physiology of infant-initiated breastfeeding. Anecdotally, many mothers report that their babies need to nurse nearly nonstop from late afternoon into the evening. Carrying the baby on their body may help. "Nursing marathons" may be frustrating for mothers, but the very frequent sucking during "marathons" seems to be highly important to the baby for food, for emotional reasons, for the sucking itself, for comfort, and/or for unknown reasons. Expectations that reassure us that the baby is progressing normally are identified in Table 8-1.

As previously noted, the newborn's sleep cycle is about 60–90 minutes (Bergman, 2013; Ludington-Hoe et al., 2006). Breastfed babies' sleep duration varies across time and differs widely among individual

Table 8-1 REASSURING SIGNS OF NORMAL PROGRESS IN THE FIRST WEEK

Reassuring Signs	Rationale
Baby is skin to skin on mother's chest many hours a day for at least 60–90 minutes or until self-wakening.	Skin-to-skin touch increases milk production and keeps baby close to mother's breast, and self-regulated sleep cycles support normal mental and physical development.
Baby is in mother's arms most of the time, and sleeps calmly and safely within arm's reach (in sensory proximity) when not being held.	Holding is comforting and increases oxytocin responses, which aid digestion and milk production and facilitate bonding and development. Unattended sleep is a risk factor.
Baby is alert ~10 hours a day, cues for feeds at least 8 or more times, and is obviously satiated after feeds.	An alert baby cues the mother to indicate that he is hungry and then that he is satisfied.
Baby rarely cries; mother responds quickly to early feeding cues before active crying begins.	Crying is a late sign of hunger and raises stress hormones in both mother and baby.
Baby actively suckles at least 140 minutes per day, 5–16 times with audible swallowing; and releases the breast spontaneously.	At least that amount of time at breast is needed to obtain sufficient milk (de Carvalho, Robertson, Merkatz et al., 1982; Kert, 2007). Swallowing reflects milk intake (Riordan, Gill-Hopple, & Angeron, 2005).
After feeds, mother's nipple is comfortable, wet, and intact; breasts are softer after feeds than before; and both mother and baby are comfortable, relaxed, and possibly drowsy.	Nipple creasing, pain, damage, and/or milk stasis suggest poor milk transfer. Hormones foster relaxation and calmness in both.
Baby and mother are satisfied with feedings.	Mothers accurately report problems with feedings.
Baby's mucous membranes are wet and skin turgor is elastic and responsive. Gently pinched skin does not remain above the normal surface (tenting).	The absence of tenting after pinching indicates that infant is sufficiently hydrated.
By the end of the first week, baby passes three to five or more loose, yellow stools per day.	Frequent stool output is one indicator of adequate nutrient intake (Nommsen-Rivers et al., 2008).
By the end of the first week, infant has six or more soaking wet diapers per day; urine is clear (not dark or concentrated).	Urine output is an indicator of adequate hydration after the first few days.
Mother reports that her milk "came in."	Mothers know their bodies.
Mother is confident in her ability to calm and feed her baby.	Confidence is an indicator of normal maternal role acquisition.

babies, ranging from 9 to 17 hours of sleep out of the 24-hour day (Galland et al., 2012), with approximately 10 hours of wakefulness (at 4 weeks) (Quillin & Glenn, 2004). Mothers get more restful quiet sleep when breastfeeding exclusively (Doan et al., 2007) and safely bedsharing (Quillin & Glenn, 2004). For the infant, each completed self-directed sleep cycle (including a period of quiet sleep) plays an important role in memory processing and neurodevelopment (Peirano et al., 2003). The hormones released in both the mother's and baby's bodies enhance and facilitate bonding and calm, restorative sleep (Uvnas-Moberg & Eriksson, 1996). Therefore, *safe* bedsharing facilitates breastfeeding, maternal rest and relaxation, and infant well-being. See the later discussion of sleeping, sudden infant death syndrome (SIDS), and bedsharing for more information on safety during bedsharing.

Common Problems in the Early Days and Weeks

Preventing problems is always easier than fixing a problem later. Prenatal breastfeeding education (Dyson et al., 2005), evidence-based hospital policies, professional education, peer support, controlling the marketing of infant formula, and mother-friendly care during labor (CDC, 2013b; Hodnett et al., 2007) establish the foundation for a smooth postpartum course. Immediate uninterrupted and sustained skin-to-skin contact beginning moments after birth and for many hours every day is the most effective and evidence-based strategy to normalize mother–baby behavior; support normal lactogenesis; avoid breast and nipple pain; assure abundant milk production; assure adequate nutrition, hydration, and comfort for the newborn; and enhance the mother's confidence and ability to breastfeed and care for her baby (Anderson et al., 2003; Dumas et al., 2013).

Baby Is Not Latching, Sucking, or Feeding Effectively

Babies are born with the inherent ability to move or crawl to the mother's breast, latch on, and begin effective feeding within about an hour after birth (Widstrom et al., 2011). When the baby is unable to latch and suck normally, everyone involved (mother, professional, and the baby) becomes frustrated. Until recently, most professionals believed that "breast refusal" was primarily due to maternal factors, including flat or inverted nipples, overfull or engorged breasts, poor positioning, or "nipple confusion" resulting from the baby learning to suck on an artificial teat or pacifier. Certainly the mother's breast shape, size, and configuration play a role in the baby's ability to latch and feed comfortably. However, as knowledge and skills improve, lactation consultants have begun to look more closely at other events and conditions that can compromise the infant's ability to latch on the breast and suckle.

The following conditions can lead to early latch and suck problems:

- Immaturity or prematurity, illness, or birth injuries (Hughes et al., 1999)
- Facial or jaw asymmetry (Wall & Glass, 2006)
- Jaundice, and/or facial anomalies such as tongue-tie or cleft lip or palate (Genna, 2013)
- Birth practices, induction of labor, and medications administered to the mother during labor:
  ◄ Epidural anesthesia or analgesia (Beilin et al., 2005; Dozier et al., 2012; Jordan et al., 2005; Montgomery & Hale, 2006; Torvaldsen et al., 2006)
  ◄ Instrument delivery (Baumgarder et al., 2003; Hall et al., 2002)
  ◄ Long, difficult labor (Dewey et al., 2003; Smith, 2007)
  ◄ Cesarean surgical birth (Evans et al., 2003; Karlstrom et al., 2007; Preer et al., 2012)
  ◄ Induction of labor, especially prior to 39 completed weeks' gestation (American Congress of Obstetricians and Gynecologists, 2013; Grivell et al., 2012)

If the baby cannot latch because of *prematurity, illness, or facial or oral structural anomalies*, collaboration with other professionals is necessary. While diagnosis and treatment plans are being developed, the lactation consultant should assist the mother to collect her milk frequently by hand-expression and/or pumping, and feed it to the baby using an open cup or other carefully selected non-teat device (WHO & UNICEF, 2009). The lactation consultant's close monitoring of the baby's development of sucking abilities, the mother's milk production, and the mother's relationship with her baby including her emotional status plays a central role in successful long-term breastfeeding (Genna, 2013).

If the baby is not latching because he is *"sleepy" or drugged from birth medications* (Wiklund et al., 2009), patience and sufficient calories (expressed colostrum or breastmilk) will buy time until the drugs are metabolized and the baby can smoothly coordinate sucking, swallowing, and breathing. Keep the mother and baby together, in skin-to-skin contact, as close to continuously as possible. Be patient, because the age and maturity of the baby, dosage and combination of drugs, and other birth interventions can all affect the baby's ability to recover and begin to breastfeed well. Some babies require several days to several weeks to recover fully. Be patient with the mother as well, because mothers who receive epidural anesthesia in labor may not exhibit the normal reduction in anxiety and aggression and increasing socialization that occur with an unmedicated birth (Jonas et al., 2008).

If the baby *can latch in only one posture or position or on only one breast*, help the mother to use that posture, position, or breast most often and at frequent intervals. Express milk from the other breast to avoid problems related to milk stasis. With patience and sufficient calories, most babies will gradually improve in skill and be able to breastfeed in other postures, in other positions, and from both breasts within a fairly short time (Genna, 2013). Increasing professional interest in therapeutic modalities such as physical or occupational therapy (Wall & Glass, 2006), chiropractic treatment or cranial–sacral therapy, or osteopathic manipulative therapy (Fraval, 1998) is occurring, as these strategies may be helpful in resolving structural or postural asymmetries in collaboration with the baby's primary care provider.

If the baby cannot latch because of the *mother's breast or nipple size or structure*, then gentle mechanical strategies may alter the breast or nipple shape sufficiently to allow latching and sucking. These strategies include, but are not limited to, brief use of a breast pump or "nipple extender" device to draw out the nipple, massage to soften the breast, shaping the nipple and areola complex, breast support, and short-term use of a thin silicone nipple shield (Chertok et al., 2006; Genna, 2009). Follow the mother–baby dyad closely if any of these devices are being used, and discontinue their use when the baby can latch and suck effectively.

If the baby *latches or sucks in a way that causes pain or nipple damage, or insufficient milk intake*, the first strategy is to remove the baby from the breast and try again using a different technique or position (Walker, 2011). A persistently painful latch indicates an infant sucking problem that needs further investigation. Suboptimal latch and suck cause pain for the mother and leave milk in her breast, which then compromises milk production and reduces

infant milk intake. Normally, the nipple tip rests deeply in the baby's mouth, and may move an average of 4 mm anterior of the hard palate–soft palate junction (Jacobs et al., 2007). Figure 8-1 shows a breastfeeding "seal" on the breast. The tongue cups around the nipple, comfortably extending the nipple back into the baby's mouth.

A deep latch assures full drainage of the milk stored in the breast (Mizuno et al., 2008). If the baby takes only the nipple tip, the upward movement of the baby's tongue during sucking will compress the nipple tip against the hard palate, causing nipple pain and damage, and restrict flow through the milk ducts, resulting in milk retention in the breast and an underfed baby (Geddes, 2007). A repositioning of the baby farther onto the breast, and/or facilitating the baby's self-directed deep attachment, may quickly result in an effective, comfortable latch (Cadwell, 2007). If a comfortable, effective latch is not achieved in a few tries, it may be counterproductive to continue attempts to latch to the point of causing nipple damage. Fear of nipple pain and damage can quickly inhibit the mother's motivation to continue (Thorley, 2005). At that point, further careful investigation of the cause(s) of poor latch will direct further strategies for resolution. In any case, the lactation consultant should continue to help the mother by assuring ongoing milk production, observing and documenting

Figure 8-1 BREASTFEEDING "SEAL" ON BREAST.

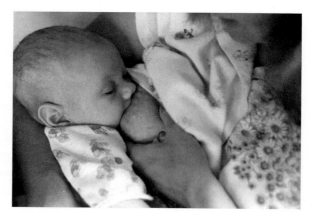

changes in the baby, and supporting and reinforcing the mother's motivation and confidence.

Some babies cannot latch and breastfeed comfortably because of *birth injuries*, including nerve injuries or damage such as brachial plexus injury/brachial palsy; fractures of the skull, clavicle, or other bones; wounds, bruises, or lacerations of the scalp, face, oropharynx, or elsewhere; swellings including cephalhematoma and caput succedaneum; muscle abnormalities including torticollis; and/or major severe complications such as subgaleal hemorrhage or intracranial hemorrhage (Parker, 2005, 2006). A baby with any of these conditions may have no outward signs or symptoms; moderate to severe pain with severe crying or crying unrelated to hunger; difficulty in some positions at breast; and/or difficulty feeding, regardless of the method used. The breastfeeding mother's instincts may serve her well in the case of hidden injuries, as she is acutely aware of even subtle aspects of her baby's behavior. Mothers' reports are reliable, and should be investigated thoroughly.

Torticollis

Torticollis is a positional deformity that is usually the result of a cramped intrauterine environment; as a result, the baby develops asymmetrical mandibles and/or tilted jaws that can make latching on to the mother's breast difficult. With torticollis, the baby consistently turns his head to one side (usually right) and tilts to the other side (usually left) because of tight muscles. Other signs are a misalignment of the eyes and ears, one ear cupped forward, and asymmetry of the jaws (see Color Plates 41, 42, 43). Assessing for torticollis is covered in the *Infant Assessment* chapter. Typically the baby prefers to breastfeed on one side and in one position, but may have other feeding difficulties as well (Wall & Glass, 2006). Use of seated baby carriers—a popular practice among today's parents—exacerbates the condition because it confines the baby's head position.

Since the 1992 "Back to Sleep" campaign to prevent SIDS (by reducing prone sleep) was initiated, the incidence of torticollis has increased among parents who do not bedshare. Before this campaign, infants often slept prone and stretched the tight neck muscle over time by turning their head from one side to the other; thus the condition resolved on its own. If torticollis is suspected, the lactation consultant should work closely with parents and refer them to the baby's primary provider and physical therapists.

Table 8-2 lists general behaviors through which to assess breastfeeding. Other evidence-based breastfeeding tools that measure breastfeeding are identified in the *Infant Assessment* chapter.

Table 8-2 ASSESSING A BREASTFEEDING

Behavior to Assess	Criteria	Rationale
Rooting	Searches with mouth and face, turns face toward breast	Readiness to feed; intact nerve responses
Angle of gape	120–160 degree angle of jaw	Allows deep latch
Shape of cheeks	Full and rounded, no dimpling or puckering	Normal pressures in mouth
Tongue placement	Under the tongue, extends past lower gum ridge, may extend past lower lip	When tongue is down, milk flows comfortably and well
Audible swallows	Quiet "ta" sound every suck or every few sucks	No clicks, slurps, smacking that indicate loss of seal
Mouth "sealed" on breast (see Figure 8-1)	Tongue cupped around breast; lips flanged; can't easily pull off	Seal indicates adequate intraoral pressures for milk flow

Table 8-2 ASSESSING A BREASTFEEDING (*CONTINUED*)

Behavior to Assess	Criteria	Rationale
Smooth rhythm of suckle/swallow/breathe	Long bursts of sucking with swallows and breathing; short pauses	Coordination needed for adequate intake
Comfortable nipple and breast	May feel nipple extend and stretch; no pain or pinching	Pain indicates poor latch or other problem
Nipple shape postfeed	Same shape as before feed; wet	Distortion indicates poor latch or suck
Breast fullness postfeed	Softer after feed than before; may not be "empty"	No change in fullness indicates lack of milk transfer

Supplementation Guidelines and Cautions

If the baby cannot breastfeed directly *for any reason*, he still must be fed. Supplementation should be undertaken only if there is an acceptable medical reason present, the mother gives fully informed consent, and the therapy is carried out in collaboration with the baby's primary care provider. The Academy of Breastfeeding Medicine's (2009) Clinical Protocol #3 and WHO's (2009) *Acceptable Medical Reasons for Use of Breast-milk Substitutes* should form the evidence basis for any medically necessary supplementation.

The full-term infant is born with additional extracellular fluid that helps maintain infant hydration in the first few days of life. After that time, neonates will experience low blood sugar disturbances, jaundice, and dehydration and eventually starvation if they are not fed. In this situation, the lactation consultant must remain in close contact with the baby's primary care provider and other professionals to investigate the cause and develop strategies for remediation of the underlying problem.

The easiest and least risky form of supplementation is to have the mother express some colostrum onto a small spoon, and spoon-feed it to her baby. Hand-expressing colostrum and milk is an essential skill for all mothers to learn, and for all healthcare professionals to be able to perform (Becker et al., 2011). The supplement itself should follow the WHO hierarchy discussed in this section; the *method* of supplementation should start with the least complicated device for the shortest time

with the goal being to establish or restore direct breastfeeding. For example, expressed colostrum fed with a small spoon may progress to the mother's own milk expressed or pumped and fed with an open cup, dropper, or tube feeding device. Continue attempts at direct breastfeeding many times a day until the baby is effectively and comfortably breastfeeding directly.

Supplemental Feeding

If the baby cannot breastfeed directly, follow WHO's hierarchy for what to feed the baby:

1. Expressed breastmilk from the infant's own mother
2. Breastmilk from a healthy wet nurse
3. Pasteurized donor human milk from a human-milk bank
4. A breastmilk substitute fed with a cup (WHO & UNICEF, 2003)

If a breastmilk substitute (formula) is unavoidable, WHO and UNICEF (2003) recommend an infant formula prepared in accordance with applicable Codex Alimentarius standards. Ready-to-use preparations are the least risky option. Concentrated formula must be diluted with clean water before use according to the container or package directions. Powdered formula is the riskiest option, and should be carefully prepared according to WHO (2007) guidelines. Reconstituted powdered formula is not sterile; furthermore, it provides an ideal environment for the growth of pathogens. Errors in adding too much or too little water can be made, especially by the low-literacy or non-English-speaking caregiver. Parents who need to use formula should be taught (through one-to-one education, not in a group class) how to safely prepare and use it after their baby is born. Formula preparation guidelines can be found at http://www.who.int/foodsafety/publications/micro/pif2007/en/. Prices of formula vary widely, so families should do comparative shopping. Information on formula recalls can be found at http://www.fda.gov.

Formula supplements can be fed by small cup, spoon, or bottle-and-teat (nipple)—that is, using any of the same devices used to feed breastmilk. Cups are least likely to alter infant suck in ways that compromise breastfeeding. If bottles and teats are chosen, select a nipple that allows the baby to suck, swallow, and breathe at a comfortable pace without choking or collapsing the nipple (Wolf & Glass, 1992).

It is unsafe to heat formula in a microwave because the heat is not distributed evenly and can burn the baby. Propping the bottle is dangerous because the baby may aspirate formula while sleeping. Moreover, lying flat puts the infant at risk for ear infections because pooled milk in the pharynx is a medium for bacterial growth. The baby should be held and cuddled during all feeds and for a short while afterward. Paced bottle-feeding is a helpful strategy (Kassing, 2001).

Encourage the mother to keep the baby in skin-to-skin contact on her chest, support the milk supply, continue attempts at breastfeeding, and keep the dyad together in a calm, supportive environment. Carefully document these situations to assist the family and other professionals, and provide future researchers with data central to investigating the causes of and solutions to persistent breast refusal or failure to latch on. A history of feeding difficulty may be a sign of significant and serious infant illness (Weber, Clinical Signs Study Group, 2008).

Nipple Pain

Nipple pain is a common, early postpartum concern and a primary cause of early discontinuation of breastfeeding that can affect the mother's entire relationship with her baby (McClellan et al., 2012). Nipple pain can result from physical (mechanical) trauma, infection, or other conditions. The pain can range from mild tenderness to stinging, itching, burning, stabbing, aching, sharp, dull, and even excruciating pain; and can occur at the start of the feed, occur throughout the feed, persist long after the feed, or even occur between feeds. The quality, characteristics, and duration of the pain may help identify the cause and direct the resolution. Most nipple pain falls into two general categories: early onset, which is primarily mechanical in origin, and late onset, which is more likely related to infection.

Early-Onset Nipple Pain

Pain that occurs during the first week postpartum, usually peaking between the third and seventh days, is classified as early onset (Wagner et al., 2013). Typically, the pain occurs as the baby latches on to the breast and may last for 20–30 seconds or even for the entire feed if the latch is shallow or suboptimal (Wilson-Clay & Hoover, 2013). Color Plate 44 shows a close-up of changes in nipple skin condition with transient soreness with mechanical-origin nipple pain. Early nipple pain may have diverse roots and should be investigated promptly and thoroughly (McClellan et al., 2012).

Most early nipple pain is mechanical in origin, caused by inappropriate or abrasive pressures on the nipple skin, and not from infection or organic conditions. One feature of mechanical pain is a changed shape of the nipple (peaked, wedge shaped, white crease across the tip, wounds on the frontal surface) after the baby releases the nipple (see Figure 8-2). In a normal feed, the nipple should come out of the baby's mouth intact, in the same shape as before the feed began (Figure 8-3), and possibly wet with milk or saliva.

Mechanical pain is nearly always related to something the infant is doing in or with his mouth, either in compensation for or consequence of a suboptimal latch or suck, such as in the newborn with tongue-tie or unusually strong sucking pressure (McClellan et al., 2008) or deliberately (as in the older child experimenting with biting during

Figure 8-2 CREASED NIPPLE POST FEED.

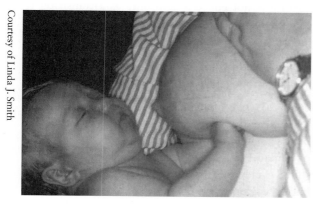

Figure 8-3 NORMAL NIPPLE POST FEED.

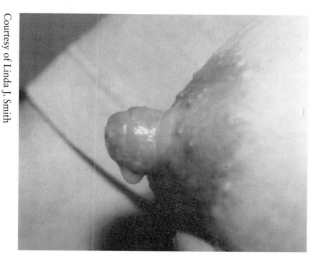

no single ideal nipple position for effective breast-feeding in normal term infants (Jacobs et al., 2007). Mothers should expect a stretching sensation in the nipple during feeding, as the human nipple stretches to more than twice its resting length in the baby's mouth (Ardran et al., 1958). When *sensation* becomes *pain* may be difficult to assess. An objective sign of excess or unusual mechanical pressure is the shape of the mother's nipple post feed. Because mechanical trauma is caused by or associated with poor latch and/or poor suck, the first remedy is correcting positioning and latch (Blair et al., 2003; Enkin et al., 2000). Poor latch and poor suck quickly result in inadequate infant milk intake and milk retention in the breast. Milk flows fastest during the downward motion of the baby's jaw and when the posterior tongue drops (Geddes, 2007); therefore, a baby who clamps his jaws tightly onto the breast is limiting milk flow. If mechanical nipple pain or damage occurs, it is very likely the infant is obtaining inadequate milk and milk stasis is increasing, causing further consequences to milk production and breast comfort.

Tongue-tie, or ankyloglossia, which is the presence of a short or tight lingual frenulum that restricts tongue movement necessary for comfortable and effective breastfeeding, can cause severe nipple pain and damage, and functionally compromises feeding ability of the newborn, resulting in early weaning, failure to thrive, and nipple damage (see Color Plate 51). Surgically releasing a restrictive tongue-tie by an incision in the frenulum is effective and widely accepted (Emond et al., 2013). Frenotomy performed by a qualified provider quickly relieves nipple pain (Buryk et al., 2011; Geddes et al., 2008; Srinivasan et al., 2006), improves latch and milk transfer (Griffiths, 2004), and fosters longer exclusive breastfeeding (Amir et al., 2006; Ricke et al., 2005). Tongue-tie is discussed in greater detail in the *Low Intake in the Breastfed Infant* chapter. The frenotomy procedure is described in Lawrence and Lawrence (2011, Appendix P, p. 1025).

Anatomic variations of the infant's oral space, of nipple size, or of nipple elasticity can cause mechanical pain and damage. Lactation consultants report nipple pain and trauma associated with a high

nursing). A shallow latch places the nipple tip too far anterior in the baby's mouth, causing friction of the nipple surface by the tongue as it presses the nipple against the hard palate with resulting pain and damage. It is thought that nipple pain and damage from improper placement of the nipple in the baby's mouth can occur quickly (Widstrom & Thingstrom-Paulsson, 1993), even during the first feeding; however, newer research indicates there is or "bubble-shaped" palate in the infant (Snyder, 1995). Very large or fibrous nipples that are significantly bigger than the infant's oral space can cause pain or be damaged until the baby's mouth grows larger and can accommodate the mother's nipple and areola comfortably (Stark, 1993). A retracted or inverted nipple, even one that is optimally positioned in the baby's mouth, may rub on the baby's palate during feeds for a time.

Resolving Early-Onset/Mechanical Nipple Pain

A "normal-looking" latch or suck pattern that causes nipple distortion and discomfort is *not* a normal latch or suck pattern. The first strategy is to release the baby from the breast and start over. It often helps to put the baby skin to skin on the mother's chest in a ventral position, with guidance from the mother by moving her breast and/or nipple to meet his mouth, allowing the baby to self-attach (Smillie, 2007). Holding the baby in different positions (vertically, horizontally, or at a 45-degree angle) may improve the latch or suck. If one position results in comfortable feeding with good milk transfer, use that position more than others.

A poor latch and suck that continues to damage the nipple is not helping either the mother or the baby. A flattened, creased, crushed nipple indicates that the milk ducts are being compressed, which restricts milk flow, leaves milk in the breast, and fails to transfer milk to the baby. If repositioning does not resolve the nipple pain and distortion fairly quickly, *do not keep trying for extended periods* because severe nipple damage can occur. Help the mother express or pump her milk and feed her baby with a cup or other device for a few feeds, or even a few days while the situation is investigated further.

Limiting the length or frequency of feeds does not prevent nipple pain or damage, because the *quality* of the feed is more likely to be the cause of the pain and/or injury than the *quantity* of nursing sessions. Limiting time at breast reduces milk flow to the infant, resulting in underfeeding for the infant and milk retention in the breast for the mother. Use of pacifiers and feeding bottles is associated

with painful nipples at hospital discharge (Centuori et al., 1999). In general, feeding bottles should be used as a last and temporary resort if direct breastfeeding is not effective and only as a transition to direct breastfeeding. If bottles are elected, careful choice of shape, flow rate, and technique (Kassing, 2001) is essential to minimize potential risks.

Currently, there are no peer-reviewed policies, protocols, or guidelines for nipple shield use (Eglash et al., 2010). Many clinicians, however, believe that placing a nipple shield (silicone) over the nipple briefly may protect the nipple from further abrasion or damage. If such a device is used, make sure the shield is cleaned thoroughly after every use, and fits both the nipple and the baby's mouth. Some mothers have found that wearing breast shells between feedings protects wounded skin from clothing rubbing on the wound. These devices do not hasten healing, however. If nipple pain persists or returns when the baby again latches onto the breast directly, continue expressing milk to maintain milk production, and seek further evaluation of the baby.

If the nipple skin is cracked, abraded, or wounded, rinse the nipple skin with clean water after every feed, just as you would clean broken skin elsewhere on the body. Cracked skin can quickly become infected with bacteria and/or yeast, and infected wounds are more painful and heal slowly. When the skin is abraded, frequent hand washing, especially before handling the breasts and nipples, will reduce risk of infection. If the skin is broken, consider applying a thin coating of a topical (non-neomycin-based) antibiotic to prevent infection with *Staphylococcus aureus* (Livingstone & Stringer, 1999). There are no reported adverse effects of a topical antibiotic on the infant.

Avoid use of nipple ointments, creams, antiseptics, tea bags, wound dressings, food-based oils, gels, and other topical remedies that were once recommended to prevent or treat sore nipples. Studies comparing various ointments and other preparations have yielded mixed results and according to one fairly recent and rigorous systematic review by Morland-Schultz and Hill (2005), no single topical agent was more effective than others in reducing nipple discomfort/pain. Furthermore, cases of severe contact dermatitis have been reported after use of various nipple creams, so caution is advised whenever a topical product is suggested to the mother.

If no infection is present in or on the nipple skin, air-blocking products may increase the mother's comfort. For example, purified lanolin is advertised as being able to create a moisture barrier that prevents evaporation, thereby allowing healing from within. A recent clinical trial (Abou-Dakn et al., 2011) compared purified hospital grade lanolin to expressed breast milk, in combination with education, in the treatment of damaged and painful nipples. This single-blind study ($n = 84$) demonstrated significant positive effects of the lanolin on pain (absolute risk reduction 0.61) and nipple trauma healing time (absolute risk reduction 0.43) on day 3 of treatment. Hydrogels, another air-blocking product, are glycerin-based or water-based nonadhesive patches that are designed to be placed over the nipple between feeds to prevent drying (Dennis et al., 2008). Rubbing expressed mothers milk (EMM) into broken nipple skin is widely recommended to aid healing based on the hypothesis that antibodies, inflammatory factors, and anti-inflammatory factors such as bifidus and lactoferrin will prevent trauma or help the healing process, but evidence to support its healing properties is not supportive (Abou-Dakn et al, 2011; Morland-Schultz & Hill, 2005).

Any known infection present in cracked, cut, or broken skin must be treated before any ointments, creams, or gels are applied. Keep in mind that two people are exposed to the product whenever it is used on the mother's nipples. What might be comforting for the mother could expose the infant to unnecessary risk. Furthermore, if a product must be removed completely from the nipple to avoid infant exposure, the care provider should consider whether some other strategy might be more appropriate, as removing the product may cause more damage to the nipple than any healing or pain relief from its use. Table 8-3 provides a clinical care plan for sore nipples.

It is evident that further research is needed in the area of treatment for early nipple pain and trauma. However, double-blind randomized controlled trials of treatments for nipple pain are usually not done because it is difficult, if not impossible, for the mother *not* to know which treatment she is using

---

Table 8-3 CLINICAL CARE PLAN FOR SORE NIPPLES

Assessment	Rationale	Interventions
Nipples are sensitive with no visible color changes and no skin breakdown.	Nipples are sensitive in early breastfeeding. Nipple skin stretches during feeds.	Assure deep latch. Reassure that stretching sensation is normal. Monitor daily.
Pain at latch-on that diminishes within a few seconds.	Stretching is a new sensation. Baby draws breast deeper into mouth as feed progresses.	Assure deep latch. Reassure that stretching sensation is normal. Monitor closely.
Pain at latch-on that persists during most or all of the feed.	Shallow latch or possible suck problem. Baby may be pulling tongue back (humping) due to a variety of oral conditions.	Massage to trigger let-down may help. Assure deep latch, or remove baby then reposition with deeper latch. If nothing relieves pain, hand-express and cup-feed while oral conditions are evaluated.
Stabbing or shooting pain radiating out from the nipple during, after, or between feeds.	Pain seems to follow the course of the 4th intercostal nerve. Could be trauma from gumming or biting, or infection.	Careful evaluation in collaboration with primary care providers. Assure deep latch. Evaluate suck and oral anatomy. Investigate possible infection.

(continues)

Table 8-3 CLINICAL CARE PLAN FOR SORE NIPPLES (CONTINUED)

Assessment	Rationale	Interventions
Cracks in nipple skin, abrasions on nipple tip.	Friction of nipple on baby's hard palate due to shallow latch or sucking problem.	Assure deep latch. Investigate baby's mouth and suck. Rinse skin with clean water, wash hands frequently, apply air-occluding preparation to prevent scab formation. Anti-inflamatory meds may help. Follow closely.
Nipple pain plus baby makes clicking sound while sucking.	Tongue is losing contact with nipple during suck-swallow sequence.	Check for tongue-tie or other oral anatomic variation. Assure deep latch, try other positions. Refer and collaborate if oral anatomy is abnormal.
Nipple tip is blanched (white, almost waxy in appearance) after feeds; may turn red or blue after feeds.	Probably nipple vasospasm (Reynaud's phenomenon). Previous nipple injury, poor blood flow to nipple.	Keep nipple and breast warm. Prescribed vasodilators may help. Mother may have vasospasms in other extremeties.
Inflamed skin on nipple and/or areola. Pain continues throughout feed and even between feeds and with pumping.	Possible infection - bacterial, yeast, or both. Possible contact dermatitis from creams or ointments.	Rinse with water before and after feeds. Collaborate with primary care provider(s) for diagnosis and treatment. Hand-express and cup-feed if direct feeds are too painful. Anti-inflammatory medications may help.
Blisters, lesions, cracks that do not heal.	Probable infection with yeast, bacteria, or both.	Collaborate with primary care provider(s) for diagnosis and treatment. Investigate other family members for yeast or bacterial infections.

on her nipples. However, single-blind clinical trials that incorporate other methods of prospective clinical trials, such as intention to treat and large samples (e.g., the previously mentioned study by Abou-Dakn et al., 2011), can provide useful evidence related to current therapies for this important problem that impacts early breastfeeding experiences for so many mothers.

Sudden Nipple Pain After a Period of Comfortable Breastfeeding

Sudden or late-onset nipple pain usually indicates an infection (fungal, bacterial, viral, or—very rarely—parasitic) or inflammatory process; a skin or vascular disorder such as psoriasis; or an allergic reaction, including eczema. Sudden-onset pain can also be caused by ineffective nursing techniques (allowing the baby to slide down onto the nipple tip or clamp down), or nipple vasospasm (Raynaud's phenomenon) (Barrett et al., 2013). In very rare cases, sudden-onset nipple pain or changes can be a malignancy. Nipple skin infections are usually shared by the baby (or babies) and require appropriate diagnosis and simultaneous treatment of all infected skin surfaces, often with prescription medications. Anything that has come into contact with the baby's mouth must be thoroughly cleaned and disinfected, including pacifiers, teething products, and nipples. These and other breast-related disorders are covered in more detail in the *Breast-Related Problems* chapter.

Engorgement + Milk Stasis = Involution

Engorgement is a confusing term that is often applied to any type of breast fullness, including edema, milk stasis, or both. Normal onset of lactogenesis II involves the marshaling of lymph and a rapid increase in lactose synthesis that changes the composition of the secreted milk, causing the onset of copious milk production. This process typically is felt by mothers around 60 hours after birth (range 24–102 hours) (Arthur et al., 1989; Kulski & Hartmann, 1981). *Edema*, an accumulation of abnormal quantities of fluid in the interstitial spaces, may be present already or occur simultaneously with the rapid rise in milk volume under certain conditions, and is usually short-lived. *Milk stasis* or breastmilk retention is an uncomfortable breast fullness that can occur at any time during lactation when excess milk remains in the breast, causing distension of the alveoli and distortion of the individual secretory cells. Milk stasis is caused by ineffective and/or infrequent removal of milk from the breast, resulting in overfullness. Given that the milk storage capacity of the breasts is variable, some breasts will reach an overfull, distended state more quickly than others. Milk storage capacities in mothers who are exclusively breastfeeding range from 81 to 606 mL per breast (Daly et al., 1993; Kent et al., 2006), and capacities may change during the duration of breastfeeding (Ramsay et al., 2006).

Milk Stasis

Milk stasis is easier to prevent than to correct later. The best prevention and resolution for *milk stasis* comprises early, frequent, and effective breastfeeding by any means, preferably a well-positioned baby with a normal, effective latch and suck response (Enkin et al., 2000; Snowden et al., 2001). The causes of milk stasis can include poor suck, scheduled as opposed

to cue-based feeds, milk synthesis that exceeds the baby's ability to remove available milk, and factors that keep the baby away from the breast. Regardless of the causes, the result is the same: milk is retained in the breast. Depending on the storage capacity of each individual breast, at some point the breast's capacity to store milk is exceeded and the process of involution begins. First, components of the milk itself exert a feedback inhibition on the mammary secretory epithelial cells (lactocytes), resulting in a slower rate of milk synthesis (Daly et al., 1993). If milk is not removed, eventually the physical distension of the alveoli causes further disruption of milk synthesis (Cregan & Hartmann, 1999).

Removal of retained milk will reverse these processes as long as milk removal is begun soon after stasis occurs. Unrelieved milk stasis triggers mammary involution. At some point in time, involution becomes irreversible as the lactocytes, which are necessary for milk synthesis, are deactivated (or destroyed through apoptosis) for that particular lactation cycle (Neville & Neifert, 1983; Wilde et al., 1999). It is unknown when the point of irreversibility is reached in women. Milk stasis can also lead to plugged ducts and inflammatory reactions in the breast, then to infectious mastitis, and then, if not corrected, to breast abscess (Walker, 2011). Milk stasis is primarily a mechanical problem; therefore, a mechanical solution is needed. The core strategy in addressing all forms of milk stasis is frequent, thorough removal of milk from the breast, preferably by the baby, by hand-expression, and/or by pumping.

When milk stasis occurs for more than a few hours, for any reason and especially in the first few days after birth, it is crucial to assure frequent and adequate milk removal both for the baby's sake and to assure long-term lactation functional capacity of the breast. The rate of growth of mammary tissue necessary for ongoing milk synthesis slows after a few weeks. Milk production on day 6 is significantly associated with milk production at week 6 (Hill & Aldag, 2005). Therefore, the top priority is removing milk from the breast, which then can be provided to the baby.

Hand expression is more effective (Ohyama et al., 2010; Parker et al., 2012) and often more comfortable compared with pumping, especially during the first 48 hours postpartum. Short, frequent expression or pumping periods may be more effective than long sessions. Pump or express until at least two milk-ejection reflexes (letdown) are observed, then continue until drops of milk no longer flow for 2 minutes (Engstrom et al., 2007). Empty breasts may secrete milk rapidly (up to 2 ounces or 58 mL per hour per breast), so be prepared to repeat the process frequently, especially if the breasts have relatively small storage capacity. On average, breasts make milk at a rate of 1 ounce (30 mL) per breast per hour (Kent, 2007).

Edema

Breast edema is common, generally short lived, and sometimes devastating. Edema in the tissue surrounding the milk ducts (interstitial) appears to inhibit full dilation of the milk ducts during the milk-ejection reflex, thus causing or exacerbating milk stasis in the breast. Lactation consultants have reported an apparent increase in breast and areolar edema following administration of IV fluids during labor and it has been documented by research (Nommsen-Rivers et al., 2010). It is possible that overhydration during labor leads to dilution of plasma protein, resulting in increased interstitial fluid in the breast after birth (Smith & Kroeger, 2010). The total amount of intravenous fluids given and the flow rate at which they are delivered may play a role in breast edema (Chantry et al., 2011; Nommsen-Rivers et al., 2010).

To resolve this problem, first assure skin-to-skin contact and allow the infant to self-attach. If the baby clearly cannot do so, then use hand expression to remove some milk and feed it to the baby by spoon or open cup. If the edema is severe enough to prevent adequate milk removal (by any means), then it must be reduced before further attempts at milk removal. Application of cold packs for about 20 minutes followed by removing the cold packs for at least the same length of time (Walker, 2011); gentle massage to mobilize lymph (Chikly, 2004); anti-inflammatory medications; reverse-pressure softening using the flower hold (Cotterman, 2004) (see Figure 8-4); or areola compression (Miller & Riordan, 2004) are suggested (but still experimental) strategies to reduce edema and increase milk flow (International Lactation Consultants Association [ILCA], 2014). Applying heat to swollen breast tissue is *not* appropriate. Once milk is flowing freely, milk removal can be accomplished by any method, preferably the baby's direct breastfeeding.

Figure 8-4 REVERSE PRESSURE SOFTENING BY FLOWER HOLD BASED ON JEAN COTTERMAN'S THEORY.

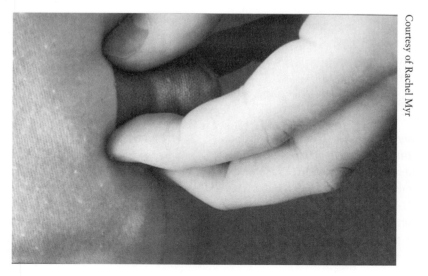

Courtesy of Rachel Myr

Milk Supply/Milk Production

"Not enough milk" is a major worry during the first few weeks postpartum, and it is one of the most common reasons given by mothers for early weaning and for supplementation. Actually, milk *production* insufficiency is quite rare. Mammalian survival has depended for millennia on sufficient breastmilk production to meet the needs of the young. If actual milk insufficiency occurred frequently, the species' survival would be in jeopardy.

Unrealistic expectations of infant behavior are major issues for mothers and professionals alike. Babies need frequent feeds because their small stomach capacity parallels lactation secretion patterns, as outlined earlier in this chapter. Expecting breasts or babies to sleep or go for long stretches between large meals is physiologically unrealistic, inappropriate, and counterproductive. Unethical marketing of infant formula continues to play a major role in fostering "milk supply" insecurities among families and even professionals.

Any event, behavior, custom, or practice that keeps the baby away from the breast or causes milk to remain in the breast for long periods (more than 4–6 hours) has the potential to inhibit milk production. These factors include, but are not limited to, scheduled feeds, use of bottles without corresponding expression of milk, use of pacifiers so that suckling time at the breast markedly decreases (see the section on pacifiers), and/or maternal or infant illness (Table 8-4).

Table 8-4 CONCERNS OR WORRIES ABOUT MILK SUPPLY

Stated Concern or Worry	What Is Probably or Actually Happening	What to Do About This
Baby is fussy, irritable, cries or whimpers frequently	Probably hungry for milk, sucking, mother, and/or all of the above. If not hungry and being carried, then possibly sick or injured.	Breastfeed again. Increase carrying and skin-to-skin contact. Check for poor latch or poor suck or scheduled feeds.
Baby sucks fist or roots again soon after a feed.	Probably hungry again, or low intake in previous feed.	Breastfeed again. Increase carrying and skin-to-skin contact. Check for poor latch or poor suck or scheduled feeds.
Baby shakes head, can't stay latched, comes off nipple frequently.	Breasts too full; suck problem and/or tongue-tie.	Express milk and feed by cup and get baby's suck evaluated.
Baby has consistently long (>30 minutes per side) or short (<5 minutes per side) feeds; falls asleep but doesn't release breast.	May be normal if baby is thriving and healthy. If baby is not thriving, or mother is exasperated, seek skilled help.	Express milk and feed by cup while baby is evaluated thoroughly.
Baby eagerly takes formula or pumped milk from a bottle right after a feeding.	Normal if suck is poor; may be a very rapid-flow nipple, and baby can't control the flow of milk easily.	Express milk and feed by cup while baby and mother are evaluated thoroughly.
Mother does not feel the let-down (milk-ejection) reflex.	Multiple let-downs occur during feeds but mothers may not sense any, or only the first (Ramsay et al., 2006).	Reassure and encourage mother to watch and listen for infant swallowing or milk flowing during pumping.

(continues)

Table 8-4 CONCERNS OR WORRIES ABOUT MILK SUPPLY (*CONTINUED*)

Stated Concern or Worry	What Is Probably or Actually Happening	What to Do About This
Breasts still full and hard after feeds.	Poor milk transfer; often because of poor latch, poor infant suck, and/or edema.	Express or pump milk; investigate infant suck.
Breasts are soft most of the time.	Normal.	Reassure.
Can't pump much milk.	Some mothers do not release milk to any pump.	Breastfeed; hand-express or try a different pump.
Baby wants to breastfeed "constantly."	Probably normal or unrealistic expectation of infant behavior.	Observe; track length and duration of feeds and infant output; follow up.
Previous breast surgery.	Surgery may affect lactation capacity.	Follow closely especially in the first week postpartum.
Breasts too small (or large).	Probably a cultural myth; rarely is a true insufficiency.	Evaluate and reassure; refer to mother-support groups.

Most mothers have sufficient lactation capacity to synthesize at least one-third more milk than their baby typically takes (Daly et al., 1996). However, if the breasts are not drained of about two-thirds of the milk most of the time by the baby's suckling or expressing, the rate of milk synthesis slows down to match the lowered demand; therefore, total daily production falls. Breast storage capacity also matters. If a mother has smaller milk storage capacity, her baby will need to feed more frequently to obtain all the milk he needs. Mothers with a large storage capacity may be able to provide larger feeds at longer intervals (if the baby is willing). If a baby cannot remove sufficient milk from the breast, milk synthesis will quickly diminish unless the mother begins pumping or expressing milk. Regular milk removal will maintain the mother's milk supply while the causes of her baby's poor suck are investigated and resolved.

Temporary Low Milk Production and Delayed Onset of Lactogenesis

The onset of lactogenesis II (the onset of copious milk secretion, or "milk coming in") occurs on average 30–40 hours after the delivery of the placenta

that triggers a sharp drop in circulating progesterone. Retained placental fragments can inhibit the fall of progesterone, thereby delaying onset of lactogenesis II (Neifert et al., 1981). During lactogenesis II, lactose synthesis rapidly increases, drawing water into what has been colostrum and resulting in a sweeter and less viscous fluid referred to as "transitional milk." Mothers perceive this event on average about 50 to 60 hours postbirth (range 24–102 hours), after the increased rate of synthesis is well under way and as their breasts fill with milk.

Delayed onset of lactogenesis II is associated with several factors: cesarean birth and high levels of stress to the mother and fetus during birth (Chapman & Perez-Escamilla, 1999; Chen et al., 1998; Dewey, 2001; Nommsen-Rivers et al., 2010; Scott et al., 2007), premature delivery, insulin-dependent diabetes mellitus, obesity, and endocrine disturbances. Delayed onset of lactogenesis II is a predictor of the cessation of any or exclusive breastfeeding (Brownell et al., 2012). Whether the delay is a maternal physiological response, due to delayed or ineffective suckling, or a combination of factors, has not yet been clearly established. Early, frequent, and effective breastfeeding appears to be the most important factor in establishing normal lactation

(Evans et al., 1995). Prolactin bursts associated with the infant suckling or breast pumping support the continued growth of secretory tissue for several weeks or months after birth (Cox et al., 1999).

Very few women are physically unable to make sufficient milk for one baby. Neville and Morton (2001) categorize failed lactogenesis as (1) preglandular, owing to a retained placenta or lack of pituitary prolactin; (2) glandular, caused by surgical procedures or insufficient mammary tissue; or (3) postglandular, caused by ineffective or infrequent milk removal. They observe that the latter category has received insufficient attention. Studies have also reported breast hypoplasia as a marker of lactation insufficiency (Huggins et al., 2000). See Table 8-5.

Too Much Milk (Oversupply/ Overproduction)

Some women make far more milk than their baby can comfortably accommodate, which can be almost as big a problem as not making enough milk. In such a case, the baby chokes, twists, and pulls back to escape the sudden flow of milk upon letdown. The mother's breasts leak to the point of interfering with daily activities, resulting in wet clothes and embarrassment in public places. Babies may have a problem with suckle–swallow–breathe coordination—in other words, this may be a baby problem, not primarily a maternal problem.

Usually overproduction problems diminish as the supply-and-demand mechanism adjusts itself. There are several approaches to dealing with a baby who chokes or gags because of high breastmilk volume or rapid flow: deliberately reduce milk volume and/or carefully investigate suckle–swallow–breathe problems in the baby. Given that "oversupply" can mask an infant problem, be sure to investigate the baby's ability to feed before attempting to alter milk production (Genna, 2013). The baby's suckling coordination almost always improves over time: by about 6 to 8 weeks post birth, the baby

Table 8-5 STRATEGIES TO INCREASE MILK PRODUCTION

Strategy	Rationale
Breastfeed on cue; at least 8–16 sessions per day.	This is how breastfeeding works.
Drain each breast thoroughly at least once a day.	Empty breasts make more milk rapidly.
Empty the breast(s) more often.	Milk is made rapidly when breast is emptiest and slower as the breast fills with milk. Milk stasis causes build-up of inhibiting factors; pressure of retained milk distorts cell function.
No long periods (> 5 hours) without milk removal.	Five hours is longer than most babies go between feeds; overfull breasts cause slower milk production.
Change or add method(s) of milk removal.	Babies with effective suck are best; hand-expression, hospital-grade pumps, other pumps.
Increase diameter of pump flange.	Larger diameter flanges allow duct expansion and more flow.
Massage breasts gently.	Mechanically compresses alveoli (Jones, Dimmock, & Spencer, 2001)
Stop hormonal medications.	Estrogen suppresses lactation; progesterone may also.
Check endocrine levels.	Endocrine system affects lactation.
Check for pregnancy.	Pregnancy will reduce milk volume and change composition.
Use lactation-enhancing drugs as a last resort.	Drugs have side effects including psychological ones.

should have overcome birth-related difficulties. Furthermore, the mother's milk supply will almost always regulate itself to what the baby takes within about 6 to 8 weeks postpartum. If the baby consistently chokes when the mother's milk lets down or has difficulty handling fast-flowing milk, carefully evaluate the baby before interpreting this situation as an oversupply issue. A baby with true gastroesophageal reflux may have some of the same symptoms (see *The Ill Child* chapter).

After careful evaluation of the baby by the lactation consultant and primary care providers and assurance that the mother is breastfeeding her normal baby on cue without pumping or otherwise altering the mother–baby nursing rhythms, the mother may wish to employ some management changes.

- Use only one breast at each feeding, for several feedings in a row over several hours. This strategy is based on autocrine control of milk synthesis. Do not try to make the baby take the second breast.
- Pump or express milk carefully, only enough to relieve distension. Do not attempt to empty the breast.
- Experiment with nursing in different positions, especially with the baby higher than the breast (mother reclining, baby facing downward). Some babies will nurse in one position much more comfortably than others, at least in the early weeks of life.
- Chart the baby's behavior at breast over a few days. If one position or breast results in better nursing sessions, use those positions more often. Check the baby for birth injuries.

If milk production greatly exceeds the baby's need for an extended period (more than a few weeks), carefully investigate the mother–baby dyad's feeding patterns looking for pacifier use, scheduled feeds (length and/or frequency), separation during nighttime sleeping, hours regularly spent apart, milk expression during separations, and family health and social issues. Also refer the mother to a provider who can thoroughly evaluate her endocrine function and other health factors. If the mother's milk production is so high that she is experiencing clogged milk ducts or mastitis, then reducing milk production may be necessary. If excess milk production (more than 60 mL per hour) continues, a referral to the mother's physician for consideration of pharmacologic reduction of milk synthesis is appropriate (Livingstone, 1996; Wilson-Clay & Hoover, 2013).

Effects of Pharmaceutical Agents on Milk Supply

The lactation consultant should always ask the mother if she is taking any prescription or nonprescription drugs, herbal remedies, homeopathic preparations, or other substances. Estrogen-containing contraceptives will quickly reduce milk supply. Some women will experience a reduction in supply from progestin-only preparations if they are used prior to 6 weeks postbirth (see the *Drug Therapy and Breastfeeding* chapter). Some herbs are inappropriate to take during lactation. Consuming encapsulated placenta reintroduces estrogen and progesterone, which suppresses milk synthesis.

The Academy of Breastfeeding Medicine Clinical Protocol #9 reviews the effects of prescribed and nonprescribed galactagogues. It makes the following recommendation: "Prior to the use of a galactagogue, thorough evaluation should be performed of the entire feeding process by a lactation expert" (Academy of Breastfeeding Medicine, 2011).

Dopamine antagonist drugs used for treating gastroesophageal reflux are known to raise serum prolactin levels, although circulating prolactin plays more of a permissive role than a regulatory role in milk synthesis. Metoclopramide (Reglan) and domperidone (Motilium) are used to increase a mother's low milk supply, especially when she has given birth prematurely (da Silva et al., 2001). Both metoclopramide and domperidone pass into milk with no measurable effects on the infant. Unlike domperidone, metoclopramide affects

Table 8-6 STRATEGIES TO HELP REDUCE OR LOWER MILK PRODUCTION

Strategy	Rationale
Allow up to two-thirds of the milk to remain in the breast unless doing so causes discomfort.	Feedback inhibition of lactation (properties of the milk itself) down-regulates the rate of milk synthesis.
Let the baby finish the first side first; don't press him to take the second side.	Infant appetite usually regulates milk production.
Express or pump the full breast, removing less than two-thirds of the milk in the breast. Save the milk for future use.	Avoid overdistension and pain. Collected milk can be used later.
Use lactation-inhibiting drugs as a last resort.	Drugs have side effects; some permanently affect lactation.

nervous system and is associated with maternal depression in long-term (more than 4 weeks) use. (See the *Drug Therapy and Breastfeeding* chapter for a detailed discussion of these drugs.)

Breast Massage

Massage of the lactating breasts is not the same technique as manual expression of milk, and can be used alone or combined with milk expression. Several techniques have been described or taught by various authors or sources. Morton reported that use of hand techniques (breast massage) during pumping increases both milk production and caloric content in milk being collected for premature babies (Morton, Hall, Wong, et al., 2009; Morton, Wong, Hall, et al., 2012).

Bolman et al. (2013) reported that Russian techniques of breast massage and hand expression are effective therapies for milk stasis, engorgement, plugged ducts, and mastitis. Jones et al. (2001) conducted a randomized controlled trial of methods of milk expression following preterm delivery and found that double-pumping with massage increased milk volume but not fat concentrations. Foda et al. (2004) studied Oketani massage and found higher levels of lipids after expression. Lymph drainage massage anecdotally shows promise when edema is present. Massage may be helpful as long as it is performed gently, by the mother herself or a skilled

clinician, and in combination with regular and frequent milk removal by any means, preferably the baby (Table 8-7).

Nausea and Other Negative Feelings During the Milk-Ejection

Maternal nausea while breastfeeding is uncommon but distressing, and is most likely due to high levels of oxytocin and other hormones active during milk ejection. Some mothers have found relief by eating before breastfeeding or using acupressure techniques (Walker, 2011). Dysphoric milk-ejection reflex (D-MER) has been reported in several journals. Heise and Wiessinger (2011) describe D-MER as an abrupt emotional "drop" that occurs in some women just before milk release and continues for a few minutes. The brief negative feelings range in severity from wistfulness to self-loathing, and appear to have a physiological cause. Heise and Wiessinger (2011) suggest that an abrupt drop in dopamine may occur when milk release is triggered, resulting in a real or relatively brief dopamine deficit for affected women. Clinicians can support women with D-MER in several ways; often, simply knowing that it is a recognized phenomenon makes the condition tolerable.

Table 8-7 BREAST MASSAGE TECHNIQUES

Description or Technique	Author, Source, Date
"Massage the milk producing cells and ducts. Start at the top of the breast. Press firmly into the chest wall. Move fingers in a circular motion on one spot on the skin. Stroke the breast area from the top of the breast to the nipple with a light tickle-like stroke. Shake the breast while leaning forward so that gravity will help the milk eject."	Marmet C. Lactation Institute, 1978–1998.
"The mother sits in a chair and someone standing behind her briskly rubs the knuckles of a fist from the base of the mother's neck to the bottom of her shoulder blades on both sides of her spine."	La Leche League, traditional.
"Gentle tactile stimulation of mammary and nipple tissue using a hand action that rolled the knuckles downward over the breast, beginning at the ribs and working towards the areola."	Spencer et al., 1998.
"When the baby is nibbling at the breast and no longer drinking with the breast. *Do not roll your fingers along the breast toward the baby, just squeeze.* Not so hard that it hurts, and try not to change the shape of the areola (the part of the breast near the baby's mouth). With the compression, the baby should start drinking again with the 'open mouth wide—*pause*—then close mouth' type of suck. *Use compression while the baby is sucking* but not drinking! Keep the pressure up until the baby no longer drinks even with the compression, and then release the pressure. Often the baby will stop sucking altogether when the pressure is released, but will start again shortly as milk starts to flow again. If the baby does not stop sucking with the release of pressure, wait a short time before compressing again. The reason for releasing the pressure is to allow your hand to rest, and to allow milk to start flowing to the baby again. The baby, if he stops sucking when you release the pressure, will start again when he starts to taste milk."	Newman, 2005.
Octane massage is performed by midwives with special training and technique. "Connective tissue massage developed by the midwife, Stoma Octane, involving manual separation of adhesions between the breast base and the major fascia of the pectoral muscles with the aim of helping to restore and maintain natural breast contour and normal breast function. The most salient characteristics of the Octane method are the following: (1) the massage causes no discomfort or pain to the mother, (2) the mother will suddenly feel general relief and comfort, (3) lactation is enhanced regardless of the size or shape of the mother's breasts and nipples, (4) deformities such as inversion, flattening, or cracking of the nipples are rectified and (5) nipple injuries and mastitis are prevented." Commentary by Hiroko Hong, La Leche League International, *Leaven* 43(1), 2007.	Oketani, 1985; described by Fonda et al., 2004.
Lymph drainage therapy is gentle massage of the lymphatic drainage channels in the breast, thought to move stagnated fluid, reduce edema, and improve cellular function. Dr. Chicly teaches this technique to mothers for self-care and to physical therapists and other qualified therapists.	Bruno Chicly, DOES (Chicly, 2004).

Table 8-7 BREAST MASSAGE TECHNIQUES (CONTINUED)

Description or Technique	Author, Source, Date
"Breast massage performed during consults includes techniques using both hands to massage all around the breast. A common approach includes rolling the breast between both hands . . . or using the backs of fists as if gently kneading. The massage is often in a rhythmic motion. It can include general circular motions and gentle vibratory hand motions on the breast. Alternatively, both hands can be placed together around the areola and then slid toward the base of the breast with or without a gentle rotation of the breasts: to the right and back, and then repeated to the left and back. Another common technique is fingertip massage, also described as 'dancing fingers.' This technique is done by placing the finger tips over the affected area and moving them in high frequency, repetitive, up and down motions. Another fingertip approach is gentle vibration with the fingers placed over the affected area and oscillated back and forth. A similar effect is achieved by using the whole palm in the same vibrating motion.	Bolman et al., 2013.
If the breasts are swollen, as in engorgement and mastitis, massage is often combined with steps facilitating fluid mobilization. The mother is reclined. Gentle stroking hand motions across the breast are performed, starting at the areola and directed toward the axillae. Clinicians speculate that this practice promotes fluid drainage through the axillary lymph nodes, where 75% of the lymphatic drainage for the breast occurs."	
Hand techniques increase caloric content and milk production in addition to pumping.	http://newborns.stanford.edu/Breastfeeding/MaxProduction.html

Clothing, Leaking, Bras, and Breast Pads

A breastfeeding mother's clothing should allow frequent, easy access to her breasts. Beyond ease of access to the breasts, no special garments are needed. A well-fitting bra is not a therapeutic device, yet may increase the mother's comfort, especially if her breasts are large or heavy. Any bra or other clothing should be loose enough to avoid constricting or compressing any part of the breast or upper body. Sleep bras, if used, should fit very loosely.

Excessive leaking that requires the use of bra pads (breast pads) is often an artifact of scheduled feeds. In the early weeks postpartum, most women synthesize more milk than their baby requires. By around 6 weeks, daily milk production has adjusted itself to the baby's needs, with sufficient residual milk volume to meet short-term increased needs. The milk-ejection reflex is triggered by infant cues and other activities associated with breastfeeding.

If worn, absorbent pads or milk-blocking devices should be comfortable, nonirritating, replaced when wet, and they should leave no residue that could be ingested by the baby. Direct pressure for a few seconds on a leaking breast, such as by crossed arms, is usually sufficient to temporarily inhibit leaking during milk ejection. Feeding the baby on cue and around the clock help prevent leaking.

Infant Concerns

Pacifiers

Pacifiers are mother-substitutes that are notorious for undermining exclusive breastfeeding, especially during the first 6 months of the baby's life (Mitchell et al., 2006; Nelson et al., 2005; Santo et al., 2007). Pacifiers given before 4 weeks and used most days are significantly associated with shorter duration of breastfeeding (Mauch et al., 2012). The most common uses of a pacifier are to soothe, put the baby to sleep, and keep the baby quiet (Mauch et al., 2012), and to postpone or stretch out the time between breastfeeds (Barros et al., 1995). Breastfed infants who use a pacifier frequently have approximately one fewer breastfeeding per 24 hours ($P \leq 0.01$) than those who did not use a pacifier (Aarts et al., 1999). Given that milk production is directly linked to frequent effective feeds, this reduction in the infants' total time at breast contributes to shorter and less exclusive breastfeeding among pacifier users (Howard et al., 1999; Vogel et al., 2001).

Routine and nontherapeutic use of pacifiers has been linked to the following:

- Injuries to the face (Keim et al., 2012)
- Dental and orthodontic problems (Peres et al., 2007)
- Accidents and injuries including fatal choking (Mattos-Graner et al., 2001)
- Increased oral thrush and other infections (Mattos-Graner et al., 2001)
- Delayed or altered speech development, behavior, and brain development (Lehtonen et al., 1998; Paul et al., 1996)
- Deficits in attachment and maturation (Barros et al., 1997; Gale & Martyn, 1996)

Despite the risks, pacifiers are used by 50% to 80% of breastfeeding mothers (Howard et al., 1999). Pacifier use is often suggested by a person older than the mother, such as a female relative or healthcare professional (Mauch et al., 2012)—possibly an artifact of past beliefs about babies' or infants' needs related to formula-feeding practices. Use of pacifiers is more common in populations of lower socioeconomic status (Mathur et al., 1990) and in those experiencing breastfeeding problems (Righard & Alade, 1997; Santo et al., 2007). Step 8 of the Baby-Friendly Hospital Initiative (WHO & UNICEF, 2009) specifies: "Give no pacifiers or artificial nipples to breastfeeding infants."

Pacifier use has been recommended as a strategy to reduce risk of SIDS (Hauck, 2006; Hauck et al., 2005) on the basis of case-control studies that appeared to show an association between lack of pacifier use on the infant's last night and an increased risk of SIDS. The AAP's Task Force on Sudden Infant Death Syndrome (2011) recommended the following:

- Consider offering a pacifier at nap time and bedtime. Although the mechanism is yet unclear, studies have reported a protective effect of pacifiers on the incidence of SIDS. The protective effect persists throughout the sleep period, even if the pacifier falls out of the infant's mouth.
- Use the pacifier when putting the infant down for sleep. It does not need to be reinserted once the infant falls asleep. If the infant refuses the pacifier, he or she should not be forced to take it. In those cases, parents can try to offer the pacifier again when the infant is a little older.
- For breastfed infants, delay pacifier introduction until breastfeeding has been firmly established, usually by 3 to 4 weeks of age.

The mechanism by which pacifiers might reduce the risk of SIDS, or by their absence increase this risk, remains unknown. The quality of the research supporting the recommendation of universal use of pacifiers has been challenged by other researchers. Pacifiers generally fall out within 5–30 minutes of the infant's falling asleep (Franco et al., 2000; Weiss & Kerbl, 2001), leading to the speculation that other factors, including the frequent attention of a responsible adult who replaces the pacifier, may be the actual protective mechanism (Fleming et al., 1999).

Sucking, swallowing, and breathing are intimately related, with each function affecting the others (Wolf & Glass, 1992). Sucking may affect respiratory centers in the brain; therefore, sucking may have a role in eliciting or maintaining breathing. Pollard studied nighttime non-nutritive sucking in infants aged 1 to 5 months using infrared cameras. Babies who slept with their mothers sucked on their mother's breasts, their mothers' fingers, their own fingers, or pacifiers. If the babies were sleeping separately from mother, they sucked on their own fingers or pacifiers. The routine pacifier-users rarely sucked their digits. Digit sucking has state-modulating effects and may be suppressed by pacifier use (Pollard et al., 1999).

The American Academy of Pediatrics AAP Breastfeeding Policy (AAP, 2012) recommends, "Given the documentation that early use of pacifiers may be associated with less successful breastfeeding, pacifier use in the neonatal period should be limited to specific medical situations. These include uses for pain relief, as a calming agent, or as part of structured program for enhancing oral motor function." Pacifiers should not be routinely used until after breastfeeding is well established, at approximately 3 to 4 weeks of age. Two Cochrane reviews of pacifiers' effect on breastfeeding did not find conclusive evidence that pacifier use reduced the duration of breastfeeding up to 4 months (Jaafar et al., 2011), and evidence to assess the short-term breastfeeding difficulties faced by mothers and the long-term effects of pacifiers on infants' health is lacking (Jaafar et al., 2012). Given the lack of evidence of benefit and the documented risks of pacifiers to the course of breastfeeding (Howard et al., 2003), breastfeeding mothers should be cautioned to avoid pacifiers except in limited situations.

Stooling Patterns

The stools of the breastfed newborn go through several predictable, observable changes and can be used as a partial indicator of milk intake (Gartner et al., 2005; ILCA, 2014; Nommsen-Rivers et al., 2008). Black, tarry stools (meconium) are passed in the first 2 days after birth. With each subsequent milk feed, the stool gradually lightens in color, changing from dark to greenish to yellow, and becomes softer and more liquid (Table 8-8). Stools may contain small curds, or have a mushy consistency that becomes firmer over time. Color ranges from greenish-yellow to mustard-yellow, and the odor is a characteristic sweet, "yeasty," or slightly cheesy odor. By 2 weeks, breastfed babies' fecal flora is very different from that of formula-fed infants. Formula-fed children have fecal flora similar to that of the adult, in which coliforms and enterococci predominate, whereas the flora of the breastfed baby is dominated by lactobacilli and bifidobacteria (Penders et al., 2006).

Table 8-8 STOOLING PATTERNS OF EXCLUSIVELY BREASTFED BABIES

Time Period	# per Day	Appearance/Color	Amount
0–2 days	2–4	Meconium (black, thick tarry)	Scant to copious
3–4[*] days	2–5	Black to green to yellow, looser	Increasing volume
4–7 days	2–6+	Yellow, seedy, runny to loose	Copious by day 6 (4–8 stools/day)
1–6 weeks	3–8+	Yellow, seedy, runny to loose	Copious
6 weeks to 6 months	3–5+; may skip days	Yellow; soft; may thicken over time because of milk compositional changes	Copious, may be passed less often
6 months and onward		Loose; color and aroma may change as family foods are added	

[*]Fewer than 4 stools per day on or after day 4 should be investigated carefully.

In the early weeks of lactation, the whey–casein ratio of human milk is 90:10 (90% whey, 10% casein). Whey is the liquid portion of the milk, which is full of immune factors and low in calcium and minerals. This early composition suits the newborn's greater need for immune protection than minerals for long bone growth. By about 6 weeks, the stools become firmer and are usually passed slightly less often, reflecting the change in the whey–casein ratio to approximately 80:20. The gradual increase in casein relative to whey results in slightly thicker, more formed stools (more like toothpaste or soft peanut butter) that may be passed less often. By the middle of the infant's first year, the whey–casein ratio has evolved to 60:40 or even 50:50—exactly paralleling the infant's increasing bone and muscle development and mobility and developing immune competence (Kunz & Lonnerdal, 1992). Shrago et al. (2006) studied stools of exclusively breastfed babies over the first 2 weeks of life and reported an average of 4 stools per day (range: 0.8–7.2) in first 5 days; the first yellow stool appeared on day 4 (range: day 3–15). Frequent feeds were correlated with the appearance of yellow stool and more feeds per day: the sooner yellow stools appeared, the faster babies gained weight. Nommsen-Rivers et al. (2008) reported a significant relationship between diaper output and breastfeeding adequacy, but this relationship was not strong enough to be used as a screening tool. Fewer than 4 stools on day 4 in combination with delay in onset of copious milk may be used as a screening tool.

If breastfeeding is not exclusive (e.g., when the child begins eating family food, or if infant formula is given), stools become darker, with larger and firmer curds, and with a stronger odor. The formula-fed infant tends to pass larger, more copious, more odorous, but less frequent stools (Quinlan et al., 1995). As the proportion of solid foods increases, stools will reflect the new foods with a change in odor, color, and consistency. Sometimes portions of undigested food may be visible in the stool (Bekkali et al., 2009).

In the first 4 to 6 weeks, newborns pass loose stools many times each day. If more than 24 hours passes without a stool, the child should be seen by a healthcare provider and adequate caloric intake assessed in other ways (Neifert, 2001). Lack of sufficient milk intake is the most common reason for lack of stooling; therefore, more attention to frequent effective breastfeeding and/or increasing milk intake should quickly increase infant output. A healthy, thriving exclusively breastfed child older than 6 weeks may stool only a few times a week or even less often. As long as the stool is soft and profuse and the infant is otherwise thriving and content, almost any pattern is possible. Stooling patterns alone are not the best indicator of health or well-being, and must be considered in the broader context of the infant's overall growth and demeanor. If unusual stool patterns persist, the lactation consultant should collaborate with the baby's primary care provider to investigate other diseases or conditions. Hirschsprung's disease, cystic fibrosis, infant botulism, cow-milk allergy (Daher et al., 2001; Vanderhoof et al., 2001), and other bowel disorders may underlie unusual bowel patterns (see *The Ill Child* chapter).

Hyperbilirubinemia

Nurses and lactation consultants are a part of the management of infants on all levels of care, including monitoring bilirubin levels. AAP guidelines mandate that every baby be screened for bilirubin levels after 24 hours of life regardless of symptoms of jaundice and other symptoms. Normal and abnormal levels are determined by a nomogram, a graph that depicts risk zones based on the baby's age in hours and the bilirubin level (see the *Jaundice and the Breastfed Baby* chapter). The Academy of Breastfeeding Medicine's (2010) Clinical Protocol #22 specifically addresses risk zones in the breastfed baby. Immediate and uninterrupted skin-to-skin contact following birth and frequent ad-lib nursing around the clock with maximum skin contact will reduce risk of jaundice, hypoglycemia, engorgement, and other breastfeeding problems. If the baby clearly cannot breastfeed immediately after birth, the mother should begin expressing colostrum within 2 hours (Parker et al., 2012) and provide it to the baby with a non-teat device (e.g., spoon, small cup).

Many babies are exposed to painful procedures such as blood tests. Ideally, these procedures will be done with the baby nursing at breast, on the mother's body, or at least being held in the mother's arms. If the mother is not available or the procedure requires restraining the baby, expressed colostrum given to the baby by spoon, dropper, or syringe is an effective pain reliever (Okan et al., 2010). See Figure 8-5.

Prolonged, elevated bilirubin levels (greater than 5 mg/dL [85 μmol/L]) in the otherwise healthy, thriving breastfed infant during the third week or even into the second month of life are common. They require no intervention beyond observation and assurance of adequate feeding (Gartner & Herschel, 2001) while remaining in contact with the baby's primary care provider.

If the baby is or becomes jaundiced after hospital discharge, review the information in the *Jaundice and the Breastfed Baby* chapter. The lactation consultant should stay in close contact with the baby's primary care provider and carefully monitor and assist with breastfeeding. Keep the mother and baby in skin-to-skin contact and close together many hours each day; assure adequate milk transfer during direct breastfeeding with careful observation and confirmation via an electronic scale; monitor the quality and quantity of direct breastfeeding; and

help the mother express and feed her milk by alternative means if direct breastfeeding is not meeting the baby's caloric needs. Continue skin-to-skin contact and attempts at direct breastfeeding until the baby is effectively and comfortably obtaining milk and the jaundice has resolved.

Crying and Colic

Breastfed babies who are nursed on cue and held and carried many hours a day and night rarely cry. An infant cries to signal a need, which may be for food, comfort, warmth, the mother's presence (Christensson et al., 1995), pain, illness, or fear. Crying increases stress, increases blood pressure and the potential for brain bleeds (Anderson, 1989), and releases potent chemicals that can alter and even damage the baby's brain (Christensson et al., 1992; Michelsson et al., 1996; Schore, 2001). It is never appropriate to "let a baby cry it out," make a baby cry to "teach him a lesson," or deliberately ignore a baby's cries. Prompt response reduces the baby's stress, enhances parental enjoyment of the baby, and increases parents' confidence in their new role. When parents and caregivers quickly respond to the baby's signals, a long, secure, and trusting relationship begins to develop and parents become more skilled in reading their baby's cues.

Before an assessment of colic is made, all other causes of crying should be investigated and ruled out, especially hunger, illness and injury, other foods or fluids including formula, and lack of enough carrying and touch. Crying is a *late* sign of hunger (Gartner et al., 2005). Reinforcing the mother's prompt response to her baby's feeding cues is always appropriate and eliminates most cases of hunger-induced crying. Lack of knowledge about normal (frequent and sometimes clustered) feeding and sleep patterns of breastfed babies has led many mothers and even professionals to identify a baby's cries as "colic" when in fact the child was simply hungry or needed to be held or carried more.

The newborn's stomach capacity is about 20 mL at birth, which is smaller than previously assumed. Frequent feeds of approximately 1 ounce (30 mL) every hour are probably biologically normal.

Figure 8-5 A Mother Breastfeeding a Baby While the Nurse Does a Heel Stick.

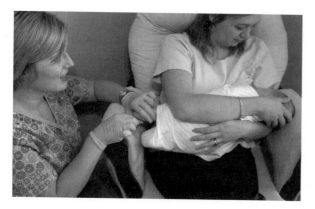

Giving larger fluid volumes at longer intervals may be stressful or even painful (Bergman, 2013). Attempting to enforce a strict schedule for feeds (day or night) is inappropriate and can result in serious underfeeding, dehydration, failure to thrive (Aney, 1998), reduction in milk supply, and undermining of the mother's confidence in caring for her baby. Breastfeeding should be the first strategy to soothe infant cries, because it instantly and automatically brings the infant his mother's presence, food, comfort, warmth, natural endorphins, and immune protection (Carbajal et al., 2003; Gray et al., 2002).

Wessel's (1954) 3-3-3 definition of colic (crying more than 3 hours a day, more than 3 days a week, and lasting more than 3 weeks) helps distinguish colic from hunger or other temporary illness or conditions. Unlike other cries, colic usually is characterized by a high-pitched wail or scream, as if the baby is in severe pain (St James-Roberts, 1999). Colic appears to be the result of sudden spasmodic abdominal cramping, with knees drawn up and sometimes a distended abdomen. Food protein hypersensitivity or allergy is the primary cause of true colic (Gupta, 2007). Infection with *Helicobacter pylori* may be a cause of some infant colic (Ali & Borei, 2013). Disturbances in parental or maternal–child interactions may contribute to colic (Gupta, 2002) and parental expectations may play a role. Canivet et al. (2005) recommend providing closer attention, information, and support to very young women, women who do not cohabit with the father, and women with high trait anxiety. Some "colic" is actually the baby's understandable and normal protest when sick, hungry, or separated from his mother, and/or as a result of a "sleep training" scheme.

When investigating causes for persistent crying and colic (in collaboration with primary care providers), first carefully document everything consumed by the infant and mother for several days. Smoking, including maternal smoking during pregnancy (Sondergaard et al., 2003), may play a role in colic, and has other serious negative consequences for the infant (Fleming & Blair, 2007).

Cow-milk protein allergy or intolerance can also appear as gastroesophageal reflux related to cow-milk protein allergy (Cavataio et al., 2000; Salvatore & Vandenplas, 2002). If the child is sensitive to cow-milk protein, he is likely also sensitive to other foods or allergens (Iacono et al., 1998). Cow milk has been shown to be the single most commonly ingested allergen in infants (Greer et al., 2008). Cow milk is the major source of protein in most manufactured infant formula. Direct ingestion (from whole milk or infant formula) causes the worst symptoms; intake via mother's milk also occurs. Other less common allergens include legumes (including soy-based formula and peanuts), beef, chicken and eggs, grains such as corn and wheat, and high-acid fruits and vegetables. Babies who develop colic in response to foods in the breastfeeding mother's diet often exhibit allergic symptoms when exposed to the same foods later in life. Dietary supplements taken by the baby or mother can also cause infant distress.

After ruling out hunger and illness, the lactation consultant may help the mother identify or rule out an allergic response to cow milk or other allergens. For the breastfed baby younger than 6 months, the following steps are helpful:

- Purify the baby's diet. Ensure that the baby gets nothing other than mother's milk by direct breastfeeding for at least 2 to 3 weeks. Avoid all bottles (even those containing mother's expressed milk), teats and pacifiers, vitamins, and supplements. If the baby has already begun to take other supplements or table foods, those items are the most likely offenders. Make sure the baby is breastfed on cue around the clock during this time.

- At the same time, ask the mother to begin keeping a detailed written diary of her food and beverage intake, any medications or supplements taken by her or the baby, the baby's breastfeeding patterns, and the baby's behavior. Include any unusual events affecting the family. Continue keeping this diary for several weeks.

- Examine the food and behavior diary carefully for emerging patterns, including the mother's cravings, foods avoided or disliked, large quantities or regular ingestion of common allergens (especially cow milk or dairy products), and maternal symptoms of allergies.

- If no discernable pattern emerges in a few weeks, consult with a professional allergist, pediatric gastroenterologist, or other specialist for further evaluation.

If the baby is truly sensitive to cow-milk protein or another component of cow milk, it may take several days to weeks for the offending substance to be cleared from the baby's body. Estep and Kulczycki (2000) report that bovine immunoglobulin G (IgG) antibody levels were markedly higher in the milk of mothers of colicky babies than in the milk of mothers whose babies were not colicky. Bovine IgG has a long half-life, and its presence in high concentrations may require an extended period of elimination. If the mother's avoidance of cow milk clearly relieves her baby's colic symptoms, she may need to continue to avoid all dairy products while consuming nondairy sources of calcium or nondairy calcium-containing supplements (Carroccio et al., 2000; Iacono et al., 1998). Soy protein is also a common allergen, is present in many formulas, and is not recommended for babies with documented allergy to cow milk (Greer et al., 2008).

Food intolerances in exclusively breastfed babies are one sign of underlying atopic (allergic) disease, which is attributable to a combination of heredity and exposure. When a baby's symptoms are relieved by the mother avoiding one trigger, keep looking. A single trigger is often the "tip of the iceberg," and other triggers are likely to be found. Before suggesting that the mother make major changes in her diet and the household environment, a referral to an allergist or comparable specialist is appropriate. Meanwhile, the mother can keep a detailed hourly diary of all foods that she eats, and the baby's reactions. After 2 to 3 weeks, patterns may emerge that will be useful diagnostic tools for the family's primary care providers. As the mother eliminates known triggers of the baby's distress, her own health may improve as well.

Various remedies for colic, reflux, and/or persistent crying (after increasing physical contact and ruling out hunger and allergies as discussed previously) have been proposed, including the following:

- Increased carrying on the back or chest (Barr et al., 1991, 1999)
- Carrying the baby in the prone position on the parent's arm
- Giving oral probiotics (*Lactobacillus reuteri* DSM 17938) (Szajewska et al., 2013)
- Spinal manipulation (chiropractic treatment) (Miller et al., 2012; Wiberg et al., 1999)

Mothering a baby who cries for hours a day can exhaust and undermine the confidence of any mother (Pauli-Pott et al., 2000) and shorten the duration of breastfeeding (Howard et al., 2006). Lactation consultants should stay in close contact with mothers of colicky breastfed babies as they investigate possible causes of the baby's distress, if for no other reason than to provide the mother with emotional support during these difficult times. Encourage and support the mother to provide more skin-to-skin contact, breastfeeding, and breastmilk, all of which are comforting to the baby. Even unsuccessful attempts to comfort the baby are valuable, because abandoning the baby to its pain is worse. Weaning the baby to infant formula will almost certainly make the baby's distress even worse.

Regurgitation

Do neonates regurgitate less often if they are breastfed? Most regurgitations in the early newborn period are essentially benign and are related to neither food allergy nor anatomic or functional intestinal obstruction. One study reported no difference in spitting up between breastfed and formula-fed babies, but studied the babies only for the first 2 days of life. In general, spitting up is related to posture (gravity works) and/or overfeeding, and is more of a laundry problem than a medical/health issue.

Multiple Infants

An increase in the number of women delaying childbirth until after age 30 and advances in techniques to treat infertility have contributed to a large increase in the number of multiple births in the last decade (Martin, 2007). Lactation consultants are likely to work with these families, as these women choose to breastfeed at about the same rate as women giving birth to single infants (Bowers & Gromada, 2005; Leonard, 2007).

Many expectant parents are uncertain whether breastfeeding is possible following a multiple birth, and their decisions regarding infant feeding are often influenced by information received from healthcare providers. Parents of multiples may be reassured that breastfeeding two or more infants is possible. Reports have even described mothers' experiences of breastfeeding conjoined twins (Bains, 2006; LaFleur & Niesen, 1996). Many mothers of twins, triplets, and quadruplets (Berlin, 2007) have breastfed for a year and longer. Research and case studies have demonstrated that most mothers of multiples are capable of producing most or all of the milk that two to five infants require (Auer & Gromada, 1998; Berlin, 2007; Bleyl, 2001; Mead et al., 1992; Saint et al., 1986; Szucs et al., 2009).

Breastfeeding is especially important for twins, triplets, and other higher-order multiples. In addition to offering optimal nutrition and immunological protection to these often preterm or otherwise compromised infants, breastfeeding helps ensure frequent mother–infant interaction with each baby. Although the frequency of feedings may be overwhelming for many new mothers, multiples' frequent feedings give a mother many daily opportunities to sit or lie down to rest while breastfeeding (Gromada, 2007).

Figure 8-6 shows comfortable positions for nursing two infants simultaneously. Note that pillows support the mother's body and arms and help hold the babies in position. The pillows can be bed pillows strategically placed to help cradle the babies or special "nursing pillows" designed for nursing twins.

Full-Term Twins or Triplets

Full-term or late preterm (near-term) multiple infants have the same needs as any full-term singleton; the mother's role, however, is more complex because she must meet the needs of two or more newborns. In addition, the mother of multiples is more likely to have experienced complications

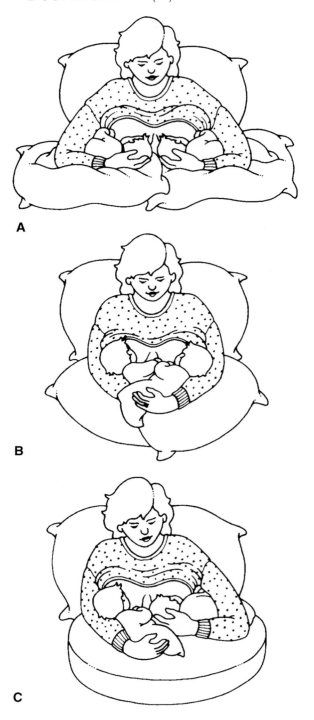

Figure 8-6 POSTIONS FOR NURSING TWINS. (A) DOUBLE CLUTCH. (B) DOUBEL CRADLE. (C) CRADLE-CLUTCH.

A

B

C

of pregnancy and childbirth, and she may require more time to recover physically. Manual expression of breastmilk is effective in the first 2 days, especially if the mother is too ill to pump; after that, pumping plus massage/expression yields more milk than pumping alone.

Mothers of multiples need help and support with early feedings, as they feel overwhelmed when first trying to figure out how to manage feedings with more than one infant. Some are anxious to initiate simultaneous feedings, as they have heard it saves time. However, it is important to first assess each infant at breast separately, as it is not unusual for one or more of the babies to breastfeed poorly even when the infants are born at term. Ongoing, individual assessment is particularly important for late preterm (near-term) multiples, even when they are basically stable and able to be with their mother, as feeding difficulties, hypoglycemia, and hyperbilirubinemia are more common among these newborns (Jain, 2007).

Preterm or Ill Multiples

When multiple infants are born prematurely or have other medical complications, direct breastfeeding may be delayed for days or weeks. The lactation consultant should advise the mother to begin expressing milk for her infants within 2 hours of giving birth (Bowers & Gromada, 2005; Parker et al., 2012). If a mother has experienced complications, she may need assistance when expressing milk (Gromada & Spangler, 1998).

The more skin-to-skin contact (kangaroo care) that the mother can provide, the better for both mother and baby. Current research supports the importance of immediate, sustained, and nearly 24-hour skin-to-skin care for vulnerable babies (Ludington-Hoe, 2011; Moore et al., 2012; Samra et al., 2013).

Simultaneous pumping using a hospital-grade electric pump along with massage is the most effective way to obtain maximum amounts of milk and to maintain lactation (Morton et al., 2012) (see the *Breast Pumps and Other Technologies* chapter). Anticipatory guidance for any expectant mother of multiples should include helping the mother to find a breast-pump rental location in her area. Specific

encouragement is welcome: "What a gift your milk is for your baby!" "To your baby, even 2 mL of your milk is significant." "There are 3 million antibodies in every drop!"

When direct breastfeeding is initiated for two or more preterm or ill newborns following days or weeks of pumping, the lactation consultant is responsible for assisting the mother in developing an individualized, evidence-based plan for transitioning each multiple to the breast. For instance, Auer and Gromada (1998) described the approach of a mother of quadruplets who used interim bottle-feedings with each baby until she increased milk production. As with other aspects of breastfeeding, strategies for transitioning two or more infants to direct breastfeeding should look at each infant's signs, or cues, that the individual infant may be ready to progress. In addition, the process of transitioning multiple infants to direct breastfeeding may take time, and a mother may become discouraged. However, one study found preterm twins eventually progressed to full, direct breastfeeding at rates comparable to term infants (Liang et al., 1997). Regular skin-to-skin contact sessions between a mother and one or more of her babies helps "normalize" the transition period, and skin contact with one baby at a time often facilitates the transition to direct breastfeeding due to baby-led latching.

Putting It All Together

Caring for and breastfeeding multiple newborns require a different kind of organization by the mother than caring for a single newborn or two infants of different ages (Bowers & Gromada, 2005). Encourage the mother to keep simple 24-hour charts for each infant's daily activities, especially those related to feeding and intake, until lactation is well established and adequate weight gain for each infant indicates the multiples are able to breastfeed effectively. The charts should record the number of breastfeedings, any pumping sessions and/or alternative feedings, and the number of wet diapers and stools for each infant. Maintaining individual charts reassures the mother that all babies are receiving sufficient nutrients. Smart phone applications can help with charting feeds.

Whether a mother or her babies are ready for simultaneous feedings in the immediate postpartum period or not, a demonstration of the various single and simultaneous feeding positions will help a mother realize that she has many choices for comfortable breastfeeding. Simultaneous feedings can save time, and many mothers feed two babies at once during the first few weeks postpartum; however, some mothers and many multiples need more time to learn to work together for simultaneous feedings (Bowers & Gromada, 2005). Also, a mother may need someone to support each infant's head during individual latch-on until she and her infants become more comfortable with simultaneous feeding. Some mothers or infants indicate a preference for individual feedings, which give a mother the opportunity to enjoy some one-on-one time with each child. Perhaps the most common scenario is a combination of simultaneous and single feedings.

In addition to an interest in simultaneous feedings, many mothers have questions about a feeding rotation and when to alternate breasts and babies. Almost any feeding rotation will work when all infants breastfeed on cue. Most mothers offer one breast per feeding. They may then alternate breasts every feeding or alternate only every 24 hours, which often is easier to remember. Mothers of odd-number sets, such as triplets, may have to alternate babies and breasts more frequently than every 24 hours. Some mothers assign each of twins a particular breast, but alternating babies and breasts appears to have more advantages unless one baby consistently cues to feed from a particular breast. Also, assigning a breast, which allows each infant to self-regulate production in that particular breast, may be a useful strategy when a mother experiences an "overactive" milk-ejection reflex and/or milk overproduction with one or more infants exhibiting signs of lactose overload, or if one or more infants has frequent refluxes or has actual gastroesophageal reflux disorder (GERD).

The caregiver must remain sensitive to infant differences when a mother is forming an attachment, or bond, with each infant. Because humans are designed to form an attachment with one person at a time, the attachment process is more complex. It is also more likely to be disrupted with multiples, particularly if the twin or triplet birth was not discovered until shortly before the infants' birth or if one infant is sicker than the others (Gromada, 2007). Healthcare providers are in a position to help parents see and relate to each baby as an individual, rather than as part of a multiple unit. Promoting attachment behaviors, such as skin-to-skin contact during an infant's hospitalization and once the baby is discharged home, is especially important with a multiple that has been less able to interact or establish eye contact with parents because of postnatal complications or illness. The healthcare provider can point out each infant's unique qualities while helping the mother breastfeed and get to know her offspring.

Household help is not a luxury for mothers recuperating from a multiple pregnancy and birth, as they must feed and care for, and form attachments with, more than one neonate simultaneously. Another pair of hands and ongoing assistance with household chores allows a mother to spend more time and energy breastfeeding and meeting the other needs of her infants. As taking care of babies is more fun than cleaning and cooking, the mother (and father) should make it clear that the helper is expected to assume household tasks, while the mother feeds and takes care of the babies. If the mother has older children, she may grieve for the loss of special time with that child or children. Assistance with the multiples may allow her some important "alone time" with older children. During holidays, family members should not expect the mother of multiples to do anything other than show up, smile, and go home with some leftovers.

A lack of physical and emotional support, feelings of isolation, sleep deprivation, and other stressors associated with the care of multiple infants may contribute to the higher risk for postpartum mood or anxiety disorders in these mothers (Leonard, 1998). Because of the negative effects such a problem may exert on breastfeeding and attachment, healthcare providers should be aware of their increased likelihood and assess mothers of multiples for these disorders.

Needs, problems, and solutions vary with each multiple-birth situation. However, practical strategies to promote effective breastfeeding with multiple infants and maternal recovery may include the following ideas:

- Develop both short- and long-term breast-feeding goals with a mother to help her think of breastfeeding as a commitment and to get through the often overwhelming first few weeks or months of frequent feedings and/or pumping sessions.
- Link the mother with other women who have successfully breastfed multiples. Show the mother how to position and stabilize two infants for simultaneous feedings using pillows. Whether using pillows available at home or a special nursing pillow, each baby should be positioned so that the hips are significantly lower than the head. (This may be especially important for preterm or late preterm twins who are at greater risk for reflux or GERD.) The mother in Figure 8-6c is using a special pillow designed for feeding multiples. This pillow is longer and wider, which gives it a deeper "shelf" than some of the nursing pillows used for a single infant.
- Review the basics of breastfeeding, maintenance of milk production, and advantages of breastfeeding with the mother of multiples during the hectic early weeks and months of breastfeeding.
- Help the mother develop a plan to alternate infants and breasts as needed. She may get ample advice from others, so encourage her to figure out what works best for her. If the babies are stooling, gaining weight, and happy, things are going fairly well.
- Suggest that the mother create a "breastfeeding station" that she supplies with nutritious liquids and foods, breast pads, infant wipes, children's books (if she has older children), a cell or portable telephone, and a television remote.
- Emphasize the need for housekeeping help for at least several months.

- Recommend that the mother advise any helpers that she expects them to be supportive of breastfeeding.
- Encourage parents to ask well-wishers who want to "do something" for the family to help by delivering a meal, cleaning the house or running errands, or sending food. The care of multiples leaves little time to prepare food, and the caloric needs of a mother who is breastfeeding multiple infants are greater than those of a mother who is breastfeeding a single infant. Suggestions for nutritious and convenient homemade foods may be helpful.

Partial Breastfeeding and Human Milk Feeding

Because mothers of multiple infants are more likely to be affected by complications or other factors that may interfere with effective early breastfeeding and milk production, they are more likely to supplement or complement breastfeeding with formula, even though this may be more challenging than exclusive breastfeeding. Complementing may take the form of "topping off" an occasional or daily breastfeeding, or it may involve replacing one or more breastfeedings with an alternative feeding.

With guidance from a lactation consultant who respects the overwhelming amount of infant care the mother faces daily and the lack of time to work on resolving problems, most mothers will be able to decrease the use of alternative feedings in favor of direct breastfeedings. Some mothers continue to offer an alternative feeding on a daily or weekly basis to have help with feedings or to sleep without interruption for a few hours. Many mothers prefer to express their own milk for feedings. Caution the mother that milk production might decrease if the total number of breastfeedings or pumping sessions dips below 8 to 10 in 24 hours.

Alternative feeding methods to provide expressed human milk have become more common with the increased availability of hospital-grade, electric breast pumps. Mothers of higher-order multiples find it helpful to pump, as it can be daunting to directly breastfeed three or more babies (Gromada, 2007).

Mothers have maintained lactation and human milk feeding without the use of other supplements for several months. Pumping leaves the door open to later direct breastfeeding. Multiples wean as individuals; they may stop breastfeeding at about the same time or one may wean before the other(s).

Breastfeeding During Pregnancy and Tandem Nursing

The risk of a subsequent pregnancy occurring during the first 6 months of exclusive or full breastfeeding is extremely low (Van der Wijden et al., 2003). The key points here are "fully breastfeeding" and "in the first 6 months." Globally, more than 50% of women will become pregnant while still breastfeeding their youngest child. When asked, many of these mothers report that the emotional needs of the child served as their principal motivation to continue breastfeeding, followed by their belief in child-led weaning.

A mother who conceives while breastfeeding may experience any or all of the following:

- Nipple and/or breast tenderness: Hormonal changes may cause sudden onset of nipple or breast pain that appears to be hormonal in nature. The usual remedies for breast or nipple pain are often ineffectual.
- Maternal fatigue: The hormones of early pregnancy often impel women to want to sleep, although this is difficult for the mother of an active toddler to do. The fatigue is related to hormonal changes of pregnancy, not to continued breastfeeding, and it will diminish as the pregnancy progresses. Pregnant women with young children, whether breastfeeding or not, should be encouraged to nap when the child naps.
- Decline in milk supply and number of feedings: About 70% of mothers report a decrease in their milk production during a subsequent pregnancy. Most nursing children breastfeed less often than they did as infants. As the pregnancy progresses, the milk volume

usually declines. Sometimes the child will wean during this period. If already talking, the toddler may complain that the milk is "all gone" or that it takes "too long to get it."

- Change in taste of milk: As the hormones of pregnancy (especially estrogen) begin to affect the breast secretory tissue, lactose in the milk will decrease while sodium increases, changing the taste of the breastmilk. The talking nursling may state quite clearly how the milk tastes or simply indicate by his actions that it is not the same.
- Uterine contractions: Women experience uterine contractions during breastfeeding. There is no documented danger to the mother or fetus when mothers breastfeed through a healthy pregnancy uncomplicated by risk factors for preterm labor (Moscone & Moore, 1993). Little is known about the effect of breastfeeding during pregnancy in the presence of such risk factors.
- Weaning: Some nursing children wean before their sibling is born, presumably because of the decline in milk volume, the milk's change in taste, and/or the mother's urging to wean. As the mother's body changes shape, her lap will also disappear, which may bother the nursing child. The child may wean spontaneously if the mother responds to the child's request to breastfeed but does not offer breastfeeding first.

A maternal history of preterm labor and birth with a previous pregnancy, repeated spontaneous abortion, "incompetent" cervix, current multiple gestation, or other risks for preterm labor and birth should be taken into consideration when contemplating continued breastfeeding through the pregnancy. The mother who continues to breastfeed during a subsequent pregnancy will need to eat a nutritious diet; she may take supplemental vitamins as a precaution. In one study (Moscone & Moore, 1993), most mothers reported continued good general health throughout their pregnancy as well as healthy outcomes in the new baby.

Tandem nursing refers to the situation when a mother continues breastfeeding her child through a subsequent pregnancy including after the new baby is born. The well-referenced book on this topic is *Adventures in Tandem Nursing* by Hillary Flower (2003). In La Leche League circles before this book was published, tandem nursing was called "nursing siblings who are not twins."

A mother who breastfeeds during pregnancy and/ or continues into tandem nursing may face criticism from her family, friends, and healthcare providers. The lactation consultant may be asked for her opinion after the mother has been told by her physician that she must wean her child—even in the absence of indicators that continuing to breastfeed is a risk for the mother or her developing fetus. In developing countries, traditional beliefs about weaning when the mother's pregnancy is confirmed may also reduce the frequency of breastfeeding during a subsequent pregnancy. The lactation consultant or nurse who openly accepts individual decisions and behavior of breastfeeding women can be helpful in providing information and guidance that supports the mother's decisions.

Sleeping, SIDS, and Bedsharing

Throughout history and around the world, mothers and babies have always slept together, especially in the early months of exclusive breastfeeding. Anthropologic studies confirm that mother–infant bedsharing represents the most biologically appropriate sleeping arrangement for humans and is both ancient and ubiquitous because breastfeeding is not easily managed without it (Gettler & McKenna, 2011). At least 75% of breastfeeding mothers sleep with their babies all or part of the night in Western nations (Huang et al., 2013; McKenna & McDade, 2005). According to Hrdy (1999), mothers are the environment for species such as primates. Bedsharing results in more and longer breastfeeding episodes (Blair & Ball, 2004; McKenna et al., 1997), more frequent suckling (Ball et al., 2006), more maternal touching and looking, and faster and more frequent maternal responses (Baddock et al., 2006). Mothers get more sleep when they are bedsharing (Quillin & Glenn, 2004) and exclusively breastfeeding (Doan et al., 2007). Sleep is fragmented

in virtually all new mothers (Campbell, 1986), and most postpartum women take several naps per day (Montgomery-Downs et al., 2010). Babies do not begin consolidating their sleep into circadian rhythms and contiguous blocks of time until well into the second 6 months of life (Middlemiss, 2004; Parmelee et al., 1964). Unfortunately, most studies on infant sleep have examined the babies in an unnatural, separate sleep location instead of sleeping next to their mothers (Gettler & McKenna, 2011). Recent studies have confirmed the normalcy and importance of the mother's physical and emotional availability to her baby during sleep (Teti et al., 2010).

Despite the historical, biological, and cultural traditions of shared sleeping, concerns about infant deaths from suffocation or overlying and from sudden infant death syndrome confuse parents, causing heated "where should the baby sleep" debates. The terms *bedsharing* and *co-sleeping* are poorly defined in the research literature (Chantry et al., 2006). Delineating safe versus unsafe conditions of shared sleep is critical to breastfeeding, because the majority of exclusively breastfeeding mothers will bring their babies into their bed for all or some sleeping sessions (Ball & Volpe, 2012; Lahr et al., 2007; Russell et al., 2013). No one sleep location can be assumed, because breastfeeding mothers typically use several strategies during the night and for naps (Ball & Volpe, 2012; McKenna & Volpe, 2007; Russell et al., 2013).

Much of the SIDS and infant mortality literature conflates SIDS and suffocation, and fails to take into account the responsible breastfeeding mother's exquisite sensitivity to her baby even while she is asleep. Infrared research studies conducted in sleep laboratories have established that breastfeeding mothers arise to a level of awareness that allows for infant monitoring without remembering that they have done so (Mosko et al., 1997).

The chief concern about bedsharing is smothering or rollover deaths.

Smothering (Rollover Concerns)

Smothering or other sudden unexplained infant death (SUID or SUDI) may be labeled "SIDS," even though other causes or risk or causative factors may be present. If a baby is found dead in a crib, the crib is usually not blamed for the death unless the crib was a clearly causative factor. However, if a baby is discovered dead in an adult bed, the adult and/or the bed is often blamed for the baby's death. The vast majority of "overlying" (smothering) deaths involve alcohol or drug use by the bed partner (Blair et al., 1999; Gessner et al., 2001); a bed partner other than the baby's parent (Hauck et al., 2003), or an unsafe surface such as a couch or sofa (Blair et al., 2006). *Unsafe sleep surfaces* can trap a baby in a dangerous position. Couches, some cribs, reclining chairs, and other surfaces that are not firm, flat, and clean are risky surfaces, especially if the infant is out of visual and sensory distance of a responsible adult (Ball et al., 2012; Carpenter et al., 2004). *Entrapment* deaths usually involve wedging of the infant between two objects or spaces between objects.

A critical issue is that breastfeeding mother–baby dyads sleep differently from formula-feeding mothers and all other people. Breastfeeding mothers instinctively adopt a protective posture with the baby facing the mother, side-lying, with the baby's head at breast level ("cuddle-curl"; Figure 8-7). The mother's arm above the baby's head prevents the baby from creeping up onto pillows, while the mother's bent lower leg prevents the baby from scooting down to the foot of the bed (Baddock et al., 2006; Richard et al., 1996).

When bedsharing, mother and baby demonstrate more mutual arousals, more maternal touching and looking, increased breastfeeding, and faster and more frequent maternal responses (Baddock et al., 2007).

Figure 8-7 Protective Posture: Safe Bedsharing Supports Breastfeeding.

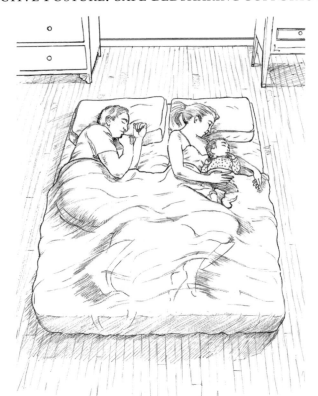

Reprinted with permission from Platypus Media, LLC. Illustration from "Sleeping With Your Baby: A Parent's Guide to Cosleeping," by James J. McKenna, PhD (Platypus Media, 2006). Illustration by Andrew Barthelmes.

Some guidelines recommend that a mother stay awake during feeds and return her baby to a crib for sleep; however, the hormones of breastfeeding induce relaxation and drowsiness in mother and baby, which is a major advantage of breastfeeding (Levine et al., 2007). By 6 weeks of attempting to breastfeed without bedsharing, a majority of breastfeeding mothers manage night feeds by (1) supplementing with formula, which *reduces* maternal sleep (Doan et al., 2007); (2) trying a sleep-training scheme such as feeding water in a darkened room; or (3) sleeping next to their babies (Ball, 2003). The first two strategies undermine exclusive breastfeeding for 6 months and have other major negative outcomes. Safe bedsharing extends the duration of any breastfeeding and lengthens the period of exclusive breastfeeding (McKenna et al., 1997; Santos et al., 2009). Sleep training schemes and forcing the baby to "cry it out" to "teach him to sleep longer" are devastatingly harmful to the baby and detrimental to the mother–baby relationship (Kendall-Tackett, 2013; Middlemiss et al., 2012).

The Academy of Breastfeeding Medicine's (2008) Protocol #6 is very clear: there is currently not enough evidence to support routine recommendations against "all bedsharing" to reduce risks of SIDS or smothering. If the mother does not bedshare, then the baby should sleep supine in a safe crib within visual and sensory distance of a responsible adult (Task Force on Sudden Infant Death Syndrome, 2011).

SIDS

SIDS is a diagnosis of exclusion, meaning other possible causes of death were ruled out during autopsy or investigation. Major risk factors for SIDS identified in 1991 were maternal smoking, prone position, and formula-feeding (Mitchell et al., 1991). The triple-risk theory of SIDS postulates that only when all three risk factors are present does SIDS occur: (1) a vulnerable infant, (2) a critical developmental period in homeostatic control, and (3) one or more exogenous stressors (Filiano & Kinney, 1994). Further research has identified maternal smoking during pregnancy as a major risk factor in nearly

every epidemiological study of SIDS, and it may account for at least 50% to 80% of all SIDS-related deaths (Fleming & Blair, 2007; Zhang & Wang, 2013). Smokers in the household, daily exposure to secondhand smoke, and all-night bedsharing with a smoker increase the risks to the infant (Lahr et al., 2005; Zhang & Wang, 2013), even if the smoker is a breastfeeding mother or smokes outside the house. Prone position continues to be a risk factor for SIDS (Moon et al., 2007). In earlier studies, formula-feeding was found to double the risks of SIDS (McVea et al., 2000). In a more rigorous meta-analysis, formula-feeding was found to be associated with at least a 56% increase in SIDS deaths (Hauck et al., 2011), possibly because of decreased arousability (Horne et al., 2004), more infections (Horne et al., 2002), and/or other factors. SIDS deaths, by definition, are *not* caused by smothering, overlying, entrapment, or suffocation.

Lactation consultants would be wise to assume a breastfeeding mother is bedsharing with her baby at least part of the time at night or for naps, and to make sure safety issues are discussed thoroughly. The book *Sweet Sleep* by La Leche League provides in-depth, well-referenced information specifically for breastfeeding families (La Leche League International et al., 2014). Parents need factual, evidence-based information about specific risks of unsafe bedsharing conditions, unsafe cribs, and other practices that increase risks to their baby (McKenna, 2007). See Table 8-9.

Clinical Implications

Even when new mothers have adequate knowledge about breastfeeding and have abundant social and clinical support, most will still benefit from a visit by a skillful breastfeeding advisor during the early postpartum period. Early and close follow-up by healthcare professionals skilled in breastfeeding should begin at birth and continue within 48 hours of release from hospital care or 3 to 5 days after birth (AAP, 2012) and again several days later (Wagner et al., 2013). An in-person evaluation at 72 to 96 hours postpartum is especially important (Dewey et al., 2003; Wagner et al., 2013). Assessing and

---

Table 8-9 SAFETY ISSUES FOR BREASTFEEDING AND BED SHARING

Do Practice Safety During Bed Sharing If	*Do Not* Bed Share All Night If
Bed partners:	**Bed partners:**
Breastfeeding mother	Formula feeding (never breastfed) mother
Conscious decision by both parents to bed share	Accidental bed sharing
Nonsmoking (never smoke)	Any tobacco smoking, even outside
Sober and drug free	Alcohol and/or drug use
Parents of the baby	Nonparents; siblings
No pets	Animals
Baby's position:	**Baby's position:**
Baby on his back (supine)	Baby in prone or side-lying position
Baby unwrapped, free to wiggle and move arms and legs	Baby swaddled or bundled in a blanket
Bedding/sleep surface:	**Bedding/sleep surface:**
Firm, flat, clean mattress	Couch or sofa; arm chair; soft or saggy mattress; waterbed
No holes, spaces, or places that could trap baby	Holes, spaces, or places that could trap baby
Tightly fitting sheets under baby	Loose sheets or blankets under baby
No pillows or blankets near baby's face	Pillows or blankets around baby
No thick duvets or comforters	Thick covers on or over baby
Room comfortable temperature, not overheated	Overheated room

---

reinforcing expected milestones and screening for breastfeeding problems is an integral part of postpartum visits. According to adult education principles, this is a "teaching moment" in which the parents are highly receptive to information that helps them deal with practical life dilemmas.

Priority teaching for parents includes the following points:

- Keep the baby physically close, maximize skin-to-skin contact, and feed on cue around the clock.
- Be sure the baby is actually getting milk. Listen for audible swallowing. Let the baby finish the first breast before offering the second so that the baby will receive the creamier milk as the feeding progresses. Watch the baby for cues that he is finished with the feed.
- Do not limit the frequency or duration of feeds. Give no other fluids or foods, or oral objects (pacifiers).

- Provide a phone number to call with questions or concerns, especially if the mother thinks the baby is not feeding well, or any nipple or breast pain occurs.
- Reinforce the mother's skill in breastfeeding with comments such as "You are making lots of good milk for your baby," "You are very responsive to your baby's need to be close and breastfed often," or "You look so comfortable and peaceful holding your baby skin to skin!"

ACKNOWLEDGMENTS

The author of this key chapter of *Breastfeeding and Human Lactation* acknowledges, thanks, and lauds Jan Riordan. Jan's vision, creativity, energy, and skillful blending of the art and science of lactation support began with her writing scholarly guidance papers for nurses and health professionals more than 3 decades ago. Jan played a vital role in guiding and shaping the emerging lactation consultant profession as a member of the founding Board of Directors of the International Board of Lactation Consultant Examiners and as its president for several years. I am honored to have been invited to write this chapter for the past three editions, and to carry on Jan's tradition of educating and mentoring the next generation of skilled lactation consultants.

SUMMARY

The postpartum period is the time of transition from pregnancy to life with a child. Understanding normal patterns of breastfeeding helps providers of lactation support—peers, mother support groups, and consultants—identify problems and answer questions from parents and other professionals. Even when all is going well, mothers can benefit from additional support from peers, mother support groups, and lactation professionals.

KEY CONCEPTS

- The breastfeeding mother–baby dyad is a single psychobiological organism. The concept that "separation is harmful" replaces and supersedes the earlier understanding that "contact is advantageous."
- Breastfeeding is robust—trust that breastfeeding will work.
- The number of feedings and the duration of feeding vary widely from mother to mother. However, reassuring signs of adequate infant intake include 8 to 12 or more effective feeds per day, profuse daily infant stools after day 4, and comfortable maternal breasts.
- The breastfed infant has a biological need to feed approximately hourly and take small amounts per feed in the early weeks. Parents should be reassured that this pattern is normal expected behavior.
- Abundant ongoing milk production depends on frequent, thorough removal of milk from the breast by the baby or by alternative means. Milk production calibrates to meet the infant's needs by about 6 weeks. About one-third of the milk available remains in the breasts over and above the baby's typical daily intake.
- Expecting babies to sleep alone or go for long stretches between large feeds is physiologically unrealistic, inappropriate, and counterproductive.
- Edema and milk stasis are two different phenomena and can occur simultaneously. The best prevention is immediate breastfeeding in the first hour after birth, and frequent effective breastfeeding thereafter.
- "Too much" or "too little" milk is often an indicator of an underlying infant suckling problem. Before reducing milk volume, rule out infant factors.
- If a baby cannot latch and comfortably feed, keep the baby in nearly continuous skin-to-skin contact and help the mother express milk for the baby. Follow the family until the baby is feeding well.
- Early-onset nipple pain is often "mechanical" pain, related to improper infant latch or suck, nipple stretching and compression, or irritation from devices. Sudden-onset nipple pain after comfortable breastfeeding is often a sign of infection from bacteria, yeasts, or other organisms.
- The majority of topical preparations do not prevent nipple pain nor speed healing. Gentle massage can increase milk flow during pumping or expressing milk.
- Pacifiers interfere with breastfeeding, and should be avoided except in short-term, therapeutic situations.
- Infant stools change from black, tarry meconium to green and then to profuse, soft, yellow stools over the first week after birth. In the first month or so, stools are passed every day. Over time, stools may become thicker and passed less often because of milk compositional changes.
- Jaundice is often a marker for poor feeding. Continued breastfeeding and/or feeding expressed milk is recommended for jaundiced infants.

- Breastfed babies who are fed on cue and held and carried many hours a day rarely cry. Crying is a late sign of distress and/or hunger. Crying is harmful for babies, and every effort should be made to immediately comfort or feed the baby.
- Sensitivity or allergy to cow-milk protein is a frequent cause of colic. Allergy to cow-milk protein or other foods calls for skilled and careful dietary management.
- Multiple infants have the same needs as any singleton. The mother's role is more complex in such cases because she must meet the needs of two or more newborns, and she is more likely to have had complications of pregnancy and childbirth, including requiring more time to recover physically.
- The risk of a subsequent pregnancy occurring during the first 6 months of exclusive or full breastfeeding is extremely low.

INTERNET RESOURCES

Academy of Breastfeeding Medicine (ABM): www.bfmed.org

American Academy of Pediatrics (AAP): www.aap.org

Center for Evidence-Based Medicine: www.cebm.net

Cochrane database/reviews of research on breastfeeding topics: www.cochrane.org

International Lactation Consultant Association (ILCA): www.ilca.org

La Leche League International (LLLI): www.lalecheleague.org

Medline/PubMed: www.ncbi.nlm.nih.gov/entrez/query.fcgi

U.S. Centers for Disease Control and Prevention: www.cdc.gov/breastfeeding

REFERENCES

Aarts C, Hörnell A, Kylberg E, et al. Breastfeeding patterns in relation to thumb sucking and pacifier use. *Pediatrics.* 1999;104(4):e50.

Abou-Dakn M, Fluhr JW, Gensch M, Wöckel A. Positive effect of HPA lanolin versus expressed breastmilk on painful and damaged nipples during lactation. *Skin Pharmacol Physiol.* 2011;24:27–35. doi:10.1159/000318228.

Academy of Breastfeeding Medicine. ABM clinical protocol #6: guideline on co-sleeping and breastfeeding. Revision, March 2008. *Breastfeed Med.* 2008;3(1):38–43. doi: 10.1089/bfm.2007.9979.

Academy of Breastfeeding Medicine. ABM clinical protocol #3: hospital guidelines for the use of supplementary feedings in the healthy term breastfed neonate, revised 2009. *Breastfeed Med.* 2009;4(3):175–182. doi: 10.1089/bfm.2009.9991.

Academy of Breastfeeding Medicine. ABM clinical protocol #22: guidelines for management of jaundice in the breastfeeding infant equal to or greater than 35 weeks' gestation. *Breastfeed Med.* 2010;5(2):87–93.

Academy of Breastfeeding Medicine. ABM clinical protocol #9: use of galactogogues in initiating or augmenting the rate of maternal milk secretion. *Breastfeed Med.* 2011;6(1). doi: 10.1089/bfm.2011.9998.

Ali AS, Borei MB. *Helicobacter pylori* and Egyptian infantile colic. *J Egypt Soc Parasitol.* 2013;43(2):327–332.

American Academy of Pediatrics (AAP). Breastfeeding and the use of human milk. *Pediatrics.* 2012;129(3): e827–e841. doi: 10.1542/peds.2011-3552.

American Congress of Obstetricians and Gynecologists. Committee opinion no 579: definition of term pregnancy. *Obstet Gynecol.* 2013;122(5):1139–1140. doi: 10.1097/01.AOG.0000437385.88715.4a.

Amir LH, James JP, Donath SM. Reliability of the Hazelbaker assessment tool for lingual frenulum function. *Int Breastfeed J.* 2006;1(1):3.

Anderson GC. Risk in mother–infant separation post-birth. *Image J Nurs Sch.* 1989;21:196–198.

Anderson GC, Moore E, Hepworth J, Bergman N. Early skin-to-skin contact for mothers and their healthy newborn infants. *Cochrane Database Syst Rev.* 2003;2:CD003519.

Aney M. Babywise advice linked to dehydration, failure-to-thrive. *AAP News.* 1998;14(4):21.

Ardran GM, Kemp FH, Lind J. A cineradiographic study of breast feeding. *Br J Radiol.* 1958;31(363):156–162.

Arthur PG, Smith M, Hartmann PE. Milk lactose, citrate, and glucose as markers of lactogenesis in normal and diabetic women. *J Pediatr Gastroenterol Nutr.* 1989;9(4):488–496.

Auer C, Gromada KK. A case report of breastfeeding quadruplets: factors perceived as affecting breast-feeding. *J Hum Lact.* 1998;14(2):135–141.

Baddock SA, Galland BC, Bolton DP, et al. Differences in infant and parent behaviors during routine bed sharing compared with cot sleeping in the home setting. *Pediatrics.* 2006;117(5):1599–1607.

Baddock SA, Galland BC, Taylor BJ, Bolton DP. Sleep arrangements and behavior of bed-sharing families in the home setting. *Pediatrics.* 2007;119(1):e200–e207.

Bains C. Breastfeeding a challenging dance: lots of patience required to help newborns nurse. *Winnipeg Free Press.* November 11, 2006:6.

Ball HL. Breastfeeding, bed-sharing, and infant sleep. *Birth.* 2003;30(3):181–188.

Ball HL, Moya E, Fairley L, et al. Infant care practices related to sudden infant death syndrome in South Asian and White British families in the UK. *Paediatr Perinatal Epidemiol.* 2012;26(1):3–12. doi: 10.1111/j.1365-3016.2011.01217.x.

Ball HL, Volpe LE. Sudden infant death syndrome (SIDS) risk reduction and infant sleep location: moving the discussion forward. *Soc Sci Med.* 2012. doi: 10.1016/j.socscimed.2012.03.025.

Ball HL, Ward-Platt MP, Heslop E, et al. Randomised trial of infant sleep location on the postnatal ward. *Arch Dis Child.* 2006;91(12):1005–1010.

Barr RG, McMullan SJ, Spiess H, et al. Carrying as colic "therapy": a randomized controlled trial. *Pediatrics.* 1991;87(5):623–630.

Barr RG, Young SN, Wright JH, et al. Differential calming responses to sucrose taste in crying infants with and without colic. *Pediatrics.* 1999;103(5):e68.

Barrett ME, Heller MM, Stone HF, Murase JE. Raynaud phenomenon of the nipple in breastfeeding mothers: an underdiagnosed cause of nipple pain. *JAMA Dermatol.* 2013;149(3):300–306.

Barros FC, Victora CG, Morris SS, et al. Breast feeding, pacifier use and infant development at 12 months of age: a birth cohort study in Brazil. *Paediatr Perinat Epidemiol.* 1997;11(4):441–450.

Barros FC, Victora CG, Semer TC, et al. Use of pacifiers is associated with decreased breast-feeding duration. *Pediatrics.* 1995;95(4):497–499.

Baumgarder DJ, Muehl P, Fischer M, Pribbenow B. Effect of labor epidural anesthesia on breast-feeding of healthy full-term newborns delivered vaginally. *J Am Board Fam Pract.* 2003;16(1):7–13.

Becker GE, Cooney F, Smith HA. Methods of milk expression for lactating women. *Cochrane Database Syst Rev.* 2011;12:CD006170. doi: 10.1002/14651858.CD006170.pub3.

Beilin Y, Bodian CA, Weiser J, et al. Effect of labor epidural analgesia with and without fentanyl on infant breast-feeding: a prospective, randomized, double-blind study. *Anesthesiology.* 2005;103(6):1211–1217.

Bekkali N, Hamers SL, Reitsma JB, et al. Infant stool form scale: development and results. *J Pediatr.* 2009;154(4):e521–e526. doi: 10.1016/j.jpeds.2008.10.010.

Bergman NJ. Neonatal stomach volume and physiology suggest feeding at 1-h intervals. *Acta Paediatr.* 2013. doi: 10.1111/apa.12291.

Berlin CM. "Exclusive" breastfeeding of quadruplets. *Breastfeed Med.* 2007;2(2):125–126.

Blair A, Cadwell K, Turner-Maffei C, Brimdyr K. The relationship between positioning, the breastfeeding dynamic, the latching process and pain in breast-feeding mothers with sore nipples. *Breastfeed Rev.* 2003;11(2):5–10.

Blair PS, Ball HL. The prevalence and characteristics associated with parent-infant bed-sharing in England. *Arch Dis Child.* 2004;89(12):1106–1110.

Blair PS, Fleming PJ, Smith IJ, et al. Babies sleeping with parents: case-control study of factors influencing the risk of the sudden infant death syndrome. CESDI SUDI research group. *BMJ.* 1999;319(7223):1457–1461.

Blair PS, Sidebotham P, Berry PJ, et al. Major epidemiological changes in sudden infant death syndrome: a 20-year population-based study in the UK. *Lancet.* 2006;367(9507):314–319.

Bleyl J. Breastfeeding triplets: Personal reflections. In: Blickstein I, Keith L, eds. *Iatrogenic multiple pregnancy: clinical implications.* New York, NY: Parthenon; 2001: 259–264.

Bolman M, Saju L, Oganesyan K, et al. Recapturing the art of therapeutic breast massage during breastfeeding. *J Hum Lact.* 2013. doi: 10.1177/0890334413475527.

Bowers NA, Gromada KK. *Care of the multiple-birth family: pregnancy and birth.* White Plains, NY: March of Dimes; 2005.

Brownell E, Howard CR, Lawrence RA, Dozier AM. Delayed onset lactogenesis II predicts the cessation of any or exclusive breastfeeding. *J Pediatr.* 2012;161(4): 608–614. doi: 10.1016/j.jpeds.2012.03.035.

Buryk M, Bloom D, Shope T. Efficacy of neonatal release of ankyloglossia: a randomized trial. *Pediatrics.* 2011. doi: 10.1542/peds.2011-0077.

Cadwell K. Latching-on and suckling of the healthy term neonate: breastfeeding assessment. *J Midwifery Womens Health.* 2007;52(6):638–642.

Campbell I. Postpartum sleep patterns of mother-baby pairs. *Midwifery.* 1986;2(4):193–201.

Canivet CA, Ostergren PO, Rosén AS, et al. Infantile colic and the role of trait anxiety during pregnancy in relation to psychosocial and socioeconomic factors. *Scand J Public Health.* 2005;33(1):26–34.

Carbajal R, Veerapen S, Couderc S, et al. Analgesic effect of breast feeding in term neonates: randomised controlled trial. *BMJ.* 2003;326(7379):13.

Carpenter RG, Irgens LM, Blair PS, et al. Sudden unexplained infant death in 20 regions in Europe: case control study. *Lancet.* 2004;363(9404):185–191.

Carroccio A, Montalto G, Custro N, et al. Evidence of very delayed clinical reactions to cow's milk in cow's milk-intolerant patients. *Allergy.* 2000;55(6):574–579.

Cavataio F, Carroccio A, Iacono G. Milk-induced reflux in infants less than one year of age. *J Pediatr Gastroenterol Nutr.* 2000;30(suppl):S36–S44.

Centers for Disease Control and Prevention (CDC). *Breastfeeding report card—United States, 2007–2013.* Atlanta, GA: CDC; 2013a.

Centers for Disease Control and Prevention (CDC). *Strategies to prevent obesity and other chronic diseases: the CDC guide to strategies to support breastfeeding mothers and babies.* Atlanta, GA: Department of Health and Human Services; 2013b.

Centuori S, Burmaz T, Ronfani L, et al. Nipple care, sore nipples, and breast-feeding: a randomized trial. *J Hum Lact.* 1999;15(2):125–130.

Chantry CJ, Nommsen-Rivers LA, Peerson JM, et al. Excess weight loss in first-born breastfed newborns relates to maternal intrapartum fluid balance. *Pediatrics.* 2011; 127(1):e171–e179. doi: 10.1542/peds.2009-2663.

Chantry C, et al. *ABM protocol #6: guideline on cosleeping and breastfeeding.* New Rochelle, NY: Academy of Breast-feeding Medicine; 2006.

Chapman DJ, Perez-Escamilla R. Identification of risk factors for delayed onset of lactation. *J Am Diet Assoc.* 1999;99(4):450–454; quiz 455–456.

Chen DC, Nommsen-Rivers L, Dewey KG, Lönnerdal B. Stress during labor and delivery and early lactation performance. *Am J Clin Nutr.* 1998;68(2):335–344.

Chertok IR, Schneider J, Blackburn S. A pilot study of maternal and term infant outcomes associated with ultra-thin nipple shield use. *J Obstet Gynecol Neonatal Nurs.* 2006;35(2):265–272.

Chikly B. *Silent waves: theory and practice of lymph drainage therapy*, 2nd ed. Scottsdale, AZ: IHH Publishing; 2004.

Christensson K, Cabrera T, Christensson E, et al. Separation distress call in the human neonate in the absence of maternal body contact. *Acta Paediatr.* 1995;84(5): 468–473.

Christensson K, Siles C, Moreno L, et al. Temperature, metabolic adaptation and crying in healthy full-term newborns cared for skin-to-skin or in a cot. *Acta Paediatr.* 1992;81(6–7):488–493.

Coons S, Guilleminault C. Development of sleep–wake patterns and non-rapid eye movement sleep stages during the first six months of life in normal infants. *Pediatrics.* 1982;69(6):793–798.

Coons S, Guilleminault C. Development of consolidated sleep and wakeful periods in relation to the day/night cycle in infancy. *Dev Med Child Neurol.* 1984;26(2):169–176.

Cotterman KJ. Reverse pressure softening: a simple tool to prepare areola for easier latching during engorgement. *J Hum Lact.* 2004;20(2):227–237.

Cox DB, Kent JC, Casey TM, et al. Breast growth and the urinary excretion of lactose during human pregnancy and early lactation: endocrine relationships. *Exp Physiol.* 1999;84(2):421–434.

Cregan MD, Hartmann PE. Computerized breast measurement from conception to weaning: clinical implications. *J Hum Lact.* 1999;15(2):89–96.

Daher S, Tahan S, Solé D, et al. Cow's milk protein intolerance and chronic constipation in children. *Pediatr Allergy Immunol.* 2001;12(6):339–342.

Daly SE, Kent JC, Owens RA, Hartmann PE. Frequency and degree of milk removal and the short-term control

of human milk synthesis. *Exp Physiol.* 1996;81(5): 861–875.

Daly SE, Owens RA, Hartmann PE. The short-term synthesis and infant-regulated removal of milk in lactating women. *Exp Physiol.* 1993;78(2):209–220.

da Silva OP, Knoppert DC, Angelini MM, Forret PA. Effect of domperidone on milk production in mothers of premature infants: a randomized, double-blind placebo controlled trial. *Can Med Assoc J.* 2001;164:17–21.

de Carvalho M, Robertson S, Merkatz R, Klaus M. et al. Milk intake and frequency of feeding in breast fed infants. *Early Hum Dev.* 1982;7(2):155–163.

Dennis C, Allen K, McCormick F, Renfrew M. Interventions for treating painful nipples among breast-feeding women (Protocol). *Cochrane Database Syst Rev.* 2008;4:CD007366. doi: 10.1002/14651858. CD007366.

Dewey KG. Maternal and fetal stress are associated with impaired lactogenesis in humans. *J Nutr.* 2001;131(11):3012S–3015S.

Dewey KG, Nommsen-Rivers LA, Heinig MJ, Cohen RJ. Risk factors for suboptimal infant breastfeeding behavior, delayed onset of lactation, and excess neonatal weight loss. *Pediatrics.* 2003;112(3 Pt 1):607–619.

Doan T, Gardiner A, Gay CL, Lee KA. Breast-feeding increases sleep duration of new parents. *J Perinat Neonatal Nurs.* 2007;21(3):200–206.

Dozier AM, Howard CR, Brownell EA, et al. Labor epidural anesthesia, obstetric factors and breastfeeding cessation. *Matern Child Health J.* 2012. doi: 10.1007/s10995-012-1045-4.

Dumas L, Lepage M, Bystrova K, et al. Influence of skin-to-skin contact and rooming-in on early mother–infant interaction: a randomized controlled trial. *Clin Nurs Res.* 2013. doi: 10.1177/1054773812468316.

Dyson L, McCormick F, Renfrew MJ. Interventions for promoting the initiation of breastfeeding. *Cochrane Database Syst Rev.* 2005;2:CD001688.

Eglash A, Ziemer AL, Chevalier A. Health professionals' attitudes and use of nipple shields for breastfeeding women. *Breastfeed Med.* 2010;5(4):147–151. doi: 10.1089/bfm.2010.0006.

Emond A, Ingram J, Johnson D, et al. Randomised controlled trial of early frenotomy in breastfed infants with mild–moderate tongue-tie. *Arch Dis Child Fetal Neonatal Ed.* 2013. doi: 10.1136/archdischild-2013-305031.

Engstrom JL, Meier PP, Jegier B, et al. Comparison of milk output from the right and left breasts during simultaneous pumping in mothers of very low birthweight infants. *Breastfeed Med.* 2007;2(2):83–91.

Enkin M, Keirse M, Neilson J, et al. *A guide to effective care in pregnancy and birth*, 3rd ed. New York, NY: Oxford University Press; 2000.

Estep DC, Kulczycki A Jr. Treatment of infant colic with amino acid-based infant formula: a preliminary study. *Acta Paediatr.* 2000;89(1):22–27.

Evans KC, Evans RG, Royal R, et al. Effect of caesarean section on breast milk transfer to the normal term newborn over the first week of life. *Arch Dis Child Fetal Neonatal Ed.* 2003;88(5):F380–F382.

Evans K, Evans R, Simmer K. Effect of the method of breast feeding on breast engorgement, mastitis and infantile colic. *Acta Paediatr.* 1995;84:849.

Filiano JJ, Kinney HC. A perspective on neuropathologic findings in victims of the sudden infant death syndrome: the triple-risk model. *Biol Neonate.* 1994;65 (3–4):194–197.

Fleming P, Blair PS. Sudden infant death syndrome and parental smoking. *Early Hum Dev.* 2007;83(11):721–725.

Fleming PJ, Blair PS, Pollard K, et al. Pacifier use and sudden infant death syndrome: results from the CESDI/SUDI case control study. *Arch Dis Child.* 1999;81(2):112–116.

Flower H. *Adventures in tandem nursing.* Schaumburg, IL: La Leche League International; 2003.

Foda MI, Kawashima T, Nakamura S, et al. Composition of milk obtained from unmassaged versus massaged breasts of lactating mothers. *J Pediatr Gastroenterol Nutr.* 2004;38(5):484–487.

Franco P, Scaillet S, Wermenbol V, et al. The influence of a pacifier on infants' arousals from sleep. *J Pediatr.* 2000;136(6):775–779.

Fraval MM. A pilot study: osteopathic treatment of infants with a sucking dysfunction. *J Am Acad Osteopath.* 1998;8(2):25–33.

Galbally M, Lewis AJ, McEgan K, et al. Breastfeeding and infant sleep patterns: an Australian population study. *J Paediatr Child Health.* 2013;49(2):E147–E152. doi: 10.1111/jpc.12089.

Gale CR, Martyn CN. Breastfeeding, dummy use, and adult intelligence. *Lancet.* 1996;347(9008):1072–1075.

Galland BC, Taylor BJ, Elder DE, Herbison P. Normal sleep patterns in infants and children: a systematic review of observational studies. *Sleep Med Rev.* 2012;16(3): 213–222. doi: 10.1016/j.smrv.2011.06.001.

Gartner LM, Herschel M. Jaundice and breastfeeding. *Pediatr Clin North Am.* 2001;48(2):389–399.

Gartner LM, Morton J, Lawrence RA, et al. Breastfeeding and the use of human milk. *Pediatrics.* 2005;115(2): 496–506.

Geddes DT. Inside the lactating breast: the latest anatomy research. *J Midwifery Womens Health.* 2007;52(6): 556–563.

Geddes DT, Langton DB, Gollow I, et al. Frenulotomy for breastfeeding infants with ankyloglossia: effect on milk removal and sucking mechanism as imaged by ultrasound. *Pediatrics.* 2008;122(1):e188–e194. doi: 10.1542/peds.2007-2553.

Genna CW. *Selecting and using breastfeeding tools.* Amarillo, TX: Hale; 2009.

Genna CW. *Supporting sucking skills in breastfeeding infants,* 2nd ed. Burlington, MA: Jones & Bartlett Learning; 2013.

Gessner BD, Ives GC, Perham-Hester KA. Association between sudden infant death syndrome and prone sleep position, bed sharing, and sleeping outside an infant crib in Alaska. *Pediatrics.* 2001;108(4):923–927.

Gettler LT, McKenna JJ. Evolutionary perspectives on mother–infant sleep proximity and breastfeeding in a laboratory setting. *Am J Phys Anthropol.* 2011;144(3): 454–462. doi: 10.1002/ajpa.21426.

Gray L, Miller LW, Philipp BL, Blass EM. Breastfeeding is analgesic in healthy newborns. *Pediatrics.* 2002;109(4): 590–593.

Greer FR, Sicherer SH, Burks AW. Effects of early nutritional interventions on the development of atopic disease in infants and children: the role of maternal dietary restriction, breastfeeding, timing of introduction of complementary foods, and hydrolyzed formulas. *Pediatrics.* 2008;121(1):183–191.

Griffiths DM. Do tongue ties affect breastfeeding? *J Hum Lact.* 2004;20(4):409–414.

Grivell RM, Reilly AJ, Oakey H, et al. Maternal and neonatal outcomes following induction of labor: a cohort study. *Acta Obstet Gynecol Scand.* 2012;91(2):198–203. doi: 10.1111/j.1600-0412.2011.01298.x.

Gromada KK. *Mothering multiples,* 3rd rev. ed. Schaumburg, IL: La Leche League International; 2007.

Gromada KK, Spangler AK. Breastfeeding twins and higher-order multiples. *J Obstet Gynecol Neonatal Nurs.* 1998;27(4):441–449.

Gupta SK. Is colic a gastrointestinal disorder? *Curr Opin Pediatr.* 2002;14(5):588–592.

Gupta SK. Update on infantile colic and management options. *Curr Opin Investig Drugs.* 2007;8(11): 921–926.

Hall RT, Mercer AM, Teasley SL, et al. A breast-feeding assessment score to evaluate the risk for cessation of breast-feeding by 7 to 10 days of age. *J Pediatr.* 2002;141(5):659–664.

Hauck FR. Pacifiers and sudden infant death syndrome: what should we recommend? *Pediatrics.* 2006;117(5): 1811–1812.

Hauck FR, Herman SM, Donovan M, et al. Sleep environment and the risk of sudden infant death syndrome in an urban population: the Chicago Infant Mortality Study. *Pediatrics.* 2003;111(5 Pt 2):1207–1214.

Hauck FR, Omojokun OO, Siadaty MS. Do pacifiers reduce the risk of sudden infant death syndrome? A meta-analysis. *Pediatrics.* 2005;116(5):e716–e723.

Hauck FR, Thompson JMD, Tanabe KO, et al. Breastfeeding and reduced risk of sudden infant death syndrome: a meta-analysis. *Pediatrics.* 2011. doi: 10.1542/peds.2010-3000.

Heise AM, Wiessinger D. Dysphoric milk ejection reflex: a case report. *Int Breastfeed J.* 2011;6(1):6. doi: 10.1186/1746-4358-6-6.

Hill PD, Aldag JC. Milk volume on day 4 and income predictive of lactation adequacy at 6 weeks of mothers of nonnursing preterm infants. *J Perinat Neonatal Nurs.* 2005;19(3):273–282.

Hodnett E, Gates S, Hofmeyr GJ, Sakala C. Continuous support for women during childbirth. *Cochrane Database Syst Rev.* 2007;3:CD003766.

Horne RS, Osborne A, Vitkovic J, et al. Arousal from sleep in infants is impaired following an infection. *Early Hum Dev.* 2002;66(2): 89–100.

Horne RS, Parslow PM, Ferens D, et al. Comparison of evoked arousability in breast and formula fed infants. *Arch Dis Child.* 2004;89(1):22–25.

Howard CR, Howard FM, Lanphear B, et al. The effects of early pacifier use on breastfeeding duration. *Pediatrics.* 1999;103(3):E33.

Howard CR, Howard FM, Lanphear B, et al. Randomized clinical trial of pacifier use and bottle-feeding or cupfeeding and their effect on breastfeeding. *Pediatrics.* 2003;111(3):511–518.

Howard CR, Lanphear N, Lanphear BP, et al. Parental responses to infant crying and colic: the effect on breastfeeding duration. 2006;1(3):146–155.

Hrdy SB. *Mother nature: a history of mothers, infants, and natural selection.* New York, NY: Pantheon Books; 1999.

Huang Y, Hauck FR, Signore C, et al. Influence of bedsharing activity on breastfeeding duration among US mothers. *JAMA Pediatrics.* 2013. doi: 10.1001/jamapediatrics.2013.2632.

Huggins KE, Petok ES, Mireles O. Markers of lactation insufficiency: a study of 34 mothers. In: Auerbach KG, ed. *Current issues in clinical lactation 2000.* Sudbury, MA: Jones and Bartlett; 2000:25–35.

Hughes CA, Harley EH, Milmoe G, et al. Birth trauma in the head and neck. *Arch Otolaryngol Head Neck Surg.* 1999;125(2):193–199.

Iacono G, Cavataio F, Montalto G, et al. Persistent cow's milk protein intolerance in infants: the changing faces of the same disease. *Clin Exp Allergy.* 1998;28(7):817–823.

International Lactation Consultants Association (ILCA). *Clinical guidelines for the establishment of exclusive breastfeeding.* Raleigh, NC: International Lactation Consultant Association; 2014.

Jaafar SH, Jahanfar S, Angolkar M, Ho JJ. Pacifier use versus no pacifier use in breastfeeding term infants for increasing duration of breastfeeding. *Cochrane Database Syst Rev.* 2011;3:CD007202. doi: 10.1002/14651858.CD007202.pub2.

Jaafar SH, Jahanfar S, Angolkar M, Ho JJ. Effect of restricted pacifier use in breastfeeding term infants for increasing duration of breastfeeding. *Cochrane Database Syst Rev.* 2012;7:CD007202. doi: 10.1002/14651858.CD007202.pub3.

Jacobs LA, Dickinson JE, Hart PD, et al. Normal nipple position in term infants measured on breastfeeding ultrasound. *J Hum Lact.* 2007;23(1):52–59.

Jain L. Morbidity and mortality in late-preterm infants: more than just transient tachypnea! *J Pediatr.* 2007;151(5):445–446.

Jenni OG, Deboer T, Achermann P. Development of the 24-h rest–activity pattern in human infants. *Infant Behav Dev.* 2006;29(2):143–152. doi: 10.1016/j.infbeh.2005.11.001.

Jonas W, Nissen E, Ransjo-Arvidson AB, et al. Influence of oxytocin or epidural analgesia on personality profile in breastfeeding women: a comparative study. *Arch Womens Ment Health.* 2008;11(5–6):335–345. doi: 10.1007/s00737-008-0027-4.

Jones E, Dimmock PW, Spencer SA. A randomised controlled trial to compare methods of milk expression after preterm delivery. *Arch Dis Child Fetal Neonatal Ed.* 2001;85(2):F91–F95.

Jordan S, Emery S, Bradshaw C, et al. The impact of intrapartum analgesia on infant feeding. *BJOG.* 2005;112(7):927–934.

Karlstrom A, Engström-Olofsson R, Norbergh KG, et al. Postoperative pain after cesarean birth affects breastfeeding and infant care. *JOGNN.* 2007;36:430–440.

Kassing D. Bottle-feeding as a tool to reinforce breastfeeding. *J Hum Lact.* 2001;18(1):56–60.

Keim SA, Fletcher EN, TePoel MRW, McKenzie LB. Injuries associated with bottles, pacifiers, and sippy cups in the United States, 1991–2010. *Pediatrics.* 2012. doi: 10.1542/peds.2011-3348.

Kendall-Tackett K. Why cry-it-out and sleep-training techniques are bad for babies. *Clin Lact.* 2013;4(2): 53–54.

Kent JC. How breastfeeding works. *J Midwifery Womens Health.* 2007;52(6):564–570.

Kent JC, Mitoulas LR, Cregan MD, et al. Volume and frequency of breastfeedings and fat content of breast milk throughout the day. *Pediatrics.* 2006;117(3):e387–e395. doi: 10.1542/peds.2005-1417.

Kulski JK, Hartmann PE. Changes in human milk composition during the initiation of lactation. *Aust J Exp Biol Med Sci.* 1981;59(1):101–114.

Kunz C, Lonnerdal B. Re-evaluation of the whey protein/casein ratio of human milk. *Acta Paediatr.* 1992;81(2):107–112.

LaFleur EA, Niesen KM. Breastfeeding conjoined twins. *J Obstet Gynecol Neonatal Nurs.* 1996;25(3):241–244.

Lahr MB, Rosenberg KD, Lapidus JA. Bedsharing and maternal smoking in a population-based survey of new mothers. *Pediatrics.* 2005;116(4):e530–e542.

Lahr MB, Rosenberg KD, Lapidus JA. Maternal–infant bedsharing: risk factors for bedsharing in a population-based survey of new mothers and implications for SIDS risk reduction. *Matern Child Health J.* 2007;11(3): 277–286.

La Leche League International, Wiessinger D, West D, et al. *Sweet sleep: nighttime and naptime strategies for the breastfeeding family.* New York, NY: Random House/Ballantine Books; 2014.

Lawrence RA, Lawrence RM. *Breastfeeding: a guide for the medical profession.* 7th ed. St. Louis, MO: Elsevier Mosby; 2011.

Lehtonen J, Könönen M, Purhonen M, et al. The effect of nursing on the brain activity of the newborn. *J Pediatr.* 1998;132(4):646–651.

Leonard LG. Depression and anxiety disorders during multiple pregnancy and parenthood. *J Obstet Gynecol Neonatal Nurs.* 1998;27(3):329–337.

Leonard LG. *Breastfeeding multiples.* Vancouver, BC: British Columbia Reproductive Care Program; 2007.

Levine A, Zagoory-Sharon O, Feldman R, Weller A. Oxytocin during pregnancy and early postpartum: individual patterns and maternal–fetal attachment. *Peptides.* 2007; 28(6):1162–1169.

Liang R, Gunn AJ, Gunn TR. Can preterm twins breast feed successfully? *N Z Med J.* 1997;110(1045):209–212.

Livingstone V. Too much of a good thing: maternal and infant hyperlactation syndromes. *Can Fam Physician.* 1996;42:89–99.

Livingstone V, Stringer LJ. The treatment of *Staphylococcus aureus* infected sore nipples: a randomized comparative study. *J Hum Lact.* 1999;15(3):241–246.

Ludington-Hoe SM. Evidence-based review of physiologic effects of kangaroo care. *Curr Women Health Rev.* 2011; 7(3):243–253. doi: 10.2174/157340411796355162.

Ludington-Hoe SM, Johnson MW, Morgan K, et al. Neurophysiologic assessment of neonatal sleep organization: preliminary results of a randomized, controlled trial of skin contact with preterm infants. *Pediatrics.* 2006;117(5):e909–e923.

Marmet C, Lactation Institute. Marmet Technique. 1978. CA: Encino.

Martin J. *Births: final data for 2005.* Hyattsville, MD: National Center for Health Statistics; 2007.

Mathur GP, Mathur S, Khanduja GS. Non-nutritive suckling and use of pacifiers. *Indian Pediatr.* 1990;27(11): 1187–1189.

Mattos-Graner RO, Corrêa MS, Latorre MR, et al. Mutans streptococci oral colonization in 12–30-month-old Brazilian children over a one-year follow-up period. *J Public Health Dent.* 2001;61(3):161–167.

Mauch CE, Scott JA, Magarey AM, Daniels LA. Predictors of and reasons for pacifier use in first-time mothers: an observational study. *BMC Pediatr.* 2012;12:7. doi: 10.1186/1471-2431-12-7.

McClellan H, Geddes D, Kent J, et al. Infants of mothers with persistent nipple pain exert strong sucking vacuums. *Acta Paediatr.* 2008;97(9):1205–1209. doi: 10.1111/j.1651-2227.2008.00882.x.

McClellan HL, Hepworth AR, Garbin CP, et al. Nipple pain during breastfeeding with or without visible trauma. *J Hum Lact.* 2012. doi: 10.1177/ 0890334412444464.

McKenna JJ. *Sleeping with your baby: a parents' guide to cosleeping.* Washington, DC: Platypus Media; 2007.

McKenna JJ, Ball HL, Gettler LT. Mother–infant cosleeping, breastfeeding and sudden infant death syndrome: what biological anthropology has discovered about normal infant sleep and pediatric sleep medicine. *Am J Phys Anthropol.* 2007;45(suppl):133–161. doi: 10.1002/ ajpa.20736.

McKenna JJ, McDade T. Why babies should never sleep alone: a review of the co-sleeping controversy in relation to SIDS, bedsharing and breast feeding. *Paediatr Respir Rev.* 2005;6(2):134–152.

McKenna JJ, Mosko SS, Richard CA. Bedsharing promotes breastfeeding. *Pediatrics.* 1997;100(2 Pt 1):214–219.

McKenna JJ, Volpe LE. Sleeping with baby: an Internet-based sampling of parental experiences, choices, perceptions, and interpretations in a western industrialized context. *Infant Child Develop.* 2007;16(4):359–385. doi: 10.1002/icd.525.

McVea KL, Turner PD, Peppler DK. The role of breastfeeding in sudden infant death syndrome. *J Hum Lact.* 2000;16(1):13–20.

Mead LJ, Chuffo R, Lawlor-Klean P, Meier PP. Breastfeeding success with preterm quadruplets. *J Obstet Gynecol Neonatal Nurs.* 1992;21(3):221–227.

Michelsson K, Christensson K, Rothgänger H, Winberg J. Crying in separated and non-separated newborns: sound spectrographic analysis. *Acta Paediatr.* 1996; 85(4):471–475.

Middlemiss W. Infant sleep: a review of normative and problematic sleep and interventions. *Early Child Develop Care.* 2004;174(1):99–122. doi: 10.1080/ 0300443032000153516.

Middlemiss W, Granger DA, Goldberg WA, Nathans L. Asynchrony of mother–infant hypothalamic–pituitary–adrenal axis activity following extinction of infant crying responses induced during the transition to sleep. *Early Hum Develop.* 2012;88(4):227–232.

Miller JE, Newell D, Bolton JE. Efficacy of chiropractic manual therapy on infant colic: a pragmatic single-blind, randomized controlled trial. *J Manipulative Physiol Ther.* 2012;35(8):600–607. doi: 10.1016/j. jmpt.2012.09.010.

Miller V, Riordan J. Treating postpartum breast edema with areolar compression. *J Hum Lact.* 2004;20:223–226.

Mitchell EA, Blair PS, L'Hoir MP. Should pacifiers be recommended to prevent sudden infant death syndrome? *Pediatrics.* 2006;117(5):1755–1758.

Mitchell EA, Scragg R, Stewart AW, et al. Results from the first year of the New Zealand cot death study. *N Z Med J.* 1991;104(906):71–76.

Mizuno K, Nishida Y, Mizuno N, et al. The important role of deep attachment in the uniform drainage of breast milk from mammary lobe. *Acta Pædiatr.* 2008;97(9):1200–1204.

Montgomery A, Hale TW. ABM clinical protocol #15: analgesia and anesthesia for the breastfeeding mother. *Breastfeed Med.* 2006;1(4):271–277.

Montgomery-Downs HE, Insana SP, Clegg-Kraynok MM, Mancini LM. Normative longitudinal maternal sleep: the first 4 postpartum months. *Am J Obstet Gynecol.* 2010;203(5):e461–e467. doi: 10.1016/j. ajog.2010.06.057.

Moon RY, Horne RS, Hauck FR. Sudden infant death syndrome. *Lancet.* 2007;370(9598):1578–1587.

Moore ER, Anderson GC, Bergman N, Dowswell T. Early skin-to-skin contact for mothers and their healthy newborn infants. *Cochrane Database Syst Rev.* 2012;5:CD003519. doi: 10.1002/14651858. CD003519.pub3.

Morland-Schultz K, Hill PD. Prevention of and therapies for nipple pain: a systematic review. *J Obstet Gynecol Neonatal Nurs.* 2005 Jul-Aug;34(4):428–437.

Morton J, Hall JY, Wong RJ, et al. Combining hand techniques with electric pumping increases milk production in mothers of preterm infants. *J Perinatol.* 2009. doi: 10.1038/jp.2009.87.

Morton J, Wong RJ, Hall JY, et al. Combining hand techniques with electric pumping increases the caloric content of milk in mothers of preterm infants. *J Perinatol.* 2012;32(10):791–796. doi: 10.1038/jp.2011.195.

Moscone SR, Moore MJ. Breastfeeding during pregnancy. *J Hum Lact.* 1993;9(2):83–88.

Mosko S, Richard C, McKenna J. Infant arousals during mother-infant bed sharing: implications for infant sleep and sudden infant death syndrome research. *Pediatrics.* 1997;100(5):841–849.

Neifert MR. Prevention of breastfeeding tragedies. *Pediatr Clin North Am.* 2001;48(2):273–297.

Neifert MR, McDonough SL, Neville MC. Failure of lactogenesis associated with placental retention. *Am J Obstet Gynecol.* 1981;140(4):477–478.

Nelson EA, Yu LM, Williams S. International Child Care Practices study: breastfeeding and pacifier use. *J Hum Lact.* 2005;21(3):289–295.

Neville MC, Morton J. Physiology and endocrine changes underlying human lactogenesis II. *J Nutr.* 2001;131(11):3005S–3008S.

Neville MC, Neifert M. *Lactation: physiology, nutrition and breastfeeding.* New York, NY: Plenum Press; 1983.

Nommsen-Rivers LA, Chantry CJ, Peerson JM, et al. Delayed onset of lactogenesis among first-time mothers is related to maternal obesity and factors associated with ineffective breastfeeding. *Am J Clin Nutri.* 2010;92(3):574–584. doi: 10.3945/ajcn.2010.29192.

Nommsen-Rivers LA, Heinig MJ, Cohen RJ, Dewey KG. Newborn wet and soiled diaper counts and timing of onset of lactation as indicators of breastfeeding inadequacy. *J Hum Lact.* 2008;24(1):27–33. doi: 10.1177/0890334407311538.

Odom EC, Li R, Scanlon KS, et al. Reasons for earlier than desired cessation of breastfeeding. *Pediatrics.* 2013;131(3):e726–e732. doi: 10.1542/peds.2012-1295.

Ohyama M, Watabe H, Hayasaka Y. Manual expression and electric breast pumping in the first 48 h after delivery. *Pediatr Int.* 2010;52(1):39–43. doi: 10.1111/j.1442-200X.2009.02910.x.

Okan F, Ozdil A, Bulbul A, et al. Analgesic effects of skin-to-skin contact and breastfeeding in procedural pain in healthy term neonates. *Ann Trop Paediatr.* 2010;30(2):119–128. doi: 10.1179/146532810X12703902516121.

Parker LA. Part 1: early recognition and treatment of birth trauma: injuries to the head and face. *Adv Neonatal Care.* 2005;5(6):288–297; quiz 298–300.

Parker LA. Part 2: birth trauma: injuries to the intra-abdominal organs, peripheral nerves, and skeletal system. *Adv Neonatal Care.* 2006;6(1):7–14.

Parker LA, Sullivan S, Krueger C, et al. Effect of early breast milk expression on milk volume and timing of lactogenesis stage II among mothers of very low birth weight infants: a pilot study. *J Perinatol.* 2012;32(3):205–209. doi: 10.1038/jp.2011.78.

Parmelee AH Jr, Wenner WH, Schulz HR. Infant sleep patterns: from birth to 16 weeks of age. *J Pediatr.* 1964;65:576–582.

Paul K, Dittrichova J, Papousek H. Infant feeding behavior: development in patterns and motivation. *Dev Psychobiol.* 1996;29(7):563–576.

Pauli-Pott U, Becker K, Mertesacker T, Beckmann D. Infants with "colic": mothers' perspectives on the crying problem. *J Psychosom Res.* 2000;48(2):125–132.

Peirano P, Algarin C, Uauy R. Sleep–wake states and their regulatory mechanisms throughout early human development. *J Pediatr.* 2003;143(4 suppl):S70–S79. doi: S0022347603004049.

Penders J, Thijs C, Vink C, et al. Factors influencing the composition of the intestinal microbiota in early infancy. *Pediatrics.* 2006;118(2):511–521.

Peres KG, De Oliveira Latorre Mdo R, et al. Social and biological early life influences on the prevalence of open bite in Brazilian 6-year-olds. *Int J Paediatr Dent.* 2007;17(1):41–49.

Pollard K, Fleming P, Young J, et al. Night-time non-nutritive sucking in infants aged 1 to 5 months: relationship with infant state, breastfeeding, and bed-sharing versus room-sharing. *Early Hum Dev.* 1999;56(2–3):185–204.

Preer GL, Newby PK, Philipp BL. Weight loss in exclusively breastfed infants delivered by cesarean birth. *J Hum Lact.* 2012;28(2):153–158. doi: 10.1177/0890334411434177.

Quillin SI, Glenn LL. Interaction between feeding method and co-sleeping on maternal–newborn sleep. *J Obstet Gynecol Neonatal Nurs.* 2004;33(5):580–588.

Quinlan PT, Lockton S, Irwin J, Lucas AL. The relationship between stool hardness and stool composition in breast- and formula-fed infants. *J Pediatr Gastroenterol Nutr.* 1995;20(1):81–90.

Ramsay DT, Mitoulas LR, Kent JC, et al. The use of ultrasound to characterize milk ejection in women using an electric breast pump. *J Hum Lact.* 2005;21(4):421–428.

Ramsay DT, Mitoulas LR, Kent JC, et al. Milk flow rates can be used to identify and investigate milk ejection in women expressing breast milk using an electric breast pump. *Breastfeed Med.* 2006;1(1):14–23.

Richard C, Mosko S, McKenna J, Drummond S. Sleeping position, orientation, and proximity in bedsharing infants and mothers. *Sleep.* 1996;19(9):685–690.

Ricke LA, Baker NJ, Madlon-Kay DJ, DeFor TA. Newborn tongue-tie: prevalence and effect on breast-feeding. *J Am Board Fam Pract.* 2005;18(1):1–7.

Righard L, Alade MO. Breastfeeding and the use of pacifiers. *Birth.* 1997;24(2):116–120.

Riordan J, Gill-Hopple J, Angeron J. Indicators of effective breastfeeding and estimates of breast milk intake. *J Hum Lact.* 2005;21:406–412.

Russell CK, Robinson L, Ball HL. Infant sleep development: location, feeding and expectations in the postnatal period. *Open Sleep J.* 2013;6(suppl 1 M9):68076. doi: 10.2174/1874620901306010068.

Saint L, Maggiore P, Hartmann PE. Yield and nutrient content of milk in eight women breast-feeding twins and one woman breast-feeding triplets. *Br J Nutr.* 1986;56(1):49–58.

Salvatore S, Vandenplas Y. Gastroesophageal reflux and cow milk allergy: is there a link? *Pediatrics.* 2002;110(5):972–984.

Samra NM, El Tawee A, Cadwell K. Effect of intermittent kangaroo mother care on weight gain of low birth weight neonates with delayed weight gain. *J Perinatal Educ.* 2013;22(4):194–200.

Santo LC, de Oliveira LD, Giugliani ER. Factors associated with low incidence of exclusive breastfeeding for the first 6 months. *Birth.* 2007;34(3):212–219.

Santos IS, Mota DM, Matijasevich A, et al. Bed-sharing at 3 months and breast-feeding at 1 year in southern Brazil. *J Pediatr.* 2009;155(4):505–509. doi: 10.1016/j.jpeds.2009.04.037.

Schore AN. Effects of a secure attachment relationship on right brain development, affect regulation, and infant mental health. *Infant Mental Health J.* 2001;22(1):7–66.

Scott JA, Binns CW, Oddy WH. Predictors of delayed onset of lactation. *Matern Child Nutr.* 2007;3(3):186–193.

Shrago LC, Reifsnider E, Insel K. The Neonatal Bowel Output Study: indicators of adequate breast milk intake in neonates. *Pediatr Nurs.* 2006;32(3):195–201.

Smillie CMM. *Baby-led breastfeeding: the mother-baby dance* [DVD]. Geddes Production; 2007.

Smith LJ. Impact of birthing practices on the breastfeeding dyad. *J Midwifery Womens Health.* 2007;52(6): 621–630.

Smith LJ, Kroeger M. *Impact of birthing practices on breastfeeding,* 2nd ed. Sudbury, MA: Jones and Bartlett; 2010.

Snowden HM, Renfrew MJ, Woolridge MW. Treatments for breast engorgement during lactation. *Cochrane Database Syst Rev.* 2001;2:CD000046.

Snyder JB. *Variation in infant palatal structure and breastfeeding.* Pasadena, CA: Pacific Oaks College; 1995.

Sondergaard C, Olsen J, Friis-Haschè E, et al. Psychosocial distress during pregnancy and the risk of infantile colic: a follow-up study. *Acta Paediatr.* 2003;92(7):811–816.

Spencer SA, Jones E, Dobson J, et al. *Breastfeeding: a multimedia learning resource for healthcare professionals.* Bradford, UK: Matrix Multimedia; 1998.

Srinivasan A, Dobrich C, Mitnick H, Feldman P. Ankyloglossia in breastfeeding infants: the effect of frenotomy on maternal nipple pain and latch. *Breastfeed Med.* 2006;1icine,1(4):216–224. doi:10.1089/bfm.2006.1.216.

Stark Y. *Human nipples: function and anatomical variations in relationship to breastfeeding.* Pasadena, CA: Pacific Oaks College; 1993.

St James-Roberts I. What is distinct about infants' "colic" cries? *Arch Dis Child.* 1999;80(1):56–61; discussion 62.

Szajewska H, Gyrczuk E, Horvath A. *Lactobacillus reuteri* DSM 17938 for the management of infantile colic in breastfed infants: a randomized, double-blind, placebo-controlled trial. *J Pediatr.* 2013;162(2): 257–262. doi: 10.1016/j.jpeds.2012.08.004.

Szucs KA, Axline SE, Rosenman MB. Quintuplets and a mother's determination to provide human milk: it takes a village to raise a baby—how about five? *J Hum Lact.* 2009;25(1):79–84. doi: 10.1177/0890334408328385.

Task Force on Sudden Infant Death Syndrome. SIDS and other sleep-related infant deaths: expansion of recommendations for a safe infant sleeping environment. *Pediatrics.* 2011. doi: 10.1542/peds.2011-2284.

Teti DM, Kim BR, Mayer G, Countermine M. Maternal emotional availability at bedtime predicts infant sleep quality. *J Fam Psychol.* 2010;24(3):307–315. doi: 10.1037/a0019306.

Thorley V. Latch and the fear response: overcoming an obstacle to successful breastfeeding. *Breastfeed Rev.* 2005;13(1):9–11.

Torvaldsen S, Roberts CL, Simpson JM, et al. Intrapartum epidural analgesia and breastfeeding: a prospective cohort study. *Int Breastfeed J.* 2006;1:24.

Uvnas-Moberg K, Eriksson M. Breastfeeding: physiological, endocrine and behavioural adaptations caused by oxytocin and local neurogenic activity in the nipple and mammary gland. *Acta Paediatr.* 1996;85(5):525–530.

Vanderhoof JA, Perry D, Hanner TL, Young RJ. Allergic constipation: association with infantile milk allergy. *Clin Pediatr (Phila).* 2001;40(7):399–402.

Van der Wijden C, Kleijnen J, Van den Berk T. Lactational amenorrhea for family planning. *Cochrane Database Syst Rev.* 2003;4:CD001329.

Vogel AM, Hutchison BL, Mitchell EA. The impact of pacifier use on breastfeeding: a prospective cohort study. *J Paediatr Child Health.* 2001;37(1):58–63.

Wagner EA, Chantry CJ, Dewey KG, Nommsen-Rivers LA. Breastfeeding concerns at 3 and 7 days postpartum and feeding status at 2 months. *Pediatrics*. 2013. doi: 10.1542/peds.2013-0724.

Walker M. *Breastfeeding management for the clinician: using the evidence*, 2nd ed. Sudbury, MA: Jones and Bartlett; 2011.

Wall V, Glass R. Mandibular asymmetry and breastfeeding problems: experience from 11 cases. *J Hum Lact*. 2006;22(3):328–334.

Weber MW, Clinical Signs Study Group. Clinical signs that predict severe illness in children under age 2 months: a multicenter study. *Lancet*. 2008;371:135–142.

Weiss PP, Kerbl R. The relatively short duration that a child retains a pacifier in the mouth during sleep: implications for sudden infant death syndrome. *Eur J Pediatr*. 2001;160(1):60.

Wessel MA, Cobb JC, Jackson EB, et al. Paroxysmal fussing in infancy, sometimes called colic. *Pediatrics*. 1954; 14(5):421–435.

Wiberg JM, Nordsteen J, Nilsson N. The short-term effect of spinal manipulation in the treatment of infantile colic: a randomized controlled clinical trial with a blinded observer. *J Manipulative Physiol Ther*. 1999;22(8): 517–522.

Widstrom AM, Lilja G, Aaltomaa-Michalias P, et al. Newborn behaviour to locate the breast when skin-to-skin: a possible method for enabling early self-regulation. *Acta Paediatr*. 2011;100(1):79–85. doi: 10.1111/j.1651-2227.2010.01983.x.

Widstrom AM, Thingstrom-Paulsson J. The position of the tongue during rooting reflexes elicited in newborn infants before the first suckle. *Acta Paediatr*. 1993; 82(3):281–283.

Wiklund I, Norman M, Uvnas-Moberg K, et al. Epidural analgesia: breast-feeding success and related factors. *Midwifery*. 2009;25(2):e31–e38. doi: 10.1016/j. midw.2007.07.005.

Wilde CJ, Knight CH, Flint DJ. Control of milk secretion and apoptosis during mammary involution. *J Mammary Gland Biol Neoplasia*. 1999;4(2):129–36.

Wilson-Clay B, Hoover K. *The breastfeeding atlas*, 5th ed. Manchaca, TX: LactNews; 2013.

Wolf LS, Glass RB. *Feeding and swallowing disorders in infancy: assessment and management*. Tucson, AZ: Therapy Skill Builders; 1992.

World Health Organization (WHO). *Safe preparation, storage and handling of powdered infant formula*. Geneva, Switzerland: WHO; 2007.

World Health Organization (WHO). *Acceptable medical reasons for use of breast-milk substitutes*. Vol. WHO/NMH/NHD/ 09.01 WHO/FCH/CAH/09.01. Geneva, Switzerland: WHO; 2009.

World Health Organization (WHO), United Nations Childrens Fund (UNICEF). *Global strategy for infant and young child feeding*. Geneva, Switzerland: WHO; 2003.

World Health Organization (WHO), United Nations Childrens Fund (UNICEF). *Baby-Friendly Hospital Initiative: revised, updated and expanded for integrated care*. Geneva, Switzerland: WHO; 2009.

Zhang K, Wang X. Maternal smoking and increased risk of sudden infant death syndrome: a meta-analysis. *Leg Med (Tokyo)*. 2013;15(3):115–121. doi: 10.1016/j. legalmed.2012.10.007.

Chapter 9

Breast-Related Problems

Karen Wambach

Introduction

An ounce of prevention is worth a pound of intervention. Many difficulties women encounter while breastfeeding can be prevented by self-care measures and breastfeeding education. When a woman fully understands how her body works, she is at less risk for frustration and failure when she encounters a barrier to breastfeeding. This chapter deals with specific breast problems and identifies how health professionals can help.

Clinicians who work with breastfeeding women agree that breast and nipple problems often present barriers to breastfeeding. During prenatal visits, women should be screened for anatomic variations in the breasts, areolae, or nipples and lack of breast enlargement. Any of these issues, coupled with previous breastfeeding difficulties, can be high-risk indicators for breastfeeding problems.

Before discussing the more clinical aspects of breast-related problems, including surgery, it is important to address the emotional significance of the female breasts. Breasts are part of a woman's internalized body image that she develops around adolescence and carries with her for the rest of her life. The breasts represent a woman's deepest sense of womanhood. Any change in her breasts (e.g., breast surgery) threatens this feminine internal view of self and creates disequilibrium. When a woman's breasts are altered by illness or infection, both her femininity and her ability to breastfeed can be threatened.

Nipple Variations

Inverted or Flat Nipples

Two types of nipple inversion are distinguished: (1) retractile/umbilicated, where the nipple can be pulled out (everted); and (2) invaginated ("true" inversion), where the nipple cannot be everted or can be everted only with great difficulty. Han and Hung (1999) identified three grades of inversions for the purpose of differentiating surgical correction techniques for each:

- Grade I: Similar to the retractile/umbilicated type noted previously. The nipple pulls out easily (everts) and maintains projection without traction.
- Grade II: Also can be manually everted, but not as easily as Grade I and tends to retract.
- Grade III: The nipple is severely inverted and retracted, is very difficult to evert, and promptly retracts after eversion.

Congenital inversion probably results from a failure of the underlying mesenchyme to proliferate and move the nipple out of its normally depressed position. In a study of prevalence of the condition, approximately 3% of Korean women ($n = 1625$) had nipple inversion. Most of these cases were retractile

(73% to 92%) and occurred bilaterally (Park et al., 1999) (see Color Plates 47 and 48).

Retractile inversion sometimes resolves itself from the beginning to the end of pregnancy. In many cases, the degree of inversion is such that it does not affect the ability of the baby to grasp the areolar tissue and draw the nipple into the mouth, although this action might take longer. Lactation consultants have observed that women who have markedly inverted nipples early in their first pregnancy and who breastfeed have much less inversion with subsequent pregnancies. In some cases, these women have reported that their nipples, which initially inverted between feedings with the first baby, no longer do so with second and later infants.

The degree to which inverted nipples are an impediment to breastfeeding reflects the belief that they prevent breastfeeding. How the nipple looks when it is not in the baby's mouth, however, does not always predict how well it functions. In most cases, as long as the mother with inverted nipples positions the baby well back on the areola so that the entire nipple is placed deep enough in the baby's mouth, there is no reason why she should forgo breastfeeding. During suckling, the nipple elongates to double its resting length (Smith et al., 1988). Such reactivity to infant suckling helps to explain by inference why the degree of inversion appears to lessen after weeks or months of repeated suckling by the infant.

Although many women are able to successfully breastfeed despite inverted nipples, some evidence suggests that breastfeeding difficulty can occur with adverse outcomes. In a prospective cohort study (Vazirinejad et al., 2009), 100 healthy term neonates were followed from birth to day 7 after being separated into two groups: 50 neonates born to mothers with specified breast variations (inverted nipples [14%], flat nipples [54%], large nipples [34%], and large breasts [24%]) and 50 neonates born to mothers without breast or nipple variations. Mean weight gain differences in the first 7 days were significantly greater in those neonates whose mother did not have breast variations ($t = 7.5$, $df = 49$, $p < 0.01$). Although this study had limitations including absence of breast/nipple measurements, scientific definitions for breast variations,

lack of data on infant outcome according to the type of breast variation, and follow-up on duration of breastfeeding, it provides evidence of a relationship between breast variations and neonatal short-term outcomes. Clearly, breast and nipple assessment is important both prenatally and postnatally.

When the clinician examines the mother's breasts and nipples in the third trimester of pregnancy, discussion about breastfeeding can continue. If the mother has flat or inverted nipples at that time, she can be taught that following birth, massage and stimulation of the nipple prior to nursing can evert the nipple and facilitate latch-on. The infant also stretches the nipples during feedings. Hoffman's exercises (exercises of the nipples during pregnancy) and breast shells—two traditional methods for treating inverted nipples— appear to be ineffective and are no longer recommended (Alexander et al., 1992). Commercial "nipple enhancers or everters" designed to evert flat or inverted nipples are available for purchase; some industry-funded "trials" have reported benefits from these products. For example, Maternal Concepts reported on its hospital trial of the Evert-It Nipple Enhancer, stating that women found it easy to use and clean, as well as effective in pulling out everted nipples (see http://www .maternalconcepts.com/index.pl?p=products/evert -it&id=1ba61620a59ae9c5bc63d2c4f5c40f47).

The first intervention for treating a retractable, inverted, or flat nipple should be to stimulate and shape the nipple just before the feeding. For a flat nipple (not inverted), massage the nipple or apply a cold cloth to help the nipple to evert outward. For an inverted nipple, instruct the mother to shape her nipple by placing her thumb about 1.5 to 2 inches behind the nipple (with her fingers beneath) and pulling back into her chest. This works best in a side-lying position. Any pump can be used to help pull out the nipple immediately before the infant feeds. Placing a silicone nipple shield (described in the *Breast Pumps and Other Technologies* chapter) on the inverted nipple is another method of dealing with the problem of the baby not being able to latch onto the breast because of nipple inversion. The baby can usually ingest sufficient milk through the thin shield, and at the same time his suckling stimulates the mother's nipples.

For severe inversion (invaginated or Grade III), surgical intervention is available and techniques are improving to reduce damage to the lactiferous sinuses/ducts. Shiau et al. (2011) reported successful breastfeeding in three cases following surgical correction using a telescope method. More recently, a minimally invasive gradual traction technique was used in 169 cases, with 42 patients successfully breastfeeding during the study follow-up period (Mu et al., 2012). Women with documented severe inversion and breastfeeding difficulty may opt to explore surgical treatment with an appropriate medical practitioner, generally a plastic surgeon.

Absence of Nipple Pore Openings

Very rarely, duct pore openings on the mother's nipple are absent. Two cases have been reported. In one case, the mother's right breast became abnormally enlarged starting in her third month of pregnancy. Following delivery of her baby, this breast became extremely engorged and she was unable to express any milk from it. An ultrasound revealed that the mother had no nipple pores and no ducts leading from the nipple to the larger ducts, which caused extreme enlargement of the right breast. (Her left breast was normal.) Cosmetic surgery was offered to this mother, but because she was newly emigrated from India and had no insurance, she refused the surgery (V. Miller, personal communication, June 2003). The other reported case was similar. Despite many attempts to breastfeed and then to pump, a Korean mother was unable to express even one drop of breastmilk.

Large or Elongated Nipples

Nipples come in assorted sizes and shapes and, like all anatomic structures, are genetically influenced. Clinicians report that Asian women are more likely to have unusually long nipples. Generally, nipples that are larger or longer than normal are less likely to cause problems in breastfeeding than are inverted or flat nipples. In fact, they are often viewed as an anatomic gift that will make breastfeeding easier. Although this is true in many cases, exceptionally long or large nipples (see Color Plate 45) may detract from breastfeeding, especially if the infant is small. Infants of mothers with extra-long nipples have been observed to gag after latch-on and to slide back toward the nipple tip (see Color Plate 46), which in some cases causes the mother to develop sore nipples. The Vazirinejad et al. (2009) study mentioned earlier documented lower weight gain in the first 7 days of life among neonates whose mothers had breast/nipple variations, including large nipples.

Plugged Ducts

No one knows the specific cause of plugged ducts, but they are usually found in mothers who have an abundant milk supply and who do not adequately drain each breast. Pathological changes within the breast that cause the plug are vaguely referred to in the literature as a stasis, clogging of milk, or local accumulations of milk or dead cells that have been shed. A plugged duct is indicated by either of these two sets of symptoms: (1) complaints of tenderness, heat, and possible redness in one area of the breast, or (2) if the plug is located in a duct close to the skin, a palpable lump of well-defined margins without a generalized fever. Sometimes, a tiny white milk plug can be seen at the opening of the duct on the nipple. One mother described it as "little bits of a hard white substance" that is just beneath the surface of milk duct outlets. Color Plate 11 shows a milk plug.

Incomplete drainage caused by a skipped feeding or a constricting bra, poor nutrition, and stress have all been implicated in the development of plugged ducts, but a cause-and-effect relationship has never been substantiated. Assessment should include a review of these possibilities with the mother and a review of events leading up to the plugged duct, especially if the mother repeatedly experiences this problem. There is no need to prescribe an antibiotic to treat a plugged duct unless fever and mastitis develop.

Clinicians have observed that the frequency of plugged ducts increases during the winter season. Although the reason for this is not clear, it may be related to the restricting effects of winter clothing or simply to the cold weather. There is also some

---

BOX 9-1 SELF-CARE FOR TREATING A PLUGGED DUCT

- Continue to breastfeed often. Begin feeding on the affected breast to promote drainage.
- Depress the breast during the feed to prevent plugged ducts (Fetherston, 1998).
- Massage the affected breast before and during feeding to stimulate flow of milk. Support the breast with a cupped hand and use firm massage, starting at the periphery of the breast, using thumb to encourage flow of milk while baby suckles. (Another option is to massage the breast in a hot shower or bath.) Outside of the shower, try using an electric vibrator (on low setting).
- Soak the affected breast(s) by leaning over a basin of warm water, and gently massage them.
- Change position of the infant during feedings to ensure drainage of all the sinuses and ductules in the breast. At least one position should result in the baby's nose being pointed toward the site of the plugged duct.
- Avoid any constricting clothing, such as an underwire bra or the straps on a baby carrier.
- Lecithin, 1600 mg daily is recommended for alleviation and prevention of clogged milk ducts, especially for women in whom it recurs (Scott, 2005).

---

evidence that, whereas some women are predisposed to developing plugged ducts, others never encounter it through multiple breastfeeding experiences. Plugged ducts can also lead to mastitis, especially if ignored or untreated. Box 9-1 presents self-care measures to recommend to a mother with a plugged duct.

In acute situations, briskly massaging the breast may effectively dislodge the blocked milk. A recent description of therapeutic hand massage by Bolman et al. (2013) advocated for this technique's use in women with plugged ducts and mastitis. The two main principles of therapeutic hand massage are (1) encouraging mobilization of fluid with massage toward the axillae to facilitate lymph circulation and (2) alternating massage and hand expression to facilitate milk removal (p. 331). In the case of plugged duct, massage and expression are alternated and a finger from the nonmassaging hand provides gentle but firm pressure moving around the edges of the plug to assist in its release.

Other therapies for plugged ducts and associated difficulties include therapeutic ultrasound by chiropractors as reported by Lavigne and Gleberzon (2012). Recent research in China (Zhao et al., 2014) has suggested that the six-step recanalization manual

therapy (SSRMT) is a low-cost and effective treatment for plugged ducts. SSRMT consists of (1) preparation, (2) clearing the plugged duct outlets, (3) nipple manipulation, (4) pushing and pressing the areola, (5) pushing and kneading the breast, and (6) checking for residual milk stasis. A large ($n = 3497$) observational trial of a single SSRMT treatment resulted in 3189 (91.2%), 173 (4.9%), and 83 (2.4%) patients achieving Grade I (complete resolution), Grade II (marked improvement), and Grade III (improvement) responses, respectively, with only 52 (1.5%) showing unresponsiveness. For the 308 (8.8% of total) non-Grade I patients, a second SSRMT given three days later resulted in Grade I, II, and III responses in 267 (7.6% of total), 28 (0.8%), and 13 (0.4%) patients, respectively, and no patients were absolutely unresponsive. More experimental research is needed to provide evidence of effectiveness of such therapies in more diverse populations.

If a mother has chronically recurring plugged ducts, some physicians may elect to open the duct with a sterile needlelike instrument. After this is done, the milk may forcibly shoot out from the duct, giving the mother relief; the "plug" that is released may also consist of strings of coalesced milk. This procedure can be followed by recurring pain in the affected area and should be performed only in extreme cases.

Mastitis

Lactation mastitis can develop during the early postpartum weeks after the mother leaves the hospital, and overall it is most commonly observed during the first 3 to 6 months of breastfeeding. Nurses and lactation consultants who practice in a clinic may be the first to speak with the mother whose symptoms suggest early-stage mastitis. The advice dispensed during this initial call can prevent this condition from advancing to an abscess, especially if the mother mistakenly thinks she should stop breastfeeding or has already done so. In fact, breastfeeding usually helps to clear up the inflammation or infection, and nursing will not harm the baby.

Mastitis is usually a benign, self-limiting condition, with few consequences for the suckling infant. The initial symptoms of puerperal mastitis are fatigue, localized breast tenderness, headache, and flulike muscle aches (Wambach, 2003). If a breastfeeding mother complains that she has the "flu," the first consideration is to rule out infectious mastitis. Typically, fever, a rapid pulse, and the appearance of a hot, reddened, and tender area on the breast follow fatigue, headache, and muscular aching (see Color Plate 19). The infection is usually unilateral and located in one area (usually in the upper outer breast quadrant because most of the breast tissue is there), although it can occur in any area of the breast (Wambach, 2003). It can occasionally occur in both breasts simultaneously and may involve a large portion of the breast.

In worldwide studies published within the last 20 years, the incidence of lactation mastitis ranged from 4% to 27% depending on the methods, especially subject selection, used in the study (Amir et al., 2007; Fetherston, 1995; Foxman et al., 2002; Vogel et al., 1999). Mastitis is most likely to occur in the first several weeks after delivery (Amir, 1999; Amir et al., 2007; Potter, 2005; Wambach, 2003). About one-third of the cases in long-term breastfeeding mothers occur after the infant is 6 months

old (Riordan & Nichols, 1990). The risk of mastitis is higher among women who have breastfed previously, especially those with a history of mastitis (Foxman et al., 2002; Wambach, 2003)—a finding that contradicts the enduring myth that mastitis results from inexperience with breastfeeding. Symptoms last approximately 2 to 5 days. Breast pain and redness peak on days 2 and 3 and return to normal by day 5. Fatigue is the slowest symptom to dissipate.

A number of risk factors predispose a woman to mastitis:

- Stress and fatigue (Fetherston, 1998; Riordan & Nichols, 1990). Mothers who have mastitis rate stress and fatigue as major factors leading to the infection; typically they describe themselves as exhausted as a result of circumstances above and beyond the normal stresses of taking care of the infant—for example, getting ready for holiday celebrations.
- Cracked or fissured nipples, and nipple pain (Amir et al., 2007; Fetherston, 1998; Foxman et al., 1994; Vogel et al., 1999). A breakdown in the epidermis provides an avenue of entry into the breast tissue, although breakdown is not a prerequisite for a breast infection. Mastitis from sore, cracked nipples usually occurs in the first few weeks postpartum.
- Plugged or blocked ducts (Fetherston, 1998). Some women repeatedly develop plugged ducts, some of which lead to a full-blown infection. It is not uncommon to be able to see this plug as a white "head" and to feel pressure and tenderness around the plug. Gentle massage above the area of tenderness while the baby is breastfeeding from that breast may help, particularly if the plug is newly formed.
- Ample milk supply or decrease in number of feedings (Vogel et al., 1999). Women with an abundant milk supply experience more plugged ducts (and subsequent mastitis) than women with a normal supply.
- Engorgement and stasis. A decrease in the frequency of feedings presents the potential for engorgement or milk stasis. Infrequent feedings and milk stasis are frequently

mentioned in the literature as being associated with mastitis, but little evidence exists to support this contention. In fact, at least one researcher (Foxman et al., 2002) discovered that women without a history of mastitis who fed 6 or fewer times per day had a rate of mastitis five times lower than those who fed 10 or more times per day. The daily use of a pacifier was associated with a *reduced* risk for mastitis in another study (Vogel et al., 1999)—just the opposite of conventional wisdom. Although it is logical to assume that the natural washing mechanism associated with breastmilk removal helps remove bacteria, bacteria can adhere to the epithelial cells lining the duct especially if the woman experiences breast trauma (Fetherston, 2001). Moreover, the presence of bacteria in milk is normal and breastmilk is not a good medium for bacterial growth.

Other conditions, such as breast trauma, constriction from tight bra or sleeping position (Fetherston, 1998), use of a manual pump (Foxman et al., 2002), poor maternal nutrition, and vigorous exercise (particularly of the upper arms and chest) have been mentioned anecdotally as factors leading up to mastitis. These factors also should be noted in the assessment and history in the event that they predispose the mother to mastitis.

Treatment for Mastitis

The treatments for hastening recovery include continued breastfeeding, application of moist heat, increased fluids, bed rest, pain medication (acetaminophen, ibuprofen) and judicious use of antibiotics (Amir et al., 2014). Table 9-1 lists recommended antibiotics.

It is well established in the medical literature that mastitis is most commonly associated with the presence of *Staphylococcus aureus*. However, if a culture is done, bacteria normally present on the skin (coagulase-negative staphylococci, non-B-hemolytic streptococci) may be the only isolates in the milk culture. Osterman and Rahm (2000) compared mastitis symptoms according to bacteria found in a milk culture by dividing a sample of women with mastitis into two groups: Group A had only the bacteria normally present on the skin, whereas Group B's culture contained potential pathogenic bacteria. The only differences in symptoms between the two groups were that women with pathogenic bacteria in their milk were more likely to have sore nipples before the mastitis and to develop the mastitis earlier post delivery than those with normal bacteria. There were no differences in other symptoms such as fever and shivering.

Only rarely is a streptococcal bacterium involved. When it is, this pathogen may be present in breastmilk without causing clinical mastitis.

Table 9-1 SELECTED ANTIBIOTICS FOR MASTITIS

Generic Name	Trade Name	Adult Dosage Ranges
Penicillinase-Resistant Penicillins		
Amoxicillin + clavulanate	Augmentin	875 mg BID
Dicloxacillin	Dycill	500 mg QID
Flucloxacillin	Flucil	500 mg QID
Cephalosporins		
Cephalexin	Keflex	500 mg QID
Used in Penicillin Allergy		
Clindamycin	Cleocin	300 mg TID
Trimethoprim-sulfamethoxazole	Bactrim or Septra	160 mg/800 mg BID

Treatment with antibiotics can eradicate the organism from the milk (Oliver et al., 2000). Although untreated cases heal almost as quickly as treated ones, the standard antibiotic for lactation mastitis is a penicillinase-resistant penicillin or a cephalosporin that covers *S. aureus* for 10 to 14 days. If symptoms do not begin to subside after 48 hours of treatment, milk cultures may be obtained to rule out methicillin-resistant *S. aureus* (MRSA), which has become a more frequently encountered infection (Amir et al., 2014).

For chronic mastitis, erythromycin at low doses (regular 250–500 mg doses every 6 hours) or trimethoprim-sulfamethoxazole (Bactrim, Septra) over a longer period of time has been recommended (Cantlie, 1988). Unfortunately, staphylococci rapidly develop resistance against erythromycin. Trimethoprim-sulfamethoxazole and erythromycin are also options when the mother is allergic to penicillin. In a case report, trimethoprim-sulfamethoxazole (2 tablets per day for 10 days) was effective in preventing recurrence of mastitis in a patient with multiple incidents of mastitis who was allergic to penicillin (Hoffman & Auerbach, 1986). These medications can be taken during breastfeeding without known untoward reactions in the infant.

Eglash and Proctor (2007) reported a case of bacterial lactiferous duct infection. The initial antibiotic choice was clindamycin 300 mg every 6 hours. Two weeks later, the patient reported a lack of improvement and a painful right nipple crack that was worsening. The woman was treated with 14 days of fluconazole in addition to clindamycin. Two weeks later, she reported feeling no better, and she was taken off clindamycin and fluconazole and treated with azithromycin 500 mg daily for 5 days. One week later, the patient called to report that the nipple cracks were healing, and she had less breast pain. After 2 more weeks of azithromycin, the patient called to say that all of her pain was resolved, her nipple crack was almost healed, and she was fully nursing her baby. The authors concluded that lactating women with chronic breast pain who have suspected bacterial lactiferous duct infection might need 4–8 weeks of an antibiotic that will cover *S. aureus.*

In the dairy industry, giving antioxidants such as vitamin E to cows is commonly recognized as a means of preventing mastitis. Echinacea, one of the most popular herbal remedies, also stimulates the immune system and may help to keep the infection in check (Binns, 2000). In addition, mothers with mastitis have reported taking vitamin C supplements (Wambach, 2003) to fight infection.

Another alternative treatment for mastitis is the application of a solution of bacteriocin nisin to the nipple and areola. Nisin, a food-grade antimicrobial peptide produced by strains of *Lactococcus lactis,* shows promise as an alternative to antibiotics for the treatment of staphylococcal mastitis (Fernandez et al., 2008).

Oxytocin nasal spray and acupuncture are used to treat mastitis in Sweden at the discretion of the midwife. Oxytocin nasal spray, which is used in the belief that drainage of the breast will be aided by the contractile effect of oxytocin on the lactiferous ducts, has been shown to hasten recovery from mastitis (Kvist et al., 2007). In the same study, acupuncture relieved the severity of symptoms but did not reduce the number of contact days needed with healthcare services for inflammatory symptoms to subside (Kvist et al., 2007).

A mother with mastitis feels ill and is often emotional and discouraged (Amir & Lumley, 2006). She may ask, "Why does this have to happen to me?" and she may contemplate weaning. In addition, her supply of milk in the affected breast may be diminished for several weeks following the infection. She needs mothering herself—a role that the lactation specialist can assume as she reassures the mother that the infection will eventually resolve. To stop or limit breastfeeding will only increase the risk of infection or recurrence. Tender loving care goes a long way in helping the mother through this difficult time. She also needs specific advice and a plan for care (Table 9-2) as well as a long-term plan for self-care. A considerable number of mothers develop mastitis more than once during the course of lactation (Wambach, 2003). Therefore, certain women may be prone to the condition, and prevention is important. Review with the mother all the possible factors that preceded and may have contributed to

Table 9-2 MASTITIS TEACHING PLAN

Content/Goal	Teaching
Prevention	
Reduction of stress and fatigue related to childbearing responsibilities	Prioritize tasks from most important to least important.
	Encourage other family members to assist in routine household tasks. Hire household help if possible.
	Delay return to job as long as possible.
	Hold one informal open house for friends and relatives to see new baby. Use voicemail to filter calls. Turn down social invitations. Ignore e-mail.
	Take day naps when infant sleeps.
Plugged ducts	Breastfeed often (at least 8 to 12 times per day).
	Massage any reddened area of breast, especially while breastfeeding.
Change in number of feedings	Pump or express milk if a feeding is skipped.
Engorgement/stasis	Pump or express milk if breasts become overfull or distended.
	Wear bras without support underwires.
Care if Mastitis Occurs	
Self-care and relief of discomfort	Recognize early signs and symptoms: redness, fatigue, fever, chills.
	Rest with infant and fluids at bedside.
	Continue frequent breastfeedings.
Medical care	Monitor oral temperature.
	Place moist, warm packs at place of infection and over nipple.
	Expect slightly reduced milk supply in affected breast post infection.
	Take antibiotics if needed. (They may not be necessary if fever is already subsiding.)
	Take antipyretic to reduce fever.

her bout(s) of mastitis. Then encourage the mother to seek medical help early if symptoms recur. Some mothers, especially if they are experienced long-term breastfeeders, do not consult their physicians, even though their mastitis warrants medical attention.

Types and Severity of Mastitis

Attempts have been made to classify types of mastitis. Generally, the distinctions are based on severity of symptoms and whether antibiotics should be started. Gibberd (1953), for instance, described two types of mastitis: cellulitis and adenitis. Cellulitis is thought to involve the interlobular connective tissue that has been infected by the introduction of bacteria through cracked nipples; it is treated with antibiotics. In adenitis, the breast ducts are presumably blocked, and the clinical symptoms are less severe. Treatment involves getting the milk flowing with heat, expression, and pumping. Antibiotics are used only if the infection is not resolving (Livingstone, 1990).

Subclinical lactation mastitis is a condition described by Willumsen et al. (2000). While testing breastmilk of women in Bangladesh and Tanzania to determine vitamin A levels, Willumsen and colleagues (2000) found one-fourth of the women tested had both a raised sodium–potassium ratio and elevated interleukin-8 (IL-8), indicating an infection without clinical symptoms. Fetherston

(2001) challenged the idea of a subclinical infection by pointing out that a high sodium level in breastmilk without other symptoms is not a reliable indicator for an infection or a subclinical infection. There are known confounding factors when sodium is normally higher, such as initiation of lactation, involution, and pregnancy. Subclinical mastitis is presumably associated with an increase in the HIV load in breastmilk and could lead to higher rates of mother-to-child transmission of HIV (see the *Viral Infections and Breastfeeding* chapter).

Infectious versus noninfectious mastitis is another proposed classification. Noninfectious mastitis occurs when milk is not removed from the breast and milk production subsequently slows; infection results if this milk stasis remains unresolved (i.e., the milk is not "washed" out of the breasts) (World Health Organization [WHO], 2000). Thomsen et al. (1985) proposed three classifications of mastitis—milk stasis, noninfectious inflammation, and infectious mastitis—based on leukocyte counts in milk from the infected breast. They recommended that antibiotic treatment be used only for infectious mastitis, the most severe classification.

Although this taxonomy might be helpful in theory, laboratory studies on mastitic milk are seldom done in practice. By the time the mother reports the problem to a healthcare provider, she usually has been ill for several hours, if not a day or two; the peak of the infectious process may have already passed, and she is getting well by the time she seeks medical treatment. There are other drawbacks to this classification

as well: (1) leukocyte counts do not always correspond with bacterial counts (Fetherston, 2001), (2) the milk sample must be collected before any antibiotics are started, (3) laboratory studies take several days, and (4) the testing expense may not be covered by health insurance. Whatever the classification of mastitis, the mother suffering from symptoms clearly needs to be treated. If she has repeated mastitis, a culture of her milk and a review of risk factors are indicated (Amir et al., 2014).

Breastmilk composition changes during a breast infection (Table 9-3) (Fetherston, Lai, & Hartmann, 2006). Levels of some anti-inflammatory components, such as lactoferrin and secretory immunoglobulin A (sIgA), rise to protect the baby from untoward effects from consuming mastitic milk (Buescher & Hair, 2001). Elevated levels of sodium and chloride caused by the temporary opening of the normally tight junctions between secretory cells in the paracellular pathways cause the breastmilk to taste salty. Sodium, chloride, and lactose are increased even when women have recovered from systemic symptoms. After the resolution of mastitis, the affected breast undergoes a temporary "resting" phase and usually produces less milk than it did before the infection.

In determining how a breast infection should be treated, it would be helpful to know the severity of the infection. With that point in mind, investigators (Fetherston et al., 2006) measured levels of serum C-reactive protein and compared them with mastitis symptoms, because C-reactive protein is a

Table 9-3 BREAST MILK COMPONENTS IN MASTITIS COMPARED WITH "HEALTHY" ASYMPTOMATIC BREASTS

Milk Component	Mastitic Breast (estimated mean)	"Healthy" Breast (estimated mean)
Sodium (mmol/L)	21.8	14
Chloride (mmol/L)	30	21
Lactose (mmol/L)	159	174
Glucose (mmol/L)	1.39	1.6
Lactoferrin (g/L)	3.45	3.2
sIgA (g/L)	1.22	1.25

Source: Data from Fetherston CM, Lai CT, Hartmann PE. Relationships between symptoms and changes in breast during lactation mastitis. *Breastfeed Med.* 2006;3;136–145.

marker of infection. They found that although an increasing severity of breast and systemic symptoms in mastitis was predictive of an increase of serum C-reactive protein in milk and blood, the presence of serum C-reactive protein in similar concentrations in both the mastitic and asymptomatic breasts suggests it is of little use in making a differential diagnosis between infective versus noninfective forms of mastitis. More recently, experts have agreed that this type of testing is likely of little value and suggested that "inflammation" is the more useful diagnosis as opposed to "infection" (Amir et al., 2014).

When a lactating woman has recurrent mastitis that does not respond to antibiotic therapy, inflammatory carcinoma must be ruled out. Inflammatory breast cancer can be mistaken for mastitis because the symptoms of an inflamed, edematous breast are similar. Breast cancer differs from mastitis in that inflammatory carcinoma rarely produces fever, there is no palpable mass, and the symptoms do not respond to antibiotic treatment. A woman with suspected breast cancer should be referred to a surgeon experienced in this area who will perform a biopsy and other laboratory diagnostic tests to determine if inflammatory carcinoma is present (Merchant, 2002). If it is, lactation is a secondary consideration, as the mother will need intensive treatments that will preclude lactation.

Breast Abscess

A small percentage (5% to 10%) of breast infections develop into abscesses (Kinlay et al., 1998). This incidence is decreasing probably because healthcare providers are more educated in prevention of abscess (Vogel et al., 1999). Amir et al. (2004) reported 3% of the women with mastitis in her sample developed an abscess, also noting the lower incidence than previously reported in the literature.

An abscess, like a boil, is basically a collection of pus that must be drained (see Color Plates 13, 16, and 17). Kataria and colleagues presented a review of treatment methods (2013). For small abscesses (3 cm or less) the recommended first line of treatment is fine-needle aspiration, single or repeated, preferably under ultrasound guidance. Percutaneous aspiration without ultrasound guidance is also a choice for these small abscesses, especially in facilities without ultrasound. For abscesses greater than 3 cm, a percutaneous suction catheter can be placed for 3 to 7 days and appears to be effective, low in complications, and cosmetically acceptable. An oral antibiotic effective against penicillin-resistant staphylococci for 10 days is used in combination with the aspiration. For a larger abscess, the physician makes an incision and drains the area. A drain is placed in the incision to promote drainage; in addition, manual expression helps to eliminate pus and milk. The incision heals from the inside out within a week or two. Oral antibiotics are also used with this treatment (Kataria et al., 2013). Dr. Susan Love (2000) recommended that her patients go home and rest; start taking daily showers (after 24 hours) and letting the water run over the breast to wash away bacteria; and then put a fresh dressing on the incision.

Dermatoses of the Breast

Dermatoses of the breast (skin rashes and lesions on the nipple–areolar complex and surrounding breast) are not uncommon, are particularly distressing if they are painful, and often prove difficult to diagnose. Thus the lactation specialist who sees these conditions should consider referring the mother to a dermatologist or other medical practitioner familiar with dermatoses to evaluate and diagnose such conditions (Barrett et al., 2013a). Differential diagnoses for dermatoses include atopic dermatitis, irritant contact dermatitis, allergic contact dermatitis, psoriasis, bacterial and yeast infections (discussed following this section), herpes simplex virus (HSV) infections, and Raynaud's phenomenon of the nipples (Barrett et al., 2013a).

Eczema most commonly affects the areolae of lactating mothers. This painful, burning, itching dermatitis is accompanied by redness, eruption of vesicles, and crusting and oozing papules in an acute erythematous eruption (Barrett et al., 2013a). It also can be a chronic problem, taking the form of a dry erythematous (red) and scaling dermatitis. Eczematous conditions fall into three main categories: (1) endogenous atopic dermatitis occurs in those with a predisposition to eczema; (2) irritant contact dermatitis occurs from direct chemical damage to the skin (e.g., soaps or chlorine); and (3) allergic contact dermatitis is a delayed hypersensitivity reaction to an allergen present in a topical agent that is applied to the nipples (e.g., solid food introduction to the infant, or topical agents such as lanolin, antibiotics, chamomile, vitamin E, fragrances) (Barrett et al., 2013a).

Topical corticosteroid ointments are the mainstay of treatment for eczema, including low- or medium-strength cortisone ointment twice a day for 2 weeks (category V or VI) (Barrett et al., 2013a). The ointment should be carefully wiped off the nipple area *before* the feeding and applied to the affected areas *after* the baby has fed. Topical antibiotics such as mupriocin, polysporin, and fusidic acid have been shown to reduce bacterial count and clinical severity. If symptoms develop soon after the baby starts eating solid foods, the mother should identify and eliminate any infant foods that might have contributed to the onset of eczema. Rinsing the affected nipple and areola with the mother's own expressed milk or with water, then patting the area dry, is also helpful (Barankin & Gross, 2004).

Amir (1993) described a case in which a breastfeeding mother with celiac disease developed red, scaly, and cracked nipples. The mother appeared to have eczema, possibly infected, involving most of both breasts. A topical steroid ointment (betamethasone dipropionate 0.05% [Diprosone]) was applied four times daily and a topical antibiotic was used twice daily. Two weeks later, the eczema had resolved, and the mother was able to continue breastfeeding without pain.

Box 9-2 presents interventions that will help prevent, alleviate, or treat such disorders. One should always be cautious in the case of slow-resolving or nonresolving of eczema of the breast: Paget's disease—a type of breast cancer—resembles nipple eczema.

In women with a history of psoriasis, flare-ups involving the nipple are common due to irritation from infant latch-on and suckling (Barrett et al., 2013a). In such a case, the lesion presents as "well-demarcated, erythematous plaques with fine micaceous scales" (Barrett et al., 2013a, p. 333). Treatment consists of topical steroids, which are applied using the same guidelines as for eczema. Calcipotriene can also be used and is safe during lactation as long as the daily body surface area coverage is less than 20% (Hale, 2010). For systemic therapy, phototherapy with ultraviolet B light is a safe option. Biologic agents thought to be moderately safe include etanercept, adalimubab, infliximab, alefacept, and ustekinumab, but evidence on their use in this indication is limited (Hale, 2010).

Bacterial infections present with complaints of deep, dull aching breast pain during or after feedings, breast tenderness with deep touch, bilateral pain, and burning. Mothers with suspected *S. aureus* infection should be treated with oral antibiotics (e.g., cephalexin, amoxicillin, or dicloxacillin for at least 2 weeks), as these agents are more effective in preventing mastitis development and reducing pain (Barrett et al., 2013a). Color Plate 8 and Color Plate

---

BOX 9-2 INTERVENTIONS FOR BREAST AND NIPPLE RASHES AND INFECTIONS

- Discontinue irritant.
- Take frequent showers.
- Wear all-cotton bras.
- Expose breasts to sunlight (15 minutes) and to air.
- Apply a medicated cream on the affected area twice a day. (Bactroban, an antifungal, antibacterial, and hydrocortisone combination, is available over the counter.) Remove cream with clean cotton swab if used on nipple or areola.
- Rinse nipple-areola area with warm water after each feeding. Pat dry, then air-dry with hair dryer on the low setting.

38 depict cracked nipples with a possible bacterial infection. In Color Plate 38 the mother's nipple had possible impetigo with raised red pimple-like bumps, cracking at the nipple base, and yellow crusting at the tips of the nipples.

Herpes simplex viral infection of the nipple or areola is a very painful condition that often presents as tiny vesicles on a reddened nipple and areola. As the vesicles heal, they form scabs. The baby may or may not have similar perioral skin lesions. This condition requires referral to a physician, who should evaluate and treat the mother. Culture of the lesion should be taken during its early stages before the lesion begins to dry and heal over. Treatment will depend on laboratory results of a culture of the lesion and maternal serum antibody titers. If the lesion is herpes simplex, it is advisable for the mother to pump her milk until the lesions are healed. The mother should be treated with an antiviral medication (acyclovir 800 mg three times daily for 5 to 7 days). For more discussion on herpes simplex virus, see the *Viral Infections and Breastfeeding* chapter.

Breastfeeding mothers, like everyone else, can develop a painful contact dermatitis from poison ivy, especially during summer months. Poison ivy does not spread by person-to-person but by direct contact with the oils on the leaf of the plant. When the body responds with vesicles, the fluids in the vesicles will not spread the poison ivy; therefore direct contact with the mother's rash will not hurt or harm the baby. However, if you have ever had poison ivy you know how extremely uncomfortable it can be. If the vesicles are on the breasts, direct contact by a nursing baby can be unbearable. The mother herself should be the one who decides if it is too uncomfortable to breastfeed; this is different for each person. Poison ivy is treated with 1% hydrocortisone applied to the affected area or by oral prednisone. Bowers' (2004) description of her experience with breastfeeding poison ivy is helpful to LCs.

Raynaud's phenomenon of the nipple is described as a vasospasm of the arterioles causing intermittent ischemia. In breast vasospasm, the nipple appears blanched after the feeding, sometimes turning blue or red before returning to its normal color. The mother feels extreme pain during the "spasm."

Raynaud's phenomenon is more prevalent in women, and there usually is a family history. Furthermore, women who have a history of Raynaud's phenomenon of the hands are at risk for development of the syndrome in the nipples.

This diagnosis should be considered if a nursing mother has experienced nipple pain for more than 4 weeks with multiple failed rounds of antifungal/antibiotic treatment (Barrett et al., 2013b). The breast pain associated with Raynaud's phenomenon is severe and throbbing and is often mistaken for *Candida albicans* infection. In a report of 12 mothers with this condition, eight mothers and their infants received multiple courses of antifungal therapy without relief before the diagnosis of Raynaud's phenomenon was made (Anderson et al., 2004). Three of the mothers reported a history of breast surgery. Another report (Morino & Winn, 2007) of a breastfeeding mother with Raynaud's phenomenon concluded that there was a definite association between the woman's symptoms and her emotional stress.

To diagnose Raynaud's phenomenon accurately, symptoms of cold stimuli, classic triphasic color change (white, blue, and red) in the nipples, or biphasic color change (white and blue) must be present (Anderson et al., 2004). Treatment includes avoiding cold temperatures, keeping the breasts and nipples warm, avoiding vasoconstrictive drugs, and taking nifedipine 30 to 60 mg/day for 2 weeks (Barrett et al., 2013b). Treatment with nifedipine has been reported to be effective for treating vasospasm without side effects (Anderson et al., 2004; Garrison, 2002; Page & McKenna, 2006). This agent is a calcium-channel blocker and vasodilator used to treat hypertension; its transfer through breastmilk to the baby is not significant (Penny & Lewis, 1989). Prompt treatment will allow mothers to continue to breastfeed pain free while avoiding unnecessary antifungal therapy.

Candidiasis (Thrush)

When a mother has persistently sore nipples, candidiasis (also referred to as candidosis) is likely. The yeast *Candida albicans* (also called *Monilia* or thrush) is the likely cause when this infection occurs orally.

Candida thrives in the warm, moist areas of the infant's mouth and on the mother's nipples. The infant's mouth can become infected during vaginal birth and can then infect the mother's breast and nipple during breastfeeding. Candidiasis should be suspected if the mother has been breastfeeding without discomfort and then rapidly develops extremely sore nipples, burning or itching, and burning, shooting, or stabbing nipple pain that radiates to the chest wall (Barrett et al., 2013a).

Although *Candida* is naturally occurring yeast that lives in the mucous membranes of the gastrointestinal and genitourinary tract and on the skin, the use of antibiotics promotes its overgrowth (candidiasis); consequently, infants and women who have received antibiotic therapy are more susceptible to candidiasis (Chetwynd et al., 2002). Mothers with vaginal candidiasis and nipple trauma are also predisposed to candidiasis of the breast.

In checking for candidiasis, inspect the woman's breasts for inflammation of the nipples and areolae. The inflammation is usually a striking deep pink, sometimes with tiny blisters (see Color Plate 12). The mother will complain of severe tenderness and discomfort, especially during and immediately after feedings. The baby may have a diaper rash, with raised, red, sore-looking pustules or red, scalded-looking buttocks. Also examine the child's mouth carefully for white patches surrounded by diffuse redness. The absence of symptoms in the child's mouth, however, does not rule out thrush, because the infant may be asymptomatic. Conversely, thrush symptoms in the baby (fussiness, refusing breast) can go unnoticed or be attributed to something else. Whenever any woman has recurrent yeast infections, her sexual partner should be considered a potential reservoir of infection. Pacifiers and bottle nipples are another source of recurrent thrush infection; they may harbor persistent oral *Candida* colonization and should be replaced or boiled after each exposure in the infant's mouth.

Candidiasis is a "family" disease; it spreads quickly among family members, especially with intimate contact involving warm, moist areas of the body, as is the case with breastfeeding and with sexual contact. Candidiasis that develops during breastfeeding can persist and recur unless all areas of possible infection in the baby, mother, and her sex partner are treated promptly and aggressively. The infant's mouth and anal area, as well as the mother's breasts (nipples and areola) and vagina, are prime sites for *Candida* infection; all should be treated simultaneously if warranted.

Diagnosis

Historically, candidiasis was most often diagnosed based on history, physical examination of the baby, and, to a lesser degree, physical examination of the mother (Brent, 2001). In Brent's survey of 312 members of the Academy for Breastfeeding Medicine, use of laboratory tests and cultures was reported to be infrequent (i.e., only 7% of providers used such methods), supposedly because cultures of the fungus would take days to grow and were difficult to differentiate from normal skin colonization.

To offset the well-recognized lack of evidence regarding accurate diagnosis of candidosis, Morrill and colleagues (2003, 2004, 2005) conducted research on detection of *Candida* on the nipple and areolar skin and in breastmilk, diagnosis of mammary candidosis, and risk factors for candidosis. First, a new culture technique for detecting *Candida* in breastmilk was developed by Morrill et al. (2003) because the natural inhibition of *Candida* growth by lactoferrin in the milk samples can result in false-negative cultures. By adding iron to the breastmilk, the ability to detect *Candida* growth was increased two- to three-fold, which markedly reduced the likelihood of false-negative culture results. Morrill and team (2004) also evaluated the sensitivity, specificity, and positive predictive value (PPV) of signs (shiny or flaky skin of nipple/areola) and symptoms (burning pain of nipple/areola, sore but not burning nipples, stabbing breast pain, and nonstabbing breast pain) of mammary candidosis reported by lactating women at 2 and 9 weeks postpartum, based on laboratory confirmation of the presence of *Candida* on the nipple/areola or in breastmilk at 2 weeks postpartum. The positive predictive value for colonization was highest when three or more signs and symptoms occurred simultaneously or when flaky or shiny skin of the nipple/areola was reported together or in combination with breast pain.

Finally, in a prospective study of 100 lactating and 40 non-pregnant, nonlactating women (controls), the team of researchers led by Morrill (2005) sought to document risk factors for *Candida* colonization and the relationship between *Candida* colonization and breastfeeding at 9 weeks postpartum. None of the non-pregnant control subjects tested positive for *Candida*, somewhat contradictory to the assumption that *Candida* is normally present in many people. Risk factors for colonization of mother were bottle use in the first 2 weeks postpartum and pregnancy duration of longer than 40 weeks. Risk factors for the infant were bottle use in the first 2 weeks postpartum and presence of siblings. Among women who tested positive at 2 weeks, 43% were still breastfeeding at 9 weeks postpartum compared to 69% who did not test positive ($P < 0.05$). The authors concluded that use of signs and symptoms could be helpful to clinicians in determining the need for cultures and for immediate treatment while awaiting culture results. Their risk factor research suggested that avoidance of bottle use in the early postpartum period may reduce risk of mammary candidosis. Furthermore, such preventive practice may help to decrease early termination of breastfeeding due to infection and pain.

An Alternative View of Candidiasis

In 2008, Hale questioned the presumption that sore and inflamed nipples with pain radiating into the axilla were due to infection with *Candida albicans*, as most studies had not actually found culturable *Candida* present in breastmilk. It was assumed that researchers were unable to grow *C. albicans* from breastmilk because the fungus was destroyed or its growth inhibited by agents present in human milk such as lactoferrin. Owing to these assumptions, studies of ductal *Candida* infection in breastfeeding women have been limited. It now appears that the original data were inaccurate. *C. albicans* is a normal fungal organism found on all human skin. As many as 80% to 90% of infants have culturable *Candida* present in their mouths. According to Hale, many

of the original studies did not sufficiently clean the mother's nipple; thus the source of the *Candida* may have actually been the saliva from the infant's mouth, rather than growth on the mother's nipple.

Yet Another View of Candidiasis

Another view of this common breast infection is that coinfection with *S. aureus* and *C. albicans* or other *Candida* species in the lactating nipple and breast may lead to inflammation and pain. A large, prospective study ($n = 360$ nulliparous women) conducted by Amir and colleagues (2013) in Australia investigated *Candida* species and *S. aureus* and the development of "nipple and breast thrush." The women in the study were followed from 36 weeks' gestation (baseline) to 8 weeks postpartum, completing seven data collections (including the baseline). The main outcome was a case definition of nipple and breast thrush based on the presence of a combination of burning nipple pain and breast pain by 4 weeks postpartum. Microbial (via culture) and molecular (via polymerase chain reaction [PCR]) samples were obtained from maternal nasal/nipple/breastmilk/vagina and baby nasal/oral sites for analysis for *Candida* and *S. aureus*. Self-report data were collected for previous *S. aureus* and *Candida* infections, breastfeeding problems, and health problems.

According to the researchers, women with the case definition of thrush were more likely to have *Candida* species in their nipple/breastmilk/baby oral samples (54%) compared to other women (36%, $p = 0.014$). *S. aureus* was also common in nipple/breastmilk/baby samples of women with (82%) and without (79%, $p = 0.597$) these symptoms. Univariate and multivariate time-to-event analysis examined predictors of thrush up to and including the time of data collection; the presence of *Candida* and nipple damage significantly and independently predicted thrush, but the presence of *S. aureus* did not.

In summary, this first prospective cohort study provided evidence that *Candida* plays a role in nipple and breast pain in lactating women but that burning nipple pain is common and a diagnosis of *Candida* infection should consider alternative differential diagnoses. The authors called for future randomized clinical trials to investigate treatment or clearance of *Candida* infection.

Treatment

Despite the availability of antifungal medications, few clinical trials have investigated their effectiveness in treating candidiasis of the lactating dyad. Clinical trials with healthy versus immunocompromised infants are even more rare.

A small (*n* = 34) randomized study in two U.S. military clinics compared nystatin and fluconazole oral suspensions for treatment of oral candidiasis in otherwise healthy infants (Groins et al., 2002). Clinical cures with nystatin were achieved in 6 of 19 patients (32%) and with fluconazole in 15 of 15 patients (100%). Microbiologic cures with nystatin at 10 days were observed in 1 of 18 infants (5.6%) and with fluconazole at 7 days in 11 of 15 infants (73%), with 10 of these 11 cures (91%) being apparent by day 3. Breastfeeding mothers of the infants, regardless of the study group, were prescribed nystatin cream for application to their nipples twice daily for the duration of the infant's treatment. The authors did not report on the outcomes for mothers in this study.

Thomassen et al. (1998) reported that treatment for mothers with mammary candidosis symptoms with 50 mg of fluconazole was ineffective. Chetwynd et al. (2002) suggested that higher dosing (100 mg) of fluconazole for a longer duration (several weeks) might be necessary for treatment.

Generally, treatment of candidiasis for the infant includes placing an antifungal medication (e.g., nystatin) in the infant's mouth with a medicine dropper after feedings and swabbing it over the mucosa, gums, and tongue. The mother applies an antifungal topical cream or lotion to her nipples and breast before and after each feeding and to the infant's entire diaper area if any redness is visible. The mother may also have vaginal yeast infection and, if she does, she should simultaneously use an antifungal intravaginal preparation. Clotrimazole (Gyne-Lotrimin) is an over-the-counter drug in the United States that is available as a vaginal suppository or as a cream but is not sold as a gel.

Other recommendations that can be made to the mother on a case-by-case basis include the following:

- "Air dry" the nipples and, if possible, expose them directly to the sun for a few minutes twice a day.
- Throw away disposable breast pads as soon as they become wet.
- Dry the external genitalia with a hair dryer on a warm setting.
- Wear 100% cotton underpants and bras that can be washed in very hot water and/or bleach to kill spores.
- Avoid baths with other members of the family.
- Restrict consumption of alcohol, cheese, bread, wheat products, sugar, and honey.
- Take 1 tablet acidophilus daily (40 million to 1 billion viable units, found at health food stores) for 2 weeks beyond the disappearance of symptoms.
- Use condoms during coitus because crossinfection with a sexual partner is possible (Wilson-Clay & Hoover, 2008).

Nystatin is the most commonly used medication for candidiasis, although its effectiveness is poor according to some reports (Chetwynd et al., 2002; Groins et al., 2002), and occasionally it can cause gastrointestinal symptoms in the baby. Its use should be limited to never-treated cases of thrush. Nystatin oral suspension is painted on the baby's oral mucosa and tongue with a large cotton swab after every breastfeeding. In the case of frank thrush and persistent candidiasis, fluconazole is safe and effective, and should be prescribed for both the mother and the infant. The amount of fluconazole that transfers through the mother's milk is not sufficient to treat the baby. One expert breastfeeding physician recommends that treatment of mother and infant be based on a holistic assessment of the case, as well as the assumption that *Candida* is a problem of host that causes overgrowth of the fungus (N. Powers, personal communication, 2007):

- If the mother has symptoms and the baby never had obvious oral thrush, the baby is not considered particularly "susceptible," so do *not* treat the baby.

- If the baby has obvious thrush and the mother has symptoms, treat *both.*
- If the baby has obvious thrush and the mother has no symptoms, treat both or treat the baby, and have the mother call immediately if she develops symptoms.

Another treatment consists of painting ketoconazole suspension on the breast twice a day for 5 days, followed by prolonged nystatin application. If the mother has allergies, the healthcare provider must be aware that Seldane (terfenadine) should *not* be taken in conjunction with the antifungal drugs ketoconazole or itraconazole or the antibiotic erythromycin. Mixing these drugs can lead to a life-threatening interaction.

Table 9-4 lists recommended dosages for commonly used antifungal medications. Dr. Jack Newman's All Purpose Nipple Ointment (Newman & Pitman, 2000) is a combination nipple ointment of antifungal and cortisone agents.

After taking an antifungal medication, mothers need encouragement and follow-up; they may not get immediate relief from pain. In fact, after starting treatment, the pain may become worse

Table 9-4 Selected Antifungal Preparations

Drug Name	Preparations	Usual Dosage
Clotrimazole (Lotrimin, Mycelex)	Creams, solutions, vaginal cream, and vaginal tablets.	Skin cream: Apply twice daily. Vaginal cream or tablet: 100 mg/day for 7 days or 200 mg/day for 3 days.
Gentian violet	Dilute solution 0.25% or 0.5%.	Topical: Infant: 2 to 3 times over several days. Do not repeat.
Fluconazole (Diflucan)	Oral.	Adult: 400 mg loading dose, then 100 mg twice daily for at least 2 weeks until pain free for a week. Pediatric: Loading dose of 6–12 mg/kg; then 3–6 mg/kg.
Ketoconazole (Nizoral)	Oral tablets.	Adult: 200–400 mg/day, given in single dose. Pediatric: Children weighing less than 20 kg, 50 mg/day; children weighing 20–40 kg, 100 mg/day.
Miconazole (Monistat)	Skin cream or lotion, vaginal cream, and vaginal suppositories.	Vaginal cream or suppository: 100 mg/day for 7 days. Skin cream or lotion: Apply 3 to 4 times per day.
Nystatin (Mycostatin)	Suspensions, cream, powders, ointment, and vaginal suppositories; *Candida* resistance to nystatin is growing.	Oral: Adult: 1.5–2.4 million into units/day divided 3 to 4 doses. Infant: 400,000–800,000 units/day divided into 3 to 4 doses. Topical: 1 million units applied twice a day. Duration of therapy: at least 2 days after symptoms disappear. Vaginal: 1–2 million units/day.
Newman's All Purpose Nipple Ointment	Ointment mixed by a pharmacist. Clotrimazole can be left out if 10% dosage is not available. Use until pain free.	Mupirocin 2% ointment (15 gm); Nystatin 100,000 unit/ml ointment (15 gm); Clotrimazole 10% vaginal cream (15 gm); Betamethasone 0.1% ointment (15 gm).

before it begins to fade. If nystatin does not clear the fungal infection, other antifungal medications—such as miconazole (Monistat), clotrimazole (Gyne-Lotrimin), naftifine (Naftin), or oxiconazole (Oxistat)—should be tried (Johnstone & Marcinak, 1990). For early cases, suggest that after feedings the mother try warm vinegar soaks (1 part vinegar, 4 parts water) followed by air drying and an antifungal preparation (La Leche League International, 2000).

Gentian violet, an old-fashioned antifungal drug, may be used as a second line of treatment following failure of other antifungal treatments. A well-known drawback of this remedy is that gentian violet stains anything with which it comes into contact, although blotting with alcohol and then a detergent solution helps to remove the dye. The more significant and dangerous side effect of gentian violet is irritation laryngotracheitis secondary to this agent and ulceration of the infant's oral mucous membrane necessitating endotracheal tube placement (Utter, 1990). A case study (Baca et al., 2001) described a very serious case of obstructive feeding tube placement secondary to refusal of the infant to breastfeed. Given the availability of other antifungals with few side effects, the authors recommended extreme caution and consideration in prescribing gentian violet.

Another recommendation from Dr. Nancy Powers is to "treat" anything that comes into contact with the baby's mouth (pacifiers, nipples, teethers, or toys) or the mother's breasts (breast-pump parts, bras, breast pads) to destroy the heat-resistant spores. This treatment can be accomplished by soaking articles in a vinegar-and-water solution for 30 minutes, boiling the articles for 20 minutes, or sterilizing pump parts in microwaveable bags sold for pumps. Likewise, Dr. Christina Smillie, a pediatrician who treats only breastfeeding patients, views *Candida* as a normal flora that is everywhere, and suggests that treatment of candidiasis should focus on restoring the skin to health so that the mother can resist infection.

It is not clear whether expressed milk of a mother with candidiasis should be saved and frozen for later use. Freezing deactivates yeast but does not kill it. Generally, it is advisable to tell mothers with candidiasis who are pumping not to freeze their milk until they have completed a course of medication treatment and are symptom free. In the situation where the mother has a large supply of stored milk, and both mother and infant are symptomatic, home pasteurization of the stored milk may be considered.

In one case of candidiasis infection of the breast (see Color Plate 12), the infant remained symptom free for the entire 4-month period, whereas the mother had repeated episodes of candidiasis. Within 4 days after resolving the painful blistering and redness, she experienced a new flare-up. After four such episodes in 4 months, she obtained medication for both her infant and herself; after 5 days of treatments after *every* suckling episode, she was symptom free and remained so (Johnstone & Marcinak, 1990).

Other Breast Pain

In some cases, pressure on the brachial plexus can result in shooting pain in the breast. Identifying the cause of this pressure (e.g., a badly fitting bra or baby-carrier straps that are pulled too tightly across the mother's back) is a key to alleviating such pain.

Women have also reported feeling shooting pain that coincided with powerful ejection of milk. Such episodes are most likely to occur in the first month of the breastfeeding course. When the milk-ejection reflex subsides, the pain often subsides as well. This temporary pain tends to occur more often in primiparous women; in many cases, the mothers who have experienced it with a first breastfeeding baby do not experience a recurrence with later infants. This pain may reflect distension of the milk ducts, which is more obvious in the early first breastfeeding course than during later periods.

In cases in which the mother reports very intense pain coincidental with a vigorous milk-ejection response, the caregiver should encourage the mother to gently massage her breasts before putting the baby to breast to enhance the likelihood of some initial leaking of milk before the baby's active suckling stimulates milk ejection. When the milk begins to drip freely, sprays, and then subsides, subsequent suckling is less likely to result in such intense discomfort. By the end of the first month, such pain is usually no longer present when the milk-ejection reflex is activated.

Milk Blister

Infrequently, a milk blister—a whitish, tender area—develops on the upper areola. Nipple-pore milk that has been sealed over by the epidermis and has triggered an inflammatory response probably causes a milk blister. This obstruction then prevents the duct system from draining, so milk build-up behind the occlusion causes symptoms of a blocked duct (Noble, 1991). The spot may be white or yellow, depending on how long it has been present. The skin on and around the area may be reddened (see Color Plate 11).

Persistent and very painful during feeding, a milk blister can remain for several days or weeks and then spontaneously heal by a peeling away of the epithelium over the affected area. If it does not spontaneously heal, an optional treatment is to break the epithelial tissue using a sterile needle, sometimes along with sterile tweezers and small sharp scissors to entirely remove the excess skin. Aspiration may be necessary to draw out the fluid. Compressing around the areola to express out any stringy plugs may help to prevent future blisters from arising (Newman & Pitman, 2000). One mother who had a nipple probe for a chronically plugged duct and blister developed a lot of pain and insisted on weaning to get relief.

A less invasive treatment is rubbing the area with a damp cloth after softening the skin by immersion in warm water. With ice packs, an analgesic to relieve discomfort, and a topical antibiotic, breastfeeding can continue and healing is rapid.

In addition to the larger blister, tiny blisters that appear to have a whitish fluid, possibly milk, may appear on nipples. These blisters are sore and painful. Vitamin E ointment (applied sparingly and wiped off before feedings) and wearing breast shells (to relieve the pressure from clothing on the nipples) can relieve discomfort and possibly aid healing.

Mammoplasty

Breast augmentation and reduction are increasingly common surgical procedures. Whereas augmentation is performed for cosmetic effect, reduction of very large breasts is often undertaken to reduce discomfort from neck and back pain and owing to the need to "feel normal" (Grassley, 2002).

Sooner or later, the clinician will see a client who has had breast augmentation or reduction and who wants to know whether she will be able to breastfeed her baby. The ability to breastfeed after these surgeries depends on the type of surgery, the specific technique used, whether neural pathways were severed, and the amount of breast tissue removed. Generally speaking, full breastfeeding is possible with augmentation surgery but usually not after reduction surgery, unless feedings are supplemented; however, exceptions occur in both instances. An explanation of the differences in the operative procedures is crucial to understanding the subsequent effect on lactation.

Gigantomastia

Gigantomastia of pregnancy is a rare (1 in 100,000), debilitating condition characterized by massive enlargement of breasts that results in tissue necrosis, ulceration, and infection (Swelstad et al., 2006). Because it appears in the early weeks of pregnancy, most believe this condition has a hormonal cause, although the exact mechanism is unknown. A literature review showed that approximately one-third of women with this problem eventually undergo breast reduction or a mastectomy (Swelstad et al., 2006). An inferior pedicle technique can be successfully performed in women with gigantomastia (Lacerna et al., 2005).

A case study in the United Arab Emirates described a woman who presented at 18 weeks' gestation with extreme growth of her breasts since 14 weeks' gestation (John & Rangwala, 2009). She had two previous pregnancies without excessive breast growth and reportedly lactated with her first baby for 11 months. During the remainder of the pregnancy, she was managed conservatively with analgesics, bromocriptine, and breast support. At 25 weeks' gestation, she was admitted to the hospital due to difficulty walking and breathing. She delivered her infant at 32 weeks without complication. During the postpartum period, she continued treatment with bromocriptine, did not breastfeed, and had bilateral reduction mammoplasty 1 year after giving birth with a reported satisfactory outcome and cosmetic results.

In another case study, Antevski and colleagues (2010) reported on a 24-year-old woman, gravida 2, at 28 weeks' gestation, with a total breast weight of 33 kg, complicated by infection, ulcerations, and subsequent hemorrhage. A bilateral simple mastectomy, without complication, was performed as a life-saving procedure to prevent fatal complications.

Other cases reported in the literature have resulted in termination of the pregnancy to prevent further complications. Obviously this condition is rare but extremely debilitating to women and their families.

Breast Reduction

The ability to breastfeed after breast reduction depends on whether the surgeon leaves nerve pathways and blood supply intact or the tissue is removed without regard for these structures (Soderstrom, 1993). Given that adipose tissue of the breast is inseparably connected to glandular tissue, breast reduction cannot be done by simply removing the adipose tissue (Nickell & Skelton, 2005; Ramsay et al., 2005). Women with the least amount of glandular tissue removed have a greater opportunity to lactate (Marshall et al., 1994), particularly if the fourth intercostal nerve that branches to the breast and areola is left intact (see the *Anatomy and Physiology of Lactation* chapter).

The two techniques used for breast reduction are the *pedicle technique* and the *free-nipple technique*. The pedicle technique can be located superiorly, laterally, medially, or inferiorly. A systematic review of the literature on breast reduction reported that breastfeeding "success" rates following use of the pedicle technique varied from 16% to 100% (Thibaudeau et al., 2010). The inferior pedicle technique is commonly used in women of childbearing age. The nipple and areola remain attached to the breast gland on a pedicle, and the tissue is "reduced." A wedge is removed from the sides of the underside of the breast (Figure 9-1). Because the breast, its ducts, its blood supply, and some nerves remain intact, breastfeeding is possible after this operation but the success of breastfeeding cannot be predicted with certainty.

The free-nipple technique (auto-transplantation of the nipple) involves removing the nipple and areola entirely from the breast and preserving it in saline (much like a graft) while the additional breast tissue (usually fatty tissue) is removed. The nipple and areola are then stitched back in place. This technique is used for women with extremely large breasts; it is designed to reduce risks and complications and to position the nipple approximately on the substantially resculpted breast. Breastfeeding is possible with the pedicle technique, but it is much less likely with the free-nipple technique, because the blood supply of the nipple and areola is completely severed and damage to the nerves occurs (Tairych et al., 2000).

Breast reduction may interfere with the ability to breastfeed, but variations reported in the cumulative research evidence make it difficult to provide solid evidence-based information to women. According to Thibaudeau and colleagues' (2010) systematic review, studies on the impact of breast reduction on lactation vary greatly in their definitions of "breastfeeding" (ranging from any breastfeeding to exclusive breastfeeding) and "breastfeeding success" (ranging from any breastfeeding on day 1 to breastfeeding beyond 6 months), sample size, design (control/comparison group versus none), and surgical techniques. Thibaudeau et al. (2010) systematically reviewed 26 studies conducted between 1957 and 2007 relative to surgical technique, study characteristics, and breastfeeding rates and use of supplementation. They calculated overall breastfeeding rates using the total number of women who had children post mammoplasty. Those rates

Figure 9-1 Breast Reduction. (A) Wedge of breast tissue removed, areloa areola pulled up, gap closed. (B) Excess tissue removed, skin closed with stitches. (C) Postoperative appearance.

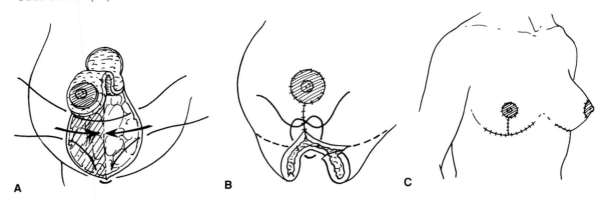

A   B   C

were then compared to published data from North America (United States and Canada).

According to Thibaudeau et al. (2010), of the 2911 women who had children post mammoplasty, 1827 (63%) met the criteria for success in breastfeeding as defined by the researchers of the individual studies. Success rates varied across studies from 0% to 100%. Reasons for unsuccessful breastfeeding or not attempting to breastfeed, as described in nine of the studies, included lack of encouragement (30%); insufficient milk (19%); painful nipple, infection, and medications (14%); personal or occupational concerns (8%); breast engorgement or delayed lactation (6%); breast surgery (2%); baby unable to latch (2%); and other reasons. Across three of the studies, 54 reasons for supplementation were reported, including insufficient milk (76%); personal/occupational issues (13%); other reasons including nipple trauma, infant refusal, and nervous mother (7%); and doctor's recommendation (4%).

Four of the studies compared different pedicle methods' effects on breastfeeding ability. No significant differences in breastfeeding ability were found, except in the study by Chiummariello et al. (as cited in Thibaudeau et al., 2010), who found that at 3 weeks postpartum breastfeeding rates were higher among those women who had breast reduction via the superior pedicle technique (61%) compared to the inferior (43%), medial (48%), and

lateral (55%) techniques. The quantity of resected glandular tissue and sensitivity of the nipple–areolar complex were not associated with breastfeeding success, as described in three of the studies that examined these variables.

Four studies compared breastfeeding rates in women post reduction with controls who had no breast surgery. Two studies indicated that controls had superior breastfeeding rates compared to those women who had reduction surgery. In the two other studies with controls, there were no significant differences by group in breastfeeding rates and need for supplementation. However, the control group was composed of women with macromastia, which might explain the lack of differences: women with large breasts may have difficulty breastfeeding due to decreased nipple–areolar sensitivity.

Finally, Thibaudeau and colleagues (2010) compared rates of breastfeeding in the studies to rates of breastfeeding in North America in 2001. They found that the majority of studies cited rates similar to those reported in 2001.

The authors of this systematic review concluded that consensus on a definition of "successful breastfeeding" is needed by plastic surgeons; they recommended adoption of the WHO definition—namely, 6 months of exclusive breastfeeding. They also recommended that the term *lactation* be used to refer to the ability to produce and express milk from the breast. Furthermore, Thibaudeau and colleagues (2010) recommended that the pedicle technique be used for breast reduction in patients who want to preserve the ability to lactate. They also suggested that future research follow women to the recommended 6 months of exclusive breastfeeding, as the majority of studies performed to date have followed patients only for the first month postpartum.

Reduction mammoplasty is a necessary surgical procedure for many childbearing-age women. Women with heavy, pendulous breasts report back, neck, and shoulder pain. They may feel depressed and stigmatized, and experience negative comments from both men and women about their breast size, including cruel jokes during their adolescence (Grassley, 2002; Guthrie et al., 1998). Recent research by Nguyen et al. (2013) indicated that young women (younger than age 21) who underwent breast reduction sustained long-term symptom resolution of shoulder pain (94.7%), breast pain (92.0%), and intertrigo-inflammation of the skin under the breasts (88.6%). Other improvements were reported in psychosocial areas such as improved quality of life and physical activity. The majority of these young women rated their surgery as successful and would recommend it to friends or family. Unfortunately, 67.2% of patients reported self-perceived decreased nipple sensitivity and 65.2% reported difficulties breastfeeding (decreased milk production, unilateral milk production, and latching problems because of an inverted nipple).

Clinical Implications of Breast Reduction

The lactation specialist should encourage women to breastfeed following reduction mammoplasty, providing evidence-based information about the likelihood of successful lactation and about options for supplemental feedings. As is true for all new mothers, women who have undergone such surgical procedures should be encouraged to initiate skin-to-skin contact and breastfeeding as soon as possible after birth and to continue to frequently stimulate the breasts through direct feeding at the breast. Infant intake and output should be monitored carefully, as well as infant weight loss/gain. If supplementation becomes necessary, use of a supplemental

feeder at the breast can provide breast stimulation and close proximity to the infant to build and maintain a close mother–baby relationship.

It is important for plastic surgeons who work with childbearing-age women to openly discuss their patients' plans for future lactation. Given increased knowledge about the impact of reduction mammoplasty on lactation ability and the importance of human milk for infant health, plastic surgeons are interested in preserving lactation ability and should discuss future lactation potential preoperatively. However, the women in one older study (Souto et al., 2003) reported that almost 80% of their surgeons indicated that breast reduction would not affect lactation. Most of these women were young and desired to have children in the future. Only half of them worried about not being able to breastfeed. Plastic surgeons must provide full information to their patients for complete informed consent.

Mastopexy

Mastopexy, much like a facelift, is a "breastlift"— a very common cosmetic surgery where sagging breasts (ptosis of the breast) are uplifted and made firmer (Figure 9-2). Breastfeeding is commonly thought to lead to breast ptosis and may influence women's decisions about breastfeeding.

Rinker and colleagues (2010), recognizing the lack of clear information on the causes of ptosis, studied 132 patients to identify antecedents of this condition. Using logistic regression for analysis, they found that age, history of significant weight loss (50 pounds), higher body mass index, larger bra cup size, number of pregnancies, and smoking history were significant risk factors for breast ptosis ($P = 0.05$). History of breastfeeding, weight gain during pregnancy, and lack of participation in regular upper-body exercise were not significant risk factors for ptosis.

Given this information, it is not surprising that most mastopexy procedures are done post childbearing. Nevertheless, some childbearing-age women do undergo the procedure, either alone or in conjunction with breast augmentation. The operation involves removing excess skin and breast tissue

Figure 9-2 BREAST "LIFT" OR MASTOPEXY. (A) SKIN EDGES PULLED TOGETHER. (B) EXCESS TISSUE REMOVED. (C) POSTOPERATIVE APPEARANCE.

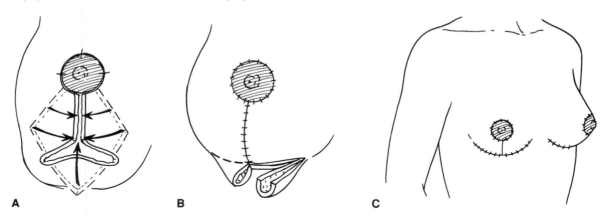

and elevating the nipple. Although there may be a slight loss of sensation in the nipple or areola, the mastopexy "theoretically" should not affect the ability to breastfeed.

Breast Augmentation

Breast augmentation is the most common aesthetic surgical procedure in the United States, with more than 300,000 of these surgeries being performed in 2011 (Hidalgo & Spector, 2014). Because of its popularity, lactation consultants are likely to have clients who have undergone this procedure (Figure 9-3). In 2006, the U.S. Food and Drug Administration (FDA) lifted a 14-year ban on the use of silicone gel breast implants after decades of contentious debate and litigation following complaints and lawsuits in the 1970s and 1980s that the devices ruptured and became hard and painful and that some women developed cancer and autoimmune diseases. Today, approximately 60% of implants used in the United States are silicone gel filled (Hidalgo & Spector, 2014). The FDA has published information for women on important considerations in choosing breast implants along with risk information (see the Internet Resources at the end of this chapter).

A number of techniques are used to enlarge the breasts. First, different locations may be used as implant pockets, each of which has its own reported advantages. The subpectoral pocket allows for better mammography visualization; the subfascial pocket protects against capsular contracture; and the subglandular pocket, which has disadvantages of risk for capsular contracture and mammography challenges,

Figure 9-3 BREAST AUGMENTATION. MOST COMMON INCISIONS INCLUDE THE AXILLARY, PERIAREOLAR, AND UNDER THE BREAST (INFAMAMMARY).

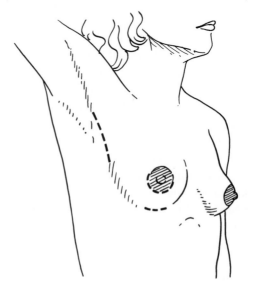

may be best for large or very low breasts. Currently, there are five incision options for augmentation (Hidalgo & Spector, 2014):

1. An *axillary enlargement* is done by making an incision underneath the arm and placing the implant below the gland or muscle. This approach has the advantage of scar avoidance. This type of implantation is ideal for young women with good shape and volume of breast tissue. It is more common for surgeons to place saline implants under the muscle, where it interferes less with mammograms; in addition, these incisions do not interfere with sentinel lymph node biopsy (Figure 9-4).

2. In the *periareolar technique*, an incision is made around the nipple–areola complex. Plastic surgeons contend that this incision provides good exposure of the implant pocket (subglandular or submuscular) and ensures that the scar is less visible than in the inframammary procedure. However, these incisions are associated with decreased nipple sensation and lactation difficulty (Hurst, 1996; Neifert et al., 1990).

3. The *inframammary technique* is the most popular choice today and is preferred for postpartum patients with atrophic breast tissue. This procedure calls for an incision to be made under the breast and for the implant (generally a larger form-stable implant) to be placed under the breast tissue or muscle. One disadvantage of this technique is that the scar may be very visible unless it is placed in the inframammary crease.

4. *Transabdominal insertion* of implants is possible for women who "have good breast shape, desire smaller implants, and are 'short-waisted,' have low breast position, or both" (Hidalgo & Spector, 2014, p. 572e).

5. *Periumbilical (superior) umbilical incisions* are used infrequently for insertion of saline implants subpectorally.

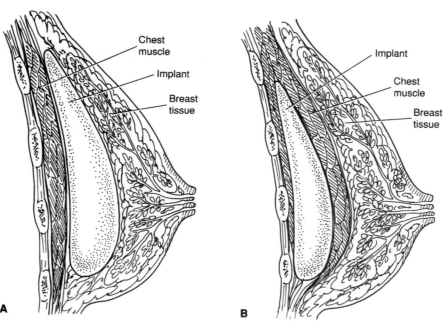

Figure 9-4 LOCATION OF BREAST IMPLANT. (A) IMPLANT PLACED BETWEEN BREAST AND MUSCLES. (B) IMPLANT PLACED UNDER MUSCLES.

Although augmentation supposedly has less impact on future lactation ability compared to reduction mammoplasty, women who have undergone previous breast augmentation surgery have a greater risk of lactation insufficiency as compared with women who had not had such surgery. Hughes and Owen (1993) interviewed 26 women with augmentation surgery and found that only one-third were successful with breastfeeding. Neifert et al. (1990), Hurst (1996), and Hill et al. (2004) reported similar findings.

Furthermore, women who had periareolar and transareolar incisions had greater incidence of lactation insufficiency. Neifert et al. (1990) studied 319 primiparous women who were breastfeeding healthy, full-term infants. The mothers with periareolar incisions were more than four times as likely to have insufficient milk compared to those with no breast surgery. Women with breast incisions in other locations had no statistically significant increase in risk compared with those who never had breast surgery. In Hurst's (1996) study of 42 women who had augmentation surgery, 64% had insufficient lactation. Of the women who had periareolar surgery, none lactated sufficiently, compared with 50% who made sufficient milk if they had submaxillary or axillary augmentation.

More recent studies of breastfeeding following augmentation surgery also demonstrate impaired lactation in women who have undergone these procedures. Cruz and Korchin (2010) compared women who had augmentation ($n = 107$) to women of similar age and BMI who had hypoplastic breasts and had children before their breast augmentation consultation ($n = 105$). Significant differences were noted between the two groups in terms of self-reported successful breastfeeding, defined as breastfeeding for the initial 2 weeks after giving birth: 88% of the control group was successful, while only 63% of the study group reported success ($p < 0.05$). The rate of supplementation with formula was also significantly higher in the study group compared to the control group (46% versus 27%; $p < 0.05$). Unlike in the earlier research by Hurst (1996), there was no significant difference in breastfeeding success or need to supplement based on periareolar

versus inframammary incisions. Within the study group, only 2% of the women reported loss of nipple sensation and there was no significant difference between the incision types.

In addition to insufficient milk production issues, reports of galactorrhea, galactocele formation, and extreme engorgement have been reported in the literature, some occurring soon after breast augmentation surgery under the hormonal influence of birth control pills (i.e., without pregnancy) and some following pregnancy (Acarturk et al., 2005; Caputy & Flowers, 1994; Deloach et al., 1994; Tung & Carr, 2011; Yang et al., 2012). Thus, augmentation can lead to other lactation-related types of problems that women should be made aware of before having surgery. Furthermore, it is essential for the healthcare provider to discuss the potential impact of surgery on adequacy of breastmilk production. Some women who have had augmentation surgery become upset that their surgeons did not discuss with them the surgery's negative impact on breastfeeding. These women are also angry with themselves for proceeding with the surgery without having been completely informed. Because childbearing and lactation may not have been a priority at the time of breast surgery, many did not ask the surgeon about their future ability to breastfeed (Hughes & Owen, 1993).

Breast Lumps and Surgery

What happens if a breastfeeding mother develops a lump or nodule in her breast? Warnings issued by organizations such as the American Cancer Society have made American women keenly aware of breast lumps, and the woman discovering one is usually anxious and perhaps frightened. However, a breast lump in a lactating woman is most often a galactocele, a milk-filled lacteal cyst caused by plugged milk in the ducts (Sabate et al., 2007; Stevens et al., 1997). A galactocele is usually tender and will atrophy rather rapidly and disappear in a matter of days.

Fine-needle aspiration of a galactocele is both diagnostic and therapeutic (Sabate et al., 2007). To aspirate a cyst, the physician first cleans and anesthetizes the skin, immobilizes the mass with his or her hand, and inserts a 20- to 22-gauge needle to draw out fluid. This procedure collapses the cyst and solves the problem.

Cysts are almost never malignant. If the lump does not resolve or reduce in size, the mother should be examined and biopsied. The type of biopsy will depend on the size and palpability of the lump. If a biopsy is necessary, one of the following methods is used (Love, 2000). (In the two types of nonsurgical biopsies where needles are used, a single stitch may be needed to close the incision.)

- A fine-needle biopsy draws out a few cells.
- Larger-gauge hollow needles are used to remove a small piece of the lump (called a core or "tru-cut" biopsy).
- In surgical or "open" biopsies, the surgeon takes out a large piece of the lump or removes it entirely.

Stereotactic biopsy has become standard procedure to excise microcalcifications. In this procedure, the breast is suspended through an opening on the surgical table and a mammogram is performed to locate the exact position of calcifications, which are biopsied.

Most diagnostic procedures are performed on an outpatient basis either in a free-standing ambulatory clinic or in a minor operating room. Using the lowest dose possible of local anesthetic (usually Lidocaine) and breastfeeding just before the biopsy minimizes the amount of anesthetic the infant might ingest. The time at which the mother resumes breastfeeding depends on her comfort level and the type of procedure used, but she certainly should be able to resume within 12 hours. Although the area will be tender, resuming feeds needs to be weighed against the discomfort of engorgement and listening to the cries of an unhappy child. If breastfeeding is not resumed within 12 hours, the mother should pump her breasts to relieve the intramammary pressure. Too much milk pressure and stasis could lead to undue stress on the surgical site and infection.

Some surgeons prefer that the mother discontinue nursing either completely before the surgery or at least stop feedings from the affected breast. Milk can leak and mix with blood, which makes a "messy" surgery. Love (2000) suggests that if the mother is thinking of weaning anyway, this point is probably a good time to do so. Otherwise, the mother should look for another surgeon.

Many mothers have shared their breastfeeding experiences after breast surgery in La Leche League's publications, which are a rich source of clinical information. One mother (Hart, 1980) had a lump removed as an outpatient. The following day, her breast started swelling with stored milk because her baby had not nursed from that breast. After expressing milk by hand for 12 days, she began feeding her infant again on the affected breast. Her milk supply in the affected breast returned, though for 2 to 3 days nursing was uncomfortable.

Another woman (Paster, 1986) underwent a breast biopsy under general anesthesia for a lump that was deep within her breast. By 12 hours after the procedure, she was able to nurse on the affected side. Although painful at first, by the second or third day, breastfeeding was quite tolerable. This mother found that putting pressure (splinting) on the dressing helped to allay the feeling that the baby would pull the incision apart. At first, there was some lessening of milk production because about 25% of the ducts had been disturbed. Subsequently, the mother nursed another baby without noticing any difference in milk production in the affected breast.

In a third case (Resico, 1990), the nipple was cut during surgery from top to bottom and lifted to remove a golf ball–sized lump. The surgeon suggested that the mother not attempt to breastfeed when she became pregnant, because he thought he had severed milk ducts during surgery. Surprisingly, the mother was able to breastfeed from that breast. This suggests one of two possibilities: either some of the ducts were not actually severed, or it is possible for milk ducts to recanalize after having been severed.

Galactoceles

Galactoceles—milk-filled cysts in the lactating breast—are the most common benign lesion of the lactating breast, although they more frequently occur after cessation of breastfeeding, when milk is retained and becomes stagnant within the breast (Sabate et al., 2007). The etiology of galactoceles is thought to be an inflammation or infection-induced blockage of the mammary ducts. This condition can also occur in infants and children, albeit infrequently (Vlahovic et al., 2012; Welch et al., 2004). Galactoceles can mimic other lesions of the breast, both benign and malignant. Ultrasound is generally used in the diagnosis, along with needle aspiration of milk. Needle aspiration also is an effective treatment in most patients with galactoceles (Rampaul et al., 2005; Sabate et al., 2007; Sawhney et al., 2002; Wang et al., 2007).

Case studies in the literature provide descriptions from which clinicians can become informed about galactoceles. Bevin and Persok (1993) described a case in which a mother had a palpable chronic galactocele behind the left areola for 10 years, during which time she breastfed several children. The left breast was the site of many plugged ducts, breast infections (some requiring antibiotics), and a breast abscess. At various stages, 10 to 20 mL of milky fluid was aspirated, but the lump refilled quickly. No single treatment was helpful. However, on one occasion, antibiotic treatment caused the galactocele to disappear temporarily. Optimal management of a galactocele has yet to be determined.

A more recent case report from London was quite unusual (Rampaul et al., 2005), as it described multiple galactoceles in both axillae of a lactating woman. A 31-year-old woman presented with a 1-week history of bilateral swellings of the axillae, having been diagnosed with bilateral hidradenitis suppurativa (a chronic skin inflammation marked by the presence of blackheads and one or more red, tender bumps) 4 years earlier. She was 3 weeks postpartum, with engorged lactating breasts. Both axillae were swollen with numerous discrete palpable lumps, each measuring about 1.5 cm within each axilla. Ultrasonography revealed multiple thin-walled cysts. A cyst in the upper outer quadrant of the left breast was also present and on aspiration was shown to contain milk. The axillary cysts were not aspirated, as they were identical on imaging to the breast galactocele. This woman also experienced an episode of milk secretion bilaterally

in the axillae that spontaneously resolved, though there were no accessory nipples on examination. It was thought that the prior episodes of hidradenitis may have acted as a nidus (site of infection) in this case and the cause of the galactoceles.

As noted previously, galactoceles have also been reported in the literature in women who have undergone breast augmentation (Acarturk et al., 2005; Tung & Carr, 2011). In the case described by Acarturk et al., massive engorgement started in the last month of pregnancy and caused major discomfort; the woman did not attempt lactation. Although the authors attributed the engorgement to bilateral galactocele formation, there is no description of ultrasonic examination or needle aspiration of the breasts.

Fibrocystic Changes of the Breast

Fibrocystic changes (FCCs) constitute the most frequent benign breast disease (BBD) (Guray & Sahin, 2006). Many other names have been used to describe FCCs over the years, including fibrocystic disease, cystic mastopathy, chronic cystic disease, and mazoplasia. Because this process is observed clinically in as many as 50% of women and histologically in 90% of women, however, the term *fibrocystic changes* has become the label of choice.

FCCs are made up of cysts (macro and micro) and solid lesions, including adenosis, epithelial hyperplasia with or without atypia, apocrine metaplasia, radial scarring, and papillomas (Guray & Sahin, 2006). Lumps (palpable masses) and pain are common symptoms of FCCs. Cysts—also called fibroadenomas—are fluid-filled round or ovoid structures that are found in as many as one-third of women between 35 and 50 years old. Although most are subclinical "microcysts," palpable (gross) cystic changes, which generally present as a simple cyst, are encountered in 20% to 25% of cases (Guray & Sahin, 2006). Fibroadenomas can vary from the size of a pea to the size of a lemon.

Ultrasound and needle aspiration accurately confirm the diagnosis. If no fluid can be aspirated, a fibroadenoma is likely. Tissue is sent to the laboratory to confirm the diagnosis. Fibroadenomas are harmless in themselves and, if the woman is lactating, most surgeons choose to delay surgery at least until lactation ceases and the child is completely weaned. A mother with persistent benign breast disease is commonly advised to reduce or eliminate her consumption of caffeine (e.g., coffee, tea, cola, chocolate) and to take vitamin E supplements.

Little is known about the relationship between benign breast disease and women's reproductive function, even though BBD is prevalent in young women. Bernardi and colleagues (2012) examined the relationship between breastfeeding and such disease in a sample of 105 women with BBD and 98 controls. The most frequent BBD was fibroadenoma (55%), followed by FCCs (19%), intraductal papilloma (6%), and inflammatory breast disorders (5%). Duration of breastfeeding was not significantly different between controls and BBD types. Among women with fibroadenomas, breastfeeding duration was positively correlated with the number of benign lesions ($p < 0.05$).

In an unusual case study in the recent literature, Aksoy et al. (2013) described hematemesis in a healthy newborn. The mother had fibrocystic breast changes, and the blood most likely came from a cyst. The authors of the case study emphasized that lactation specialists and physicians should be aware of this rare condition, and fibrocystic breast changes of the mother should be included in the differential diagnosis of newborns with hematemesis.

Bleeding from the Breast

Red-tinged, pink, or rusty breastmilk is relatively rare, but it does occur and causes concern because it signals the presence of blood. O'Callaghan (1981) described 37 cases of this syndrome in Australian women. Most of these women reported that their breast discharge was either red or brown. The earliest appearance of the discolored milk occurred during the fourth month of pregnancy and was associated with antenatal breast expression in a little more than half of the mothers. Dairy farmers report similar rusty milk from cows calving for the first time and suggest that the reason is slight internal bleeding from edema during the cow's first engorgement.

The earliest published research on this condition was by Merlob and colleagues in 1990. These Israeli neonatologists prospectively studied 7774 live births over a period of 2 years (1986–1988). Eight mothers had this atypical breast discharge, a prevalence rate of 1 per 971 live births (0.1%). The phenomenon was characterized by early appearance (frequently shortly after giving birth), with normal bacteriologic and cytologic testing, disappearance in 2 to 5 days without adverse effects on the mothers and their babies, no recurrence after cessation, and occurrence in the previous pregnancies (3 of the 5 multipara).

The term *rusty pipe syndrome* was first used at a La Leche League conference in 1990 by Chele Marmet. Marmet had worked with mothers whose milk appeared brown or rusty looking, like rusty water emitted from pipes that have not been used for a long while—hence the nickname. The syndrome appears during the early stages of lactogenesis, is not associated with any discomfort, and is thought to be caused by increased vascularization of rapidly developing alveolae, which are easily traumatized, resulting in blood escaping into breast secretions (Sabate et al., 2007). A recent case study by Faridi et al. (2013) further described two mothers who presented with rusty pipe syndrome between March 2012 and May 2012. With proper counseling, the mothers were able to successfully breastfeed.

Bright-red bleeding from the breast in the absence of nipple soreness or cracking indicates that the mother should be assessed for the possibility of an intraductal papilloma (Sabate et al., 2007). This small, benign, wartlike growth on the lining of the duct bleeds as it erodes the tissue. Usually no mass or tumor is palpable, and the condition may or may not be associated with moderate pain and discomfort. Often the bleeding stops spontaneously without any treatment. If bleeding continues, however, the woman should be medically evaluated. She can pump her breasts to maintain lactation (on a low setting) until the cause of the bleeding is identified. Cytologic evaluation, mammography, and ultrasound can be useful diagnostic tools in these cases (Berens, 2002). The physician will probably remove the tissue surgically to confirm that it is an intraductal papilloma and not something more serious, such as intraductal cancer. In any case, the lactation consultant can reassure the mother that the infant is not harmed by the intake of small amounts of serosanguinous discharge. Larger amounts may lead to the infant regurgitating the blood.

Breast Cancer

Breast cancer is the most common malignancy among women and overall the most common malignancy in the United States (National Cancer Institute [NCI], 2014b). Approximately 12.3% of women will be diagnosed with breast cancer at some point during their lifetime, based on 2008–2010 data. Pregnancy-associated breast cancer (PABC) is defined as breast cancer occurring anytime during gestation, during lactation, or within 1 year after delivery. Breast cancer is the most common cancer in pregnant and postpartum women, being diagnosed in about 1 in 3000 pregnant women. The average patient is between 32 and 38 years of age; thus, because many women today are choosing to delay childbearing, it is likely that the incidence of breast cancer during pregnancy will increase (NCI, 2014a).

Breast cancer in lactating women is a clinical issue. New technology can detect even tiny precancerous calcifications that require further investigation. More women choose to breastfeed now, especially those who become pregnant later in life.

Breastfeeding is one of the few potentially modifiable factors that can help prevent breast cancer. Two large meta-analyses examining the effect of breastfeeding on the development of breast cancer concluded that breastfeeding provides a protective function against breast cancer (Bernier et al., 2000; Collaborative Group on Hormonal Factors in Breast Cancer, 2002). Studies suggest that the inverse association between breast cancer and breastfeeding exists mainly among premenopausal women (Katsouyanni et al., 1996; Newcomb et al., 1994; Yang et al., 1997), particularly among those who breastfed for a long time (Katsouyanni et al., 1996; Newcomb et al., 1994; United Kingdom National

Case-Control Study Group, 1993; Zheng et al., 2001) and gave birth at an early age (Brinton et al., 1995; Yoo et al., 1992).

For a woman who is at risk for breast cancer, prolonged breastfeeding may at least delay its occurrence before menopause. According to the estimates published by the Collaborative Group on Hormonal Factors in Breast Cancer (2002), if women in developed countries had 2.5 children on average, but breastfed each child for 6 months longer than the current average, about 5% of breast cancers would be prevented each year, and 11% of breast cancers might be prevented yearly if each child were breastfed for an 12 additional months.

An older study on women in fishing villages near Hong Kong who customarily breastfeed only with the right breast is probably the most dramatic example of the protective effect of breast cancer. These women had a fourfold increased risk of cancer in the unsuckled breast (Ing et al., 1977).

More recently, Daniels et al. (2004) provided evidence of the association between lifestyle, religious value systems, and risk factors for breast cancer. Their group surveyed 848 non-Hispanic white females from Utah, the state with the lowest female malignant breast cancer incidence rate in the United States, partly due to low rates among women of the Church of Latter-Day Saints (LDS or Mormon), to determine the association between selected breast cancer risk factors and religious preference and religiosity. Parity, prevalence of breastfeeding, and lifetime total duration of breastfeeding were highest among LDS-affiliated women who attended church weekly. Average months of breastfeeding per child was greater among weekly church attendees, regardless of religious preference. Oral contraceptive use and total duration of hormone replacement therapy use were greatest among individuals of any religion attending church less than weekly and among those with no religious preference. These findings provided strong support for the role of breastfeeding and parity in the relatively low breast cancer incidence rates previously identified among female LDS members in Utah.

Breastfeeding's protective effect may arise because it reduces the number of ovulations proportionally to breastfeeding duration and intensity, and because it causes a woman to maintain lower estrogen levels than if she were menstruating. In addition, breastfeeding can reduce concentrations of endogenous and exogenous carcinogens present in the ductal and lobular epithelial cells (Helewa et al., 2002).

Although lactation lowers the risk of developing breast cancer, it *does not prevent* the development of a malignant cancer in the breast during lactation. Pregnancy-associated breast cancers are often advanced at the time of diagnosis and estrogen-receptor negative, but they carry a similar prognosis to other breast cancers when matched for stage and age (Woo et al., 2003). Some sources suggest that cancer diagnosed during lactation likely was present during pregnancy, so that a delay in detection and treatment up to 19 months could result from lactation (Yang et al., 2006).

Diagnosis of Breast Cancer

Difficulties in evaluating the breast during pregnancy and lactation may be due to the increased density, glandularity, and water content of the lactating breast. The sensitivity of conventional mammography has been questioned in a review of past research (Woo et al., 2003), and ultrasound is currently considered the most appropriate diagnostic approach in pregnancy and lactation (Sabate et al., 2007). Some research has demonstrated improvement in tumor detection via mammography despite the density of the breast in a pregnant or lactating woman (Yang et al., 2006). Research has also indicated that magnetic resonance imaging (MRI) is useful in detecting breast carcinoma in lactating women (Espinosa et al., 2005), although this technique is not recommended in pregnant women due to the risk of contrast crossing the placenta and entering the fetus (Sabate et al., 2007). When MRI is used, because a small amount of gadolinium is excreted into breastmilk, full bilateral expression is performed prior to the exam and breastfeeding is not recommended for 24 hours after the examination (Sabate et al., 2007).

Core needle biopsy (CNB) is now the standard procedure for assessing breast masses during pregnancy and lactation due to its safety, cost-effectiveness, ability to make a precise diagnosis, and avoidance of surgical biopsy. Because of the increased vascularity of the lactating breast, the risk of bleeding is slightly increased with CNB. There is also risk of infection due to ductal dilation, milk production, and breastfeeding trauma; likewise, the risk of milk fistula formation is increased with this type of biopsy. These risks are minimized by stopping breastfeeding prior to undergoing biopsy, paying close attention to hemostasis, and performing the procedure with strict asepsis (Sabate et al., 2007). Some sources also recommend inhibiting lactation using ice packs, binding, and/or lactation suppression medication (Woo et al., 2003).

Descriptions of breast cancer during lactation that are useful to the clinician working with breastfeeding mothers are still not common in the literature. A dated but important description was given by Petok (1995), who described several cases of breast carcinoma seen in her consulting practice: lobular carcinoma, ductal carcinoma, and inflammatory breast cancer. Most of these women came for treatment of what they called a plugged duct and described a large lump in the breast that had persisted for 1 to 2 weeks. The lumps were 4 to 6 cm in diameter and were irregularly shaped. One mass felt like two firm lumps clustered together. The lumps did not change after feedings or after the usual treatments for a plugged duct (e.g., hot compresses, frequent feedings, breast massage, pumping). Only one woman reported feeling pain at the site of the lump. In one woman, slight redness showed on the side of the breast opposite the lump. The redness lasted only a few days and then disappeared, although the lump did not change. This woman later developed peau d'orange (dimples on the breast similar to those on an orange peel). All of the infants were breastfeeding and gaining weight. None of the infants rejected the cancerous breast, as has been described in the literature (Hadary et al., 1995; Saber, 1996), although one did show a preference for the noncancerous breast. After diagnosis of breast cancer, two of the three women weaned their infants before beginning chemotherapy. The third woman continued to breastfeed for 4 months, despite the objections of her physician, before initiating chemotherapy.

Petok (1995) recommended referring the lactating mother to a physician for evaluation for the following reasons:

- Any mass that shows no decrease in size after 72 hours of treatment
- Afebrile mastitis-like symptoms that are unresolved after a course of antibiotics
- Recurrent mastitis or plugged ducts that appear at the same location

The initial referral is usually to a primary physician, who then refers the patient to a general surgeon. Hesitation to refer out of fear of causing unnecessary concern by mentioning referral to rule out a tumor in a breastfeeding mother is unwise.

One of the myths about breastfeeding and breast cancer is that a baby can receive cancer-causing viral particles in human milk. This is not true: there is no evidence that breastfeeding after treatment for breast cancer carries any health risk to the child (Helewa et al., 2002). There is neither an increase nor a decrease in incidence of breast cancer in breastfed daughters of women who have had breast cancer (Michels et al., 2001).

Rejection of the breast without apparent reason may be an early warning sign of breast cancer (as noted earlier). Although it is true that most of the time an infant rejects the breast for another reason, close surveillance and perhaps also a search for an occult breast carcinoma in the involved breast may enable earlier diagnosis and improved prognosis.

Treatment of Breast Cancer During Lactation

If a positive diagnosis of breast carcinoma is made, breastfeeding should be interrupted and treatment begun. Women receiving chemotherapy for breast cancer or for any other cancer should not breastfeed. All chemotherapeutic drugs cross into the milk. Although their levels are low in milk, these compounds are potent antimetabolites, and they are potentially toxic to the infant.

Breast-conserving procedures (e.g., lumpectomy) are now very common surgical treatments for breast cancer. Radiation therapy often follows breast-conserving procedures or may be used alone depending on the cancer grade. Radiation may cause damage to the milk-producing structures of the breast. Nevertheless, Leal et al. (2013) described lactation following radiation therapy in approximately 50% of patients, although milk volume was reduced. Lactation was not impacted in the nonaffected breast.

Lactation Following Breast Cancer

Approximately 7% of fertile women treated for mammary carcinoma subsequently become pregnant, usually within the first 5 years. Their survival rate is the same as for women who were never pregnant (Deemarsky & Semiglazov, 1987; Donegan & Spratt, 1988). According to a comprehensive review of studies of pregnancy-associated breast cancer by Woo et al. (2003), outcome and survival rates are similar for both pregnant and non-pregnant women who are of similar age and disease stage at the time of diagnosis. In some studies, a so-called healthy mother effect was observed in which former cancer patients who become pregnant had a better 10-year survival rate than their matched controls. Overall, future pregnancies seemed safe for these mothers unless the cancer was estrogen-receptor positive and was not cured.

As long as the woman with a history of breast carcinoma remains clinically free of cancer, there is no therapeutic benefit in interrupting the pregnancy. If advanced cancer is diagnosed in the first or second trimester, however, treatment choices will be limited due to risks to the fetus. In such a case, termination may be considered.

Women who have undergone treatment (surgery, radiation, chemotherapy) for breast cancer and later became pregnant and gave birth report common experiences (David, 1985; Green, 1989; Higgins & Haffty, 1994; Leal et al., 2013; Tralins, 1995; Varsos & Yahalom, 1991):

- There is little or no enlargement of the treated breast during pregnancy.
- The ability to lactate and breastfeed from the untreated breast is normal, but there is less likelihood of having a full milk supply from the treated breast and possibly absence of lactation.

- Difficulty with latch-on sometimes occurs because the nipple on the breast may not extend as completely as might be expected.
- There is less likelihood of an absence of lactation with a circumareolar incision; lactation from the treated breast is less likely to occur in centrally located lesions (Higgins & Haffty, 1994).
- The interval from the time of treatment to the time of delivery does not appear to adversely affect lactation from the treated breast.

Women with estrogen- or progesterone-positive breast cancer are candidates for antiestrogen therapy such as tamoxifen, which stops estrogen from binding to estrogen receptors and stimulating cancer cell growth. Tamoxifen is not recommended during pregnancy or lactation. It inhibits milk production and has a long half-life (Helewa et al., 2002). Significant risks to the infant from exposure to tamoxifen probably outweigh the benefits of breastfeeding.

Women who have experienced breast cancer obviously have many concerns, including fears of reoccurrence of cancer. In addition, women of childbearing age have many psychosocial issues related to their fertility, contraceptive choices, pregnancy, and breastfeeding following breast cancer. Connell et al. (2006) conducted a qualitative study of 13 women with breast cancer in Australia, interviewing them multiple times over a period of 18 months. Concerns related to breastfeeding among women who became pregnant during the study included fears and anxiety of further breast cancer activation and difficulty in detecting breast cancer. These fears, understandable as they may be, conflicted with the women's desire to be a good mother (i.e., breastfeeding is best for the baby). Certainly, the lactation consultant and other healthcare providers who counsel women with a history of breast cancer must be aware of the potential for such fears and anxiety and ready to provide information and support for the woman.

Breast Screening

Noninvasive screening of the breast is extensively used to detect breast abnormalities in nonlactating women, especially breast cancer, so as to diagnose and treat them at an early stage. Types of screening techniques are listed here.

Mammogram

A *screening mammogram* is used to look for breast disease in women who appear to have no breast problems; it is essentially an X-ray of the breast. Some discomfort is felt from flattening the breasts, but it is necessary for an accurate evaluation. A *diagnostic mammogram* is the same as a screening procedure except it may include additional views to magnify suspicious areas to obtain a better analysis of breast tissue. Women with implants will receive a diagnostic mammogram.

Breast Magnetic Resonance Imaging

MRI uses a magnetic field and pulses of radio wave energy to see what is inside the breast without having to perform surgery. MRI of the breast has no known health hazards and shows clear images of dense breasts and implants. The woman lies on her stomach with both breasts hanging freely into a cushioned recess containing a breast coil receiver; she must remain still for up to 15 minutes while images are obtained. MRI is expensive and is not recommended by itself for early detection of breast cancer, although it may be used in conjunction with other techniques.

Breast Ultrasound

Also known as sonography, ultrasound is a method in which high-frequency sound waves are used to "look inside" the breast. A handheld instrument placed on the skin transmits the sound waves through the breast. Echoes from the sound waves are picked up and translated into a computer image. This technology is generally used to evaluate breast problems that are found during a physical exam and after viewing mammogram results. There is no exposure to radiation during this test. An objective, reliable, noninvasive technique, ultrasound is also used to study the breast's anatomic structures and patterns of breastmilk flow.

Thermography Imaging

Thermography imaging maps and measures the heat on the surface of the breast with the use of a heat-sensing camera. It is based on the premise that temperature rises in areas with increased blood flow and metabolism, which could be interpreted as a problem. This technology is not an effective screening tool for early detection of breast cancer, especially in lactating women, who have a much higher level of breast blood flow and temperature than those who are not lactating.

Clinical Implications

With abscess drainage, lump removal, or biopsy, there is usually no reason why the mother should stop breastfeeding. In fact, irrigating a biopsy wound with the many antimicrobial and anti-inflammatory factors found in human milk may facilitate healing. Even when a breast abscess is surgically drained, the mother can breastfeed on the unaffected side and possibly on the affected side, if the incision is far enough from the nipple so that the baby's mouth does not touch it when he breastfeeds. Sometimes the baby feeds only from the unaffected breast while waiting for the affected breast to heal, and the mother hand-expresses or pumps milk from the affected side.

If the wound is left open to drain, breastfeeding can be "messy," because milk and other body fluids may leak from the ducts for as long as 4 weeks or more. The mother should be prepared to replace soiled dressings with clean pads. Milk leaking from the wound may slow healing. As a result, the mother is at risk for a breast infection or a milk cyst; a low-dose prophylactic antibiotic is sometimes prescribed to help the woman avoid infection. A silicone nipple shield with the teat cut off (leaving a doughnut ring of silicone over her nipple) will hold down the bandage and keep the baby's mouth off it. Wounds closer to the nipple–areola complex and in the lower part of the breast usually take longer to heal. If the problems persist, gradual weaning from the affected side might be necessary while the baby feeds from the unaffected side.

Usually the mother resumes breastfeeding on the affected breast when the drain or stitches are removed and when she can tolerate it. A child's reaction to being prevented from feeding from the affected breast (sometimes his "favorite" breast)

varies. Some infants cooperate without a fuss; others are distraught and actively fight to breastfeed there.

Any woman contemplating breast surgery needs to be fully informed about the procedure and the different techniques that are available. A chart that shows the anatomy and lactation functions of the breast is indispensable for explaining the possible effects of surgery. If the patient is highly motivated to breastfeed, it is the clinician's responsibility to counsel her and suggest techniques that will be less disruptive to breastfeeding than other options. If the surgery is very likely to disrupt breastfeeding, that likelihood should be made clear to the woman before the operation. At the same time, it is almost impossible to predict whether breastfeeding will be successful. If supplements become necessary, a feeding tube could be used, thereby allowing the infant to suckle at the breast while receiving a supplement and stimulating milk production.

ACKNOWLEDGMENT

I have had the honor of working with Jan Riordan, the founding editor of *Breastfeeding and Human Lactation*, for many years! I appreciate her mentorship, professionalism, and passion for supporting breastfeeding women while advancing scholarship in this special area of knowledge and clinical practice. This chapter was originally authored by Jan, and I commend her for the thoroughness and evidence-based principles used in the writing. I am proud to take the reins on this chapter and many more in the text, along with my editorship of the text.

SUMMARY

Breast-related problems account for a substantial proportion of clinical breastfeeding counseling. The overuse of antibiotics that leads to candidiasis, the surge in the popularity of cosmetic breast surgery, and digital mammography are human-made barriers to breastfeeding that are unique to affluent countries.

Most of what lactation consultants do for their clients is to give of themselves—the therapeutic self. Therefore, when a mother faces surgery or other procedures on her breasts that are painful and that might also potentially alter or scar her breasts, it is the lactation consultant's responsibility to encourage her to talk, to openly express her feelings, and to answer her questions—and perhaps anticipate her unspoken fears—as completely as possible.

Women have the right to be fully informed about any medical procedure, especially a surgical one, because the outcome is apt to be irreversible. Part of the health professional's responsibility is to act as a client advocate. The client should know all options available to her (including the right to refuse surgery) and all probable outcomes before consenting to a medical procedure.

KEY CONCEPTS

- Breastfeeding knowledge prevents problems that can be common barriers to breastfeeding.
- A woman's feminine identity is closely related to her breasts. Any changes or issues, including those due to illness, disease, or breastfeeding, hold an emotional significance to her.
- Inverted nipples need not impede breastfeeding, provided a mother receives accurate information and assistance in learning effective intervention techniques. The degree of inversion typically lessens as breastfeeding continues.
- The size and length of nipples vary greatly among women and are genetically influenced. Unusually long nipples can make it difficult for a small infant to breastfeed.
- Recurrent plugged milk ducts plague some mothers, whereas other mothers never experience one. There is no conclusive evidence that shows one particular cause for this problem, but it is commonly thought that a constricting bra, poor nutrition, stress, and an inadequately drained breast are contributing factors.
- A red, tender spot in the breast that is warm to the touch characterizes a plugged milk duct. This palpable lump with well-defined margins occurs close to the surface of the skin or can be located deeper in the breast.

- A breast infection or mastitis may or may not be the result of a plugged duct. This condition is characterized by the symptoms of a plugged duct, but will include a flulike muscular aching and fever.
- Mastitis is usually treated with a penicillinase-resistant penicillin or a cephalosporin that covers *Staphylococcus aureus* (the bacteria usually present) for 6 to 10 days. Trimethoprim-sulfamethoxazole and erythromycin are used to treat chronic mastitis.
- Breastfeeding mothers can experience unexplained rashes, eczema, and herpes lesions on the breast that are painful and can hinder breastfeeding. Accurate diagnosis and use of medications help to resolve the problem.
- *Candida* is a yeast naturally found in the mucous membranes of the gastrointestinal and genitourinary tract. Use of antibiotics promotes its overgrowth, which can result in symptoms that include pain in the mother's breast and vagina and symptoms in the baby's mouth and diaper area. Oral and topical antifungal medications are prescribed for such infections. Sometimes, the mother's sexual partner requires treatment as well.
- A breast vasospasm causes extreme breast or nipple pain and is often referred to as a variation of Raynaud's phenomenon, which affects fingers and toes. Exposure to the cold may trigger painful nipple blanching, after which the nipple can experience a color change from white to blue to red. Treatment includes a vasodilator, nifedipine, and use of heat to relieve pain.
- A milk blister can cause extreme pain when the epidermis seals over the ductal opening and prevents milk from draining. If this blockage does not resolve naturally, it is possible to manually remove the excess skin to promote healing.
- Breast augmentation is now commonplace in U.S. society. Silicone gel is again being used for breast implants (as many as 60% of augmentations today). Breast augmentation is less likely to impede breastfeeding than is

breast reduction, but insufficient milk volume is a problem for many women following such surgery. Women who have had previous breast surgery have a threefold higher risk of lactation insufficiency when compared with women who have not had surgery.

- A breast lump in a lactating woman is typically caused by a galactocele, a milk-filled lacteal cyst. Although seldom malignant, a lump that does not resolve itself should be biopsied. After the biopsy, breastfeeding can usually resume within 12 hours.

- Fibrocystic changes are the most frequent benign disorder of the breast. A cyst (also called a fibroadenoma) is a smooth, round lump that moves easily when palpated and is harmless; it is common in women with benign breast disease. A needle aspiration will confirm the diagnosis.

- Slight bleeding from the breast occurs in a small percentage of women, sometimes during pregnancy or upon the birth of the baby. The breast discharge can appear pink to dark red or brown. It is painless, and if it continues during lactogenesis, it is not harmful for the baby to ingest.

- Bleeding from the breast that appears bright red with no other explanation could be an indication of intraductal papilloma, a small, benign, wartlike growth on the lining of the duct. After medical evaluation, a physician may elect to surgically remove the tissue, to confirm that it is not intraductal cancer.

- Pregnancy-associated breast cancer is defined as breast cancer occurring anytime during gestation, during lactation, or within 1 year after delivery. Breast cancer is the most common cancer in pregnant and postpartum women, affecting about 1 in 3000 pregnant women.

- Premenopausal women who breastfed may have at least some protection from breast cancer based on how many children they have, how long each child was nursed, and what age the mother was when she gave birth.

- Breastfeeding's protective effect relative to breast cancer may derive from the reduction in the number of ovulations and lower estrogen levels. Breastfeeding also reduces the concentration of carcinogens present in the ductal and lobular epithelial cells in the breast.

- Although the condition is rare, lactating breasts can develop breast cancer. Diagnosis, even with today's improved technologies, is often delayed due to difficulty in palpating a lump and lack of sensitivity of mammography due to the density, glandularity, and water content of the lactating breast.

- A breastfeeding mother who has a lump that does not show change during the normal course of breastfeeding over a 72-hour period should have it evaluated.

- Breastfeeding mothers who suffer from recurring bouts of mastitis or a plugged duct that occurs in the same location should be evaluated.

- A mother diagnosed with breast cancer will not harm her baby by continuing to breastfeed. When chemotherapy begins, however, the infant must be weaned. All chemotherapeutic drugs cross into the milk and are potentially toxic to the infant. Women who have been treated for breast cancer may go on to have normal, uneventful pregnancies, although lactation in the treated breast may be abnormal.

- After breast surgery, breastfeeding can resume as soon as the mother becomes comfortable with it. Until then, a breast pump can be used to relieve discomfort and to stimulate the milk supply.

- Breast surgery has many implications for a breastfeeding mother and baby. Healthcare professionals must provide accurate and realistic information and support for the mother who must contemplate breast surgery. The lactation consultant, in particular, must act as an advocate for the breastfeeding mother and baby as the mother evaluates all possible options available to her.

INTERNET RESOURCES

Breast Implant Information

United States Food and Drug Administration: http://www.fda.gov/medicaldevices /productsandmedicalprocedures/implants andprosthetics/breastimplants/default.htm).

Breast Cancer in Pregnancy and Lactation

Centers for Disease Control and Prevention: http://www.cdc.gov/cancer/breast

National Cancer Institute: http://www.cancer .gov/cancertopics/pdq/treatment/breast -cancer-and-pregnancy/Patient

American Cancer Society: http://www.cancer .org/cancer/breastcancer/moreinformation /pregnancy-and-breast-cancer

Breast Surgery Information for Healthcare Providers and Mothers

Breastfeeding After Reduction (BFAR): http://www.bfar.org/index.shtml

American Society of Plastic Surgeons: http://www.plasticsurgery.org

Thrush and Other Breastfeeding Information for Mothers and Parents

The Bump: http://pregnant.thebump.com/new -mom-new-dad/baby-symptoms-conditions /articles/thrush-baby.aspx

REFERENCES

Acarturk S, Gencel E, Tuncer I. An uncommon complication of secondary augmentation mammoplasty: bilaterally massive engorgement of breast after pregnancy attributable to postinfection and blockage of mammary ducts. *Aesth Plast Surg.* 2005;29: 274–279.

Aksoy HT, Eras Z, Erdeve O, Dilmen U. A rare cause of hematemesis in newborn: fibrocystic breast disease of mother. *Breastfeed Med.* 2013 Aug;8(4):418–20. doi: 10.1089/bfm.2013.0031.

Alexander JM, Grant AM, Campbell MJ. Randomised controlled trial of breast shells and Hoffman's exercises for inverted and non-protractile nipples. *Br Med J.* 1992;304:1030–1032.

Amir LH. Eczema of the nipple and breast: a case report. *J Hum Lact.* 1993;9:173–175.

Amir LH. An audit of mastitis in the emergency department. *J Hum Lact.* 1999;15:221–124.

Amir LH, Donath SM, Garland SM, et al. Does *Candida* and/ or *Staphylococcus* play a role in nipple and breast pain in lactation? A cohort study in Melbourne, Australia. *BMJ Open.* 2013;3:e002351. doi: 10.1136/bmjopen-2012-002351.

Amir LH, Forster D, Lumley J, et al. A descriptive study of mastitis in Australian breastfeeding women: incidence and determinants. *BMC Public Health.* 2007;7: 62–71.

Amir LH, Forster D, McLachlan H, et al. Incidence of breast abscess in lactating women: report from an Australian cohort. *BJOG: Int J Obstet Gyn.* 2004;111:1378–1381.

Amir LH, Lumley J. Women's experiences of mastitis: I have never felt worse. *Aus Fam Phys.* 2006;35:745–747.

Amir LH, Trupin S, Kvist LJ. Diagnosis and treatment of mastitis in breastfeeding women. *J Hum Lact.* 2014;30: 10–13.

Anderson JE, Held N, Wright K. Raynaud's phenomenon of the nipple: a treatable cause of painful breast-feeding. *Pediatrics.* 2004;113:e360–e364.

Antevski BM, Smilevski DA, Stojovski MZ, et al. Extreme gigantomastia in pregnancy: case report and review of literature. *J Pediatr (Rio J).* 2010;86(3):239–244. doi: 10.2223/JPED.2002.

Baca D, Drexler C, Cullen E. Obstructive laryngotracheitis secondary to gentian violet exposure. *Clin Pediatr.* 2001;40:233–236.

Barankin B, Gross MS. Nipple and areolar eczema in the breastfeeding women. *J Cutan Med Surg.* 2004;8(2): 126–130.

Barrett ME, Heller MM, Stone HF, et al. Dermatoses of the breast in lactation. *Dermatol Ther.* 2013a;26:331–336.

Barrett ME, Heller MM, Stone HF, et al. Raynaud phenomenon of the nipple in breastfeeding mothers: an underdiagnosed cause of nipple pain. *JAMA Dermatol.* 2013b;149(3):300–306.

Berens PD. Prenatal, intrapartum, and postpartum support of the lactating mother. In: Schanler RJ, ed. Breastfeeding, part II: the management of breastfeeding. *Pediatr Clin North Am.* 2002;48:365–375.

Bernardi S, Londero AP, Bertozzi S, et al. Breast-feeding and benign breast disease. *J Obstet Gynaecol.* 2012;32(1): 58–61. doi: 10.3109/01443615.2011.613496.

Bernier MO, Plu-Bureau G, Bossard N, et al. Breastfeeding and risk of breast cancer: a meta-analysis of published studies. *Hum Reprod Update.* 2000;6:374–386.

Bevin TH, Persok CK. Breastfeeding difficulties and a breast abscess associated with a galactocele: a case report. *J Hum Lact.* 1993;9:177–178.

Binns SE. Light-mediated antifungal activity of echinacea extracts. *Planta Med.* 2000;66(3):241–244.

Bolman M, Saju L, Oganesyan K, et al. Recapturing the art of therapeutic breast massage during breastfeeding. *J Hum Lact*. 2013;29:328–331. doi: 10.1177/0890334413475527.

Bowers, M. Isabel and the angry itch: does poison ivy really mean weaning? *Mothering*. 124:68, 2004.

Brent NB. Thrush in the breastfeeding dyad: results of a survey on diagnosis and treatment. *Clin Pediatr*. 2001;40: 503–506.

Brinton LA, Potischman NA, Swanson CA, et al. Breastfeeding and cancer risk. *Cancer Causes Control*. 1995;6: 199–208.

Buescher ES, Hair PS. Human milk anti-inflammatory component content during acute mastitis. *Cell Immunol*. 2001;210:87–95.

Cantlie HB. Treatment of acute puerperal mastitis and breast abscess. *Can Fam Physician*. 1988;34: 2221–2226.

Caputy CG, Flowers RS. Copious lactation following augmentation mammoplasty: an uncommon but not rare condition. *Aesth Plast Surg*. 1994;18:393–397.

Chetwynd EM, Ives TJ, Payne PM, et al. Fluconazole for postpartum *Candida* mastitis and infant thrush. *J Hum Lact*. 2002;18:168–171.

Collaborative Group on Hormonal Factors in Breast Cancer. Breast cancer and breastfeeding: collaborative reanalysis of individual data from 47 epidemiological studies in 30 countries, including 50,302 women with breast cancer and 96,973 women without the disease. *Lancet*. 2002;360:187–195.

Connell S, Patterson C, Newman B. A qualitative analysis of reproductive issues raised by young Australian women with breast cancer. *Health Care Women Int*. 2006;27: 94–110.

Cruz N, Korchin L. Breast-feeding after vertical mammoplasty with medial pedicle. *Plast Reconstr Surg*. 2010; 114(4):890–894.

Daniels M, Merrill RM, Lyon JL, et al. Associations between breast cancer risk factors and religious practices in Utah. *Prev Med*. 2004;38:28–38.

David FC. Lactation following primary radiation therapy for carcinoma of the breast [letter]. *Int J Radiat Oncol Biol Phys*. 1985;11:1425.

Deemarsky LJ, Semiglazov VF. Cancer of the breast and pregnancy. In: Ariel IM, Cleary JB, eds. *Breast cancer: diagnosis and treatment*. New York, NY: McGraw-Hill; 1987:475–488.

Deloach ED, Lord SA, Ruf LE. Unilateral galactocele following augmentation mammoplasty. *Ann Plast Surg*. 1994; 33:68–71.

Donegan WL, Spratt JS. *Cancer of the Breast*. Philadelphia, PA: W. B. Saunders; 1988:685–687.

Eglash A, Proctor R. A breastfeeding mother with chronic breast pain. *Breastfeed Med*. 2007;2(2):99–104.

Espinosa LA, Daniel BL, Vidarsson L, et al. The lactating breast: contrast-enhanced MR imaging of normal tissue and cancer. *Radiology*. 2005;237(2):429–436.

Faridi MM, Dewan P, Batra P. Rusty pipe syndrome: counseling a key intervention. *Breastfeed Rev*. 2013;21(3): 27–30.

Fernandez L, Delgado S, Herrero H, et al. The bacteriocin nisin, an effective agent for the treatment of staphylococcal mastitis during lactation. *J Hum Lact*. 2008;24:311–316.

Fetherston C. Factors influencing the initiation and duration of breastfeeding in a private Western Australian maternity hospital. *Breastfeed Rev*. 1995;3:9–14.

Fetherston C. Risk factors for lactation mastitis. *J Hum Lact*. 1998;14:101–109.

Fetherston C. Mastitis in lactating women: physiology or pathology? *Breastfeed Rev*. 2001;9(1):5–12.

Fetherston CM, Lai CT, Hartmann PE. Relationships between symptoms and changes in breast physiology during lactation mastitis. *Breastfeed Med*. 2006;3:136–145.

Fetherston C, Wells JI, Hartmann PE. Severity of mastitis symptoms as a predictor of C-reactive protein in milk and blood during lactation. *Breastfeed Med*. 2006;1(3): 127–135.

Foxman B, D'Arcy H, Gillespie B, et al. Lactation mastitis: occurrence and medical management among 946 breastfeeding women in the United States. *Am J Epidemiol*. 2002;155:103–114.

Foxman B, Schwartz K, Looman SJ. Breastfeeding practices and lactation mastitis. *Soc Sci Med*. 1994;38:755–761.

Garrison CP. Nipple vasospasm, Raynaud's syndrome and nifedipine. *J Hum Lact*. 2002;18:382–385.

Gibberd GF. Sporadic and epidemic puerperal breast infections. *Am J Obstet Gynecol*. 1953;65:1038–1041.

Grassley JS. Breast reduction surgery. *AWHONN Lifelines*. 2002;6:244–249.

Green JP. Post-irradiation lactation [letter]. *Int J Radiat Oncol Biol Phys*. 1989;17:244.

Groins RA, Ascher D, Waecker N, et al. Comparison of fluconazole and nystatin oral suspensions for treatment of oral candidiasis in infants. *Pediatr Infect Dis J*. 2002;21: 1165–1167.

Guray M, Sahin AA. Benign breast diseases: classification, diagnosis, and management. *Oncologist* 2006;11: 435–449.

Guthrie E, Bradbury E, Davenport P, et al. Psychosocial status of women requesting breast reduction surgery as compared with a control group of large-breasted women. *J Psychosom Res*. 1998;45(4):331–339.

Hadary A, Zidan J, Oren M. The milk-rejection sign and earlier detection of breast cancer. *Harefuah*. 1995;128: 680–681.

Hale T. *Candida albicans*: is it really in the breast? ILCA Conference and Annual Meeting; Las Vegas, NV; July 23–27, 2008.

Hale T. *Medications and mothers' milk*, 14th ed. Amarillo, TX: Hale Publications; 2010.

Han S, Hung Y. Nipple inversion: its grading and surgical correction. *Plast Reconstr Surg*. 1999;104(2):389–395.

Hart J. Nursing after breast surgery. *La Leche League News.* 1980;22:10.

Helewa M, Levesque P, Provencher D. Breast cancer, pregnancy, and breastfeeding. *J Obstet Gynecol Canada.* 2002; 111:164–171.

Hidalgo D, Spector J. Breast augmentation. *Plast Reconstr Surg.* 2014;133:567e–583e.

Higgins S, Haffty BG. Pregnancy and lactation after breast-conserving therapy for early stage breast cancer. *Cancer.* 1994;73:2175–2180.

Hill P, Wilhelm PA, Aldag JC, et al. Breast augmentation and lactation outcome. *MCN.* 2004;29:238–242.

Hoffman KL, Auerbach KG. Long-term antibiotic prophylaxis for recurrent mastitis. *J Hum Lact.* 1986;1:72–75.

Hughes V, Owen J. Is breast-feeding possible after breast surgery? *MCN.* 1993;18:213–217.

Hurst N. Lactation after augmentation mammoplasty. *Obstet Gynecol.* 1996;87:30–34.

Ing R, Ho JHC, Petrakis NL. Unilateral breast-feeding and breast cancer. *Lancet.* 1977;2:124–127.

John MK, Rangwala TH. Gestational gigantomastia. *BMJ Case Rep.* 2009. doi: 10.1136/bcr.11.2008.1177 PMCID: PMC3027370.

Johnstone HA, Marcinak JF. Candidiasis in the breast-feeding mother and infant. *JOGNN.* 1990;19:171–173.

Kataria K, Srivastava A, Dhar A. Management of lactational mastitis and breast abscesses: review of current knowledge and practice. *Indian J Surg.* 2013 Dec;75(6): 430–5. doi: 10.1007/s12262-012-0776-1. Epub 2012 Dec 12.

Katsouyanni K, Lipworth L, Trichopoulou A, et al. A case-control study of lactation and cancer of the breast. *Br J Cancer.* 1996;73:814–818.

Kinlay JR, O'Connell DL, Kinlay S. Incidence of mastitis in breastfeeding women during the six months after delivery: a prospective cohort study. *Med J Aust.* 1998;169(6):310–312.

Kvist LJ, Hall-Lord ML, Rydhstroem H, et al. A randomized-controlled trial in Sweden of acupuncture and care interventions for the relief of inflammatory symptoms of the breast during lactation. *Midwifery.* 2007;23: 184–195.

Lacerna M, Spears J, Mitra A, et al. Avoiding free nipple grafts during reduction mammoplasty in patients with gigantomastia. *Ann Plast Surg.* 2005;55:21–24.

La Leche League International. *Treating thrush.* Schaumburg, IL: La Leche League; 2000.

Lavigne V, Gleberzon BJ. Ultrasound as a treatment of mammary blocked duct among 25 postpartum lactating women: a retrospective case series. *J Chiropr Med.* 2012;11(3):170–178. doi: 10.1016/j.jcm.2012.05.011.

Leal SC, Stuart SR, Carvalho Hde A. Breast irradiation and lactation: a review. *Expert Rev Anticancer Ther.* 2013; 13(2):159–164. doi: 10.1586/era.12.178.

Livingstone V. Problem-solving formula for failure to thrive in breast-fed infants. *Can Fam Phys.* 1990;36:1541–1545.

Love SM. *Dr. Susan Love's breast book,* 3rd ed. Cambridge, MA: Perseus; 2000:95–100.

Marmet C. Breast assessment: a model for evaluating breast structure and function. La Leche League International Annual Seminar for Physicians; Boston, MA; July 1990.

Marshall DR, Callan PP, Nicholson W. Breastfeeding after reduction mammoplasty. *Br J Plast Surg.* 1994;47: 167–169.

Maternal Concepts. http://www.maternalconcepts.com. Accessed June 10, 2014.

Merchant DJ. Inflammation of the breast. *Obstetrics Gynecol Clin North Amer.* 2002;29:89–102.

Merlob P, Aloni R, Präger H, et al. Bloodstained maternal milk: prevalence, characteristics and counselling. *Eur Obs Gynecol Reprod Biol.* 1990;35(2):153–157.

Michels K, Trichopoulos D, Rosner BA, et al. Being breastfed in infancy and breast cancer incidence in adult life: results from the two Nurses' Health Studies. *Am J Epidemiol.* 2001;153:275–283.

Morino C, Winn S. Raynaud's phenomenon of the nipples: an elusive diagnosis. *J Hum Lact.* 2007;23:191–193.

Morrill JF, Heinig MJ, Pappagianis D, et al. Diagnostic value of signs and symptoms of mammary candidosis among lactating women. *J Hum Lact.* 2004;20:288–295.

Morrill JF, Heinig MJ, Pappagianis D, et al. Risk factors for mammary candidosis among lactating women. *JOGNN.* 2005;34:37–45.

Morrill JF, Pappagianis D, Heinig MJ, et al. Detecting *Candida albicans* in human milk. *J Clin Microb.* 2003;41: 475–478.

Mu D, Luan J, Mu L, et al. A minimally invasive gradual traction technique for inverted nipple correction. *Aesth Plast Surg.* 2012;36:1151–1154. doi: 10.1007/s00266-012-9959-1.

National Cancer Institute (NCI), National Institutes of Health. Breast cancer treatment and pregnancy (PDQ®). 2014b. http://www.cancer.gov/cancertopics /pdq/treatment/breast-cancer-and-pregnancy /HealthProfessional.

National Cancer Institute (NCI), National Institutes of Health. SEER stat fact sheets: breast cancer. 2014a. http://seer.cancer.gov/statfacts/html/breast.html.

Neifert M, DeMarzo S, Seacat J, et al. The influence of breast surgery, breast appearance, and pregnancy-induced breast changes on lactation sufficiency as measured by infant weight gain. *Birth.* 1990;17:31–38.

Newcomb PA, Storer BE, Longnecker MP, et al. Lactation and a reduced risk of premenopausal breast cancer. *N Engl J Med.* 1994;330:81–87.

Newman J, Pitman T. *The ultimate breastfeeding book of answers.* Roseville, CA: Prima; 2000.

Nguyen JT, Palladino H, Sonnema AJ, et al. Long-term satisfaction of reduction mammoplasty for bilateral symptomatic macromastia in younger patients. *J Adolesc Health.* 2013 Jul;53(1):112–117. doi: 10.1016/j.jadohealth.2013.01.025.

Nickell WB, Skelton J. Breast fat and fallacies: more than 100 years of anatomical fantasy. *J Hum Lact.* 2005;21: 126–130.

Noble R. Milk under the skin (milk blister): a simple problem causing other breast conditions. *Breastfeed Rev.* 1991;2: 118–119.

O'Callaghan MA. Atypical discharge from the breast during pregnancy and/or lactation. *Aust NZ J Obstet Gynaecol.* 1981;21:214–216.

Oliver WJ, Bond DW, Boswell TC, et al. Neonatal group B streptococcal disease associated with infected breast milk. *Arch Dis Child Fetal Neonatal Ed.* 2000;83:48–49.

Osterman KL, Rahm V. Lactation mastitis: bacterial cultivation of breast milk, symptoms, treatment and outcome. *J Hum Lact.* 2000;16:297–302.

Page SM, McKenna DS. Vasospasm of the nipple presenting as painful lactation. *Obstet Gynecol.* 2006;208: 806–808.

Park HS, Yoon CH, Kim HJ. The prevalence of congenital inverted nipple. *Aesth Plast Surg.* 1999;23:1446.

Paster BA. Surgery on the nursing breast. *New Beginnings.* 1986;2:92.

Penny WJ, Lewis MJ. Nifedipine is excreted in human milk. *Eur J Clin Pharmacol.* 1989;36:427–428.

Petok ES. Breast cancer and breastfeeding: five cases. *J Hum Lact.* 1995;11:205–209.

Potter B. A multi-method approach to measuring mastitis incidence. *Comm Pract.* 2005;78:169–173.

Rampaul RS, Chakrabarti J, Burrell H, et al. A tale of two axillae. *Breast J.* 2005;11:160–161.

Ramsay D, Kent JC, Hartmann RA, et al. Anatomy of the lactating human breast redefined with ultrasound imaging. *J Anatomy.* 2005;206(6):525–534.

Resico S. Nursing after breast surgery. *New Beginnings.* 1990; 6:118.

Rinker B. Veneracion M, Walsh CP. Breast ptosis: causes and cure. *Ann Plast Surg.* 2010;64:579–584.

Riordan J, Nichols F. A descriptive study of lactation mastitis in long-term breastfeeding women. *J Hum Lact.* 1990; 6:53–58.

Sabate JM, Clotet M, Torrubia S, et al. Radiologic evaluation of breast disorders related to pregnancy and lactation. *RadioGraphics.* 2007;27:S101–S124.

Saber A. The milk rejection sign: a natural tumor marker. *Am Surg.* 1996;62:998–999.

Sawhney S, Petkovska L, Ramadan S, et al. Sonographic appearances of galactoceles. *J Clin Ultrasound.* 2002;30: 18–22.

Scott CR. Lecithin: It isn't just for plugged milk ducts and mastitis anymore. Alleviating mastitis and plugged milk ducts. Midwifery Today, Winter, 2005;76:26–27.

Shiau J, Chin C, Lin M. Correction of severely inverted nipple with telescope method. *Aesth Plast Surg.* 2011;35: 1137–1142. doi: 10.1007/s00266-011-9739-3.

Smith WL, Erenberg A, Nowak A. Imaging evaluation of the human nipple during breastfeeding. *Am J Dis Child.* 1988;142:76–78.

Soderstrom B. Helping the woman who has had breast surgery: a literature review. *J Hum Lact.* 1993;9: 169–171.

Souto GC, Giugliani ER, Giugliani C, et al. The impact of breast reduction surgery on breastfeeding performance. *J Hum Lact.* 2003;19:43–49.

Stevens K, Burrell HC, Evans AJ, et al. The ultrasound appearances of galactoceles. *Br J Radiol.* 1997;70: 239–241.

Swelstad MR, Swelstad BB, Rao VK, et al. Management of gestational gigantomastia. *Plast Reconstr Surg.* 2006; 118:840–848.

Tairych G, Worseg A, Kuzbari R, et al. A comparison of long-term outcomes of 6 techniques of breast reduction. *Handchir Mikrochir Plast Chir.* 2000;32:159e65.

Thibaudeau S, Sinno H, Williams B. The effects of breast reduction on successful breastfeeding: a systematic review. *J Plast Reconstr Aesthetic Surg.* 2010;63: 1688e–1693e.

Thomassen P, Johansson VA, Wassberg C, et al. Breastfeeding, pain and infection. *Gynecol Obstet Invest.* 1998;46:73–74.

Thomsen AD, Espersen T, Maigaard S. Course and treatment of milk stasis, noninfectious inflammation of the breast, and infectious mastitis in nursing women. *Am J Obstet Gynecol.* 1985;149:492–495.

Tralins AH. Lactation after conservative breast surgery combined with radiation therapy. *Am J Clin Oncol.* 1995;18: 40–43.

Tung A, Carr N. Postaugmentation galactocele: a case report and review of literature. *Ann Plast Surg.* 2011;67(6): 668–670. doi: 10.1097/SAP.0b013e3182069b3c.

United Kingdom National Case-Control Study Group. Breast feeding and risk of breast cancer in young women. *Br Med J.* 1993;307:17–20.

Utter AR. Gentian violet treatment for thrush: can its use cause breastfeeding problems? *J Hum Lact.* 1990;6: 178–180.

Varsos G, Yahalom J. Lactation following conservation surgery and radiotherapy for breast cancer. *J Surg Oncol.* 1991; 46:141–144.

Vazirinejad R, Darakhashan S, Esmaelli A, Hadadian S. The effect of maternal breast variations on neonatal weight gain in the first seven days of life. *Int Breastfeed J.* 2009; 4:13. doi: 10.1186/1746-4358-4-13.

Vlahovic A, Djuricic S, Todorovic S, et al. Galactocele in male infants: report of two cases and review of the literature. *Eur J Pediatr Surg.* 2012;22(3):246–250. doi: 10.1055/ s-0032-1308694.

Vogel A, Hutchison BL, Mitchell EA. Mastitis in the first year postpartum. *Birth.* 1999;26:218–225.

Wambach KA. Lactation mastitis: a descriptive study. *J Hum Lact.* 2003;19:24–34.

Wang IY, Lee JH, Kim KT. Galactocele as a changing axillary lump in a pregnant woman. *Arch Gynecol Obstet*. 2007; 276:379–382.

Welch ST, Babcock DS, Ballard ET. Sonography of pediatric male breast masses: gynecomastia and beyond. *Pediatr Radiol*. 2004;34:952–957.

Willumsen JF, Filteau SM, Coutsoudis A, et al. Subclinical mastitis as a risk factor for mother–infant HIV transmission. *Adv Exp Med Biol*. 2000;478:211–223.

Wilson-Clay B, Hoover K. *The breastfeeding atlas*. Austin, TX: LactNews Press; 2008.

Woo JC, Yu T, Hurd TC. Breast cancer in pregnancy. *Arch Surg*. 2003;138:91–98.

World Health Organization (WHO). *Mastitis: causes and management*. Geneva, Switzerland: WHO; 2000.

Yang E, Lee K, Pyon J, et al. Treatment algorithm of galactorrhea after augmentation mammoplasty. *Ann Plast Surg*. 2012;69:247Y249.

Yang PS, Yang TL, Liu CL, et al. A case-control study of breast cancer in Taiwan: a low-incidence area. *Br J Cancer*. 1997;75:752–756.

Yang WT, Dryden MJ, Gwyn K, et al. Imaging of breast cancer diagnosed and treated with chemotherapy during pregnancy. *Radiology*. 2006;239:52–60.

Yoo K-Y, Tajima K, Kuroishi T, et al. Independent protective effect of lactation against breast cancer: a case-control study in Japan. *Am J Epidemiol*. 1992;135: 726–733.

Zhao C, Tang R, Wang J, et al. Six-step recanalization manual therapy: a novel method for treating plugged ducts in lactating women. *J Hum Lact*. May 7, 2014. [Epub ahead of print.]

Zheng T, Holford TR, Mayne ST, et al. Lactation and breast cancer risk: a case-control study in Connecticut. *Br J Cancer*. 2001;84:1472–1476.

Low Intake in the Breastfed Infant: Maternal and Infant Considerations

Nancy G. Powers

Introduction

Low intake of breastmilk relative to the infant's needs is the common denominator for a number of different clinical end points. There are numerous causes of low intake and, in turn, numerous outcomes. The complex interrelationship of factors is illustrated in Figures 10-1 and 10-2, which contrast the normal and abnormal situations. Table 10-1 lists various authors' methods of organizing and approaching a conceptual framework for low intake and poor growth in the breastfed infant; however, none of these frameworks are able to encompass the interactions of all potential factors.

Infant intake and maternal milk production are often similar to "the chicken and the egg" problem—which comes first? *Production* is the term used by researchers to indicate the amount of milk produced in response to infant intake, not including any extra expressed milk (Daly et al., 1993). *Perceived insufficient milk supply (PIMS)* is the belief that a mother is not producing enough milk for her infant—when, in reality, there is no objective documentation of milk production, either normal or low (Gatti, 2008). However, in the early postpartum days, delayed secretory activation (also called lactogenesis II) may cause PIMS and create vulnerability to actual low milk supply if supplements

are unnecessarily introduced (Chen et al., 1998). During subsequent breastfeeding, at any time that the mother perceives "insufficient milk," the introduction of supplementary fluids or foods will cause negative feedback on milk production, lowering the actual amounts available. If the infant receives a low volume of intake from breastfeeding but is given supplementation, then the infant will gain weight normally, but the mother's milk supply will decline further. The mother will likely be concerned about low supply, but health professionals may dismiss the concern because the infant is growing well.

During delayed lactogenesis, if the infant does not receive supplementation, low intake may result in excessive weight loss; the excessive weight loss, in turn, may decrease the baby's energy for feeding, causing a secondary low milk production. If the infant is ill and has an increased caloric expenditure, the mother's production may technically be "normal" (for a healthy baby), but her child is not thriving.

Slow weight gain in the breastfed infant is a major concern for both parents and health professionals. When the breastfed infant is not gaining weight normally, the infant is the "identified patient." However, to evaluate the situation, both mother and infant must be assessed for their contribution

359

Figure 10-1 POSITIVE CYCLE OF MILK AND WEIGHT GAIN.

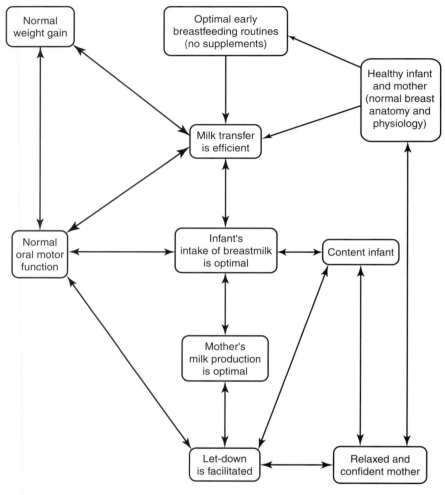

Source: Modified from Powers NG. Slow weight gain and low milk supply in the breastfeeding dyad. *Clin Perinatol.*1999;26(2):399–430, with permission from Elsevier.

to the breastfeeding relationship. In most cases, by careful history taking and examination, along with breastfeeding observation, the astute clinician will be able to develop a differential diagnosis for the dyad, which then allows specific management for the individual case.

The groundwork for optimal feeding with sufficient milk intake is laid during the first days and weeks of breastfeeding and lactation. The critical importance of mother and baby staying together, the baby having unrestricted access to the breast, the "proper" latch (which can prevent

Figure 10-2 NEGATIVE CYCLE OF LOW INTAKE AND LOW MILK SUPPLY.

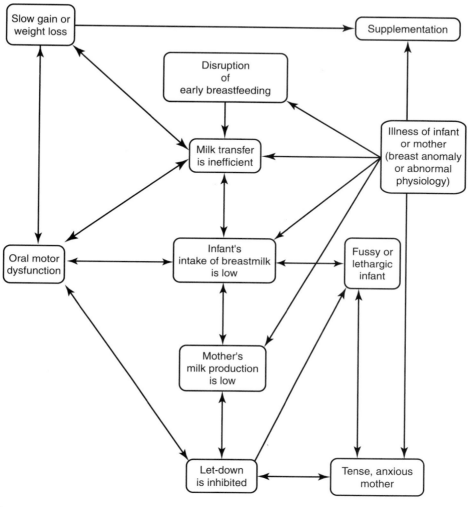

Source: Modified from Powers NG. Slow weight gain and low milk supply in the breastfeeding dyad. *Clin Perinatol*.1999;26(2):399–430, with permission from Elsevier.

most common problems), and the avoidance of other foods and liquids for the baby are addressed in other chapters of this text. Issues related to milk production and milk synthesis in mothers of pre-term infants are likewise considered elsewhere. The current discussion of low intake in the breastfed infant will begin with some general information regarding normal intake and growth patterns of healthy term babies. We will then move beyond the basics of early breastfeeding to examine more complex issues and interactions between mother and infant, as well as anatomic or physiologic variations, health status, medications, and psychosocial and medical factors.

Table 10-1 ASSORTED SCHEMA FOR POOR INFANT GROWTH DURING BREASTFEEDING

Scheme	Concepts	Authors
Rate of gain	Slow gain vs. impending failure to thrive vs. growth failure	Desmarais, 1990
		Lawrence, 2005
Chronology	Newborn vs. infant 6 weeks to 6 months vs. infant over 6 months	Lukefahr, 1990
Energy balance	Decreased intake vs. increased losses vs. increased metabolic demands	Lawrence, 2005
Behavioral	Content vs. fretful	Davies, 1978
		Habbick, 1984
Etiology	Maternal vs. infant	Lawrence, 2005
		Neifert, 1983
Etiology	Primary vs. secondary	Desmarais, 1990
Etiology	Medical vs. psychosocial/cultural	Lawrence, 2005
Compartmental	Milk synthesis vs. milk removal vs. milk intake	Livingstone, 2002, 2005
	Subcategories of each: preglandular, glandular, postglandular	
Occurrence	Common vs. rare	Powers, 1999
Appearance at presentation	Apparently healthy vs. known illness	Powers, 1999

Global Standards for Optimal Growth: The WHO Child Growth Standards

In 2006, the World Health Organization (WHO) released long-awaited, updated global growth standards derived from the Multicenter Growth Reference Study (MGRS). The MGRS was nearly 15 years long—including planning, data collection, and data analysis. All of the planning, methodology, and results are posted on the WHO website (WHO Child Growth Standards, www.who.int /childgrowth/en/) and published as a supplement to the *Food and Nutrition Bulletin* (de Onis et al., 2004). The new standards were developed from a large and detailed prospective study of infant growth and developmental milestones among *optimally breastfed* infants (see study definition, to follow) in Brazil, Ghana, India, Norway, Oman, and the United States. The MGRS data were gathered on more than 8000 children between 1997 and 2003.

For purposes of the longitudinal study, the definition of breastfeeding required the following practices: exclusive or predominant breastfeeding for at least 4 months, introduction of appropriate complementary foods by 6 months, and continued partial breastfeeding for at least 12 months. Six gross motor milestones were included to correlate physical growth with developmental progress.

The study resulted in the following conclusions:

- Breastfeeding is the biological norm.
- Children all over the world grow and develop very similarly when optimally fed with human milk.
- Nutritional and environmental factors have greater influence than genetic factors on child growth.

The WHO standards for height, weight, and body mass index (BMI) are now "prescriptive" (demonstrating how children should grow) instead of "descriptive" (describing how children actually have grown in a given environment). The results are summarized in Box 10-1 (de Onis et al., 2007). These standards apply to children from birth to age 5 years. The new growth charts are split into more age categories than were previously available,

---

BOX 10-1 RESULTS OF THE MULTICENTER GROWTH REFERENCES STUDY (MGRS)

- Breastfeeding is the biological norm.
- Children all over the world grow and develop very similarly when optimally fed with human milk.
- Nutritional and environmental factors have greater influence than genetic factors on child growth.
- Global standards for height, weight, and BMI are now "prescriptive" (demonstrating how children should grow).
- Normal, optimally growing children are somewhat lower in weight and slightly taller than our previous standards have reflected.
- The new standards will generate higher rates of undernutrition from birth to 6 months of age.
- The new standards will generate lower rates of undernutrition after 6 months of age.
- The new standards will generate higher rates of overweight and obesity.

Source: Data from de Onis M et al. Comparison of the WHO child growth standards and the CDC 2000 growth charts. *J Nutr.* 2007;137: 144–148

Figure 10-3 WHO CHILD GROWTH STANDARDS FOR BOYS, BIRTH TO 6 MONTHS (WEIGHT-FOR-AGE PERCENTILES).

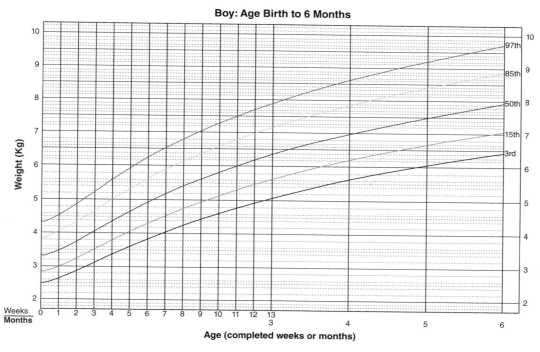

Boy: Age Birth to 6 Months

Source: World Health Organization. Child growth standards: weight-for-age: birth to 6 months, 2013. Available at: http://www.who.int /childgrowth/standards/chts_wfa_boys_p/en/index.html. Accessed May 17, 2013. Used with permission.

with a birth-to-6-month chart that details more frequent measurements (i.e., weekly for the first 3 months) than older charts (Figures 10-3 and 10-4). Compared to previous growth charts (Figure 10-5), the new growth standards are likely to increase the prevalence of children labeled as underweight (in the 0- to 6-month age range), to increase the prevalence of overweight in selected

Figure 10-4 WHO CHILD GROWTH STANDARDS FOR BOYS, BIRTH TO 2 YEARS (WEIGHT-FOR-AGE PERCENTILES).

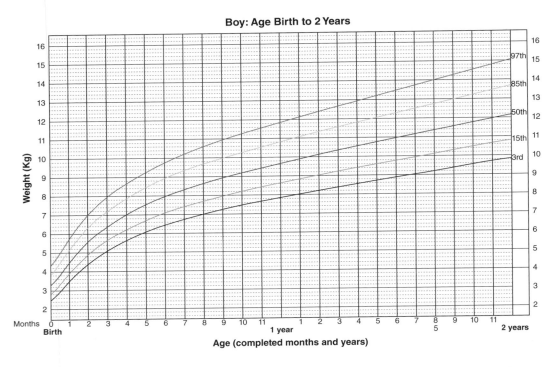

Source: World Health Organization. Child growth standards: weight-for-age: birth to 6 months, 2013. Available at: http://www.who.int /childgrowth/standards/chts_wfa_boys_p/en/index.html. Accessed May 17, 2013. Used with permission.

populations, and to result in an overall increase in rates of stunting (low length/height for age) when compared to results with older growth charts (see again Box 10-1).

When the growth standards were released in 2006, WHO anticipated that their implementation would require significant amounts of new training for health workers; the WHO goal was for the majority of countries to have adopted the new standards by the year 2010. The most recent reports (de Onis, 2011; de Onis et al., 2012) indicated that 125 countries had adopted the standards, another 25 were considering adopting them, and 30 had not adopted them. However, the fact that a country had adopted the growth standards did not necessarily mean that the standards had been fully implemented. For, example, the United States had adopted the standards by 2011, but the American Academy of Pediatrics (AAP) website was still featuring the older 2000 growth charts in early 2013; the Centers for Disease Prevention and Control (CDC) had *both* the 2000 growth charts and the WHO growth standards available on its website at that time. Everyone working with infants and children is encouraged to use the WHO standards by downloading the growth charts from the WHO website (www.who .int/childgrowth/standards/en/).

Because the WHO growth standards are not fully implemented in many settings, the following section will review some of the problems with the previous growth charts.

Figure 10-5 CDC 2000 GROWTH CHART FOR BOYS, BIRTH TO 36 MONTHS, (LENGTH-FOR-AGE AND WEIGHT-FOR-AGE PERCENTILES).

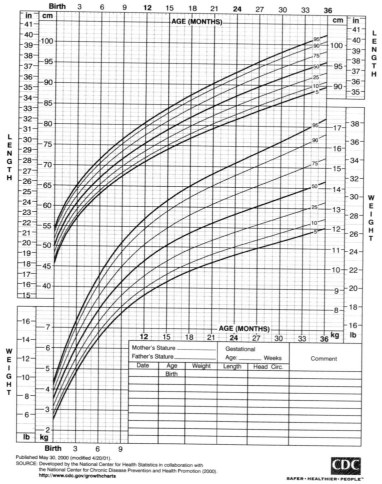

Source: Centers for Disease Control and Prevention, Growth Charts. Available at: http://www.cdc.gov/growthcharts/clinical_charts.htm#Set1. Accessed May 17, 2013.

Older Growth Curves Are Now Outdated

The growth charts previously used in the United States and subsequently adopted in 99 other countries were published in the year 2000 by the CDC (www.cdc.gov/growthcharts). How do these charts compare to the WHO Child Growth Standards? The CDC curves are descriptive: they include a cross section of infants and children in five nutritional surveys conducted between 1963 and 1994. The CDC charts represent only infants from the United States. They include very few infants and children with optimal breastfeeding practices. In addition, there are no actual measurements taken between birth and 2 months of age.

While the CDC curves represented an improvement from previous growth charts, the methodology is obviously quite different from that employed for the MGRS. There has been a detailed analysis of the differences between the WHO Child Growth Standards and the 2000 CDC Growth Charts (de Onis et al., 2007). The CDC charts reflect a heavier and somewhat shorter sample than the WHO sample. Compare Figures 10-3 and 10-4 to Figure 10-5 to see how the WHO and CDC growth charts differ, and see Table 10-2 for a detailed summary of differences in methodology used to generate the two sets of curves.

Table 10-2 COMPARISON OF 2006 WHO CHILD GROWTH STANDARDS AND 2000 CDC GROWTH CHARTS

	WHO Child Growth Standards for Infants and Young Children	2000 CDC Growth Charts
Population—locations and dates	Global and diverse, from 1997 to 2003	United States only, primarily children of northern European descent from 1963 to 1994
Population—number of study subjects	• 882—longitudinal study (birth to 24 months) • 6669—cross-section study (2 to 5 years)	• Cross-sectional data • Data from 10 different data sets • Number of subjects varies for different ages of subjects
Population—nutrition	Optimal prescribed nutrition: • Exclusive or predominant breastfeeding for at least 4 months (longitudinal sample) or at least 3 months (cross-sectional sample) • Introduction of appropriate complementary foods by 6 months • Continued partial breastfeeding for at least 12 months	Observed nutrition in the United States: • Only 50% of children were *ever breastfed* • No information about exclusive breastfeeding • Very few infants were breastfed beyond 6 months of age
Population—environmental factors	• Strict criteria for site selection that would support optimal feeding routines • Other criteria that minimize environmental exposure to infectious diseases or environmental contaminants	• No environmental criteria
Population—health factors	Low-risk population • No maternal smoking (prenatal or postnatal) • Availability of energy-dense complementary foods • Socioeconomic conditions favorable to growth	Mixed population • No exclusion for smoking • Some data sets were collected from low-income populations
Data sampling (measurements)	Frequent sampling in the first 2 months	No sampling between birth and 2 months
Motor milestones	Included to assess association of physical growth and motor developmental	No measurement of development milestones

Sources: Data from Onis et al., 2007; Dewey, 2001.

Using Growth Charts for Management of Individual Patients

When using any growth chart, it is important to understand that the data have been gathered on a population basis. For any given child, we may see a pattern that does not exactly follow the lines on the charts. Each child must be evaluated individually according to his or her health status, activity level, development, family traits, and other individual considerations, before jumping to conclusions based solely on numbers on a graph.

Infants and young children actually grow in a stair-step pattern (termed *saltation*) over the short term, characterized by short bursts of growth in weight and stature that are separated by periods of quiescence. Growth charts, however, are "smoothed" over the time period to give the curved appearance we have grown to expect. In general, infants and young children will tend to follow along a particular percentile for each measurement (stature, weight, head circumference) over time but a number of exceptions can occur. These types of changes are usually gradual and can be explained if a good history is taken.

Problematic patterns with growth are represented by actual weight loss (never normal in a young child), by a flat line in growth with crossing of several percentiles for weight, and by lack of growth in stature or head circumference. Low caloric intake will first result in loss of percentiles for weight, and if sustained will be followed by loss of percentiles for length/height; very prolonged malnutrition will result in decreased head growth. If there is concern about the growth pattern of the child, make careful measurements yourself to double-check the accuracy, look at the overall health of the child, take into consideration the size of the parents, and work with a clinician who has experience evaluating child growth (typically, a pediatrician or a health worker who has been trained in a course such as *Training Course on Child Growth Assessment* by WHO; www.who.int/childgrowth/training/en/). Some children with abnormal growth will have a medical problem as the cause of their growth failure.

The Relationship of Newborn Weight Loss to Onset of Lactation

The events of secretory activation (lactogenesis II) are set in motion by the delivery of the placenta. There is wide individual variation in the rapidity of onset of copious milk secretion among women: some women take up to 2 weeks to produce the volume of milk that other women produce on the second or third day (Neville et al., 1988).

A large comprehensive observational study in the United States carried out by Dewey et al. (2003) studied primiparous and multiparous women (and their infants) who were breastfeeding. The study revealed that the average weight loss for breast-fed infants (supplemented with less than 60 mL (2 ounces) total of non-breastmilk fluids) in the first 3 days of life was 5.5% ± 3.8% of their birth weight. "Excess weight loss" was defined as an infant losing 10% or more of the birth weight. Twelve percent of the newborns were in the "excess" category. Only 5% of infants gained weight in the first 3 days of life. Onset of lactation (OL), as perceived by the mother, occurred in less than 72 hours postpartum in 59% of women. However, 33% of primiparas had OL later than 72 hours postpartum. Late OL (more than 72 hours) was associated with seven times greater risk of excess infant weight loss than normal onset of lactation. A retrospective study of "level I" newborns found 6% of newborn infants had weight loss of 10% or greater during the hospital stay (Flaherman et al., 2010).

A smaller study of infants born in a U.S. Baby-Friendly Hospital showed a mean weight loss of 4.9%, but 19.8% of infants lost more than 7% from birth weight and *no infants lost more than 10%* (Grossman et al., 2012). These authors suggested that "baby-friendly" practices that optimized early breastfeeding experiences are associated with only moderate weight loss among breastfed infants (either exclusively breastfed or breastfed for more than 50% of feedings).

At the same hospital 2 years earlier, there had been a study of a cohort of 200 women who underwent cesarean section (C-section). Among the infants born after C-section, there was a median weight loss of 7.1% of birth weight, with 6.5% losing 10% or more from birth weight. The greatest association with weight loss was found to be among those babies whose C-section birth was not preceded by labor (e.g., repeat C-section) (Preer et al., 2012).

In a prospective study in Switzerland, where mean duration of hospital stay was 5.5 days, there was a 2.4% incidence of weight loss of 10% or more of birth weight. Of the infants with weight loss of 10% or greater, there was a 27% incidence of serum sodium values greater than 150 mm/L—a condition considered "severe hyponatremia" (Konetzny et al., 2009.) In contrast, in a retrospective case study over 12 years in Jamaica, where the modal length of hospital stay for mothers was 24 hours, readmission of neonates with hypernatremic dehydration (mean sodium level at presentation was 164.8 mm/L) was "an uncommon" occurrence (24 infants in 12 years) but was associated with severe morbidity and mortality including renal failure, seizures, intraventricular hemorrhage, and one death (Trotman et al., 2004).

Intravenous fluid administration during labor has been suggested as one factor associated with excessive weight loss. Some observational studies have found a relationship between higher rates of IV fluid administration and excessive infant weight loss (Chantry et al., 2011; Dewey et al., 2003; Noel-Weiss et al., 2011), but other observational studies have not (Grossman et al., 2012; Lamp & Macke, 2010). One randomized controlled trial suggested that intravenous fluid administration greater than 2500 mL to the mother during labor is a risk factor for subsequent weight loss of more than 10% of birth weight in the infant (Watson et al., 2012).

Dewey et al. (2003) developed the concept of "SIBB" (suboptimal infant breastfeeding behavior), finding that 49% of infants had SIBB in the first 24 hours after birth. SIBB had some correlation to OL/infant weight loss. SIBB on day 0 and delayed OL were significant predictors of excess infant weight loss (10% or more below birth weight). Ninety-two percent of infant cases with excess weight loss could be predicted by combining SIBB on day 0

and delayed OL—one or the other, but not necessarily both. Other risk factors identified for SIBB or excess infant weight loss were primiparity, cesarean section, flat or inverted nipples, long duration of stage II labor, total duration of labor of more than 14 hours, labor medications in multiparas, and BMI of greater than 37 kg/m^2. Heavier birth weight of infants born to primiparas was another risk factor for delayed OL. Risk factors for delayed lactogenesis, supplementation, and excess infant weight loss (10% or more below birth weight) are summarized in Boxes 10-2 and 10-3.

The woman with slower onset of milk production will likely perceive more difficulties with milk supply in the early days following childbirth (Chen et al., 1998; Segura-Millan et al., 1994). This causes anxiety, which interferes with letdown (limiting flow of colostrum) and increases the tendency to provide supplements, which then further limits milk supply. This vicious negative cycle of events, described earlier as "perceived insufficient milk," is correlated with shorter duration of breastfeeding. The cycle becomes difficult to reverse, and continues to spiral downward. In some cases, the milk supply is so low that "relactation" is required if the mother wants to continue breastfeeding (see the *Women's Health and Breastfeeding* chapter of this text regarding relactation).

Ongoing milk production is stimulated by milk removal, either by the infant or by some other means of expression, such as pumping (Peaker & Wilde, 1987). In the normal situation, higher-birth-weight babies stimulate a larger volume of milk production than do smaller babies, and the milk supply is "infant driven" (Daly et al., 1993; Dewey & Lonnerdal, 1986; Dewey et al., 1991; Kent et al., 1999, 2006). In the abnormal situation, the milk supply is not appropriately stimulated because the infant is not feeding frequently enough, is not staying at the breast for a sufficient length of time, or is ineffective at milk removal, or (rarely) because the maternal physiology is unable to respond to the stimulation of the suckling infant. Underweight or poor-quality nutrient intake in the mother has not been found to correlate with milk volumes in full lactation.

BOX 10-2 MATERNAL RISK FACTORS FOR DELAYED ONSET OF LACTATION (OL) (LATER THAN 72 HOURS POSTPARTUM)

Prenatal Factors

Excessive gestational weight gain (GWG) (Hilson et al., 2006)
Higher prepregnant BMI (Hilson, 2006)
Insulin-dependent diabetes mellitus (IDDM) with poor control (Neubauer et al., 1993)
Inverted or flat nipples (Dewey, 2003)
Obesity and excessive GWG are additive (Hilson, 2006)
Overweight and obesity (Chapman & Perez- Escamilla, 1999; Dewey, 2003; Hilson, 2006; Rasmussen & Kjolhede, 2004)
Primiparity (Chen et al., 1998; Dewey et al., 2002, 2003; Grajeda & Perez-Escamilla, 2002; Hilson, 2006)

Intrapartum Factors

High cortisol levels (during labor) in multiparas (Chen et al., 1998; Grajeda & Perez-Escamilla, 2002)
Hospital delivery (vs. home delivery) (Chen et al., 1998)
Long duration of labor (Chen et al., 1998; Dewey et al., 2003)
Maternal exhaustion during labor and delivery (Chen et al., 1998)
Prolonged duration of stage II labor (Chapman & Perez-Escamilla, 1999; Dewey et al., 2003)
Unscheduled C-section (Chen et al., 1998; Dewey et al., 2003; Grajeda & Perez-Escamilla, 2002); C-section (Dewey et al., 2003)

Postpartum Factors

Exclusive formula feeding prior to onset of lactation (OL) (Chapman & Perez-Escamilla, 1999)
Heavier baby born to a primiparous mother (Dewey et al., 2003)
No rooming in (Perez-Escamilla & Chapman, 2001)

With the current epidemic of obesity, issues regarding maternal overweight, obesity, and excessive gestational weight gain (GWG) have entered into the discussion about early lactation. A review by Rasmussen (2007) revealed the complexity inherent in this arena, including the potential biological mechanisms by which excess fat tissue may reduce milk production, animal research that shows differing effects of maternal overfeeding depending upon the timing in the life cycle, the complex interactions of physical and psychosocial factors, and issues created by the pregnancy/labor/birth process for obese women (e.g., the increased risk of cesarean section) that may confound breastfeeding outcomes.

Prepregnant obesity (based on BMI) has been found to be associated with decreased incidence of intention to breastfeed and decreased breastfeeding initiation rates (Guelinckx et al., 2012). Prepregnant overweight and obesity have been associated with slower onset of lactogenesis (Chapman & Perez-Escamilla, 1999; Chen et al., 1998; Hilson et al., 2004; Nommsen-Rivers et al., 2010). One possible mechanism underlying this relationship is the diminished response to prolactin among overweight/obese women in the first week postpartum (Rasmussen & Kjolhede, 2004). There is also evidence of a higher incidence of early cessation of breastfeeding when the mother has a higher BMI

BOX 10-3 RISK FACTORS FOR EXCESSIVE WEIGHT LOSS IN INFANTS (10% OR MORE BELOW BIRTH WEIGHT IN THE FIRST 3 DAYS OF LIFE)

Maternal Factors

Delayed onset of maternal lactation (delayed OL) over 72 hours postpartum (Dewey et al., 2003)
Primiparity, if birth unmedicated (Dewey et al., 2003)
Labor pain medications, in multiparas (Dewey et al., 2003)

Infant Factors

Smaller infant size
Suboptimal infant breastfeeding behavior (SIBB) in the first 24 hours of life (Dewey et al., 2003)
Infant stress (cord blood cortisol and glucose concentrations) (Chen et al., 1998)
Low-risk infant status at delivery (Dewey et al., 2003)*

Feeding-Related Factors

Lower mother–baby assessment (MBA) scores (Hilson et al., 2006)
*Curious result, paradoxical, hard to explain; this finding may be due to chance.

(Hilson et al., 1997). In one study, excessive pregnancy weight gain was found to be associated with shorter durations of exclusive breastfeeding among all categories of prepregnant BMI that were studied (normal, overweight, obese) (Hilson et al., 2006). This effect was additive in the women who were obese prior to pregnancy. However, a recent study using a different methodology (Bartok et al., 2012) did not find a difference in duration of breastfeeding between women in differing weight categories. Most studies have been based on populations of white women, but one study found that there was a negative association of breastfeeding with obesity in Hispanic women but not black women (Kugyelka et el., 2004). We are far from understanding the full impact of overweight, obesity, and gestational weight gain on early lactation and breastfeeding.

Initial Newborn Weight Loss and Early Weight Gain

In the first 2 to 3 days after birth, one study showed that more than 95% of full-term infants lose weight, due to loss of fat mass and nonfat mass (including fluid loss) (Roggero et al., 2010). This weight loss is probably due to a combination of hormonal changes along with a relatively low (but normal) intake of colostrum. The percent weight loss below birth weight shows large variation within term newborns, yet the significance of greater weight loss is uncertain. There is concern that formula-fed infants are overfed, raising questions about the point at which weight loss becomes pathologic in an otherwise "healthy" newborn (Mulder et al., 2010; Regnault et al., 2011).

The WHO Child Growth Standards (www.who.int/childgrowth/standards/w_velocity/en/index.html) are the most comprehensive data that we have regarding early weight gain in optimally breastfed infants. They provide detailed data for the first weeks and months (Table 10-3). Weight increment tables reveal that *75% of both boys and girls regain birth weight by 7 days of age, and 95% of both boys and girls have regained birth weight by 14 days of age.* Reviewing the absolute weight loss from that database, it becomes apparent the weight loss is less than the traditionally accepted estimates: *25% of both boys and girls weigh 6% less than their birth weight*

Table 10-3 TERM NEWBORN WEIGHT GAIN OR LOSS IN THE MULTICENTER
GROWTH REFERENCE STUDY

By Age of	Over Birth Weight	Weight Gain	Under Birth Weight	Weight Loss
7 days	75% of newborns	3% above birth weight or 4 g/kg/day	25%	–6% below birth weight or 10 g/kg/day
14 days	95% of newborns	6% above birth weight or 8 g/kg/day	5%	–1.5% below birth weight or 2 g/kg/day
Between Ages of	Weight Gain	Average		
14 to 60 days	Girls: 28–42 g/day	Girls: 39 g/day		
	Boys: 15–52 g/day	Boys: 46g/day		

Data from: World Health Organization, Weight velocity. Available at: http://www.who.int/childgrowth/standards/w_velocity/en/index.html.

by 7 days of age; 5% of babies are only 1.5% below birth weight by 14 days. The previous edition of this text stated, "Initial weight loss of more than 7% from birth weight may be an indicator of breast-feeding difficulties and requires observation and evaluation of the breastfeeding process. Weight loss of more than 10% definitely requires intervention from the physician or lactation consultant (Academy of Breastfeeding Medicine, 2002; International Lactation Consultant Association, 2005)." These former guidelines have reflected the reality of excessive weight loss encountered in environments with suboptimal breastfeeding practices. As the Baby-Friendly Hospital Initiative gains a stronger foothold in developed countries, we may be able to see our guidelines conform more closely to the numbers seen in the WHO growth standards.

In the United States, the American Academy of Pediatrics (AAP) has advocated for early follow-up of the breastfed infant. AAP guidelines (Eidelman, 2012) state that an infant released from the hospital before 48 hours of age must be seen by a health professional at 3 to 5 days of age, when infant status and maternal milk production are at a critical juncture. Infants at risk for hyperbilirubinemia may need to be seen sooner. Thereafter, the infant should be seen as necessary to reevaluate breastfeeding and monitor weight gain. Once above birth weight and gaining steadily, the baby is seen at routine health supervision intervals.

Low Intake and Low Milk Supply: Definitions and Incidence of Occurrence, Confusing Terminology, Limited Data, and Nonstandardized Research

Terminology surrounding abnormal growth can be confusing. Many texts have different definitions of the term *failure to thrive*. Most definitions of poor growth refer to deviations on growth charts, which, as discussed previously, prior to the WHO Child Growth Standards, were not suitable for breastfed infants. Some authors refer to "slow gain" or "growth failure." In clinical practice, the term *failure to thrive* often carries negative connotations that imply poor parenting, neglect, or abuse. For these reasons, we will refer to the guidelines presented in Table 10-4 and the growth charts produced by the WHO Child Growth Standards (for examples, see Figures 10-3 and 10-4), rather than any of the other jargon. If the infant falls into the category where concern is warranted, we must thoroughly evaluate the feeding process and intervene when necessary. Watchful waiting at this stage may be inappropriate, because unidentified problems often become more difficult to manage over time as the infant loses weight and the milk supply dwindles.

Table 10-4 WHEN TO EVALUATE THE NEWBORN AND YOUNG INFANT FOR GROWTH CONCERNS, BASED ON WHO GROWTH STANDARDS

Parameter	Normal: Follow Clinically	Concerning: Evaluate Medical Condition and Breastfeeding
Initial weight loss (percent below birth weight)	6% or less	7–10%
Return to birth weight	7–14 days of age	Later than 14 days of age
Average daily weight gain (after return to birth weight)	Females: 39 g Males: 46 g	Less than 30–40 g
Weight loss after immediate newborn period	None	Any amount of unexplained weight loss
Growth curve—weight	Weight follows curves of WHO Growth Standards	Completely flat or crossing percentiles downward on WHO Growth Standards at any age
Growth curve—length	Length continues on a given percentile	Crossing of percentiles downward (crossing percentiles upward may also be of medical concern)
Growth curve—head circumference	Head size continues on a given percentile	Crossing of percentiles upward or downward

Much of the data regarding definitions of sufficient or insufficient weight gain in the breastfed infant is derived from the same studies that "define" sufficient and insufficient milk production. The infant's weight gain is often used as a proxy for maternal milk supply. This means that the definition of "adequate" infant weight gain will determine the "adequacy" of the milk supply. Unfortunately, various studies have applied different definitions of adequate weight gain and used different time points to measure the babies' weights. Dewey et al. (2003) prospectively studied newborn weight loss in 280 infants. Approximately 12.5% of these infants lost 10% or more from birth weight by day 3. This initial excessive weight loss was correlated with delayed onset of lactation (see again Boxes 10-2 and 10-3). Neifert, Seacat, and colleagues (1990) found that 15% of infants gained less than 28.5 g per day after the fifth day of life. None of the infants in their study were identified as having any underlying medical problems. The cutoff point of 28.5 g per day is probably too high, as the data from de Onis et al. (2004), discussed earlier, would have predicted that 25% of normal infants would gain less than 28 g per day. Lukefahr (1990) prospectively identified 38 breastfed infants with poor growth during a 4-year period in his private practice. When the infant presented with abnormal growth at more than 1 month of age, organic causes were present in 50% of cases. It is difficult to draw conclusions, however, because these three reports have different study designs, represent different patient selection biases, and have different definitions of "insufficient" weight gain.

Approaching the issue of low intake from the maternal side is equally confusing. The definition of insufficient milk is not standardized, and there are numerous confounding variables—biological as well as cultural and psychosocial. There is also the problem of determining a meaningful control group. Selection criteria, study design, and breastfeeding definition are different for each study.

As mentioned previously, in the study by Dewey et al. (2003), 12.5% of newborns lost more than 10% of birth weight—implying that there was also a 12.5% rate of insufficient milk supply at day 3 postpartum. In four additional studies of self-selected populations of U.S. women who decided to breastfeed exclusively for at least 3 to 4 months, only a small percentage of women were unable to produce enough milk for their infants. Parity was mixed in these studies (Butte et al., 1984; Dewey et al., 1991; Neville et al., 1988; Stuff & Nichols, 1989). Neifert, Seacat, and colleagues' (1990a) study—mentioned earlier in regard to the infant—used the same results to categorize 15% of U.S. primiparas as unable to produce "sufficient milk." Table 10-5 summarizes the results of these six studies, but caution is urged in interpreting the findings; they serve to illustrate how few data we have and how definitions can bias study results.

The definition of insufficient milk, for the purposes of this chapter, is as follows: insufficient breastmilk production to sustain normal infant weight gain despite appropriate feeding routines, maternal motivation to continue breastfeeding, and skilled assistance with breastfeeding problems.

Table 10-5 FREQUENCY OF INSUFFICIENT MILK IN SELECTED REPORTS

Author	Year	Number Insufficient of Total Number of Patients	Percent
Dewey et al.	2003	30 of 240	12.5
Dewey et al.	1991	1 of 92	1
Neifert et al.	1990	48 of 319	15
Stuff & Nichols	1989	3 of 58	5
Neville et al.	1988	0 of 13	0
Butte et al.	1984	0 of 45	0

This article was published in Clinic Perinatol. 26, Powers NG. Slow weight gain and low milk supply in the breastfeeding dyad, 399–430. Copyright Elsevier 1999. Used with permission.

Abnormal Patterns of Growth: The Baby Who Appears Healthy

Inadequate Weight Gain in the First Month

Once over birth weight, the neonate who gains less than 30–40 g per day in the first 2 months of life (see Tables 10-3 and 10-4) requires thorough medical and breastfeeding evaluation (see Box 10-4 and Tables 10-6 through 10-8). Poor feeding or poor weight gain can be subtle signs of illness in young infants. It is essential to keep illness (see again Box 10-2) as part of the differential diagnosis of feeding problems or poor weight gain. Yet, in the first month of life, problems with the feeding process are by far a more common cause of poor weight gain than are organic illnesses (Lukefahr, 1990; Neifert et al., 1985). Detection and correction of the feeding problem should be addressed. Once feeding has improved, ongoing lack of weight gain may indicate underlying illness. Differential diagnosis and management are discussed later in this chapter.

The Late-Preterm Infant

Late-preterm infants, delivered at 34 to 36 weeks' gestation, more closely resemble premature than term infants due to the immaturity of most of their organ systems. Their immaturity predisposes them to the following complications: excessive sleepiness, feeding difficulties, low motor tone, dehydration, hyperbilirubinemia, apnea, hypothermia, hypoglycemia, and respiratory distress (Engle et al., 2007). Overall, the late-preterm infant is two to three times more likely to be readmitted to the hospital; if not admitted to the neonatal intensive care unit (NICU) and discharged before 48 hours of age, these children's risk of readmission may be as high as 5 to 10 times that of infants born after more than 37 weeks' gestation. Neonatal mortality (death at 0–27 days chronologic age) of late-preterm newborns is 7 times that of term newborns.

BOX 10-4 INFANT AND MATERNAL CONDITIONS THAT MAY CONTRIBUTE TO SLOW WEIGHT GAIN OR LOW MILK SUPPLY

Infant

Allergy
Ankyloglossia (tongue-tie)
Biliary atresia
Cleft lip or palate
CNS abnormality
Congenital heart disease
Cystic fibrosis
Gastrointestinal infections
Gastrointestinal malformations
Gastroesophageal reflux
Hypocalcemia
Hypovitaminosis D
Inborn errors of metabolism
Increased caloric needs from chronic disease, infection, malabsorption
Intestinal malabsorption syndrome
Neurological disorders
Oral–motor dysfunction (abnormal suck)
Prematurity
Renal disease
Rickets
Sepsis of the newborn
Thyroid disease
Urinary tract infection

Maternal

Autoimmune disease
Breast surgery
Chronic illness of any type
Connective tissue disease
Eating disorder
Hypopituitarism
Inverted nipples
Polycystic ovary syndrome
Postpartum hemorrhage
Pregnancy
Primary mammary glandular insufficiency
Psychiatric illness
Renal failure
Retained placenta
Stress
Theca lutein cyst
Thyroid disease

Table 10-6 HISTORY AND PHYSICAL FOR EVALUATION OF THE BREASTFEEDING DYAD

Infant and Maternal History	Infant Examination	Maternal Examination	Laboratory Tests
• Prenatal risk factors • Previous feeding experiences • Prenatal care • Feeding plan and education • Perinatal history, especially labor, delivery, and first feeding		• Prenatal breast exam	
• Medical problems • Medications • Past medical history, especially breast surgery, postpartum hemorrhage, endocrine disorders	• Weight and growth parameters • Vital signs • General physical exam • Neurological exam, especially motor tone • Oral–motor exam (detailed)	• Vital signs • General physical exam • Thyroid exam	• General laboratory tests as indicated; consider thyroid function tests and/or endocrine consultation (prolactin levels are rarely helpful)
• Postnatal feeding and elimination history	• Breastfeeding observation	• Breast and nipple examination • Breastfeeding observation	• Test-weight, if indicated
• Infant temperament and sleep patterns • Maternal sleep, fatigue, appetite	• State transition, self-calming behaviors • General appearance, alertness, attentiveness		
• Family history, especially atopy, diabetes, autoimmune diseases, cancer	• General exam	• General exam	
• Psychosocial history	• Mother-infant interaction	• Mother–infant interaction	• Depression screening or drug testing, if indicated
• Use of tobacco, alcohol, drugs		• Signs of milk ejection reflex	

Courtesy of Nancy G. Powers, MD.

Table 10-7 Infant Factors: Problem-Oriented Management for Slow Gain or Insufficient Milk Supply

Etiology	Management
Acute or chronic illness	• Medical management of specific entity
Ankyloglossia (short frenulum, tongue-tie)	• The presence of ankyloglossia associated with any feeding problem is usually an indication for frenotomy
Congenital anomalies	• Expression or pumping of milk to increase mother's production • Facilitate maternal let-down (relaxation techniques) • Patient attempts to latch baby at breast • Expanded definition of breastfeeding: the use of human milk by whatever feeding method is successful
Food allergy	• Maternal elimination diet; may take over 1 week for results • Maternal nutrition consultation • If severe or no response to elimination diet, refer to pediatric allergist and/or pediatric gastroenterologist
Gastroesophageal reflux	• Evaluate for maternal oversupply • Increase delivery of hindmilk (see special techniques for management) • Reduce maternal supply, if applicable • Position more upright during feeds • Frequent burping • Consider the possibility of overlapping cow's milk allergy • Medical management as indicated
Increased caloric demands	• Maximize volumes to 200 ml/kg/day if possible • Have the mother collect hindmilk • Add supplemental calories/nutrients to expressed breastmilk • See also "volume restriction" below.
Neurological conditions	• Expression or pumping of milk to increase mother's production • Chin/jaw support may be helpful • Feeding-tube device or alternative feeding method with expressed mother's milk or formula as needed for weight gain • Oral–motor therapy may be beneficial • Referral to lactation consultant • Referral to infant feeding specialist (e.g., pediatric occupational, physical, or speech therapist)
Oral–motor dysfunction	• Increased frequency of feeding • Expression or pumping of milk to increase mother's production • Feeding-tube device or alternative feeding method with expressed mother's milk or formula as needed for weight gain • Oral–motor exercises may be beneficial • Referral to lactation consultant • Referral to infant feeding specialist

Table 10-7 INFANT FACTORS: PROBLEM-ORIENTED MANAGEMENT FOR SLOW GAIN OR INSUFFICIENT MILK SUPPLY (CONTINUED)

Prematurity, stable infant	• Promote skin-to-skin contact • Minimize heat loss • Feeding-tube device or alternative feeding method with expressed mother's milk, donor milk, or formula as indicated by weight loss/gain
Volume restriction	• Additional caloric density may be indicated by supplemental means: commercial fortifier or carbohydrate or lipid • Have the mother collect hindmilk • Another alternative: skim the fat layer from stored expressed milk, then add this fat to additional expressed milk to achieve higher caloric density per given volume (approximately 8–10 calories per ml)

This article was published in Clinic Perinatol. 26, Powers NG. Slow weight gain and low milk supply in the breastfeeding dyad, 399–430. Copyright Elsevier 1999. Used with permission.

Table 10-8 MATERNAL FACTORS: PROBLEM-ORIENTED MANAGEMENT FOR SLOW GAIN OR INSUFFICIENT MILK SUPPLY

Etiology	Management
• Acute or chronic illness	• Medical management of specific entity
• Attachment difficulties	• Consistent skilled assistance with latch-on
• Nipple pain or trauma	• Expression (pumping) of milk 8 times/24 hr
• Inverted nipples	
• Breast abnormalities (breast surgery, breast trauma, insufficient glandular development)	• Follow infant weight gain closely the first month • Use feeding-tube device with formula as needed to maintain appropriate weight gain • Maximize production by proper positioning, frequent feedings, extra pumping
• Disruption of early breastfeeding	• Increase frequency of feedings • Nurse on both sides for sufficient lengths • Awaken baby at night for feedings • Household help and support for mother • Address sources of pain, anxiety, or stress
• Delayed milk ejection	• Relaxation techniques • Pain relief • Household help • Stress reduction techniques • Support groups or professional counseling • Intranasal oxytocin spray may be available via compounding pharmacy (expensive)

(continues)

Table 10-8 MATERNAL FACTORS: PROBLEM-ORIENTED MANAGEMENT FOR SLOW GAIN OR INSUFFICIENT MILK SUPPLY (*CONTINUED*)

• Hormonal alterations (pregnancy, retained placenta, thyroid disorders, theca lutein cysts, hypopituitarism)	• Continue breastfeeding, tandem nursing is an option during pregnancy • Medical management of specific entity
• Ineffective milk removal (ineffective baby or pump)	• Review proper position and latch-on; check pump pressures • Chin support, if indicated • Express milk to increase supply; better pump if indicated • Evaluation by OT/PT/speech therapist
• Maternal medications	• Change to medications with similar therapeutic effect, but which will not affect milk supply • Feed baby more frequently to increase supply • Expression (pumping) of milk 8 times/24 hr
• Nipple shields	• Express or pump milk to increase or maintain supply • Wean from shield by removing it midfeed, or gradually cutting larger hole in tip
• Psychosocial problems	• Social work involvement
• Substance use/abuse	• Determine whether continued breastfeeding is appropriate

This article was published in Clinic Perinatol. 26, Powers NG. Slow weight gain and low milk supply in the breastfeeding dyad, 399–430. Copyright Elsevier 1999. Used with permission.

Infant mortality (death between 28 days and 1 year chronologic age) of late-preterm infants is 3 times higher (Engle et al., 2007).

Shapiro-Mendoza et al. (2008) reported that when maternal complications of antepartum hemorrhage or hypertensive disorders of pregnancy were present, the late-preterm infant has 11 times the morbidity of a term infant born to a mother with no maternal complications.

Considering the significant immaturity of the late-preterm infant, it is not surprising that initiation of breastfeeding among these infants is lower than among full-term infants. In one study in the United States, the initiation rate for late-preterm infants was 8% lower than that for term infants (62% versus 70%) (Demirci et al., 2012). Given that breastfeeding was found to be statistically significantly associated with readmission (Edmonson et al., 1997; Engle et al., 2007; Shapiro-Mendoza et al., 2006; Soskolne et al., 1996) in late-preterm

infants, we may deduce that breastfeeding does not always go well with those late-preterm infants who do initiate breastfeeding. Sixty-three percent of the readmissions in this population were due to hyperbilirubinemia (Shapiro-Mendoza et al., 2006).

Oral–Motor Dysfunction (Ineffective Suckling)

When breastfed infants are put to breast frequently yet fail to effectively remove milk, two problems may be responsible (separately or in combination): the infant is not attached properly and/or some form of suckling abnormality is present. The rate and pattern of suckling are flow dependent: higher suckling rates (non-nutritive) occur with decreased flow of milk (Bowen-Jones et al., 1982; Glass & Wolf, 1994). Thus ineffective suckling results in low milk supply and low flow, which further results in less efficient suckling (see again Figure 10-2).

New research from the Hartmann Human Lactation Group (University of Perth, Australia), using ultrasound along with intraoral pressure measurements to study suckling at the breast, is elucidating some of the physiology of suckling at breast. Vacuum is responsible for milk flow as the baby's tongue drops, creating a closed chamber with negative pressure. The milk flowing from the ducts can actually be visualized on ultrasound. Non-nutritive suckling has been defined as swallowing of saliva only, while nutritive suckling occurs when milk is swallowed. This work has shown that babies have the same pattern of sucking at 3 days of age as they do at around 2 weeks, although the sucking rate becomes somewhat faster and the depth of jaw excursion increases at the second time point (Sakalidis et al., 2013).

"Oral–motor dysfunction" is a broad term encompassing abnormal motor tone and/or coordination of infant suck due to a variety of conditions. Oral–motor dysfunction may occur as an isolated and subtle finding in normal infants, often in conjunction with variations in motor tone or poor state regulation in the infant. Low-normal tone may result in weak suction and poor coordination, while high-normal tone results in clenching, biting, or vertical compression with the tongue. Infants with isolated oral–motor dysfunction can usually become proficient with at least one feeding method (bottle-, cup-, or finger-feeding). Oral–motor dysfunction will be an obvious concern when there are significant medical conditions such as neurologic abnormality or cleft lip or palate.

A variety of other sources (Drane, 1996; Glass & Wolf, 1994; Lawrence & Lawrence, 2011) provide in-depth discussion of suckling disorders. Unfortunately, much of the research on this topic is based on observations of infants on artificial nipples, and their relevance to breastfeeding is uncertain. The new research techniques using ultrasound and intraoral pressure measurements have shown that excessive negative pressure is associated with nipple pain and that babies with ankyloglossia (tongue-tie) have abnormal tongue movement (Geddes et al., 2008) (see the section on ankyloglossia later

in this chapter). Oral–motor dysfunction presents often with maternal nipple trauma and pain as well as with poor weight gain in the infant (see Figures 10-6 and 10-7). Clinically, these babies often remain calm or asleep only when at the breast. Although they appear to be asleep, when taken off the breast they cry hungrily. During active feeding, they will demonstrate a nutritive suck for only a few minutes after the initial letdown, before reverting to the non-nutritive suck (see the case study in Box 10-5). In these cases, it is frequently difficult to determine whether the initial problem was the infant's suck problem or the mother's milk supply, but odds favor the infant. In nearly all cases, maternal milk supply is determined by the baby. An assessment of the infant's oral–motor behavior by a lactation consultant or an infant feeding specialist (e.g., an occupational, physical, or speech therapist) is most helpful in this situation, although some infants will improve over time if they maintain a normal weight gain.

Gastroesophageal Reflux, Cow Milk Allergy, and Oversupply

The fussy breastfed baby may have gastroesophageal reflux disease (GERD) or cow milk allergy/sensitivity, or symptoms may be caused by maternal oversupply. Primary care physicians encounter gastroesophageal reflux and/or milk allergy with sufficient frequency that these diagnoses are commonly made. Sometimes gastroenterologists or allergists have entered the picture. One review article states that approximately half of all infants less than 1 year of age with GERD have an associated cow milk allergy. The diagnosis of cow-milk-induced GERD is made on the basis of an elimination diet and challenge (Salvador & Vandenplas, 2002). Even though breastfed infants are less likely than formula-fed infants to have reflux and/or allergy, there are occasional severe cases in breastfed infants. Cow milk allergy in the breastfed infant may require a strict elimination diet by the mother, as well as nutrition consultation for both diagnosis and management of this condition.

Figure 10-6 An Infant Who Had Low Intake and Slow Gain at 2 Months of Age Due to Oral Motor Dysfunction.

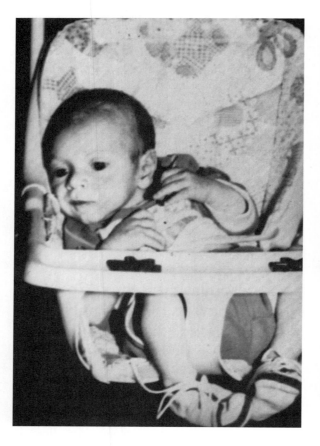

Source: Used with permission of Kathleen Auerbach.

Figure 10-7 The Same Infant as in Figure 10-6 at 4 Months of Age, Following Management of Low Intake and Low Milk Supply.

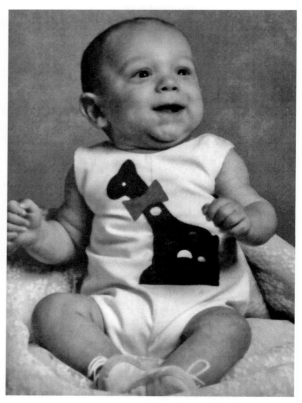

Source: Used with permission of Kathleen Auerbach.

One variation of reflux in the breastfed infant is caused by oversupply of maternal milk, with delivery of high volumes of foremilk. The typical scenario for oversupply is a very chubby baby who is fussy or colicky, has very frequent watery or foamy stools (lactose overload—not lactose intolerance), and is fussy during feedings. Rarely, one may encounter failure to thrive in such an infant. Woolridge and Fisher (1988) reported a single case in which the dyad was successfully managed by measures that increased delivery of hindmilk, improved weight gain for the baby, and gradually reduced maternal milk supply.

Nonspecific Neurologic Problems

Infant feeding problems with resultant poor weight gain may be the earliest indicator of various neurologic problems. Developmental delays and neuromuscular disorders may not become apparent for many months, but subtle abnormalities in motor tone are usually present in infancy and may

---

BOX 10-5 LOW INTAKE AND LOW MILK SUPPLY: A CASE STUDY

Figure 10-7 shows a 6-week-old infant who looked and acted passive. When he went to breast, he immediately closed his eyes and appeared to be asleep; however, he could not be put down because he continually fussed and cried when not held at breast.

Birth weight was 7 lb 11 oz (3.5 kg). At 2 weeks of age, the baby was 8% below birth weight, and the physician recommended formula supplementation by bottle. (Note: This is NOT the current recommendation!)

The baby returned to birth weight within 1 week. The mother then made the decision to go off of supplementation, but at the 6-week visit the baby was only 6 oz (180 gm) above birth weight. The baby's physical examination did not suggest any physical problems other than weak suck. At this time, referral to a lactation consultant led to supplementation with a feeding-tube device. The baby started at 1 oz (30 ml) in the feeding-tube device (at breast) during seven daytime feedings, and breastfed two or three times at night. The infant's appetite quickly increased to 2 oz (60 ml) per feeding (or 14 oz/320 ml per day) for approximately 2 weeks. After catch-up growth, the amount of supplement in the feeding tube gradually declined over the next 2 months. By 4 months of age, the infant was fully breastfeeding without supplementaton, as seen in Figure 10-8. This case was delayed in diagnosis and management. If proper intervention had occurred at 2 weeks, the intervention would probably have been of much shorter duration.

---

present as oral–motor dysfunction (see the previous section), with resultant growth problems. In the author's experience, neurologically based early breastfeeding problems are often characterized by inefficient feeding or disorganized feeding reflexes indicated by choking, brief apnea, or poor pacing of the suckle/swallow/breathe cycle. Inefficiency or disorganization typically causes very long feeding episodes during which the baby is not removing enough milk to gain weight and/or satiate the appetite. With subtle neurologic problems, these difficulties often occur across all feeding methods (breast-, bottle-, cup-, and finger-feeding); in contrast, in the infant with isolated oral–motor dysfunction, the baby can usually manage better on the bottle than on the breast.

Ankyloglossia (Tongue-Tie, Tight Frenulum)

Controversy remains regarding frenotomy for breastfeeding difficulties because of the limits of the research in this area. There is a large variation in the clinical findings associated with various types of ankyloglossia, but lack of a consistent classification system or definition for significant ankyloglossia makes comparisons among studies almost impossible. We also lack a tool that can predict the need for intervention, and only a relatively small number of subjects have been studied in randomized trials. Nevertheless, current evidence indicates that a tight (restricted) frenulum (Figure 10-8) may be associated with a variety of breastfeeding problems that show up in either mother or baby. New research techniques using ultrasound and intraoral pressure measurements have shown that babies with ankyloglossia (tongue-tie) have abnormal tongue movement (Geddes et al., 2008).

A recent systematic review (Webb et al., 2013) included 20 studies that met the researchers' criteria for data extraction from 1966 to June 2012; five of those studies were randomized controlled trials. In this systematic review, a number of objective measures of breastfeeding outcomes were studied, and results are summarized in Table 10-9. Subjective outcomes (the mothers' experiences) of breastfeeding were also published in some studies. "[G]eneral themes of improved breastfeeding

Figure 10-8 THE TWO ENDS OF THE ANKYLOGLOSSIA SPECTRUM. ON THE LEFT IS A CLASSIC THIN ANTERIOR FRENUM. NOTE THE NOTCH IN THE TONGUE TIP AND THE LIMITED HEIGHT OF THE TONGUE LIFT. ON THE RIGHT IS A THICK POSTERIOR FRENUM, VISIBLE AS A WHITE LINE IN THE POSTERIOR FLOOR OF THE MOUTH.

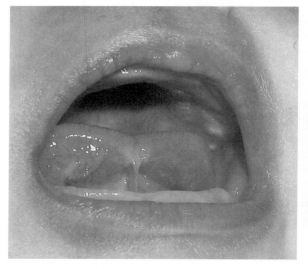
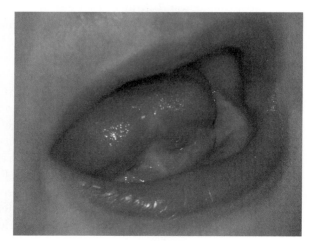

Reprinted with permission from Catherine Watson Genna.

and procedural satisfaction emerged" (Webb et al., 2013). The authors also state that subjective maternal pain scores, as used in four of the studies, consistently revealed improvement in maternal pain post frenotomy. This is important because the measure used has been shown to be reliable in many studies. However, only one of the studies included a control group, possibly allowing for treatment bias to affect the overall results.

The latest trend in the breastfeeding literature regarding frenotomy is to distinguish "anterior" from "posterior" tongue-tie. Hong et al. (2010), a group of otolaryngologists, published a retrospective chart review of frenotomy performed for breastfeeding problems in 341 patients. They distinguished between the obvious anterior tongue-tie and the more subtle and difficult-to-treat posterior tongue-tie. These authors did not use any formal classification system, but rather depended upon the judgment of the surgeon. Their results were remarkable for a higher incidence of anterior tongue-tie in males (as in previous studies) but a higher incidence of posterior tongue-tie in females. They also noted

a higher frequency of revisions needed for posterior tongue-tie. In 2011, Knox et al. published an abstract that showed a nearly equal distribution of posterior tongue-tie in males and females, using a much larger sample size (1046) than in the study by Hong et al. The Knox group used the classification system developed by Elizabeth Coryllos (Coryllos et al., 2004) and popularized in the book *Supporting Sucking Skills in Breastfeeding Infants* (Genna, 2008); see Table 10-10.

A comprehensive study by O'Callahan, Macary, and Clemente (2013) was not included in the systematic review cited previously. This report summarized the outcomes for 299 infants who underwent frenotomy for breastfeeding problems after referral to a pediatrician for assessment and treatment. Fifty-four percent of the infants were male. Although not specifically stated, the authors appeared to use the Coryllos classification system: 3% of infants had type I ankyloglossia, 12% had type II, 36% had type III, and 49% had type IV. Thus, combining types III and IV, 85% of the babies had posterior ankyloglossia in this sample.

Table 10-9 SYSTEMATIC REVIEW OF TONGUE-TIE DIVISION: OBJECTIVE MEASURES OF BREASTFEEDING OUTCOMES

Type of Measurement	Number of Studies Using This Measure	Results
LATCH scores	3 studies	Three studies showed improvement but only 2 studies showed statistically significant improvement.
Pain scores (SF-MPQ—not specific to breastfeeding pain)	Small case series significantly improved maternal nipple pain by two measures	One study showed statistically significant improvement post frenotomy compared to sham procedure (controls); $p < 0.001$.
IBFAT	1 study	Mean score improved from 9.3 ± 0.69 preintervention to 11.6 ± 0.81 post frenotomy compared to sham procedure (controls), who did not show any improvement; $p < 0.029$.
Milk production and feeding characteristics	3 studies	Significant increase in milk production, milk intake, milk transfer, and time between feeds; corresponding decrease in length of feeds per minute. $p < 0.01$ or less for these measures.
Nipple compression	1 study	Nipple compression was reduced post frenotomy based on submental ultrasonography.
Weight gain	1 study	Significant weight gain at 2 weeks post frenotomy; $p < 0.0001$.

Notes: IBFAT: infant breastfeeding assessment tool; LATCH: latch, audible swallowing, type of nipple, comfort, and hold; SF-MPQ: short-form McGill pain questionnaire.

Source: Data from Webb AN, Hao W, Hong P. The effect of tongue-tie division on breastfeeding and speech articulation: a systematic review. *International Journal of Pediatric Otorhinolaryngology.* 2013;77(5):635–646.

Table 10-10 CLASSIFICATION OF ANKYLOGLOSSIA AS IT PERTAINS TO BREASTFEEDING PROBLEMS

Type	Superior Attachment	Inferior Attachment	Characteristics of Frenulum
1	Tip of tongue	Alveolar ridge	Often thin, may be elastic
2	2–4 mm behind tongue	On or just behind alveolar ridge	Often thin, may be elastic
3	Mid-tongue	Middle of floor of mouth	Usually thicker, more fibrous, inelastic
4	Submucosal	Floor of mouth at base of tongue	Usually thick, fibrous, shiny and inelastic

Source: Coryllos E, Genna C, Salloum A. Congenital tongue-tie and its impact on breastfeeding. American Academy of Pediatrics, Breastfeeding: Best for Baby and Mother. 2004:1–11. Used with permission.

The male-to-female ratio for posterior tongue-tie was just slightly greater than 1:1—similar to the findings of the study by Knox et al. (2011). The mothers of these infants were asked to complete a Web-based questionnaire regarding mother–infant breastfeeding characteristics before and after intervention, but the completion rate was only 53%, so improvement (or lack of improvement) is difficult to judge by this measure.

One anecdotal comment by O'Callahan et al. (2013) that is echoed in another article (Edmunds et al., 2012) is that frenotomy may heal "closed" again and require revision. Revision may potentially be prevented by manipulation of the operative site ("swipe the underside and lift the tongue") after every infant feed for 5 to 14 days until the site has completely healed.

Any surgical procedure is associated with potential risks, particularly infection and bleeding. The systematic review mentioned previously (Webb et al., 2013) stated that adverse results from frenotomies have included (1) minor blood loss easily controlled by pressure, (2) recurrence of tongue-tie, and (3) rare serious injuries to the tongue or submandibular ducts.

Multiple reports from the United States and Europe have indicated that simple frenotomy is safe, with no reports of complications. However, two cases of life-threatening blood loss were reported in Nigeria when frenotomy was performed by a community health worker and a traditional birth attendant. The author emphasizes the importance of referral of infants to a properly trained health professional for performance of frenotomy (Opara & Gabriel-Job, & Opara, 2012). It is also imperative to screen for a family history of easy bleeding.

Some dentists have become educated regarding frenotomy during breastfeeding (Merdad & Mascarenhas, 2010) and are reporting use of lasers to treat tight mandibular and maxillary frenula (Kotlow, 2011).

In summary, there is now a small and growing body of evidence suggesting that (1) ankyloglossia is associated with a number of breastfeeding problems; (2) the appearance of the tongue is not related to the degree of breastfeeding impairment; (3) posterior tongue-tie may be more difficult to diagnose by initial physical examination, so it requires a high index of suspicion; and (4) if breastfeeding problems (maternal, infant, or both) are occurring in the presence of a tight frenulum, frenotomy is indicated for treatment of the breastfeeding dyad. "Due to the increasing rates of breastfeeding one could make the argument that the diagnosis of ankyloglossia in infants should be a basic competency for all primary care providers" (O'Callahan et al., 2013). In addition, otolaryngologists, oral surgeons, and dentists will need the knowledge, skills, and experience to diagnose and treat these infants.

Abnormal Patterns of Growth: The Baby with Obvious Illness

The presence of a known medical complication, such as prematurity, infection, congenital heart disease, trisomy 21, congenital abnormalities, cystic fibrosis, and other health conditions (see again Box 10-4), puts the infant at risk for poor growth. These infants often have a combination of increased metabolic demands, low endurance for feeding, and lower growth rates despite close attention to feeding routines (Combs & Marino, 1993; Jones, 1988). Although these babies need increased caloric intake, volume restrictions may be necessary. Because such infants particularly benefit from human milk, special assistance must be provided to mothers regarding maintaining milk production while creative efforts are made to get adequate calories into the baby (see the section on special techniques for management at the end of this chapter). The goal is that with improved growth, the infant will eventually nurse completely at the breast. See *The Ill Child: Breastfeeding Implications* chapter for detailed information regarding individual disorders and feeding implications.

Maternal Considerations: The Mother Who Appears Healthy

When there have been no previous known risk factors in the perinatal history, perhaps undiscovered risks are present, or some new disease process has arisen since the birth of the baby. Which factors might be present and relatively asymptomatic other than the disruption of lactation? Box 10-4 lists maternal pathology associated with low milk production and low weight gain.

Delayed Lactogenesis

As mentioned earlier in this chapter, delayed lactogenesis may contribute to early supplementation, and subsequently to a reduction in milk supply. (See again Box 10-2, which lists risk factors for delay of lactogenesis.)

Inverted Nipples

Because inverted nipples can cause difficulty with proper latch-on, milk supply obviously may be adversely affected. Dewey and colleagues (2003) found that delayed onset of lactation was approximately twice as common among women with "flat or inverted nipples." Some experts have emphasized the importance of breast examination during the third trimester, with the intent to "treat" inverted nipples with various manual or mechanical methods. One prospective study found 6.7% of pregnant nulliparas ($n = 1926$) with at least one inverted or nonprotractile nipple (Alexander et al., 1992). This study is the only one performed to assess the efficacy of various treatments. There was no difference in breastfeeding outcomes between women who received treatment versus those who received no intervention. Prenatal treatment remains controversial, but knowledgeable and supportive care after the baby is born is clearly essential.

Nipple Shields

Nipple shields are devices made of latex or silicone that cover the mother's nipple and areola, providing an artificial nipple for the infant while suckling at the breast. Nipple shields have been used to assist and maintain latch-on, to provide temporary relief from sore nipples, and to reduce rapid flow. Early studies indicated that use of such shields impaired milk removal and subsequent milk production. A review of original research regarding nipple shields concluded that the research was insufficient to conclude that nipple shields are safe or effective; rather, they should be considered an "unknown risk" (McKechnie & Eglash, 2010). Some earlier case reports and editorials (Bodley & Powers, 1996; Pessl, 1996; Sealy, 1996; Wilson-Clay, 1996) as well as one limited study in preterm infants (Meier et al., 2002) have indicated that knowledgeable professionals may choose to use a silicone (not latex) shield in selected cases, after weighing the risks versus the benefits of this intervention (see the *Breast Pumps and Other Technologies* chapter). If a silicone nipple shield is used, the mother should express her milk at the end of or between nursing sessions to ensure an adequate milk supply. Eventually, the shield is removed and milk expression is discontinued. Close follow-up of weight gain and milk supply are imperative until the shield has been discontinued.

Hormonal Alterations

Milk production depends upon an array of primary and supporting hormones (see the *Biological Specificity of Breastmilk* chapter). Thus it is not surprising to find that a variety of maternal conditions characterized by hormonal alterations will affect milk supply. Pregnancy superimposed on established lactation or retained placental fragments may decrease milk supply (Lawrence & Lawrence, 2011; Neifert et al., 1981). Hormonal characteristics of polycystic ovary syndrome and theca lutein cysts are suspected of inhibiting lactation, probably due to high circulating androgen levels (Hoover et al., 2002). Regarding oral contraceptives, individual effects will vary according to the timing during lactation, the dose of the estrogenic compound in the formulation, and the individual woman's susceptibility to the effects of estrogen. For details, see *LactMed* (2013) or the Academy of Breastfeeding Medicine's Protocol #13, "Contraception and Breastfeeding" (www.bfmed.org/Resources/Protocols.aspx), as well as the *Drug Therapy and Breastfeeding* chapter in this text.

Postpartum thyroiditis occurs in as many as 5% of new mothers and may be associated with either hyperthyroidism or hypothyroidism (Wilson & Foster, 1992). Lactation experts generally agree that thyroid disorders in lactating women can affect milk supply.

Hypopituitarism (Sheehan's syndrome) following childbirth is a rare occurrence. In this condition, postpartum hemorrhage with significant hypotension causes thrombotic infarction of the anterior pituitary and loss of those hormones. Thus prolactin is not secreted, resulting in failure of lactogenesis (Lawrence & Lawrence, 2011).

Medications and Substances

In rare situations, nonhormonal maternal medications will affect milk supply. For example, long-acting or high doses of short-acting thiazide diuretics may suppress lactation (*LactMed*, 2013). Pseudoephedrine, given as a single 60-mg dose, decreases milk production over the short term and repeated use probably interferes with lactation (*LactMed*, 2013). Bromocriptine, which reduces prolactin levels, was once used for suppression of lactation but is no longer indicated for this purpose because of risk of maternal seizures and stroke. Similarly, cabergoline suppresses lactation but has been determined to be somewhat safer for treating women with pituitary adenoma during pregnancy or lactation (*LactMed*, 2013).

Several studies have demonstrated the detrimental effects of maternal smoking on milk ejection, milk volumes, infant weight gain, and total duration of breastfeeding (Hopkinson et al., 1992; Horta et al., 1997; *LactMed*, 2013; Lawrence & Lawrence, 2011). Environmental (second-hand) smoke was shown in one study to be associated with shorter duration of breastfeeding (Horta et al., 1997). Another study revealed smoking to be a risk factor for failed breastfeeding initiation among women with severe preeclampsia (Cordero, 2012).

Alcohol blocks the release of oxytocin (blocks milk ejection), and after maternal ingestion of alcohol in the research setting, suckling-induced prolactin spikes are inhibited (Lawrence & Lawrence, 2011). In an experiment that sought to analyze the effect of smell and taste upon breastmilk ingestion, Mennella (1997) found that infants ingested less breastmilk after their mothers drank an alcoholic beverage. Another study (Mennella & Pepino, 2010) showed a blunted prolactin response to alcohol (following breast pumping) among women with a positive family history of alcoholism in a first-degree relative, and no increase in milk volume following consumption of an alcoholic beverage. The preponderance of data refutes the myth that alcohol is a galactagogue.

Breast Surgery

It is "common knowledge" among lactation consultants that breast surgery is associated with breastfeeding difficulties. This knowledge is not shared by plastic and aesthetic surgeons, whose literature conflicts with that of the breastfeeding community. These contradictory results probably result from inherent biases in the populations served. However, a systematic review of studies between 1950 and 2008, considered level I evidence, revealed that in the first month postpartum, women with reduction mammoplasty breastfed at the same rates as the general population in North America (Thibaudeau et al., 2010). The conclusion of this review was that "difficulties related to breastfeeding [among patients with reduction mammoplasty] appear to be mostly explained by psychosocial issues related to advice and coaching received by healthcare workers during breastfeeding as well as other patient personal considerations."

From the traditional viewpoint of the lactation consultant, the history of breast surgery is a critical component of the full working knowledge base about a patient, based upon previous studies with lower levels of evidence. If a complete medical history has been obtained, the practitioner should have learned of prior breast surgery. However, some women hide this information from their spouse or partner and from their healthcare provider. Others neglect to mention biopsy when asked about any previous surgery. Cosmetic breast surgery may be difficult to detect with routine physical examination.

Neifert, DeMarzo, et al. (1990) published an observational report that implicated breast surgery as a major risk factor for decreased milk production. Periareolar incision was associated with a fivefold increase in risk of "insufficient milk" as determined by infant weight gain. A retrospective chart review confirmed these results (Hurst, 1996). Recent surgical techniques for augmentation employ an axillary incision, and placement of implants underneath the pectoral muscle, which minimizes surgical damage to mammary structures and nerves. Many women with breast implants harbor anxiety about potential problems caused by previous breast surgery (especially those with silicone implants). At this time, silicone breast implants are not considered a contraindication to breastfeeding. Silicone is a ubiquitous substance, and levels are higher in cow milk and infant formula than in human milk (Semple et al., 1998).

Another important consideration for patients who have undergone breast augmentation is to take a careful history regarding size, shape, symmetry, and development of the breasts prior to surgery. Unrecognized "insufficient glandular development of the breast" (discussed in the next section) may have been the reason for undergoing augmentation.

Breast reduction always involves disruption of mammary tissue, and breastfeeding outcomes are highly variable. In a 2003 controlled cohort study by Souto et al., 49 Brazilian women status post breast reduction surgery were matched with neighborhood controls. All subjects and controls in the study had initiated breastfeeding. The mean duration of exclusive breastfeeding for the reduction group was 4 days; for controls, it was 3 months ($p < 0.001$). Women who had undergone breast reduction surgery had an 8.7 times higher risk of discontinuing exclusive breastfeeding at 1 month postpartum compared to controls; complete weaning at 4 months was 11.6 times higher. This population in Brazil appears to differ from the population in North America. More research is necessary to clarify the issues involved with breastfeeding success versus failure in women with breast surgery.

Insufficient Glandular Development of the Breast

In 1985, Neifert, Seacat, and Jobe reported "insufficient glandular development of the breasts" (sometimes referred to as "primary lactation failure") of three women. These women demonstrated several strikingly similar features. They had notable asymmetry of their breasts, and little or no breast changes during pregnancy. They were unable to nourish their infants despite maximum feeding frequency, effective milk removal, and professional breastfeeding assistance. They had normal prolactin levels. For their infants, increasing the frequency of feeding did not result in significant weight gain, and the infants required supplementation. The assumption, based on clinical findings, was that the syndrome is apparently analogous to arrested development of other organs or glands. Neifert, DeMarzo, et al. (1990) then published results of a prospective study initially designed to determine the frequency of this disorder. More than 400 women were recruited for the study, none of whom had the clinical characteristics of insufficient glandular development of the breast. The study did detect a significant number of women who had experienced breast surgery. Huggins, Petok, and Mireles (2000) published a descriptive report of 34 mothers with breast "hypoplasia." Based on Neifert, DeMarzo, et al.'s (1990) study and the experience of various lactation centers, it appears that approximately 1 out of 1000 (0.01%) lactating women may have this clinical syndrome.

When Geddes et al. (2012) studied characteristics of blood of the human lactating breast, they found that one hypoplastic breast with almost no milk production had a substantial reduction in blood flow, while in other cases the amount of blood flow did not correlate with the amount of milk produced. One research abstract reported breast hypoplasia with reduced milk production following radiation treatment for breast cancer (Abstracts from the 16th International Society for Research in Human Milk and Lactation Conference, 2012). See Figure 10-9 for further information on breast development and milk production, as well as the *Breast-Related Problems* chapter.

Stress

Labor and childbirth are stressful events. Chen and colleagues (1998) found that higher degrees of stress were associated with delayed onset of lactogenesis. New mothers also commonly experience a number of physical, social, and emotional stresses after giving birth, related to the life-changing event of

Figure 10-9 **Women with Variations of Hypoplastic Breasts. (A) Type 1 hypoplasia. (B) Type 2 hypoplasia. (C) Type 3 hypoplasia. (D) Type 4 hypoplasia.**

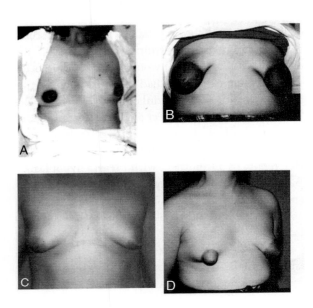

Source: Huggins KE, Petok ES, Mireles O. Markers of lactation insufficiency: a study of 34 mothers. In: Auerbach KG, ed. *Current issues in clinical lactation.* Boston, MA: Jones and Bartlett; 2000.

childbirth. These stresses are expected and should not normally interfere with breastfeeding.

Moderate to severe stress has been documented to inhibit oxytocin and subsequently interfere with milk production (see again Figure 10-2). Ruvalcaba (1987) reported some fascinating cases of sudden loss of milk and loss of milk flow in several women living in Mexico City during the 1985 earthquake. Zhu et al. (2013) described the biopsychosocial stressors that impact "onset of lactation" and subsequent duration of breastfeeding: the psychosocial stressors included stressful

life events during the first trimester of pregnancy. However, other mothers have been able to survive extreme circumstances while continuing to breastfeed their infants. A commentary by Eidelman (2013) describes a documentary about children born in a concentration camp near the end of the Holocaust to women who were marginally nourished yet delivered live-born infants and successfully breastfed them to survival.

Psychosocial Factors

Some women do not want to breastfeed but are pressured to do so by a family member. Breastfeeding rarely goes well under these circumstances. Classic psychosocial failure to thrive (the result of emotional or physical neglect or abuse) is rarely seen in the breastfed infant, but it does occur. Parental drug or alcohol abuse or domestic violence may be a factor in some of these cases. Moderate to severe postpartum depression may result in excessive anxiety about the baby, alienation of the mother from her infant, and occasionally overt abuse (Wisner et al., 2002). Two cases of Munchausen syndrome by proxy have been reported in which the infant received ipecac in expressed maternal breast milk (Berkner et al., 1988; Sutphen & Saulsbury, 1988). Hypothyroidism must be considered in the differential diagnosis of maternal depression, and postpartum psychosis is often a manifestation of bipolar disorder (Wisner et al., 2002).

Maternal Nutrition

Several studies show no significant relationship between reduced maternal intake of calories or fluids and the volume of milk produced. Poor maternal nutrition will decrease birth weight of the infant, and smaller infants stimulate lower volumes of milk production (Institute of Medicine, 1991). The lactating woman needs to maintain good nutritional status for her own health as well as for future pregnancies. Rapid weight loss in well-nourished women requires further study to determine the effects on milk volume. Much current research is focused on the effects of overweight and obesity upon lactation performance (see the earlier discussion in this chapter as well as Box 10-2) (Chapman & Perez-Escamilla, 1999; Dewey et al., 2003; Hilson et al., 1997, 2006). Obviously, a woman with an eating disorder presents nutritional and psychosocial risks to the mother–infant relationship. See the *Women's Health and Breastfeeding* chapter for further information on maternal nutrition during lactation.

Anemia

One study (Henley et al., 1995) detected an association of anemia (postpartum hemoglobin of less than 10 g/dL) with "insufficient milk syndrome" (referred to earlier in this chapter as "perceived insufficient milk supply"). Even though this association was noted, the PIMS was more closely correlated with early weaning than was anemia. More data are needed regarding anemia and its effects on breastfeeding and milk supply.

Maternal Considerations: Obvious Illness

Acute illnesses may temporarily decrease milk supply, but production should rebound after the initial insult, especially in full lactation. Insulin-dependent diabetes mellitus was associated with delayed lactogenesis and lower volumes of milk production when diabetic control was poor (Neubauer et al., 1993; Perez-Escamilla & Chapman, 2001). Occasionally, mastitis will reduce milk secretion in the affected breast for the duration of lactation. The ability of women with other chronic illnesses to breastfeed depends upon their general condition (e.g., energy level, motor abilities) and the medications that they are required to take. There is currently little information regarding the effect of specific illnesses upon volume of milk production. Each case must be assessed and managed individually. See the *Women's Health and Breastfeeding* chapter for further discussion of these issues.

History, Physical Exam, and Differential Diagnosis

History

A complete history and physical exam for both mother and infant are critical to the evaluation of low intake or insufficient milk (see again Table 10-6; see also the *Infant Assessment* chapter). Perinatal history includes prenatal risk factors, labor and childbirth, medications, interventions, and any resuscitation efforts. A complete feeding history reviews a mother's previous feeding experiences, her feeding plan for this infant, the first feeding experience after giving birth, and subsequent feeding difficulties or breast problems. Maternal past medical history and review of systems must include current routine medications, history of breast surgery, postpartum hemorrhage (risk for anemia or panhypopituitarism), or endocrine disorders. Family history and psychosocial history may also provide clues to slow weight gain due to familial conditions or family stress.

Physical Examination and Laboratory Tests

Physical examination for the mother (see again Table 10-6) is focused on areas of concern: vital signs, general skin condition, breasts, nipples, thyroid, and any other area suggested by careful history. A complete physical examination of the infant includes vital signs, weight, length, head circumference, and general examination with close attention to subtle neurological features and oral–motor exam (see also the *Infant Assessment* chapter). Observation and evaluation of a breastfeeding session by a knowledgeable, experienced practitioner is an integral part of the objective assessment.

A multidisciplinary approach is recommended, with input from the primary care provider (family physician, obstetrician, pediatrician, midwife, nurse practitioner, or physician's assistant) and lactation consultant. In some programs with formal feeding teams, a pediatric developmental team (developmental pediatrician, speech pathologist, occupational and physical therapists), a pediatric gastroenterologist, or a pediatric allergist may conduct part of the feeding evaluation. Selective use of laboratory tests may be helpful. Postpartum maternal thyroid disease is relatively common and may be asymptomatic aside from low milk production. Prolactin levels remain difficult to interpret, since they do not strictly correlate with milk volume. Prolactin levels are generally not very helpful in trying to evaluate or treat low milk supply.

Differential Diagnosis

After the history and physical examination have been completed, a differential diagnosis may be developed. Potential etiologies that can ultimately lead to a problem-oriented approach to management can be identified (see again Tables 10-7 and 10-8). Specific management suggestions are also included in the tables to assist with individualizing the treatment guidelines given here.

Clinical Management

Determining the Need for Supplementation

Many cases of slow weight gain in the breastfed infant will require a decision regarding supplementation—a term that is frequently used but rarely defined in relationship to breastfeeding. For the purposes of this chapter, and specifically for the management guidelines given in this section, the term will be used to indicate the practice of giving the breastfed infant additional nutriment other than what he obtains directly from the breast. Supplementation may also include additional nutrients to increase the caloric density of human milk feedings (e.g., human milk fortifier). Two important facets

Figure 10-10 A MOTHER AND INFANT UTILIZE A COMMERCIAL FEEDING-TUBE DEVICE IN ORDER TO DELIVER EXTRA MILK TO THE INFANT WHILE THE MOTHER IS ABLE TO FEED THE INFANT AT BREAST AND GRADUALLY INCREASE HER MILK SUPPLY.

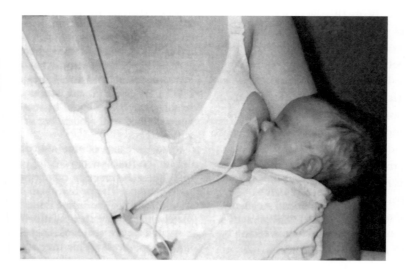

Source: Reproduced from Powers N, Slusser W. Breastfeeding update 2: clinical lactation management. *Pediatrics in Review.* 1997;18(5):147–161. Reproduced by permission of *Pediatrics in Review.*

of supplementation must be kept in mind: (1) the choice of type of supplement and (2) the choice of method for supplementation.

Management guidelines in this chapter imply a hierarchy of preferences for type and method of supplementation. The first choice for type of supplement is the mother's own expressed milk; pasteurized donor breastmilk (if indicated and if available) is the second choice; commercially manufactured infant formula is the third choice. The choice of method of supplementation has not been well studied. Various experts (personal communications) have different preferences regarding various methods to supplement the breastfed baby. Some experts prefer to use the feeding-tube device and keep the baby at the breast (see Figures 10-10 and 10-11). Other experts prefer to have the baby bottle-feed to provide a rapid restoration of caloric intake, weight gain, and increase in energy for suckling once returned to the breast. Cup-feeding has been well studied and is safe, hygienic, and practical for resource-poor settings (Howard et al., 1999, 2003). Syringe- or spoon-feeding may provide other options, depending on the specific circumstances of the case. Finger-feeding, though widely practiced, has no evidence base (see the section "Oral–Motor Dysfunction [Ineffective Suckling]" earlier in this chapter).

Effective maternal milk expression (or pumping) is a mainstay for women who are supplementing their infants. This is best accomplished by professional electric pump or skilled hand expression.

Intervention

The following management guidelines are suggested for a general approach to the slow-gaining baby. Figure 10-12 provides a flowchart of the general approach, which is an expert recommendation, but not otherwise evidence based due to a lack of research regarding specific management techniques. Despite general recommendations, individualized management is required. (See again Tables 10-7 and 10-8, which give additional suggestions in this regard.)

Figure 10-11 A Homemade Feeding-Tube Device Can Be Made from Supplies Found in an Office or Hospital. a small bottle with a slit nipple has a no. 5 French feeding tube threaded through the nipple with the hub resting in the milk. A rubber band and safety pin allow atttachment of the device to the mother's clothing.

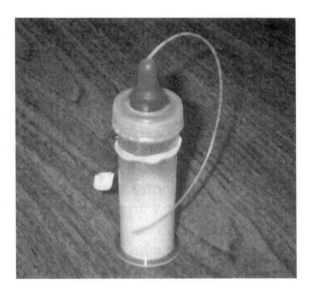

Source: Reproduced from Powers N, Slusser W. Breastfeeding update 2: clinical lactation management. *Pediatrics in Review.* 1997;18(5): 147–161. Reproduced by permission of *Pediatrics in Review.*

1. Check the basics: Double-check proper positioning and latch-on. Increase the frequency, duration, and effectiveness of feedings at the breast, if these factors are not optimal, and if the infant is alert and hungry. Alternate-breast massage and switch nursing may be used, if the infant is suckling actively during feedings. (See the section on special techniques for management of low intake or low supply later in this chapter.)

Figure 10-12 Flowchart for Assessment and Management of Newborn Weight Loss Based on Expert Opinion

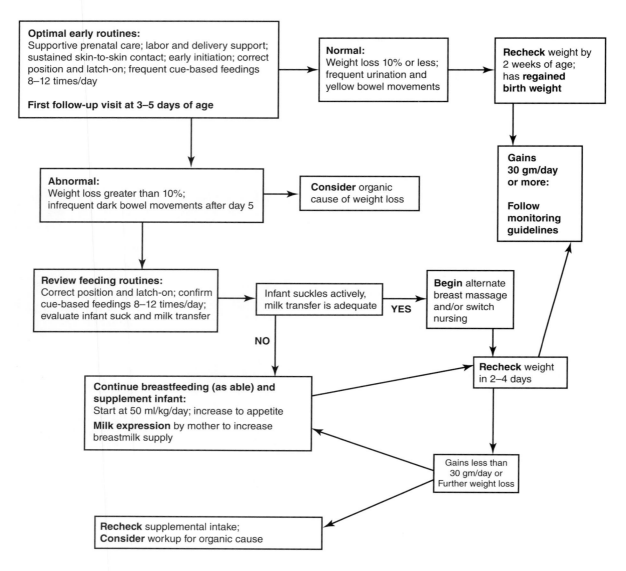

Source: Courtesy of Nancy G. Powers, MD.

2. Have the mother express breastmilk between feedings to increase her milk supply (see Box 10-6).

3. If the infant is clinically stable and exhibiting hunger cues, suggest optional supplementation with expressed breastmilk. If immediate supplementation is indicated by the flowchart in Figure 10-12 or by the clinical condition of the infant, use expressed breastmilk (or another alternative) to supplement the infant during or after breastfeeding.

Box 10-6　Measures That Encourage Increased Milk Production

- Apply moist heat to breasts a few minutes before feeding.
- Massage the breasts before and during feeding or pumping.
- Use relaxation techniques to reduce stress and enhance let down.
- Feed your baby or express milk at least 8 times every 24 hours.
- Continue frequent milk removal, even if small amounts are obtained.
- Use hand expression and "hands-on pumping."

Box 10-7　Amount of Supplement to Use for a Breastfed Baby

Once you have decided to use supplementation, it is important to specify the amount of extra milk the baby needs to gain weight.

- A general rule of thumb for normal total intake is 150 to 200 mL/kg/day of breastmilk or formula.
- If the baby is showing good hunger cues, begin with ad lib supplement feedings, following the baby's appetite. You may find that the baby initially exceeds the normal intake guidelines, but give at least the minimum amounts shown in the following table.
- If the baby is not exhibiting hunger cues, aim for a minimum of 100 mL/kg/24 hr, divided into 6 or 8 feedings (see table below). This minimum is suggested for infants who are not exhibiting hunger cues and whose stomachs are still small due to very low intake. Within 1 to 2 days, begin to push the amount of supplement up for these nondemanding babies until they start to act hungry.

Infant Weight kg (lb)	MINIMUM Daily Supplement: 100 mL/kg/day mL (oz per day)	MINIMUM Approximate per Feeding Supplement: 6–8 times/day mL (oz per feeding)
2.5 kg (5 lb 8 oz)	250 mL (8 oz)	30–40 mL (1 oz)
3.0 kg (6 lb 9 oz)	300 mL (10 oz)	35–50 mL (1–2 oz)
3.5 kg (7 lb 11 oz)	350 mL (12 oz)	40–60 mL (1.5 to 2 oz)
4.0 kg (8 lb 12 oz)	400 mL (13 oz)	50–70 mL (2–2.5 oz)
5.0 kg (11 lb)	500 mL (17 oz)	60–80 mL (2–3 oz)

---

4. Begin with ad lib supplemental feedings, following the baby's appetite. If the baby is not exhibiting hunger cues, aim for a **minimum** of 100 mL/kg/24 hr, divided into 6 to 8 feedings (see Box 10-7). *This minimum is suggested for infants who are not exhibiting hunger cues and whose stomachs are still small due to very low intake. Within 1 to 2 days, begin to push the amount of supplement up for these nondemanding babies until they start to act hungry.* Any infant may have more volume, as matched to appetite.

5. Increase the amount of supplement as indicated by infant appetite.

6. See other specific management suggestions in Tables 10-7 and 10-8.

7. Monitor and follow up with infants younger than 3 months as follows:
   a. Monitor infant weight closely, every 2 to 4 days.
   b. Verify that weight stabilizes within 2 to 4 days.
   c. Verify that weight gain begins within 4–7 days.
   d. After 7 days, verify that the infant is gaining at least 30 g/day (larger daily weight gain is preferable, and some infants gain 60 g/day or more). Once weight gain averages 30 g/day or more, recheck every 1 to 2 weeks until the infant becomes established on a consistent growth curve.
8. If maternal milk supply has not increased within 1 week, do the following:
   a. Check the frequency of milk expression.
   b. Reevaluate maternal risk factors.
   c. Consider laboratory evaluation (especially maternal thyroid) as indicated.
   d. If maternal factors are involved, manage as indicated.
   e. Consider use of a galactagogue.
   f. If maternal evaluation is negative, reevaluate the infant.
9. If the infant does not gain weight as expected, consider the following:
   a. Verify that the infant is receiving the prescribed amount of supplemental feedings. Review specific amounts with the mother and ask her to keep written records.
   b. Determine whether the infant is willing to take the minimal amount of supplementation that is recommended. If not, strongly consider an organic illness or neurologic problem.
   c. If the infant is actually ingesting the prescribed amount of supplement and still not gaining weight, evaluate the infant for illness or neurologic problems.
   d. Arrange for lab tests as indicated.
   e. Treat infant illness as indicated.
   f. If these recommendations are not effective and medical workup is under way, consider using special techniques that are discussed in the next section.

Reducing the Amount of Supplementation

As the mother's own milk production increases, the amount of other types of supplements (e.g., infant formula) will be reduced in favor of expressed breastmilk. Once maternal milk supply increases, the infant takes more milk directly from the breast and less milk by supplementary methods (infant appetite and satiety will determine this change). After the infant has attained a normal weight for age, the amount of supplementation may be reduced gradually to stimulate more milk production. This depends upon an increased frequency of breastfeeding as well as the infant being effective at milk removal. Continue to monitor weight gain while supplementation is reduced or withdrawn.

Family and Peer Support

Verbal, emotional, and physical supports are very important for a mother who is stressed by a significant feeding problem. In addition to support from family members, new mothers may find peer support in the community by checking with their physician, hospital, local breastfeeding support groups, or the Internet.

When Maternal Milk Supply Does Not Increase

Most women who seek professional help with breastfeeding are highly motivated to breastfeed their infant. Sometimes, despite appropriate intervention and conscientious attempts by the mother to follow the suggested treatment plan, her milk supply does not increase enough to fully meet the infant's needs. In some cases, her milk supply will remain at a minimal level or "dry up" completely. In these situations, the practitioner must acknowledge the emotional impact of this "failure" upon the maternal psyche: a grief reaction is common. It is often helpful for the mother to be able to talk openly with the healthcare provider or a close family member regarding her loss. If possible, they should reassure her that she did everything in her power to rectify the situation. As in any other grief situation, the passage of time will allow some degree of healing.

Special Techniques for Management of Low Intake or Low Supply

Breast Massage

Breast massage during feeding is a simple method of increasing volume and fat content of the breastmilk. It can be used before and during every feeding to increase calorie delivery to the breastfed infant.

Switch Nursing

In normal breastfeeding, the baby is allowed to finish one breast before the mother switches to the other side. Infant-led feeding usually results in optimal intake (Woolridge et al., 1990). However, for the infant who spends a large part of the feeding in a "non-nutritive" sucking pattern and is gaining weight slowly, the technique of switch nursing may be considered. Although there is no research regarding the technique, it is widely recommended. Switch nursing involves changing the baby frequently from breast to breast to facilitate more active swallowing and promote multiple letdowns during the feeding. The mother is taught to observe for a change from nutritive to non-nutritive suckling. At that point, she switches the infant to the other breast, and when non-nutritive sucking is again apparent, switches back. This pattern is repeated several times during a feeding. Switch nursing may not be useful if the baby has low endurance (due to prematurity, illness, or weight loss) or oral–motor dysfunction with an ineffective suck. If switch nursing is recommended, close follow-up of weight status is necessary.

Feeding-Tube Device

The infant can receive supplementation at the same time that he is suckling from the breast by use of a feeding-tube device that can be purchased commercially or constructed with syringes and feeding tubes (see again Figures 10-10 and 10-11). This technique provides extra volume of intake for the infant while continuing to stimulate the maternal milk supply and avoiding the potential risk of bottle preference. A feeding-tube device works well for young infants who have plenty of energy and good sucking ability but for whom the maternal milk supply has not been adequate. This device is not a good choice for infants who are sleepy or who have inefficient suckling patterns. The mother must be carefully instructed regarding the amounts of supplement to provide, as well as the general use and cleaning of such a device (see Box 10-8).

Test Weighing

Infant test weighing has become widespread, although few practitioners understand its limitations (see Box 10-9). The methodology for test weighing was developed and validated in the 1980s (Woolridge et al., 1984). Test weighing involves the use of a sensitive scale (sensitivity of 2 g or less) with digital readout and computerized integration to account for infant movement. The infant is weighed before and after feeding to determine the amount of breastmilk ingested. Weight gain in grams is approximately equal to the intake of the infant in milliliters. Test weighing on a regular office scale is not reliable and should not be done (Whitfield et al., 1981).

Breastfed infants ingest vastly different amounts of milk at each feeding: in statistical terms, they demonstrate large "feed-to-feed variability." It takes 3 days of test weighing the baby at every feed to derive an "average" feeding size for that baby. Test weighing during one feeding does not offer an adequate representation of an "average" feeding or allow calculation of overall intake (Woolridge et al., 1984).

Several studies have examined the effect of test weighing on maternal self-confidence, stress levels, and progress of the dyad toward exclusive breastfeeding. Test weighing of premature infants was not found to contribute to maternal "stress" during feeding transition (Hurst et al., 2004), nor did it contribute to more successful breastfeeding outcomes (Funkquist et al., 2010; Hall et al., 2002). In a secondary data analysis by Wilhelm et al. (2010) of term infants with birth weight more than 2500 g, higher test-weight measurements at study points (2–4 days, 2 weeks, and 6 weeks) were

BOX 10-8 GUIDELINES FOR USING A FEEDING-TUBE DEVICE

1. Begin using the device when the mother and baby are most rested and when other household or family activities are unlikely to require the mother's attention. Use will become easier with practice.
2. Refer to Box 10-7 to estimate the amount of supplement to put into the feeding-tube device. Note that most babies will take less volume per feeding in the feeding-tube device than they would from a bottle feeding.
3. Prepare the feeding and begin the feeding process before the baby becomes overly hungry or fussy. Both mother and baby should be as relaxed as possible.
4. Fill the device and position the tubing so that it extends slightly past the end of the mother's nipple. Use any kind of hypoallergenic tape to hold the tubing in place. If the baby appears to be sucking only on the end of the tubing, pull it back so that it is flush with the end of the mother's nipple.
5. Look for the appearance of air bubbles in the reservoir. This indicates that the baby is actively swallowing.
6. Be aware that most babies will take most of the fluid in the device within the first 30 minutes. Different size tubes (to increase or decrease flow) are available with some commercial devices.
7. If the baby is actively suckling but the device is flowing very slowly or not at all, look for several potential problems:
   a. The tube may be kinked so as to block the flow. Check the tubing from bottle cap to baby's mouth.
   b. The tube may be blocked inside the baby's mouth by improper placement or kinking back on itself. Relatch the baby.
   c. The feeding-tube device may have developed a vacuum. Release the unused tube, or "prime" the device by pushing on the reservoir.
   d. The cap may be screwed on too tightly, blocking the flow. Loosen the cap and squeeze the container gently to activate the flow. If the device is working properly, there should be a steady drip from the end of the tubing.
   e. If formula mixed from powder is used in the device, small clumps of unmixed formula may block the tubing. Clean the tubing with hot soapy water pushed through with a syringe.
   f. The tubing was not properly cleaned and is blocked by old supplement. Try to clean the tubing again using hot soapy water pushed through with a syringe.
8. Clean the feeding-tube device soon after the feeding is finished (refer to manufacturers' instructions). The small diameter of the tubing is easily blocked.

associated with longer duration of (any) breastfeeding. These limited studies point toward test weighing as an "optional" tool for mothers of premature infants as they transition from nasogastric feedings to breastfeeding.

In situations where infant growth is of concern, test weighing may be used at each feeding to determine the need for supplementation (Meier et al., 1990). Alternatively, test weighing in the office may be used to "confirm" one's clinical impression of low intake or to "convince" the mother that the feedings are small. When test weighing is used for management of individual cases, it is crucial to have an electronic scale and to use the proper protocol with each weight, and for caretakers to keep detailed records of weights and feedings (see Box 10-10 for a sample procedure for performing infant test weights).

BOX 10-9 PRINCIPLES OF TEST WEIGHING AN INFANT

- The scale must be accurate to 2 gm or less, with computer integration for movement and a digital read-out.
- The infant must be weighed before and after every feeding for several days to get representative values.
- Infant intake in ml is approximately equal to infant weight gain in grams.
- The typical office scale is not accurate or reliable for test weighing.
- Test weighing may be used in complicated clinical situations to monitor intake and/or adjust volume of supplementation.

Data from: Woolridge et al., 1984; Jensen & Neville, 1984; Whitfield, Kay, & Stevens, 1981.

BOX 10-10 PROCEDURE FOR INFANT TEST WEIGHING

Definition of test weighing: Weighing a baby before and after breastfeeding to determine intake.

Equipment: Digital scale with integration function that allows for movement of the infant, accurate to 2 gm (for example, Olympic Smart Scale or Medela Baby Weigh Scale).

Procedure:

- Before breastfeeding, place baby on the scale and weigh him.

This is the "before" weight. It is fine to have clothing or a blanket but the final weighing must be done with exactly the same clothing and accessories as the initial weighing.

- Mother breastfeeds the infant. Do not change diaper yet.
- Reweigh the infant, with the exact same clothes, diaper, blanket, burp cloth, etc.

This is the "after" weight. (It is possible to weigh before and after each breast, if the information is useful.)

- Subtract the first (before) weight from the second (after) weight. The difference in grams is considered the "intake" in milliliters. (Some scales automatically store the values and compute the difference for you. Refer to manufacturers' instructions.)
- If the "after" weight is smaller than the "before" weight, this means the baby has lost weight—which is possible. It also might mean that you forgot a blanket on the second weighing or that someone changed the diaper and removed weight.
- Burp cloth or clothing with any drool or emesis shall be included with the weight, to reflect original intake. (Record emesis in documentation of output.)
- If the infant receives a tube feeding at the same time as breastfeeding, subtract the amount given via tube to determine the amount of breastmilk ingested directly by breastfeeding.
- Record the intake of breastmilk and any supplement volumes.
- Parents can be taught to perform test weights for the hospital or home setting.

This allows them to start a feeding without waiting for a nurse to come and perform the test weights.

Galactagogues

Galactagogues are agents that promote milk production, such as drugs, herbs, or foods. Pharmacologic and herbal galactagogues have become widely used in the United States and Canada and are probably overused considering the relative lack of evidence regarding efficacy and safety (Academy of Breastfeeding Medicine, 2011; Anderson, 2013; Budzynska et al., 2012; Mortel & Mehta, 2013). There are only a few randomized controlled trials for these drugs. The currently recognized pharmaceutical galactagogues are dopamine antagonists that are believed to work by increasing prolactin levels. However, prolactin levels have never been correlated with milk volumes, so that link remains to be established. Current pharmaceutical galactagogues are all used "off label" (i.e., they are not approved for used as galactagogues) in the United States. Herbal galactagogues, by comparison, are not subject to regulation in the United States, so questions of dosage and purity are an issue. If a clinician has reviewed the other basic aspects of lactation/breastfeeding and then makes a decision to recommend galactagogues, there must be a serious discussion with the mother regarding the potential risks versus benefits of using the agent. The Academy of Breastfeeding Medicine (2011) does not recommend the use of any specific galactagogues and suggests an abundance of caution for practitioners who prescribe them. The details are contained in the "ABM Protocol #9: Galactogogues" (Academy of Breastfeeding Medicine, 2011, or www.bfmed .org/Resources/Protocols.aspx).

Domperidone has been used widely as a galactogogue in Canada and other countries, but is not commercially available in the United States. It was the subject of one randomized, controlled, double-blinded trial among women who were pumping breastmilk for premature infants less than 31 weeks' gestation. The study lasted for 14 days and showed a significant increase in milk volume during that time, but did not follow up beyond the 2 weeks (Campbell-Yeo et al., 2010). Another very small randomized study of six patients added very little information (Wan et al., 2008). The typical dosage used in published studies is 10 mg, given three times a day, for 4 to 10 days, with larger doses showing no advantage in increasing milk production while increasing the risk of cardiac toxicity (*LactMed*, 2013). The notable advantage of domperidone is its lack of central nervous system (CNS) side effects. The key adverse effect of concern with domperidone is a prolonged QT interval that may be seen on EKG, particularly with increased blood levels of domperidone. Such increased levels are likely to be seen with increased doses or when domperidone is combined with some substrates metabolized by CYP3A4 enzyme inhibitors, such as fluconazole, grapefruit juice, ketoconazole, macrolide antibiotics, and many other commonly used drugs (Academy of Breastfeeding Medicine, 2011).

Metoclopramide, which is readily available in the United States, has frequent CNS side effects—particularly, sedation, restlessness, agitated depression, and extrapyramidal/dystonic reactions, which are generally reversible. This agent also carries a significant warning regarding *tardive dyskinesia*, which may be irreversible. Other maternal side effects of this drug include dizziness, nausea, and sweating. If CNS side effects occur other than sedation, metoclopramide must be discontinued immediately, and symptoms typically resolve within 1 week. Small amounts of the drug enter into the milk but have not been associated with clinical effects in the infant in the studies in which infants were monitored. The recommended dose of metoclopramide is 10 mg, given two to three times a day, for 7 to 14 days (*LactMed*, 2013). There is no evidence that higher doses are useful. If there is a response to the drug, it is usually seen 4 to 7 days after starting the prescription. Prescribing metoclopramide as a galactagogue is an "off-label" use of the drug. Some studies suggest that the increased milk production induced by metoclopramide will continue in the absence of the drug, while others indicate that milk production will drop off when its use is discontinued.

Although not strictly a galactagogue, oxytocin nasal spray (40 IU/mL) is used to stimulate milk ejection if the mother's own letdown is inhibited by stress or pain. Oxytocin nasal spray is not commercially available, but like domperidone, may be specially compounded by selected pharmacies.

Foods and herbs are used in many cultures to increase milk supply. A systematic review of herbal galactagogues (Mortel & Mehta, 2013) did not reveal sufficient evidence to recommend the five substances studied in randomized controlled trials: shatavari (*Asparagus racemosus*), torbangum (*Coleus amboinicus Lour*), fenugreek tea, a Japanese multiherbal product, and milk thistle (*Silymarin marianum*).

Hindmilk

Hindmilk refers to breastmilk that is obtained toward the end of the feeding episode, as contrasted with the initial milk, called "foremilk." Fat content varies considerably from feed to feed, but within a given feeding, it rises steadily. There is no specific cutoff time for this definition, nor any specific fat percentage. The concept of foremilk and hindmilk imbalance is an artificial construct used for dyads when maternal production is significantly higher than infant intake. This might occur during early engorgement or when a mother is expressing milk for a sick infant.

As there is no precise timing during pumping, hindmilk instructions must be tailored individually to each mother. For example, a mother may be expressing 900 mL (30 oz) per day for a premature infant who is ingesting only 300 mL (10 oz) per day. In that case, during each pumping session, she could set aside two thirds of the volume for "foremilk" and one third of the volume for "hindmilk," using the hindmilk for the baby's feedings now and storing the foremilk for use at some later date when the baby can manage a larger volume of intake. Very-low-birth-weight infants who receive fortified breastmilk must also receive fortification in hindmilk. If the infant is feeding at the breast of a mother with milk volume higher than the baby's intake, delivery of hindmilk may be increased by unlimited nursing on the first breast and/or by massage of the breast during feeding. The use of hindmilk has no application if the mother's milk production is lower than the baby's required intake.

SUMMARY

Low intake of breastmilk in the breastfed infant and low maternal milk supply are significant clinical problems. Early breastfeeding follow-up by a skilled provider at 3 to 5 days after birth would allow early detection of many correctable problems that contribute to slow gain in the first month. By the time the baby's weight gain slows, the mother's milk supply has often already declined, so that both mother and infant must be evaluated and managed with a problem-oriented approach.

Infant or maternal illness, though unusual as a cause of slow weight gain, must always be considered a possibility so as not to overlook a condition that is potentially serious and/or treatable. If infant well-being requires supplementation, it is preferable to give expressed breastmilk. Once the infant gains weight and the maternal milk supply improves, the amount of supplementation can gradually be decreased and the infant returned to full feedings at the breast. Rarely, maternal anatomy or physiology will preclude a full milk supply. In these cases, the mother is supported to provide as much breastmilk as possible while acknowledging the grieving process that comes with the loss of the desired breastfeeding experience.

KEY CONCEPTS

- Numerous factors, both maternal and infant, may affect infant intake and maternal milk supply; the interrelationships of these factors are complex.
- Proper positioning and latch-on are the foundation of efficient milk transfer and infant weight gain.
- Removal of milk by the infant determines the amount of milk production, and maternal limitations on milk supply are rare.
- If infant weight is low, then intake from breastfeeding is low, and the maternal milk supply is probably also low.
- During the first several weeks of breastfeeding, individual patterns of milk supply, infant intake, and infant growth patterns vary widely.

- Maternal undernutrition is not correlated with milk production.
- Maternal overweight, obesity, and excessive pregnancy weight gain appear to be risk factors for delayed lactogenesis and early cessation of breastfeeding.
- Follow-up by a health professional must take place at 3 to 5 days postpartum, when breastfeeding progress is at a critical juncture: this may be an office visit or a home visit.
- Weight loss of more than 7% from birth weight warrants investigation of a potential feeding problem; weight loss of more than 10% from birth weight requires thorough assessment and intervention.
- Between 14 days and 60 days of age, the average newborn weight gain is 39 g/day for females and 46 g/day for males.
- The minimal acceptable average weight gain is 30 g/day during the first 2 months.
- If the infant is not gaining weight (not effectively removing milk), assume that the mother's milk supply has started to decline.
- In the first month of life, problems with the feeding process are more common than illness as a cause of poor weight gain.
- Infant illness should be suspected as a potential cause of poor feeding and poor weight gain, especially in the immediate postpartum period and after the first month of life.
- With the release of the WHO Child Growth Standards, we now have appropriate growth charts for optimally breastfed infants and young children. These standards are prescriptive and show how all babies should grow if optimally fed and nurtured.
- Taking a history and physical examination of both mother and infant, including breastfeeding observation, allow the clinician to develop a differential diagnosis for slow infant weight gain.
- Management of slow infant weight gain can be tailored to the suspected diagnosis.
- Two simple interventions for low intake—for an actively suckling infant—are breast massage during feeding and switch nursing.

- If supplementation is indicated, start with ad lib feedings. If the baby is not demonstrating hunger cues, start with 50 to 100 mL/kg/day divided into 6 to 8 feedings. This feeding rate should increase rapidly over the next few days.
- A mother's own expressed breastmilk is the preferred type of supplement.
- Supplementation can be given by feeding-tube device, cup, spoon, or bottle, depending on individual circumstances.
- As the maternal milk supply increases and the infant becomes more effective at the breast, the amount of supplementation may be decreased.
- Weighing the infant before and after feeding (test weighing) requires an electronic digital scale that is accurate to 2 g or less.
- Test weighing is generally restricted to complicated clinical situations, to management of premature infants, or to research projects.
- Medications and herbs may be an option for increasing milk production after other measures have been tried.
- Delivery of more hindmilk to the infant is one method of increasing caloric intake.
- A few women will be unable to resolve the problem of low intake and low supply; they are likely to undergo a grieving process.

INTERNET RESOURCES

Academy of Breastfeeding Medicine:
   www.bfmed.org
American Academy of Pediatrics (AAP):
   www.aap.org
Centers for Disease Control and Prevention
   (CDC): www.cdc.gov/growthcharts
International Lactation Consultant Association:
   www.ilca.org
LactMed (drugs during breastfeeding):
   http://toxnet.nlm.nih.gov
La Leche League International:
   www.lalecheleague.org

World Health Child Growth Standards:
http://www.who.int/childgrowth
/standards/w_velocity/en/index.html
World Health Organization: www.WHO.int

REFERENCES

Abstracts from the 16th International Society for Research in Human Milk and Lactation Conference. Abstract # 15. *Breastfeed Med.* 2012;7(6):556–577.

Academy of Breastfeeding Medicine. Protocol #3: hospital guidelines for the use of supplementary feedings in the healthy term breastfed neonate. 2002. Available at: http://www.bfmed.org. Accessed October 31, 2008.

Academy of Breastfeeding Medicine. ABM clinical protocol #9: use of galactogogues in initiating or augmenting the rate of maternal milk secretion (first revision January 2011). *Breastfeed Med.* 2011;6(1):41–49.

Alexander JM, Grant AM, Campbell MJ. Randomized controlled trial of breast shells and Hoffman's exercises for inverted and non-protractile nipples. *Br Med J.* 1992; 305:1030–1032.

Anderson PO. The galactogogue bandwagon. *J Hum Lact.* 2013;29(1):7–10.

Bartok CJ, Schaefer EW, Beiler JS, Paul IM. Role of body mass index and gestational weight gain in breastfeeding outcomes. *Breastfeed Med.* 2012;7(6):448–456.

Berkner P, Kastner T, Skolnick L. Chronic ipecac poisoning in infancy: a case report. *Pediatrics.* 1988;82:384–386.

Bodley V, Powers D. Long-term nipple shield use: a positive perspective. *J Hum Lact.* 1996;12:301–304.

Bowen-Jones A, Thomsen C, Drewett RF. Milk flow and sucking rates during breastfeeding. *Develop Med Child Neurol.* 1982;24:626–633.

Budzynska K, Gardner ZE, Dugoua JJ, et al. Systematic review of breastfeeding and herbs. *Breastfeed Med.* 2012;7(6):489–503.

Butte NF, Garza C, Smith EO, Nichols BL. Human milk intake and growth in exclusively breast-fed infants. *J Pediatr.* 1984;104(2):187–195.

Campbell-Yeo ML, Allen AC, Joseph KS, et al. Effect of domperidone on the composition of preterm human breast milk. *Pediatrics.* 2010;125(1):e107–e114.

Chantry CJ, Nommsen-Rivers LA, Peerson JM, et al. Excess weight loss in first-born breastfed newborns relates to maternal intrapartum fluid balance. *Pediatrics.* 2011;127(1):e171–e179.

Chapman DJ, Perez-Escamilla R. Identification of risk factors for delayed onset of lactation. *J Am Diet Assoc.* 1999;99:450–454.

Chen DC, Nommsen-Rivers L, Dewey KG, Lönnerdal B. Stress during labor and delivery and early lactation performance. *Am J Clin Nutr.* 1998;68(2):335–344.

Combs VL, Marino BL. A comparison of growth patterns in breast and bottle-fed infants with congenital heart disease. *Pediatr Nurs.* 1993;19:175–178.

Cordero L, Valentine CJ, Samuels P, et al. Breastfeeding in women with severe preeclampsia. *Breastfeed Med.* 2012;7(6):457–463.

Coryllos E, Genna C, Salloum A. Congenital tongue-tie and its impact on breastfeeding. In: American Academy of Pediatrics. *Breastfeeding: best for baby and mother.* New York, NY: American Academy of Pediatrics; 2004:1–11.

Davies DP, Evans T. The starved but contented breastfed baby. *Arch Dis Child.* 1978;53:763.

Daly SE, Owens R, Hartmann PE. The short-term synthesis and infant-regulated removal of milk in lactating women. *Exp Physiol.* 1993;78(2):209–220.

Demirci JR, Sereika SM, Bogen D. Prevalence and predictors of early breastfeeding among late preterm mother–infant dyads. *Breastfeed Med.* 2012;8(3):277–285.

de Onis M. New WHO Child Growth Standards catch on. *Bull WHO.* 2011;89:250–251.

de Onis M, Garza C, Onyango AW, Borghi E. Comparison of the WHO Child Growth Standards and the CDC 2000 growth charts. *J Nutr.* 2007;137(1):144–148.

de Onis M, Garza C, Victora CG, et al. The WHO Multicentre Growth Reference Study: planning, study design, and implementation. *Food Nutr Bull.* 2004;25(suppl 1):S15–S26.

de Onis M, Onyango A, Borghi E, et al. Worldwide implementation of the WHO Child Growth Standards. *Public Health Nutr.* 2012:1–8.

Desmarais L, Browne S. Inadequate weight gain in breastfeeding infants: assessments and resolutions. In: Auerbach KG, ed. Lactation Consultant Series. Garden City Park, NY: Avery Publishing Group; 1990.

Dewey KG, Heinig J, Nommsen LA, et al. Maternal versus infant factors related to breast milk and residual milk volume: the DARLING study. *Pediatrics.* 1991;87(6):829–837.

Dewey KG, Lonnerdal B. Infant self-regulation of breastmilk intake. *Acta Paediatr Scand.* 1986;75:893–898.

Dewey KG, Nommsen-Rivers LA, Heinig MJ, Cohen RJ. Lactogenesis and infant weight change in the first weeks of life. Adv Exp Med Biol. 2002;503:159–66.

Dewey KG, Nommsen-Rivers, LA, Heinig, MJ, Cohen, RJ. Risk factors for suboptimal infant breastfeeding behavior, delayed onset of lactation, and excess neonatal weight loss. *Pediatrics.* 2003;112:607–619.

Drane D. The effect of use of dummies and teats on orofacial development. *Breastfeed Rev.* 1996:4:59–64.

Edmonson MB, Stoddard JJ, Owens LM. Hospital readmission with feeding-related problems after early postpartum discharge of normal newborns. *JAMA.* 1997;278:299–303.

Edmunds J, Hazelbaker A, Murphy JG, Philipp BL. Roundtable discussion: tongue-tie. *J Hum Lact.* 2012;28(1):14–17.

Eidelman AI. Breastfeeding mitigates a disaster. *Breastfeed Med.* 2013:8:344–345.

Eidelman A, Section on Breastfeeding. Breastfeeding and the use of human milk. *Pediatrics*. 2012;129(3): e827–e841.

Engle WA, Tomashek KM, Wallman C, et al. "Late-preterm" infants: a population at risk. *Pediatrics*. 2007;120:1390–1401.

Flaherman VJ, Bokser S, Newman TB. First-day newborn weight loss predicts in-hospital weight nadir for breast-feeding infants. *Breastfeed Med*. 2010;5(4):165–168.

Funkquist EL, Tuvemo T, Jonsson B, et al. Influence of test weighing before/after nursing on breastfeeding in preterm infants. *Adv Neonatal Care*. 2010;10(1):33–39.

Gatti L. Maternal perceptions of insufficient milk supply in breastfeeding. *J Nurs Scholarsh*. 2008;40(4):355–363.

Geddes DT, Aljazaf KM, Kent JC, et al. Blood flow characteristics of the human lactating breast. *J Hum Lact*. 2012;28(2):145–152.

Geddes DT, Langton DB, Gollow I, et al. Frenulotomy for breastfeeding infants with ankyloglossia: effect on milk removal and sucking mechanism as imaged by ultrasound. *Pediatrics*. 2008;122(1):e188–e194.

Genna CW, ed. *Supporting sucking skills in breastfeeding infants*. Sudbury, MA: Jones and Bartlett; 2008:22–25.

Glass RP, Wolf LS. Incoordination of sucking, swallowing, and breathing as an etiology for breastfeeding difficulty. *J Hum Lact*. 1994;10(3):185–189.

Grajeda R, Perez-Escamilla R. Stress during labor and delivery is associated with delayed onset of lactation among urban Guatemalan women. *JNutr*. 2002; 132:3055–3060.

Grossman X, Chaudhuri JH, Feldman-Winter L, Merewood A. Neonatal weight loss at a US Baby-Friendly Hospital. *J Acad Nutr Diet*. 2012;112(3):410–413.

Guelinckx I, Devlieger R, Bogaerts A, et al. The effect of pre-pregnancy BMI on intention, initiation and duration of breast-feeding. *Public Health Nutr*. 2012;15(5):840–848.

Hall WA, Shearer K, Mogan J, Berkowitz J. Weighing preterm infants before and after breastfeeding: does it increase maternal confidence and competence? *MCN Am J Matern Child Nurs*. 2002;27(6):318–326.

Habbick BF, Gerrard JW. Failure to thrive in the contented breastfed baby. *Can Med Assoc J*. 1984;131:765–768.

Henley SJ, Anderson CM, Avery MD, et al. Anemia and insufficient milk in first-time mothers. *Birth*. 1995;22:87–92.

Hilson JA, Rasmussen KM, Kjolhede CL. Maternal obesity and breast-feeding success in a rural population of white women. *Am J Clin Nutr*. 1997;66:1371–1378.

Hilson JA, Rasmussen KM, Kjolhede CL. High prepregnant body mass index is associated with poor lactation outcomes among white, rural women independent of psychosocial and demographic correlates. *J Hum Lact*. 2004;20(1):18–29.

Hilson JA, Rasmussen KM, Kjolhede CL. Excessive weight gain during pregnancy is associated with earlier termination of breastfeeding among white women. *J Nutr*. 2006;136(1):140–146.

Hong P, Lago D, Seargeant J, et al. Defining ankyloglossia: a case series of anterior and posterior tongue ties. *Int J Pediatr Otorhinolaryngol*. 2010;74(9):1003–1006.

Hoover KL, Barbalinardo LH, Platia MP. Delayed lactogenesis II secondary to gestational ovarian theca lutein cysts in two normal singleton pregnancies. *J Hum Lact*. 2002;18(3):264–268.

Hopkinson JM, Schanler RJ, Fraley JK, Garza C. Milk production by mothers of premature infants: influence of cigarette smoking. *Pediatrics*. 1992;90(6):934–948.

Horta BL, Victora CG, Barros FC, et al. Environmental tobacco smoke and the breastfeeding duration. *Am J Epidemiol*. 1997;146:128–133.

Howard CR, Howard FM, Lanphear B, et al. Randomized clinical trial of pacifier use and bottle-feeding or cupfeeding and their effect on breastfeeding. *Pediatrics*. 2003;111:411–518.

Howard CR, Victora CG, Menezes AM, Barros FC. Physiologic stability of newborns during cup and bottle-feeding. *Pediatrics*. 1999;104:1204–1207.

Huggins KE, Petok ES, Mireles O. Markers of lactation insufficiency: a study of 34 mothers. In: Auerbach KG, ed. *Current issues in clinical lactation, 2000*. Sudbury, MA: Jones and Bartlett; 2000:25–36.

Hurst NM. Lactation after augmentation mammoplasty. *Obstet Gynecol*. 1996;87:30–34.

Hurst NM, Meier PP, Engstrom JL, Myatt A. Mothers performing in-home measurement of milk intake during breastfeeding of their preterm infants: maternal reactions and feeding outcomes. *J Hum Lact*. 2004;20(2):178–187.

Institute of Medicine. *Nutrition during lactation*. Washington, DC: National Academy Press; 1991.

International Lactation Consultant Association. *Clinical guidelines for the establishment of exclusive breastfeeding*. Raleigh, NC: ILCA Publications; 2005.

Jones WB. Weight gain and feeding in the neonate with cleft: a three-center study. *Cleft Palate J*. 1988;25:379–384.

Kent JC, Mitoulas L, Cox DB, et al. Breast volume and milk production during extended lactation in women. *Exp Physiol*. 1999;84(2):435–447.

Kent JC, Mitoulas LR, Cregan MD, et al. Volume and frequency of breastfeedings and fat content of breast milk throughout the day. *Pediatrics*. 2006;117(3): e387–e395.

Knox I, Amir L, Genna C, et al. Abstracts: the Academy of Breastfeeding Medicine 16th Annual International Meeting. *Breastfeed Med*. 2011;6(suppl 1):S1–S24.

Konetzny G, Bucher HU, Arlettaz R. Prevention of hypernatraemic dehydration in breastfed newborn infants by daily weighing. *Eur J Pediatr*. 2009;168(7):815–818.

Kotlow L. Diagnosis and treatment of ankyloglossia and tied maxillary fraenum in infants using Er:YAG and 1064 diode lasers. *Eur Arch Paediatr Dent*. 2011;12(2): 106–112.

Kugyelka JG, Rasmussen KM, Frongillo EA. Maternal obesity is negatively associated with breastfeeding success among Hispanic but not black women. *J Nutr.* 2004;134(7):1746–1753.

LactMed. Toxnet. Available at: http://toxnet.nlm.nih.gov. Accessed May 14, 2013.

Lamp JM, Macke JK. Relationships among intrapartum maternal fluid intake, birth type, neonatal output, and neonatal weight loss during the first 48 hours after birth. *J Obstet Gynecol Neonatal Nurs.* 2010;39(2):169–177.

Lawrence RA, Lawrence R. *Breastfeeding: a guide for the medical profession,* 7th ed. St. Louis, MO: CV Mosby; 2011.

Lawrence RA, Lawrence R. Breastfeeding—A Guide for the Medical Profession. 6th ed. St. Louis, MO: CV Mosby; 2005.

Livingstone VH. Common lactation and breast-feeding problems. In: Ismail J, ed. Manual of Breast Diseases. Lippincott Williams & Wilkins; 2002:95–134.

Livingstone V. Neonatal insufficient milk syndrome (NIMS): a bio/psycho/social classification, (poster abstract). 10th Annual Conference of the Academy of Breastfeeding Medicine; October 21, 2005; Denver, CO.

Lukefahr JL. Underlying illness associated with failure to thrive in breastfed infants. *Clin Pediatr.* 1990;29(8):468–470.

McKechnie AC, Eglash A. Nipple shields: a review of the literature. *Breastfeed Med.* 2010;5(6):309–314.

Meier PP, Brown LP, Hurst NM, et al. Nipple shields for preterm infants: effect on milk transfer and duration of breastfeeding. *J Hum Lact.* 2002;16:106–114.

Meier PP, Lysakowski TY, Engstrom JL, et al. The accuracy of test weighing for preterm infants. *J Pediatr Gastroenterol Nutr.* 1990;10(1):62–65.

Mennella JA. The human infant's suckling responses to the flavor of alcohol in mother's milk. *Alcohol Clin Exp Res.* 1997;21:581–585.

Mennella JA, Pepino MY. Breastfeeding and prolactin levels in lactating women with a family history of alcoholism. *Pediatrics.* 2010;125(5):e1162–e1170.

Merdad H, Mascarenhas AK. Ankyloglossia may cause breast-feeding, tongue mobility, and speech difficulties, with inconclusive results on treatment choices. *J Evid Based Dent Pract.* 2010;10(3):152–153.

Mortel M, Mehta SD. Systematic review of the efficacy of herbal galactogogues. *J Hum Lact.* 2013;29(2):154–162.

Mulder PJ, Johnson TS, Baker LC. Excessive weight loss in breastfed infants during the postpartum hospitalization. *J Obstet Gynecol Neonatal Nurs.* 2010;39(1):15–26.

Neifert MR, McDonough SL, Neville MC. Failure of lacto-genesis associated with placental retention. *Am J Obstet Gynecol.* 1981;140(4):477–478.

Neifert MR, Seacat JM, DeMarzo S, Young D. The association between infant weight gain and breast milk intake measured by office test weights [Abstract]. *Am J Dis Child.* 1990;144:420–421.

Neifert MR, Seacat JM, Jobe WE. Lactation failure due to insufficient glandular development of the breast. *Pediatrics.* 1985;76(5):823–828.

Neifert M, DeMarzo S, Seacat J, et al. The influence of breast surgery, breast appearance, and pregnancy-induced breast changes on lactation sufficiency as measured by infant weight gain. *Birth.* 1990;17(1):31–38.

Neifert MR. Failure to thrive. In: Neville MC, Neifert MR, eds. Lactation: Physiology, Nutrition and Breastfeeding. New York, NY: Plenum Press; 1983.

Neubauer SH, Ferris AM, Chase CG, et al. Delayed lactogenesis in women with insulin-dependent diabetes mellitus. *Am J Clin Nutr.* 1993;58:54–60.

Neville MC, Keller R, Seacat J, et al. Studies in human lactation: milk volumes in lactating women during the onset of lactation and full lactation. *Am J Clin Nutr.* 1988;48:1375–1386.

Noel-Weiss J, Woodend AK, Peterson WE, et al. An observational study of associations among maternal fluids during parturition, neonatal output, and breastfed newborn weight loss. *Int Breastfeed J.* 2011;6:9.

Nommsen-Rivers LA, Chantry CJ, Peerson JM, et al. Delayed onset of lactogenesis among first-time mothers is related to maternal obesity and factors associated with ineffective breastfeeding. *Am J Clin Nutr.* 2010;92(3):574–584.

O'Callahan C, Macary S, Clemente S. The effects of office-based frenotomy for anterior and posterior ankyloglossia on breastfeeding. *Int J Pediatr Otorhinolaryngol.* 2013;77(5):827–832.

Opara PI, Gabriel-Job N, Opara KO. Neonates presenting with severe complications of frenotomy: a case series. *J Med Case Rep.* 2012;6:77.

Peaker M, Wilde CJ. Milk secretion: autocrine control. *News Physiol Sci.* 1987;2:124–126.

Perez-Escamilla R, Chapman DJ. Validity and public health implications of maternal perception of the onset of lactation: an international analytical overview. *J Nutr.* 2001;131:3021S–3024S.

Pessl MM. Are we creating our own breastfeeding mythology? *J Hum Lact.* 1996;12:271–272.

Powers NG. Slow weight gain and low milk supply in the breastfeeding dyad. *Clinics in Perinatology.* 1999;26:399–429.

Preer GL, Newby PK, Philipp BL. Weight loss in exclusively breastfed infants delivered by cesarean birth. *J Hum Lact.* 2012;28(2):153–158.

Rasmussen KM. Association of maternal obesity before conception with poor lactation performance. *Annu Rev Nutr.* 2007;27:103–121.

Rasmussen K, Kjolhede C. Prepregnant overweight and obesity diminish the prolactin response to suckling in the first week postpartum. *Pediatrics.* 2004;113(5):e465–e471.

Regnault N, Botton J, Blanc L, et al. Determinants of neonatal weight loss in term-infants: specific association with pre-pregnancy maternal body mass index and infant feeding mode. *Arch Dis Child Fetal Neonatal Ed.* 2011;96(3):F217–F222.

Roggero P, Gianni ML, Orsi A, et al. Neonatal period: body composition changes in breast-fed full-term newborns. *Neonatology*. 2010;97(2):139–143.

Ruvalcaba RHA. Stress-induced cessation of lactation. *West J Ed*. 1987;146:228–230.

Sakalidis VS, Williams TM, Garbin CP, et al. Ultrasound imaging of infant sucking dynamics during the establishment of lactation. *J Hum Lact*. 2013;29(2):205–213.

Salvador S, Vandenplas Y. Gastroesophageal reflux and cow milk allergy: is there a link? *Pediatrics*. 2002;110:972–984.

Sealy CN. Rethinking the use of nipple shields. *J Hum Lact*. 1996;12(4):299–300.

Segura-Millan S, Dewey KG, Perez-Escamilla R. Factors associated with perceived insufficient milk in a low-income urban population from Mexico. *J Nutr*. 1994;124:202–212.

Semple JL, Lugowski SJ, Baines CJ, et al. Breast milk contamination and silicone implants: preliminary results using silicon as a proxy measurement for silicone. *Plastic Reconstr Surg*. 1998;102(2):528–533.

Shapiro-Mendoza CK, Tomashek KM, Kotelchuck M, et al. Risk factors for neonatal morbidity and mortality among "healthy" late preterm newborns. *Sem Perinatol*. 2006;30(2):54–60.

Shapiro-Mendoza CK, Tomashek KM, Kotelchuck M, et al. Effect of late-preterm birth and maternal medical conditions on newborn morbidity risk. *Pediatrics*. 2008;121:e223–e232.

Soskolne EI, Schumacher R, Fyock C, et al. The effect of early discharge and other factors on the readmission rates of newborns. *Arch Pediatr Adolesc Med*. 1996;150:373–379.

Souto GC, Giugliani ERJ, Giugliani C, Schneider MA. The impact of breast reduction surgery on breastfeeding performance. *J Hum Lact*. 2003;19(1):43–49.

Stuff JE, Nichols BL. Nutrient intake and growth performance of older infants fed human milk. *J Pediatr*. 1989;115:959–968.

Sutphen JL, Saulsbury FT. Intentional ipecac poisoning: Munchausen syndrome by proxy. *Pediatrics*. 1988;82:453–456.

Thibaudeau S, Sinno H, Williams B. The effects of breast reduction on successful breastfeeding: a systematic review. *J Plastic Reconstr Aesthet Surg*. 2010;63(10):1688–1693.

Trotman H, Lord C, Barton M, Antoine M. Hypernatraemic dehydration in Jamaican breastfed neonates: a 12-year review in a baby-friendly hospital. *Ann Trop Paediatr*. 2004;24(4):295–300.

Wan EW-X, Davey K, Page-Sharp M, et al. Dose-effect study of domperidone as a galactagogue in preterm mothers with insufficient milk supply, and its transfer into milk. *Br J Clin Pharmacol*. 2008;66(2):283–289.

Watson J, Hodnett E, Armson BA, et al. A randomized controlled trial of the effect of intrapartum intravenous fluid management on breastfed newborn weight loss. *J Obstet Gynecol Neonatal Nurs*. 2012;41(1):24–32.

Webb AN, Hao W, Hong P. The effect of tongue-tie division on breastfeeding and speech articulation: a systematic review. *Int J Pediatr Otorhinolaryngol*. 2013;77(5):635–646.

Whitfield M, Kay R, Stevens S. Validity of routine clinical test weighing as a measure of intake of breast-fed infants. *Arch Dis Child*. 1981;56:919.

WHO Multicenter Growth Reference Study Group. WHO child growth standards based on length/height, weight and age. *Acta Paediatrica Suppl*. 2006;450:76–85.

Wilhelm S, Rodehorst-Weber TK, Flanders Stepans MB, Hertzog M. The relationship between breastfeeding test weights and postpartum breastfeeding rates. *J Hum Lact*. 2010;26:168–174.

Wilson JD, Foster DW, eds. *Williams textbook of endocrinology*. Philadelphia, PA: W. B. Saunders; 1992:441–442.

Wilson-Clay B. Clinical use of silicone nipple shields. *J Hum Lact*. 1996;12:279–285.

Wisner KL, Parry BL, Piontek CM. Postpartum depression. *N Engl J Med*. 2002;347:194–199.

Woolridge MW, Fisher C. Colic, "overfeeding" and symptoms of lactose malabsorption in the breast-fed baby: a possible artifact of feed management? *Lancet*. 1988;2(8607):382–384.

Woolridge MW, Ingram JC, Baum JD. Do changes in pattern of breast usage alter the baby's nutrient intake? *Lancet*. 1990;336:395–397.

Woolridge MW, et al. Methods for the measurement of milk volume intake of the breast-fed infant. In: Jensen RG, Neville MC, eds. *Human lactation: milk components and methodologies*. New York: Plenum; 1984:5–21.

World Health Organization (WHO). Child growth standards. Available at: http://www.who.int/childgrowth/standards/w_velocity/en/index.html. Accessed April 14, 2013.

World Health Organization (WHO). Training course on child growth assessment. Available at: http://www.who.int/childgrowth/training/en/). Accessed April 30, 2013.

Zhu P, Hao J, Jiang X, et al. New insight into onset of lactation: mediating the negative effect of multiple perinatal biopsychosocial stress on breastfeeding duration. *Breastfeed Med*. 2013;8(2):151–158.

Chapter 11

Jaundice and the Breastfed Baby

Lawrence M. Gartner

Physiologic jaundice, caused by an elevation of serum unconjugated bilirubin, is a common clinical condition seen in approximately two-thirds of newborn infants. In artificially fed infants, the jaundice disappears within 1 week, and the serum bilirubin drops to adult normal levels (upper limit of 1.5 mg/dL) by 10 to 14 days of life. In the great majority of breastfed infants, serum unconjugated bilirubin elevations persist for many weeks thereafter, falling to normal values by 1 to 2 months of age. Clinical jaundice also remains present in many breastfed infants until 3 to 6 weeks of life. This normal prolongation of physiologic jaundice in the healthy, thriving breastfed infant is known as breastmilk jaundice.

Breastmilk jaundice, which was first recognized more than 40 years ago (Arias et al., 1964; Newman & Gross, 1963; Stiehm & Ryan, 1965), results from the effect of an as yet unidentified factor in human milk that promotes an increase in intestinal absorption of bilirubin (Alonso et al., 1991; Gartner et al., 1983). This factor is not found in colostrum, but rather appears only with the secretion of transitional and mature milk beginning on about the fifth day of life. This coincides with the observation that serum bilirubin concentrations of normal formula-fed and adequately breastfed infants are identical during the first 5 days of life, with the higher bilirubin values in optimally breastfed infants being seen after

the fifth day of life. Although rarely necessary, discontinuation of breastfeeding for 24 to 48 hours in infants with breastmilk jaundice results in a prompt decline in serum bilirubin. Resumption of breastfeeding increases bilirubin levels, albeit usually to lower levels than seen before discontinuation.

Because bilirubin is an effective antioxidant and newborns are deficient in naturally occurring antioxidants, it has been suggested that this mechanism for prolongation of physiologic jaundice (breastmilk jaundice) may be protective for the newborn (Dore et al., 1999; Stocker et al., 1987). To date, insufficient clinical evidence has been published to confirm this intuitive and attractive concept, but animal studies strongly support the protective effect of hyperbilirubinemia in ischemic bowel injury (Hammerman et al., 2002). In addition, adults with lifelong, low-grade unconjugated hyperbilirubinemia (Gilbert's syndrome) have been found to have significant reductions in heart disease and cancer, providing additional support for the hypothesis that bilirubin acts as an effective antioxidant (Hunt et al., 1996; Schwertner et al., 1994; Temme et al., 2001; Vítek et al., 2002).

Although most infants with breastmilk jaundice have low levels of unconjugated hyperbilirubinemia (generally less than 10 mg/dL), occasional breastfed infants have more exaggerated bilirubin levels. These higher bilirubin levels are often caused by the presence of an independent acquired or inherited disorder that results in either increased bilirubin production or reduced clearance of bilirubin.

Inadequate breastfeeding, particularly in the early days of life, can also result in elevated levels of bilirubin (Gartner, 2001). This manifestation is known as starvation jaundice of the newborn (also known as breast-nonfeeding jaundice) and is the neonatal manifestation of the adult disorder known as starvation jaundice (Whitmer & Gollan, 1983). In this condition, which is characterized by inadequate milk and caloric intake but not necessarily by dehydration, there may be a delay in bilirubin clearance resulting from low stool output (de Carvalho et al., 1985) with an increase in the intestinal absorption of unconjugated bilirubin. Exaggerated jaundice caused by poor breastfeeding should not be considered physiologic. It has been shown that in neonates who were adequately breastfed on demand, not according to a rigid time schedule, there was no difference in the percentage with an elevated level of bilirubin during the first days of life between those who were breastfed or those who were bottle-fed (Rubaltelli, 1993), nor was there a difference in the percentage of weight loss. After the fifth day of life, exaggerated hyperbilirubinemia and jaundice may be due to the combined effect of breastmilk jaundice and starvation jaundice of the newborn.

Despite the knowledge of an association between exaggerations of neonatal jaundice and breastfeeding, it would be a mistake to assume, without careful consideration, that because a neonate is breastfed and is jaundiced, breastfeeding is the sole, or main, cause of the jaundice. It would also be a mistake to believe that if the jaundice is associated with breastfeeding, it can never be harmful. This chapter discusses neonatal jaundice, its physiologic and pathologic causes, its potential risks, and its evaluation and management.

Neonatal Jaundice

Jaundice, or icterus, is defined as a yellowish color of the sclerae and skin as a result of the deposition of bilirubin, a yellow molecule, in body tissues. Bilirubin is largely derived from red blood cell lysis and the breakdown of hemoglobin into globin and heme; subsequently, heme is degraded by the enzyme heme oxygenase to produce equimolar amounts of iron, biliverdin, and carbon monoxide. Biliverdin is reduced to bilirubin by biliverdin reductase (Dennery et al., 2001).

More than half of all newborns have some degree of visible jaundice. The intensity of jaundice depends on the balance of bilirubin production and bilirubin elimination. Serum bilirubin levels in newborns are higher than those in adults for several reasons (Gartner & Lee, 1992).

Increased Bilirubin Synthesis

The fetus in utero exists in a relatively low oxygen environment, which stimulates increased erythropoiesis and produces a large fetal red cell mass to assure adequate oxygen delivery to the tissues. The fetus also has a relatively large blood volume in addition to a high hemoglobin concentration compared to an adult or older child. The hematocrit of the newborn at birth increases further in proportion to the time between birth and clamping of the umbilical cord (Shurin, 1992). This increase in transfer of blood from the placenta to the newborn upon birth ensures an adequate volume of blood to fill the expanded vascular beds (e.g., lungs, intestine) and adequate iron to meet future metabolic needs, including new hemoglobin synthesis. Thus, within a few minutes, the newborn has a much greater volume of red cells relative to body weight than does an adult or older child. In addition, the life span of the red cells formed in utero (approximately 70 to 90 days) is shorter than that of the adult (100 to 120 days). This large volume of heme combined with a shorter life span of the red cells in the circulation results in synthesis of more bilirubin per unit of body weight than in the adult.

In addition, the fetus produces red cells not only in the bone marrow but also in the liver and spleen. This very active erythropoiesis is driven by the hormone erythropoietin. Immediately after delivery of the infant into room air and the initiation of respiration, the blood oxygen level increases dramatically, resulting in a fall in erythropoietin production and complete cessation of erythropoiesis. The immature inactive red cells in the liver, spleen, and bone marrow are destroyed, producing additional bilirubin. All of the bilirubin formed in this process—unconjugated bilirubin—is insoluble in plasma, requiring that it be transported bound to serum albumin. In the fetus, the small amount of insoluble bilirubin formed is cleared from the circulation by passive diffusion across the placenta; in the newborn, it must be eliminated by another pathway.

Bilirubin Metabolism

In the newborn, the insoluble bilirubin—also referred to as unconjugated or indirect-reacting bilirubin—must enter the liver cell (hepatocyte) by a process of facilitated diffusion. In the newborn, this process is less active than in an older child or adult, reducing the rate of clearance of bilirubin from the plasma. Once in the liver, bilirubin is conjugated with glucuronic acid via the enzyme uridine diphosphate glucuronyl transferase (UGT1A1) to become water-soluble bilirubin glucuronide, a requirement for transfer from the liver cell into bile and movement into the small intestine and ultimately into stool. Bilirubin glucuronide is also called conjugated or direct-reacting bilirubin. Compared to adults, newborns' conjugating system is relatively immature, as is their uptake of bilirubin. The degree of imbalance between high bilirubin synthesis and limited liver cell uptake and conjugation of bilirubin causes the varying elevation of serum bilirubin concentration in blood and body tissues and the degree of severity of jaundice. This normal elevation of unconjugated bilirubin and the resulting visible jaundice are collectively known as physiologic jaundice of the newborn.

Intestinal Metabolism of Bilirubin

For the conjugated bilirubin to be eliminated from the body, it must be passed in the neonatal stool. However, neonates, unlike adults, have a high level of the beta-glucuronidase enzyme in their intestinal mucosa. This enzyme removes the glucuronide from the conjugated bilirubin, making the bilirubin once again water insoluble and, therefore, available for transport back across the intestinal lumen into the neonate's circulation. This process, called the enterohepatic circulation of bilirubin, contributes to neonatal jaundice. The absence of intestinal bacteria in the neonate (which in the adult convert bilirubin into other metabolites), combined with the high level of beta-glucuronidase in the intestine and the high concentration of unconjugated bilirubin, leads to a marked increase of intestinal reabsorption of bilirubin in the neonate. This, in turn, increases the quantity of bilirubin in the circulation and the load of bilirubin presented to the liver for metabolism and excretion.

Assessment of Jaundice

Traditionally, clinicians have relied on visual inspection to determine the level of jaundice in newborns. As there is a craniocaudal progression in icterus of the skin with rising levels of bilirubin, the serum level of bilirubin has been inferred from the apparent level of demarcation of jaundice on the neonate's body. Some evidence suggests that the visual inspection for the estimation of bilirubin level is unreliable and inaccurate (Moyer et al., 2000). This is particularly true in pigmented races. In this era of hospital discharge of neonates at or around 48 hours of life, it is very difficult to distinguish, simply by inspection, a pathological or abnormally high level of bilirubin from a normal level. For this reason, many experts now recommend that all neonates be screened by serum or transcutaneous level of bilirubin prior to hospital discharge and that this level be plotted on the nomogram of bilirubin level according to hours of age of the baby, as shown in Figure 11-1 (Bhutani et al., 1999). One can then readily determine into which risk category an infant falls. Significant hyperbilirubinemia, which is defined as bilirubin level greater than the 95th or 75th percentiles at any age, strongly predicts that dangerously high serum bilirubin levels can be anticipated in the immediate future. This can be a guide as to which diagnostic testing may be indicated, whether the infant ought to be discharged to home, and when the early follow-up appointment should be scheduled.

Figure 11-1 RISK DESIGNATION OF TERM AND NEAR-TERM WELL NEWBORNS BASED ON SERUM BILIRUBIN VALUES. THE HIGH-RISK ZONE IS DESIGNATED BY THE 95TH PERCENTILE TRACK. THE INTERMEDIATE-RISK ZONE IS SUBDIVIDED TO UPPER AND LOWER RISK ZONES BY THE 75TH PERCENTILE TRACK. THE LOW-RISK ZONE HAS BEEN ELECTIVELY AND STATISTICALLY DEFINED BY THE 40TH PERCENTILE TRACK. (DOTTED EXTENSIONS ARE BASED ON < 300 TSB VALUES/EPOCH.)

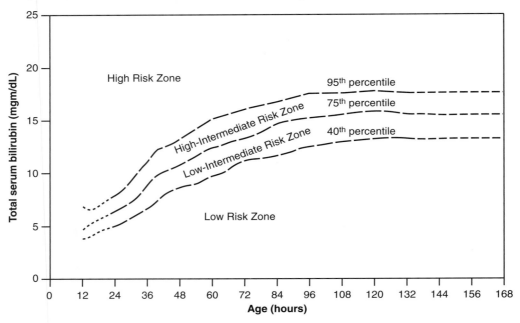

Source: Reproduced with permission from Pediatrics, Vol. 103, Page(s) 6–14, Copyright ? 1999 by the AAP.

Postnatal Pattern of Jaundice

Because of the physiological mechanisms described previously, bilirubin levels rise in neonates after birth for a few days and then, typically, fall to the adult level. In the formula-fed healthy Caucasian term infant, bilirubin levels peak on day 2 to 3, which is often after hospital discharge has taken place. In preterm neonates and in infants of some racial groups—for example, in some full-term Asians—the peak may occur later, on days 4 and 5, and usually will be higher than in the Caucasian term newborn (Brown & Wong, 1965). Jaundice will have resolved in most infants by day 7 in the formula-fed normal term neonate, and by days 10 to 21 in the preterm neonate. The pattern of jaundice in the breastfed neonate, known as breastmilk jaundice, is more prolonged.

Breastmilk Jaundice

With its onset after the fifth day of life, in association with the appearance of transitional and mature milk, breastmilk jaundice is an extension of physiologic jaundice (Gartner & Herschel, 2001). The levels of jaundice rarely become dangerously high; if so, a careful evaluation for other causes of jaundice is essential (discussed later). Breastmilk jaundice is seen in healthy, thriving neonates who have good weight gain; it may persist for many weeks. However, stools will be normal yellow in color, and the conjugated fraction of total bilirubin, which should be measured by 2 to 3 weeks of age in all infants who are still jaundiced, will be normal (less than 2 mg/dL and less than 10% of the total bilirubin).

Breastmilk jaundice is a normal physiologic phenomenon, not a disorder (Gartner & Herschel, 2001). Two-thirds of all breastfed babies have an elevation in bilirubin, and half of those have visible jaundice during the second to fourth weeks of life. As bilirubin is a potent antioxidant, modest elevations of bilirubin may possibly be beneficial.

Breastmilk jaundice has been shown to result from an increase in the intestinal absorption of bilirubin, not to an inhibitor of the conjugating enzyme, UGT1A1 (Alonso et al., 1991). An as yet unidentified substance in the milk of the majority of breastfeeding mothers is responsible for this increase in intestinal reabsorption of bilirubin (Gartner, 2001).

Gilbert's syndrome, a benign inherited condition characterized by reduced activity of the bilirubin-conjugating enzyme, has been associated with prolonged neonatal jaundice. Genetic studies of the promoter for the conjugating enzyme, UGT1A1, in a Scottish population (Monaghan et al., 1999) revealed that there is a significant association between prolonged jaundice and breastfeeding in neonates who have an increase in the number of TATA box repeats. In Asians, a DNA sequence variant (Gly 71 Arg mutation) of the UGT1A1 gene has been shown to be associated with neonatal hyperbilirubinemia (Maruo et al., 1999). Fifteen of 17 Japanese infants with prolonged jaundice in association with breastfeeding had at least one UGT1A1 mutation (Maruo et al., 2000). Two different types of mutations of the gene for the UGT1A1 enzyme are major contributors to neonatal hyperbilirubinemia in European and Japanese populations. Thus breastfeeding combined with this inherited defect in conjugation of bilirubin may result in very high levels of bilirubin and in even greater prolongation of the hyperbilirubinemia and jaundice (Kaplan et al., 2003).

Although neonatal jaundice without other signs is almost never indicative of a bacterial infection, in 7.5% of afebrile, asymptomatic jaundiced newborns (predominantly formula-fed) younger than 8 weeks of age (mean age of 12 days) presenting to an emergency department, a urinary tract infection was diagnosed (Garcia & Nager, 2002). Bacterial infection in association with hyperbilirubinemia increases the risk of bilirubin toxicity and the development of kernicterus (Volpe, 2001). A diagnostic workup for bacterial infections is indicated in jaundiced infants who have signs of sepsis, including poor feeding, lethargy, hypotonia, respiratory distress, and fever. It should be recognized, however, that these may also be early signs of bilirubin toxicity (kernicterus). In either situation, treatment to lower serum bilirubin concentrations is indicated (discussed later in this chapter).

Starvation Jaundice

Breastmilk jaundice will usually be identified after the neonate has been discharged home, as it generally presents as a prolongation of the earlier physiologic jaundice. In contrast, starvation jaundice (previously known as breastfeeding jaundice or breast-nonfeeding jaundice), may be seen in the first few days after birth, but not before 24 hours (Gartner & Herschel, 2001). Again, other causes for jaundice must be considered and ruled out. Starvation jaundice is seen in neonates who have not established feedings because of maternal or neonatal factors, or a combination of both. This condition is comparable to the starvation jaundice seen in adults with inadequate caloric intake, in whom bilirubin levels rise above baseline (Whitmer & Gollan, 1983). A 24-hour period of complete caloric deprivation is sufficient in virtually all normal adults to double the serum bilirubin to approximately 2 to 3 mg/dL, a level that is not associated with visible jaundice. In those adults with Gilbert's syndrome, clinical jaundice may be evident when they go without eating for more than 24 hours because they double their bilirubin from an already elevated serum bilirubin concentration.

For infants who have not established effective breastfeeding, whether owing to sleepiness, prematurity, poor positioning and poor latch with inadequate milk transfer, or other conditions, it is unwise to send them home until the problem is resolved (Maisels & Newman, 1998; Neifert, 1998).

Breastfeeding should be formally evaluated by a trained health professional at least twice each day in the hospital, with attention paid to position, latch, and milk transfer. Failure to correct breastfeeding problems prior to hospital discharge may result in excessive weight loss (great than 7% to 10%), dehydration, hypernatremia, and excessive and dangerous levels of bilirubin, with a catastrophic outcome possible, such as kernicterus (bilirubin encephalopathy) (Johnson et al., 2002), a permanent neurologic condition characterized by athetoid cerebral palsy and deafness. In addition to the risk of kernicterus, venous thrombosis has been reported in a few such instances (Gebara & Everett, 2001).

For neonates with jaundice and poor breastfeeding, the solution is not to stop the breastfeeding, but rather to correct the breastfeeding problem and to restore fluid and caloric intake. In some instances, expressed milk, banked human milk, or artificial milk supplementation may be required for a time. The main point is that the baby must be fed and the mother must be supported. Regardless of the etiology of the jaundice, if breastfeeding is not going well, it must be improved, not abandoned. Adequate caloric intake can prevent excessive hyperbilirubinemia even in infants with inherited defects in bilirubin conjugation (Sato et al., 2013).

Infants who develop elevated bilirubin levels in the early days of life due to starvation jaundice are also at increased risk of developing very high bilirubin levels when they enter the stage of breastmilk jaundice. If they have developed an exaggerated bilirubin pool early, that pool will multiply with mature human milk feeding due to enhanced intestinal bilirubin absorption. Conversely, good breastfeeding practices that keep early bilirubin at lower levels will prevent later excessive levels from developing.

Hyperbilirubinemia

Factors that have been associated with exaggerated hyperbilirubinemia may be categorized in the following way (Dennery et al., 2001), recognizing that there are often multiple reasons for hyperbilirubinemia in a given baby:

- Increased production of bilirubin (hemolysis)
  - ◄ Blood group incompatibility with isoimmunization (direct antibody [Coombs'] test DAT positive)
  - ◄ Inherited red blood cell abnormalities such as enzyme deficiencies (glucose-6-phosphate dehydrogenase [G6PD] deficiency) and red cell membrane defects (spherocytosis, elliptocytosis)
  - ◄ Birth "trauma" (ecchymoses, cephalhematoma, internal bleeding, subgaleal hemorrhage)
  - ◄ Genetic factors (Greek Island extraction, Asian race)
  - ◄ Prematurity (shortened erythrocyte life span)
  - ◄ Polycythemia
- Decreased elimination of bilirubin
  - ◄ Genetic variants/disorders of conjugation—Gilbert's syndrome, Crigler-Najjar syndrome, Asian race (Akaba et al., 1998)
  - ◄ Low oral intake of feedings (caloric deprivation)
  - ◄ Prematurity (immature hepatic metabolism)
  - ◄ Breastmilk feedings
- Multifactorial risks
  - ◄ Prematurity
  - ◄ Maternal diabetes
  - ◄ Urinary tract infection (Garcia & Nager, 2002)
  - ◄ Hypothyroidism
  - ◄ G6PD deficiency with Gilbert's syndrome (Kaplan, 2001)
  - ◄ Asian race (Young et al., 2001)

Bilirubin Encephalopathy

Bilirubin encephalopathy, also known as kernicterus, is a form of brain damage resulting from the entry of unconjugated bilirubin into the brain (Shapiro et al., 2006; Volpe, 2001). The damage to neurons occurs only in certain regions of the brain stem and cerebellum, particularly the basal ganglia. The initial presentation of bilirubin encephalopathy is characterized by lethargy, poor feeding, vomiting, and irregular respiration. This early stage may be reversible with prompt removal of bilirubin from the circulation and brain by exchange transfusion. If severe hyperbilirubinemia continues, the infant then manifests more severe neurologic signs characterized by opisthotonus (retrocollis), increased extensor tone of the extremities, high-pitched cry, fever, and seizures. While some infants may die in this stage, with modern intensive care most infants with bilirubin encephalopathy survive (Bhutani et al., 2005; Harris et al., 2001). Survivors of this more severe stage of bilirubin encephalopathy almost always have significant permanent neurologic damage, characterized by choreoathetoid cerebral palsy, deafness, and paralysis of upward gaze of the eyes. In the more severe forms of this disorder, the child will not be able to sit, stand, walk, swallow, talk, or have any purposeful movements of the extremities. Despite the severity of the motor disability, these children often have normal intellectual function, probably because the cerebral cortex is not affected by bilirubin.

It was believed by many that this devastating outcome of hyperbilirubinemia was no longer of concern following the introduction of preventive treatment for severe hemolytic disease of the newborn secondary to Rh incompatibility, which was a common cause of severe hyperbilirubinemia in the past. Reports of infants with this condition have made it evident that bilirubin encephalopathy continues to occur (Centers for Disease Control and Prevention, 2001), especially in (1) breastfed infants, (2) infants who may weigh as much as full-term infants but whose gestational age is less than 38 weeks, and (3) infants with large internal hemorrhage such as cephalhematomas.

An informal kernicterus registry at the University of Pennsylvania suggested that there was a rise in incidence of this devastating outcome (Johnson et al., 2002). The cause of the rise was considered multifactorial. As a result of some articles in the pediatric literature, many pediatricians and others had adopted a more liberal and permissive approach to elevated bilirubin levels. Furthermore, it was suspected that early hospital discharge of newborns combined with an increase in the number who were breastfed, without timely follow-up within the first few days after discharge, were contributing factors. Newborns were being sent home before feedings were established, without adequate assessment for the risk of significant jaundice and without appropriate and timely follow-up (Johnson et al., 2002).

For a given neonate, it is not known at what level of bilirubin, and for what duration of exposure to that level, kernicterus may occur. Certain factors may increase the risk, in addition to the level of serum bilirubin. The form of bilirubin that crosses into the brain is unconjugated bilirubin that is not bound to plasma proteins, so-called free bilirubin. Low concentrations of serum albumin or the presence in sera of any substance that competes with bilirubin for albumin-binding sites may increase the risk of free bilirubin being available to enter the brain. This mechanism was first recognized in the 1950s (Harris et al., 1958) when an association was found between prophylactic sulfisoxazole antibiotic usage in preterm neonates and kernicterus. Sulfisoxazole competes with unconjugated bilirubin for albumin-binding sites and can displace bilirubin, which then may enter the brain. Benzyl alcohol, which at one time was used frequently as a preservative in parenteral medications for newborns in intensive care nurseries, may have had the same effect. Some medications for newborns may still contain benzyl alcohol as a preservative.

The potential for displacement of bilirubin from albumin-binding sites must be considered whenever a medication is prescribed for a newborn. Sulfisoxazole (Gantrisin) administered to infants was recognized as a major cause of kernicterus in infants with hyperbilirubinemia due to its competitive binding with bilirubin on albumin (Odell et al., 1969). The commonly used antibiotic, ceftriaxone, competes for bilirubin-binding sites on albumin (Martin et al., 1993), although no cases of kernicterus are known to have been attributed to this drug.

Hemolysis also appears to increase the risk of kernicterus, although the mechanism underlying this effect remains undefined. In addition, factors affecting the integrity of the blood–brain barrier, such as asphyxia, acidosis, sepsis, or prematurity, may increase this risk. Although one must always consider the potential effect on the jaundiced neonate of drugs in breastmilk, all drugs commonly given to mothers on a prenatal or postpartum basis are safe with regard to neonatal jaundice, with the important exception of nalidixic acid, nitrofurantoin, sulfapyridine, and sulfisoxazole in mothers of infants with G6PD deficiency, because of the risk of hemolysis in the neonate (American Academy of Pediatrics [AAP], 2001). Maternal ingestion of fava beans is also dangerous to the breastfed neonate with G6PD deficiency because it is excreted in breastmilk and can cause hemolysis. Naphthalene mothballs and flakes should not be used in the home or in the clothes of any neonate because of the potential for vapors from these agents to produce hemolysis in infants with G6PD deficiency (Kaplan & Hammerman, 2004; Kaplan et al., 2000, 2001, 2004, 2005, 2006).

Recent studies have suggested that G6PD deficiency in newborns results in severe hyperbilirubinemia only when there is severe hemolysis due to exposure to an inciting hemolytic agent with gross hemolysis or when the infant with G6PD deficiency also has a second inherited factor that reduces the capacity of the liver to conjugate bilirubin, such as abnormalities in the promoter region of the gene responsible for production of glucuronyl transferase, the hepatic-conjugating enzyme (Gilbert's syndrome). In the latter group of infants, hemolysis may not be evident because it is relatively mild. Other investigators have also suggested that G6PD deficiency may in some way reduce the capacity of the liver to metabolize bilirubin. Although G6PD deficiency is relatively common worldwide, relatively few infants with it develop severe hyperbilirubinemia. Even so, it has been recommended that newborn screening for G6PD deficiency be made a routine diagnostic procedure for all jaundiced neonates.

Evaluation of Jaundice

As noted earlier, it is currently recommended by experts that all neonates be screened for their level of bilirubin prior to hospital discharge (Johnson et al., 2002). The serum bilirubin concentration combined with evaluation for various risk factors will provide guidance for future management (AAP, 2004; Newman et al., 2005).

With the availability of transcutaneous devices for the noninvasive measurement of serum bilirubin that have been shown to be as accurate as routine laboratory methods for bilirubin screening (Felc, 2005; Rubaltelli et al., 2001), this testing can be performed rapidly at the bedside. If the transcutaneous reading is 15 mg/dL or higher, confirmation with a serum bilirubin level is recommended (Bhutani et al., 2000). Every newborn should have a risk assessment for factors that might increase future bilirubin levels and a transcutaneous bilirubin before discharge. This combination of predischarge assessments is highly predictive of future need for phototherapy and other management for reduction of hyperbilirubinemia (Bhutani et al., 2013). If the bilirubin level plotted on the nomogram is at or above the 75th percentile, the neonate is at risk for significant hyperbilirubinemia and will need careful assessment; delay of hospital discharge may be appropriate.

Every hospital using transcutaneous bilirubin devices should calibrate the instrument against its standard laboratory measurement of serum bilirubin in a series of babies before relying upon the device. Variations in accuracy may occur with different providers and with infants of different ages, skin color, and physical condition. The transcutaneous bilirubin device should be used as a screening tool, and elevated levels should always be confirmed with a serum bilirubin determination.

Diagnostic Assessment

Having established that the neonate has, or is at risk for, significant hyperbilirubinemia according to the nomogram of bilirubin level for hours of age, consideration must be given to the cause of the jaundice. Therapy will be guided, to some extent, by the cause. Most cases of hyperbilirubinemia are caused, at least in part, by increased bilirubin production from hemoglobin degradation (hemolysis) (Stevenson et al., 2001). It is important to identify hemolysis because it may lead to very high levels of bilirubin and/or significant anemia. Hemolysis is also associated with an increased risk for bilirubin encephalopathy at all elevated serum bilirubin levels.

Traditional hematological tests (hematocrit, reticulocyte count, blood smear, direct antiglobulin [DAT; Coombs'] test) are generally not very helpful in making a diagnosis of hemolysis in the neonate (Herschel et al., 2002; Newman & Easterling, 1994). A clinical technique that is noninvasive and simple for estimating the rate of bilirubin production (hemolysis) is measurement of exhaled end-tidal carbon monoxide (CO), corrected for ambient CO (ETCOc) (Vreman et al., 1996). When red blood cells break down, hemoglobin is released. The heme moiety is degraded by an enzyme, heme oxygenase, to release iron, CO, and biliverdin in equimolar amounts. Biliverdin, a water-soluble nontoxic compound, is reduced to unconjugated bilirubin, a fat-soluble compound. CO is excreted as a component of expired breath. Because CO and bilirubin are produced in equimolar quantities, measurement of expired CO provides an indication of the rate of bilirubin production. A device has been developed that can be used to measure ETCOc in newborns at the bedside, quickly and noninvasively. The result obtained with this CO detector is immediately available on a data strip printout and can be plotted on a nomogram of ETCOc levels for hours of age to identify infants with excessive hemolysis.

The advantage of using ETCOc over the Coombs' test is that ETCOc will identify infants with hemolysis due to causes other than isoimmunization (Rh, ABO), such as G6PD enzyme deficiency or red cell membrane defects. Furthermore, a positive Coombs' test may be misleading as to the risk for hemolysis because many neonates with a positive test do not have significant hemolysis (Herschel et al., 2002). Other tests that may be diagnostic of hemolysis in adults are not usually helpful in neonates. The expired carbon monoxide measuring device was, unfortunately, no longer available for purchase at the time of publication of this book. At some time in the future, it may again be commercially produced.

Because the level of bilirubin reflects the balance between production and elimination, one must also consider deficiencies in the elimination of bilirubin in the neonate with hyperbilirubinemia. A common underlying cause of increased hyperbilirubinemia in the newborn is a variation in the promoter region of the gene for the conjugating enzyme (glucuronyl transferase) UGT1A1 that results in decreased activity of the conjugating enzyme. When it occurs by itself, this disorder is asymptomatic, although affected individuals may have mild unconjugated hyperbilirubinemia (Gilbert's syndrome); when it occurs in combination with even mild hemolysis or with starvation, however, bilirubin becomes significantly elevated. It has been shown that neonatal hyperbilirubinemia due to G6PD deficiency occurs in those neonates who also have Gilbert's syndrome (Kaplan, 2001).

Another reason for decreased elimination of bilirubin is an increase in the enterohepatic circulation of bilirubin (intestinal absorption) due to insufficient caloric intake (starvation jaundice) or, more commonly, due to ingestion of mature human milk (breastmilk jaundice). Increased weight loss and decreased weight gain in the first 2 weeks of life are strongly associated with increased serum bilirubin concentrations and risk for more severe hyperbilirubinemia (Chen et al., 2012).

Management of Jaundice

The reader is referred to the recent Protocol #22 of the Academy of Breastfeeding Medicine (Academy of Breastfeeding Medicine Protocol Committee, 2010), the American Academy of Pediatrics' (2004) *Clinical Practice Guideline on Management of Hyperbilirubinemia in the Newborn Infant 35 or More Weeks of Gestation*, and the technical report that accompanies the latter clinical practice guideline (Ip et al., 2004) for a detailed discussion of the management of neonatal jaundice. An update and clarification of these guidelines has been published more recently and should be consulted as well (Maisels et al., 2009).

The management of hyperbilirubinemia will depend to some extent on the cause, but ultimately reflects the level of bilirubin and the condition of the neonate. If the neonate is less than 38 weeks' gestation or has hemolysis or other medical problems, the bilirubin level for initiating phototherapy may be somewhat lower than if the neonate is full term, is healthy, and does not have any type of hemolytic disease (Figure 11-2) (AAP, 2004). Very high or rapidly rising bilirubin levels may

Figure 11-2 GUIDELINES FOR PHOTOTHERAPY.

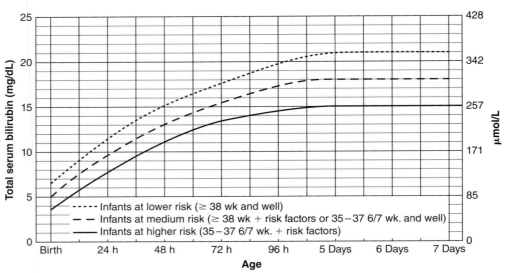

- Use total bilirubin. Do not subtract direct reacting or conjugated bilirubin.
- Risk factors = isoimmune hemolytic disease, G6PD deficiency, asphyxia, significant lethargy, temperature instability, sepsis, acidosis, or albumin < 3.0g/dL (if measured).
- For well infants 35 – 37 6/7 wk can adjust TSB levels for intervention around the medium risk line. It is an option to intervene at lower TSB levels for infants closer to 35 wks and at higher TSB levels for those closer to 37 6/7 wk.
- It is an option to provide conventional phototherapy in hospital or at home at TSB levels 2 – 3 mg/dL (35 – 50 μmol/L) below those shown but home phototherapy should not be used in any infant with risk factors.

Source: Reproduced with permission from Pediatrics, Vol. 114, Page(s) 297–316, Copyright ? 2004 by the AAP.

need to be controlled with an exchange transfusion (Figure 11-3), in which case feedings would be temporarily interrupted for the procedure. Neonates who are treated only with phototherapy should continue to be breastfed or receive other milk feedings, as good caloric intake improves the effectiveness of phototherapy.

Phototherapy of hyperbilirubinemia is based on the knowledge that light of a wavelength in the blue spectrum (450–500 nanometers) is absorbed by bilirubin and results in a change in the structure of the bilirubin molecule such that the fat-soluble, unconjugated bilirubin becomes water soluble without having to be conjugated in the liver. This stereoisomer of bilirubin, a product of light therapy, can be excreted in the stool and urine without conjugation with glucuronic acid. Phototherapy treatment of jaundice should be reserved for those infants who meet the AAP criteria for intervention (AAP,

2004; Maisels et al., 2009). When phototherapy is indicated, it should be performed intensively so that it is as effective as possible (Maisels, 1996). Home phototherapy does not have a role in treating neonates with significant hyperbilirubinemia who need close and thus frequent monitoring of bilirubin levels and who would otherwise be at risk for exchange transfusion if not properly and effectively managed with light therapy. Infants under phototherapy should be fed orally and do not need intravenous fluids unless they have signs of dehydration (Boo & Lee, 2002). Breastfeeding need not be interrupted; feeding with breastmilk may continue while a baby is in the hospital under light therapy, although the more time the infant spends under the light, the faster the bilirubin will decline. In some instances, the newborn may need to be fed while under phototherapy if the level of bilirubin is high enough that exchange transfusion might become necessary if the

Figure 11-3 GUIDELINES FOR EXCHANGE TRANSFUSION.

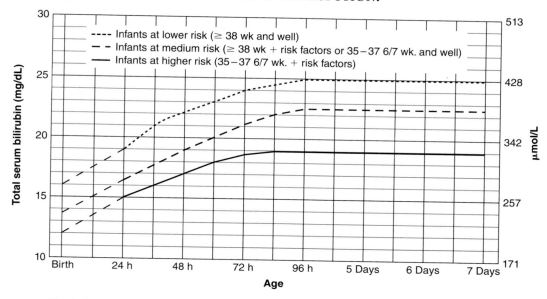

- The dashed lines for the first 24 hours indicate uncertainty due to a wide range of clinical circumstances and a range of responses to phototherapy.
- Immediate exchange transfusion is recommended if infant shows signs of acute bilirubin encephalopathy (hypertonia, arching, retrocollis, opisthotonos, fever, high-pitched cry) or if TSB is ≥ 5 mg/dL (85 μmol/L) above these lines.
- Risk factors—isoimmune hemolytic disease, G6PD deficiency, asphyxia, significant lethargy, temperature instability, sepsis, acidosis.
- Measure serum albumin and calculate B/A ratio (see legend).
- Use total bilirubin. Do not subtract direct reacting or conjugated bilirubin.
- If infant is well and 35–37 6/7 wk (median risk) can individualize TSB levels for exchange based on actual gestational age.

Source: Reproduced with permission from Pediatrics, Vol. 114, Page(s) 297–316, Copyright ? 2004 by the AAP.

hyperbilirubinemia cannot be lowered. In that case, the mother could pump and feed breastmilk. For most infants under phototherapy, interruptions of light treatment for up to 30 minutes every 2 to 3 hours will not significantly reduce the effectiveness of the phototherapy.

ACKNOWLEDGMENT

Marguerite Herschel, MD, was the original first author of this chapter in the third edition of this book. Sadly, Dr. Herschel died shortly after publication of that edition. Dr. Herschel was a marvelous and dedicated teacher and clinical researcher. Her research on neonatal jaundice is noted in this chapter.

SUMMARY

The diagnosis, assessment, and management of neonatal jaundice should take place within the context of the breastfeeding. While jaundice and breastfeeding are known to be associated, one must be very careful not to convey the wrong message to the mother and her family that breastfeeding is potentially dangerous or harmful to her baby. Mothers commonly feel guilty when their infants experience neonatal jaundice, believing they have caused the baby to be jaundiced (Hannon et al., 2001).

As emphasized in this chapter, a careful evaluation for the etiology of the hyperbilirubinemia must be made, with jaundice associated with breastfeeding being considered as a diagnosis of exclusion. In any case, regardless of the cause, breastfeeding must be optimized and supported. This often requires that the hospital caregivers not make remarks to mothers that they should supplement their babies with formula. The nurses and lactation specialists on all shifts must be knowledgeable in helping babies and their mothers achieve a proper latch and feed frequently. They should also encourage mothers to speak up to get help. Caregivers must know the right questions to ask mothers to assess the adequacy of the breastfeeding and must be able to make careful direct observations of feedings, the patterns of stools, and weight loss or gain. At least twice a day, a formal evaluation of breastfeeding for position, latch, and milk transfer should be made by a knowledgeable healthcare provider. The results of these assessments must be recorded in the infant's medical record.

Neonates with jaundice who are breastfed, just as newborns with jaundice who are artificially fed, should be approached in a global manner in the diagnostic evaluation and management of the jaundice. This will ensure the optimal outcome for the neonate and family.

KEY CONCEPTS

- Jaundice, a yellow discoloration of the sclerae and skin, is caused by the deposition of bilirubin in those tissues. Bilirubin is a product of red blood cell—specifically hemoglobin—breakdown.
- Physiologic jaundice is a common clinical condition in the majority of newborn infants that generally resolves within the first week of life in the term artificial-milk-fed neonate. Approximately 60% of all newborns will have some jaundice in the first week of life. Nearly all newborns will have some elevation of serum bilirubin concentration compared with adult normal values.
- Breastmilk jaundice, which is characterized by prolongation of physiologic jaundice, is a normal manifestation in at least one-third of breastfed infants. Approximately two-thirds

of all breastfed infants will have an elevation of serum bilirubin concentration.
- Inadequate breastfeeding may lead to jaundice, particularly in the first few days of life, but not on day 1. This condition is the neonatal manifestation of the adult disorder, starvation jaundice.
- Despite the known association of jaundice and breastfeeding, other causes for jaundice must be ruled out before attributing jaundice solely to breastfeeding.
- The level of bilirubin in a neonate resulting in neonatal jaundice is determined by the balance between production and elimination of bilirubin.
- Increased production of bilirubin, owing to increased red cell breakdown (hemolysis), may lead to very high levels of bilirubin.
- Extreme hyperbilirubinemia may result in permanent brain damage, known as bilirubin encephalopathy (kernicterus).
- To prevent severe hyperbilirubinemia and the tragic outcome of kernicterus, all neonates should be screened for bilirubin level prior to hospital discharge. Adequate breastfeeding must be documented prior to discharge. Follow-up with a healthcare provider must take place at 3 to 5 days of age or 1 to 3 days after discharge. At that visit, jaundice and breastfeeding must be assessed.

INTERNET RESOURCES

American Academy of Pediatrics. Practice guideline: management of hyperbilirubinemia in the newborn infant 35 or more weeks of gestation: http://www.aap.org (Keyword: jaundice)

REFERENCES

Academy of Breastfeeding Medicine Protocol Committee (Gartner LM, ed.). Protocol #22: guidelines for management of jaundice in the breastfeeding infant equal to or greater than 35 weeks gestation. *Breastfeed Med.* 2010;5:87–93.

Akaba K, Kimura T, Sasaki A, et al. Neonatal hyperbilirubinemia and mutation of the bilirubin uridine diphosphate-glucuronosyltransferase gene: a common missense mutation among Japanese, Koreans and Chinese. *Biochem Mol Biol Int.* 1998;46:21–26.

Alonso EM, Whitington PF, Whitington SH, et al. Enterohepatic circulation of nonconjugated bilirubin in rats fed with human milk. *J Pediatr.* 1991;118:425–430.

American Academy of Pediatrics (AAP). Clinical practice guideline on management of hyperbilirubinemia in the newborn infant 35 or more weeks of gestation. *Pediatrics.* 2004;114:297–316.

American Academy of Pediatrics (AAP), Committee on Drugs. The transfer of drugs and other chemicals into human milk. *Pediatrics.* 2001;108:776–789.

Arias IM, Gartner Lm, Seifter S, Furman M. Prolonged neonatal unconjugated hyperbilirubinemia associated with breast feeding and a steroid, pregnane-3(alpha), 20(beta)-diol, in maternal milk that inhibits glucuronide formation in vitro. *J Clin Invest.* 1964;43: 2037–2047.

Bhutani VK, Johnson LH, Keren R. Treating acute bilirubin encephalopathy before it's too late. *Contemp Pediatr.* 2005;22(5):57–74.

Bhutani VK, Johnson L, Sivieri EM. Predictive ability of a predischarge hour-specific serum bilirubin for subsequent significant hyperbilirubinemia in healthy term and near-term newborns. *Pediatrics.* 1999;103:6–14.

Bhutani VK, Stark AR, Lazzeroni LC, et al. Predischarge screening for severe neonatal hyperbilirubinemia identifies infants who need phototherapy. *J Pediatr.* 2013;162:477–482.

Bhutani VK, Gourley GR, Adler S, et al. Noninvasive measurement of total serum bilirubin in a multiracial predischarge newborn population to assess the risk of severe hyperbilirubinemia. *Pediatrics.* 2000;106:e17.

Boo NY, Lee HT. Randomized controlled trial of oral versus intravenous fluid supplementation on serum bilirubin level during phototherapy of term infants with severe hyperbilirubinemia. *J Paediatr Child Health.* 2002;38:151–155.

Brown WR, Wong HB. Ethnic group differences in plasma bilirubin levels of full-term, healthy Singapore newborns. *Pediatrics.* 1965;336:745–751.

Centers for Disease Control and Prevention. Kernicterus in full-term infants, United States, 1994–1998. *MMWR.* 2001;50:491–494.

Chen YJ, Chen WC, Chen CM. Risk factors for hyperbilirubinemia in breastfed term neonates. *Eur J Pediatr.* 2012;171:167–171.

de Carvalho M, Robertson S, Klaus M. Fecal bilirubin excretion and serum bilirubin concentrations in breast-fed and bottle-fed infants. *J Pediatr.* 1985;107:786–790.

Dennery PA, Seidman DS, Stevenson DK. Neonatal hyperbilirubinemia. *N Engl J Med.* 2001;344:581–590.

Dore S, Takahashi M, Ferris CD, et al. Bilirubin, formed by activation of heme oxygenase-2, protects neurons against oxidative stress injury. *Proc Natl Acad Sci USA.* 1999;96:2445–2450.

Felc Z. Improvement of conventional transcutaneous bilirubinometry results in term newborn infants. *Am J Perinatol.* 2005;22:173–179.

Garcia FJ, Nager AL. Jaundice as an early diagnostic sign of urinary tract infection in infancy. *Pediatrics.* 2002;109:846–851.

Gartner LM. Breastfeeding and jaundice. *J Perinatol.* 2001;21:S25–S29.

Gartner LM, Herschel M. Jaundice and breastfeeding. *Pediatr Clin North Am.* 2001;48:389–399.

Gartner LM, Lee KS. Jaundice and liver disease. In: Fanaroff AA, Martin RJ, eds. *Neonatal–perinatal medicine: diseases of the fetus and infant.* St. Louis, MO: Mosby–Year Book, 1992:1075–1104.

Gartner LM, Lee KS, Moscioni AD. Effect of milk feeding on intestinal bilirubin absorption in the rat. *J Pediatr.* 1983;103:464–471.

Gebara BM, Everett KO. Dural sinus thrombosis complicating hypernatremic dehydration in a breastfed neonate. *Clin Pediatr.* 2001;40:45–48.

Hammerman C, Goldschmidt D, Caplan MS, et al. Protective effect of bilirubin in ischemia-reperfusion injury in the rat intestine. *J Pediatr Gastro Nutr.* 2002;35:344–349.

Hannon PR, Willis SK, Scrimshaw SC. Persistence of maternal concerns surrounding neonatal jaundice. *Arch Pediatr Adolesc Med.* 2001;155:1357–1363.

Harris MC, Bernbaum JC, Polin JR, et al. Developmental follow-up of breastfed term and near-term infants with marked hyperbilirubinemia. *Pediatrics.* 2001;107:1075–1080.

Harris RC, Lucey JF, Maclean JR. Kernicterus in premature infants associated with low concentrations of bilirubin in the plasma. *Pediatrics.* 1958;21:875–884.

Herschel M, Karrison T, Wen M, et al. Evaluation of the direct antiglobulin (Coombs') test for identifying newborns at-risk for hemolysis as determined by end-tidal carbon monoxide concentration (ETCOc) and comparison of the Coombs' test with ETCOc for detecting significant jaundice. *J Perinatol.* 2002;22:341–347.

Hunt SC, Wu LL, Hopkins PN, Williams RR. Evidence for a major gene elevating serum bilirubin concentration in Utah pedigrees. *Arterioscler Thromb Vasc Biol.* 1996;16:912–917.

Ip S, Chung M, Kulig J, et al. An evidence-based review of important issues concerning neonatal hyperbilirubinemia. *Pediatrics.* 2004;114:e130–e153.

Johnson LH, Bhutani VK, Brown AK. System-based approached to management of neonatal jaundice and prevention of kernicterus. *J Pediatr.* 2002;40:396–403.

Kaplan M. Genetic interactions in the pathogenesis of neonatal hyperbilirubinemia: Gilbert's syndrome and glucose-6-phosphate dehydrogenase deficiency. *J Perinatol.* 2001;21:S30–S34.

Kaplan M, Algur N, Hammerman C. Onset of jaundice in glucose-6-phosphate dehydrogenase-deficient neonates. *Pediatrics.* 2001;108:956–959.

Kaplan M, Hammerman C. Glucose-6-phosphate dehydrogenase deficiency: a hidden risk for kernicterus. *Semin Perinatol.* 2004;28:356–364.

Kaplan M, Hammerman C, Feldman R, Brisk R. Predischarge bilirubin screening in glucose-6-phosphate dehydrogenase-deficient neonates. *Pediatrics.* 2000;105:533–537.

Kaplan M, Hammerman C, Maisels MJ. Bilirubin genetics for the nongeneticist: hereditary defects of neonatal bilirubin conjugation. *Pediatrics.* 2003;111:886–891.

Kaplan M, Herschel M, Hammerman C, et al. Hyperbilirubinemia among African American, glucose-6-phosphate dehydrogenase-deficient neonates. *Pediatrics.* 2004;114:e213–e219.

Kaplan M, Herschel M, Hammerman C, et al. Neonatal hyperbilirubinemia in African American males: the importance of glucose-6-phosphate dehydrogenase deficiency. *J Pediatr.* 2006;149:83–88.

Kaplan M, Hoyer JD, Herschel M, et al. Glucose-6-phosphate dehydrogenase activity in term and near-term male African American neonates. *Clinica Chimica Acta.* 2005;355:113–117.

Maisels MJ. Why use homeopathic doses of phototherapy? *Pediatrics.* 1996;98:283–287.

Maisels MJ, Bhutani VK, Bogen D, et al. Hyperbilirubinemia in the newborn infant greater than 35 weeks gestation: an update with clarifications. *Pediatrics.* 2009;124:1193–1198.

Maisels MJ, Newman TB. Jaundice in full-term and near-term babies who leave the hospital within 36 hours: the pediatrician's nemesis. *Clin Perinatol.* 1998;25:295–302.

Martin E, Fanconi S, Kälin P, et al. Ceftriaxone–bilirubin–albumin interactions in the neonate: an in vivo study. *Eur J Pediatr.* 1993;152:530–534.

Maruo Y, Nishizawa K, Sato H, et al. Association of neonatal hyperbilirubinemia with bilirubin UDP-glucuronosyltransferase polymorphism. *Pediatrics.* 1999;103:1224–1227.

Maruo Y, Nishizawa K, Sato H, et al. Prolonged unconjugated hyperbilirubinemia associated with breast milk and mutations of the bilirubin uridine diphosphate-glucuronosyltransferase gene. *Pediatrics.* 2000;106:e59.

Monaghan G, McLellan A, McGeehan A, et al. Gilbert's syndrome is a contributory factor in prolonged unconjugated hyperbilirubinemia of the newborn. *J Pediatr.* 1999;134:441–446.

Moyer VA, Ahn C, Sneed S. Accuracy of clinical judgment in neonatal jaundice. *Arch Pediatr Adolesc Med.* 2000;154:391–394.

Neifert MR. The optimization of breast-feeding in the perinatal period. *Clin Perinatol.* 1998;25:303–326.

Newman AJ, Gross S. Hyperbilirubinemia in breast-fed infants. *Pediatrics.* 1963;32:995–1001.

Newman TB, Easterling MJ. Yield of reticulocyte counts and blood smears in term neonates. *Clin Pediatr.* 1994;33:71–76.

Newman TB, Liljestrand P, Escobar GJ. Combining risk factors with serum bilirubin levels to predict hyperbilirubinemia in newborns. *Arch Pediatr Adolesc Med.* 2005;159:113–119.

Odell GB, Cohen SN, Kelly PC. Studies in kernicterus. II. The determination of the saturation of serum albumin with bilirubin. *J Pediatr.* 1969;74:214–230.

Rubaltelli FF. Unconjugated and conjugated bilirubin pigments during perinatal development. IV. The influence of breast-feeding on neonatal hyperbilirubinemia. *Biol Neonate.* 1993;64:104–109.

Rubaltelli FF, Gourley GR, Loskamp N, et al. Transcutaneous bilirubin measurement: a multicenter evaluation of a new device. *Pediatrics.* 2001;107:1264–1271.

Sato H, Uchida T, Toyota K, et al. Association of breast-fed neonatal hyperbilirubinemia with UGT1A1 polymorphisms: 211G>A (G71R) mutation becomes a risk factor under inadequate feeding. *J Hum Genet.* 2013;58:7–10.

Schwertner HA, Jackson WG, Tolan G. Association of low serum concentration of bilirubin with increased risk of coronary artery disease. *Clin Chem.* 1994;40:18–23.

Shapiro SM, Bhutani VK, Johnson L. Hyperbilirubinemia and kernicterus. *Clin Perinatol.* 2006;33:387–410.

Shurin SB. The blood and hematopoietic system. In: Fanaroff AA, Martin RJ, eds. *Neonatal–perinatal medicine: diseases of the fetus and infant.* St. Louis, MO: Mosby–Year Book; 1992:941–989.

Stevenson DK, Dennery PA, Hinz SR. Understanding newborn jaundice. *J Perinatol.* 2001;21:S21–S24.

Stiehm ER, Ryan J. Breast-milk jaundice. *Am J Dis Child.* 1965;109:212–216.

Stocker R, Yamamoto Y, McDonagh AF, et al. Bilirubin is an antioxidant of possible physiological importance. *Science.* 1987;235:1043–1046.

Temme EH, Zhang J, Schouten EG, Kesteloot H. Serum bilirubin and 10-year mortality risk in a Belgian population. *Cancer Causes Control.* 2001;12:887–894.

Vítek L, Jirsa M, Brodanová M, et al. Gilbert syndrome and ischemic heart disease: a protective effect of elevated bilirubin levels. *Atherosclerosis.* 2002;160:449–456.

Volpe JJ. *Neurology of the newborn,* 4th ed. Philadelphia, PA: WB Saunders; 2001:521–546.

Vreman HJ, Baxter LM, Stone RT, Stevenson DK. Evaluation of a fully automated end-tidal carbon monoxide instrument for breath analysis. *Clin Chem.* 1996;42:50–56.

Whitmer DI, Gollan JL. Mechanism and significance of fasting and dietary hyperbilirubinemia. *Semin Liver Dis.* 1983;3:42–51.

Young BWY, Chan ML, Ho HT, et al. Predicting pathologic jaundice: the Chinese perspective. *J Perinatol.* 2001;21:S73–S75.

Breast Pumps and Other Technologies

Chapter 12

Marsha Walker

Special devices have been used for hundreds of years to help breastfeeding mothers overcome various problems. Examples of someone, or something, other than a baby removing milk from the breasts are cited in medical literature as early as the mid-1500s (Fildes, 1986). Before breast pumps or other instruments were used to withdraw milk from the breasts, children, young puppies, or birth attendants were enlisted to do the job. By the 1500s, the medical literature included discussions of "sucking glasses." These devices allowed women to remove milk themselves and were recommended for relieving engorgement or expressing milk when the nipples were damaged or when mastitis was present. Sucking glasses were also thought to help evert flat and inverted nipples. For the most part, a vacuum was generated by mouth, and the devices were made of glass (Figure 12-1). Women could use a glass, glass vial, or glass bottle heated with very hot water and applied to the breast to draw out milk. French breast pumps in the 1700s resembled smoking pipes.

As technology advanced, so did breast pump materials and designs. Combinations of materials such as brass, wood, glass, pewter, and rubber were used to make pumps like the syringe pump (Figure 12-2), the long-handled lever pump (Figure 12-3), and the syringe pump with pewter flanges (Figure 12-4).

Figure 12-1 AN AMERICAN SUCKING GLASS, CIRCA 1870.

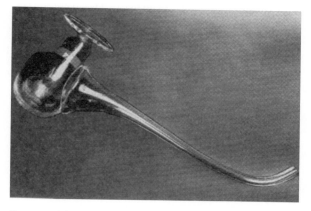

Courtesy of Canon Babysafe Ltd., Suffolk, England/Courtesy of Hollister/Ameda-Egnell

Women pump their breasts for short periods of time to solve acute problems or to donate to a human milk bank, and for extended periods to provide human milk for their babies under such circumstances as employment, induced lactation, re-lactation, compromised milk supply, maternal or infant illness, or following a preterm birth. Win et al. (2006) reported that in a study of 587 mothers, those who expressed breast milk at one or more time periods were less likely to discontinue breastfeeding

419

Figure 12-2 EXPRESSING THE BREASTS WITH A SYRINGE PUMP, CIRCA 1830.

DRAWING THE BREASTS.

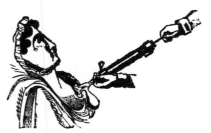

Where the breast is hard, swollen and painful, from inflammation, or the nipple sore from excoriation, the application of this instrument is attended with more ease to the patient than any other means, and she may without difficulty use it herself, by which she can regulate its action agreeably to her own sensations. The flat surface of the glass should be smeared with oil before it is put on, and the bulb preserved in a dependant position to receive the fluid. During the operation the small aperture in the brass socket must be closely covered with the finger, which being removed, admits air into the glass and causes it to be detached from the breast whenever it may be desired.

Courtesy of Canon Babysafe Ltd., Suffolk, England/Courtesy of Hollister/Ameda-Egnell

Figure 12-3 EXPRESSING BREASTMILK WITH A LONG-HANDLED LEVER PUMP, CIRCA 1830.

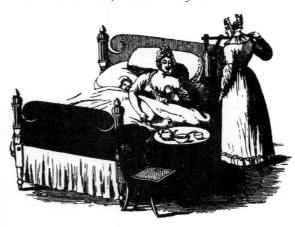

Figure 12-4 PEWTER BREAST PUMP (WEEDON), CIRCA 1830–1856.

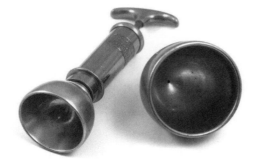

Courtesy of 'Phisick' www.phisick.com

before 6 months. In a more recent study of 903 mothers, almost all (98%) had expressed their milk at some point, with the most frequent reason being insufficient milk or to be able to make more milk (Clemons & Amir, 2010).

Binns et al. (2006) calculated that the proportion of mothers who had expressed breast milk almost doubled in the decade between 1993 and 2003. They attributed this trend to the increased encouragement of exclusive breastfeeding, a possible change in how clinicians managed early breastfeeding problems, and the availability of more efficient breast pumps. The trend for increased breast pump use was also seen in data from the Infant Feeding Practices Study II in the United States: 85% of breastfeeding mothers in the sample of 1564 women had successfully expressed breastmilk since their infant was born (Labiner-Wolfe et al., 2008). In a study by Shealy et al. (2008), 6% of the mothers exclusively pumped their milk, not feeding at the breast at all.

Buckley (2009) conducted a qualitative study of the impact of breast pump technology on lactation consultant practice and on reasons that mothers used a breast pump. A number of themes emerged from this study:

- Many mothers feel that they need a breast pump to successfully breastfeed. References and images of breast pumps flourish as an accepted and normal part of breastfeeding. Mothers see breast pumps on layette lists and on baby registries; receive pumps at baby showers; read about pumps on blogs and Internet review sites; see pump demonstrations in online videos; hear about pumps in prenatal classes; see pumps in hospital gift shops and hospital rooms; and see pumps carried in maternity stores, catalogues, and large toy stores.

- Pumps are often an easy option to turn to for addressing breastfeeding problems on a busy maternity unit that may be understaffed or not have the recommended patient-to-staff ratio of International Board Certified Lactation Consultants (IBCLCs).
- Breast pump usage has increased along with the rise in interventions used during childbirth. Many of these interventions, in combination with the increased acuity of many new mothers and infants, have contributed to the growing use of pumps during the postpartum hospital stay as well as following discharge.
- Pumps may represent a means for mothers to control the feeding situation. Pumps may be used in lieu of assessment by a lactation expert, as experts may not be available or affordable, or the mother may wish to solve problems herself.

The increase in breast pump use has also raised concerns about data quality in research. Mothers may be classified as exclusively breastfeeding in surveys even though they are not exclusively feeding at the breast. Geraghty and colleagues (2012) and Geraghty and Rasmussen (2010) suggested that data collection questions include inquiries regarding pumping and the feeding of expressed milk and that studies be conducted regarding whether expressing and feeding expressed breastmilk have any consequences for the health of mothers and infants.

Concerns of Mothers

Most mothers want a pump that works efficiently and comfortably at a reasonable cost. They want pumps that are easy to find, easy to use, and easy to clean. The amount of milk expressed and the time it takes to obtain it are the two issues most frequently mentioned by mothers when they are choosing or using a breast pump.

Satisfaction with breast pumps, however, is highly individual. In an informal survey conducted with more than 200 mothers (Walker, 1992), a pump was rated highly if it (1) worked quickly— (less than 20 minutes total), (2) obtained 2 or more ounces of milk from each breast, and (3) did not cause pain. The mothers in this survey suggested pumping techniques to speed the process and to increase the volume of milk per pumping session. Many mothers expressed the most milk before or after the first morning feeding when the breasts were reported to be fullest (and intramammary pressure was the highest); later volumes steadily decreased throughout the day. Many mothers mentioned that if they were not relaxed, or if they were uncomfortable or felt rushed, their output dropped by one-third to one-half of the usual amount.

The majority of mothers used one or more techniques to increase pumping efficiency (Walker, 1992). The two most frequently mentioned techniques were eliciting the milk-ejection reflex before starting to pump and massaging the breast while pumping. Both techniques increased pumping speed and milk output. Some mothers were able to double the amount pumped by using both of these techniques at each pumping session. Other techniques and concerns mentioned by mothers include the importance of reducing stress during pumping and how long to actually pump during each pumping session.

Elicit the Milk-Ejection Reflex First

It is interesting to note that in dairy cows, massaging the udder with a hot, wet cloth for 1 to 2 minutes before pumping begins is an effective stimulus for initiating the letdown reflex. This is done to minimize the time needed to extract milk. Human mothers have reported that using hot compresses, taking a hot shower, and breast massage before pumping help elicit the letdown reflex. Some mothers report that they are most successful if they pump one side while the baby feeds on the other breast (as with pumping in dairy cattle when all teats are milked simultaneously); if the baby elicits the milk-ejection reflex first and the mother then pumps; or if they hand-express first or massage the breast first and then pump.

Yigit and colleagues (2012) reported that significantly more milk was expressed from breasts that had been warmed prior to pumping by placement of a hot compress around the breast. Similarly, Kent and colleagues (2011) reported that use of a warmed breast shield during pumping (flange on the collection kit) resulted in a decreased amount of time necessary to remove 80% of the total milk yield and increased the percentage of available milk removed after 5 minutes of expression. It is not known whether the improved milk flow resulted from a warmed breast or a warmed nipple/areolar complex improving milk duct dilation, relaxing smooth muscles in the nipple, or relieving constrictions in the milk ducts.

Upon nipple stimulation, oxytocin is released in a pulsatile nature consisting of brief 3- to 4-second bursts of oxytocin into the bloodstream every 5 to 15 minutes. This shortens and widens the lactiferous ducts, increasing the pressure inside the breast, and is essential for maximum removal of milk from the breast (Neville, 2001). Correlations between oxytocin pulsatility on day 2 and the duration of exclusive breastfeeding suggest that development of an early pulsatile oxytocin pattern is of importance for sustained exclusive breastfeeding (Nissen et al., 1996). Oxytocin can also be released prior to the baby being placed at breast and is not solely dependent on tactile stimulation for release. It takes the baby between 54 and 60 seconds to elicit the milk-ejection reflex on the first side and 47 seconds on the second side, on average. Older research indicated that some pumps can take up to 4 minutes to elicit the milk-ejection reflex (mean 103.2 seconds ± 89.2 seconds) (Kent et al., 2003; Mitoulas et al., 2002). More recent studies using a Medela Symphony pump show that the time the pump takes to stimulate the first milk ejection as detected by breast ultrasound is approximately 90 seconds (Ramsay et al., 2006). Some pumps are electronically programmed to "stimulate" milk ejection by initially providing low vacuum and rapid cycling, then switching to a higher vacuum and lower cycling.

Massage the Breast During Pumping

Massaging during breast pumping can markedly increase milk yield. Breast massage may increase fat content and milk yield when a baby is at breast. Bowles, Stutte, and Hensley (1988) and Stutte, Bowles, and Morman (1988) found that infants gained greater amounts of weight and mothers experienced little nipple pain or painful engorgement when the breasts were massaged by quadrant in an alternating pattern with the baby's suckling bursts. Breast massage represents a form of positive pressure, which adds to the pressure created within the milk ducts during letdown, as it significantly increases the plasma oxytocin level (Yokoyama et al., 1994). The diameter of the milk ducts increases by approximately 79% after letdown, (Hartmann, 2000) with duct diameters drifting down after a 1- to 2-minute period following letdown (Hartmann, 2002). Morton and colleagues (2009) found that breast massage while pumping contributes to significantly more milk being pumped at each pumping session. Mothers who use a combination of electric pumping, hand expression, and breast massage/compression produce calorie-dense fat-rich milk that can average 26 calories per ounce, something especially important in the feeding of preterm infants.

A pump needs to remove milk quickly before the volume of milk in the ducts decreases and another letdown is necessary to reestablish the pressure gradient between breast and pump. Adding external compression probably acts as an "artificial" letdown, increasing the positive pressure within the breast and helping milk flow toward the negative pressure created in the pump. The establishment of an effective pressure gradient that can be sustained over a long-enough period of time will contribute to the optimal drainage of each breast.

Relaxation to Aid Letdown

As early as 1948, researchers described the adverse effect of a painful or distracting stimulus during nursing on the milk-ejection reflex (Newton & Newton, 1948). Pain and psychological stress can inhibit the milk-ejection reflex by reducing the number of oxytocin pulses during suckling episodes (Ueda et al., 1994). Furthermore, opiate and β-endorphin release during stress can block stimulus-related oxytocin secretion (Lawrence & Lawrence, 2010). Therefore, women may use specific relaxation techniques and visual imagery before and during pumping to facilitate letdown. Feher et al. (1989) reported using a guided relaxation audiotape to increase milk output during breast pumping among mothers of preterm infants. Keith and colleagues (2012) found that mothers of preterm infants who listened to music during pumping produced significantly more milk with higher fat content during the first 6 days of the study.

Stop Pumping as Soon as the Milk Stops Flowing

Many mothers switch to the other breast when the milk flow slows in the breast being pumped. Some mothers mention that pain is the cue for this switch, indicating a change in the pressure gradient. Auerbach (1990b) found that protracted pumping times did not significantly increase milk yield beyond a certain point. Those mothers who pumped (sequentially or simultaneously) for longer than 16 minutes averaged total milk volumes of 55 mL or less. Mitoulas et al., (2002) found that the rate of milk expression changed over the course of a 5-minute expression period, remaining constant during the first 2.5 minutes but decreasing by 5 minutes. The variation among mothers was large, with some mothers delivering almost 2 oz in the first 30 seconds and others delivering no milk by the end of 5 minutes. If it takes a particular mother 4 minutes to elicit the milk-ejection reflex, she may need a much longer time to pump than another mother who delivers 99% of the milk in her breasts within 5 minutes.

Kent and colleagues (2008) showed that mothers achieved a higher milk yield when they used the maximum comfortable vacuum on the pump, with a high milk volume being expressed during the first two milk ejections. These first two milk ejections occurred on average within the first 8 minutes after the beginning of pumping. Subsequent milk ejections resulted in minimal yields. Thus, for many mothers expressing milk, using the maximum comfortable vacuum for 8 minutes (with simultaneous pumping) may be sufficient (Ramsay et al., 2006).

Other Desirable Attributes of Breast Pumps

Breast pumps must be easy to clean, affordable, and accessible. When recommending a pump, the caregiver should give a specific name and several places to find that model to avoid acquisition of a pump that may be inappropriate or ineffective (Figure 12-5). The cost of the accessory kit and daily rental charges for an electric pump can be expensive, even with a long-term rental contract. The Affordable Care Act of 2010 requires insurers to provide breast pumps with no co-pay requirements. Some insurance carriers and health maintenance organizations

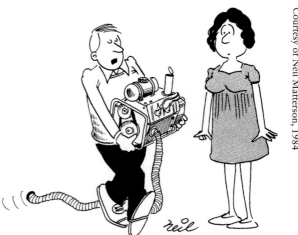

Figure 12-5 "They Didn't Actually Have a Breast Pump..."

Courtesy of Neil Matterson, 1984

cover the cost of pump rentals only while a baby is hospitalized or for only a limited period of time. Some insurers provide inappropriate breast pumps.

Clinicians should check with the insurers in their state to ascertain exactly which pumps are provided in which situations.

Box 12-1 Recommendations for the Nursing Mother Who Uses a Pump

General Pumping Recommendations

1. Read the instructions on the use and cleaning of a pump before expressing milk with any product.
2. Wash hands before each pumping session.
3. Frequency: For occasional pumping, pump during, after, or between feedings, whichever gives the best results.

   Most mothers tend to express more milk in the morning. For mothers employed outside the home, pumping should occur on a regular basis for the number of nursings that are missed.

   For premature or ill babies who are not at breast, the number of pumpings should total 8–10 or more each 24 hours for the first 14 days. Initiation of pumping should be delayed no longer than 6 hours following birth unless medically indicated. This ensures appropriate development and sensitivity of prolactin receptors. More frequent pumping will avoid the build-up of excessive backpressure of milk during engorgement.

4. Duration: With single-sided pumping, duration ranges from 10 to 15 minutes with an electric pump and 10 to 20 minutes with a manual pump. If double pumping with an electric or two battery-operated pumps, 7 to 15 minutes is optimal.

   Encourage mothers to tailor these times to their own situation.

5. Technique:
   - Elicit the milk-ejection reflex before using the pump.
   - Use only as much vacuum as is needed to maintain milk flow and remain comfortable.
   - Massage the breast in quadrants before and during pumping to increase intramammary pressure.
   - Allow enough time for pumping to avoid anxiety.
   - Use inserts or different sized flanges if needed to obtain the best fit between pump and breast.
   - Avoid long periods of uninterrupted vacuum.
   - Stop pumping when the milk flow is minimal or has ceased.

Recommendations for Specific Types of Pumps

1. Avoid pumps that use rubber bulbs to generate a vacuum.
2. Cylinder pumps:
   - When O rings are used, they must be in place for proper suction.
   - Gaskets must be removed after each use for cleaning to avoid harboring bacteria in the pump.
   - The gasket on the inner cylinder may be rolled back and forth to restore it to its original shape.
   - The pump stroke may need to be shortened as the outer cylinder fills with milk.

- The mother may need to empty the outer cylinder once or twice during pumping.
- Hand position should be palm up with the elbow held close to the body.

3. Battery-operated pumps:
   - Use alkaline batteries, not rechargable batteries.
   - Replace batteries when cycles per minute decrease.
   - Interrupt vacuum frequently to avoid nipple pain and damage if the pump does not autocycle.
   - Use an AC adapter when possible, especially if the pump generates fewer than 6 cycles per minute.
   - Consider purchasing or renting an electric pump for pumping that will continue for longer than 1 or 2 months.
   - Use two pumps simultaneously if pumping time is limited or to increase the quantity of milk obtained.
   - Choose a pump in which the vacuum can be regulated.
   - Massage the breast by quadrants during pumping.

4. Semi-automatic pumps:
   - Vacuum may be easier to control if the mother does not lift her finger completely off the hole but rolls it back and forth rhythmically so that the vacuum is efficient but not painful.

5. Automatic electric pumps:
   - Use the lowest pressure setting that is efficient. Mothers may find that changing the vacuum and/or the cycling characteristics of the pump during each expressing session may increase milk volume.
   - Use a double setup (simultaneous pumping) when time is limited in order to increase a milk supply, as well as for prematurity, maternal or infant illness, or other special situations.

Hormonal Considerations

When milk expression using a pump is necessary, the device used must be efficient enough to activate prolactin and oxytocin release sufficiently to remove milk from the breasts.

Prolactin

A steady rise in prolactin during pregnancy prepares the breasts for lactation (Neville, 1983). Prolactin levels rise during pregnancy from about 10 ng/mL in the non-pregnant state to approximately 200 ng/mL at term. Baseline levels do not drop to normal in a lactating woman, but average about 100 ng/mL at 3 months postpartum and 50 ng/mL at 6 months. Prolactin levels can double with the stimulus of suckling. After about 6 months of breastfeeding, the prolactin rise with suckling amounts to only 5 to 10 ng/mL. This is accounted for by the increased prolactin-binding capacity or sensitivity of the mammary tissue, which allows full lactation in the face of falling prolactin levels over time. The high levels of prolactin during pregnancy and early lactation may also serve to increase the number of prolactin receptors and are dependent on tactile input for stimulation and release. In spite of the importance of prolactin to lactation itself, this hormone does not directly regulate the short-term or long-term rate of milk synthesis (Cox et al., 1996). Once lactation is well established, prolactin is still required for milk synthesis to occur, but its role is permissive rather than regulatory (Cregan & Hartmann, 1999).

Prolactin concentration in the plasma is highest during sleep and lowest during the waking hours; it operates as a true circadian rhythm (Stern & Reichlin, 1990). The prolactin response is superimposed on the circadian rhythm of prolactin secretion, such that the same intensity of suckling stimulus can elevate prolactin levels more effectively at certain times of the day when the circadian input enhances the effect of the sucking stimulus (Freeman et al., 2000).

Prolactin levels remain elevated after the first weeks postpartum only if the baby is put to breast or, in the absence of breast stimulation by an infant, if a pump is used to mechanically maintain prolactin cycling. Small studies with wide variations in methodology demonstrated the ability of various older pumps to elevate prolactin levels (de Sanctis et al., 1981; Howie et al., 1980; Neifert & Seacat, 1985; Noel et al., 1974; Weichert, 1980; Zinaman et al., 1992). More recently, Hill and colleagues (2009) compared preterm pump-dependent mothers with full-term breastfeeding mothers relative to the elevation of prolactin levels. The preterm mothers who were double-pumping with a hospital-grade pump had elevated prolactin levels similar to those seen in term mothers during feedings at the breast. A study that compared the prolactin response to pumping between two electric breast pumps, the Embrace by Playtex and the Pump in Style by Medela, showed that the prolactin response was greater with the Embrace pump, but the Pump in Style extracted milk more efficiently (Hopkinson & Heird, 2009). The authors explain this as the Embrace pump stimulating the endocrine portion of the milk production system and the Pump in Style stimulating the autocrine arm of milk production. The mothers in the study alternated the use of both pumps and did not rate one pump as better than the other.

Clinical Implications

The function of infant suckling (or mechanical milk removal) varies between lactogenesis II, the onset of copious milk production, and lactogenesis III, the maintenance of abundant milk production. Lactogenesis II occurs in the absence of milk removal over the first 3 days postpartum, but milk composition and volume will not proceed along the continuum to maximum milk production and mature milk composition in the absence of frequent milk removal after that time. While suckling (or mechanical milk removal) may not be a prerequisite for lactogenesis II, it is critical for lactogenesis III. Delayed suckling by the infant, whether owing to premature delivery (Cregan et al., 2000), cesarean delivery (Sozmen, 1992), or other factors that necessitate mechanical milk removal, may affect the timing or delay the onset of lactogenesis II. Additional breast pumping after a couple of breastfeeds before the onset of lactogenesis II has not been shown to hasten the event or result in increased milk transfer to the baby at 72 hours (Chapman et al., 2001). In the absence of a baby at breast, the breasts need to be stimulated eight or more times every 24 hours. Parker and colleagues (2012) found that initiation of milk expression within 1 hour following delivery increased milk volume and decreased the time to lactogenesis II in preterm mothers of very low-birth-weight infants. Pumping only once or twice during the day and never at night, when prolactin levels are at their peak, may contribute to delayed lactogenesis II. A faltering milk supply in the following weeks may be attributed to the lack of sufficient prolactin receptors and infrequent breast stimulation while lactation is being established.

Painful over-distension of the breasts (secondary engorgement) must be prevented. As alveolar pressure rises, lactation suppression begins. Painful engorgement lasting longer than 48 hours can potentially decrease the milk supply. Therefore, if a baby cannot keep up with a suddenly increased milk supply, the mother should express her milk. When milk production begins in the absence of a baby, pumping frequency may need to be temporarily increased to prevent involution of the alveoli caused by the back-pressure of milk and the build-up of suppressor peptides that down-regulate milk volume. Wilde et al., (1995) identified this peptide and named it the feedback inhibitor of lactation (FIL).

Early breastfeeding has a critical period during which frequent nipple stimulation and milk removal are necessary to ensure a plentiful milk supply in later weeks. The clinician should offer management guidelines with this in mind, especially if mother and baby are separated. Woolridge (1995) provided a practical identification of six separate stages in the lactation process:

1. Priming (changes of pregnancy).
2. Initiation (birth and the management of early breastfeeding).
3. Calibration (the concept that milk production gets under way without the breasts actually "knowing" how much milk to make in the beginning). Over the first 3 to 5 weeks, milk output is progressively calibrated to the baby's needs, usually building up (up-regulation) but occasionally down-regulating to meet the baby's needs.
4. Maintenance (the period of exclusive breastfeeding).
5. Decline (the period after complementary foods or supplements are added).
6. Involution (weaning).

The second, third, and fourth time periods are crucial to ensuring abundant milk production. Close attention must be given to alterations that could impact the breasts' ability to calibrate their milk output to the needs of the baby.

Daly et al. (1992, 1993) have shown that the degree of breast emptying is inversely proportional to the amount of milk made to replace it; that is, the more thoroughly a breast is drained, the more milk is made. Daly and Hartmann (1995a, 1995b) noted that milk in breasts with smaller storage capacities may need to be expressed more frequently than milk in breasts with larger storage capacities, even though both types of breasts are capable of synthesizing similar amounts of milk in 24 hours. Mothers with larger storage capacities are able to express a higher volume of milk with each pumping session but not necessarily more milk in total in a 24-hour period than mothers with smaller storage capacities. The volume of milk expressed is also related to the degree of fullness of the breast, with a fuller breast yielding more milk volume when pumped (Mitoulas et al., 2002). Full breasts tend to take less time to achieve the milk-ejection reflex, with a less full breast taking up to 120 seconds (Hartmann, 2002).

Expressed milk volume tends to be higher from the right breast than the left, with these differences sometimes being quite large but remaining stable over time (Engstrom et al., 2007). Primiparous mothers and first-time breastfeeders have demonstrated the greatest differences in this regard. A possible explanation could be that the right breast preferentially receives more blood flow than the left—a fact demonstrated in a Doppler ultrasound study in women with established lactation (Aljazaf, 2004).

Oxytocin

Oxytocin is responsible for the milk-ejection reflex. By acting on the myoepithelial processes, oxytocin causes shortening of the ducts without constricting them, thereby increasing the milk pressure. Cobo et al. (1967) measured milk ejection by recording intraductal mammary pressure using a catheter placed in a mammary duct. Values were measured at 0.19 plus or minus 0.04 in/min and from 0 to 25 mm Hg on recording paper. Ductal contractions lasted about 1 minute and occurred at about 4 to 10 contractions every 10 minutes. Caldeyro-Barcia (1969) reported that intramammary pressure rose 10 mm Hg after 5 days postpartum with oxytocin release. Drewett et al., (1982) and McNeilly et al. (1983) showed, by minute-to-minute blood sampling, that oxytocin occurs in impulses at about 1-minute intervals. Thus oxytocin release is pulsatile and variable with intermittent bursts. These pressure changes cease when suckling stimulation ends. Oxytocin also responds in the same way to prenursing stimuli and mechanical nipple stimulation by a breast pump.

The milk-ejection reflex, initiated by oxytocin release, serves to increase the intraductal mammary pressure and maintain it at sufficient levels to overcome the resistance of the breast to the outflow of milk. The infant ingests approximately 30 to 35 mL of milk per milk ejection (Hartmann, 2002). Milk ducts stay dilated approximately 1.5 to 3.5 minutes following letdown (Hartmann, 2002), making it beneficial to elicit multiple letdowns during the course of a pumping session. Ramsay et al. (2006) observed that the first milk ejection of the expression period released significantly more milk than subsequent milk ejections regardless of vacuum level. In another study, the first two milk ejections produced the greatest percentage (62%) of total milk volume during breast expression with an electric breast pump (Prime et al., 2011). The rate at which milk is removed significantly declines after the initial milk ejection (Ramsay et al., 2005).

Overall, women with the highest increase in ductal diameter and with more and longer milk ejections express more milk. This may provide a partial explanation of why some mothers are able to express large amounts of milk in short periods of time, whereas others do not experience as many letdowns during pumping and thus express lesser amounts of milk.

Pumps
Mechanical Milk Removal

A pump does not pump, suck, or pull milk out of the breast. Instead, it reduces resistance to milk outflow from the alveoli, allowing the internal pressure of the breast to push out the milk. The milk-ejection reflex produces an initial rise in the intramammary pressure; because of the pulsatile nature of oxytocin release and its short half-life, periodic rises in ductal pressure maintain the pressure gradient over time.

The classic work on breast pumps conducted by Einar Egnell (1956) was based on research in dairy cattle and Egnell's own experiments with a pump that created periodic and limited phases of negative pressure. Egnell assumed that the milk-secreting alveoli of the breast and the cow udder were similar, even though the two organs are anatomically different and do not drain in the same way. He postulated that the quantity of milk secreted is regulated by the counter-pressure it exerts. This counter-pressure rises as milk fills the available space; secretion ceases when the pressure reaches 28 mm Hg. Egnell's pump created a maximum negative pressure of 200 mm Hg below atmospheric pressure (760 mm Hg).

He based this setting on previous research done with an Abt pump (on human mothers), which produced 30 periods of negative pressure per minute and was reported to rupture the nipple skin in every third breast. Placing his settings well below this level to avoid damaging the human nipple, Egnell calculated the difference between the pressure-filled alveoli and his pump's negative pressure as $760 + 28 - 560 = 228$ mm Hg. He maintained that it was the pressure within the breast that activated milk outflow.

Egnell's original pump operated in four phases per cycle, with one cycle spanning from one initiation of suction to the next initiation of suction. The four phases included (1) a period of increasing suction that is relatively short, (2) a decreasing phase of suction, (3) a resting phase, and (4) a slight amount of positive pressure when the decreased suction phase is finished. Egnell contended that mechanical pumping was safer than manual expression because he feared that the "high" positive pressure generated by "squeezing" the breast could damage the alveoli and ducts. He also speculated that manual expression would leave too much milk in the breast, a common concern in the dairy industry.

In fact, no research appears to show that increased breast damage occurs with hand expression. However, the volume of expressed milk tends to be higher when using a breast pump compared to manual expression. Paul et al. (1996) showed that use of a cylinder pump resulted in significantly higher volumes of milk expressed per session compared to hand expression. Slusher et al. (2007) compared milk volumes expressed by hand, double-collection pedal pump, and double-collection electric pump. Both pumps resulted in higher expressed milk volumes compared to hand expression, with the double-collection electric pump expressing the highest volume of milk. More recently, Slusher and colleagues (2012) showed that expressed milk volumes were larger over a 7-day period when using an electric breast pump compared to a manual pump or hand expression in 161 mothers whose infants were in a special care nursery. However, hand expression has been shown to be more effective than breast pumps in extracting colostrum during the colostral phase of milk production in the first 3 days postpartum. Ohyama and colleagues (2010) found that in mothers separated from their infants during the first 48 hours after birth, hand expression was more effective in removing colostrum than a hospital-grade electric pump. Morton and colleagues (2009) found that not only was hand expression more effective than an electric pump during the first 3 days, but mothers who hand-expressed breastmilk frequently (more than 5 times/day) in the first 3 postpartum days also had the highest volumes of expressed milk at week 2 and week 8. These studies may illustrate that vacuum by itself is not as efficient in removing thick, viscous colostrum as the compressive forces from hand expression. The choice of how to express milk (hand, pump, or both) may be dependent on the time since birth and the purpose of milk expression.

Many pump manufacturers continue to use Egnell's pressure settings as a guide. However, various pumps are still capable of generating more suction than stated in his calculations.

Vacuum

The vacuum applied to the breast by an infant during suckling is not constant. The vacuum is initiated, it rises, it is released, and it is maintained with a basal resting pressure to keep the nipple in the mouth. The vacuum stretches the teat to approximately twice its resting length, in tandem with a 70% reduction of the teat's original diameter (Smith et al., 1988; Weber et al., 1986). Speculation on the function of this vacuum ranges from thoughts that (1) the vacuum facilitates the refilling with milk of the ducts within the teat following each swallow of the infant or (2) milk is released from the teat by the vacuum caused when the infant's jaw lowers and enlarges the oral cavity (Smith et al., 1988).

In a breastfeeding ultrasound study, Jacobs et al. (2007) showed that an infant's tongue in its uppermost position (securing the nipple in contact with the palate) did not compress any milk into the oral cavity. Tongue movement downward was followed by milk exiting the nipple. An infant feeding at the breast achieves a range of 42 to 126 suck cycles per minute, with a mean of 74 sucks per minute (Bowen-Jones et al., 1982). Suction is applied over approximately half of the suck cycle (Halverson, 1944).

However, vacuum or suction is not the only force that an infant employs to extract milk from the breast. A compressive force from the tongue and jaw is also applied during the suction cycle to more effectively create milk transfer from the breast to the baby. In an ultrasound study, Woolridge (2012) identified both peristaltic movements of the tongue as well as vacuum application by infants during feedings at the breast. Both types of tongue movements may be capable of removing milk independently, but they are more likely to complement each other and act synergistically to accomplish the most efficient method of removing milk from the breast. Thus sucking seems to be a dynamic process, shifting between both peristaltic movements and vacuum-generating movements, possibly in response to the varying rate of milk release from the breast. Vacuum-generating movements of the tongue may be superimposed on the peristaltic movements of the tongue and are generated as part of the same sequence.

Computer modeling that compares breastfeeding and breast pumps has shown that there is an optimal time during the suction cycle when an infant applies the compressive peristaltic force of the tongue. This results in an asymmetric compression of the teat between the infant's tongue and hard palate. Using a model that applied symmetric peristaltic compression of the teat during a suction cycle, Zoppou et al., (1997b) found that the compressive force applied at the optimal time and speed during the suck cycle could significantly increase the mean fluid flow through the teat, whereas a compressive force applied at the wrong time in the pressure cycle restricted the flow of fluid. A compressive force applied by a breast pump approximately one-fourth of the way through the suction cycle increased the milk volume over one suction cycle by 15%, while a compressive force that compressed the teat early in the suction cycle restricted milk flow into the teat and reduced milk volume (Zoppou et al., 1997a).

Compression

Whittlestone (1978) described a breast pump that not only accommodated the simultaneous pumping of both breasts, but also adopted principles from the commercial dairy milking machines of providing a compressive force to the breast from a liner inside the pump flange that rhythmically contracted around the teat. He called this a physiologic breast-milker. Alekseev et al. (1998) found that adding the compressive stimulus changed the dynamics of milk expression. Using an experimental pump where the compressive stimulus could be switched on and off, it was found that in a 3- to 5-minute period of pumping, 50% of the milk could be removed from the breast, but when the compressive stimulus was turned off it took 1.5 to 2.0 times longer to express this volume of milk. Currently the PJ's Comfort pump from Limerick (Figure 12-6) employs a compressive liner in its flanges. The Dr. Brown's double electric pump (formerly Simplisse; Figure 12-7) also uses a compressive flange.

The Evolution of Pumps

As breastfeeding rates have increased and reasons for pumping changed, mothers and professionals have demanded products that are safe, efficient, and effective in both initiating and maintaining a good milk supply. Three broad classifications of breast pumps are discussed in this chapter: (1) hand pumps that generate suction manually, (2) battery-operated pumps with small motors that generate suction from power supplied by batteries, and (3) electric pumps in which suction is created by various types of electric motors. There is no intent to recommend any particular brand of pump. A listing of companies that sell breast pumps can be found in Appendix 12-A. More extensive descriptions and pictures of pumps can be found at the company websites.

A Comparison of Pumps

The efficiency of pumps and how well they work for mothers have received some attention in the research literature and are discussed in this section. In addition, many mothers and clinicians have turned to Internet sites that report mothers' evaluations of the various pumps they have used. A variety of websites (e.g., www.breastpumpsdirect.com /breast-pump-reviews_a/183.htm, www.epinions .com, www.viewpoints.com, and www.amazon.com)

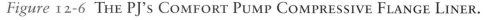

Figure 12-6 THE PJ'S COMFORT PUMP COMPRESSIVE FLANGE LINER.

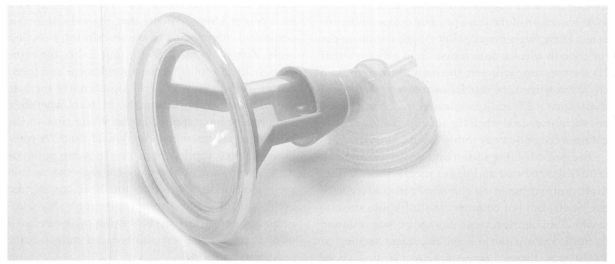

Figure 12-7 Dr. Brown's Double Electric Pump (Formerly Simplisse) with Compressive Flange.

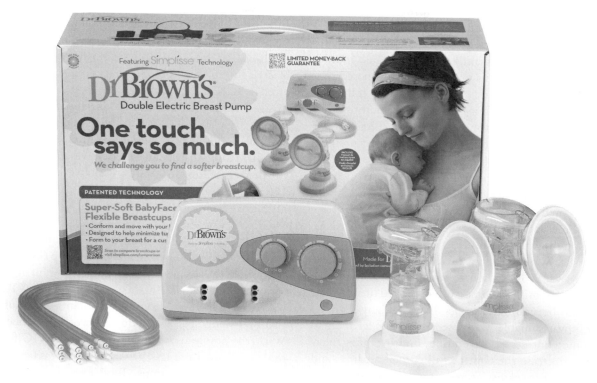

provide pump reviews. While not very scientific, these reviews run the gamut of pros and cons from a mother's perspective with some helpful hints about pump use, troubleshooting problems, and pumping situations.

Fewtrell, P. Lucas, and Collier (2001) compared the efficacy of the Avent Isis manual pump and the Egnell electric pump in mothers who delivered preterm infants less than 35 weeks' gestation. At 7 to 10 days, the mothers evaluated "consumer" characteristics of their assigned pump (ease of use, amount of suction, comfort, pleasant to use, and overall opinion of the pump). Mothers did not use or compare both pumps to each other. While these mothers rated the Avent Isis as a more comfortable pump, mothers in both groups pumped a mean of three times per day with a mean volume of less than 7 ounces per day (199 mL/day, range 57 to 323 mL, with the Avent Isis; 218 mL/day, range

126 to 341 mL, with the electric pump). It is difficult to concur with the authors' conclusions that the manual pump reflected a significant advance in pumping milk for preterm infants when milk output was so low for the amount of time spent pumping. The study did not address the ability of the pumps to initiate a milk supply or maintain milk production over a long period of time.

Fewtrell et al. (2001) compared the efficacy of the Avent Isis manual pump and the Medela Mini Electric pump in term 8-week-old babies. Each pump was tested on a single occasion, with the second pump tested 2 to 3 days after the first, and the mothers rated the pumps on the same "consumer" scale as described earlier. The sole rating factor for the mothers was whether the pump was pleasant to use, not how much milk was expressed. These data also showed that irrespective of which pump was tested as the second pump, milk volumes were increased. However, when the second pump was the Mini Electric model, milk volume was 164 mL ± 673 mL compared to 149 mL ± 671 mL with the manual pump. The value of this study remains unknown, as neither of the study pumps was used over a longer period of time or validated as being capable of sustaining milk production in a mother who is dependent on a pump for this purpose.

Bernabe-Garcia and colleagues (2012) compared the effectiveness of four manual breast pumps—Isis (Philips Avent), Harmony (Medela), Little Heart (Medela), and Evenflo—in mothers of preterm infants in a developing country. Mothers preferred the squeeze handle pumps (Isis and Harmony) over the cylinder pumps, with the Isis pump being the most preferable. Pumped milk volumes were low in some mothers (range 4.4 to 577.0 mL/day), although sufficient milk was provided for some infants. While such manual pumps may be more affordable in low-resource countries and situations, expressed milk volumes often proved insufficient for full breastmilk feedings. However, any pumped milk was valuable when used as trophic feedings to promote intestinal maturation, improve milk tolerance, decrease the time to full enteral feeding, and help protect against necrotizing enterocolitis.

Hayes et al. (2008) studied whether an electric breast pump or a manual pump would increase breastfeeding duration in mothers returning to work or school on a full-time basis. The use of an electric breast pump did not differ statistically from the use of a manual pump in terms of overall duration of breastfeeding. Although the same information and support were given to all mothers in the study, additional support was required in some cases for women in the manual pump group. Some crossover occurred, with a number of mothers in the manual pump group also using an electric pump, but with the researchers unaware of this break in protocol. The authors claimed that the findings suggest that the manual breast pump may work as well as the electric breast pump when breastfeeding is encouraged and supported among women returning to work or school. However, the findings may not warrant such a claim given that some mothers in the manual pump group also used an electric

pump, raising questions about the conclusion and whether an electric breast pump was needed due to the ineffectiveness of the manual pump.

Sisk and colleagues (2010) looked at factors that supported or hindered initiation and maintenance of breastmilk expression after the birth of a very low-birth-weight infant. Mothers who relied on small electric or manual pumps to express their milk after being discharged from the hospital reported great difficulty in establishing an effective pumping schedule and an adequate milk supply. Mothers attributed this poor outcome to the pumps being painful, tiring to use, and ineffective at emptying the breasts. Some mothers were too weak to manually pump milk, resulting in several days with no milk expression at all.

Clark and Dellaport (2011) looked at the efficacy of issuing a multiuser electric breast pump compared to a single-user electric breast pump (Medela) to mothers in the Special Supplemental Nutrition Program for Women, Infants, and Children (WIC) who were separated from their infants for more than 30 hours per week during work or school. With the single-user breast pump, less WIC formula was issued and less WIC staff time was needed to issue the breast pumps. Total formula costs for the multiuser electric pump group who chose to supplement with formula amounted to $8564.77 for the year; by comparison, among the single-user breast pump group, formula costs amounted to $5287.16 for the year. The single-user breast pump group appeared to increase the duration of offering breastmilk to the WIC participants' infants.

Wight and colleagues (2011) compared the milk production of preterm mothers who used a small multiuser breast pump (PJ's Comfort pump) with the features of a larger, more expensive multiuser breast pump. In this study, 83% of mothers using the pump achieved 350 mL or more or expressed milk per day, 66% achieved 500 mL or more per day, and 29% pumped 700 mL or more per day—volumes compatible with the ability to supply adequate amounts of milk over the long term to premature infants (Hill et al., 2005). The authors state that this pump is a viable alternative to the larger, more expensive electric pumps and provides another option for mothers of preterm infants to acquire an efficient but less expensive pump that will initiate and maintain their milk production.

Manual Hand Pumps

The various types of hand pumps rely on differing mechanisms to generate suction.

Rubber Bulb Models

Rubber bulb pumps are seldom seen in current clinical practice. Squeezing and releasing a rubber bulb generates a vacuum in these pumps. In most "bicycle horn" pumps, the rubber bulb is attached directly to the collection container. Some manufacturers separated the bulb from the collection container by modifying the angle at which it is attached to the pump or by adding a length of tubing. These modifications were thought to reduce the high potential for bacterial contamination of the bulb caused by the easy backflow of milk. Vacuum control on these pumps is extremely difficult, thus increasing the likelihood of nipple pain and damage. The "bicycle horn" pumps are inexpensive, but collect only about 0.5 ounce of milk at a

time and must be emptied frequently. (The other pumps collect milk in a bottle.) Mothers often complain of nipple pain during pumping and low milk yields, especially if they have used these pumps for more than a few weeks. Most mothers no longer see these pumps in stores, but some models may still be available online and are a poor choice in any circumstance.

Squeeze-Handle Models

Squeeze-handle models (Figures 12-8 and 12-9), such as the Avent Isis, EnHande (Hygeia), Ameda One-Hand, First Years Breastflow Manual, Medela Harmony, Dr. Brown's Handicraft (formerly Simplisse), Lansinoh Manual, and Evenflo SimplyGo Manual, involve squeezing and releasing a handle that creates suction in the pump. They are typically used for occasional pumping and are a type that can be used when no electricity is available. These pumps are easily cleaned but their operation

Figure 12-9 THE AMEDA ONE-HAND PUMP.

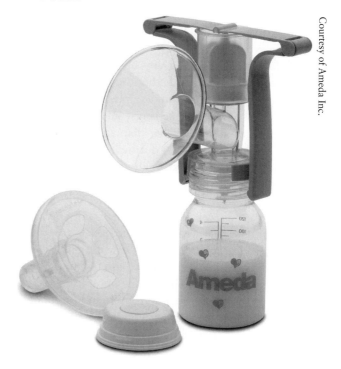

Figure 12-8 THE AVENT SQUEEZE-HANDLE MANUAL PUMP.

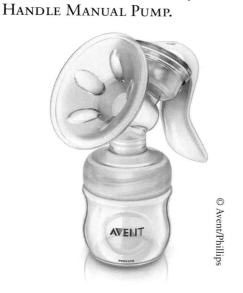

may present difficulties for women with hand or arm problems, such as arthritis or carpal tunnel syndrome. The hand and wrist can tire easily with repeated or prolonged use.

Cylinder Pumps

Cylinder-type pumps, such as the Base (Medela) and EnHande Two-Hand (Hygeia) manual pumps, generate a vacuum as a cylinder or plunger is pulled away from the body. Other cylinder-within-a-cylinder pumps are available online. The inner cylinder with the flange is placed against the breast; a gasket at the other end helps form a seal with the edge of the outer cylinder. Gaskets may need to be replaced occasionally if they dry out, shrink, or lose their ability to form a seal. Gaskets can also harbor bacteria and must be removed during cleaning, contrary to some user instructions. When placing the gasket back on the cylinder, roll it back and forth over the cylinder to help restore the shape. Some pumps come with extra gaskets.

Small plastic or silicone inserts can be placed in the inner opening to custom-fit the cylinder-type pump to the breast. Silicone liners are available for some pumps; these are designed to collapse against the breast during the suction phase to provide external positive pressure. These pumps are lightweight, not too expensive, and easily cleaned.

Before recommending any of these pumps, the clinician should check whether the pump automatically interrupts the vacuum at a preset level, if there are adjustable vacuum settings, and if the pump has a collection bottle rather than an outer cylinder where milk accumulates during pumping. Some pumps also provide an extra cylinder for milk storage or have an angled rather than a straight flange. Some mothers report that the pumps with an angled flange do not work as well as the straight pumps. As the outer cylinder fills with milk, the gasket is repeatedly dunked in the milk. Mothers who express more than 3 oz of milk at a time may have to empty these pumps more than once in a single pumping episode.

Efficiency of use varies from brand to brand. Some cylinder-type pumps can also be adapted for use on the larger electric pumps. A higher vacuum is generated as the outer cylinder fills with milk.

Mothers may need to shorten the outward stroke after collecting more than 1 oz of breastmilk. These pumps are seen less and less in actual use.

Battery-Operated Pumps

Battery-operated pumps use a small motor powered by either size AA 1.5-volt batteries or size C batteries (e.g., the Medela Mini Electric). Most have a vacuum adjustment mechanism. The vacuum in some pumps can take a relatively long time to reach its maximum level and is regulated by how frequently the vacuum is interrupted.

Some of these pumps include a button that the mother can press to release the vacuum periodically and to simulate the rhythm of a nursing baby. All take varying periods of time for the recovery of suction following each release. This limits the number of suction/release cycles per minute to as few as six and may require relatively long periods of vacuum application to the nipple. To compensate for this limitation, some mothers leave the suction on for much longer than the pump instructions recommend. Mothers in one survey mentioned 30 to 60 seconds (Walker, 1992). Four women in the same survey never interrupted the suction during the entire pumping session because they could not get the milk flow restarted following vacuum interruption. Some pumps have preset automatic cycling.

Most pumps have AC adapters to decrease battery use. A major complaint about these pumps is their short battery life, which affects pumping efficiency because fewer cycles are generated as the batteries wear down. Batteries may have to be replaced as frequently as every second or third use. Rechargeable batteries are an option, but they usually require charging each night and may not produce as many cycles per minute as alkaline batteries. AC adapters usually allow the maximum number of cycles per minute that the motor can produce. Maximum suction after each vacuum release will often continue decreasing in amount throughout the pumping session. In contrast, the Medela battery pump automatically produces 32 cycles per minute with alkaline batteries, 30 cycles per minute with rechargeable batteries, and 42 cycles per minute with the A/C adapter.

Battery pumps require only one hand to operate, and are lightweight. Some mothers use two battery-operated pumps simultaneously to decrease pumping time when they are on a tight schedule. Mothers who plan to pump for several months while at work may consider a larger personal-use pump or a long-term rental contract for an electric pump, because battery replacement can be very expensive . Some of these pumps operate with a quiet hum, but others are very noisy. These pumps are seen less frequently today.

Electric Pumps

Electric breast pumps fall into one of three categories:

- Small semi-automatic pumps
- Personal-use pumps (Figure 12-10) (lightweight portable pumps often used by employed mothers)
- Multiuser, institutionally used pumps, such as those commonly rented and/or used in the hospital

Various types of electric motors are used in this group of pumps to generate suction. Semi-automatic pumps such as the Nurture III (Bailey Medical Engineering; Figure 12-11) require the mother to cycle suction by covering and uncovering a hole in the flange base in an individualized, rhythmical pattern. These pumps maintain a constant negative pressure. Some lack a dial or mechanism to adjust the amount of suction. The actual amount of vacuum delivered to the nipple is determined by the degree of closure of the hole in the flange base. Many mothers learn to roll their finger three fourths of the way off the hole rather than lift the finger completely, so as to generate vacuum faster for the subsequent cycle by preventing complete interruption of vacuum. However, too much negative pressure, or negative pressure applied for too long a period, increases the risk of damage to the nipple and underlying vascular structures. The initiation of suction places the greatest pressure on the nipple; thus it is most desirable that a pump generate suction quickly.

Figure 12-10 Medela Pump in Style Advanced.

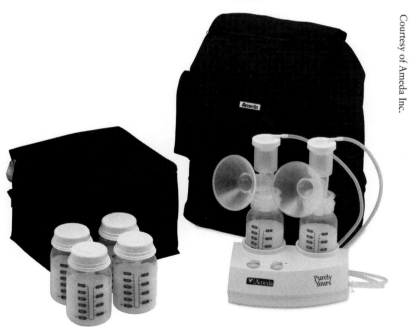

Courtesy of Ameda Inc.

Figure 12-11 THE NURTURE III, A SMALL SEMI-AUTOMATIC PUMP.

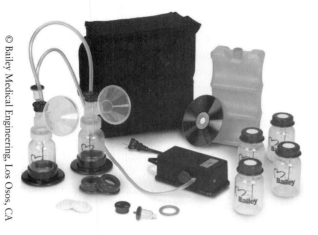

© Bailey Medical Engineering, Los Osos, CA

Automatic electric pumps are designed to cycle pressure rather than to maintain it. Because Egnell (1956) observed nipple damage when cycles were 2 seconds long (30 per minute), manufacturers increased the number of cycles so that they more closely simulate that of a nursing baby. Pressure-setting parameters on these large pumps also attempt to mimic the pressure exerted by an infant. Mean sucking pressures of most full-term infants range from −50 mm Hg to −155 mm Hg, with a maximum of −220 mm Hg (Caldeyro-Barcia, 1969). In pumps that have a preset pulsed suction (automatic pumps), there is typically a 60/40 ratio. Negative pressure is applied for 60% of the cycle; 40% of the cycle is the resting phase. The Medela Classic/Lactina pattern has a fixed number of cycles per minute (48), with "relax" times becoming longer in lower vacuum ranges. The Medela Symphony (Figure 12-12) operates with a "stimulation" phase at the start of the pumping session at 120 cycles per minute with variable adjustable vacuum of 50 to 200 mm Hg. This causes a change in the "expression" phase to 54 to 78 cycles per minute, with a vacuum ranging from 50 to 250 mm Hg. The number of cycles per minute varies in this pump according to the set vacuum, with higher vacuum levels resulting in lower cycles per minute. At the minimum vacuum of 50 mm Hg, the Symphony applies 78 cycles per minute; at the maximum vacuum of

Figure 12-12 THE MEDELA SYMPHONY PUMP.

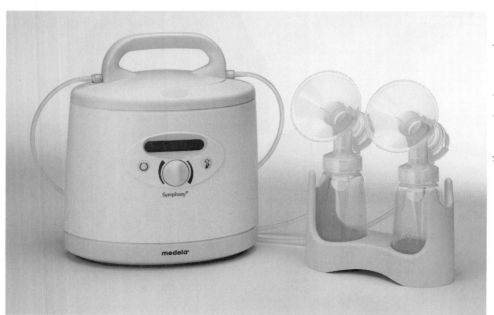

Courtesy of Medela, Inc., McHenry, IL.

250 mm Hg, 54 cycles per minute are applied. The maximum pressure that these pumps will generate at their normal (high) setting is approximately 220 to 250 mm Hg. By comparison, the Nurture III semi-automatic pump produces 220 mm Hg after about 2.5 seconds using a single collecting kit (approximately 24 cycles per minute). With the double-collecting kit, this same pump takes about 3.25 seconds to achieve this level, generating about 18 cycles per minute.

Negative pressure—a function of the volume of air in the accessory kit—increases as the collecting bottle fills with milk. The pressure generated varies with different-sized bottles (collecting containers) and from one manufacturer to another. When double-pump setups are used (with two collecting containers being filled simultaneously), the potential for very low negative pressure exists when the containers are empty; negative pressure increases as the bottles fill. Most accessory kits compensate for this factor by separating the collection containers from the power source so that the amount of air in the system remains constant regardless of the amount of fluid in the collection container. If a mother is using an accessory kit or pump without a similar feature, she can compensate by using a smaller collection bottle (Vol-u-feeders fit on some pumps), turning down the vacuum as the bottle fills, emptying the bottle more frequently, or cycling the suction more frequently on hand-operated, battery-operated, or semi-automatic pumps.

Electric pumps can be multiuser models (often referred to as hospital grade or rental grade)—such as the Symphony and Lactina (Medela), Platinum and Elite (Ameda), EnDeare and EnJoye (Hygeia), PJ's Comfort (Limerick), and Melodi (Lucina Care)—or single-user models (sometimes called personal-use pumps)—such as Pump in Style (Medela), and Purely Yours (Ameda). Personal-use (single-user) pumps are generally recommended for employed mothers or mothers who must pump frequently over a longer period of time. Multiuser hospital-grade pumps are often used for mothers of preterm infants or those mothers who will be dependent upon a pump to initiate and maintain their milk supply.

Simultaneous and/or Sequential Pumping

All of the automatic electric pumps and a few of the battery-operated pumps have collection kits that allow pumping both breasts at the same time. Over time, several studies have documented that simultaneous (SIM) and sequential (SEQ) pumping yield similar milk volumes but simultaneous pumping is done in significantly less time (Auerbach, 1990b; Groh-Wargo et al., 1995; Neifert & Seacat, 1985), Studies also demonstrate a significantly higher prolactin rise with double pumping. This finding is similar to Tyson's report (1977) of a doubling in prolactin rise when two infants were put to breast simultaneously and echoes the findings of Saint et al., (1986), who reported larger milk volumes in mothers of twins (up to double that of singleton mothers).

More recently, and with the introduction of newer pump technology, Prime and colleagues (2012) investigated whether milk removal using an electric breast pump differed for simultaneous versus sequential pumping. Simultaneous pumping resulted in a higher percentage of milk yield in a shorter period of time, an increase in the number of milk ejections, and milk with a higher cream/caloric content. The greater milk yield may be related to the increased number of milk ejections seen with simultaneous pumping.

Other aspects of simultaneous versus sequential pumping have also been studied, helping the clinician to construct pumping guidelines tailored to maximizing milk output for mothers encountering a variety of problems or situations (Table 12-1). A number of factors combine to result in optimal milk expression: vacuum generated by the pump, cycling patterns of the vacuum, compressive forces from the pump flange, compressive forces external to the pump, oxytocin pulses, sequential or simultaneous pumping, number of times per day and per week of pumping sessions, time postpartum when pumping was initiated, type of flange, proper fit of the flange, comfort, and so on (Table 12-2).

Table 12-1 METHODS OF MILK EXPRESSION: SELECTED STUDIES

Study	Findings
Neifert & Seacat, 1985 *n* = 10 term infants	Milk yield similar, volume obtained in half the time with SIM with lower vacuum levels; increased prolactin rise with SIM.
Auerbach, 1990b *n* = 25 5–35 weeks postpartum term infants	SIM = highest milk yields in 7–12 minutes; higher milk volume SEQ = 10–15 minutes to reach maximum milk yield
Groh-Wargo et al., 1995 *n* = 32 Preterm infants Pumped 3–5 times/day	SIM = 16 minutes/session; 7.6 ± 3 hours/week SEQ = 24 minutes/session; 11.1 ± 3.1 hours/week Average 28 pumping sessions/week = 400 ml/day of milk did not see increased prolactin.
Hill et al., 1996 *n* = 9 Preterm infants Pumped 5 times/day during hospital stay Pumped 8 times/day at home through day 42	SEQ 5 × 5 × 5 × 5 20 minutes total; milk volumes decreased after 25 days; proportion of prolactin at day 42 was 52% of level at day 21. Milk yield ranges 158.4 g day 3–505.8 g day 20; SIM milk volumes continued to rise over entire study time; prolactin at day 42 was 85% of level at day 21. Milk volume ranges 41.4 g day 3 to 741 g on day 41.
Hill et al., 1999 *n* = 39 Preterm infants Pumped 8 times/day	SIM 10 minutes; milk weights higher each week of the study in SIM; pumping frequency = 31 + 11.93 times/to 45 + 10.88 times. SEQ 5 × 5 × 5 × 5 for 20 minutes; pumping frequency = 28 ± 8.9 times/week to 41 ± 9.05 times/week. Hours from birth to initiation of pumping: SEQ—9.7 hours to 101 hours (4.2 days) SIM—28.28 hours to 84.3 hours (3.5 days) Milk weights inversely correlated to number of hours from birth to initiation of pumping. Milk weights positively correlated with weekly frequency of pumping and kangaroo care.
Hill et al., 2001 *n* = 39 Preterm infants 2–5 weeks postpartum	Studied median number of hours from birth to initiation of pumping and median frequency of pumping over weeks 2–5 to categorize subjects into high and low pumping frequency and early and late pumping initiation. Early initiation = 30.9 ± 11.4 hours post delivery. Late initiation = 82.0 ± 37.9 hours post delivery. Low pumping frequency group = 4.9 times/day; range = 2.6–6.14 times/day. High pumping frequency = 7.0; range 6.25–8.10 times/day. Mothers with both late initiation and low frequency had lowest milk weights. Frequency of pumping was primary influence on milk weights.

Table 12-1 METHODS OF MILK EXPRESSION: SELECTED STUDIES (*CONTINUED*)

Study	Findings
Jones et al., 2001 $n = 36$ Preterm infants 4 days total study time	Compared simultaneous and sequential pumping on milk volume and energy yield. Secondary aim: measure the effect of breast massage on milk volume and fat content. Milk yield per expression: SEQ with no massage = 51.32 ml SEQ with massage = 78.71 ml SIM with no massage = 87.69 ml SIM with massage = 125.08 ml Fat concentrations were not affected.

Key: SIM = simultaneous pumping; SEQ = sequential pumping.

Flanges

Most pumps have hard plastic shields called flanges. Some may have softer plastic or silicone flanges, soft inner liners, soft inserts, projections on the flange that compress the breast when vacuum is applied, or inserts that change the diameter of the nipple opening.

Johnson (1983) measured several aspects of flanges, including the diameters of the outer opening (flare), the inner opening, the depth of flare, and the length of the shank. She measured negative pressure at the inner opening of the flange and reported that the smaller the nipple cup, the greater the pressure exerted on the tip of the nipple. Larger and deeper flanges may provide greater stimulation of the areolar region of the breast. Zinaman (1988) repeated the same measurements on 11 manual pumps, 4 battery pumps, and 7 electric pumps. Comparing these measurements among pumps highly rated in the other studies showed that the flange's diameter ranged from 60 to 69 mm, its depth ranged from 25 to 30 mm, and the inner opening was between 21 and 26 mm for the manual pumps. A woman with a large or wide nipple may have difficulty with a flange that has a small opening or a narrow slope.

Because one size of flange may not fit all breasts, some manufacturers provide a choice in sizes of flanges (Table 12-3), silicone flange liners, or small plastic inserts that are placed at the level of the inner opening to change the diameter of the shank and inner opening. Silicone or soft plastic flange liners are supposed to cushion the pumping forces and are purported to "massage" the breast or mimic external compressive forces. Inserts placed in the flanges are designed to provide a better fit between pump and breast. The PJ's Comfort pump has only one size of flange; it is a soft silicone cup that contours to the mother's breast during pumping and provides a compressive force as well as vacuum (see Figure 12-6). The Dr. Brown's (formerly Simplisse) flange is also one size made of soft silicone that compresses the breast during pumping (see Figure 12-7).

When a vacuum is applied, the nipple and part of the areola elongate and are drawn past the inner opening and down into the shank or nipple tunnel (Biancuzzo, 1999). In general, the pump is more likely to be effective when the flange accommodates the anatomic configuration of the particular breast. However, mothers have differently sized nipples. Ziemer and Pidgeon (1993), Stark (1994), and Wilson-Clay and Hoover (2005) measured nipple diameters that ranged from less than 12 mm at the base to greater than 23 mm at the base. Wilson-Clay and Hoover (2005) also observed that nipples swell during pumping. Thus a mother with large nipples may find that a standard-size flange is too small to accommodate both the large nipple and subsequent swelling. Meier et al. (2004) observed a sample of mothers expressing milk for their preterm infants, with about half requiring a 27- to 30-mm flange (rather than a standard 23- to 24-mm flange); as lactation progressed, 77% of the mothers found

Table 12-2 COMPARISON OF PRESSURE, HORMONAL RESPONSES, AND MECHANICS AMONG VARIOUS METHODS OF BREASTMILK REMOVAL

Negative Pressure Ranges

Baby	Hand Expression	Hand Pump	Battery Pump	Electric Pump
50–241 mm Hg 50–155 mm Hg average Basal resting pressure to keep nipple in mouth 70–200 mm Hg	None	0–400 mm Hg	50–305 mm Hg	10–500 mm Hg

Positive Pressure Ranges

Breast and Milk-Ejection		Hand Expression	Hand Pump	Battery Pump	Electric Pump
Baby	Reflex				
Tongue 0.73–3.6 mm Hg	28 mm Hg when breast is full	Theoretically could exert > 760 mm Hg, which is atmospheric pressure	With compression stimulus	None to minimal	Without compression stimulus, none to minimal
Jaw 200–300 mm Hg	10–20 mm Hg with milk ejection reflex				

Hormonal Response Ranges

Baby	Hand Expression	Hand Pump	Battery Pump	Electric Pump
Prolactin basal levels up to 200 ng/ml first 10 days; 10–90 days, 60–110 ng/ml; 90–180 days, 50 ng/ml; 180 days to 1 year, 30–40 ng/ml 55–550 ng/ml	67 ng/ml 28–42 days postpartum	67 ng/ml 28–42 days postpartum	59.7 ng/ml 28–42 days postpartum	46–405 ng/ml Single pumping 92.1 ± 29.2 ng/ml Double pumping 136 ± 31.6 ng/ml
Oxytocin 5–15 units/ml 100 mU released during 10 minutes				

Mechanics

	Baby	Hand Expression	Hand Pump	Battery Pump	Electric Pump
Cycles per minute	36–126 cycles	Variable	Variable	5–60 cycles	2–84 cycles
Duration of vacuum	0.7 seconds	None	Variable	1–50 seconds	1–3 seconds
Duration of rest	0.7 seconds	Variable	Variable		
Volume of milk per suck	0.14 ml/suckle at the beginning of a feeding 0.01 ml/suckle at end of feeding				

Table 12-3 FLANGE SIZES

Company	Flange	Tunnel Diameter
Avent	One standard	22.2 mm flange with projections
Whisper Wear	One size	22.0 mm
Ameda	Custom flange	30.5 mm
	Custom flange	28.5 mm with insert
	Standard flange	25.0 mm
	Standard flange	23.0 mm with reducing insert
	Standard flange	21.0 mm with Flexishield
Medela	Personal Fit	21.0 mm small
	Personal Fit	24.0 mm standard
	Personal Fit	27.0 mm large
	Personal Fit	30.0 mm extra large
	Personal Fit	36.0 mm extra large
	Blown glass	40.0 mm

they needed a larger flange. Clinicians have observed damage on the areola presenting as suction rings or cracks at the junction of the nipple and areola from flanges that are too small. Such a misfit between flange and breast could endanger milk production if the teat were strangulated to the point where little to no milk could be expressed. Wilson-Clay and Hoover (2005) speculate that if a mother has a nipple size of approximately 20.5 mm (or the size of a U.S. nickel) or larger, she may benefit from using a pump flange that is larger than the standard size.

Lacking a clinical algorithm for nipple size and flange selection that would provide a path for decision making, some health professionals who have access to autoclaving or similar sterilizing facilities offer mothers the opportunity to try several different brands of breast pumps and flange sizes to ascertain optimal fit before they purchase or rent a pump. Some mothers find that they can achieve a good fit between a nipple that changes size during the pumping session and the use of an angled flange such as the Pumpin Pal.

Pedal Pumps

Medela manufactures breast pump pedals that generate a vacuum when the mother presses a foot down on a pedal. The leg muscles tend to be stronger than hand and arm muscles; thus this type of a pump may be useful for women with a compromised upper body, arms, or hands. The pumps run without electricity and may accommodate a number of different flange and tubing sets.

Clinical Implications Regarding Breast Pumps

The concerns of health professionals may differ considerably from those of mothers (Human Milk Banking Association of North America, 2011) and typically center on safe collection techniques and the maintenance of low bacteria counts in the expressed milk. Of equal importance are choosing the right pump for each individual situation, providing appropriate pumping instructions, and tempering all this with a consideration of the emotional toll that pumping can sometimes exact.

The professional literature includes reports of bacterial contamination of breastmilk and breast pumps. Factors related to nipple cleansing, hand washing, collection technique, type of pump, feeding method of preterm infants, pump-cleaning routines, and gestational age of the baby have all been identified as contributing to concern over high bacteria counts in expressed milk. Expressed breast milk is not sterile (el-Mohandes et al., 1993b). There is considerable disagreement over what constitutes an acceptable bacteria count, especially if the recipient of the milk is a preterm infant (Cossey et al., 2011; el-Mohandes et al., 1993a).

Historically, and with the increased use of both hand and electric pumps in the 1970s, many reports described contaminated milk as one source of neonatal bacteremia, but the reports lacked conclusive epidemiology. Hand-expressed breastmilk showed lower bacteria counts than breastmilk obtained by manual or electric pumps when pumps first began to be commonly used. Donowitz et al. (1981) reported an outbreak of *Klebsiella*-caused bacteremia in a neonatal intensive care unit (NICU). The electric breast pump was grossly contaminated and lacked proper bacterial surveillance. Once gas sterilization of pump parts was required between each mother's use of the equipment, the problem disappeared. Gransden et al. (1986) reported an outbreak of *Serratia marcescens* infection in a NICU via inadequately disinfected breast pumps (Kaneson manual and Egnell electric models). When the Egnell pump parts were autoclaved and the Kaneson pumps were washed at 80°C, the problem was resolved. Moloney et al. (1987) reported isolation of *Serratia marcescens*, *Staphylococcus aureus*, and *Streptococcus faecalis* from hand-operated and electric breast pumps. The pumps were disinfected in a hypochlorite solution as in the previous study. More recent studies have also documented the ongoing issue of bacterial contamination of expressed breastmilk in NICUs (Gras-Le et al., 2003; Mammina et al., 2008; Olver et al., 2000; Qutaishat et al., 2003; Wang et al., 2007; Youssef et al., 2002).

Faro and colleagues (2011) described a mother who reported that her breast pump parts had turned bright pink. *Serratia marcescens* has a distinctively pink coloration and was isolated from the pump parts. From the location of the pink coloration, it appeared that the mother may not have completely disassembled the pump to clean it. The mother was started on antibiotics, as this pathogen can be associated with mastitis. She also weaned the infant out

of fear that the bacteria would be transmitted to and sicken the infant.

Other approaches to reducing the bacterial count in expressed breastmilk have included expressing techniques and various breast-nipple cleansing routines. Asquith et al. (1984) noted that the bacterial content of milk is high when expression is first begun, regardless of collection technique. However, Pittard et al. (1991) found no difference in the number of heavily contaminated (more than 10,000 colony-forming units per milliliter [cfu/mL]) milk cultures when a clean versus a sterile collection container was used, or when manual versus mechanical collection techniques were employed. These researchers did not observe increased levels of bacteria in the initial milk removed from the breast.

Studies in the 1980s demonstrated that bacterial counts in the NICU could be significantly reduced by employing maternal hand washing and nipple/areola disinfection protocols (Costa, 1989; Meier & Wilks, 1987). However, Thompson et al. (1997) demonstrated that pre-expression breast cleaning with pHisoDerm and tap water were no more effective than cleaning with plain tap water in producing expressed milk that was free from bacterial contamination. No control group that refrained from breast cleaning preparations provided a basis for comparison. Because breastmilk is not sterile, some bacteria will always be present, even if they are nonpathologic. In a larger study by Law et al. (1989), no cases of infant sepsis could be linked to the particular bacteria present in expressed breastmilk feedings received by an infant who was either colonized or septic.

In the 1980s, guidelines for care of hospital breast pump equipment that included scrubbing collection kits and tubing with instrument cleaning solution after each use and autoclaving each item were implemented (Wilks & Meier, 1988). They recommended that the exterior of the pump be cleaned with antiseptic solution each day and the pump cultured monthly. The guidelines also described other factors that may influence the amount of nonpathogens that a preterm baby could tolerate—namely, the baby's clinical condition; the use of bolus feedings every 2 hours rather than continuous feedings;

the use of refrigerated rather than frozen milk to retain active anti-infective properties; and feeding the baby directly from the breast as much as possible to receive unaltered anti-infective properties, thereby further decreasing the risk of infection.

Despite these guidelines, relatively recent research indicates that contamination continues to occur. In one study, cultures were performed by D'Amico et al. (2003) in the NICU on breast pump kit attachments for the Medela Classic or Lactina that included three sites—the tubing, the small white barrier membrane, and the bottom of the collection bottle. Positive cultures were obtained from the bottom of a bottle and from the membrane area. The membrane was probably contaminated when mothers inadvertently touched it or tried to remove it for cleaning, which they had been instructed not to do. A positive culture from the bottom of the bottle suggested that collection bottles should be inverted to dry or wiped dry with a paper towel so that remaining droplets do not provide a medium for bacterial growth.

Despite the issues related to bacterial contamination of expressed milk from the mother or the NICU environment, human milk is considered the preferred nutrition for all infants, with rare exceptions. Guidelines to assess and improve quality and safety of milk expression, collection, transfer, storage, and readying for use in NICUs are routinely followed, and efforts to improve these procedures are ongoing (Cossey et al., 2011).

Each year many pumps change or add features that reduce the chance of milk backflow and contamination. Some models now have in-line air filters in the pump; some use overflow bottles; and others have filters and/or protection against overflow in the accessory kit. Some have a completely closed collection system (Ameda), deemed the optimal manner in which to prevent contamination (Human Milk Banking Association of North America, 2011; Slusser & Frantz, 2001). When choosing a pump for milk collection for term or preterm babies, the professional should know whether and how the pump or accessory kit guards against contamination. This consideration is especially important if the pump is operated by more than one user.

Cleaning Pumps

Mothers should generally follow the cleaning instructions provided with the pump. For most purposes, the combination of hot soapy water, thorough rinsing, avoidance of abrasives, and air drying is sufficient to clean pump parts that come in contact with the milk. If the tubing for electric pumps develops condensation, the tubing can be spun like a lasso to move out water droplets. Many mothers find it easier to remove the flanges and collection bottles from the tubing and run the pump for a few minutes—a technique that pulls in air and air dries the tubing. Alcohol can also be injected down the disconnected tubing to dry it and reduce the likelihood of contamination. Tubing can be boiled, although doing so may cause the tubing to become opaque, making it more difficult to see condensation or milk droplets if present. Collection bottles should be inverted to dry or wiped dry with a clean paper towel.

Pump parts can be stored in a lightly covered container (Gilks et al., 2007). Sterilizing or disinfecting pump parts can be accomplished by boiling the parts, using an electric sterilizer, placing the parts in a sterilizer bag made for the microwave, or using a dishwasher with a high-temperature sanitizing cycle. Cloth towels should be avoided to either dry or store pump parts. Harsh chemicals and abrasive scrubbing should not be used so that small scratches are not created that could harbor bacteria or mold.

Mothers sharing an electric pump (such as in a NICU or workplace) may wish to wipe the outside of the pump with a germicidal solution prior to each use. Mothers should make sure to disassemble the pump parts/collection kits completely to make sure that all surfaces are properly cleaned.

Maternal Concerns and Education Needs

Morse and Bottorff (1988) observed 61 nursing mothers and their emotional experiences related to expressing milk. Many were surprised that the ability to express their milk was not automatic. They often found that verbal and written instructions were unclear and confusing; many learned by trial and error. Mothers in this study emphasized that "instructions for one mother did not necessarily work for all." Some were embarrassed and others were frustrated when they obtained only small amounts of milk. Although success with expression increased a mother's self-confidence, women who perceived expression to be an important aspect of breastfeeding, but who were unable to express milk, displayed heightened feelings of inadequacy. The authors suggest modifying how expression is taught to include not only explicit how-to's but also encouragement of private exploratory practice and the use of humor by the instructor (when appropriate) to reduce embarrassment. Although not directly related to milk expression, a more recent study of women's reasons for weaning earlier than intended found that women felt pumping was no longer worth the effort that it required (Odom et al., 2013). Odom and her team also recommended the need for direct support from providers in relation to breastmilk expression as well as workplace support for continued breastfeeding.

Many mothers receive only the instructions that come with the pump to use as a guide in learning milk expression and handling. These instructions vary widely in their recommendations for pumping techniques and even for the cleaning of the pump. Further confusion is possible if a mother uses more than one type of pump, especially if she fails to read all of the instructions carefully or if the instructions from one manufacturer conflict with those from another.

The concerns of mothers are rarely addressed in the professional literature on breast pumps and milk expression. Clinicians must remember that the best pump will do little for a mother whose emotional needs are not met and who lacks the guidelines necessary to use the equipment properly for optimal results.

When Pumps Cause Problems

In the United States, breast pumps are class II medical devices regulated by the U.S. Food and Drug Administration (FDA) within the FDA's Center for Devices and Radiological Health. The FDA maintains a medical product reporting program, called MedWatch, that enables consumers and healthcare providers to report problems with these devices. Problems with breast pumps could include defective parts, poor labeling, malfunction of the pump, nipple damage or pain, or being ineffective at removing milk, and should always be reported to the manufacturer. It may be difficult to separate a pump that is ineffective or painful from how the pump is being used or simply if the flanges are too small for the mother. Few adverse events are reported to the FDA; in fact, more reports of injuries and malfunctions are reported on Internet websites than to the FDA (Brown et al., 2005). In addition, problems can be reported to the FDA online at the FDA's website (www.fda.gov).

Some mothers give their used pumps to other mothers, borrow used pumps, or purchase previously used breast pumps to save money. This practice has the potential for improper functioning and cross-contamination (Box 12-2). Use of single-user devices by multiple women also typically invalidates the manufacturer's warranty. Most single-user pumps are open systems and may not have any protective barrier to prevent cross-contamination when multiple users share the device. A borrowed pump can be ineffective or break, necessitating the purchase of a replacement pump. Because pumps have a limited lifetime, some mothers who borrow or purchase previously used pumps may put their milk supply at risk because the device cannot operate at its optimum. If the pump motor is worn out from extended use, it may not generate a strong enough vacuum.

Sample Guidelines for Pumping

The healthcare professional needs to base pumping recommendations on many factors and to take into account each mother's situation. For example, a mother whose premature infant is younger than 30 weeks' gestation and is not taking oral feedings needs instructions very different from those provided to a mother who is pumping during her hours

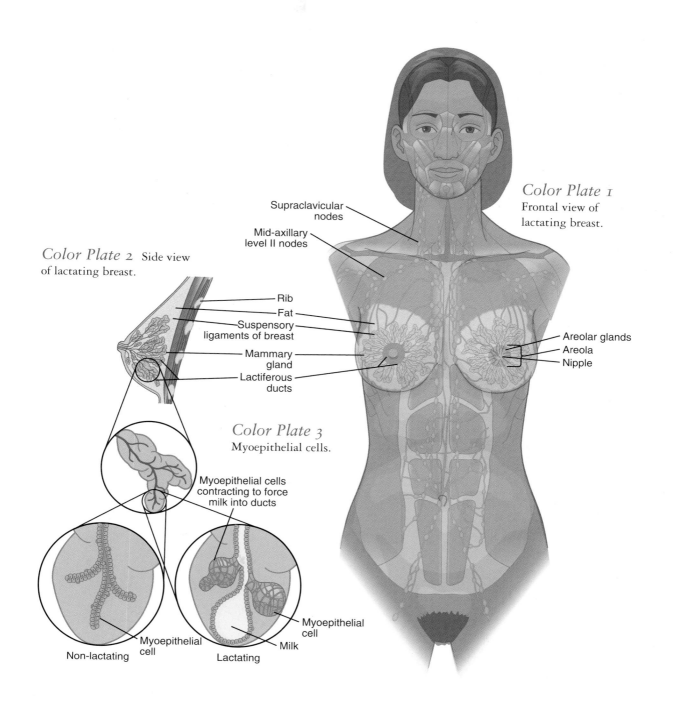

Supraclavicular nodes

Mid-axillary level II nodes

Color Plate 1 Frontal view of lactating breast.

Rib

Fat

Suspensory ligaments of breast

Mammary gland

Lactiferous ducts

Areolar glands

Areola

Nipple

Color Plate 2 Side view of lactating breast.

Color Plate 3 Myoepithelial cells.

Myoepithelial cells contracting to force milk into ducts

Myoepithelial cell

Myoepithelial cell

Non-lactating

Milk

Lactating

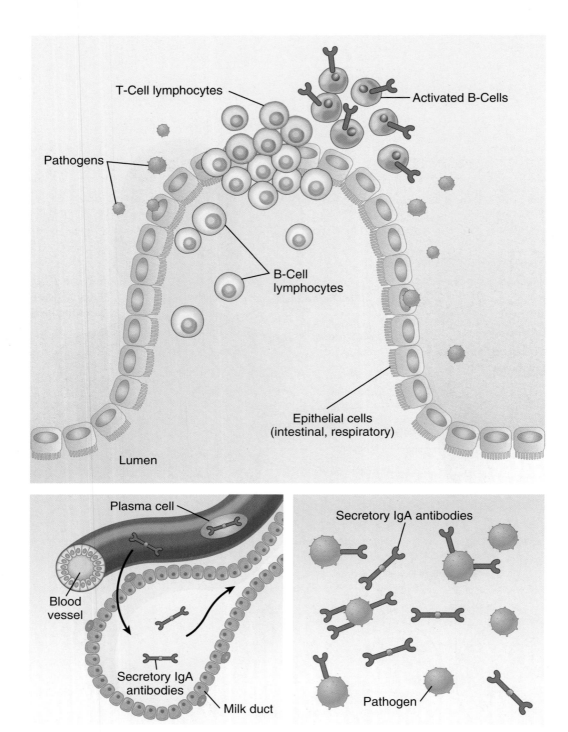

Color Plate 4 Balt and galt migration. B cells originate in the epithelium of the mother's intestinal tract or respiratory tract. Theseb-cell lymphocytes are sensitized by microbial antigens from bacteria in the mother's intestines and activated by a chemical from t-cell lymphocytes. The sensitized b cells migrate to the mother's breast by a special "homing" system (galt or balt) described in the text. Once there, they can secrete iga that enters into breastmilk. When the infant consumes the milk, it coats his intestinal walls, providing protection. The b-cell lymphocytes can also travel in milk to the baby and secrete iga antibodies in the infant's own intestinal tract. Either way, the infant has secretory iga antibodies against the specific bacteria he will most likely encounter in his environment.

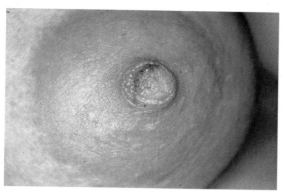

Color Plate 5 Nipple bruised and cracked from poor positioning. This trauma occurred on postpartum day 1. It was corrected by lifting the baby out of the mother's lap and into her arms and turning the baby so that his entire body faced the mother.

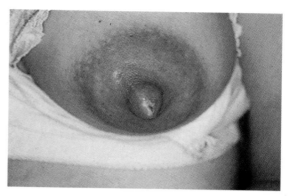

Color Plate 6 Sore nipple with trauma from poor positioning. The white streak across the face of the nipple is a sign that the baby's lower jaw was too close to the tip of the nipple. Positioning the baby centrally across the mother's torso resulted in the baby driving his chin in closer to the breast rather than to the nipple.
Reprinted with permission from Barbara Wilson-Clay.

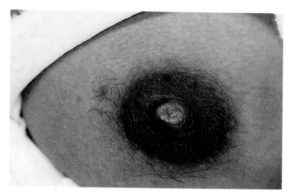

Color Plate 7 Nipple fissure that resulted from use of a poorly designed breast pump for three days. Even short-term use of a poorly designed pump can cause significant nipple damage.
Reprinted with permission from Catherine Watson Genna.

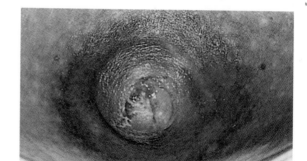

Color Plate 8 Badly cracked nipple with possible bacterial infection. Such trauma can become an entry point for bacterial invasion and subsequent inflammation or infection.
Reprinted with permission from Kay Hoover.

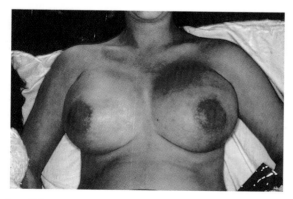

Color Plate 9 Extreme engorgement. Engorgement occurred 30 to 36 hours postpartum, secondary to ineffective and infrequent breastfeeding and no expression or pumping when the infant did not obtain milk.
Reprinted with permission from Chele Marmet, Lactation Institute.

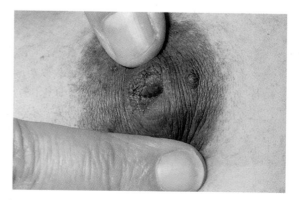

Color Plate 10 Abraded folded nipple. The abrasion occurred when the nipple tissue remained wet between feedings; air-drying after each breastfeeding resolved the problem.

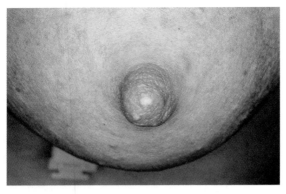

Color Plate 11 Milk plugs at nipple pores, often charachterized by acute pain. When milk is released from the duct, relief is immediate.

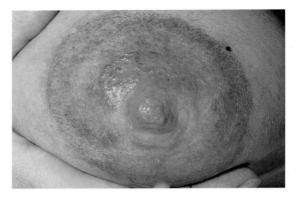

Color Plate 12 Candidiasis (thrush) of the breast. This mother experienced four separate episodes in which her breasts, but not the baby's mouth, were treated. Within one week of simultaneous treatment of mother and baby, neither the baby's mouth nor the mother's breasts were infected.

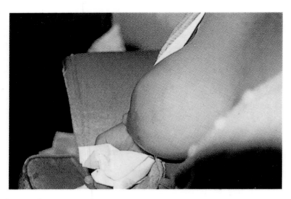

Color Plate 13 Breast abscess prior to excision. A breast abscess will often present with generalized redness. When the affected area is palpated, it is hot and hard to the touch.
Reprinted with permission from Barbara Wilson-Clay.

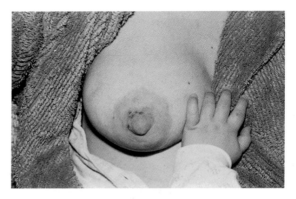

Color Plate 14 Herpes on the areola. A thirteen-month-old nursing toddler contracted oral herpes by using a playmate's contaminated rattle; the mother was the infected. The breast lesion appeared soon after the baby's infection was identified.
Reprinted with permission from Chele Marmet, Lactation Institute.

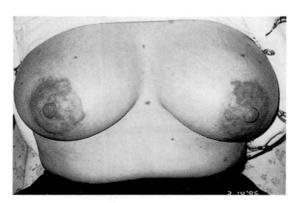

Color Plate 15 Psoriasis of the nipples. Although previous lesions had occurred on her breasts (But never on her nipples areolae), this mother developed psoriasis on her nipples within a week of her baby's birth. When the baby latched on at the beginning of each breastfeeding session, she felt pain, which gradually subsided as the feeding progressed.
Reprinted with permision from Karen Foard.

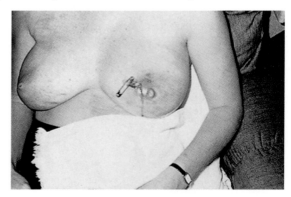

Color Plate 16 Breast abscess with Iodoform gauze drain inplace; the safety pin is not holding the drain in place.
Reprinted with permission from Donna Corrieri.

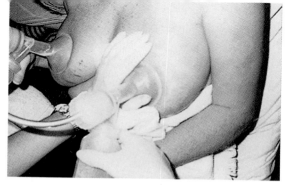

Color Plate 17 Pumping the breast following abcess drainage. When a mother cannot put a baby to breast following treatment for a breast abscess, pumping may be necessary. The lc's gloved hand is placing gentle, even pressure over the area of the abcess drain to create a seal, in order to pump both breasts simultaneously and comfortably.
Reprinted with permission from Donna Corrieri.

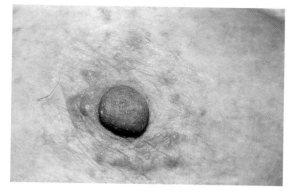

Color Plate 18 Poison ivy on the areola.
Reprinted with permission from Kay Hoover.

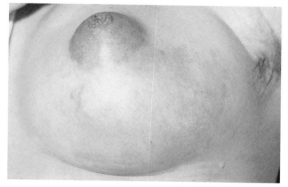

Color Plate 19 Mastitis involving the lower outer quadrant of the breast. The mother was placed on intravenous antibiotics in the hospital, and lactation continued throughout the iv therapy. Her baby was housed with her during her hospitalization.

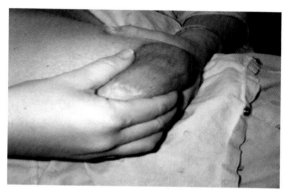

Color Plate 20 This mother is displacing breast edema (different from engorgement) by applying pressure from the areola backwards toward the chest wall, rotating the fingers around the "clock" and moving back, holding the pressure until the tissue becomes soft. The procedure can take a few minutes to 30 minutes depending on the severity of the edema.

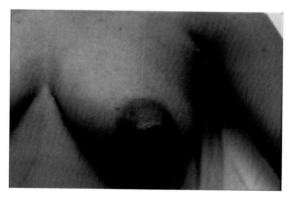

Color Plate 21 Auxillary breast and nipple tissue. A common site for additional breast or nipple tissue. In the absence of stimulation, milk production and tissue swelling ceases.

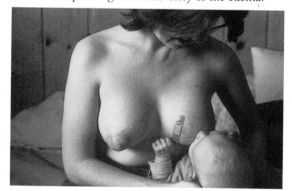

Color Plate 22 Breastfeeding following biopsy for a benign tumor. The mother, with a totally breastfed infant, is shown four months postpartum. The tumor was discovered during lactation two weeks prior to biopsy. The baby is breastfeeding four hours after biopsy, the mother keeping the baby's hand away from the biopsy incision area.
Reprinted with permission from Chele Marmet, Lactation Institute.

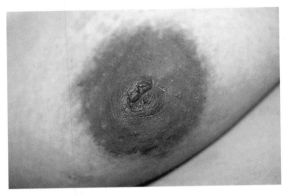

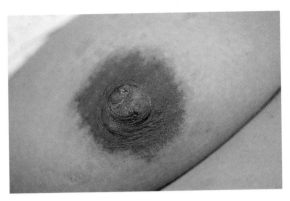

Color Plate 23 Nipple inversion. The mother had successfully breastfed her previous baby using both breasts.

Color Plate 24 Nipple eversion. Following gentle suction with a hand breast bump, the nipple completely everted.

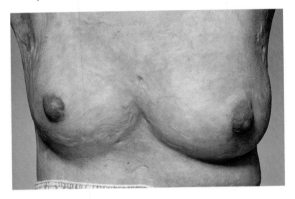

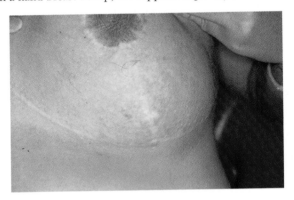

Color Plate 25 Burn scars on breast. This mother sustained third-degree burns as a child and experienced numerous subsequent reconstructive surgeries, including one to reconstruct her nipples. Although the breast tissue was difficult to compress because of extensive scar tissue, the baby was able to breastfeed.

Color Plate 26 Breast-reduction scars. This mother has breast surgery at age 28, two years before her first pregnancy; her bra size Changed from a 32hh to a 36b prior to her first pregnancy. The nipples were not entirely detached, but both areaolae were reduced in size and repositioned on the breast. Following surgery, the left breast had heightened sensation; the right nipple had no sensation at all. Some milk was obtained from each breast.
Reprinted with permission from Chele Marmet, Lactation Institute.

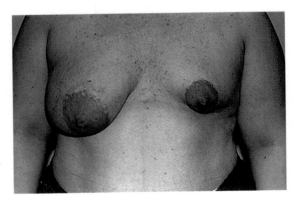

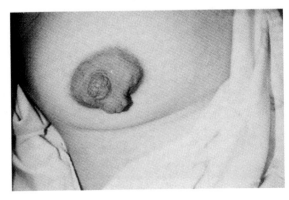

Color Plate 27 Significantly different breast size and shape, suggestive of primary breast insufficiency; this mother was referred for a lactation consultation for inadequate milk supply.
Reprinted with permission from Kay Hoover.

Color Plate 28 Double nipple on the same breast. His mother's baby needed to gape widely enough to take both nipples into his mouth.
Reprinted with permission from Linda Stewart.

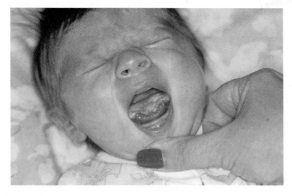

Color Plate 29 Oral candidiasis (thrush). When first seen, the baby was fifteen days old; the gums and inner cheeks were as involved as his tongue. The mother's nipples were also inflamed. After four weeks of intermittent treatment, neither the baby's mouth nor the mother's breasts were infected.
Reprinted with permission from Chele Marmet, Lactation Institute.

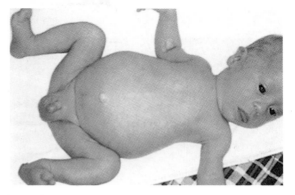

Color Plate 30 Baby with down syndrome. Note the small genitalia characteristic of a child with down syndrome. Poor head and neck control, weak jaw and other motor abilities, and a poor suck often require special assistance while the baby is learning how to suckle the breast.
Reprinted with permission from Chele Marmet, Lactation Institute.

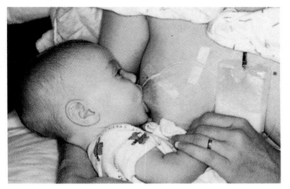

Color Plate 31 Baby with ftt. At birth, this baby weighed 8 obs 12 oz. When referred to the lc at 4 1/2 months, he still weighed only 10 lbs 11 oz. He avidly sucked his own fingers and slept for long periods; when put to the breast, he was extremely lethargic. In addition, he sucked in his cheeks, generating no effective negative pressure on the breast.
Reprinted with permission from Jane Bradshaw.

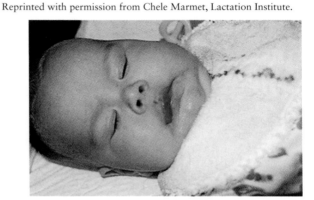

Color Plate 32 Hemangioma of the infant's lip. Although it may appear to be troublesome, this condition did not cause feeding problems for the baby.
Reprinted with permission from Barbara Wilson-Clay.

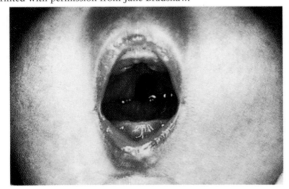

Color Plate 33 Cleft of the soft palate. Such a cleft can occur without a cleft of the lip.
Reprinted with permission from Jane Bradshaw.

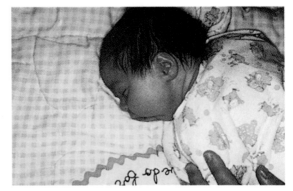

Color Plate 34 Baby with pierre robin syndrome. This syndrome is characterized by a severely receded chin, which can require special assistance and creative positioning to help the baby latch on. Other characteristics of this syndrome, such as cleft palate, may also render breastfeeding difficult or impossible to achieve for varying lengths of time.
Reprinted with permission from Jane Bradshaw.

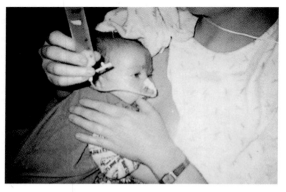

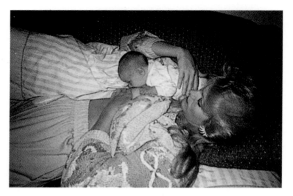

Color Plate 35 Baby being fed by ng tube while at breast. Sometimes a baby unable to feed directly can be fed with a nasogastric tube. doing so while holding her baby next to her breast and allowing the baby to suck on a finger or thumb can help the mother to normalize this feeding situation.

Reprinted with permission from Jane Bradshaw.

Color Plate 36 Baby breastfeeding in over-the-shoulder positioning of the baby. Mother lying on back with baby approaching breast from over her shoulder.

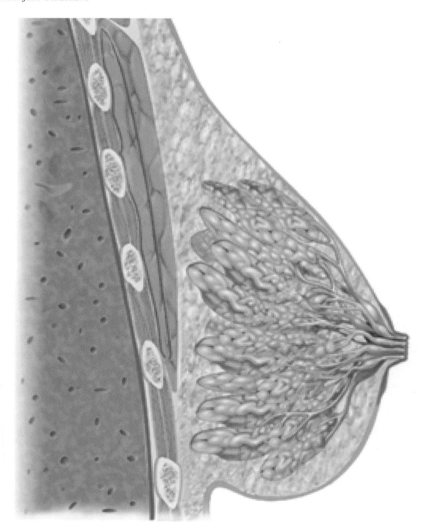

Color Plate 37 Artist's drawing of the anatomy of the inside of the breast.

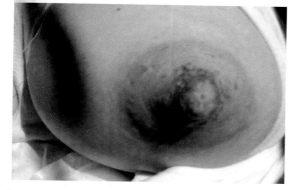

Color Plate 38 Staph infection (impetigo). Raised red pimple-like "bumps," cracking at nipple base with yellow crustingat nipple tips.
Reprinted with permission from Vonie Miller.

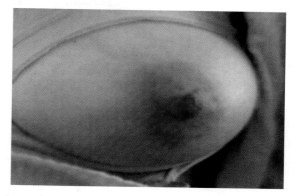

Color Plate 39 Vasopasm and skin tag. This nipple Demonstrates the purple phase of color change association with nipple vasospasm. An incidental finding is the small skin tag seen between 12 to 1 o'clock.
Reprinted with permission from Nancy Powers.

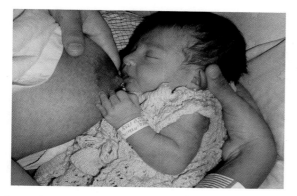

Color Plate 40 Late preterm infant. Late preterm infants are placced on the regular postpartum unit with their mothers. Most late preterm infants require more time and effort to help them breastfeed because they are smaller and less mature neurologically.

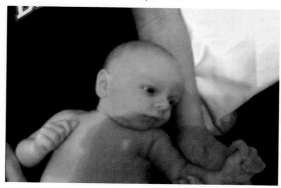

Color Plate 41 Torticollis, head turned to left. This infant This infant with congenital muscular torticollis shows several class if findings shown in plates 41 through 43. The shortened and tightened sternocleidomastoid muscle causes the infant routinely to assume a "position of comfort" with his head tilted to the left. Often there will be secondary changes to the shape of the skull, positional plaigiocephaly.
Reprinted with permission from Nancy Powers.

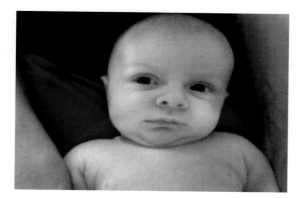

Color Plate 42 Torticollis, jaw to side. In this photo, the same infant demonstrates obvious jaw asymmetry, with the left side slanting more acutely toward the ear while the right side is rounder and fuller. This is caused by the pressure of the baby's face and jaw against the left shoulder in utero. It will usually be accompanied by asymmetry of the gums as well.
Reprinted with permission from Nancy Powers.

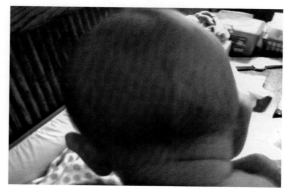

Color Plate 43 Torticollis, left ear out. The same infant as in the previous two photos demonstrates the left ear protrududing further from the skull than the right side. It is also slightly larger. Compression of the ear against the shoulder in untero is responsible for overgrowth of the ear. This finding is most easily appreciated from the posterior view.
Reprinted with permission from Nancy Powers.

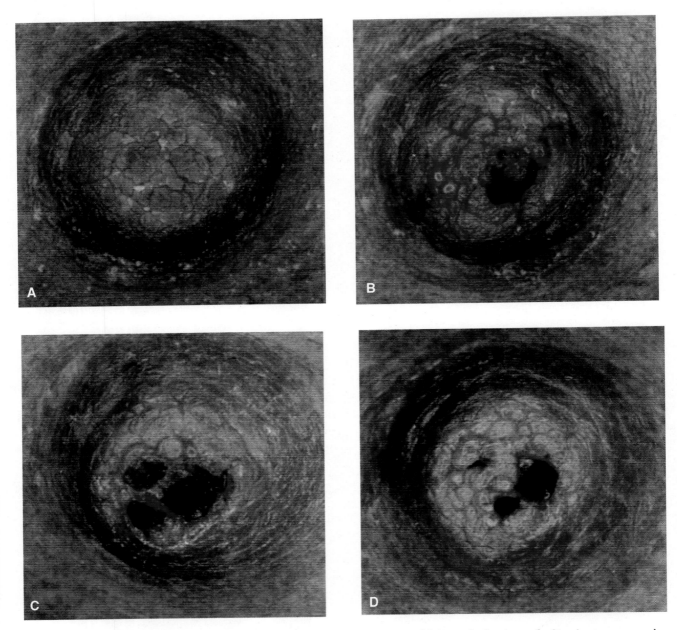

Color Plate 44 Nipple healing. (a) day 1. Nipple skin condition the day of delivery before breastfeeding has commenced. Note the white flecks on the skin. (b) day 3. Two small areas that appear to be blisters can be noted at the 7 o'clock position. (c) day 5. A fissure on the nipple skin and eschar formation can be seen. (d) day 7. Eschar remains adhered to the surface of the nipple. Nipple condition improved. (magnification factor of 22.)

Used with permission from Ziemer M, Pidgeon J. Skin changes and pain in the nipple during the first week of lactation. *JOGNN*. 1993;22:247–256.

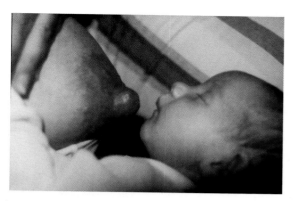

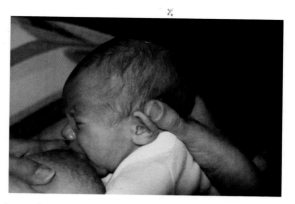

Color Plate 45 Large nipples. Unusually large nipples can cause latch on problems at first but tend to resolve as the baby grows.
Used with permission from Barbara Wilson-Clay and Kay Hoover.

Color Plate 46 Gagging due to large nipple. Large nipples can cause gagging in early breastfeeds until the baby matures.
Used with permission from Barbara Wilson-Clay and Kay Hoover.

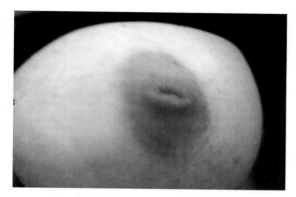

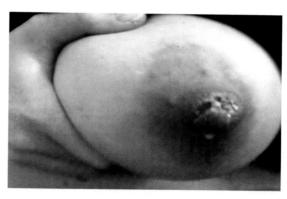

Color Plate 47 Inverted nipple. This patient has bilateral significantly inverted nipples that evert during milk expression with a breast pump, but immediately return to the inverted state. In this photo, the right nipple/areplar complex is erythematous from pumping her breastmilk postpartum.
Reprinted with permission from Nancy Powers.

Color Plate 48 Deep crack in inverted nipple. The same patient as previous photo show a deep crack on the left nipple that would not heal because the inversion kept the tissue "buried" without air or light. The nipple everted only immediately after applying the breast pump.
Reprinted with permission from Nancy Powers.

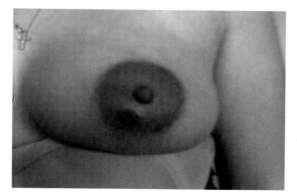

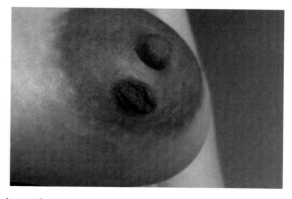

Color Plate 49 A large pigmented lesion appears on the areola to the left of the nipple. The referring clinicial was uncertain what to recommend.

Color Plate 50 Upon closer inspection, the lesion appears soft and deflated, but will erect with tactile stimulation. This lesion qas surgically removed during pregnancy to help avoid interference with breastfeeding. It is a large sumernumerary nipple.

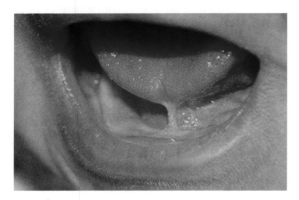

Color Plate 5 1 Tongue-tie.
Reprinted with permission from Linda Smith.

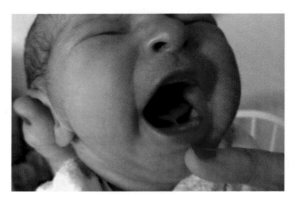

Color Plate 5 2 Side view of tongue-tie. Exists in many variations. Accordingly, tongue movement and suckling ability can present with a variety of different clinical effects for mother and/or baby.
Reprinted with permission from Nancy Powers.

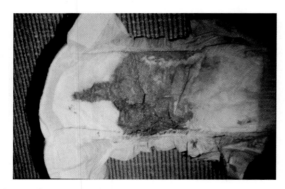

Color Plate 5 3 Normal yellow, frothy stool of exclusively breastfed baby at two months old.

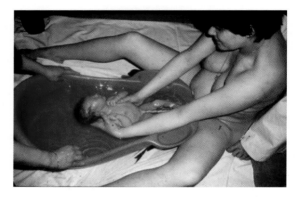

Color Plate 5 4 Natural birth.

of employment, or one who is expressing milk only occasionally. The mother of the premature infant needs a pump that has the following characteristics:

- Removes milk quickly
- Pumps both breasts simultaneously
- Promotes physiologic prolactin cycling
- Mimics the sucking action of an infant
- Obtains milk with a high energy content
- Has an easily controlled vacuum
- Permits the vacuum to be applied for short periods of time to avoid tissue damage
- Produces high milk yield
- Is easy to use
- Is heat resistant for sterilization
- Has a collection kit that is easily assembled and cleaned
- Is durable (will not stop working or break easily)
- Is economical
- Is accessible

A reasonable option for long-term pumping is an electric pump with a double collecting kit that is rented on a long-term basis. The mother should begin pumping as soon after the birth as possible (preferably within the first hour or at least within the first 6 hours) and do so at least eight times each 24 hours (Hill et al., 1996). Hand expression and hand techniques should be combined with early pumping for mothers of preterm infants.

The mother who has a healthy 2- to 3-month-old infant and is returning to full-time employment outside the home may have different needs. This mother could consider a long-term lease on an electric pump or the purchase of a personal-use pump. A mother with carpal tunnel syndrome; arthritis; or other hand, wrist, arm, or shoulder problems may need to use an electric pump rather than a manual or battery-operated pump to avoid exacerbation of her symptoms.

A mother who expresses only small amounts of milk or who has a low milk supply should be advised to elicit the milk-ejection reflex by baby suckling, looking at a picture of her baby, listening to guided relaxation tapes or music, or practicing slow chest breathing before applying the pump, and to massage the breast by quadrants throughout the pumping session. She may need to sit in a quiet area that permits relaxation with a minimum of interruptions. Pumping early in the morning or on the opposite breast while the baby is nursing may

---

BOX 12-2 FDA POLICY ON USED BREAST PUMPS

Should I Buy a Used Breast Pump or Share a Breast Pump?

You should never buy a used breast pump or share a breast pump.

Only FDA-cleared, hospital-grade pumps should be used by more than one person.

With the exception of hospital-grade pumps, the FDA considers breast pumps single-use devices. That means that a breast pump should only be used by one woman because there is no way to guarantee the pump can be cleaned and disinfected between uses by different women.

The money you may save by buying a used pump is not worth the health risks to you or your baby. Breast pumps that are reused by different mothers can carry infectious diseases, such as HIV or hepatitis.

Buying a used breast pump or sharing a breast pump may be a violation of the manufacturer's warranty, and you may not be able to get help from the manufacturer if you have a problem with the pump.

Source: U.S. Food and Drug Administration, Center for Devices and Radiological Health. Breast Pumps—Choosing a Breast Pump. 2007. Available at: http://www.fda.gov/cdrh/breastpumps/choosing.html#4.

also prove helpful. Flange size should be checked to assure that the mother is using a flange that will accommodate the nipple throughout the pumping session. She could also be advised to pump after each breastfeeding to drain the breasts as much as possible.

Some mothers find the use of synthetic oxytocin nasal spray helpful in eliciting the milk-ejection reflex. While it may not increase overall volume of milk pumped (Fewtrell et al., 2006), its use may help individual mothers overcome delayed milk ejection and reduce pumping time. This preparation can be obtained by prescription from a compounding pharmacy.

Common Pumping Problems

The most common pumping problems seen by clinicians are sore nipples, obtaining only small amounts of milk per pumping session, erratic or delayed milk-ejection reflex, and dwindling milk supply over a long-term course of pumping (Walker, 1987).

Sore nipples caused by breast pumps can be minimized by using the lowest amount of vacuum that works to obtain milk; eliciting the milk-ejection reflex before applying the vacuum; interrupting the vacuum frequently to avoid or decrease pain while still maintaining milk flow; switching from side to side frequently as the milk flow slows (when using single-sided pumping); ensuring proper flange fit with an inner opening that is not too small for the nipple entering it or too large to be effective; and pumping for shorter periods of time. Some mothers find that lubricating the pump flange with a small amount of olive oil is soothing.

Obtaining only small amounts of milk per pumping session is a frustrating and common problem. Mothers may complain that the milk drips but does not spray out and that it takes more than 45 minutes to accumulate 0.5 to 1 oz. As a result of this frustration, pump vacuum levels are often increased. This contributes more to sore nipples than to increased milk yields. To elicit the milk-ejection reflex, some mothers have reported using a hot shower or hot compresses, using breast massage

or hand expression, or establishing a pumping routine (activities performed prior to each pumping session that elicit milk flow).

Increasing fluid intake does not usually increase milk yield. Some mothers pump whenever they experience a spontaneous milk ejection. Timing pumping sessions may also help, particularly if some women find it difficult to obtain much milk immediately after the baby has fed. Pumping midway between feedings may help this situation. Morning pumping sessions also tend to yield more milk. Mothers who are employed on a full-time basis report that pumping sessions early in the week also tend to yield more milk than pumping sessions later in the week (Auerbach & Guss, 1984).

Oxytocin nasal spray has been used prior to each pumping session as a temporary boost to milk ejection. While it is no longer available from manufacturers as a nasal spray, compounding pharmacies can purchase oxytocin and mix it into the nasal spray form (Gross, 1995). Oxytocin has been used by mothers during the first week of pumping following a preterm birth with significant results. In one study, milk production increased by a factor of 3.5 for primiparous mothers and by a factor of 2.5 for multiparous mothers compared to mothers not using oxytocin nasal spray prior to each pumping session (Ruis et al., 1981). In contrast, Fewtrell et al. (2006), in a randomized double-blind trial of oxytocin nasal spray versus placebo in the first 5 days after birth of a preterm infant, found no significant difference in milk production, milk weight, or milk fat content.

Some mothers are able to increase their milk production through the use of what is popularly called power pumping, cluster pumping, or super pumping. In this technique, a mother pumps for as long as it takes to elicit the first milk-ejection reflex and removes the milk made available during the time the milk ducts stay dilated. As much as 45% of the milk available in the breast is released during the first milk letdown period (Ramsay et al., 2006), which may last no longer than 5 minutes. The mother then pumps again in 10–15 minutes or so to once more take advantage of the first and largest milk-ejection reflex of a pumping session.

She may cluster this pattern for a period of time during the day.

Mothers should massage and compress each breast while pumping to create a more efficient pressure gradient. They can also warm the breast and the pump flange to increase milk yield. Sometimes these interventions cease working, in which case the mother can be advised to change to a completely different pump. A different suction curve may better suit such a mother.

Today, medicine and technology are saving infants as young as 23 weeks' gestational age. Mothers wishing to breastfeed extremely preterm infants will be pumping milk for many months. They can encounter difficulties maintaining an optimal milk supply through artificial means. A flexible pumping plan should be developed for optimal milk production (Auerbach & Walker, 1994; Hill et al., 1999; Walker, 2012). Faltering milk production is not unusual with extended pumping. In addition to the guidelines in this chapter, other interventions for a faltering milk supply (Gabay, 2002) include the use of metoclopromide (Ehrenkranz & Ackerman, 1986; Toppare et al., 1994), acupuncture (Clavey, 1996), domperidone (da Silva et al., 2001; Jantarasaengaram & Sreewapa, 2012; Wan et al., 2008), human growth hormone (Gunn et al., 1996), fenugreek (Turkyilmaz et al., 2011), and recombinant human prolactin (Powe et al., 2010, 2011).

Factors other than the type of equipment used also affect milk flow. Morse and Bottorff (1988) have stated that "understanding the complex feelings towards expressing and the experimental nature of learning to express has important implications for the way that expression is taught." An erratic or delayed milk-ejection reflex is common when a mother must respond to a mechanical device rather than her baby, particularly when she is first learning to use a pump. If the milk-ejection reflex is not triggered quickly, the nipples and breast tissue are exposed to high levels of vacuum over an inefficient pressure gradient. This can result in low milk yields, sore nipples, and frustration with the pumping process.

Although pumps are capable of eliciting milk ejection and their instructions often advise applying the pump for this purpose, some women will have difficulty releasing their milk. This problem may be caused by inhibitory messages received by the hypothalamus. Embarrassment, tension, fear of failure, pain, fatigue, and anxiety may block the neurochemical pathways required for milk ejection. If these factors appear to interfere with milk ejection, ask the mother how she feels about pumping. A negative attitude does little to contribute to milk flow. One mother, when offered the option of double pumping, said it made her feel like a cow; single-sided pumping was more appealing to her. When the clinician knows the mother's feelings and attitudes about pumping, guidelines can be individually created for each situation.

It is not unusual for the milk-ejection reflex to take longer to trigger as the lactation course increases. This is common both with a baby at breast and with long-term pumping. What works early in lactation may change over time. Some mothers report improved results later in lactation, after they change to a different pump or use a different flange that fits the breast better.

Expressing milk has different meanings for each mother. Some women see it as a way to continue providing breastmilk in their absence, especially in families with a history of allergies. Some mothers prefer to express milk by hand because they obtain as much milk in as quick a time as they do when using a pump. Other mothers view pumping as part of a grief-like reaction that is reinforced every 2 to 3 hours when they must use a pump in the absence of a baby at breast. Sound pump recommendations, pumping instructions based on a clear understanding of the anatomy and physiology of the breast, and knowledge of the lactation process will enable many women to give their infant the best possible nutritional and emotional start.

Nipple Shields

Nipple shields appeared in the medical literature as early as the mid-1600s. Scultetus, an early physician, described shields made of silver and used so that "nurses may suckle the infants without trouble which, when children were breast-fed until long after their front teeth were cut, must have been very necessary" (as cited in Bennion, 1979). Shields were first used to evert flat nipples and protect nipples from the cold and rubbing against clothing between feedings. Between the 1500s and 1800s, a variety of other functions for shields were also described:

- To cover flat nipples
- To prevent sore or ulcerated nipples
- To treat cracked, sore, or infected nipples
- To protect clothing from milk leakage
- To be used as a base for attaching an artificial nipple or cow's teat

In historical usage, shields were made of lead (which caused brain damage in babies), wax, wood, gum elastic, pewter, tin, horn, bone, ivory, silver, and glass. The gum elastic shield in Figure 12-13 was used for babies to nurse on. Maygrier (1833) stated, "This mode is difficult and generally the child is unwilling."

The design of nipple shields has changed little since the 1500s. By the 1800s, however, rubber shields began appearing. The Maw's shield (Figure 12-14) was constructed with a rubber lining, a glass shank, and a rubber teat. In the 1980s, this design was still used with a glass or plastic shank and a rubber teat (Davol). Rubber versions of the silver and wood shields also began appearing. The early shields were composed of thick rubber with a firm nipple cone (The Mexican Hat, Macarthy's Surgical). One U.S. version, the Breast-Eze, consisted of a modified rubber nipple on a rubber base with thick rubber ribs lining the inside to help "stimulate" the breast. This design was reported to be very painful to use. Over time, the rubber shields gradually became thinner (Evenflo) and were replaced with the thin latex (Lewin Woolf, Griptight) and ultrathin silicone (Canon Babysafe, Medela, Ameda, Avent) versions seen today (Figure 12-15).

Early nipple shield use generated poor outcomes in many babies due to misuse, misunderstanding, and the very thick nature of the device that prevented mothers from feeling the baby at breast (which probably reduced prolactin levels) and contributed to overall poor milk transfer. The barrier that the thick shield created between

Figure 12-13 EARLY NIPPLE SHIELDS, CIRCA 1883.

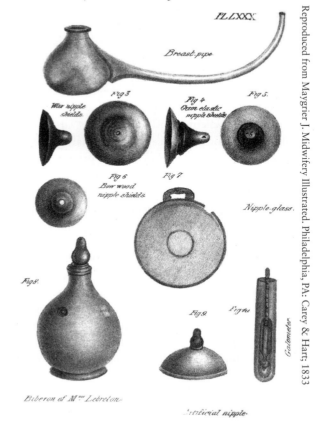

Reproduced from Maygrier J. Midwifery Illustrated. Philadelphia, PA: Carey & Hart; 1833

Figure 12-14 NIPPLE SHIELD AND BREAST GLASS, CIRCA 1864.

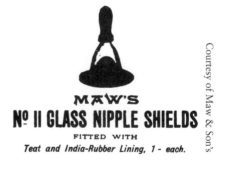

Courtesy of Maw & Son's

Figure 12-15 Modern Silicone Nipple Shields (Left) and Breast Shells (Right).

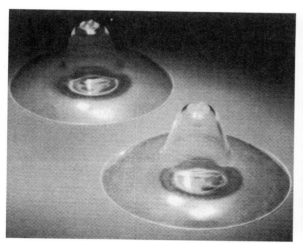
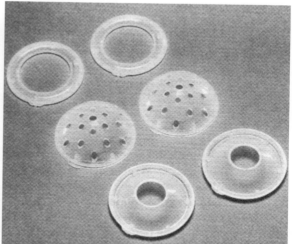

the baby's mouth and teat exceeded the limits of the mechanical requirements for milk removal. Such devices became destructive to the course of lactation and risky to the health of the baby (Desmarais & Browne, 1990).

Selected Review of the Literature on Nipple Shields

Woolridge, Baum, and Drewett (1980) studied the effect of the all-rubber shield (Macarthy-Mexican Hat) and a thin latex shield on the suckling patterns and milk intake of 5- to 8-day-old babies of mothers with problem-free lactation experiences. The Macarthy-Mexican Hat reduced milk transfer by 58% and changed infant suckling patterns by increasing the suckling rate and the time spent pausing. This is a pattern typically seen when milk flow decreases. The thin latex shield reduced milk intake by 22% and had no significant effect on suckling patterns. This thin shield was being tested as part of an apparatus in a new system for measuring milk flow and composition during breastfeeding. The babies observed in this study had no difficulty latching onto their mothers' nipples, and no nipple soreness was reported by the mothers in the study.

Theoretically, if these problems existed, milk transfer and suckling patterns could be further compromised with the continued use of a thick shield. Using the same thin latex shield, Jackson et al. (1987) showed a 29% decrease in milk transfer during their study of nutrient intake in healthy, full-term newborns.

Amatayakul et al. (1987) measured plasma prolactin and cortisol levels in mothers, with and without a thin latex nipple shield in place. They found that prolactin and cortisol levels were unaffected by the shield but that milk transfer was decreased by 42% when the shield was in place during feedings. They postulated that this effect on milk volume was attributable to an interference with oxytocin release.

Auerbach (1990a) studied changes in pumped milk volume with and without the use of a thin silicone shield (Cannon Babysafe). Twenty-five mothers used a breast pump (Medela electric model) to provide milk samples, which prevented any change in infant suckling patterns from affecting milk volume amounts. Milk volume was significantly reduced when a shield was in place. Seventy-one percent of the total milk obtained was recorded when no shield was used. Pumping without a shield resulted in mean volumes five to seven times greater than when a shield was in place.

Chertok (2009) examined weight gain in 54 term infants with and without the use of ultrathin silicone nipple shields. Infant weight gain was similar in maternal–infant dyads using nipple shields for 2 months compared to those not using shields. A majority of the mothers (89.8%) reported a positive experience with the shield, and 67.3% of the mothers stated that the nipple shield helped prevent breastfeeding abandonment.

Key to good outcomes is the use of ultrathin silicone shields, critical assessment by a skilled lactation consultant, and continuous follow-up. Eglash and colleagues (2010) reported that nipple shield use is a common recommendation among health professionals. In their survey of 490 health professionals, most providers used nipple shields to facilitate latching in infants less than 35 weeks' gestation. Shields have also been used for latch assistance in term infants, infants with oral anomalies, and infants with upper airway dysfunction or anomalies. Babies who otherwise may have been unable to breastfeed have benefited from the judicious use of this device.

Hanna and colleagues (2012) explored the satisfaction and breastfeeding experiences of mothers with early breastfeeding problems who used ultrathin silicone nipple shields. The majority of the 81 mothers found the shield to be extremely helpful. In this study, mothers who otherwise would have abandoned breastfeeding found that the shield helped them continue to nurse their infants, with 31% still breastfeeding at 6 months.

Despite these results, much of the published research on nipple shields is not considered definitive (McKechnie & Eglash, 2010) due to lack of prospective, randomized controlled trials of shield use; references to old studies; use of samples of babies with no feeding problems; small samples; and sometimes measurement only a single feeding (Table 12-4).

Types of Shields

Rubber Shields
Rubber shields are seldom, if ever, seen today and should not be used.

Standard Bottle Nipples or Bottle Nipples Attached to a Glass or Plastic Base
These types of shields place the baby and his mouth 1 to 2 inches away from the mother's nipple, significantly altering positioning at breast. This does

Table 12-4 Nipple Shield Research

Study	Description
Brigham, 1996	Reviewed 51 mothers, with 81% reporting positive outcomes in resolving breastfeeding problems.
Bodley & Powers, 1996	In 10 cases weight gain was appropriate during and following the period of nipple shield use.
Woodworth & Frank, 1996	Shield used for breast refusal.
Wilson-Clay, 1996	Experiences of 32 mothers using shields to resolve breastfeeding problems.
Clum & Primomo, 1996	9 of 15 preterm infants consumed 50% more milk at breast with an ultrathin shield than without a shield.
Meier et al., 2000	34 preterm infants showed increased milk transfer with a shield; 3.9 ml without the shield and 18.4 ml with the shield.
Chertok et al., 2006	32 mothers demonstrated no significant difference in hormonal levels and infant milk intake with and without ultrathin nipple shield use.
Chertok, 2009	Infant weight gain was similar for infants using shields compared with those not using shields. Maternal satisfaction was confirmed.

Table 12-4 NIPPLE SHIELD RESEARCH (CONTINUED)

Study	Description
Eglash, Zeimer, & Chevalier, 2010	Maternal response to nipple shields was that they were helpful. Mothers rated lack of follow-up by providers as their greatest concern with nipple shield use.
McKechnie & Eglash, 2010	A review of the literature on nipple shield use showed that the body of evidence did not include well-designed mixed methods studies or large prospective trials of shield use.
Hanna, Wilson, & Norwood, 2012	Shields were shown to help mothers who otherwise might have abandoned breastfeeding. Problems with latch and nipple pain and anomalies were helped with the use of shields.

not permit compression of the milk sinuses or skin-to-skin stimulation of the nipple–areolar complex and may alter prolactin cycling. Milk may pool in the base, which holds the artificial nipple, and never reach the baby, or simply leak out the sides. These devices are seldom seen and should not be used, nor should an artificial nipple itself be placed over a mother's nipple.

Latex and Silicone Shields

These devices are extremely thin, flexible shields with the nipple portion being firmer. Because the silicone is so thin, more stimulation reaches the areola, and milk volume is not as seriously depleted as with the other designs (Auerbach, 1990a). Because of the increasing reports of latex allergy in the general population, latex-containing shields should be avoided. Silicone shields are available in a number of sizes (Table 12-5).

Shield Selection and Instructions

There is little in the literature regarding shield selection and instructions for use. If the height of the teat of a shield is greater than the length from the junction of the hard and soft palate to the lips, then the infant's jaw closure and tongue compression will fall on the shaft of the teat, and not over the breast. Wilson-Clay and Hoover (2005) also recommend that the base diameter should fit the mother's nipple and that better results occur with the shortest teat height and smallest base diameter. A summary of instructions includes the following:

- Apply the shield by turning it almost inside out.
- Moisten the edges to help it adhere better or warm the shield with hot water.
- Drip expressed milk onto the outside of the teat to encourage the baby.
- Hand-express a little milk into the teat if necessary.
- Use alternate massage to help drain the breast.
- Run tubing inside or outside of the shield for supplementation.
- The baby's mouth must not close on the shaft of the teat.

Table 12-5 SILICONE SHIELDS

Product	Diameter (in.)	Height of Nipple (in.)	Width of Nipple (in.)	Number of Holes
Avent	2 6/8	7/8	5/8 at tip, 1 at base	3
Medela Standard	2 6/8	7/8	5/8 at tip, 1 at base	4
Medela Extra Small	2 6/8	6/8	3/8 at tip, 5/8 at base	3
Ameda	2 5/8	7/8	4/8 at tip, 7/8 at base	5

- The latch should be checked to see that the baby is not just suckling on the tip of the teat.
- The shield should be washed in hot soapy water after each use and rinsed well.
- If yeast is present on the areola, the shield should be boiled.
- Some mothers may need more than one shield.
- Perform a weight check of the infant about every 3 days until the mother's milk supply is stable and the baby is gaining weight well.
- Check the breasts for plugged ducts and areas that are not draining well.

Weaning from the Shield

Recommendations regarding weaning from the nipple shield include the following:

- There is no set time for weaning; extended use of the ultrathin silicone shield has not been shown to be detrimental.

- Mothers start by just placing the baby skin-to-skin next to the nipple, starting the feed with the shield and removing it, and gradually trying feeds without the shield.
- The shield should not be cut.

Responsibilities

The healthcare professional has the following responsibilities regarding breastfeeding women and nipple shields:

- Document all of your encounters and instructions and communicate these to the primary healthcare provider.
- Understand the risks and advantages of using such a device (Box 12-3).
- Assess the situation before recommending a shield (Auerbach, 1989). Shields used as a quick fix to ensure infant feedings before early discharge act as "Band-Aid therapy"— that is, they cover up the problem without addressing the cause. Identify and take steps

---

BOX 12-3 QUICK GUIDE TO NIPPLE SHIELD USE

What Shields Do

- Therapeutically supply oral stimulation not provided by mother's nipples
- Create a nipple shape in infant's mouth
- Allow extraction of milk by expression with minimal suction and negative pressure
- Help compensate for weak infant suction
- Present a stable nipple shape that remains during pauses in suckling bursts
- Maintain the nipple in a protruded position
- Raise the rate of milk flow

What Shields Will Not Do

- Correct milk transfer problems or weight gain if the mother has inadequate milk volume
- Fix damaged nipples if the cause is not discovered and remedied
- Replace skilled intervention and close follow-up

Advantages of Nipple Shields

- Permit learning to feed at breast
- Allow supplementation at breast (i.e., thread tubing under or alongside of the shield)
- Encourage nipple protractility
- Will not overwhelm mother with gadgets
- Prevent baby fighting the breast

Disadvantages of Nipple Shields

- Used as a substitute for skilled care
- Used as a quick fix
- May exacerbate original problem
- May lead to insufficient milk volume, inadequate weight gain, weaning
- Prevent proper extension of the nipple back into the baby's mouth (Minchin, 1985)
- May pinch the nipple and areola, causing abrasion, pain, skin breakdown, and internal trauma to the breast if not applied properly
- Create nipple shield addiction (DeNicola, 1986), after which the baby will not feed at breast without the shield in place
- Predispose the nipple to damage when the baby is put to breast without the shield, as he may chew rather than suckle
- Discarded as a useful intervention in selected situations

Possible Indications for Nipple Shield Use

Latch Difficulty

- Nipple anomalies (flat, retracted, fibrous, inelastic)
- Mismatch between small baby mouth and large nipple
- Baby from heavily medicated mother
- Birth trauma (vacuum extraction, forceps)
- Oral aversion (vigorous suctioning)
- Artificial nipple preference (pacifiers, bottles)
- Transition baby from bottle to breast
- Baby with weak or disorganized suckle (slips off nipple, preterm, neurological problems)
- Baby with high or low tone
- Delay in putting baby to breast

Oral Cavity Problems

- Cleft palate
- Channel palate (Turner's syndrome, formerly intubated)
- Bubble palate
- Lack of fat pads (preterm, SGA)
- Low threshold mouth
- Poor central grooving of the tongue
- Micrognathia (recessed jaw)

Upper Airway Problems

- Tracheomalacia
- Laryngomalacia

Damaged Nipples

- When all else fails and mother states she is going to quit breastfeeding to correct the problem rather than issuing a shield as the initial therapy.

- Ensure that the mother will receive close follow-up during the time the shield is in use.
- Realize that the risks of nipple shield use have legal implications for the hospital and/ or professional who recommend them (Bornmann, 1986).
- Provide proper instructions and referrals if a shield is used as an interim recommendation to assist with breastfeeding. If a mother is discharged from the hospital using a shield, a community referral must be made to a lactation consultant or the nurse practitioner at the pediatrician's office for daily follow-up. Weight checks may need to be obtained twice a week. The pediatrician should be alerted to the problem that required use of the shield in the first place and should be aware of suggestions for discontinuing its use.

Breast Shells

Breast shells are two-piece plastic devices worn over the nipple and areola to evert flat or retracted nipples. Historically, these shells were called nipple glasses (Figure 12-15) and were used to protect the mother's clothing from leaking milk, or were applied if the mother had "too much" milk. Some brands are still marketed as devices for catching leaked milk between feedings. Currently, shells are not recommended for this use, although many mothers find them helpful for collecting drip milk from one breast while nursing or pumping on the opposite side. Some clinicians also recommend their use for engorgement, as their gentle pressure encourages milk to leak and for areolar edema to create a circular pit that exposes the nipple. The milk collected between feedings must be discarded because of potential high bacteria counts. If drip milk is collected during a feeding or pumping session, it can be stored as usual.

Inverted nipples are identified when the areola is compressed behind the base of the nipple and the nipple retreats into the surrounding skin.

This is caused by the presence of the original invagination of the mammary dimple. In the past, breast shells were worn prenatally for increasingly longer periods of time throughout the day and removed at night. The constant gentle pressure around the base of the nipple was thought to release the adhesions anchoring the nipple, thus allowing it to protrude when the baby latches onto the breast. Shells can be worn between feedings, after the baby is born, if nipple flattening or retraction is identified postpartum, or if the nipples still need correction. Research has indicated that little correction of the nipple actually took place prenatally and that some women do not like using these devices (Alexander et al., 1992). Consequently, most clinicians no longer recommend prenatal use of this product.

Several brands of shells are available, all of which have a dome that is placed over a base through which the nipple protrudes when worn under a bra. Depending on the brand, the dome may have one or many ventilation holes. The domes with only one or two holes may not provide adequate air circulation to the nipple and areola. The retained moisture and heat (especially in hot weather) can create a miniature greenhouse effect that promotes soreness and skin breakdown. Extra holes can be drilled in the top of the dome. Some brands have many holes in the dome to help with this problem. Another form of breast shell with a wider base has been used for sore nipples to keep air circulating around them and to prevent them from adhering to a bra. Currently, most clinicians seldom recommend these devices.

Feeding-Tube Devices

Judicious use of feeding-tube devices enables many mothers and babies to breastfeed who otherwise would have lost this unique opportunity. Such devices consist of a container to hold breastmilk or formula and a length of thin tubing that runs from the container to the mother's nipple. The tube is secured in place by nonallergenic tape or run under the nursing bra or nipple shield, and as the baby suckles at breast, supplement is simultaneously delivered. Providing milk in this manner may be a novel idea to the mother. Careful explanations should include how the feeding-tube device is used and the expected outcomes. Some mothers are put off by the thought of feeding their babies in what they consider a "non-natural" way that at first appears complicated. Explaining that the device is a temporary aid in establishing the baby at breast while ensuring adequate nutrition helps the mother to accept tube feeding. Several commercial devices are on the market; in addition, noncommercial devices can be constructed from bottles or syringes and tubing.

Lact-Aid

Developed in 1971 for nursing the adopted baby, the Lact-Aid device created a breastfeeding experience for those mothers and babies who previously had no choice in terms of feeding methods. It is a closed system consisting of a presterilized, disposable 4-oz bag to hold milk—with a cap through which a length of fine tubing extends to the nipple. The bag hangs around the mother's neck on a cord. Air is squeezed out of the bag to facilitate milk flow. Powdered formulas will not flow readily through the device.

Supplemental Nutrition System (Medela)

The Supplemental Nutrition System device consists of a 5-oz plastic bottle with a cap through which a length of tubing is secured to each breast. This two-tube unit allows the tubing to be set up on both breasts at the same time and comes with three different sizes of tubing. The vented system has a cap with notches for pinching off both tubes while setting up the unit and securing one tube while the baby is feeding from the other side. Flow rates are influenced by the size of the tubing used (small, medium, large), the height of the bottle, and whether the opposite tube is pinched off during the feeding. A smaller version is also available with only one tube.

Situations for Use

Feeding-tube devices can be recommended and used in many situations where other measures have failed or in an effort to prevent further complications.

Infant Situations

Candidates for feeding-tube devices include the following infants:

- Babies with weak, disorganized, or dysfunctional suckling
- Infants with insufficient weight gain or weight loss
- Some infants with oral anomalies
- Preterm infants

Maternal Situations

Mothers can benefit from the use of feeding-tube devices in the following situations:

- Adoptive nursing (induced lactation) mothers (Auerbach & Avery, 1981; Sutherland & Auerbach, 1985)
- Re-lactation—meaning inducing a milk supply after a separation or interruption of breastfeeding (Auerbach & Avery, 1980; Bose et al., 1981)
- Breast surgery, especially breast reduction mammaplasty that involved moving the nipple
- Primary or secondary lactation insufficiency—not enough functional breast tissue to support a full milk supply (Neifert & Seacat, 1985) or to increase faltering milk production
- Severe nipple trauma
- Illness, surgery, or hospitalization

Generally, a feeding-tube device is used to maintain a mother's milk supply, to deliver sufficient or extra nutrients to the baby, and to create a behavior-modification situation that shapes the baby's suckling pattern to one suitable for obtaining milk from the breast (or prevents the suckling pattern from changing). These devices allow feedings to be done at breast when formerly, in certain situations, bottles with artificial nipples were used. Because these devices are used only in special situations, it is imperative that the professional who recommends their use follow up closely (daily if necessary) to ensure adequate milk intake by the baby, to validate correct use by the mother, and to wean from the device when it is appropriate to do so.

A baby using a feeding tube at breast must be able to latch on and execute some form of suckling. For babies who are unable at first to do this because of complete nipple confusion, strong extensor positioning, hypotonia, or lethargy, finger-feeding with the device can be used as an interim measure (Bull & Barger, 1987), followed by attempts to feed at breast. To do so, the mother places a tube on the pad of her index finger or whichever finger is closest in size to her nipple. She then allows the baby to draw the finger into his mouth. Correct suckling will cause the milk to flow and will reward the desired behavior; no milk is removed if the baby bites the finger like an artificial nipple. While this also allows the father or other caregiver to feed the baby, some babies become unable to feed at breast because of the strong stimulus that the firm finger provides. Finger-feeding in this manner may prevent improper suckling patterns from being reinforced and move the baby to breast faster than if artificial nipples are used to feed the baby, but care must be taken that babies do not become so accustomed to this form of feeding that they are unwilling to suckle at breast. A number of finger-feeding devices are marketed, such as the Hazelbaker FingerFeeder (Aidan & Eva) and the SuppleMate (Maternal Concepts).

When considering feeding-tube devices, the clinician should note the following guidelines:

- These devices can be used to temporarily assist the baby at breast but are generally not necessary if the baby is gaining weight adequately.
- In situations of adoptive nursing; breast reduction surgery; primary lactation insufficiency; and certain genetic, anatomic, or neurologic problems in an infant, these feeding devices may require long-term use with or without breast pumping.
- Close follow-up is mandatory with short- or long-term use.

- Because the baby controls the flow, he will not aspirate or be overwhelmed by the fluid he receives. When he swallows or releases the vacuum, the milk flows backward and the baby must initiate another suckle to start the flow. If the infant cannot initially do this, the bottle or bag of supplement can be squeezed or the plunger of the syringe can be pushed slightly. The milk will not continuously drip or flow as with a bottle and artificial nipple.
- Risks of use include "addiction" to the device by the clinician, mother, and/or baby. The mother and baby should be weaned from the device as quickly as is appropriate. Some mothers may have difficulty believing that they can support a milk supply without the device and not trust themselves to provide for the baby. The clinician should avoid routine use of tube-feeding devices except where necessary. Some clever babies learn to suckle only on the tube, in which case it should be placed so it does not extend beyond the end of the mother's nipple. If the baby has become accustomed to the feel of the tubing, it can be moved to the corner of his mouth and gradually removed. One mother finally taped a 1-inch length of the tube to her areola and withdrew it after her baby latched on.
- One or both tubes can be secured on either side of the areola or the top or bottom, whichever gives the best results.
- The clutch position may be easier to use at first because the mother has greater control of the infant's head.
- A gavage setup with a No. 5 feeding-tube can be used as a feeding device.
- Tubing from a butterfly needle can also be used, as it is smaller and softer than gavage tubing (Edgehouse & Radzyminski, 1990).
- A baby can also be fed by dropper, spoon, cup, or bowl if tubing is not available.
- Powdered formulas and special formulas may clog the smaller tubes if the formula is not mixed well. Larger sizes of tubing may be necessary to prevent clogging.

- The device should be rinsed in cold water after each use and then filled with warm soapy water that is squeezed through the tubing and rinsed well. Sterilization can be done once a day, usually by placing it in boiling water for 20 minutes.
- Feeding in public may be more difficult or obvious. The mother may prefer to use alternatives to tube feeding when she is away from home.

SUMMARY

Just as the healthcare professional must base recommendations for use of breast pumps on various factors, the same holds true for the temporary use of other breastfeeding technologies. Too often a breastfeeding mother may see a device advertised as an aid to breastfeeding and assume that she needs to use it. If she then attempts to do so without thoroughly understanding its risks and benefits, actual and presumed, she could unwittingly interfere with the lactation course and the baby's ability to breastfeed. This is particularly true if the mother obtains the device from a person or institution that lacks a specialist in lactation management.

Nipple shields are the devices most apt to be used when they are not necessary—in part because of their wide availability and in part because of their attractiveness in busy hospitals or practices, where healthcare workers offer the devices because they appear to "make the baby nurse." Thus, when a healthcare provider considers offering the device to a mother, careful instructions and emphasis on the temporary nature of the use of the device must accompany it.

Feeding-tube devices are more complex and, therefore, potentially more off-putting than either breast shells or nipple shields. Mothers who insist on using these devices because they are convinced that their own milk supplies are inadequate to support appropriate infant growth need careful follow-up. Too often, the mother misinterprets the instructions or reads only enough to know how to put the device together and to clean it. The manner in which the device should be used is rarely completely understood from a single reading of the instructions that accompany the device. Healthcare providers or counselors who recommend the inappropriate use of feeding-tube devices can potentially interrupt the breastfeeding relationship or cause further problems. In addition, observation and assessment of the mother and infant as they breastfeed both with and without the device is a necessity if the healthcare provider is to make appropriate recommendations for an optimal outcome. In most cases, the nature of the problem that requires assistance of a feeding-tube device is such that the mother's anxiety level is high and the need to provide additional nutrition for the baby is critical. The lactation consultant, nurse, or other healthcare worker can expect that working with such a mother and baby will be time consuming and will require many more hours of follow-up time than is the case for other situations.

In all cases where any breastfeeding device or pump is used, the benefits of such technology must be weighed against the risks of interfering in the breastfeeding relationship. Anticipating the emotional response of mothers to devices and discussing them in a straightforward manner will assist the healthcare provider in determining whether and when to suggest a particular technology, as well as how to help the mother stop using it when it is no longer necessary. As with all other care, the use of a breastfeeding device of any kind must first be found to "do no harm."

KEY CONCEPTS

- Examples of mothers using a device to remove milk from the breasts are cited in the medical literature as early as the mid-1500s. Historically, a variety of devices were typically used to relieve engorgement or to express milk because of damaged nipples or mastitis.
- Today women express breastmilk on a short-term basis to solve acute problems, but they also pump on a long-term basis to provide human milk for their babies following a pre-term birth or during periods of employment, illness, induced lactation, or re-lactation.

- Mothers list the following criteria as important when choosing a breast pump: (1) quick and effective in removing milk, (2) comfortable to use, (3) reasonably priced, and (4) easy to find, use, and clean.

- To increase pumping efficiency, mothers use two techniques: (1) elicitation of the milk-ejection reflex before pumping and (2) massage of the breasts while pumping. Research and literature from the dairy industry support both techniques.

- Other factors that contribute to pumping efficiency include using relaxation techniques and visual imagery and applying warm, moist heat to the breasts before and during pumping. To avoid breast or nipple injury, it is recommended that the pump be removed as soon as the milk stops flowing.

- Considering the bewildering array of breast pumps in the marketplace today, a caregiver recommending one to a new mother should give a specific name and several places to find it. Prices vary considerably depending upon where the pump is purchased.

- When expressing milk, the device used must be efficient enough to activate prolactin and oxytocin release. The volume of milk expressed is also related to the degree of fullness of the breast, with a fuller breast yielding more milk volume when pumped. Full breasts tend to take less time to achieve the milk-ejection reflex, with a less full breast taking up to 120 seconds.

- Stage III of lactogenesis is dependent upon early and regular stimulation of the nipple and regular removal of milk from the breasts. Lactogenesis II occurs in the absence of milk removal, but lactogenesis III can be inhibited without regular milk removal. The amount of milk produced depends on the rate at which the breast is emptied.

- A breast pump does not pump, suck, or pull milk out of the breast. It reduces resistance to milk outflow from the alveoli, allowing the internal pressure of the breast to push out the milk.

- Einar Egnell was a pioneer in breast pump design and based his design on research from the dairy industry. He designed a pump that created periodic and limited phases of negative pressure and that operated in four phases per cycle. Many pump manufacturers still use Egnell's pressure settings as a guide in current breast pump design.

- W. G. Whittlestone found that providing a compressive force to the breast from a liner inside the pump flange enhanced the dynamics of milk expression. This compression is analogous to a baby's tongue and jaw compressing the teat between the tongue and hard palate during the suction cycle. Some pumps currently offer a soft flange that collapses over the teat when suction is applied, whereas others with a hard plastic flange offer an insert or liner that is intended to serve the same purpose.

- Breast pumps are divided into three broad classifications: (1) manual hand pumps, (2) battery-operated pumps, and (3) electric pumps.

- Manual hand pumps are easy to find, easy to use, and inexpensive. Some are more effective than others in expressing milk. These pumps are typically used on a short-term or occasional basis. The hand and wrist can tire easily with their repeated use. Because of nipple pain and low milk yields, the old-fashioned "bicycle horn" pump is not recommended.

- Battery-operated pumps use a small motor to create a vacuum that is usually adjustable. Most have a button the mother presses to release the vacuum in a rhythmic pattern to simulate the rhythm of a nursing baby. These pumps are lightweight, easy to find and use, and are relatively inexpensive, but have the disadvantage of a short battery life. Some have AC adapters. The time each pump takes to achieve optimal suction varies, and those that require up to 30 seconds can cause nipple pain.

- Electric pumps include some models that are small and semi-automatic and use a small motor to create a vacuum that is adjustable. Most have an open hole in the flange that the mother covers and uncovers with her fingertip to create a rhythmic pattern to simulate the rhythm of a nursing baby. These pumps are moderately priced and most can do double pumping.

- Automatic electric pumps are designed to cycle pressure rather than maintain it. Pressure setting parameters are established to mimic a nursing infant. Pumps are now designed with adjustable cycling rates up to 120 cycles per minute; vacuum pressure adjusts up to 250 mm Hg. These pumps are considered the most effective of all pumps and use double-collection kits. They cost more and are heavier than their handheld counterparts.

- All automatic electric pumps and some of the smaller semi-automatic pumps offer double-collection kits that allow both breasts to be pumped simultaneously. Research has shown that prolactin levels are significantly higher and maximum milk yield occurs with double pumping.

- Product manufacturers offer flanges in different sizes to accommodate the anatomic configuration of a particular breast. If a nipple swells during pumping, the mother with a larger nipple may find that a standard-size flange is too small to accommodate both the large nipple and subsequent swelling. Those mothers whose nipples are larger than 20.5 mm (the size of a U.S. nickel) may benefit from a larger-sized flange.

- Expressed breastmilk is not sterile, and there is considerable disagreement over what constitutes an acceptable bacteria count, especially when pumping for a preterm infant. Many factors play a part in determining the bacteria level, including nipple cleaning, hand washing, collection techniques, type of pump, feeding method of preterm infant, pump-cleaning routines, and gestational age of infant. Some bacteria will always be present and are nonpathogenic. Healthy term

infants can tolerate some pathogens and relatively high levels of nonpathogenic bacteria. By comparison, preterm or high-risk infants may be at greater risk from the same levels of bacterial presence.

- Electric breast pumps with multiple users are associated with greater infection risks, and healthcare facilities must take the necessary precautions to prevent contamination.

- Colostrum and breastmilk inhibit bacterial growth at different rates in both full-term and preterm milk. Milk storage guidelines and practices differ depending on the health of the infant.

- Mothers who choose to discontinue pumping for their hospitalized infants often cite insufficient milk collection as the primary reason and complain that pumping is too time consuming.

- Mothers pumping for a hospitalized infant need much clinical encouragement and emotional support to ease embarrassment and frustration and gain understanding of the significance of collecting breastmilk for their hospitalized infant.

- Breast pumps are considered to be medical devices by the FDA and as such are regulated within the FDA's Center for Devices and Radiological Health. This government agency maintains a medical product reporting program to record problems with breast pumps as encountered by consumers and clinicians.

- The issue of mothers selling and buying used breast pumps remains pertinent. The FDA advises that certain risks are presented by breast pumps that are reused by different mothers if these devices are not properly cleaned and sterilized. It is not recommended that a pump that is labeled as a single-user pump be reused or resold.

- Common pumping problems include sore nipples, low milk yield, erratic or delayed milk-ejection reflex, and dwindling milk supply over a long-term course of pumping.

- An erratic or delayed milk-ejection reflex can have an overwhelming impact on effective milk expression. A mother's negative feelings about pumping, such as embarrassment, tension, fear of failure, pain, fatigue, and anxiety, can inhibit the neurochemical pathways required for milk ejection. When a clinician knows a mother's feelings and attitudes about pumping, guidelines can be individually created for her specific situation.

- Early nipple shields generated poor outcomes. The thickness of material created a barrier that prevented a mother from feeling her baby at the breast and inhibited milk transfer.

- Nipple shields fell into disfavor when the ramifications of their use were recognized as destructive to the course of lactation and risky to the health of the baby.

- More beneficial outcomes are associated with the use of ultrathin silicone nipple shields. Use of all other types of nipple shields, including latex, is not recommended. Critical assessment and continuous follow-up by a skilled lactation consultant is essential when these devices are employed. Babies who otherwise may have been unable to breastfeed have benefited from the judicious use of this tool.

- Nipple shields can therapeutically supply oral stimulation not provided by mother's nipples, create a nipple shape in an infant's mouth, and allow extraction of milk by expression with minimal suction. With negative pressure inside the shield tip keeping milk available, the shield may compensate for weak infant suck, present a stable nipple shape that is retained during pauses in sucking bursts, maintain the nipple in a protruded position, and impact the rate of milk transfer.

- The disadvantages of nipple shields include their use as a substitute for skilled care or a quick fix. Use of these devices may lead to insufficient milk volume, inadequate weight gain or weaning, and a nipple shield

addiction after which the baby will not feed without the shield in place. They may also predispose the nipple to damage when the baby is put to breast without the shield, as he may chew rather than suckle.

- The proper size of nipple shield must be used. The teat height should not exceed the length of the infant's mouth from the juncture of the hard and soft palates to lip closure. The base diameter should fit the mother's nipple. Better results occur with the shortest teat height and smallest base diameter.

- Breast shells are two-piece plastic devices worn over the nipple and areola to evert flat or inverted nipples. Historically, these shells were called nipple glasses and were used to protect the mother's clothes from leaking milk, or used if the mother had "too much milk." Milk collected in the shells must be discarded due to potential bacterial growth.

- Historically, when worn prenatally, breast shells were designed to create a constant gentle pressure around the base of the inverted nipple and were thought to release the adhesions anchoring the nipple. Research has since shown that little correction of the nipple actually happens prenatally.

- Although breast shells have been used to provide air circulation around sore nipples and to keep a bra from adhering to the nipple, most clinicians today seldom recommend these devices.

- Designed to supplement feedings at the breast, feeding-tube devices can enable many mothers and babies to breastfeed when they would otherwise have to use an alternate feeding method without the baby at the breast.

- Feeding-tube devices consist of a container to hold breastmilk or formula and a length of thin tubing that runs from the container to the mother's nipple. The tube is secured in place with nonallergenic tape.

- The use of a feeding-tube device is indicated for babies with weak, disorganized, or dysfunctional sucking. A partial list of candidates for such feeding includes those babies who are preterm, hypertonic, or hypotonic; babies who have Down syndrome, cardiac problems, nipple preference, neurological impairment, or cleft lip or palate; and infants who have experienced perinatal asphyxia; low, slow, or no weight gain; or weight loss due to ineffective suckling.

- The feeding-tube device is useful in maternal situations such as adoptive nursing and for mothers who are re-lactating, have undergone breast surgery, suffer from primary lactation insufficiency, have severe nipple trauma, are suffering from an illness, or are undergoing surgery or hospitalization.
- With finger-feeding, a mother places the tube on the pad of her index finger or whichever finger is closest in size to her nipple. The baby draws the finger into his mouth and, with correct suckling, causes the milk to flow. This method also allows the father or other caregiver to feed the baby.
- Finger-feeding can also be used to take the edge off the baby's hunger before putting him to the breast and to help transition a baby to nursing at the breast.
- When a feeding-tube device is employed, the clinician must closely follow the progress in short- or long-term use. Risks of use include "addiction" to the device by the clinician, mother, and/or baby. The mother and baby should be weaned from the device as quickly as is appropriate.
- Healthcare professionals must judiciously use devices and other technologies that are designed to aid in breastfeeding. As with all care, the use of a breastfeeding device of any kind must be found to "do no harm"; thereafter its benefits must outweigh the risks it represents for the breastfeeding relationship to be truly supported.

RESOURCES FOR MOTHERS

Berggren K. *Working without weaning.* Amarillo, TX: Hale; 2006.

Casemore S. *Exclusively pumping breast milk: a guide to providing expressed breast milk for your baby.* Bath, ON: Gray Lion; 2004.

Colburn-Smith C, Serrette A. *The milk memos: how real moms learned to mix business with babies—and how you can, too.* New York: Tarcher; 2007.

Freeman P, Mannel R. ILCA's inside track: milk expression and pumping. *J Hum Lact.* 2007;23(3):281–282.

Pryor G, Huggins K. *Nursing mother, working mother.* Rev. ed. Boston, MA: Harvard Common Press; 2007.

Pumpin' Pal's pocket guide to breast pumping: a how-to breast pumping guide for new moms and working moms. Exeter, DEV, United Kingdom: Pumpin' Pal; 2006.

Stafford S. *Pumping breast milk successfully.* Lincoln, NE: iUniverse; 2003.

RESOURCES FOR HEALTHCARE PROVIDERS

Rhode Island Breastfeeding Coalition. Breast pump selection criteria. http://www.ribreastfeeding.org/uploads/7/6/7/6/7676852/ribc_breast_pump_selection_criteria.pdf

Walker M. *Pumps and pumping protocols.* Amarillo, TX: Hale; 2012.

Watson-Genna C. *Selecting and using breastfeeding tools.* Amarillo, TX: Hale; 2009.

INTERNET RESOURCES

Websites for Mothers Who Are Pumping
http://groups.yahoo.com/group/epers
http://messageboards.ivillage.com/iv-ppexcluspump
Hand-Expressing and Pumping Videos
http://newborns.stanford.edu/Breastfeeding/
Low Milk Supply Website
http://www.lowmilksupply.org/increasingmilk.shtml
Websites That Review Breast Pumps
http://www.breastpumpcomparisons.com/
www.amazon.com

www.epinions.com
www.viewpoints.com

REFERENCES

Alekseev NP, Ilyin VI, Yaroslavski VK, et al. Compression stimuli increase the efficacy of breast pump function. *Eur J Obstet Gynecol Reproduct Biol.* 1998;77:131–139.

Alexander JM, Grant AM, Campbell MJ. Randomized controlled trial of breast shells and Hoffman's exercises for inverted and non-protractile nipples. *Br Med J.* 1992;304(6833):1030–1032.

Aljazaf KMNH. *Ultrasound imaging in the analysis of the blood supply and blood flow in the human lactating breast.* [Dissertation]. Medical Imaging Science, Curtin University of Technology; Perth, Australia; 2004.

Amatayakul K, Vutyavanich T, Tanthayaphinant O, et al. Serum prolactin and cortisol levels after suckling for varying periods of time and the effect of a nipple shield. *Acta Obstet Gynecol Scand.* 1987;66:47–51.

Asquith M, Pedrotti PW, Harrod JR, et al. The bacterial content of breast milk after early initiation of expression using a standard technique. *J Pediatr Gastroenterol Nutr.* 1984;3:104–107.

Auerbach KG. Using nipple shields appropriately. *Rental Roundup.* 1989;6:4–5.

Auerbach KG. The effect of nipple shields on maternal milk volume. *JOGNN.* 1990a;19:419–427.

Auerbach KG. Sequential and simultaneous breast pumping: a comparison. *Int J Nurs Stud.* 1990b;27:257–265.

Auerbach KG, Avery JL. Relactation: a study of 366 cases. *Pediatrics.* 1980;65:236–242.

Auerbach KG, Avery JL. Induced lactation: a study of adoptive nursing by 240 women. *Am J Dis Child.* 1981;135:340–343.

Auerbach KG, Guss E. Maternal employment and breastfeeding: a study of 567 women's experiences. *Am J Dis Child.* 1984;138:958–960.

Auerbach KG, Walker M. When the mother of a premature infant uses a breast pump: what every NICU nurse needs to know. *Neonatal Network.* 1994;13:23–29.

Bennion E. *Antique medical instruments.* Berkeley, CA: University of California; 1979:271.

Bernabe-Garcia M, Lopez-Alarcon M, Villegas-Silva R, et al. Effectiveness of four manual breast pumps for mothers after preterm delivery in a developing country. *J Am Coll Nutr.* 2012;31:63–69.

Biancuzzo M. Selecting pumps for breastfeeding mothers. *JOGNN.* 1999;28:417–426.

Binns CW, Win NN, Zhao Y, Scott JA. Trends in the expression of breastmilk 1993–2003. *Breastfeed Rev.* 2006;14:5–9.

Bodley V, Powers D. Long-term nipple shield use: a positive perspective. *J Hum Lact.* 1996;12:301–304.

Bornmann P. *Legal considerations and the lactation consultant— USA, Unit 3* (Lactation Consultant Series). Garden City Park, NY: Avery Publishing Group; 1986.

Bose C, D'Ercole AJ, Lester AG, et al. Relactation by mothers of sick and premature infants. *Pediatrics.* 1981;67: 565–568.

Bowen-Jones A, Thompson C, Drewett RF. Milk flow and sucking rates during breast-feeding. *Dev Med Child Neurol.* 1982;24:626–633.

Bowles B, Stutte P, Hensley J. Alternate massage in breast-feeding. *Genesis.* 1988;9:5–9.

Brigham M. Mothers' reports of the outcome of nipple shield use. *J Hum Lact.* 1996;12:291–297.

Brown SL, Bright RA, Dwyer DE, Foxman B. Breast pump adverse events: reports to the Food and Drug Administration. *J Hum Lact.* 2005;21:169–174.

Buckley KM. A double-edged sword: lactation consultants' perceptions of the impact of breast pumps on the practice of breastfeeding. *J Perinat Educ.* 2009;18:13–22.

Bull P, Barger J. Fingerfeeding with the SNS. *Rental Roundup.* 1987;4:2–3.

Caldeyro-Barcia R. Milk-ejection in women. In: Reynolds M, Folley S, eds. *Lactogenesis: the initiation of milk secretion at parturition.* Philadelphia, PA: University of Pennsylvania Press; 1969: 229–243.

Chapman, D, Young S, Ferris AM, Pérez-Escamilla R. Impact of breast pumping on lactogenesis stage II after cesarean delivery: a randomized clinical trial. *Pediatrics.* 2001;107(6):e94. Available at: http://www .pediatrics.org/cgi/content/full/107/6/e94. Accessed October 30, 2007.

Chertok IR. Reexamination of ultra-thin nipple shield use, infant growth and maternal satisfaction. *J Clin Nurs.* 2009;18:2949–2955.

Chertok IR, Schneider J, Blackburn S. A pilot study of maternal and term infant outcomes associated with ultrathin nipple shield use. *J Obstet Gynecol Neonatal Nurs.* 2006;35:265–272.

Clark A, Dellaport, J. Development of a WIC single-user electric breast pump protocol. *Breastfeed Med.* 2011;6:37–40.

Clavey S. The use of acupuncture for the treatment of insufficient lactation (Que Ru). *Am J Acupuncture.* 1996;24:35–46.

Clemons SN, Amir LH. Breastfeeding women's experience of expressing: a descriptive study. *J Hum Lact.* 2010;26:258–265.

Clum D, Primomo J. Use of a silicone nipple shield with premature infants. *J Hum Lact.* 1996;12:287–290.

Cobo E, De Bernal MM, Gaitan E, Quintero CA. Neurohypophyseal hormone release in the human: II. Experimental study during lactation. *Am J Obstet Gynecol.* 1967;97:519–529.

Cossey V, Jeurissen A, Thelissen MJ, et al. Expressed breast milk on a neonatal unit: a hazard analysis and critical control points approach. *Am J Infect Control.* 2011;39(10):832–838.

Costa K. A comparison of colony counts of breast milk using two methods of breast cleansing. *JOGNN.* 1989;18:231–236.

Cox DB, Owens RA, Hartmann PE. Blood and milk prolactin and the rate of milk synthesis in women. *Exp Physiol.* 1996;81:1007–1020.

Cregan MD, de Mello TR, Hartmann PE. Preterm delivery and breast expression: consequences for initiating lactation. *Adv Exp Med Biol.* 2000;478:427–428.

Cregan MD, Hartmann PE. Computerized breast measurement from conception to weaning: clinical implications. *J Hum Lact.* 1999;15:89–96.

Daly SEJ, Hartmann PE. Infant demand and milk supply. Part 1: infant demand and milk production in lactating women. *J Hum Lact.* 1995a;11:21–26.

Daly SEJ, Hartmann PE. Infant demand and milk supply. Part 2: the short-term control of milk synthesis in lactating women. *J Hum Lact.* 1995b;11:27–37.

Daly SEJ, Kent JC, Huynh DQ, et al. The determination of short-term breast volume changes and the rate of synthesis of human milk using computerized breast measurement. *Exp Phys.* 1992;77:79–87.

Daly SEJ, Owens RA, Hartmann PE. The short-term synthesis and infant regulated removal of milk in lactating women. *Exp Phys.* 1993;78:209–220.

D'Amico CJ, DiNardo CA, Krystofiak S. Preventing contamination of breast pump kit attachments in the NICU. *J Perinatal Neonatal Nurs.* 2003;17:150–157.

da Silva OP, Knoppert DC, Angelini MM, Forret PA. Effect of domperidone on milk production in mothers of premature newborns: a randomized double-blind, placebo-controlled trial. *Can Med Assoc J.* 2001;164:17–21.

de Sanctis V, Vitali U, Atti G, et al. Comparison of prolactin response to suckling and breast pump aspiration in lactating mothers. *La Ric Clin Lab.* 1981;11:81–85.

DeNicola M. One case of nipple shield addiction. J Hum Lact. 1986;2:28–29.

Desmarais L, Browne S. *Inadequate weight gain in breastfeeding infants: assessments and resolutions, Unit 8* (Lactation Consultant Series). Garden City Park, NY: Avery Publishing Group; 1990.

Donowitz L, Marsik FJ, Fisher KA, Wenzel RP. Contaminated breast milk: a source of *Klebsiella* bacteremia in a newborn intensive care unit. *Rev Infect Dis.* 1981;3:716–720.

Drewett R, Bowen-Jones A, Dogterom J. Oxytocin levels during breastfeeding in established lactation. *Horm Behav.* 1982;16:245–248.

Edgehouse L, Radzyminski S. A device for supplementing breast-feeding. *MCN.* 1990;15:34–35.

Eglash A, Ziemer AL, Chevalier A. Health professionals' attitudes and use of nipple shields for breastfeeding women. *Breastfeed Med.* 2010;5:147–151.

Egnell E. The mechanics of different methods of emptying the female breast. *J Swe Med Assoc.* 1956;40:1–8.

Ehrenkranz RA, Ackerman BA. Metoclopramide effect on faltering milk production by mothers of premature infants. *Pediatrics.* 1986;78:614–620.

el-Mohandes AE, Keiser JF, Johnson LA, et al. Aerobes isolated in fecal microflora of infants in the intensive care nursery: relationship to human milk use and systemic sepsis. *Am J Infect Control.* 1993a;21:231–234.

el-Mohandes AE, Schatz V, Keiser JF, Jackson BJ. Bacterial contaminants of collected and frozen human milk used in an intensive care nursery. *Am J Infect Control.* 1993b;21:226–230.

Engstrom JL, Meier PP, Jegier B, et al. Comparison of milk output from the right and left breasts during simultaneous pumping in mothers of very low birthweight infants. *Breastfeed Med.* 2007;2:83–91.

Faro J, Katz A, Berens P, Ross PJ. Premature termination of nursing secondary to *Serratia marcescens* breast pump contamination. *Obstet Gynecol.* 2011;117:485–486.

Feher S, Berger LR, Johnson JD, Wilde JB. Increased breast-milk production for premature infants with a relaxation/imagery audiotape. *Pediatrics.* 1989;83:57–60.

Fewtrell MS, Lucas P, Collier S. Randomized trial comparing the efficacy of a novel manual breast pump with a standard electric breast pump in mothers who delivered preterm infants. *Pediatrics.* 2001;107:1291–1297.

Fewtrell M, Lucas P, Collier S, Lucas A. Randomized study comparing the efficacy of a novel manual breast pump with a mini-electric breast pump in mothers of term infants. *J Hum Lact.* 2001;17:126–131.

Fewtrell MS, Loh KL, Blake A, et al. Randomised, double blind trial of oxytocin nasal spray in mothers expressing breast milk for preterm infants. *Arch Dis Child Fetal Neonatal Ed.* 2006;91:F169–F174.

Fildes V. *Breasts, bottles, and babies.* Edinburgh: Edinburgh University; 1986:141–143.

Freeman ME, Kanyicska B, Lerant A, Nagy G. Prolactin structure, function, and regulation of secretion. *Physiol Rev.* 2000;80:1523–1631.

Gabay MP. Galactagogues: medications that induce lactation. *J Hum Lact.* 2002;18:274–279.

Geraghty SR, Rasmussen KM. Redefining "breastfeeding" initiation and duration in the age of breastmilk pumping. *Breastfeed Med.* 2010;5:135–137.

Geraghty SR, Sucharew H, Rasmussen KM. Trends in breastfeeding: it is not only at the breast anymore. *Matern Child Nutr.* 2012; ahead of print. doi: 10.1111/j.1740-8709.2012.00416.x.

Gilks J, Gould D, Price E. Decontaminating breast pump collection kits for use on a neonatal unit: review of current practice and the literature. *J Neonatal Nurs.* 2007;13:191–198.

Gransden W, Webster M, French GL, Phillips I. An outbreak of *Serratia marcescens* transmitted by contaminated breast pumps in a special care baby unit. *J Hosp Infect.* 1986;7:149–154.

Gras-Le GC, Lepelletier D, Debillon T, et al. Contamination of a milk bank pasteuriser causing a Pseudomonas aeruginosa outbreak in a neonatal intensive care unit. *Arch Dis Child Fetal Neonatal Ed.* 2003;88:F434–F435.

Groh-Wargo S, Toth A, Mahoney K, et al. The utility of a bilateral breast pumping system for mothers of premature infants. *Neonat Network.* 1995;14:31–36.

Gross MS. [Letter]. *ILCA Globe.* 1995;3:5.

Gunn AJ, Gunn TR, Rabone DL, et al. Growth hormone increases breast milk volumes in mothers of preterm infants. *Pediatrics.* 1996;98:279–282.

Halverson HM. Mechanisms of early infant feeding. *J Gen Psych.* 1944;64:185–223.

Hanna S, Wilson M, Norwood S. A description of breastfeeding outcomes among U.S. mothers using nipple shields. *Midwifery.* 2012; ahead of print.

Hartmann P. *Human lactation: current research and clinical implications.* Presented at Australian Lactation Consultants' Association Conference; Melbourne, Australia; October 12–15, 2000.

Hartmann P. New insights into breast physiology and breast expression and development of the Symphony breast pump. In: *Human lactation: the science of the art series* [CD]. Baar, Switzerland: Medela AG, Medical Technology; 2002.

Hayes DK, Prince CB, Espinueva V, et al. Comparison of manual and electric breast pumps among WIC women returning to work or school in Hawaii. *Breastfeed Med.* 2008;3:3–10.

Hill PD, Aldag JC, Chatterton RT. The effect of sequential and simultaneous breast pumping on milk volume and prolactin levels: a pilot study. *J Hum Lact.* 1996;12:193–239.

Hill PD, Aldag JC, Chatterton RT. Effects of pumping style on milk production in mothers of non-nursing preterm infants. *J Hum Lact.* 1999;15:209–216.

Hill PD, Aldag JC, Chatterton RT. Initiation and frequency of pumping and milk production in mothers of non-nursing preterm infants. *J Hum Lact.* 2001; 17:9–13.

Hill PD, Aldag JC, Chatterton RT, Zinaman M. Comparison of milk output between mothers of preterm and term infants: the first 6 weeks after birth. *J Hum Lact.* 2005;21:22–30.

Hill PD, Aldag JC, Demirtas H, et al. Association of serum prolactin and oxytocin with milk production in mothers of preterm and term infants. *Biol Res Nurs.* 2009:10:340–349.

Hopkinson J, Heird W. Maternal response to two electric breast pumps. *Breastfeed Med.* 2009;4:17–23.

Howie P, McNeilly AS, McArdle T, et al. The relationship between suckling-induced prolactin response and lactogenesis. *J Clin Endocrinol Metab.* 1980;50:670–673.

Human Milk Banking Association of North America. *Best practice for expressing, storing and handling human milk in hospitals, homes and child care settings,* 3rd ed. Fort Worth, TX: Human Milk Banking Association of North America; 2011.

Jackson D, Woolridge MW, Imong SM, et al. The automatic sampling shield: a device for sampling suckled breast milk. *Early Hum Dev.* 1987;15:295–306.

Jacobs LA, Dickinson JE, Hart PD, et al. Normal nipple position in term infants measured on breastfeeding ultrasound. *J Hum Lact.* 2007;23:52–59.

Jantarasaengaram S, Sreewapa P. Effects of domperidone on augmentation of lactation following cesarean delivery at full term. *Int J Gynecol Obstet.* 2012;116:240–243.

Johnson CA. An evaluation of breast pumps currently available on the American market. *Clin Pediatr.* 1983;22:40–45.

Jones E, Dimmock PW, Spencer SA. A randomized controlled trial to compare methods of milk expression after preterm delivery. *Arch Dis Child Fetal Neonatal Ed.* 2001;85:F91–F95.

Keith DR, Weaver BS, Vogel RL. The effect of music-based listening interventions on the volume, fat content, and caloric content of breast milk produced by mothers of premature and critically ill infants. *Adv Neonatal Care.* 2012;12:112–119.

Kent JC, Geddes DT, Hepworth AR, Hartmann PE. Effect of warm breastshields on breast milk pumping. *J Hum Lact.* 2011;27:331–338.

Kent JC, Mitoulas LR, Cregan MD, et al. Importance of vacuum for breastmilk expression. *Breastfeed Med.* 2008;3:11–19.

Kent JC, Ramsay DT, Doherty D, et al. Response of breasts to different stimulation patterns of an electric pump. *J Hum Lact.* 2003;19:179–186.

Labiner-Wolfe J, Fein SB, Shealy KR, Wang C. Prevalence of breast milk expression and associated factors. *Pediatr.* 2008;122(suppl 2):S63–S68.

Law BJ, Urias BA, Lertzman J, et al. Is ingestion of milk-associated bacteria by premature infants fed raw human milk controlled by routine bacteriologic screening? *J Clin Microbiol.* 1989;27:1560–1566.

Lawrence RA, Lawrence RM. *Breastfeeding: a guide for the medical profession,* 7th ed. St. Louis, MO: Mosby; 2010.

Mammina C, Di Carlo P, Cipolla D, et al. Nosocomial colonization due to imipenem-resistant Pseudomonas aeruginosa epidemiologically linked to breast milk feeding in a neonatal intensive care unit. *Acta Pharmacol Sin.* 2008;29:1486–1492.

Maygrier J. *Midwifery illustrated.* Philadelphia, PA: Carey & Hart; 1833:173.

McKechnie AC, Eglash A. Nipple shields: a review of the literature. *Breastfeed Med.* 2010;5:309–314.

McNeilly AS, Robinson IC, Houston MJ, Howie PW. Release of oxytocin and prolactin response to suckling. *Br Med J.* 1983;286:646–647.

Meier PP, Brown LP, Hurst NM. Nipple shields for preterm infants: effect on milk transfer and duration of breastfeeding. *J Hum Lact.* 2000;16:106–114.

Meier P, Motyhowski J, Zuleger J. Choosing a correctly-fitted breast shield for milk expression. *Medela Messenger.* 2004;21:8–9.

Meier P, Wilks S. The bacteria in expressed mothers' milk. *MCN.* 1987;12:420–423.

Minchin M. Breastfeeding Matters. Victoria, Australia: Alma Publications; 1985:142–145.

Mitoulas LR, Lai CT, Gurrin LC. Efficacy of breast milk expression using an electric breast pump. *J Hum Lact.* 2002;18:344–352.

Moloney A, Quoraishi AH, Parry P, Hall V. A bacteriological examination of breast pumps. *J Hosp Infect.* 1987;9:169–174.

Morse J, Bottorff J. The emotional experience of breast expression. *J Nurs Midwifery.* 1988;33:165–170.

Morton J, Hall JY, Wong RJ, et al. Combining hand techniques with electric pumping increases milk production in mothers of preterm infants. *J Perinatol.* 2009;29:757–764.

Neifert M, Seacat J. *Milk yield and prolactin rise with simultaneous breast pumping.* Presented at Ambulatory Pediatric Association Meeting; Washington, DC; May 7–10, 1985.

Neville M. Regulation of mammary development and lactation. In: Neville M, Neifert M, eds. *Lactation: physiology, nutrition and breast-feeding.* New York, NY: Plenum; 1983:118.

Neville MC. Anatomy and physiology of lactation. *Pediatr Clin North Am.* 2001;48(1):13–34.

Newton M, Newton N. The let-down reflex in human lactation. *J Pediatr.* 1948;33:698–704.

Nissen E, Uvnäs-Moberg K, Svensson K, et al. Different patterns of oxytocin, prolactin, but not cortisol release during breastfeeding in women delivered by cesarean section or by the vaginal route. *Early Hum Dev.* 1996;45:103–118.

Noel G, Suh H, Frantz A. Prolactin release during nursing and breast stimulation in postpartum and nonpostpartum subjects. *J Clin Endocrinol Metab.* 1974;38:413–423.

Odom EC, Li R, Scanlon KS, et al. Reasons for earlier than desired cessation of breastfeeding. *Pediatrics.* 2013;131(3):e726–e732.

Ohyama M, Watabe H, Hayasaka Y. Manual expression and electric breast pumping in the first 48 hours after delivery. *Pediatr Int.* 2010;52:39–43.

Olver WJ, Bond DW, Boswell TC, Watkin SL. Neonatal group B streptococcal disease associated with infected breast milk. *Arch Dis Child Fetal Neonatal Ed.* 2000;83:F48–F49.

Parker LA, Sullivan S, Krueger C, et al. Effect of early breast milk expression on milk volume and timing of lactogenesis state II among mothers of very low birth weight infants: a pilot study. *J Perinatol.* 2012;32:205–209.

Paul VK, Singh M, Deorari AK, et al. Manual and pump methods of expression of breast milk. *Indian J Pediatr.* 1996;63:87–92.

Pittard W, Geddes KM, Brown S, et al. Bacterial contamination of human milk: container type and method of expression. *Am J Perinatol.* 1991;8:25–27.

Powe CE, Allen M, Puopolo KM, et al. Recombinant human prolactin for the treatment of lactation insufficiency. *Clin Endocrinol.* 2010;73:645–653.

Powe CE, Puopolo KM, Newburg DS, et al. Effects of recombinant human prolactin on breastmilk composition. *Pediatrics.* 2011;127:e359–e366.

Prime DK, Garbin CP, Hartmann PE, Kent JC. Simultaneous breast expression in breastfeeding women is more efficacious than sequential breast expression. *Breastfeed Med.* 2012; ahead of print.

Prime DK, Geddes DT, Hepworth AR, et al. Comparison of the patterns of milk ejection during repeated breast expression sessions in women. *Breastfeed Med.* 2011;6:183–190.

Qutaishat SS, Stemper ME, Spencer SK, et al. Transmission of Salmonella enterica serotype typhimurium DT104 to infants through mother's breast milk. *Peds.* 2003;111:1442–1446.

Ramsay DT, Mitoulas LR, Kent JC, et al. The use of ultrasound to characterize milk ejection on women using an electric breast pump. *J Hum Lact.* 2005;21:421–428.

Ramsay DT, Mitoulas LR, Kent JC, et al. Milk flow rates can be used to identify and investigate milk ejection in women expressing breast milk using an electric breast pump. *Breastfeed Med.* 2006;1:14–23.

Ruis H, Rolland R, Doesburg W, et al. Oxytocin enhances onset of lactation among mothers delivering prematurely. *Br Med J.* 1981;283:340–342.

Saint L, Maggiore P, Hartmann P. Yield and nutrient content of milk in eight women breast-feeding twins and one woman breast-feeding triplets. *Br J Nutr.* 1986;56:49–58.

Shealy KR, Scanlon KS, Labiner-Wolfe J, et al. Characteristics of breastfeeding practices among US mothers. *Pediatrics.* 2008;122(suppl 2):S50–S55.

Sisk P, Quandt S, Parson N, Tucker J. Breast milk expression and maintenance in mothers of very low birth weight infants: supports and barriers. *J Hum Lact.* 2010;26:368–375.

Slusher T, Slusher IL, Biomdo M, et al. Electric breast pump use increases maternal milk volume in African nurseries. *J Trop Pediatr.* 2007;53:125–130.

Slusher TM, Slusher IL, Keating EM, et al. Comparison of maternal milk (breastmilk) expression in an African nursery. *Breastfeed Med.* 2012;7:107–111.

Slusser W, Frantz K. High-technology breastfeeding. Part II: the management of breastfeeding. *Pediatr Clin North Am.* 2001;48:505–516.

Smith W, Erenberg A, Nowak A. Imaging evaluation of the human nipple during breastfeeding. *Am J Dis Child.* 1988;142:76–78.

Sozmen M. Effects of early suckling of cesarean-born babies on lactation. *Biol Neonate.* 1992;62:67–68.

Stark Y. *Human nipples: function and anatomical variations in relationship to breastfeeding* [Master's thesis]. Pasadena, CA: Pacific Oaks College; 1994.

Stern JM, Reichlin S. Prolactin circadian rhythm persists throughout lactation in women. *Neuroendocrinology.* 1990;51:31–37.

Stutte P, Bowles B, Morman G. The effects of breast massage on volume and fat content of human milk. *Genesis.* 1988;10:22–25.

Sutherland A, Auerbach KG. *Relactation and induced lactation, Unit 1* (Lactation Consultant Series). Garden City Park, NY: Avery Publishing Group; 1985.

Thompson N, Pickler RH, Munro C, Shotwell J. Contamination in expressed breast milk following breast cleansing. *J Hum Lact.* 1997;13:127–130.

Toppare MF, Laleli Y, senses D, et al. Metoclopramide for breast milk production. *Nutr Res.* 1994;14:1019–1029.

Turkyilmaz C, Onal E, Hirfanoglu IM, et al. The effect of galactagogue herbal tea on breast milk production and short-term catch up of birth weight in the first week of life. *J Altern Complement Med.* 2011;17:139–142.

Tyson J. Nursing and prolactin secretion: principal determinants in the mediation of puerperal infertility. In: Crosignani P, Robyn C, eds. *Prolactin and human reproduction.* New York: Academic; 1977:97–108.

Ueda T, Yokoyama Y, Irahara M, Aono T. Influence of psychological stress on suckling-induced pulsatile oxytocin release. *Obstet Gynecol.* 1994;84:259–262.

Walker M. How to evaluate breast pumps. *MCN.* 1987;12:270–276.

Walker M. *Breast pump survey.* Unpublished manuscript; 1992.

Walker M. *Pumps and pumping protocols.* Amarillo, TX: Hale; 2012.

Wan EW, Davey K, Page-Sharp M, et al. Dose-effect of domperidone as a galactagogue in preterm mothers with insufficient milk supply and its transfer into milk. *Br J Clin Pharmacol.* 2008.66:283–289.

Wang LY, Chen CT, Liu WH, Wang YH. Recurrent neonatal group B streptococcal disease associated with infected breast milk. *Clin Pediatr.* 2007;46:547–549.

Weber F, Woolridge MW, Baum JD. An ultrasonographic study of the organization of sucking and swallowing by newborn infants. *Dev Med Child Neurol.* 1986;28:19–24.

Weichert C. Prolactin cycling and the management of breastfeeding failure. *Adv Pediatr.* 1980;27:391–407.

Whittlestone W. The physiologic breastmilker. *NS Fam Phys.* 1978;5:1–3.

Wight N, Turfler K, Grassley J, Spencer B. Evaluation of milk production with a multi-user, electric double pump with a soft flange in mothers of very low birth weight (VLBW) (<1500 gm, ≤31 wk gest) NICU infants: a pilot study. *Breastfeed Med.* 2011;6(suppl 1):S21–S22.

Wilde CJ, Prentice A, Peaker M. Breast-feeding: matching supply with demand in human lactation. *Proc Nutr Soc.* 1995;54:401–406.

Wilks S, Meier P. Helping mothers express milk suitable for preterm and high-risk infant feeding. *MCN.* 1988;13:121–123.

Wilson-Clay B. Clinical use of silicone nipple shields. J Hum Lact. 1996;12:279–285.

Wilson-Clay B, Hoover K. *The breastfeeding atlas,* 3rd ed. Austin, TX: LactNews Press; 2005.

Win NN, Binns CW, Zhao Y, Binns CW, Zhao Y. Breastfeeding duration in mothers who express breast milk: a cohort study. *Int Breastfeed J.* 2006;1:28.

Woodworth M, Frank E. Transitioning to the breast at six weeks: use of a nipple shield. *J Hum Lact.* 1996;12:305–307.

Woolridge MW. Breastfeeding: physiology into practice. In: Davies DP, ed. *Nutrition in child health: Proceedings of conference jointly organized by the Royal College of Physicians of London and the British Paediatric Association.* London, UK: RCPL Press; 1995:13–31.

Woolridge, M. *The mechanics of infant feeding revisited: fresh ultrasound studies of breastfeeding and bottle-feeding. Do babies extract milk from the breast using peristalsis, suction or a combination of both?* Presented at International Lactation Consultant Association conference; Orlando, FL; July 25–29, 2012.

Woolridge M, Baum J, Drewett R. Effect of a traditional and of a new nipple shield on sucking patterns and milk flow. *Early Hum Dev.* 1980;4:357–364.

Yigit F, Cigdem Z, Temizsoy E, et al. Does warming the breasts affect the amount of breastmilk production? *Breastfeed Med.* 2012; ahead of print. doi: 10.1089/bfm.2011.0142.

Yokoyama Y, Ueda T, Irahara M, Aono T. Releases of oxytocin and prolactin during breast massage and suckling in puerperal women. *Eur J Obstet Gynecol Reprod Biol.* 1994;53:17–20.

Youssef RF, Darcy E, Barone A, Borja MT, Leggiadro RJ. Expressed breast milk as a source of neonatal sepsis. *Pediatr Infect Dis J.* 2002;21:888–889.

Ziemer M, Pidgeon J. Skin changes and pain in the nipple during the first week of lactation. *JOGNN.* 1993;22:247–256.

Zinaman M. Breast pumps: ensuring mothers' success. *Contemp Obstet Gynecol.* 1988;32:55–62.

Zinaman M, Hughes V, Queenan JT, et al. Acute prolactin, oxytocin response and milk yield to infant suckling and artificial methods of expression in lactating women. *Pediatrics.* 1992;89:437–440.

Zoppou C, Barry SI, Mercer GN. Comparing breastfeeding and breast pumps using a computer model. *J Hum Lact.* 1997a;13:195–202.

Zoppou C, Barry SI, Mercer GN. Dynamics of human milk extraction: a comparative study of breast feeding and breast pumping. *Bull Math Biol.* 1997b;59:953–973.

Manufacturers and Distributors of Breast Pumps and Feeding Equipment

Breast Pumps

Ameda
475 Half Day Road
Lincolnshire, IL 60069
866-99-AMEDA
www.ameda.com

Bailey Medical
2216 Sunset Drive
Los Osos, CA 93402
800-413-3216
www.baileymed.com

Handi-craft
Dr. Brown's (formerly Simplisse)
support@simplisse.com
877-962-2525
www.simplisse.com

Hygeia II Medical Group, Inc.
1600 East Orangethorpe Ave.
Fullerton, CA 92831
888-PUMP-4-MOM (888-786-7466) or 714-515-7571
www.hygeiababy.com

Lansinoh Laboratories, Inc.
333 North Fairfax Street, Suite 400
Alexandria, VA 22314
800-292-4794
www.lansinoh.com

Limerick, Inc.
2150 N. Glenoaks Blvd.
Burbank, CA 91504-4327
877-LIMERIC (877-546-3742)
www.limerickinc.com

Lucina Care
1500 West Cypress Creek Road, Suite 410
Fort Lauderdale, FL 33309
888-809-9750
info@lucinacare.com

Medela, Inc.— Breastfeeding
P.O. Box 660
1101 Corporate Drive
McHenry, IL 60050
800-435-8316
www.medelabreastfeedingus.com

Philips Avent
P.O. Box 77900
1070 MX
Amsterdam, Netherlands
800-542-8368
www.usa.philips.com/c/avent-baby-breastfeeding/28523/cat/en/

Playtex Baby
Energizer Personal Care
890 Mountain Ave.
New Providence, NJ 07974
888-310-4290
www.playtexbaby.com

The First Years
1111 W. 22nd Street, Suite 320
Oak Brook, IL 60523
1-800-704-8697
www.thefirstyears.com

Finger-Feeding Devices

Hazelbaker FingerFeeder
614-451-1154
www.fingerfeeder.com

SuppleMate
Maternal Concepts
130 N. Public Street
Elmwood, WI 54740
800-310-5817
www.maternalconcepts.com

Equipment

Pumpin Pal
1-877-466-8283
www.pumpinpal.com/

Hands-Free Pumping Bras

http://www.handsfreepumpbra.com/
http://simplewishes.com/

Chapter 13

The Use of Human Milk and Breastfeeding in the Neonatal Intensive Care Unit

Diane L. Spatz

Introduction

Human milk is the preferred form of nutrition for all infants. Advances in neonatal care have resulted in the survival of very preterm (less than 32 weeks' gestation) infants, presenting a challenging context for the establishment of breastfeeding. The American Academy of Pediatrics (AAP, 2012) clearly states that preterm infants should receive human milk, and if the mother's own milk is not available, that donor milk should be used. The importance of human milk in the management of preterm infants is well recognized (AAP, 2012) and has been reported to improve host defenses, digestion and absorption of nutrients, gastrointestinal function, neurodevelopmental outcomes, and maternal psychological well-being (AAP, 2012). Yet mothers of preterm infants encounter numerous, well-documented barriers to breastfeeding that are not experienced by mothers of healthy term infants (Callen et al., 2005; Meier, 2001).

To improve these breastfeeding outcomes, clinicians must use evidence-based strategies that target specific barriers to breastfeeding initiation and duration for mothers and their preterm infants. Numerous scientific reports have focused on delineating and studying these barriers as part of an effort to develop strategies to optimize breastfeeding outcomes (Baker & Rasmussen, 1997; Blaymore Bier et al., 1997; Cregan et al., 2002; Edwards & Spatz, 2010; Hedberg Nyqvist & Ewald, 1999; Hurst et al., 1998; Jaeger et al., 1997; Jones & Spencer, 2007; Killersreiter et al., 2001; Lau et al., 2003; Nyqvist et al., 1999; Ortenstrand et al., 2001; Pietschnig et al., 2000; Pinelli et al., 2001; Spatz, 2004; Wheeler et al., 1999). Compared to term infants, preterm infants have maturity-dependent physiologic and metabolic differences that require integration. Similarly, mothers of preterm infants face unique physiologic and emotional challenges, such as maintaining lactation for several weeks and coping with extreme vulnerability about infant intake during breastfeeding.

Informed Decision: Human Milk as a Medical Intervention

Human milk should be viewed as a medical intervention for infants in the neonatal intensive care unit (NICU). Evidence for the benefits of human milk feeding for NICU-treated infants continues to accumulate (Table 13-1). Specific bioactive factors, such as secretory IgA, lactoferrin, lysozyme, oligosaccharides, nucleotides, cytokines, growth factors, enzymes, antioxidants, and cellular components present in human milk, have been implicated in reports of decreased rates of infections (sepsis, respiratory, gastrointestinal, and urinary tract) in premature infants fed human milk compared with those fed commercial formula (Akisu et al., 1998; Bernt & Walker, 1999;

Table 13-1 BENEFITS OF HUMAN MILK FEEDING FOR PRETERM INFANTS

Host Defense

- Cellular functions (Blumer et al., 2007; Garofalo & Goldman, 1998; Hanson, 1999)
- Bioactive factors (Akisu et al., 1998; Bernt & Walker, 1999; Henderson et al., 2001; Newburg et al., 2005; Newburg & Walker, 2007)
  - ◀ Secretory IgA (Eibl et al., 1988; Paramasivam et al., 2006)
  - ◀ Cytokines (Fituch et al., 2001; Ustundag et al., 2005)
  - ◀ Lactoferrin (Fituch et al., 2001; Goldblum et al., 1989; Hutchens et al., 1991; van der Strate et al., 2001; Ward et al., 2005)
- Enzymes (Henderson et al., 2001)
- Reduced risk and severity of morbidities (Contreras-Lemus et al., 1992; Furman et al., 2003; Hylander et al., 1998; Hylander et al., 2001; Kosloske, 2001; Lucas & Cole, 1990; Schanler et al., 1999)

Gastrointestinal

- Hormones (Armand et al., 1996; Elmlinger et al., 2007)
- Lactase activity (Kunz & Rudloff, 1993; Shulman et al., 1998b)
- Growth factors (Diaz-Gomez et al., 1997; Sangild et al., 2002)
  - ◀ Epidermal growth factor (Xiao et al., 2002)
  - ◀ Insulin-like growth factors (Elmlinger et al., 2007)
- Improved feeding tolerance (Aggett et al., 2006; Moody et al., 2000; Schanler et al., 1999; Schmolzer et al., 2006; Shulman et al., 1998b)

Nutrition

- Amino acids (Moro et al., 1989; van den Berg et al., 2005)
- Lipid profile (Charpak & Ruiz, 2007; Genzel-Boroviczeny et al., 1997; Heird, 2001; Peterson et al., 1998; Saarela et al., 2005)
- Antioxidants (Korchazhkina et al., 2006; Shoji & Koletzko, 2007)
- Glutamine, taurine (Bernt & Walker, 1999; Rassin et al., 1983; van den Berg et al., 2005)

Neurodevelopment

- Omega-3 fatty acids (Farquharson et al., 1995; Heird, 2001; Lauritzen et al., 2005; Luukkainen et al., 1995)
- Cholesterol (Boehm et al., 1995; Singhal et al., 2004; Woltil et al., 1995)
- Improved visual acuity (Birch et al., 1992; Birch et al., 1993; Jorgensen et al., 1996; Uauy et al., 1992; Uauy & Hoffman, 2000)
- Enhanced neurocognitive outcomes (Amin et al., 2000; Bier et al., 2002; Lucas et al., 1998; Lucas et al., 1994; Vohr et al., 2006, 2007; Wang et al., 2003)
- Maternal–infant bonding (Aguayo, 2001; Flacking et al., 2007; Hildebrandt & Gundert-Remy, 1983; Wheeler et al., 1999)

Hamosh, 2001; Hylander et al., 1998; Levy et al., 2009; Newburg et al., 2005; Newburg & Walker, 2007; Paramasivam et al., 2006; Schanler et al., 1999), Patel and colleagues (2013) found that for every increase of 10 mL/kg/day in the average daily dose of human milk, the odds of developing sepsis were reduced by 19% ($p = 0.008$).

More recently, stem cells have been discovered in human milk; these cells have the ability to develop into many different types of tissue (e.g., bone, neuronal) (Hassiotou et al., 2013), Gastrointestinal effects of feeding human milk include enhanced intestinal lactase activity (Shulman et al., 1998a), more rapid gastric emptying (Ewer & Yu, 1996), and a decrease in intestinal permeability early in life (Shulman et al., 1998b), compared with feeding preterm formula. Taylor and colleagues (2009) found that infants who receive the majority (more than 75%) of their feedings as human milk have a significantly lower intestinal permeability as compared to infants who receive minimal or no human milk (less than 25% or none of their feedings). Furthermore, a dose-related response within the first month was observed, suggesting that 100% human milk feeds are critical during the first 30 days after birth (Taylor et al., 2009). When human milk is fed to an infant, insulin-like growth factors and insulin-like growth factor proteins appear to arrive in the infant's bowel intact and are able to exert promotive effects, providing further evidence of the critical role of human milk in the early development of preterm infants (Elmlinger et al., 2007).

The feeding of human milk has been associated with improved cognitive and motor development at 3, 7, 12, 18, and 30 months (Bier et al., 2002; Vohr et al., 2006, 2007; Wang et al., 2003), greater intellectual performance scores at 7.5 to 8.0 years of age (Lucas et al., 1998), and faster brain stem maturation (Amin et al., 2000) compared with formula-feeding in former preterm infants. Human milk-fed infants have been found to have enhanced visual acuity (Birch et al., 1992, 1993; Jorgensen et al., 1996; Uauy & Hoffman, 2000) and less incidence and severity of retinopathy of prematurity (Hylander et al., 2001) compared to preterm formula-fed infants—possibly due to the presence of very-long-chain polyunsaturated fatty acids and antioxidant activity in human milk (Koletzko et al., 2001).

Preterm infants are at high risk for protracted oxidative stress, and human milk feeding can at least partially protect them from this problem (Ledo et al., 2009). Newer research has underscored the antioxidant capacity of human milk and shown that the infant's exposure to these antioxidants differs depending on whether the milk comprises colostrum, transition milk, or mature milk (Lugonja et al., 2013; Zarban et al., 2009). These data suggest that using colostrum for feeding premature infants in the first days of life is vital, especially considering the oxidative-stress diseases that NICU-treated infants are at risk of developing (e.g., bronchopulmonary dysplasia [BPD], retinopathy of prematurity [ROP], and necrotizing enterocolitis [NEC]) (Lugonja et al., 2013; Zarban et al., 2009). Libster and colleagues (2009) found a gender-differentiated response in the protective effects of human milk against severe acute lung disease, with girls being more protected from this outcome. Infants fed human milk also have decreased rates of rehospitalization after discharge as well as improved body composition in adolescence (Schanler, 2011). Finally, the provision of the mother's own milk to her infant allows the mother to have a distinct role in the care of her infant, at a time when many of the infant's needs are being met by the nursing and medical NICU staff (Meier et al., 1993).

Studies comparing human milk composition of mothers delivering prematurely compared to those delivering at term have shown specific differences, at least during the first few weeks following delivery (Gross et al., 1980). The higher concentrations in preterm milk compared to term milk of several components, including secretory immunoglobulin A (sIgA) and other anti-infective properties (Ballabio et al., 2007; Britton, 1986); oligosaccharides (Miller et al., 1994); protein (Butte et al., 1984); fat (Luukkainen et al., 1994); and sodium, chloride, and iron (Lemons et al., 1982; Torres et al., 2006), has led some to speculate that the mother's milk adapts to the greater nutriment needs of her preterm infant. Mehta and Petrova (2011) found that human milk from mothers of preterm infants was higher in IgA, lysozyme, and adinopectin. Researchers in Spain noted that preterm delivery influenced the immune composition (i.e., IgA, epidermal growth factor [EGF], and cytokines) of colostrum, transitional, and mature milk, with milk samples from mothers of infants born between 30 and 37 weeks' gestation being higher in most all factors studied (Castellotte et al., 2011). By comparison, milk from mothers whose infants were born before 30 weeks' gestation was low in IgA and some cytokines (Castellotte et al., 2011). These differences aside, Mehta and Petrova (2011) found that the milk of mothers of preterm infants has cytokine content equal to that in the milk of term mothers. Cytokines are beneficial to the regional and systemic immune response of preterm infants (Mehta & Petrova, 2011).

Researchers examining the influence of gestational age at delivery and duration of lactation on the changing macronutrient composition of preterm milk have theorized that these compositional differences are a result of the interruption of the gestational developmental processes occurring in the mammary gland (Maas et al., 1998). Research by Bauer and Gerss (2011) demonstrated that amounts of fat, carbohydrates, and proteins are all significantly higher in the milk of mothers who deliver preterm infants. Furthermore, these researchers noted that the differences persisted for 8 weeks post delivery and that composition was gestational age specific (i.e., younger gestational age = higher macronutrient content) (Bauer & Gerss, 2011). Researchers in Spain found that fat content was higher in very preterm (before 30 weeks) milk samples than in preterm and term milk samples (Moltó-Puigmartí et al., 2011). Medium-chain fatty acid concentrations were also highest in the very preterm colostrum and transitional milk (Moltó-Puigmartí et al., 2011).

Whatever the etiology of these compositional differences, the clinical significance of these gestationally dependent differences in milk composition is apparent when short- and long-term health outcomes are compared for preterm infants receiving either human milk or formula-feedings. These outcomes, summarized in Table 13-1, suggest that human milk may provide optimal "nutritional programming" for preterm infants and may be protective against several prematurity-related health conditions (Dvorak et al., 2003; Furman et al., 2003; Schanler & Atkinson, 1999; Schmolzer et al., 2006).

Yet despite these profound benefits, studies have shown the rate of linear growth and bone mineralization is negatively affected in preterm infants fed unfortified human milk (Nicholl & Gamsu, 1999; Schanler et al., 1999). Commercial fortifiers providing mineral supplementation of mother's own milk have been demonstrated to normalize these indices

(Kuschel & Harding, 1998 [2003]; Schanler, 1998). Given these findings, current recommendations include the provision of fortified mother's own milk as the preferred feeding for preterm infants (AAP, 2013).

Mothers of Preterm Infants

A focus on the experiences of mothers of preterm infants reveals a time-dependent process involving varying degrees of alienation and separation from the woman's infant (Jackson et al., 2003), powerlessness related to her infant's daily care needs (Bialoskurski et al., 2002), and a delay in her transition to motherhood (Flacking et al., 2007; Shin & White-Traut, 2007). The ability to provide her milk and breastfeed has been described as a contribution to infant care that only the mother can make and as one aspect of care that does not have to be forfeited in the event of preterm birth. These clinical impressions have been confirmed in several qualitative studies of mothers of preterm infants interviewed during their infant's hospitalization (Bernaix et al., 2006; Sweet, 2006) and following discharge (Flacking et al., 2007; Kavanaugh et al., 1997). These women, who received evidence-based in-hospital breastfeeding services, reported that "the rewards outweigh the efforts" in describing their breastfeeding experiences during the first month that their infants were home (Kavanaugh et al., 1997, p. 19).

The mothers from Kavanaugh et al.'s study (1997) delineated and exemplified five rewards of breastfeeding their preterm infants. The most frequently reported reward was "knowing that they had given their infants a good start in life" (p. 17), with references to the health benefits of breastfeeding for premature babies, followed by the mothers' enjoyment of the physical closeness and intimacy of breastfeeding, and their perception that their infants "preferred" the breast to bottle-feedings of expressed milk. A fourth reward was "making a unique contribution to infant care" (p. 17), although mothers circumscribed this reward to the NICU stay, when other caretaking opportunities were limited. Finally, the mothers felt that, even with the extra effort of feeding and continued milk expression in the home, breastfeeding was "convenient" for them. Qualitative research by Rossman and colleagues (2013) underscored that when women are provided with the evidence regarding expressing milk for their infant that they "have faith in their milk" to be the best thing for their child (p. 361).

Mothers of very preterm infants in various geographic and cultural environments reveal an incongruity related to their breastfeeding expectations and the realities they faced within the context of the NICU experience. Australian mothers viewed their expressed breastmilk as an object, more easily scrutinized and examined by themselves and by others (Sweet, 2006). Swedish mothers described emotional swings from exhaustion to relief, secure to insecure, and viewing breastfeeding as reciprocal as well as nonreciprocal (Flacking et al., 2007). These altered expectations were validated in a cohort of women in a Midwestern U.S. NICU (Bernaix et al., 2006). Yet the process of breastfeeding and providing breastmilk for their infants was universally described as an experience that strengthened the bonds between mother and preterm infant.

Thus the literature suggests that breastfeeding and the provision of human milk affords unique advantages for this vulnerable population that complement the health benefits of breastfeeding for mothers of term healthy infants. These important findings provide scientific justification for the allocation of resources to improve breastfeeding outcomes for this vulnerable population.

Rates of Breastfeeding Initiation and Duration

Recent research from Denmark (Maastrup, 2014), noted high (85%) breastfeeding rates for NICU-treated infants at discharge, with 68% of these infants being exclusively breastfed and 17% being partially breastfed. A recent study published in the United States reported human milk feeding rates for very-low-birth-weight (VLBW) infants at discharge as being between 37% and 61% (Brownell et al., 2013). At these authors' institution, which has a well-established breastfeeding support system,

60% of infants were receiving any (non-exclusive) human milk at discharge.

Another institution with a well-established breastfeeding support program reported a 98% pumping initiation rate, but at discharge 60.7% of NICU-treated infants were not on human milk (Bigger et al., 2014). Of the 39.3% of infants receiving human milk at discharge, 24.2% were exclusively breastfeeding and 15.1% were receiving partial human milk feeding. These researchers argue that human milk at discharge is not the critical indicator—that it is more important that infants receive a high dose of human milk during the early feeding period (Bigger et al., 2014).

Another institution with a well-established and comprehensive lactation program including unit-based Breastfeeding Resource Nurses reported a 99% pumping initiation rate for mothers of critically ill infants (Edwards & Spatz, 2010). Data from this institution indicate that of all infants delivered in-house in the Special Delivery Unit, 81% were discharged on human milk (42% exclusive and 39% fortified or partial human milk) (Children's Hospital of Philadelphia data, 2013).

Overall, however, human milk feeding rates at NICU discharge continue to be lower in the United States than in other countries. For example, researchers in Italy noted statistically significant higher rates of human milk feeding at discharge compared to infants in the Vermont Oxford Network (VON) data set (De Nisi et al., 2009). Furthermore, research examining VON NICUs and nurse staffing found that NICUs with better staffing and more experienced nurses had more parents who received breastfeeding support ($p < 0.05$) (Hallowell et al., 2014). Additionally, NICUs with more BSN-prepared nurses had more VLBW infants discharged on human milk ($p < 0.01$) (Hallowell et al., 2014).

Thus it appears that breastmilk feeding rates continue to be variable across the United States and the world. Human milk feeding rates appear to be increasing among the NICU-treated population, however, and it is clear that if comprehensive evidence lactation services are provided, human milk feeding rates both initially and at discharge will improve.

Evidence-Based Lactation Support Services

Research demonstrates that counseling mothers of preterm infants (regardless of their initial feeding intentions) can increase the incidence of lactation initiation and breastmilk feeding without increasing maternal stress and anxiety (Miracle et al., 2004; Sisk et al., 2006). Several publications have provided models for provision of breastfeeding services in the NICU (Hurst et al., 1998; Jones, 1995; Meier et al., 1993, 2004; Spatz, 2005). Specific interventions are organized within a four-phase temporal model: (1) expression and collection of mothers' milk; (2) gavage feeding of mothers' milk; (3) in-hospital breastfeeding; and (4) postdischarge breastfeeding management. A central feature of this model is that breastfeeding services are directed or coordinated by a nurse and/or physician with expertise in both lactation and intensive preterm infant care.

Making an Informed Decision

All mothers who are hospitalized for preterm labor should be approached by a health professional to provide specific infant feeding information. Emphasizing the importance of sharing evidence-based health benefits of breastfeeding with parents allows for an informed decision about feeding method (Meier, 2001; Meier & Brown, 1997; Rodriguez et al., 2005). If the mother has already given birth, breastfeeding should be discussed as soon after delivery as the mother is able to converse. The clinician should use specific information about the baby—such as maturity or health condition—and share with the mother research-based information that is relevant to her baby's situation.

Alternatives to Exclusive, Long-Term Breastfeeding

Many mothers, especially those who had not intended to breastfeed, remain indecisive or reluctant to begin milk expression if they feel they must make a commitment to exclusive breastfeeding for several months. Additionally, healthcare providers or family members may have advised them that breastfeeding is "too much" for them at a time when they are consumed with discomfort, anxiety, stress, and fatigue. These women should be encouraged to begin milk expression immediately after birth when the hormonal milieu is optimal so their infants can receive colostrum. Mothers should be told that they can cease milk expression at any time if they desire, and that professional help is available to help them discontinue pumping.

When women are indecisive and their initial plans include a day-by-day commitment to breastfeeding, several issues can help women make these important choices. For example, mothers who are unenthusiastic about pumping often ask how long they must provide milk for their infants. The practitioner can use infant milestones to place these recommendations in a more pragmatic time frame for the mother. For example, a mother can be told that the most important time for the preterm infant is the introduction and advancement of early feedings, and that her colostrum is ideal for this purpose. This translates into milk expression for approximately 1 week. The clinician can add that providing milk until term-corrected age for the infant is especially beneficial because of the unique nature of the lipids in preterm milk. Most mothers are willing to consider short-term "contracts" of this nature when they understand the day-by-day importance of their milk for their infant.

Some mothers will express milk with a breast pump, but do not want to feed their infants at the breast. The practitioner can introduce this option by stating: "Some women decide that they will use a breast pump to express milk and then feed it to their babies by bottle. Is this something that you would consider?" This approach informs mothers and reassures them that other women have chosen this option. Honoring mothers' wishes is important, yet families must understand that human milk is an intervention that will optimize the health and developmental outcomes of the NICU graduate.

Models for Hospital-Based Lactation Support Services

A variety of hospital-based breastfeeding support services have been developed in recent years and serve as models for clinical areas choosing to improve their services. It is important to note that NICUs exist in both birth hospitals and children's hospitals, and that the needs may be different across institutions. Furthermore, the role of breastfeeding support in the NICU cannot just fall on a lactation consultant. Hallowell and colleagues (2014) in a study of NICUs across the United States found that 49% of NICUs did not have dedicated lactation consultant staff and that NICUs with more BSN-prepared nurses had more VLBW infants discharged on human milk. Clearly, nurses play a critical role in providing evidence-based lactation support and care (Spatz, 2010).

The Breastfeeding Resource Nurse (BRN) model at the Children's Hospital of Philadelphia (CHOP) was established to enhance the provision of evidence-based lactation support and care (Spatz, 2005). BRNs take a 2-day course focused on the provision of human milk to and breastfeeding of vulnerable infants. Cricco-Lizza (2009), who conducted an ethnography at CHOP following implementation of the BRN program, found that nurses who had received the educational course viewed their role in lactation support markedly differently and observed that in the NICU, the bedside nurse must continually advocate for human milk and breastfeeding.

Other reports also emphasize education of all health professionals as a means to improve breastfeeding outcomes in the NICU (Pineda et al., 2009). One educational program increased human milk feeding initiation by 11% and improved the number of infants directly feeding at the breast (Pineda et al., 2009). In a similar pre-intervention/post-intervention evaluation report, the "BEST Program" was noted to increase human milk feeding rates in the NICU from 74% to 82% (Montgomery et al., 2008).

The Mothers' Milk Club at Rush-Presbyterian Hospital in Chicago utilizes a peer-support group model in providing breastfeeding support to mothers of hospitalized preterm infants (Meier, 2001). Mothers meet once a week to discuss issues related to breast pumping, expressed-breastmilk feeding, and initiation and progression of breastfeeding in the hospital and post discharge. Meier et al. (2013) further describe the role of the breastfeeding peer counselor in not only providing direct lactation care and support in the NICU, but also serving as a research assistant. In the Rush-Presbyterian Hospital program, the peer counseling program evolved from a volunteer program to a paid breastfeeding peer counselor, with an increasing number of peer counselors being recruited as the program expanded. Similar mother-to-mother support groups have reported effective results in reducing maternal stress and increasing perceived social support (Preyde & Ardal, 2003). Trained peer counselors utilized in the NICU and post hospitalization have also been shown to improve breastfeeding outcomes (Agrasada et al., 2005; Merewood et al., 2006).

In September 2011, a NICU Baby-Friendly Summit was held in Sweden to discuss modification of the Baby-Friendly Hospital Initiative (BFHI) for the preterm infant. The Nordic/Canadian model proposed may be an effective model for some countries, but not all (Nyqvist et al., 2013). The proposed model focuses on achieving direct breastfeeding at the breast and avoiding the use of bottles. These recommendations may not be practical in all NICUs, and they may not be attractive to the mother who is interested in providing milk for her infant but not direct breastfeeding.

Spatz (2004) has outlined 10 steps to promote and protect human milk feeding and breastfeeding in vulnerable infants. These 10 steps have been implemented in many NICUs across the United States as well as other countries worldwide. The World Health Organization (WHO) does not plan to change the original BFHI, however, so each country will be required to determine if and how it will evaluate "baby-friendly care in the NICU." At the time of this text's writing, Baby-Friendly USA had established a taskforce to develop guidelines for implementation of a human milk/breastfeeding model for NICU care in the United States.

Regardless of the model or combination of approaches used in a specific clinical environment, without the provision of evidence-based rationale for specific lactation management and breastfeeding policies and procedures to all staff involved, compliance will be less than optimal. Specifically, this information should include factual verbal, written, and multimedia materials and alternatives to exclusive, long-term breastfeeding for women who do not want to make these commitments. Both CHOP's program and the Rush-Presbyterian Hospital program use DVDs that emphasize the critical role of human milk for NICU infants regardless of the mother's prior decisions related to infant feeding. For critically ill infants, it is essential to emphasize the provision of human milk versus breastfeeding per se. All mothers should be given the opportunity to make the informed decision to provide milk for their infants. As health professionals, tailoring our interventions based on the mother's feeding plans and goals will allow for individualized strategies to ensure that these goals are realized.

Finally, a primary source of support for breastfeeding can be other family members. One qualitative study examined the management styles observed in breastfeeding families of preterm infants (Krouse, 2002). Families were described as facilitating (positive and proactive), maintaining (passive and adaptive), or obstructing (negative and feeling out of control) in their management styles related to breastfeeding. Although this small sample of families received intensive breastfeeding support services, the diversity in management styles observed highlights the complexity in providing effective interventions to assist mothers in meeting their breastfeeding goals. A qualitative study conducted in Australia further underscored the importance of fathers in the provision of breastfeeding support (Sweet & Darbyshire, 2009). In this study, fathers were important in supporting mothers expressing milk in the NICU, but often verbalized being more comfortable with the idea of feeding expressed milk

in the bottle versus the baby feeding directly at the breast. A systematic review of five qualitative and two mixed-method studies found that from the parents' perspective, coherent and accurate education and reinforcement are essential (Alves et al., 2013). The relationship between the family and the healthcare professional could serve as either a facilitator or a barrier to milk expression in the NICU.

Initiation and Maintenance of Milk Supply

Mothers of preterm infants must initiate and maintain lactation with a breast pump until their infants are able to regulate intake from the breast. The pump-dependent state experienced by these mothers adds to their burdensome schedule and may last several weeks to several months. Mothers need evidence-based instruction and emotional support to persevere with their breastfeeding goals during this time.

Principles of Milk Expression

Little is known about the differences, if any, in the physiologic responses of maternal lactation following preterm compared to term gestation, or the effects of the NICU environment. Few studies have focused on the mother's physiologic response to exclusive, long-term breast pump use (Chatterton et al., 2000; Cregan et al., 2002; Hartmann & Cregan, 2001). Thus the principles of lactation that have been studied for the healthy population are commonly applied to the mother who initiates and maintains lactation with a breast pump. Although giving birth prematurely does not appear to limit milk production, several factors surrounding the birth experience—prolonged bed rest, maternal complications, fatigue, stress, and irregular breast emptying—are documented prolactin inhibitors and can adversely affect milk volume. In high-risk pregnancies, a variety of conditions may exist that alter the normal progression and hormonal responses characteristic to pregnancy. A shortened gestation may prevent specific hormones from reaching their maximum levels and, therefore, alter, delay, or prevent the normal onset of lactogenesis. It is speculated that a shortened gestation may result in a blunted or minimized response in the oxytocin, prolactin, and opiate effects on the maternal brain. Additionally, the immediate and prolonged separation of the mother from her preterm infant limits the close, physical contact associated with the stimulation of these lactogenic hormones (Carter & Altemus, 1997; Uvnas-Moberg, 1998).

A growing body of evidence indicates that mothers need to begin pumping with a hospital-grade double pump as soon as possible after giving birth (Hill et al., 1999; Hopkinson, 1988). A randomized, controlled trial conducted by Parker and colleagues (2012) found that women who pumped within 1 hour of birth (as compared to 6 hours) had significantly earlier lactogenesis II as well as more milk at 3 weeks post delivery. Factors shown to optimize milk yield include frequent milk expression of adequate duration to promote complete breast emptying (Hill et al., 2001). Clinically, advising mothers to express milk more frequently (e.g., 8–10 times daily) during the first week to 10 days post birth may result in a milk volume approximating 750–1000 mL per day. Theoretically this practice may stimulate mammary alveolar growth during a time when circulating lactogenic hormones are elevated (Bialoskurski et al., 2002). Some (Groh-Wargo et al., 1995; Prime et al., 2012), but not all studies (Fewtrell et al., 2001; Hill et al., 1999) have shown an advantage to simultaneous compared to sequential breast pumping. The predictors for risk of insufficient milk production at week 12 postpartum among mothers of preterm infants include multiple birth, week 6 inadequate milk supply, maternal age younger than 29 years, and intended length of lactation less than 34 weeks (Hill et al., 2007).

Selecting a Breast Pump

Studies by Hartmann and colleagues have provided objective determination of major parameters of breast pump efficacy—namely, time to milk ejection, amount of milk removed, and rate of milk removal (Aljazaf et al., 2003; Daly et al., 1993; Daly et al., 1996). Mothers who initiate long-term milk expression need a hospital-grade electric breast pump and, as studies have demonstrated (Hill et al., 1999; Slusher et al., 2003), benefit from a double-collection kit. Furthermore, in a U.S. survey of 1844 women, researchers found that mothers who used battery-operated pumps were more likely to experience injury and problems and that mothers who used hand pumps also encountered more problems (Qi et al., 2014).

To optimize milk production and ensure increased access to colostrum, mothers should have access to a pump that has a specifically designed pumping pattern for the lactation initiation and maintenance phases (Premie Plus®). Meier and colleagues (2012) conducted a randomized control trial comparing this initiation-phase pattern to the standard breast pump pattern and found that the new pattern increased the efficiency of colostrum removal from the breast. In addition, mothers utilizing this pattern were more likely to have the milk volumes expected of mothers of exclusively breastfed term infants at 5 to 6 days postpartum (i.e., 500–600 mL/day).

Despite the fact that the Affordable Care Act (ACA) now requires insurance companies to provide coverage for breast pumps, mothers may not have access to the appropriate pump. The National Breastfeeding Center (2014) used the Verden's group policy search tool to examine breastfeeding policies of 100 nationwide insurers, focusing on two major areas: services and pumps. Only 4 out 100 insurers earned a grade of "A" on their breastfeeding implementation, and the majority of insurers failed to meet the minimum standards of the ACA.

The healthcare provider should proactively provide prescriptions and/or letters of medical necessity (like that shown in Figure 13-1) to facilitate the mother's access to an appropriate hospital-grade pump. It is also helpful to have a packet of evidence-based materials, such as the following documents, that parents can use to challenge insurers' decisions:

- An official letter on institutional letterhead that is specific to the infant's condition and the mother's breastfeeding needs
- Research reports that demonstrate the superiority of electric breast pumps (Becker et al., 2008)

Figure 13-1 SAMPLE LETTER TO REQUEST THIRD-PARTY PAYMENT FOR BREAST PUMP RENTAL.

NURSING STANDARDS MANUAL 22:2:b

BREASTFEEDING ASSISTANCE FOR THE NEW AND HIGH-RISK INFANT

Appendix B

Date: _____

Patient: _____

Name of Policy Holder: _____

Policy Number: _____

_____ delivery the high-risk infant, _____ on _____ , and the child is premature or too ill to nurse directly at the breast. However, it is well established that breastmilk provides optimal infant nutrition for the first year breasts in order to establish and maintain a milk supply and to provide breastmilk for her hospitalized newborn until the baby can ultimately breastfeed at the breast.

The intermittent electric breast pump is by far the most efficient, effective, and physiological means of simulating the suckling action of a normal infant. Inexpensive manual, battery-operated, or small electric breast pumps are not effective for maintenance of lactation, as they are designed for occasional use. An electric breast pump such as the Medela Symphony® breast pump is essential for maintenance of lactation whenever a child is unable to breastfeed at the breast. Such pumps cost approximately $1300 and thus are far more economical to rent.

The electric breast pump will be necessary until the infant is able to take all required nutrition by nursing at the breast. An electric breast pump is not a convenience for the mother. It is a medical necessity in the best interest of the child.

Sincerely,

_____

(MD Signature/Neonatologist)

- Official statements and/or data that endorse the importance and health outcomes of human milk feeding for preterm infants (such as the AAP's position statement)

In terms of outcomes, research by Jeiger and colleagues (2010) found that the cost of providing 100 mL of human milk is less than $2 per day or, with maternal opportunity cost factored in, $2.60 to $6.18. When considering the cost of electric breast pumps compared to the actual cost of formula, pumps are actually more economical.

Milk Expression Technique

The mother's milk expression technique can influence the composition and bacterial content of her milk. Lipids provide at least 50% of the calories in human milk, and lipid concentration increases over a single milk expression (Daly et al., 1993;

Woodward et al., 1989). The last few drops of milk are very high in lipid, and can contribute a substantial proportion of the calories in the entire milk sample. Mothers should be advised of this relationship and encouraged to continue pumping until milk ceases to flow. Generally, 10–15 minutes of pumping per session is sufficient, but this may vary from woman to woman, and once lactation is established, some mothers may find that less time is required to achieve breast emptying.

The distribution of lipid in expressed milk is uneven in not only changing fat content as the breast is emptied, but also because milk fat (cream) rises to the top on the storage container after expression. Mothers should be advised to mix the milk thoroughly but gently before distributing into sterile storage containers. If the milk is not mixed, the infant can receive feedings with markedly different fat and caloric values, affecting metabolic processes and overall weight gain (Valentine et al., 1994). An exception to this principle is the intentional feeding of hindmilk only, which is discussed later in this chapter.

Milk Expression Schedule

The actual number of daily milk expressions will depend on each mother's breastfeeding goals. Mothers who need to produce maximal volumes of milk to achieve their goals should plan to express milk eight times per day to establish supply. Included in this group are women who want to breastfeed exclusively at the time of infant discharge, provide hindmilk for infant feedings, and/or have given birth to multiples.

The NICU staff can modify the nursery environment to enhance the probability that mothers will pump more frequently and consistently. Enabling mothers to remain at their infants' bedside while expressing milk with the electric breast pump (Meier, 2001) promotes frequent stimulation and sends a strong message to the mother regarding the importance placed (by the staff) on providing her milk to her infant. This arrangement also provides an opportunity for the mother to see, touch, or hold her infant while expressing milk. Bedside

pumping incorporates the scientific literature on the use of relaxation and imagery in enhancing milk volume (Feher et al., 1989), and is convenient for the mother and staff. Additionally, the expectation that mothers will provide milk while in the NICU highlights their indispensable role in infant care. Anecdotally, mothers have reported that they express more milk at their babies' bedsides, and combined with skin-to-skin care and non-nutritive sucking at the breast, that bedside pumping gives them a purpose for frequent and lengthy NICU visits. Interestingly, qualitative research conducted by Hurst and colleagues (2013) found that mothers view the breast pump as both a wedge and a link to their infants.

Pumping Records

Keeping a log of pumping frequency and milk volumes expressed allows the mother to monitor her progress. Documenting the time, duration, and amount of milk expressed (Figure 13-2) provides useful information to the mother that can be shared with the NICU staff for assessment of milk volume maintenance. Logs can be kept in a written format or electronically. It is critical that the bedside nurse monitor the mother's pumping schedule and volumes daily. If the staff nurse understands maternal milk production, she can assist the mother in modifying her pumping schedule (to be explained later) based on her individual milk synthesis rate.

Maintaining Maternal Milk Volume

Expressed Milk Volume Guidelines

An arbitrary guideline categorizing levels of 24-hour milk volume is useful to determine the need for appropriate intervention (Box 13-1). Most preterm infants will require at least 500 mL/24 hours at the time of discharge. Providing specific guidelines will help each mother assess her individual breastfeeding goals and need for more (or less) frequent pumping. As previously mentioned, encouraging mothers to maintain a pumping record will allow an accurate

Figure 13-2 SAMPLE OF PUMPING RECORD.

⭐ **Mom's Pumping Log Goal:** 8 pumpings in 24 hours, 500 to 1,000 mls in 24 hours

Date	Medications?	Location	Start time	End time	Type of pump	Single or double	Amount pumped

BOX 13-1 GUIDELINE FOR EXPRESSED MILK VOLUMES FOR MOTHERS OF HOSPITALIZED INFANTS

By day 10 to 14 following delivery, milk volume is:

Ideal	> 750 ml/24 hr
Borderline	350–500 ml/24 hr
Low	< 350 ml/24 hr

accounting of each mother's individual milk expression pattern and need for appropriate interventions. In the event that a mother does not achieve a minimum milk volume of 350 mL/24 hours by 10 to 14 days following delivery, strategies to stimulate milk synthesis should be initiated immediately. The maternal hormonal milieu is believed to confer maximum responsivity to stimulate lactation during the first few weeks after giving birth. Later attempts to increase milk production may be less successful.

Based on research demonstrating the variability from mother to mother regarding the rate of milk synthesis (Daly & Hartmann, 1995b), mothers can be advised whether extending the nonpumping interval at night is appropriate or not. Calculating the volume attained at a pumping and dividing that volume by the interval (in hours) between milk expressions provides an estimate of the rate of milk synthesis. Calculating milk synthesis rates over a 24-hour period provides a picture of the mother's overall milk synthesis rate. Milk synthesis rates are calculated by taking the volume obtained divided by the number of hours since the last milk expression (e.g., 90 cc divided by 3 hours = 30 cc/hr). Studies have found that mothers with large milk storage capacities are able to maintain fairly consistent milk synthesis rates despite longer intervals between breast emptying (Kent et al., 1999). This is an invaluable benefit for mothers who must maintain their milk volumes over a long period of time.

Preventing Low Milk Volume

Milk expression guidelines as previously described are based on observational studies demonstrating that mothers who pump early and often following delivery experience higher milk yields (Hill et al., 1999). Yet despite the best efforts of some mothers, persistent low milk volumes occur—or milk production decreases over the many weeks following preterm delivery. Due to a lack of research, little is known about the physiology of long-term milk expression for mothers who are separated from their infants for extended periods following delivery. Therefore, strategies to manage low milk volume for mothers of preterm infants have focused on pharmacologic and nonpharmacologic enhancement of prolactin secretion (Budd et al., 1993; Emery, 1996; Milsom et al., 1998; Novak et al., 2000). Obtaining a thorough history from the mother is vital to provide appropriate interventions to manage low milk volume. Information regarding maternal medication use, history of breast surgery, infertility, thyroid conditions, polycystic ovarian syndrome, extended bed rest prior to delivery, and previous breastfeeding experience will provide a clearer picture of potential risk factors and possible effective interventions. Box 13-2 outlines the assessment and strategies to increase low maternal milk volume.

The use of certain maternal medications, including oral contraceptives, may diminish milk volume in mothers of preterm infants who are expressing milk with a breast pump. Although obstetricians usually advise women that progestin-only contraceptives will not interfere with lactation, mothers' experiences indicate that this may not be true for a less-established "vulnerable" milk supply. Anecdotally, mothers report that milk volume diminishes markedly within days of starting oral contraceptives, but returns to baseline shortly after they are discontinued. This phenomenon needs to be explored in controlled studies. In the interim, clinicians should ask about oral contraceptive use if mothers report a rapid decline in a previously adequate volume. Some nonprescription medications, such as pseudoephedrine (Aljazaf et al., 2003), have been associated with a 30% decrease in maternal milk volume. Because some mothers do not consider oral contraceptives and over-the-counter medications to be of concern when breastfeeding, it is best to ask about these groups of medications specifically. See the *Drug Therapy and Breastfeeding* chapter for additional information

---

BOX 13-2 ASSESSMENT OF AND STRATEGIES TO INCREASE/PREVENT LOW MILK VOLUME

- Obtain lactation risk history (e.g., breast surgery, endocrine disease, previous insufficient lactation).
- Review recent milk expression patterns.
- Ensure frequent milk expression (> six times per day).
- Encourage periodic breast massage concurrent with pumping to facilitate breast emptying.
- Minimize nonpumping intervals of >6 hours in a 24-hour period.
- Check efficiency/comfort of pump and fit of pump flange.
- Determine maternal medication use (including OTC drugs, birth control pills).
- Consider maternal stress, depression, and sleep deprivation.
- Recommend 5–6 hours uninterrupted sleep.
- Strategize ways to minimize steps in pumping routine and activities of daily living.
- Maximize maternal/infant contact.
- Suggest pumping at the infant's bedside.
- Encourage frequent and extended skin-to-skin holding of infant.
- Consider initiation of pharmacologic (e.g., metoclopramide, domperidone).

on medication/contraceptive use in breastfeeding mothers.

Most mothers of preterm infants experience a decrease in milk volume during the second month of milk expression (Hill et al., 1995; Hurst et al., 1998). Although no published studies have examined the physiology of this phenomenon, data from studies of term infants may offer some insight. Studies (Daly & Hartmann, 1995a, 1995b) have documented that maternal milk volume is limited primarily by infant demand, rather than a finite capacity of the mother to produce milk. These findings suggest that, over days or weeks, the milk expression procedure may be ineffective in stimulating an optimal milk supply for mothers of preterm infants. In particular, a breast pump does not mimic the infant's physical closeness and responsiveness that may be essential for optimal hormonal regulation of milk volume. Thus, encouraging infant contact during and after milk expression in the NICU may represent a promising intervention in preventing and improving low milk volume.

Human Milk Management

Hospitals should ensure that a comprehensive human milk management system exists to ensure the safe storage and delivery of milk to the infant. Procedures for pumping, labeling, and storage of milk are essential. In addition, the hospital must invest in equipment to support human milk management. Provision of food-grade collection containers for the mother as well as an adequate number of refrigerators and freezers to store milk are essential components of care. All too often, mothers are told to store their expressed milk at home because of insufficient storage space in the NICU freezer. However, this approach would not be recommended for medications or blood—and expressed milk should be no exception. When milk is out of sight of the NICU staff, there is no assurance that it has remained completely frozen and/or unopened before it is subsequently fed to small preterm infants. Additionally, considerations should be made to ensure that stored milk cannot be tampered with. Ideally, all milk should be stored in locked refrigerators and freezers or the units themselves be in an area of restricted access.

Human milk is not sterile (el-Mohandes et al., 1993; Thompson et al., 1997). However, it is extremely important to provide mothers with instructions regarding good hand washing and meticulous cleaning of pump equipment so as to prevent colonization of the equipment with pathogens other than normal skin flora (Jones, 2011). Milk collection and storage guidelines are summarized in Box 13-3. All pump parts should be disassembled and washed with hot soapy water and rinsed thoroughly after each use.

Box 13-3 Guidelines for Collection and Storage of Mother's Own Milk for NICU Infant Feeding

1. Wash hands and scrub under fingernails prior to each milk expression. Wipe the nipple area with water only (no soap) prior to each pumping.
2. Collect and store expressed milk in glass (Pyrex) or hard plastic (polypropylene) containers. Plastic bags are not recommended for milk storage for NICU infants.
3. Wash all milk collection equipment coming in contact with the breast milk with hot soapy water and rinse thoroughly following each use. Disassemble all parts prior to cleaning. Use a bottle brush to clean small crevices.
4. Sterilize milk collection equipment once a day by either boiling parts in water for 15–20 minutes or using a microwave sterilizing bag.
5. Label each bottle with infant's name, medical record number, date, and time of pumping. List any current maternal medications on the label.

Pump pieces can also be sterilized once per day to minimize the risk of contamination.

Glass (Pyrex) and rigid plastic (polypropylene) containers are preferable for storage of human milk, as both provide for stability of water-soluble constituents and immunoglobulin A and are easy to handle (Goldblum et al., 1981; Williamson & Murti, 1996). Flexible polyethylene bags are not recommended for milk collection and storage owing to the significantly greater loss of cells (Goldblum et al., 1981) and chance of leakage during storage and handling. The temperature at which milk is stored is based on the duration of time until the infant receives the milk for feeding. Box 13-4 summarizes the criteria to determine the proper storage temperature to be used for human milk; the impact of various temperatures on milk constituents is also outlined.

Quality Control Issues

Mothers of hospitalized infants play a vital role in the human milk management process by ensuring correct labeling of each milk container with the infant's name, medical record number, date and time of collection, and use of any maternal medications. If the milk is to be transferred to another container by the nurse or other designated NICU staff prior to feeding, each individual syringe and bottle should be labeled appropriately. Human milk is a living fluid, not unlike blood, and it should be handled as such. Proper hand washing and/or wearing gloves during handling should be practiced to avoid potential bacterial contamination of the milk. Countertops and surfaces used for milk preparation should be wiped down with an appropriate antibacterial cleaner prior to preparation activities.

Every effort should be made to adhere to stringent quality control standards to minimize potential errors in which infants receive another mother's milk. Considering the risk of possible transmission of viruses (e.g., cytomegalovirus, hepatitis C, human immunodeficiency virus) via unpasteurized donor breastmilk, administering another mother's milk to an infant is a serious error. Proper labeling of milk collection/preparation containers with the infant's name and medical record number and verification of this information (checked with another nurse) against infant's name band before feeding is an effective procedure to avoid potential errors.

Oral Care and Initiation of Enteral Feeds

During the time that an infant is on NPO status, colostrum, transitional, and/or mature milk can be used for oral care. Rodriguez et al. (2010) established the safety of this practice for VLBW infants and provided the theoretical evidence for its usage (Gephart & Weller, 2014). The National Association of Neonatal Nurses has also published a descriptive article on implementation of a human milk oral care program. When the infant's mouth is coated with human milk, the infant benefits from the immunobiological components and antimicrobial nature of human milk. In addition, human milk has a sweet flavor, and infants have sweet receptors on their tongue; thus oral care is pleasurable for the infant. Edwards and Spatz (2010) include oral care in their transition to breast pathway to facilitate future transition to at-breast feeds. Oral care with human milk may help to counteract some of the negative oral stimuli that NICU-resident infants receive. In addition, teaching parents to perform oral care with human milk is another way to involve parents in their child's care at a time where they may not be able to hold their infant and, therefore, may feel very helpless (Figure 13-3).

Skin-to-Skin Care

Worldwide, studies have documented many benefits of skin-to-skin (STS), or kangaroo, care: promoting physiologic stability in preterm and high-risk infants (Bauer et al., 1997; Bier et al., 1996; Bohnhorst et al., 2001; Browne, 2004; Cattaneo et al., 1998; Charpak et al., 2005; Dodd, 2005; Gazzolo et al., 2000; Tornhage et al., 1998; Whitelaw & Liestol, 1994), analgesia during heel sticks (Ludington-Hoe et al., 2005), strengthening maternal–infant interaction (Korja et al., 2008), accelerating autonomic

Box 13-4   Guidelines to Minimize/Prevent Bacterial Growth of Mother's Own Milk for Infant Feeding

Milk Collection

- Instruct mother on proper collection technique including hand washing and maintenance of pumping equipment (see Box 13-3).

Milk Storage

- Use fresh, unrefrigerated milk within 4 hours of milk expression.
- Refrigerate milk immediately following expression when the infant will be fed within 96 hours.
- Freeze milk when infant is not being fed or the mother is unable to deliver the milk to the hospital within 96 hours of expression.
- Store each collection in a separate bottle. When pumping both breasts at the same time, two bottles can be combined into one.
- Ensure fresh/frozen milk is transported to the hospital on ice, in an insulated cooler to avoid thawing or warming.
- Thawed milk should not be refrozen.

Thawing

- Milk should be thawed in a waterless machine.
- Label milk with date and time thawed.

Milk Preparation

- Designate optimal physical space in the NICU for milk preparation.
- Gloves should be worn by staff when preparing or handling milk.
- When preparing feedings for more than one infant at a time, wash hands or change gloves, and wipe down counter between preparations.

Fortification

- Add fortification per physician's order ensuring complete mixing.
- Avoid vigorous shaking of milk to prevent disruption of milk fat membrane integrity (can result in adherence of milk fat to feeding tubes, bottles, etc.).
- Feed milk within 24 hours of addition of fortifier to expressed mother's milk (EMM).

Warming

- EMM should be warmed to body temperature prior to feeding in electric warming units.
- Use of unattended warm water baths for warming purposes should be discouraged as milk could be warmed to high temperatures resulting in changes in milk constituents.

Feeding

- For continuous milk infusions, limit infusion time to 4 hours.
- Avoid use of additional extension tubing for gavage feeding of EMM.

Figure 13-3 FATHER DOING ORAL CARE. ORAL CARE WITH COLOSTRUM AND HUMAN MILK CAN INVOLVE THE WHOLE FAMILY.

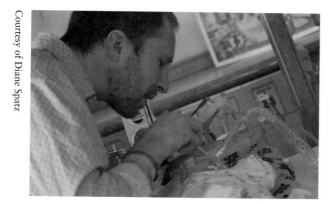

Courtesy of Diane Spatz

and neurobehavioral maturation in the infant (Feldman & Eidelman, 2003), and improving sleep patterns (Ludington-Hoe et al., 2006). Furthermore, the duration of breastfeeding appears to be longer for STS-recipient infants than for incubator controls (Charpak et al., 2001; Ludington-Hoe et al., 1994). In one study, mothers who participated in STS care had a significantly greater increase in milk volume between 2 and 4 weeks than mothers who did not practice STS care (Hurst et al., 1997). Furthermore, Hurst et al. speculated that STS holding may trigger the production of maternal milk antibodies to specific pathogens in the infant's environment through mechanisms in the enteromammary pathway. Additionally, STS holding has been positively correlated with improved maintenance of milk expression as evidenced by continued pumping frequency (Lau et al., 2007).

Mothers whose infants are in STS care have reported observing their infants' rooting and mouthing movements, and moving toward the nipple during STS sessions (Hurst et al., 1997). Mothers frequently note feelings of milk ejection, leaking, and expressing higher milk volumes immediately following STS care. Interestingly, the administration of exogenous oxytocin nasal spray prior to pumping does not result in significant improvement of milk production (Fewtrell et al., 2006). The apparent effects from the release of endogenous oxytocin are validated in studies of positive social interactions during the developing maternal–infant relationship (Uvnas-Moberg, 1997). During social interactions, oxytocin can be released by sensory stimuli perceived as positive, including touch, warmth, and odors (Uvnas-Moberg, 1998). Because the release of oxytocin can become conditioned to emotional states and mental images, the actions of this peptide may provide an additional explanation for the long-term benefits of positive experiences.

The conditioning of the oxytocin-release response for the mother of a critically ill infant, at least initially, is related to experiences far removed from her infant, such as entering the NICU, turning on an electric breast pump, or walking into the entry of the hospital. How best to "normalize" this conditioning to its proper maternal–infant orientation is one of the challenges clinicians must face when working with this vulnerable population—and STS holding may provide an early antidote (Feldman et al., 2002).

Recent research from Sweden demonstrated that kangaroo mother care improved breastfeeding outcomes for very preterm infants (less 32 weeks' gestation). This group of researchers concluded that this STS contact had empowering effects on the process of breastfeeding (Flacking et al., 2011). In addition, a randomized controlled trial conducted in the United States found improved breastfeeding outcomes for mothers who participated in STS contact. Mother–infant dyads who participated in such patterns of care breastfed significantly longer (5.08 months) compared to the control group (2.05 months); these dyads also had higher rates of exclusive breastfeeding. The mean time that mother–infant dyads participated in STS contact each day was 4.47 hours (Hake-Brooks & Anderson, 2008).

Although a complete review of procedures for STS holding is beyond the scope of this chapter, several principles can be summarized:

- Infants can be safely placed in STS care while very small and mechanically ventilated (Gale et al., 1993; Legault & Goulet, 1995; Tornhage et al., 1999).
- There is no scientific reason to restrict the duration of STS care, unless an infant becomes physiologically unstable while on the mother's chest. Typically, a STS care session is ended based on the mother's availability, rather than infant criteria.
- The position of the infant in STS care is important in maintaining physiologic stability, and recliners are ideal in achieving this position. The infant should be placed upright between the mother's breasts, with the side of the face against the internal surface of one breast (Figure 13-4). The recliner is angled back to allow the infant's body to remain at a 45- to 60-degree angle from the floor. A mirror positioned to allow the mother to observe her infant's face is helpful during these sessions.
- STS sessions of 2 or more hours are ideal, and it is not uncommon for infants to display

behaviors that suggest autonomic instability when returned to the incubator following STS care (Kirsten et al., 2001).

Optimization of Human Milk for Feeding

The scientific literature supports feeding of fresh (unfrozen) milk when possible, because the anti-infective properties are maximally preserved (Hamosh, 2001; Hamosh et al., 1996; Jones, 2011). Ideally, preterm infants should receive at least one daily feeding of milk that has been pumped at the bedside and fed without refrigeration. Such milk retains all of the anti-infective properties and has been subjected to minimal handling and temperature changes. Many mothers will ensure that their infants have fresh milk available for feedings if they understand the rationale behind this practice. The staff can support this plan by developing a sequence of feeding the milk so it can be used within 96 hours of expression and/or alternated with frozen milk when necessary. Additionally, it is important to emphasize to the mother that frozen milk retains most of the anti-infective properties and is nutritionally superior to formula.

Volume Restriction Status

Special considerations regarding the feeding of expressed mother's milk (EMM) to preterm infants are based on the infant's fluid restrictive status at a time of greatest nutritional need. Although full feeding volume status for preterm infants is routinely considered to be a daily volume of 150 cc/kg/day, human milk-fed infants usually tolerate much higher volumes—up to 200 cc/kg/day (Schanler, 2001). The ability to handle a greater volume has been attributed to the faster gastric emptying rates observed with human milk (Moody et al., 2000). However, to achieve optimal bone mineralization at a vulnerable time in the preterm infant's development, human milk fortifiers are routinely mixed with the milk to provide greater intake of specific minerals, such as calcium and phosphorus (Sankaran et al., 1996; Wauben, Atkinson, Grad et al., 1998).

Figure 13-4 SKIN-TO-SKIN CARE IN THE NICU.

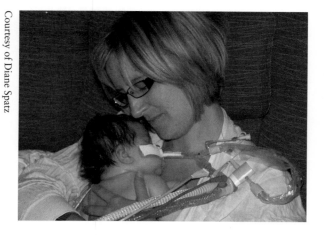

Commercial Nutritional Additives

Unfortified EMM is deficient in protein and selected minerals needed to support optimal growth and bone mineralization for small preterm infants (Schanler, 1998; Schanler, Hurst, & Lau, 1999; Schanler, Shulman, & Lau, 1999; Simmer et al., 1997). Thus, for most preterm infants, these additional nutrients are provided in the form of commercial milk fortifiers. Table 13-2 lists commercially available fortifiers.

Studies evaluating the effects of nutrient fortification on some of the general host defense properties of human milk have shown no effect on the concentrations of IgA (Jocson et al., 1997; Quan et al., 1994), and bacterial growth was not affected during 4 hours (Jocson et al., 1997) and 6 hours (Telang et al., 2005) at room temperature and decreased over 24 hours (Jocson et al., 1997) and 72 hours (Santiago et al., 2005) at refrigerator temperature. However, recent research on Enfamil human milk fortifier (HMF) demonstrated that acidification of the milk from the fortifier led to a 76% decrease in white blood cells and a 56% decrease in lipase activity in the human milk (Erickson et al., 2013). Additionally, adding HMF and additional protein to human milk increases the osmolarity to more than 400 mOsm/L, which exceeds the recommended threshold (Kreissl et al., 2013). For this reason, it is not recommended that HMF and additional protein be used together. The results of these studies under simulated nursery conditions suggests that current practice should include limiting storage to 4 hours at room temperature and 24 hours in the refrigerator once fortification is added to the milk.

A better option for fortification of human milk is HMF made from human milk, such as Prolacta Plus. Adding HMF made from human milk does not negatively affect the antibacterial activity of the milk, although bovine protein–based fortifier is almost totally inhibited (Chan et al., 2007). Furthermore, infants receiving an exclusively human milk diet have significantly lower rates of necrotizing enterocolitis (NEC; $p = 0.02$) and NEC requiring surgical intervention ($p = 0.007$) (Sullivan et al., 2010).

Table 13-2 COMPOSITION OF COMMERCIALLY AVAILABLE HUMAN MILK FORTIFIERS*

	Type of Fortifier			
	Enfamil Human Milk Fortifier** (amounts in 4 vials to be added to 100 mL human milk)	**Similac Human Milk Fortifier*** (amounts in 4 packets to be added to 100 mL human milk)	**Prolacta+4**[†] (amounts in 20 mL of liquid fortifier to be added to 80 mL human milk)	**Prolacta6** [†] (amounts in 30 mL of liquid fortifier to be added to 70 mL human milk)
Calories	30	14	29.2	43.8
Proteins (g)	2.2	1.00	1.2	1.8
Fat (g)	2.3	0.36	1.8	2.7
Carbohydrate (g)	<1.2	1.80	2.0	3.0
Calcium (mg)	116	117	108.4	120.0
Phosphorus (mg)	63	67	62.0	70.8
Magnesium (mg)	1.84	7.0	4.2	5.4
Iron (mg)	1.76	0.35	0.2	0.2

*Only selected nutrients and minerals are displayed in this table.

**Values presented by Mead Johnson Nutrition, retrieved from http://www.enfamil.com/app/iwp/enf10/content.do?dm=enf&id=/Consumer_Home3/FeedingSolutions/EnfamilHumanMilkFortifier2&iwpst=B2C&ls=0&csred=1&r=3500313837#second.

***Values presented by Abbott Nutrition, retrieved from http://abbottnutrition.com/products/similac-human-milk-fortifier.

[†]Values presented by Prolacta Bioscience, retrieved from http://www.prolacta.com/fortifier.php.

Researchers have also reported that despite the cost of the product (approximately $5.63/mL), an exclusively human milk–based diet offers cost savings. They report a decrease in length of stay by 3.9 NICU days and an $8167.17 cost savings for every extremely preterm infant ($p < 0.0001$) (Ganapathy et al., 2012).

Hindmilk Feeding

The feeding of the hindmilk-only fraction of EMM has received considerable attention among clinicians (Griffin et al., 2000; Ogechi et al., 2007; Valentine et al., 1994). The lipid and caloric content of hindmilk is greater than that of foremilk or composite milk (e.g., a full pumping that includes both foremilk and hindmilk). By fractionating the hindmilk portion of a milk expression, mothers can provide high-lipid, high-calorie milk that promotes accelerated infant growth (Ogechi et al., 2007; Slusher et al., 2003; Valentine et al., 1994). Although hindmilk feeding holds remarkable potential for preterm infant nutrition, this technique has not yet been subjected to randomized controlled trials.

There is tremendous within- and between-mother variation in breastmilk lipid content. Thus a standard procedure for collection of hindmilk does not ensure a standard outcome. Clinically, the lipid and caloric content of milk can be estimated with the creamatocrit, a technique that involves centrifuging a milk specimen that has been drawn into a capillary tube (Lucas et al., 1978; Polberger & Lonnerdal, 1993). The creamatocrit, or the percentage of total volume in the capillary tube that is equivalent to lipid, can be converted to an estimate of lipid and caloric content using one of the published regression graphs (Table 13-3). However,

creamatocrits performed in this manner represent only a relative estimate of lipid and calories. A more accurate quantification of lipid and caloric content requires that the creamatocrit be standardized with one of the direct measures of total milk lipid, such as the Folch technique (Jensen, 1989).

Hindmilk and commercial fortifiers and additives are not interchangeable—a point that is often misunderstood. Although commercial fortifiers provide small amounts of calories in the form of carbohydrates, their primary purpose is to supplement essential minerals, such as calcium and phosphorus, which are needed in higher concentrations than are present in human milk. In contrast, hindmilk does not "concentrate" these nutrients (Valentine et al., 1994), but does provide an extremely efficient energy source by concentrating the endogenous milk lipids. Thus the use of hindmilk does not replace the need for mineral supplementation, and commercial fortifiers are a relatively inefficient means of supplying extra calories.

Finally, the needs of the mother must be considered whenever her composite milk is not used exclusively. It is easy for mothers to infer that their milk is not "adequate" for their infants when it must be fortified or fractionated for hindmilk feedings. Mothers should be informed that their milk is ideal with respect to immunologic and nutritional properties—but the rapid growth of their very small infants requires temporary supplementation with commercial human milk fortifiers and/or hindmilk.

Lactoengineering of own mother's milk (OMM) through a combination of hindmilk and creamatocrit measures can be empowering for mothers of preterm infants (Griffin et al., 2000; Jennings et al., 1997). Specifically, mothers are assisted in expressing milk with a creamatocrit value that

Table 13-3 CREAMATOCRIT READINGS AND ASSOCIATED FAT/CALORIC CONTENT OF HUMAN MILK

Creamatocrit	3	4	5	6	7	8	9	10	11
Cal/oz	15.7	17.8	20	22.1	24.3	26.4	28.5	30.7	32.8
% of calories–fat	22	37	44	48.2	52.1	56	58.2	60.4	62.6

Adapted from Lucas et al., 1978.

meets their individual infant's growth needs. When their infants demonstrate the desired weight gain pattern, mothers recognize that their milk modifications supported the desired growth.

The Future of Human Milk Optimization: Human Milk Nutrient Analysis

Newer technology has been demonstrated to be superior to the current practice of using the creamatocrit to analyze human milk content. Human milk nutrient analyzers (HMAs) use mid- or near-infrared spectroscopy to determine not only fat and caloric density, but also protein and carbohydrate content of human milk. A major potential barrier to widespread implementation of this technology is cost. Table 13-4 lists the commercially available HMAs and their costs.

Researchers have noted that creamatocrit analysis overestimates fat and caloric content as compared to using an HMA (O'Neill et al., 2013). Furthermore, research primarily conducted outside the United States has demonstrated that not only are HMAs accurate, but the current standard fortification practices also fail to meet the recommendations for protein intake (Arslanoglu et al., 2010; Corvaglia et al., 2010; Rochow et al., 2013). Ideally, to optimize nutrition for infants in the NICU, targeted fortification should occur. However, implementation of a targeted fortification program requires practitioners to understand the nuances of human milk and hospital administrators to be willing to invest in the cost of HMAs as well as personnel. Rochow and colleagues (2103) found that in 650 pooled samples of human milk, all samples required the adjustment of at least one macronutrient.

Methods of Milk Delivery

A series of studies provides strong scientific support for the administration of EMM by intermittent rather than slow-infusion continuous gavage (Brennan-Behm et al., 1994; Schanler et al., 1999).

Table 13-4 COMMERCIALLY AVAILABLE HUMAN MILK NUTRIENT ANALYZERS

	Cost	Application	Research Publications
Miris Human Milk Analyzer	€13,000 ($17,013)	• 60 seconds/measurement • 1–3 mL samples • Key features: small size, robustness, easy handling	Yes
SpectraStar Neonatal Analyzer	$49,500	• 10–60 seconds/measurement • 1 mL samples • Key features: one-button operation, automatic calculation reported for nutritional supplementation	Yes
Calais Human Milk Analyzer	$59,000	• <60 seconds/measurement • 8 mL samples • Key features: automatically homogenizes sample before analysis, auto-rinse cycle for easy cleaning	No
MilkoScan FT1	Not being sold for use with human milk	• 30 seconds/measurement • 8 mL samples	No
Milkoscope Julie Z7 Automatic	Price listing not available		No

In particular, milk lipids that make up 50% to 60% of the calories in EMM adhere to the lumen of infusion tubings, and their loss results in a relatively dilute, low-calorie feeding (Brennan-Behm et al., 1994). The greatest lipid loss occurs during the slowest infusion rates (Greer et al., 1984; Stocks et al., 1985). Clinically, this means that the smallest babies, for whom caloric requirements are the highest, will receive EMM by the slowest infusion rates, resulting in a low-calorie milk. For this reason, EMM should be administered by slow intermittent bolus, rather than by continuous gavage infusion.

Warming Milk for Feeding

Rapid heating, especially microwaving, has been demonstrated to adversely affect both the immunologic and nutritional properties of EMM (Hamosh et al., 1996; Quan et al., 1992). Refrigerated EMM should be gradually warmed (over 30 minutes) to approximately body temperature before being fed to small preterm infants (Newman et al., 2000). For the smallest infants, the feeding volume can be withdrawn into a syringe that is placed in the infant's incubator for gradual warming.

Maternal Medication Use

Preterm infants, especially those with an extremely low birth weight, have immature metabolic and excretory pathways. This can pose a risk when the mother is taking medications that are present in her breastmilk. Of course, one must also consider the risk of the infant not receiving the mother's own milk. When the mother is taking medications, it is essential to make an informed risk–benefit assessment using reference tools specifically for medications in mother's milk, such as the Hale book *Medications and Mother's Milk* (2012) or Lactmed (http://toxnet.nlm.nih.gov/cgi-bin/sis/htmlgen?LACT). Although a detailed description of these issues is beyond the scope of this chapter, several principles should be considered when a mother of a preterm infant must take medications:

- The medication should be considered "safe" for healthy term infants (AAP, 2013).

- Extra caution is needed when lipid-rich hindmilk is being fed; medications that are lipophilic may cross readily into the milk.

Only healthcare professionals who have expertise in lactation, pharmacology, and neonatal care should provide advice concerning the safety of medications for small preterm infants. When in doubt about a specific medication, or a combination of medications, a national expert should be consulted. In all instances, any information about maternal medications should be reviewed with the neonatologist who is responsible for the infant's care, and mothers should record any medications consumed on the individual milk container.

Transmission of Viruses and Other Pathogens via EMM

Transmission of viruses (Jim et al., 2004; Omarsdottir et al., 2007; Yasuda et al., 2003) and other pathogens (Arias-Camison, 2003; Byrne et al., 2006; Kotiw et al., 2003) in breastmilk have been described. Several studies have reported cytomegalovirus (CMV) seropositive rates between 52% and 97% in mothers of preterm infants (Doctor et al., 2005; Hamprecht et al., 2001; Jim et al., 2004), with CMV-positive breastmilk rates as high as 38% to 70% being documented. Yet despite these high rates, rates of postnatal asymptomatic and symptomatic CMV infections in preterm infants are low—25% and 1% to 5%, respectively (Miron et al., 2005; Mussi-Pinhata et al., 2004; Schanler, 2005). Nevertheless, given the vulnerability of the very preterm immune-compromised infant, consideration of exposure to high viral loads is of concern.

One goal is the elimination of CMV from a mother's breastmilk without damaging protective constituents. Studies of freezing techniques to eliminate this virus have yielded inconclusive results (Curtis et al., 2005; Hamprecht et al., 2004; Sharland et al., 2002) and have not shown complete viral inactivation. As no recommendations related to CMV and breastmilk feeding in very preterm infants exist, some clinicians have suggested using freeze-thawed milk combined with at least some fresh milk feeding each day for the most vulnerable infants to minimize possible exposure. Additionally, it is speculated that the exclusivity of EMM feeding may be protective against CMV infection given the "enveloping" characteristic of the virus. As it happens, this same characteristic exists with HIV and may be a factor in the protection provided by exclusive human milk feedings of infants of HIV-positive women compared to mixed feedings.

Group B streptococcus (GBS) is the most common cause of sepsis in newborns, and preterm infants are more susceptible to infection than term infants. Breastmilk feeding has been implicated as a source of several reports of infant GBS infection (Arias-Camison, 2003; Byrne et al., 2006; Kotiw et al., 2003; Olver et al., 2000). Additionally, methicillin-resistant *Staphylococcus aureus* (MRSA) has been isolated from EMM (Behari et al., 2004; Gastelum et al., 2005; Novak et al., 2000). Several explanations for the etiology of these infections were put forth, including the development of a more virulent strain of GBS following the use of prophylactic antibiotics in labor; early introduction of mixed feedings/human milk fortifier; and high bacterial load during mastitis episode. Recommendations for management included infant blood and EMM cultures to document transmission and the withholding of EMM until adequate therapy is achieved (Byrne et al., 2006; Kotiw et al., 2003). Interestingly, in a study of 161 mothers of infants born at less than 30 weeks' gestation, weekly milk cultures (from 1 to 11 weeks) were not predictive of infection (Schanler, 2005).

Non-nutritive Sucking at the Breast

Early oral experiences may influence later oral feeding development. Many clinicians specializing in feeding disorders report a high percentage of their patients as former preterm infants. This is not surprising given the amount of negative oral insults experienced by these infants, such as intubation, suctioning, and insertion of feeding tubes. Thus the provision of positive oral experiences early in their development may counteract some of the negative effects by these negative, but necessary, procedures. Non-nutritive suckling and suckling at the emptied maternal breast provides a positive experience for preterm infants.

There are no universally established criteria for the initiation of breastfeeding (or bottle-feeding, for that matter) for preterm infants. Although a minimum body weight or gestational age (commonly 34 weeks) has been used, more recent practice has been to consider each infant's individual abilities when determining the initiation of oral feeding, be that breast or bottle (Lau & Hurst, 1999; McGrath & Braescu, 2004; Medoff-Cooper, 2000; Simpson et al., 2002). Whereas judging the ability to breastfeed has been based on the infant's achievement of consuming a prescribed milk volume by bottle, evidence-based research has proved this practice inappropriate. In neonatal units where infants are allowed non-nutritive sucking at the emptied breast (Meier, 2001; Narayanan et al., 1991), the idea of "when to initiate" breastfeeding has been reconceptualized.

Controlled clinical trials have demonstrated many benefits of non-nutritive sucking (NNS) with a pacifier for preterm infants (Pinelli & Symington, 2005). In addition, in a small study, it was noted that infants respond to the odor of human milk by increasing the frequency of non-nutritive sucking (Bingham et al., 2007). Therefore preterm infants should be given opportunities for suckling at the mother's recently pumped breast, an experience that may also maximize the mother's milk production (Figure 13-5). Initiating NNS at the emptied breast provides a maternal stimulus that is different from routine breast pump use and, as such, may increase milk yield. Additionally, mothers receive instant reinforcement from infants' behaviors that reflect enjoyment and physiologic stability while at the breast. For the infant, the ability to "taste" the milk allows for optimal oral stimulation during a time when the oral cavity is bypassed via oral–gastric tube feedings. Another sensory experience—smell—may also condition the infant for breastfeeding, as evidenced in a randomized study of preterm

Figure 13-5 NON-NUTRITIVE SUCKING AT THE BREAST.

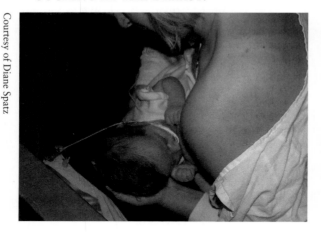

Figure 13-6 INFANT WITH NCPAP TUBES AT THE BREAST.

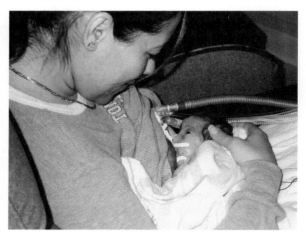

With permission, Rush Mothers' Milk Club, Rush-Presbyterian St. Luke's Medical Center, Chicago.

infants (30–33 weeks) exposed to their mother's own milk odor immediately following early breastfeeding attempts (Raimbault et al., 2007). During each breastfeeding session, infants exposed to the milk odor displayed longer sucking bouts and bursts, and also consumed more milk than the control (exposed to water) infants.

For a small (weight less than 1000 g) infant, the mother completely expresses milk from the breast just prior to the infant being placed in STS care at the breast. The infant should be supported in the football hold or across the chest, so that the infant's entire ventral surface is in direct contact with the lateral aspect of the mother's breast. The infant's temperature can be monitored noninvasively if this is a concern—however, the same criteria and outcomes utilized for STS holding should apply during suckling at the emptied breast (Dodd, 2005). Although the infant should be held in proximity with the breast, no attempt should be made to "position" the infant's mouth and gums over the nipple and areola. Instead, licking and suckling on the nipple tip is all that is expected of very small preterm infants. In one NICU, NNS is begun as soon as small infants are extubated (Meier, 2001). Infants on NCPAP can participate in NNS; positioning across the lap with NCPAP tubing directed upward and over the breast is most effective (Figure 13-6). For larger infants, the

mother can combine NNS at the emptied breast with administering her freshly expressed milk by gavage.

These early opportunities for the infant to suckle at the emptied breast allow the mother to observe the infant's behavior and developing signs for readiness to oral feeding. In this way, the mother can provide invaluable input into the plan of care as it relates to advancement of oral feeding. For this reason, a specific postnatal/gestational age or body weight is not used as the criteria for advancing oral feedings (Nyqvist et al., 1999; Sidell & Froman, 1994). Observations made by the mother and nursing staff during early STS holding and suckling sessions allow for the development of an individualized plan of care regarding initiation and progression of oral feeding (Nyqvist. Ewald, & Sjödén, 1996; Shaker & Woida, 2007). As feeding at breast advances in the NICU, two principal topics should be discussed: the science and practice of initiating and advancing direct breastfeedings, and the measurement and facilitation of milk transfer.

The Science of Early Breastfeeding

Studies have demonstrated that preterm infants serving as their own controls have more stable measures of transcutaneous oxygen pressure and body temperature during breastfeeding as compared to bottle-feeding (Blaymore Bier et al., 1997; Meier, 1988; Meier & Anderson, 1987), but less milk is transferred during breastfeeding than measured during bottle-feeding (Blaymore Bier et al., 1997; Furman & Minich, 2004; Martell et al., 1993; Meier & Brown, 1996). Table 13-5 summarizes the literature to date regarding breastfeeding behavior in preterm infants. These data suggest that the more stable patterns of oxygenation for breastfeeding than for bottle-feeding are a result of less interruption of breathing during breastfeeding—possibly as a result of a slower rate of milk flow during breastfeeding. To safely project a bolus of milk through the pharynx, an infant must coordinate sucking, swallowing, and breathing. Infant oral-motor skills must not only be adequate for sucking, but sucking must also be intricately coordinated with both swallowing and breathing (Gewolb et al., 2001). Considering the preterm infant's novice skills, the restricted milk flow experienced during breastfeeding may be a more optimal environment for development of oral-motor skills.

To test this theory, Meier and Brown (1996) studied a cohort of clinically stable preterm infants who served as their own controls for serial breastfeeding and bottle-feedings from the time of oral feeding initiation until NICU discharge. The following variables were monitored and recorded continuously on an eight-channel polygraph: sucking event, respiratory event, body temperature, and oxygen saturation during each feeding session. Volume of milk intake was measured by test-weighing. Previous research in Meier's laboratory had validated the instruments that were used for the measurement of sucking (deMonterice et al., 1992) and milk intake (Kavanaugh et al., 1989; Meier et al., 1990) in this research. The results revealed that during bottle-feedings, preterm infants frequently did not breathe during sucking bursts; instead, they alternated short bursts of sucking with pauses during which they breathed rapidly. Oxygen saturation measures in response to this suck–breathe patterning varied. For most, but not all, infants who maintained short sucking bursts (e.g., minimal durations of not breathing), oxygen saturation remained relatively stable. For infants who attempted longer sucking bursts, or for those who demonstrated long durations of suspended breathing followed by short sucking bursts, oxygen saturation declined significantly. Examples of these patterns of suck–breathe coordination are depicted in Figure 13-7. During breastfeeding episodes, these same infants integrated breathing within sucking bursts (Figure 13-8). A maturational trend was seen, in which less mature infants demonstrated brief episodes of suspended breathing within long sucking bursts. As the infants approached 34 to 35 weeks' gestation, the suck–breathe patterning approximated a ratio of 1:1.

These findings are consistent with those of previous researchers who described more stable patterns of oxygenation during breastfeedings than during bottle-feedings for preterm infants. However, these findings explain the mechanism for this stability: less interruption in breathing during breastfeeding. Meier (Meier & Brown, 1996) concluded that differences in suck–breathe patterning for bottle-feeding and breastfeeding may be due to the infant's ability to control the flow of milk during breastfeeding by subtle alterations in the suck mechanism. These alterations, which consist of the infant's manipulation of intrasuck and intersuck intervals to accommodate breathing, may not be clinically apparent, but were detected during this research (Figure 13-8). Infants did not demonstrate similar suck–breathe patterning during bottle-feedings until they were several weeks older.

In a large cohort (*n* = 71) of Swedish preterm infants, breastfeeding was studied prospectively from initiation until discharge (Hedberg Nyqvist & Ewald, 1999). In this Swedish hospital setting, where early maternal contact was encouraged, infants demonstrated rooting, areolar grasp, and latching on as early as 28 weeks; nutritive sucking (as defined by intake of 5 mL or greater volume) from 30.6 weeks; and repeated swallowing at 31 weeks. In a smaller cohort (*n* = 26), Nyqvist and colleagues (2001) used surface electrodes to record the oral behavior during breastfeeding of preterm infants. The preterm infants (mean gestational

Table 13-5 STUDIES RELATED TO PHYSIOLOGIC EFFECTS OF BREASTFEEDING IN PRETERM INFANTS

Reference	Design/Sample (N)	Measures	Findings	Limitations
Meier, 1988	Crossover; healthy preterm (5)	Respiratory rate PaO$_2$ Heart rate Temperature	tcPO$_2$ patterns were more stable and body temperature increased during Bfing compared to Bot.	Small sample size Milk intake was not measured
Martell et al., 1993	Crossover; preterm infants Breastfed (16) Bottle-fed (46)	Milk intake measured: Bf—test weights @ 3 min. intervals Bot—ingested vol. during each SU period	Shorter feeding duration w/Bot compared to Bf.	Only six infants were studied at all time periods—no explanation given—one possibility, infants were unable to sustain attachment to the breast for the initial attempts
Bier et al., 1993	Crossover; preterm (20); 9 infants ≥ 1 morbidities associated w/ prematurity	Respiratory rate PaO$_2$ Heart rate Temperature Test weights NOMAS scores	No diff. in PaO$_2$ during Bf; 21% vs. 38% in Bf vs. Bot in O$_2$ desaturation (< 90%); Milk intake during Bf < during Bot; No diff. in temp, feeding duration, NOMAS scores.	
Nyqvist, Sjödén, & Ewald, 1999	Observational; healthy preterm infants (71)	Describe the development of feeding behavior; Time to full oral feeds	1st experience Bf @ median 33.7 wks PMA; 51% of infants observed on 1st day of Bf intro; all but 2 infants showed rooting behavior.	Total duration of latch and SU during each session and vigor of sucking behavior were not assessed; focus of study on infant behavior, not milk intake
Dowling, 1999	Crossover; healthy preterm (8)	Sucking parameters Respiratory rate PaO$_2$ Heart rate Test weight	SU bursts longer for Bot than Bf; no difference in SU rate between Bot and Bf; 10 Bf & 1 Bot feeding were not included due to no milk intake.	Only one type of Bot nipple was tested; effect of orthodontic nipple on the time to full Bf/duration of Bf not reported

Table 13-5 Studies Related to Physiologic Effects of Breastfeeding in Preterm Infants (*CONTINUED*)

Reference	Design/Sample (N)	Measures	Findings	Limitations
Meier et al., 2000	Crossover, healthy preterm (34)	Milk transfer as measured by test weights w/ and w/o nipple shield (NS); duration of NS use; duration of Bfing	Mean milk transfer significantly greater for feedings w/NS (18.4 vs. 3.9 ml), with all infants consuming more milk w/NS in place; mean duration NS use 32.5 d. Mean duration of Bfing 169.4 days; No significant association between % of time NS used and Bfing duration.	Maternal nipple characteristics were not reported
Chen et al., 2000	Crossover, healthy preterm (25)	PaO_2 Heart rate Respiratory rate Body temperature	PaO_2 and body temp significantly higher during Bfing; 2 episodes of apnea and 20 episodes of $PaO_2 <$ 90% during Bot, none during Bf.	Milk intake was not measured
Nyqvist et al., 2001	Observational; preterm (26)	SU and SW behavior as measured by electromyography (EMG)	Agreement between direct observations of SU and EMG data were high. Considerable variation between infants in extent of mouthing. No association with maturational level for any oral behavioral components.	Milk intake was not measured
Furman & Minich, 2004	Observational; preterm Breastfed (35) Bottle-fed (70)	A modified version PIBBS (Nyqvist, Sjödén, & Ewald, 1999)	At 35 wks corrected age, Bfing compared to Bot took in smaller volumes (6.5 vs. 30.5 ml, P < .001), fed less efficiently.	Only 1 feeding session was observed for each infant; no subjective/objective measure of maternal milk ejection noted

Figure 13-7 Polygraphic Recording of Suck/Breathe Pattern and Oxygenation. (A) Polygraphic recording demonstrating suck/breathe patterning and oxygenation during bottle-feeding for a preterm infant. In this recording, the infant alternates short sucking bursts with breathing but does not breathe within sucking burst. Oxygen saturation remains stable. (B) Polygraphic recording demonstrating suck/breathe patterning and oxygenation during bottle-feeding for a preterm infant. oxygen saturation fluctuates, with values as low as 78% during short sucking bursts.

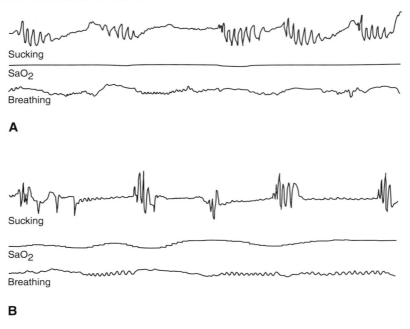

Reproduced by permission of Royal Society of Medicine Press, London

age: 32.5 ± 2.1; range: 26.7 to 36) showed a wide variation in sucking behavior, both in duration and intensity. Analyses of possible factors influencing the infants' oral feeding behavior revealed only one significant association: Infants with a greater post-natal age had a higher mean duration of sucks ($r = 0.39$, $P < 0.05$).

The results of these studies demonstrate the infant's sucking ability at the breast and physiologic stability during breastfeeding. Thus, waiting to initiate breastfeeding until the infant demonstrates the ability to consume entire bottle-feedings is not a research-based criterion of readiness to breastfeed. Additionally, these early "practice" sessions may have other benefits, as evidenced in a small cohort of preterm bottle-feeding infants, whereby a regimen of oral stimulation for 10 days prior to the initiation of oral feedings resulted in some, but not all, oral–motor functions (Fucile et al., 2005). For clinical purposes, all infants should be monitored for physiologic stability during early oral feedings, regardless of method.

Progression of In-Hospital Breastfeeding

When infants are placed at the breast for daily NNS opportunities, the transition to "nutritive feedings" can be a natural progression appropriate to the infant's individual abilities. When it is determined

Figure 13-8 POLYGRAPHIC RECORDING DEMONSTRATING SUCK/BREATHE PATTERNING AND OXYGENATION DURING BREASTFEEDING FOR AN INFANT OF 33 WEEKS' GESTATIONAL AGE. THE INFANT BREATHES WITHIN THIS LONG (104 SUCKS) SUCKLING BURST UNTIL PHASE A, WHEN BREATHING IS INTERRUPTED FOR SEVERAL SUCKS. IN PHASE B, THE INFANT ALTERS THE DURATION AND AMPLITUDE OF INDIVIDUAL SUCKS, APPARENTLY TO REINSTITUTE A MORE REGULAR BREATHING PATTERN, WHICH CONTINUES THROUGH THE REMAINDER OF THE BURST.

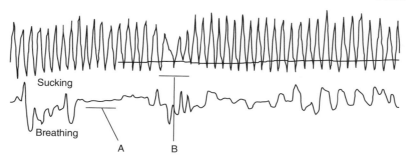

Reproduced by permission of Royal Society of Medicine Press, London

that the infant should consume some "low-flow" milk, the mother can express some, but not all, of the milk from the breast. In this way, the preterm infant is introduced to small droplets of milk that do not necessitate prolonged closure of the airway for swallowing. As the infant matures, the mother can regulate the milk flow by pumping the amount of milk necessary to reduce the postmilk ejection flow. When the infant demonstrates the ability to coordinate sucking and breathing, the mother no longer needs to express milk prior to the feeding. This progressive increase in the rate of flow during breastfeeding is consistent with observations from studies in which suction and expression pressures were measured during low-flow bottle feedings for low-birth-weight infants (Lau et al., 1997; Scheel et al., 2005). Data from these studies suggest that less mature preterm infants can initiate feedings safely, provided that milk flow is restricted.

The preterm infant should be breastfed in a position that affords support to the head and neck, such as the football or the across-the-lap hold. The head of the preterm infant is heavy in relation to the weak musculature of the neck, and undirected head movements can easily collapse the airway, with resultant apnea and bradycardia. Use of these positions will also compensate for the preterm infant's

disadvantage in extracting milk from the breast. Specifically, the data from NNS and bottle-feeding studies reveal that suction pressures are maturationally dependent (Hafström & Kjellmer, 2000; Lau et al., 2000). With this limitation, the small preterm infant needs to be "placed" and "kept" on the nipple, because the limited suction pressures do not permit the infant to draw the nipple into the intraoral cavity to achieve milk extraction (Figure 13-9).

Measuring Milk Transfer

Factors Influencing Milk Transfer During Breastfeeding

Milk transfer during breastfeeding is dependent upon sufficient maternal milk secretion and ejection concurrent with proficient infant oral–motor skills. Table 13-6 provides an algorithm of the various components essential to achieve milk transfer during breastfeeding and the possible outcomes in the absence of each of these components. Upon examining this diagram, it becomes apparent that the mother contributes important elements (milk synthesis/ejection and maternal nipple/areolar attributes) and the infant equally vital components

Figure 13-9 PROVIDING SUPPORT OF THE INFANT'S HEAD AND SUPPORT OF THE BREAST DURING BREASTFEEDING.

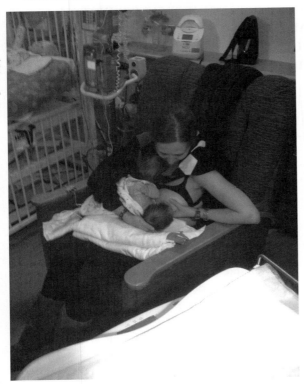

Courtesy of Diane Spatz

(effective suck/swallow). Mothers and their preterm infants may experience problems with any or all of these components. Conversely, because these components are interactive, a problem with one, such as ineffective suckling, can be compensated for by adequacy in the other components. Application of this framework to intake-related questions and problems is essential in determining the appropriate clinical intervention.

For example, most but not all preterm infants have ineffective and/or marginally effective suckling during early breastfeeding experiences. Typically, these infants suckle in short bursts and fall asleep quickly at the breast (Kavanaugh et al., 1995; Nyqvist, Ewald, & Sjödén, 1996; Nyqvist, Rubertsson, et al., 1996). Recently, feeding efficiency was compared in 35 breastfeeding and 70 bottle-feeding VLBW (less than 1500 g) infants (Furman & Minich, 2004). A single feeding observation at a mean corrected age of 35 ± 1 weeks was performed for each infant in the study. Breastfeeding as compared with bottle-feeding infants transferred smaller milk volumes (median 6.5 mL versus 30.5 mL, $P < 0.001$), fed less efficiently (median 0.6 mL/min versus 2.2 mL/min, $P < 0.001$), and spent less time with sucking bursts (mean 33% versus 55%, $P < 0.001$). One limitation to this study was a lack of objective or subjective evidence of maternal milk ejection during breastfeeding sessions. Maternal milk volume and ejection can compensate for marginally effective infant sucking. Anecdotally, it is not uncommon for some mothers whose milk-ejection response has become conditioned to the higher suction pressures experienced with the mechanical breast pump to have difficulty eliciting milk ejection during early breastfeeding attempts.

To document the progression of breastfeeding behavior observed for each individual mother–infant dyad, several tools have been used, varying from simple approximation based on the observer's assessment (Jenson et al., 1994; Mulford, 1992) to detailed observations using checklists or coding forms (Nyqvist, Rubertsson, et al., 1996). The Preterm Infant Breastfeeding Behavior Scale (PIBBS) is a tool developed specifically for mothers of preterm infants (Nyqvist, Ewald, & Sjödén, 1996). It was developed from observations of preterm behavior in collaboration between observers and mothers. By observing her infant in a more systematic way using the PIBBS, the mother develops greater sensitivity to her infant's behavioral pattern at the breast and is able to develop his capacity for nutritive suckling without restrictions of breastfeeding frequency or duration of breastfeeding sessions, irrespective of maturational level or age (see Appendix 13-A).

Several years ago, Hurst at Texas Children's Hospital developed a checklist to document specific behaviors and observations made by the nurse or lactation consultant during a breastfeeding session in the NICU (Figure 13-10). This form was developed because existing breastfeeding tools lacked key components necessary to effectively evaluate the infant and maternal contributions to the dyad in the preterm population. Inclusion of this documentation in the infant's medical record provides pertinent

Table 13-6 ALGORITHM OF ESSENTIAL COMPONENTS OF MILK TRANSFER DURING BREASTFEEDING

	Essential Components								Outcome
	Maternal Components					Infant Components			
	MS*	+ ME	+ MA	→	SU	+ SW	=		MT
Clinical States									
1.	+	+	+		+	+	=		Adequate
2.	−	+	+		+	+	=		Insufficient*
3.	+	−	+		+	+	=		Insufficient
4.	+	+	−		+	+	=		Insufficient**
5.	+	+	+		−	+	=		Insufficient†
6.	+	+	+		+	−	=		Insufficient†

Clinical Interventions

No intervention required (1)

Interventions to increase MS required (2)

Strategies to elicit ME are required to facilitate milk flow (3)

Interventions to facilitate attachment to the maternal nipple (e.g., nipple shield) (4)

Strategies to improve infant SU response (5)

Strategies to improve infant SW ability (6)

Key: MA = maternal nipple/areolar attributes; ME = milk ejection; MS = milk synthesis; MT = milk transfer; SU = infant expression or suction or combination of both; SW = infant swallow
*May be sufficient for the preterm infant considering lower milk volume needs.
**May be sufficient if infant can achieve sustained attachment despite MA.
†May be sufficient if attachment to breast and MS + ME are adequate.

information regarding the preterm infant's progress with breastfeeding, which is then conveyed to the entire healthcare team. This checklist of key components provides an evaluation of the infant's sucking behavior and activity, as well as the mother's milk-ejection response and average pumped milk volume. This tool is not used to place a "score" on the feeding session, but rather provides information about relevant aspects of the contributions made by each member of the breastfeeding dyad, allowing for appropriate interventions to be utilized.

Methods to Estimate Milk Transfer

Along with these key components observed during feeding, it is important to evaluate milk transfer once the preterm infant has been introduced to unrestricted milk flow during breastfeeding. Mothers and healthcare professionals are unable to use clinical indices to accurately estimate milk intake for preterm infants (Kavanaugh et al., 1995; Meier et al., 1996). However, clinicians are concerned that more accurate measures of milk intake are either too stressful for mothers or unnecessary for preterm infants (Meier, 1995; Walker, 1995). Similarly, many care providers are unaware that accurate measurement of milk intake for preterm infants is possible.

Test-weighing procedures, whereby the clothed infant is weighed before and after feeding (the difference in weight equals the volume consumed) provides an accurate measure of milk intake for clinical and research settings (Meier et al., 1994, 1996; Scanlon et al., 2002). Using test-weights, 1 g of weight gain approximates 1 mL of milk intake. When performed correctly, test-weighing is accepted as the technique of choice in clinical

Figure 13-10 PREMIE Breastfeeding Assessment.

PREMIE Breastfeeding Assessment

Recent Oral Feeding

Number of PO feeding attempts/d during previous 24 hours (circle one): None   1   3–5   8
Type of PO feeding attempt: Breast (#)_____   Bottle (#)_____
If bottle-fed, % of prescribed volume taken_____
If breastfed, was additional milk given via bottle or gavage pc: Yes____ No____

Maternal Nipple Attributes (Prior to Feeding)
(Check appropriate items.)
- ☐ Prominent
- ☐ Flat
- ☐ Inverted
- ☐ Other, describe:_____

Assessment of Breastfeeding Session:
(Check appropriate items.)

Predominant infant behavior
- ☐ Quiet/active alert
- ☐ Drowsy
- ☐ Deep sleep/crying

Rooting
- ☐ Obvious rooting w/ minimal stimulation
- ☐ Some rooting w/ stimulation
- ☐ No rooting

Effective latch-on
- ☐ Maintains effective latch
- ☐ Attempts latch, slips off or holds nipple in mouth
- ☐ No latch achieved

Milk ejection
- ☐ Obvious objective or subjective signs
- ☐ Possible signs, uncertain or not noticed
- ☐ No objective or subjective signs

Infant suck
- ☐ Rhythmic sucking
- ☐ Arrhythmic sucking
- ☐ No sucking

Evident swallowing
- ☐ Smooth swallowing
- ☐ Strained swallowing
- ☐ No swallowing

Nipple shield used? If so, which size: ☐ Small   ☐ Newborn

Maternal Milk Volume
Average pumped volume nearest to the time of the current feeding session_____(ml)

Milk Transfer
Infant weight prior to feeding_____(gm)   Following feeding_____(gm)
Total milk transfer during feeding (postfeed weight – prefeed weight)_____(gm)

With permission, The Lactation Support Program, Texas Children's Hospital.

situations whereby milk intake needs to be measured accurately (Scanlon et al., 2002).

Test-weighing should be introduced in the NICU when it appears that milk transfer has occurred or discharge is imminent. For smaller preterm infants, the test-weight estimate permits individualized complementation of breastfeedings, so that 24-hour fluid and caloric requirements can be met. For larger infants awaiting NICU discharge, test-weights can be used to diagnose milk-transfer problems. For example, the infant may suckle marginally, but the mother's milk volume may be adequate. It is impossible to know whether the mother's milk flow can compensate for the infant's suck unless the volume of intake is measured.

Strategies to Facilitate Milk Transfer

Seldom does significant milk transfer occur during the first few breastfeeding sessions for preterm infants (Furman & Minich, 2004). However, as NICU discharge approaches, consistently small volumes of intake become a concern that must be evaluated. Selected problems of milk transfer are particularly common among preterm infants.

The single most important factor for mothers who will be breastfeeding a preterm infant at home is maintaining a milk supply that exceeds the baby's requirements at hospital discharge (Hill et al., 1997; Lawrence, 2001; Meier, 2001). With an adequate milk supply, the infant's immature sucking pattern may be less problematic. Mothers can plan for this by expressing their milk an extra time or two in the week before their baby's discharge. For mothers who have a borderline milk supply as NICU discharge approaches, the clinician should consider a regimen of metoclopramide (Emery, 1996) or domperidone. Research conducted outside the United States demonstrates that domperidone is the preferred medication, with no side effects being reported when this medication was used in mothers with infants in the NICU and the mothers' milk supply increasing by 267% (Campbell-Yeo et al., 2010; Campbell-Yeo et al., 2006). A multicenter clinical trial (the EMPOWER trial) of the use of domperidone to augment milk yield is currently ongoing (Asztalos et al., 2012). Theoretically, the prolactin stimulus from this medication will be maintained by the infant's direct breastfeeding in the home.

Mothers should be reminded to express milk with the electric breast pump after each breastfeeding in the hospital. NICU staff and mothers seldom appreciate that a preterm infant cannot substitute for the breast stimulation provided by the electric breast pump, especially if the infant consumes only small milk volumes. Mothers frequently question how to coordinate milk expression with demand feedings because they are concerned their breasts will be empty when their infants awake to feed. An appropriate strategy in this situation is to emphasize the priority of maintaining milk yield by maintaining complete breast emptying during their transition to exclusive breastfeeding.

Many mothers of preterm infants deny feeling the sensations of milk ejection both when using the electric pump and when feeding their infants at breast. Thus it is often difficult to evaluate the synchronization of milk ejection and infant sucking. One strategy that may be useful in evaluating the milk-ejection response is to instruct the mother to uncover the opposite breast during a breastfeeding session and observe the spontaneous dripping of milk during milk ejection. Typically, mothers experience a delay in milk ejection when infants are placed at the breast because the women are conditioned to the sensations of the breast pump. It is not uncommon for milk flow to begin just as the preterm infant falls asleep at the breast. If this situation persists for more than a few feedings, the mother can use the electric breast pump to initiate the milk flow. This can be done by placing the infant at one breast and the pump at the other, or by first initiating the milk flow with the breast pump and then placing the infant at breast.

Sustaining Attachment to the Maternal Breast

The sucking pattern of the healthy term infant is characterized by the rhythmic alternation of two types of pressure: negative (suction) and positive (compression) pressure (Dubignon & Campbell,

1969; Sameroff, 1967). Suction defines the negative intraoral pressure generated as the infant draws milk into the mouth, whereas compression is the positive pressure resulting from the compression and/or stripping of the nipple between the tongue and the hard palate as milk is ejected into the mouth (Ardran et al., 1958; Nowak et al., 1994, 1995; Waterland et al., 1998). The majority of milk transfer problems for preterm infants can be traced to immaturity and inconsistency in suckling (Kavanaugh et al., 1995; Meier & Brown, 1996). The relatively low suction pressures and the infant's inconsistent, irregular sucking bursts do not sustain the milk flow needed for effective milk transfer or, in many cases, do not allow for sustained attachment to the maternal breast. These phenomena appear to be maturationally dependent. Until the infant achieves term-corrected age, strategies to increase the effectiveness of sucking to achieve sustained attachment to the breast are often necessary.

Weak sucking pressures (-2.5 to -15 mm Hg) measured in preterm infants may result in difficulties maintaining attachment to the maternal breast (Lau et al., 1997). Bottle-feeding studies by Lau and colleagues (1997, 2000) concluded that sucking ability does not need to be at a mature level before preterm infants are introduced to oral feeding. In these studies, preterm infants were able to transfer milk during bottle-feeding via compression only, using little or no suction pressure. Therefore the provision of a rigid nipple may allow the infant the ability to transfer milk without the need to generate suction pressure, utilizing instead the compression component of infant feeding. Interestingly, preterm infants have been shown to modify their sucking skills to maintain a rate of transfer that is compatible with the level of suck/swallow/breathe coordination they have attained at a particular time (Scheel et al., 2005).

This theoretical basis may explain reports of improved milk transfer during breastfeeding in preterm infants using a thin, silicone nipple shield placed over the mother's nipple to facilitate sustained attachment (Clum & Primomo, 1996; Meier et al., 2000). A study of 34 preterm infants (Meier et al., 2000) revealed a significantly greater increase in milk transfer with the shield than during previous breastfeeding without the shield (18.4 mL versus 3.9 mL, $P = 0.0001$). In a retrospective study of 15 preterm infants, the nipple shield was introduced following at least five failed attempts to achieve breast attachment or milk transfer without the nipple shield (Clum & Primomo, 1996). Nine of the 15 infants consumed at least half or greater of the prescribed feeding amount with the nipple shield. Clinical indications for nipple shield use among this group included the inability of the infant to sustain attachment to the breast, holding the nipple in the mouth while falling asleep, and maternal nipple characteristics.

The results of these studies (Clum & Primomo, 1996; Meier et al., 2000) raise further questions as to the underlying etiology of the nipple shield's effect on infant and maternal breastfeeding responses. One possible explanation could be that the nipple shield provides a uniform rigid structure that extends deeper into the infant's oral cavity, thereby creating greater tactile stimulation (Figure 13-11). As a result of this stimulation, the infant responds by compression or compression/suction and sustained breast attachment. Consequently, a sustained attachment and compression of the shield results in

Figure 13-11 PRETERM INFANT AT THE BREAST WITH NIPPLE SHIELD IN PLACE.

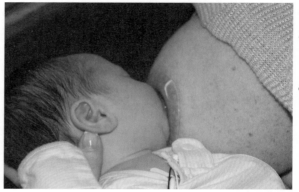

stimulation of the underlying nipple/areolar tissue, providing a stimulus for activation of the maternal milk-ejection reflex and improved milk flow and transfer. These responses are only speculative, however, as maternal nipple/areolar attributes and/or infant suction pressures were not measured in these studies. Although an ideal nipple shield for preterm infants has yet to be designed, the smallest, thinnest shield available is indicated for these babies.

The nipple shield is extremely well accepted by mothers, because it often represents the first breastfeeding experience in which the infant remains awake, sucks eagerly, and consumes measurable volumes of milk. However, mothers are concerned about providing the gentle pressure necessary to keep the infants correctly positioned over the areola, because of the plastic nature of shield. Thus mothers need to be shown how to support the breast with the shield in place so that the infant can achieve an effective sucking position while keeping the shield away from the nose.

Clinicians often assume that preterm infants do not take as much milk with the shield in place as they would without its use. This concern seems to be based on the Auerbach 1990 data that demonstrated reduced milk transfer when mothers of term infants expressed milk with a breast pump with a nipple shield in place (as cited in Auerbach, 1992). Although this study addressed an important concept, the findings cannot be applied indiscriminately to infants, as milk transfer was measured for milk expression with a breast pump—not infant feeding. Preterm infants, when they are unable to transfer milk during breastfeeding prior to nipple shield use, actually increase milk intake when the shield is in place. Similarly, concern that use of the shield will reduce the milk yield over time is not applicable in this situation. Preterm infants who feed longer and more eagerly with the shield in place provide considerably more breast stimulation than breastfeeding without the shield.

Some clinicians suggest that other feeding techniques, such as cup- or finger-feedings, should be used as an alternative to the nipple shield. This approach appears to reflect an unscientific bias against the nipple shield, and is especially problematic because use of the shield means that the infant can feed at the breast. Mothers of preterm infants, who may have spent weeks or months expressing milk, prefer to feed their babies at the breast, even if it entails temporary nipple shield use. Use of the shield also saves time for mothers, because they do not need to offer a complement after breastfeeding, as is the case with a cup- or finger-feeding.

Finally, the duration of nipple shield use is a common concern, in that clinicians frequently ask how to "wean" babies from the shield. Data indicate that for a sample of preterm, low-birth-weight infants who received the same research-based breastfeeding services, duration of breastfeeding was twice as long for the group of infants who were breastfed with the shield (Meier et al., 2000). Thus common concerns that use of the nipple shield decreases the milk supply and shortens the duration of breastfeeding are not supported by the available research for preterm infants.

If the nipple shield is effective in correcting milk transfer problems in the hospital, its use should be continued after NICU discharge. Additionally, there is no scientific reason for recommending that infants be "weaned" from the shield as soon as possible. Typically, the infant will require the shield for adequate milk transfer until he reaches approximately term-corrected age. For most mothers, this coincides with 2 to 3 weeks of nipple shield use, a period over time the infant's intake and weight gain can be monitored regularly. Mothers have described their individual approaches to discontinuing the shield, but in no case should they be advised to cut back or tamper with the integrity of the shield. Serial test-weights are helpful to most mothers as they transfer from the shield to feeding at the breast without the shield.

In addition to the nipple shield, other breastfeeding devices are frequently recommended to measure and facilitate milk transfer. A supplemental nurser can be helpful for the mother who has a limited milk supply and whose infant is able to achieve sustained attachment and sucking mechanism at the breast. This device is especially helpful for borderline preterm infants (more than 34 weeks' gestation) who are still premature with respect to the ability to extract adequate volumes of milk. Providing they are able to sustain attachment, these infants can receive the extra milk they need with a supplemental nurser while feeding at the breast.

Discharge Planning for Postdischarge Breastfeeding

Unlike term healthy infants, preterm infants do not demonstrate predictable, easily detectible hunger cues until close to their term-corrected age (Kavanaugh et al., 1995; Nyqvist et al., 1999; Ross & Browne, 2002), and mothers report difficulty in recognizing these behaviors (Reyna et al., 2006). Thus infants may consume minimal volumes at a breastfeeding and still sleep for several hours, if undisturbed. The use of test-weights permits the emergence of demand feeding behaviors, while retaining a safeguard against slow weight gain and dehydration in the days before NICU discharge.

Research from the Netherlands demonstrates that early discharge with tube-feedings at home is associated with longer breastfeeding duration (Meerlo-Habing et al., 2009). In this study, infants were sent home on tube-feeding with follow-up from specialized pediatric nurses, which significantly increased breastfeeding duration. The results showed that 64% of infants who were discharged with tube-feedings were breastfeeding at 4 months after discharge, compared to only 37% of the control group. If a mother's goal is to breastfeed her child, she should be encouraged to consider taking the infant home on a feeding tube and with a scale to measure milk transfer.

When the infant has demonstrated the ability to consume all feedings orally, the neonatologist or neonatal nurse practitioner can prescribe a 24-hour minimal milk intake for the infant. The 24-hour volume can then be subdivided into 6- or 8-hour volumes to permit a modified demand-feeding schedule. For example, if an infant weighing 1700 g needs a minimum of 300 mL per day, the mother and nurse can plan to feed 100 mL every 8 hours. Then, the infant is allowed to "demand," but must receive the prescribed 100 mL volume within an 8-hour period. Test-weights are measured with each breastfeeding, and the volume of complements and/or supplements is recorded. Thus, if the infant consumes 15 mL, 12 mL, and 18 mL within a period of 2 hours, the infant has been given the opportunity to self-regulate sleep and feeding. However, the infant still must consume the remaining 55 mL over the next 6 hours. NICU nurses can help mothers implement this plan in the days before infant discharge, so that mothers develop an understanding of how the infant coordinates sleep and feeding.

Many mothers of preterm infants—both borderline babies and those who are smaller—find it reassuring to measure milk intake and/or serial weight gain in the first days after infant discharge (Hurst et al., 2004). A portable, battery-operated scale that mothers can rent and perform test-weights and/or daily weights in the home is ideal for this purpose. The scale, which weighs to the nearest 2 g and automatically calculates milk intake from the prefeed and postfeed weights, has been demonstrated to measure milk intake accurately for term and preterm infants (Meier et al., 1994). Such a scale can be a useful adjunct to breastfeeding management for mothers and preterm infants during the first week or two after discharge. However, mothers should be introduced to the proper use of the scale during the days prior to NICU discharge.

The United States is different from most developed countries in that preterm infants are typically discharged from the NICU before their expected birth dates, whether or not breastfeeding has been well established. In contrast, in some European countries, preterm infants are discharged only when weight gain on exclusive breastfeeding has been documented, which may be several weeks later than in the United States (Akerstrom et al., 2007; Flacking et al., 2003; Nyqvist et al., 1999). In developing countries, preterm infants are frequently discharged at lower weights, but many of these infants are small for gestational age (Ramasethu et al., 1993) and/or maintained in skin-to-skin care in the home (Bergman & Jurisoo, 1994; Cattaneo et al., 1998; Charpak et al., 1994; Whitelaw & Liestol, 1994).

When these data are considered in combination, it appears that preterm infants remain at risk for under-consumption of milk by exclusive at-breast feeding until approximately term-corrected age (Meier & Brown, 1996). This implication is suggested by the low incidence of exclusive at-breast feeding in the early weeks after NICU discharge in the United States (Furman et al., 1998; Hill et al., 1997); the longer hospitalization in European countries so that exclusive at-breast feeding is established (Nyqvist et al., 1999); and the slow weight gain on exclusive breastfeedings in the first 2 to 4 weeks after hospital discharge in developing countries. This commonality probably reflects a problem with the maturationally dependent "infant suckling" component of milk transfer, often expressed by mothers as "getting enough."

Getting Enough: Determining Need for Extra Milk Feedings

Studies from the United States have examined the phenomenon of "getting enough" for mothers and preterm infants (Hill et al., 1997; Kavanaugh et al., 1995). However, clinicians who work primarily with term, healthy infants do not always comprehend the difference between "getting enough" and "insufficient milk supply." As a result, mothers of preterm infants are frequently told to breastfeed their babies and/or pump more frequently—interventions that focus on the milk volume component of milk transfer. These recommendations are inappropriate for most mothers of preterm infants who describe problems with "getting enough." These women report that they can express adequate volumes of milk with the breast pump, but perceive that their infants do not take all of the milk available to them. Thus effective interventions must focus on the infant suckling component of milk transfer. This distinction has important research and practice implications.

The most fundamental research issue is that the accepted nomenclature for describing and classifying amount of breastfeeding does not fit the breastfeeding patterns for this population (Meier &

Brown, 1997). For example, most mothers of preterm infants complement at-breast feedings with their own expressed milk during the early weeks at home (Hurst et al., 2004; Wooldridge & Hall, 2003), but the Labbok and Krasovec schema does not accurately capture this pattern. If this pattern is categorized as "exclusive breastfeeding," it overestimates mothers' successes and misrepresents data on duration of breastfeeding. Thus evidence-based criteria to categorize the amount of breastfeeding for these mothers must be developed and standardized.

Research addressing the early postdischarge period must also include methods that accurately and reliably distinguish between insufficient maternal milk supply and the infant's ability to consume adequate milk volumes (Hill et al., 1997; Meier & Brown, 1997). These studies must incorporate available technology to measure milk volume and infant intake during breastfeeding, rather than relying on checklists or clinical indices that have been demonstrated to be inaccurate and/or unreliable. Similarly, other studies in which milk intake during breastfeeding was not measured have related slow weight gain and/or the need for continued milk fortification postdischarge to address deficiencies in the mother's milk (Chan et al., 1994; Hall et al., 1993; Wauben et al., 1998). The value of nutrient enrichment of mother's own milk post discharge also remains unclear (Zachariassen et al., 2011). Fortification of mother's own milk for very preterm infants has not been found to influence breastfeeding duration (Zachariassen et al., 2011). The question remains whether it is necessary, as the fortification in the Zachariassen et al. study did not improve growth of infants at 1 year of age compared to infants fed unfortified human milk.

Methods to Deliver Extra Milk Feedings Away from the Breast

In most NICUs in the United States, the most common method of oral feeding when the mother is not available is by bottle. Several investigators have suggested that the differences in sucking patterns required during breastfeeding compared to bottle-feeding contribute to difficulties transitioning to exclusive breastfeeding. Alternative feeding devices are frequently recommended by clinicians to avoid "nipple confusion" (Cronenwett et al., 1992; Lang et al., 1994; Neifert et al., 1995). Reports suggest that one such alternative feeding method—cup-feeding—is safe when performed by experts (Lang et al., 1994; Rocha et al., 2002), but few controlled clinical trials have established increased breastfeeding prevalence when these devices are employed (Dowling et al., 2002; Rocha et al., 2002). An interesting finding in one study revealed the oral mechanisms used by preterm infants during cup-feeding to be "sipping" rather than "lapping" in the majority of the 15 cup-feeding sessions for eight preterm (mean gestational age at birth = 30.6 weeks) infants (Dowling et al., 2002). Additionally, a significant amount (38.5%) of milk spillage during cup-feeding was reported by Dowling et al. (2002) and others (Aloysius & Hickson, 2007).

Postdischarge Breastfeeding Management

Strategies that have been demonstrated to improve breastfeeding outcomes both prior to and following infant discharge include skin-to-skin contact, prefeed and postfeed weights at home, peer counseling, and postdischarge lactation support (Ahmed & Sands, 2010). Several key principles must be understood and incorporated into postdischarge breastfeeding plans for preterm infants:

- The practitioner must recognize that the clinical indices of intake used for healthy term infants, such as breastfeeding behaviors, wet diapers, frequency of stools, and sleep patterns, are not accurate or reliable for preterm infants. For example, a preterm infant may remain "hydrated," but still not consume enough milk to grow.
- Preterm infants may not consistently "demand," so mothers must not be told, "You'll know when your baby is hungry."

- These infants should not be awakened more frequently than every 3 hours to breastfeed because sleep interruption interferes with growth hormone release, retarding weight gain.
- Mothers of preterm infants are not reassured with nonspecific comments such as "Trust your body." It is important to accept that mothers' concerns about intake are real, and not just a reflection of their NICU experience.

In summary, mothers of preterm infants need a safety net during the first weeks at home until their infants have demonstrated the ability to gain weight on exclusive breastfeedings. Milk transfer must be monitored regularly, such as every 48 to 72 hours, and accurately at this time, either through frequent visits to the primary care provider for serial growth measures or by in-home test-weighing.

Care must be taken to listen to these women and their feelings of vulnerability with respect to infant intake. They must not be hurried through these processes or told that they are not breastfeeding "correctly." For example, if a mother feels that she needs to give bottle supplements of her expressed milk in the first few days, she should not be warned about "nipple confusion" or told that alternative feedings should be used. Instead, her ability to determine and advocate what she feels is best for her infant must be interpreted as a sign of strength. It is important to remember that breastfeeding is only one activity that these women must deal with; their babies are vulnerable to many conditions, and mothers need time to sort out care priorities.

Similarly, mothers should be encouraged to continue the breastfeeding strategies that worked in the hospital until their infants have demonstrated an acceptable pattern of growth for at least a week or two. For many women, these devices will include a nipple shield and/or in-home weighing, and there are no data to support withdrawing these aids before the mother is ready. Finally, the mother needs access to both consumer-support groups and a professional who is experienced with breastfeeding for preterm infants when discharge approaches.

Acknowledgment

The author gratefully acknowledges the authors of the previous version of this chapter, Nancy Hurst and Paula Meier.

Summary

Breastfeeding for preterm infants and mothers is different from breastfeeding for healthy populations in many important ways. The vast body of research in this area suggests that these differences are physiologic, biologic, metabolic, and emotional, and that they are common across a variety of national boundaries and cultures. The challenge to researchers and clinicians who work with mothers and preterm infants is to continue to generate new studies and practices that incorporate findings from these scientific publications. Only research-based practices can address the many barriers to breastfeeding initiation and duration for this at-risk population.

Key Concepts

- Studies indicate that preterm infants are not just "small term infants" with respect to breastfeeding management. Therefore evidence-based strategies that target specific barriers for this vulnerable population should be used.
- Human milk may provide optimal "nutritional programming" for preterm infants, and may be protective against several prematurity-related conditions.
- Based on current research related to the superiority of human milk for preterm infants, parents should be provided with accurate information to help them make an informed choice about providing mother's own milk for their preterm infant.
- Mothers providing breastmilk for their preterm infants should be praised for their efforts regardless of the length of time of their commitments.
- Although giving birth prematurely does not appear to limit milk production, several factors surrounding the birth experience are documented prolactin inhibitors and can adversely affect milk volume.
- The mother's milk-expression technique can influence the composition and the bacterial count of the milk to be fed to her infant.
- Documenting the time, duration, and amount of milk expressed provides useful information to the mother that can be shared with the NICU staff for assessment of milk volume maintenance.
- It has been speculated that skin-to-skin holding may trigger the production of maternal milk antibodies to specific pathogens in the preterm infant's environment through mechanisms in the enteromammary pathway.
- Proper NICU procedures should be developed and adhered to so as to minimize bacterial growth and possible changes in milk constituents during storage and feeding.
- Special consideration regarding the feeding of expressed mother's milk to preterm infants is based on the infant's fluid restrictive status at a time of greatest nutritional need.
- Unfortified expressed mother's milk is deficient in protein and selected minerals needed to support optimal growth and bone mineralization for small preterm infants.
- Lactoengineering of expressed mother's milk through a combination of hindmilk and creamatocrit measures can impact the caloric density of the milk provided to preterm infants, as well as empower these infants' mothers.
- Early oral feeding experiences may influence later oral feeding development in preterm infants.
- There are no universally established criteria for the initiation of breastfeeding (or bottle-feeding, for that matter) for preterm infants.
- In NICUs where infants are allowed nonnutritive suckling at the emptied breast, the mother is afforded valuable observation of

her infant's behavior and developing signs for readiness to oral feeding.

- Delayed initiation of breastfeeding until the infant demonstrates the ability to consume entire bottle-feedings is not an evidence-based criterion of readiness to breastfeed.
- Milk transfer during breastfeeding depends on sufficient maternal milk secretion and ejection concurrent with proficient infant oral–motor skills.
- Test-weighing procedures provide the most accurate measure of milk intake in clinical and research settings.
- The single most important factor for mothers who will be breastfeeding a preterm infant at home is maintaining a milk supply that exceeds the infant's requirements at hospital discharge.
- The majority of milk transfer problems for preterm infants are related to immaturity and inconsistency in suckling.
- For preterm infants who are unable to sustain attachment to the maternal breast and/or transfer milk, the nipple shield has proved an effective strategy as a milk transfer device.
- Preterm infants remain at risk for under-consumption of milk by exclusive at-breast feeding until they reach term-corrected age.
- Mothers' concerns regarding their preterm infants' ability to "get enough" milk during breastfeeding are real and should not be dismissed.

INTERNET RESOURCES

- Children's Hospital of Philadelphia Breastfeeding and Lactation operates a website that provides health professional and parent information as well as brief video content: http://www.chop.edu/service/breastfeeding-and-lactation/home.html
- Congenital Heart Information Network (CHIN) is an international organization that provides reliable information, support services, and resources to families of children with congenital heart defects and acquired heart disease: www.tchin.org
- La Leche League International provides parent and professional materials on breastfeeding a preterm infant: www.lalecheleague.org
- National Organization of Mothers of Twins Clubs, Inc. (NOMOTC), founded in 1960, is a group providing support, education, and information for mothers of twins: www.nomotc.org
- Premature Baby Premature Child is a volunteer-run website providing parents with information about caring for premature infants: www.prematurity.org
- Rush Mothers' Milk Club is a website that provides resources for families and health professionals as well as research updates: http://www.rushmothersmilkclub.com/
- Supporting Premature Infant Nutrition is part of the University of California–San Diego website and provides resources for both families and health professionals: http://health.ucsd.edu/specialties/obgyn/maternity/newborn/nicu/spin/Pages/default.aspx

REFERENCES

Aggett PJ, Agostoni C, Axelsson I, et al. Feeding preterm infants after hospital discharge: a commentary by the ESPGHAN Committee on Nutrition. *J Pediatr Gastroenterol Nutr.* 2006;42(5):596–603.

Agrasada GV, Gustafsson J, Kylberg E, Ewald U. Postnatal peer counselling on exclusive breastfeeding of low-birthweight infants: a randomized, controlled trial. *Acta Paediatr.* 2005;94(8):1109–1115.

Aguayo J. Maternal lactation for preterm newborn infants. *Early Hum Dev.* 2001;65(suppl):S19–S29.

Ahmed AH, Sands LP. Effect of pre- and postdischarge interventions on breastfeeding outcomes and weight gain among premature infants. *J Obstet Gynecol Neonatal Nurs.* 2010;39(1):53–63. doi: 10.1111/j.1552-6909.2009.01088.x.Review.

Akerstrom S, Asplund I, Norman M. Successful breastfeeding after discharge of preterm and sick newborn infants. *Acta Paediatr.* 2007;96(10):1450–1454.

Akisu M, Kültürsay N, Ozkayin N, et al. Platelet-activating factor levels in term and preterm human milk. *Biol Neonate.* 1998;74(4):289–293.

Aljazaf K, Hale TW, Ilett KF, et al. Pseudoephedrine: effects on milk production in women and estimation of infant exposure via breastmilk. *Br J Clin Pharmacol.* 2003;56(1):18–24.

Aloysius A, Hickson M. Evaluation of paladai cup feeding in breast-fed preterm infants compared with bottle feeding. *Early Hum Dev.* 2007;83(9):619–621.

Alves E, Rodrigues C, Fraga S, et al. Parents' views on factors that help or hinder breast milk supply in neonatal care units: systematic review. *Arch Dis Child Fetal Neonatal Ed.* 2013;98(6):F511–F517. doi: 10.1136/archdis-child-2013-304029.

American Academy of Pediatrics (AAP), Section on Breastfeeding. Breastfeeding and the use of human milk. *Pediatrics.* 2012;129(3). doi: 10.1542/peds.2011-3552.

American Academy of Pediatrics (AAP). The transfer of drugs and therapeutics into human milk: an update on selected topics. *Pediatrics.* 2013;132:e796–e809.

Amin SB, Merle KS, Orlando MS, et al. Brainstem maturation in premature infants as a function of enteral feeding type. *Pediatrics.* 2000;106(2 Pt 1):318–322.

Ardran GM, Kemp FH, Lind J. A cineradiographic study of breastfeeding. *Br J Radiol.* 1958;31:156–162.

Arias-Camison JM. Late onset group B streptococcal infection from maternal expressed breast milk in a very low birth weight infant. *J Perinatol.* 2003;23(8):691–692.

Armand M, Hamosh M, Mehta NR, et al. Effect of human milk or formula on gastric function and fat digestion in the premature infant. *Pediatr Res.* 1996;40(3):429–437.

Arslanoglu S, Moro GE, Ziegler EE, WAPM Working Group on Nutrition. Optimization of human milk fortification for preterm infants: new concepts and recommendations. *J Perinat Med.* 2010;38(3):233–238. doi: 10.1515/JPM.2010.073.

Asztalos EV, Campbell-Yeo M, daSilva OP, et al. Enhancing breast milk production with domperidone in mothers of preterm neonates (EMPOWER trial). *BMC Pregnancy Childbirth.* 2012;12:87. doi: 10.1186/1471-2393-12-87.

Auerbach KG. Re: "Changes in nutritive sucking patterns with increasing gestational age." *Nurs Res.* 1992;41(2):126–127.

Baker BJ, Rasmussen TW. Organizing and documenting lactation support of NICU families. *J Obstet Gynecol Neonatal Nurs.* 1997;26(5):515–521.

Ballabio C, Bertino E, Coscia A, et al. Immunoglobulin-A profile in breast milk from mothers delivering full term and preterm infants. *Int J Immunopathol Pharmacol.* 2007;20(1):119–128.

Bauer J, Gerss J. Longitudinal analysis of macronutrients and minerals in human milk produced by mothers of preterm infants. *J Clin Nutr.* 2011;30(2):215–200. doi: 10.1016/j.clnu.2010.080003.

Bauer K, Uhrig C, Sperling P, et al. Body temperatures and oxygen consumption during skin-to-skin (kangaroo) care in stable preterm infants weighing less than 1500 grams. *J Pediatr.* 1997;130:240–244.

Becker GE, McCormick FM, Renfrew MJ. Methods of milk expression for lactating women. *Cochrane Database Syst Rev.* 2008;4:CD006170.

Behari P, Englund J, Alcasid G, et al. Transmission of methicillin-resistant *Staphylococcus aureus* to preterm infants through breast milk. *Infect Control Hosp Epidemiol.* 2004;25(9):778–780.

Bergman NJ, Jurisoo LA. The "kangaroo-method" for treating low birth weight babies in a developing country. *Tropic Doct.* 1994;24(2):57–60.

Bernaix LW, Schmidt CA, Jamerson PA, et al. The NICU experience of lactation and its relationship to family management style. *Am J Matern Child Nurs.* 2006;31(2):95–100.

Bernt KM, Walker WA. Human milk as a carrier of biochemical messages. *Acta Paediatr Suppl.* 1999;88(430):27–41.

Bialoskurski MM, Cox CL, Wiggins RD. The relationship between maternal needs and priorities in a neonatal intensive care environment. *J Adv Nurs.* 2002;37(1):62–69.

Bier JA, Ferguson A, Anderson L, et al. Breast-feeding of very low birth weight infants. *J Pediatr.* 1993;123(5):773–778.

Bier JA, Ferguson AE, Morales Y, et al. Comparison of skin-to-skin contact with standard contact in low-birth-weight infants who are breast-fed. *Arch Pediatr Adolesc Med.* 1996;150(12):1265–1269.

Bier JA, Oliver T, Ferguson AE, Vohr BR. Human milk improves cognitive and motor development of premature infants during infancy. *J Hum Lact.* 2002;18(4):361–367.

Bigger HR, Fogg LJ, Patel A, et al. Quality indicators for human milk use in very low-birthweight infants: are we measuring what we should be measuring? *J Perinatol.* 2014;34(4):287–291. doi: 10.1038/jp.2014.5. Epub February 13, 2014.

Bingham PM, Churchill D, Ashikaga T. Breast milk odor via olfactometer for tube-fed, premature infants. *Behav Res Meth.* 2007;39(3):630–634.

Birch E, Birch DG, Hoffman DR, Uauy R. Dietary essential fatty acid supply and visual acuity development. *Invest Ophthalmol Vis Sci.* 1992;33(11):3242–3253.

Birch E, Birch D, Hoffman D, et al. Breast-feeding and optimal visual development. *J Pediatr Ophthalmol Strabismus.* 1993;30(1):33–38.

Blaymore Bier JA, Ferguson AE, Morales Y, et al. Breastfeeding infants who were extremely low birth weight. *Pediatrics.* 1997;100(6):E3.

Blumer N, Pfefferle PI, Renz H. Development of mucosal immune function in the intrauterine and early postnatal environment. *Curr Opin Gastroenterol.* 2007;23(6):655–660.

Boehm G, Moro G, Müller DM, et al. Fecal cholesterol excretion in preterm infants fed breast milk or formula with different cholesterol contents. *Acta Paediatr.* 1995;84(3):240–244.

Bohnhorst B, Heyne T, Peter CS, Poets CF. Skin-to-skin (kangaroo) care, respiratory control, and thermoregulation. *J Pediatr.* 2001;138(2):193–197.

Brennan-Behm M , Carlson GE, Meier P, Engstrom J. Caloric loss from expressed mother's milk during continuous gavage infusion. *Neonatal Netw.* 1994;13(2):27–32.

Britton JR. Milk protein quality in mothers delivering prematurely: implications for infants in the intensive care unit nursery setting. *J Pediatr Gastroenterol Nutr.* 1986;5(1):116–121.

Browne JV. Early relationship environments: physiology of skin-to-skin contact for parents and their preterm infants. *Clin Perinatol.* 2004;31(2):287–298.

Brownell EA, Lussier MM, Hagadorn JI, et al. Independent predictors of human milk receipt at neonatal intensive care unit discharge. *Am J Perinatol.* Epub December 17, 2013.

Budd SC, Erdman SH, Long DM, et al. Improved lactation with metoclopramide: a case report. *Clin Pediatr (Phila).* 1993;32(1):53–57.

Butte NF, Garza C, Johnson CA, et al. Longitudinal changes in milk composition of mothers delivering preterm and term infants. *Early Hum Dev.* 1984;9:153–162.

Byrne PA, Miller C, Justus K. Neonatal group B streptococcal infection related to breast milk. *Breastfeed Med.* 2006;1(4):263–270.

Callen J, Pinelli J, Atkinson S, Saigal S. Qualitative analysis of barriers to breastfeeding in very-low-birthweight infants in the hospital and postdischarge. *Adv Neonatal Care.* 2005;5(2):93–103.

Campbell-Yeo ML, Allen AC, Joseph KS, et al. Effect of domperidone on the composition of preterm human breast milk. *Pediatrics.* 2010;125(1):e107–e114. doi: 10.1542/peds.2008-3441. Epub December 14, 2009.

Campbell-Yeo ML, Allen AC, Joseph KS, et al. Study protocol: a double blind placebo controlled trial examining the effect of domperidone on the composition of breast milk [NCT00308334]. *BMC Pregnancy Childbirth.* 2006;6:17.

Carter CS, Altemus M. Integrative functions of lactational hormones in social behavior and stress management. *Ann N Y Acad Sci.* 1997;807:164–174.

Castellote C, Casillas R, Ramírez-Santana C, et al. Premature delivery influences the immunological composition of colostrum and transitional and mature human milk. *J Nutr.* 2011;141(6):1181–1187. doi: 10.3945/jn.110.133652.

Cattaneo A, Davanzo R, Worku B, et al. Kangaroo mother care for low birthweight infants: a randomized controlled trial in different settings. *Acta Paediatr.* 1998;87(9):976–985.

Chan GM, Borschel MW, Jacobs JR. Effects of human milk or formula feeding on the growth, behavior, and protein status of preterm infants discharged from the newborn intensive care unit. *Am J Clin Nutr.* 1994;60(5):710–716.

Chan GM, Lee ML, Rechtman DJ. Effects of a human milk-derived human milk fortifier on the antibacterial actions of human milk. *Breastfeed Med.* 2007;2(4):205–208.

Charpak N, Ruiz J. Breast milk composition in a cohort of pre-term infants' mothers followed in an ambulatory programme in Colombia. *Acta Paediatr.* 2007;96(12):1755–1759.

Charpak N, Ruiz JG, Zupan J, et al. Kangaroo mother care: 25 years after. *Acta Paediatr.* 2005;94(5):514–522.

Charpak N, Ruiz-Pelaez JG, Charpak Y. Rey-Martinez Kangaroo Mother Program: an alternative way of caring for low birth weight infants? One year mortality in a two cohort study. *Pediatrics.* 1994; 94(6 Pt 1):804–810.

Charpak N, Ruiz-Pelaez JG, Figueroa de C Z, Charpak Y. A randomized, controlled trial of kangaroo mother care: results of follow-up at 1 year of corrected age. *Pediatrics.* 2001;108(5):1072–1079.

Chatterton RT Jr, Hill PD, Aldag JC, et al. Relation of plasma oxytocin and prolactin concentrations to milk production in mothers of preterm infants: influence of stress. *J Clin Endocrinol Metab.* 2000;85(10):3661–3668.

Chen CH, Wang TM, Chang HM, Chi CS. The effect of breast- and bottle-feeding on oxygen saturation and body temperature in preterm infants. *J Hum Lact.* 2000;16(1):21–27.

Clum D, Primomo J. Use of a silicone nipple shield with premature infants. *J Hum Lact.* 1996;12(4):287–290.

Contreras-Lemus J, Flores-Huerta S, Cisneros-Silva I, et al. Morbidity reduction in preterm newborns fed with milk of their own mothers. *Bol Med Hosp Infant Mex.* 1992;49(10):671–677.

Corvaglia L, Aceti A, Paoletti V, et al. Standard fortification of preterm human milk fails to meet recommended protein intake: bedside evaluation by near-infrared-reflectance-analysis. *Early Hum Dev.* 2010;86(4):237–240. doi: 10.1016/j.earlhumdev.2010.04.001.

Cregan MD, De Mello TR, Kershaw D, et al. Initiation of lactation in women after preterm delivery. *Acta Obstet Gynecol Scand.* 2002;81(9):870–877.

Cricco-Lizza R. Formative infant feeding experiences and education of NICU nurses. *Am J Matern Child Nurs.* 2009;34(4):236–242.

Cronenwett L, Stukel T, Kearney M, et al. Single daily bottle use in the early weeks postpartum and breast-feeding outcomes. *Pediatrics.* 1992;90(5):760–766.

Curtis N, Chau L, Garland S, et al. Cytomegalovirus remains viable in naturally infected breast milk despite being frozen for 10 days. *Arch Dis Child Fetal Neonatal Ed.* 2005;90(6):F529–F530.

Daly SE, Di Rosso A, Owens RA, Hartmann PE. Degree of breast emptying explains changes in the fat content, but not fatty acid composition, of human milk. *Exp Physiol.* 1993;78(6):741–755.

Daly SE, Hartmann PE. Infant demand and milk supply. Part 1: infant demand and milk production in lactating women. *J Hum Lact.* 1995a;11(1):21–26.

Daly SE, Hartmann PE. Infant demand and milk supply. Part 2: the short-term control of milk synthesis in lactating women. *J Hum Lact.* 1995b;11(1):27–37.

Daly SE, Kent JC, Owens RA, Hartmann PE. Frequency and degree of milk removal and the short-term control of human milk synthesis. *Exp Physiol.* 1996;81(5):861–875.

deMonterice D, Meier PP, Engstrom JL, et al. Concurrent validity of a new instrument for measuring nutritive sucking in preterm infants. *Nurs Res.* 1992;41(6):342–346.

De Nisi G, Berti M, Malossi R, et al. Comparison of neonatal intensive care: Trento area versus Vermont Oxford Network. *Ital J Pediatr.* 2009;35(1):5. doi: 10.1186/1824-7288-35-5.

Diaz-Gomez NM, Domenech E, Barroso F. Breast-feeding and growth factors in preterm newborn infants. *J Pediatr Gastroenterol Nutr.* 1997;24(3):322–327.

Doctor S, Friedman S, Dunn MS, et al. Cytomegalovirus transmission to extremely low-birthweight infants through breast milk. *Acta Paediatr.* 2005;94(1):53–58.

Dodd V. Implications of kangaroo care for growth and development in preterm infants. *J Obstet Gynecol Neonatal Nurs.* 2005;34(2):218–232.

Dowling DA. Physiological responses of preterm infants to breast-feeding and bottle-feeding with the orthodontic nipple. *Nurs Res.* 1999;48(2):78–85.

Dowling DA, Meier PP, DiFiore JM, Blatz M, Martin RJ. Cup-feeding for preterm infants: mechanics and safety. *J Hum Lact.* 2002 Feb;18(1):13-20.

Dubignon J, Campbell D. Sucking in the newborn during a feed. *J Exp Child Psychol.* 1969;7(2):282–298.

Dvorak B, Fituch CC, Williams CS, et al. Increased epidermal growth factor levels in human milk of mothers with extremely premature infants. *Pediatr Res.* 2003;54(1):15–19.

Edwards TE, Spatz, DL. An innovative model for achieving breastfeeding success in infants with complex surgical anomalies. *J Perinat Neonatal Nurs.* 2010;24(3):254–255. doi: 10.1097/JPN.0b013e3181e8d517.

Eibl MM, Wolf HM, Fürnkranz H, Rosenkranz A. Prevention of necrotizing enterocolitis in low-birth-weight infants by IgA-IgG feeding. *N Engl J Med.* 1988;319(1):1–7.

Elmlinger MW, Hochhaus F, Loui A, et al. Insulin-like growth factors and binding proteins in early milk from mothers of preterm and term infants. *Horm Res.* 2007;68(3):124–131.

el-Mohandes AE, Schatz V, Keiser JF, Jackson BJ. Bacterial contaminants of collected and frozen human milk used in an intensive care nursery. *Am J Infect Control.* 1993;21(5):226–230.

Emery MM. Galactogogues: drugs to induce lactation. *J Hum Lact.* 1996;12:55–57.

Erickson T, Gill G, Chan GM. The effects of acidification on human milk's cellular and nutritional content. *J Perinatol.* 2013;33:371–373.

Ewer AK, Yu VY. Gastric emptying in pre-term infants: the effect of breast milk fortifier. *Acta Paediatr.* 1996;85(9):1112–1115.

Farquharson J, Jamieson EC, Abbasi KA, et al. Effect of diet on the fatty acid composition of the major phospholipids of infant cerebral cortex. *Arch Dis Child.* 1995;72(3):198–203.

Feher SD, Berger LR, Johnson JD, Wilde JB. Increasing breast milk production for premature infants with a relaxation/imagery audiotape. *Pediatrics.* 1989;83(1):57–60.

Feldman R, Eidelman AI. Skin-to-skin contact (kangaroo care) accelerates autonomic and neurobehavioural maturation in preterm infants. *Dev Med Child Neurol.* 2003;45(4):274–281.

Feldman R, Eidelman AI, Sirota L, Weller A. Comparison of skin-to-skin (kangaroo) and traditional care: parenting outcomes and preterm infant development. *Pediatrics.* 2002;110(1 Pt 1):16–26.

Fewtrell MS, Loh KL, Blake A, et al. Randomised, double blind trial of oxytocin nasal spray in mothers expressing breast milk for preterm infants. *Arch Dis Child Fetal Neonatal Ed.* 2006;91(3):F169–F174.

Fewtrell M, Lucas P, Collier S, Lucas A. Randomized study comparing the efficacy of a novel manual breast pump with a mini-electric breast pump in mothers of term infants. *J Hum Lact.* 2001;17(2):126–131.

Fituch CC, Palkowetz KH, Hurst NM, et al. Interlukin-10 concentration in milk of mothers delivering extremely low birth weight infants. *Pediatr Res.* 2001;49(4):398A.

Flacking R, Ewald U, Starrin B. "I wanted to do a good job": experiences of "becoming a mother" and breastfeeding in mothers of very preterm infants after discharge from a neonatal unit. *Soc Sci Med.* 2007;64:2405–2416.

Flacking R, Ewald U, Wallin L. Positive effect on kangaroo mother care on long-term breastfeeding in very preterm infants. *J Obstet Gynecol Neonatal Nurs.* 2011;40(2):190–197. doi: 10.1111/j.1552-6909.2011.01226.x.

Flacking R, Nyqvist KH, Ewald U, Wallin L. Long-term duration of breastfeeding in Swedish low birth weight infants. *J Hum Lact.* 2003;19(2):157–165.

Fucile S, Gisel EG, Lau C. Effect of an oral stimulation program on sucking skill maturation of preterm infants. *Dev Med Child Neurol.* 2005;47(3):158–162.

Furman L, Minich N. Efficiency of breastfeeding as compared to bottle-feeding in very low birth weight (VLBW, <1.5 kg) infants. *J Perinatol.* 2004;24(11):706–713.

Furman L, Minich NM, Hack M. Breastfeeding of very low birth weight infants. *J Hum Lact.* 1998;14(1):29–34.

Furman L, Taylor G, Minich N, Hack M. The effect of maternal milk on neonatal morbidity of very low-birth-weight infants. *Arch Pediatr Adolesc Med.* 2003;157(1):66–71.

Gale G, Franck L, Lund C. Skin-to-skin (kangaroo) holding of the intubated premature infant. *Neonatal Netw.* 1993;12(6):49–57.

Ganapathy V1, Hay JW, Kim JH. Costs of necrotizing enterocolitis and cost-effectiveness of exclusively human milk-based products in feeding extremely premature infants. *Breastfeed Med.* 2012;7(1):29–37. doi: 10.1089/bfm.2011.0002.

Garofalo RP, Goldman AS. Cytokines, chemokines, and colony-stimulating factors in human milk: the 1997 update. *Biol Neonate.* 1998;74(2):134–142.

Gastelum DT, Dassey D, Mascola L, et al. Transmission of community-associated methicillin-resistant *Staphylococcus aureus* from breast milk in the neonatal intensive care unit. *Pediatr Infect Dis J.* 2005;24(12):1122–1124.

Gazzolo D, Masetti P, Meli M. Kangaroo care improves post-extubation cardiorespiratory parameters in infants after open heart surgery. *Acta Paediatr.* 2000;89(6):728–729.

Genzel-Boroviczeny O, Wahle J, Koletzko B. Fatty acid composition of human milk during the 1st month after term and preterm delivery. *Eur J Pediatr.* 1997;156(2):142–147.

Gephart SM, Weller M. Colostrum as oral immune therapy. *Adv Neonatal Care.* 2014;14(1):44–51.

Gewolb IH, Bosma JF, Taciak VL, Vice FL. Abnormal developmental patterns of suck and swallow rhythms during feeding in preterm infants with bronchopulmonary dysplasia. *Dev Med Child Neurol.* 2001;43(7):454–459.

Goldblum RM, Garza C, Johnson CA, et al. Human milk banking I: effects of container upon immunologic factors in mature milk. *Nutr Res.* 1981;1:449–459.

Goldblum RM, Schanler RJ, Garza C, Goldman AS. Human milk feeding enhances the urinary excretion of immunologic factors in low birth weight infants. *Pediatr Res.* 1989;25(2):184–188.

Greer FR, McCormick A, Loker J. Changes in fat concentration of human milk during delivery by intermittent bolus and continuous mechanical pump infusion. *J Pediatr.* 1984;105(5):745–749.

Griffin TL, Meier PP, Bradford LP, et al. Mothers' performing creamatocrit measures in the NICU: accuracy, reactions, and cost. *J Obstet Gynecol Neonatal Nurs.* 2000; 29(3):249–257.

Groh-Wargo S, Toth A, Mahoney K, et al. The utility of a bilateral breast pumping system for mothers of premature infants. *Neonatal Netw.* 1995;14(8):31–36.

Gross SJ, David RJ, Bauman L, Tomarelli RM. Nutritional composition of milk produced by mothers delivering preterm. *J Pediatr.* 1980;96(4):641–644.

Hafström M, Kjellmer I. Non-nutritive sucking by infants exposed to pethidine in utero. *Acta Paediatr.* 2000; 89(10):1196–1200.

Hale TW. *Medications and mother's milk.* Amarillo, TX: Pharmasoft; 2012.

Hall RT, Wheeler RE, Rippetoe LE. Calcium and phosphorus supplementation after initial hospital discharge in breast-fed infants of less than 1800 grams birth weight. *J Perinatol.* 1993;13(4):272–278.

Hallowell SG, Spatz DL, Hanlon AL, et al. Characteristics of the NICU work environment associated with breast-feeding support. *Adv Neonatal Care.* 2014;14(4): 290-300. doi: 10.1097/ANC.0000000000000102.

Hake-Brooks SJ, Anderson GC. Kangaroo care and breastfeeding of mother–preterm infant dyads 0–18 months: a randomized, controlled trial. *Neonatal Netw.* 2008; 27(3):151–159.

Hamosh M. Bioactive factors in human milk. *Pediatr Clin North Am.* 2001;48(1):69–86.

Hamosh M, Ellis LA, Pollock DR, et al. Breastfeeding and the working mother: effect of time and temperature of short-term storage on proteolysis, lipolysis, and bacterial growth in milk. *Pediatrics.* 1996;97(4):492–498.

Hamprecht K, Maschmann J, Müller D, et al. Cytomegalovirus (CMV) inactivation in breast milk: reassessment of pasteurization and freeze-thawing. *Pediatr Res.* 2004; 56(4):529–535.

Hamprecht K, Maschmann J, Vochem M, et al. Epidemiology of transmission of cytomegalovirus from mother to preterm infant by breastfeeding. *Lancet.* 2001;357(9255): 513–518.

Hanson LA. Human milk and host defense: immediate and long-term effects. *Acta Paediatr Suppl.* 1999;88(430): 42–46.

Hartmann P, Cregan M. Lactogenesis and the effects of insulin-dependent diabetes mellitus and prematurity. *J Nutr.* 2001;131(11):3016S–3020S.

Hassiotou F, Geddes DT, Hartmann PE. Cells in human milk: state of the science. *J Hum Lact.* 2013;29(2):171–182. doi: 10.1177/0890334413477242.

Hedberg Nyqvist K, Ewald U. Infant and maternal factors in the development of breastfeeding behaviour and breastfeeding outcome in preterm infants. *Acta Paediatr.* 1999;88(11):1194–1203.

Heird WC. The role of polyunsaturated fatty acids in term and preterm infants and breastfeeding mothers. *Pediatr Clin North Am.* 2001;48(1):173–188.

Henderson TR, Hamosh M, Armand M, et al. Gastric proteolysis in preterm infants fed mother's milk or formula. *Adv Exp Med Biol.* 2001;501:403–408.

Hildebrandt R, Gundert-Remy U. Lack of pharmacological active saliva levels of caffeine in breast-fed infants. *Pediatr Pharmacol (NY).* 1983;3(3-4):237–244.

Hill PD, Aldag JC, Chatterton RT. Effects of pumping style on milk production in mothers of non-nursing preterm infants. *J Hum Lact.* 1999;15(3):209–216.

Hill PD, Aldag JC, Chatterton RT. Initiation and frequency of pumping and milk production in mothers of non-nursing preterm infants. *J Hum Lact.* 2001 Feb;17(1):9-13.

Hill PD, Aldag JC, Zinaman M, Chatterton RT. Predictors of preterm infant feeding methods and perceived insufficient milk supply at week 12 postpartum. *J Hum Lact.* 2007;23(1):32–38, 39–43.

Hill PD, Andersen JL, Ledbetter RJ. Delayed initiation of breast-feeding the preterm infant. *J Perinat Neonatal Nurs.* 1995;9(2):10–20.

Hill PD, Ledbetter RJ, Kavanaugh KL. Breastfeeding patterns of low-birth-weight infants after hospital discharge. *J Obstet Gynecol Neonatal Nurs.* 1997;26(2):189–197.

Hopkinson JM, Schanler RJ, Garza C. Milk production by mothers of premature infants. *Pediatrics.* 1988;81(6):815–820.

Hurst N, Engebretson J, Mahoney JS. Providing mother's own milk in the context of the NICU: a paradoxical experience. *J Hum Lact.* 2013;29(3):366–373. doi: 10.1177/0890334413485640.

Hurst NM, Meier PP, Engstrom JL, Myatt A. Mothers performing in-home measurement of milk intake during breastfeeding of their preterm infants: maternal reactions and feeding outcomes. *J Hum Lact.* 2004;20(2):178–187.

Hurst NM, Myatt A, Schanler RJ. Growth and development of a hospital-based lactation program and mother's own milk bank. *J Obstet Gynecol Neonatal Nurs.* 1998;27(5):503–510.

Hurst NM, Valentine CJ, Renfro L, et al. Skin-to-skin holding in the neonatal intensive care unit influences maternal milk volume. *J Perinatol.* 1997;17(3):213–217.

Hutchens TW, Henry JF, Yip TT, et al. Origin of intact lactoferrin and its DNA-binding fragments found in the urine of human milk-fed preterm infants: evaluation by stable isotopic enrichment. *Pediatr Res.* 1991;29(3):243–250.

Hylander MA, Strobino DM, Dhanireddy R. Human milk feedings and infection among very low birth weight infants. *Pediatrics.* 1998;102(3):E38.

Hylander MA, Strobino DM, Pezzullo JC, Dhanireddy R. Association of human milk feedings with a reduction in retinopathy of prematurity among very low birth-weight infants. *J Perinatol.* 2001;21(6):356–362.

Jackson K, Ternestedt BM, Schollin J. From alienation to familiarity: experiences of parents of preterm infants during the first 18 months of life. *J Adv Nurs.* 2003;43(2):120–129.

Jaeger MC, Lawson M, Filteau S. The impact of prematurity and neonatal illness on the decision to breast-feed. *J Adv Nurs.* 1997;25(4):729–737.

Jeiger, Meier, Engstrom, McBride. The initial maternal cost of providing 100 mL of human milk for very low birth weight infants in the neonatal intensive care unit. *Breastfeed Med.* 2010;5(2):71–77. doi: 10.1089/bfm.2009.0063.

Jennings T, Meier W, Meier P. High lipid and caloric content in milk from mothers of preterm infants. *Pediatr Res.* 1997;41:233A.

Jensen RG. *The lipids of human milk.* Boca Raton, FL: CRC Press; 1989.

Jenson D, Wallace S, Kelsay P. LATCH: a breastfeeding charting system and documentation tool. *J Gynecol Obstet Neonatal Nurs.* 1994;23:27–32.

Jim WT, Shu CH, Chiu NC, et al. Transmission of cytomegalovirus from mothers to preterm infants by breast milk. *Pediatr Infect Dis J.* 2004;23(9):848–851.

Jocson MA, Mason EO, Schanler RJ. The effects of nutrient fortification and varying storage conditions on host defense properties of human milk. *Pediatrics.* 1997;100(2 Pt 1):240–243.

Jones E. Strategies to promote preterm breastfeeding. *Mod Midwife.* 1995;5(3):8–11.

Jones E, Spencer SA. Optimising the provision of human milk for preterm infants. *Arch Dis Child Fetal Neonatal Ed.* 2007;92(4):F236–F238.

Jones F. *Best practice for expressing, storing and handling human milk in hospitals, homes, and child care settings,* 3rd ed. Fort Worth, TX: Human Milk Banking Association of North America; 2011.

Jorgensen MH, Hernell O, Lund P, et al. Visual acuity and erythrocyte docosahexaenoic acid status in breast-fed and formula-fed term infants during the first four months of life. *Lipids.* 1996;31(1):99–105.

Kavanaugh K, Mead L, Meier P, Mangurten HH. Getting enough: mothers' concerns about breastfeeding a preterm infant after discharge. *J Obstet Gynecol Neonatal Nurs.* 1995;24(1):23–32.

Kavanaugh K, Meier PP, Engstrom JL. Reliability of weighing procedures for preterm infants. *Nurs Res.* 1989;38(3):178–179.

Kavanaugh K, Meier P, Zimmermann B, Mead L. The rewards outweigh the efforts: breastfeeding outcomes for mothers of preterm infants. *J Hum Lact.* 1997;13(1):15–21.

Kent J, Mitoulas L, Cox D, et al. Breast volume and milk production during extended lactation in women. *Exp Phys.* 1999;84:435–447.

Killersreiter B, Grimmer I, Buhrer C, et al. Early cessation of breast milk feeding in very low birthweight infants. *Early Hum Dev.* 2001;60(3):193–205.

Kirsten GF, Bergman NJ, Hann FM. Kangaroo mother care in the nursery. *Pediatr Clin North Am.* 2001;48(2):443–452.

Koletzko B, Agostoni C, Carlson SE, et al. Long chain polyunsaturated fatty acids (LC-PUFA) and perinatal development. *Acta Paediatr.* 2001;90:460–464.

Korchazhkina O, Jones E, Czauderna M, Spencer SA. Effects of exclusive formula or breast milk feeding on oxidative stress in healthy preterm infants. *Arch Dis Child.* 2006;91(4):327–329.

Korja R, Maunu J, Kirjavainen J, et al. Mother–infant interaction is influenced by the amount of holding in preterm infants. *Early Hum Dev.* 2008;84(4):257–267.

Kosloske AM. Breastmilk decreases the risk of neonatal necrotizing enterocolitis. *Adv Nutr Res.* 2001;10:123–137.

Kotiw M, Zhang GW, Daggard G, et al. Late-onset and recurrent neonatal Group B streptococcal disease associated with breast-milk transmission. *Pediatr Dev Pathol.* 2003;6(3):251–256.

Kreissl A, Zwiauer V, Repa A, et al. Effect of fortifiers and additional protein on the osmolarity of human milk: is it still safe for the premature infant? *J Pediatr Gastroenterol Nutr.* 2013;57(4):432–437. doi: 10.1097/MPG.0b013e3182a208c7.

Krouse AM. The family management of breastfeeding low birth weight infants. *J Hum Lact.* 2002;18(2):155–165.

Kunz C, Rudloff S. Biological functions of oligosaccharides in human milk. *Acta Paediatr.* 1993;82:903–912.

Kuschel C, Harding J. Multicomponent fortification of human milk for promoting growth in premature infants. *Cochrane Database Syst Rev.* 1998(revised 2003);3;CD000343. doi: 10.1002/14651858.CD000343.pub2.

Lang S, Lawrence CJ, Orme RL. Cup feeding: an alternative method of infant feeding. *Arch Dis Child.* 1994;71(4):365–369.

Lau C, Alagugurusamy R, Schanler RJ, et al. Characterization of the developmental stages of sucking in preterm infants during bottle feeding. *Acta Paediatr.* 2000;89(7):846–852.

Lau C, Hurst N. Oral feeding in infants. *Curr Probl Pediatr.* 1999;29(4):105–124.

Lau C, Hurst NM, Smith EO, Schanler RJ. Ethnic/racial diversity, maternal stress, lactation and very low birth-weight infants. *J Perinatol.* 2007;27(7):399–408.

Lau C, Sheena HR, Shulman RJ, Schanler RJ. Oral feeding in low birth weight infants. *J Pediatr.* 1997;130(4):561–569.

Lau C, Smith EO, Schanler RJ. Coordination of suck-swallow and swallow respiration in preterm infants. *Acta Paediatr.* Jun 2003;92(6):721–727.

Lauritzen L, Jørgensen MH, Olsen SF, et al. Maternal fish oil supplementation in lactation: effect on developmental outcome in breast-fed infants. *Reprod Nutr Dev.* 2005;45(5):535–547.

Lawrence RA. Breastfeeding support benefits very-low-birthweight infants. *Arch Pediatr Adolesc Med.* 2001;155(5):543–544.

Ledo A, Arduini A, Asensi MA, et al. Human milk enhances antioxidant defenses against hydroxyl radical aggression in preterm infants. *Am J Clin Nutr.* 2009;89(1):210–215. doi: 10.3945/ajcn.2008.26845.

Legault M, Goulet C. Comparison of kangaroo and traditional methods of removing preterm infants from incubators. *J Obstet Gynecol Neonatal Nurs.* 1995;24(6):501–506.

Lemons JA, Moye L, Hall D, Simmons M. Differences in the composition of preterm and term human milk during early lactation. *Pediatr Res.* 1982;16(2):113–117.

Levy I, Comarsca J, Davidovits M, et al. Urinary tract infection in preterm infants: the protective role of breastfeeding. *Pediatr Nephrol.* 2009;24(3):527–531. doi: 10.1007/s00467-008-1007-7. Epub October 21, 2008.

Libster R, Bugna Hortoneda J, Laham FR, et al. Breastfeeding prevents severe disease in full term female infants with acute respiratory infection. *Pediatr Infect Dis J.* 2009 Feb;28(2):131–4. doi: 10.1097/INF.0b013e31818a8a82.

Lucas A, Cole TJ. Breast milk and neonatal necrotising enterocolitis. *Lancet.* 1990;336(8730):1519–1523.

Lucas A, Gibbs JA, Lyster RL, Baum JD. Creamatocrit: simple clinical technique for estimating fat concentration and energy value of human milk. *Br Med J.* 1978;1(6119):1018–1020.

Lucas A, Morley R, Cole TJ. Randomised trial of early diet in preterm babies and later intelligence quotient. *BMJ.* 1998;317(7171):1481–1487.

Lucas A, Morley R, Cole TJ, Gore SM. A randomised multi-centre study of human milk versus formula and later development in preterm infants. *Arch Dis Child Fetal Neonatal Ed.* 1994;70(2):F141–F146.

Ludington-Hoe SM, Hosseini R, Torowicz DL. Skin-to-skin contact (kangaroo care) analgesia for preterm infant heel stick. *AACN Clin Issues.* 2005;16(3):373–387.

Ludington-Hoe SM, Johnson MW, Morgan K, et al. Neurophysiologic assessment of neonatal sleep organization: preliminary results of a randomized, controlled trial of skin contact with preterm infants. *Pediatrics.* 2006;117(5):e909–e923.

Ludington-Hoe SM, Thompson C, Swinth J, et al. Kangaroo care: research results, and practice implications and guidelines. *Neonatal Netw.* 1994;13(1):19–27.

Lugonja N, Spasić SD, Laugier O, et al. Differences in direct pharmacologic effects and antioxidative properties of mature breast milk and infant formulas. *Nutrition.* 2013;29(2):431–435. doi: 10.1016/j.nut.2012.07.018.

Luukkainen P, Salo MK, Janas M, Nikkari T, et al. Fatty acid composition of plasma and red blood cell phospholipids in preterm infants from 2 weeks to 6 months postpartum. *J Pediatr Gastroenterol Nutr.* 1995;20(3):310–315.

Luukkainen P, Salo MK, Nikkari T. Changes in the fatty acid composition of preterm and term human milk from 1 week to 6 months of lactation. *J Pediatr Gastroenterol Nutr.* 1994;18(3):355–360.

Maas YG, Gerritsen J, Hart AA, et al. Development of macronutrient composition of very preterm human milk. *Br J Nutr.* 1998;80(1):35–40.

Maastrup R. Factors associated with exclusive breastfeeding of preterm infants: results from a prospective national cohort study. *PLoS One.* 2014;9(2):e89077. doi: 10.1371/journal.pone.0089077.

Marchbank T, Weaver G, Nilsen-Hamilton M, Playford RJ. Pancreatic secretory trypsin inhibitor is a major motogenic and protective factor in human breast milk. *Am J Physiol Gastrointest Liver Physiol.* 2009;296(4):G697–G703. doi: 10.1152/ajpgi.90565.2008. Epub January 15, 2009. PubMed PMID: 19147803.

Martell M, Martínez G, González M, Díaz Rosselló JL. Suction patterns in preterm infants. *J Perinat Med.* 1993;21(5):363–369.

McGrath JM, Braescu AV. State of the science: feeding readiness in the preterm infant. *J Perinat Neonatal Nurs.* 2004;18(4):353–368, 369–370.

Medoff-Cooper B. Multi-system approach to the assessment of successful feeding. *Acta Paediatr.* 2000;89(4): 393–394.

Meerlo-Habing ZE, Kosters-Boes EA, Klip H, Brand PL. Early discharge with tube feeding at home for preterm infants is associated with longer duration of breast feeding. *Arch Dis Child Fetal Neonatal Ed.* 2009 Jul;94(4):F294-7. doi: 10.1136/adc.2008.146100.

Mehta R, Petrova A. Very preterm gestation and breastmilk cytokine content during the first month of lactation. *Breastfeed Med.* 2011;6(1):21–24. doi: 10.1089/bfm.2010.0024.

Meier PP. Bottle and breast-feeding: effects on transcutaneous oxygen pressure and temperature in preterm infants. *Nurs Res.* 1988;37(1):36–41.

Meier PP. Caution needed in extrapolating from term to preterm infants: author's reply. *J Hum Lact.* 1995; 11:91.

Meier PP. Breastfeeding in the special care nursery: prematures and infants with medical problems. *Pediatr Clin North Am.* 2001;48(2):425–442.

Meier PP, Anderson GC. Responses of small preterm infants to bottle- and breast-feeding. *Am J Matern Child Nurs.* 1987;12(2):97–105.

Meier PP, Brown LP. State of the science: breastfeeding for mothers and low birth weight infants. *Nurs Clin North Am.* 1996;31(2):351–365.

Meier PP, Brown LP. Defining terminology for improved breastfeeding research. *J Nurse Midwifery.* 1997;42(1): 65–66.

Meier PP, Brown LP, Hurst NM, et al. Nipple shields for preterm infants: effect on milk transfer and duration of breastfeeding. *J Hum Lact.* 2000;16(2):106–114, 129–131.

Meier PP, Engstrom JL, Crichton CL, et al. A new scale for in-home test-weighing for mothers of preterm and high risk infants. *J Hum Lact.* 1994;10(3):163–168.

Meier PP, Engstrom JL, Fleming BA, et al. Estimating milk intake of hospitalized preterm infants who breastfeed. *J Hum Lact.* 1996;12(1):21–26.

Meier PP, Engstrom JL, Janes JE, et al. Breast pump suction patterns that mimic the human infant during breastfeeding: greater milk output in less time spent pumping for breast pump-dependent mothers with premature infants. *J Perinatol.* 2012;32(2):103–110. doi: 10.1038/jp.2011.64.

Meier PP, Engstrom JL, Mangurten HH, et al. Breastfeeding support services in the neonatal intensive-care unit. *J Obstet Gynecol Neonatal Nurs.* 1993;22(4): 338–347.

Meier PP, Engstrom JL, Mingolelli SS, et al. The Rush Mothers' Milk Club: breastfeeding interventions for mothers with very-low-birth-weight infants. *J Obstet Gynecol Neonatal Nurs.* 2004;33(2):164–174.

Meier PP, Engstrom JL, Rossman B. Breastfeeding peer counselors as direct lactation care providers in the neonatal intensive care unit. *J Hum Lact.* 2013;29(3):313–322. doi: 10.1177/0890334413482184.

Meier PP, Lysakowski TY, Engstrom JL, et al. The accuracy of test weighing for preterm infants. *J Pediatr Gastroenterol Nutr.* 1990;10(1):62–65.

Merewood A, Chamberlain LB, Cook JT, et al. The effect of peer counselors on breastfeeding rates in the neonatal intensive care unit: results of a randomized controlled trial. *Arch Pediatr Adolesc Med.* 2006;160(7):681–685.

Miller JB, Bull S, Miller J, McVeagh P. The oligosaccharide composition of human milk: temporal and individual variations in monosaccharide components. *J Pediatr Gastroenterol Nutr.* 1994;19(4):371–376.

Milsom SR, Rabone DL, Gunn AJ, Gluckman PD. Potential role for growth hormone in human lactation insufficiency. *Horm Res.* 1998;50(3):147–150.

Miracle DJ, Meier PP, Bennett PA. Mothers' decisions to change from formula to mothers' milk for very-low-birth-weight infants. *J Obstet Gynecol Neonatal Nurs.* 2004;33(6):692–703.

Miron D, Brosilow S, Felszer K, et al. Incidence and clinical manifestations of breast milk-acquired cytomegalovirus infection in low birth weight infants. *J Perinatol.* 2005;25(5):299–303.

Moltó-Puigmartí C, Castellote AI, López-Sabater MC. Additional data from our study on fatty acids variations during lactation: correlations between n-3 and n-6 PUFAs in human colostrum, transitional, and mature milk. *Clin Nutr.* 2011;30(3):402–403. doi: 10.1016/j.clnu.2011.03.006.

Montgomery D, Schmutz N, Baer VL, et al. Effects of instituting the "BEST Program" (Breast Milk Early Saves Trouble) in a level III NICU. *J Hum Lact.* 2008;24(3): 248–251. doi: 10.1177/0890334408316080.

Moody GJ, Schanler RJ, Lau C, Shulman RJ. Feeding tolerance in premature infants fed fortified human milk. *J Pediatr Gastroenterol Nutr.* 2000;30:408–412.

Moro G, Fulconis F, Minoli I, et al. Growth and plasma amino acid concentrations in very low birthweight infants fed either human milk protein fortified human milk or a whey-predominant formula. *Acta Paediatr Scand.* 1989;78(1):18–22.

Mulford C. The mother–baby assessment (MBA): an "Apgar score" for breastfeeding. *J Hum Lact.* 1992;8:79–82.

Mussi-Pinhata MM, Yamamoto AY, do Carmo Rego MA, et al. Perinatal or early-postnatal cytomegalovirus infection in preterm infants under 34 weeks gestation born to CMV-seropositive mothers within a high-seroprevalence population. *J Pediatr.* 2004;145(5):685–688.

Narayanan I, Mehta R, Choudhury DK, Jain BK. Sucking on the "emptied" breast: non-nutritive sucking with a difference. *Arch Dis Child.* 1991;66(2):241–244.

National Breastfeeding Center. Healthcare insurers graded on support for breastfeeding moms: Anthem and Aetna score highly! April 2, 2014. http://www.nbfcenter.com /PayerScorecard.html.

Neifert M, Lawrence R, Seacat J. Nipple confusion: toward a formal definition. *J Pediatr.* 1995;126(6):S125–S129.

Newburg DS, Ruiz-Palacios GM, Morrow AL. Human milk glycans protect infants against enteric pathogens. *Annu Rev Nutr.* 2005;25:37–58.

Newburg DS, Walker WA. Protection of the neonate by the innate immune system of developing gut and of human milk. *Pediatr Res.* 2007;61(1):2–8.

Newman TB, Xiong B, Gonzales VM, Escobar GJ. Prediction and prevention of extreme neonatal hyperbilirubinemia in a mature health maintenance organization. *Arch Pediatr Adolesc Med.* 2000;154(11):1140–1147.

Nicholl RM, Gamsu HR. Changes in growth and metabolism in very low birthweight infants fed with fortified breast milk. *Acta Paediatr.* 1999;88(10):1056–1061.

Novak FR, Da Silva AV, Hagler AN, Figueiredo AM. Contamination of expressed human breast milk with an epidemic multiresistant *Staphylococcus aureus* clone. *J Med Microbiol.* 2000;49(12):1109–1117.

Nowak AJ, Smith WL, Erenberg A. Imaging evaluation of artificial nipples during bottle feeding. *Arch Pediatr Adolesc Med.* 1994;148(1):40–42.

Nowak AJ, Smith WL, Erenberg A. Imaging evaluation of breast-feeding and bottle-feeding systems. *J Pediatr.* 1995;126(6):S130–134.

Nyqvist KH, Ewald U, Sjödén PO. Supporting a preterm infant's behaviour during breastfeeding: a case report. *J Hum Lact.* 1996;12(3):221–228.

Nyqvist KH, Färnstrand C, Eeg-Olofsson KE, Ewald U. Early oral behaviour in preterm infants during breastfeeding: an electromyographic study. *Acta Paediatr.* 2001;90(6):658–663.

Nyqvist KH, Häggkvist AP, Hansen MN, et al. Expansion of the Baby-Friendly Hospital Initiative Ten Steps to Successful Breastfeeding into neonatal intensive care: expert group recommendations. *J Hum Lact.* 2013; 29(3):300–309. doi: 10.1177/0890334413489775.

Nyqvist KH, Rubertsson C, Ewald U, Sjödén PO. Development of the Preterm Infant Breastfeeding Behavior Scale (PIBBS): a study of nurse–mother agreement. *J Hum Lact.* 1996;12(3):207–219.

Nyqvist KH, Sjödén PO, Ewald U. The development of preterm infants' breastfeeding behavior. *Early Hum Dev.* 1999;55(3):247–264.

Ogechi AA, William O, Fidelia BT. Hindmilk and weight gain in preterm very low-birthweight infants. *Pediatr Int.* 2007;49(2):156–160.

Olver WJ, Bond DW, Boswell TC, et al. Neonatal Group B streptococcal disease associated with infected breast milk. *Arch Dis Child Fetal Neonatal Ed.* 2000;83(1): F48–F49.

Omarsdottir S, Casper C, Zweygberg Wirgart B. Transmission of cytomegalovirus to extremely preterm infants through breast milk. *Acta Paediatr.* 2007;96(4): 492–494.

O'Neill EF, Radmacher PG, Sparks B, Adamkin DH. Creamatocrit analysis of human milk overestimates fat and energy content when compared to a human milk analyzer using mid-infrared spectroscopy. *J Pediatr Gastroenterol Nutr.* 2013;56(5):569–572. doi: 10.1097/ MPG.0b013e31828390e4.

Ortenstrand A, Winbladh B, Nordström G, Waldenström U. Early discharge of preterm infants followed by domiciliary nursing care: parents' anxiety, assessment of infant health and breastfeeding. *Acta Paediatr.* 2001;90(10):1190–1195.

Paramasivam K, Michie C, Opara E, Jewell AP. Human breast milk immunology: a review. *Int J Fertil Women's Med.* 2006;51(5):208–217.

Parker, Sullivan S, Krueger C, et al. Effect of early breast milk expression on milk volume and timing of lactogenesis stage II among mothers for very low birthweight infants: a pilot study. *J Perinatal.* 2012;32:205–209.

Patel AL, Johnson TJ, Engstrom JL, et al. Impact of early human milk on sepsis and health-care costs in very low birth weight infants. *J Perinatol.* 2013;33(7):514–519. doi: 10.1038/jp.2013.2. Epub January 31, 2013.

Peterson JA, Hamosh M, Scallan CD. Milk fat globule glycoproteins in human milk and in gastric aspirates of mother's milk-fed preterm infants. *Pediatr Res.* 1998; 44(4):499–506.

Pietschnig B, Siklossy H, Gottling A, et al. Breastfeeding rates of VLBW infants: influence of professional breastfeeding support. *Adv Exp Med Biol.* 2000;478: 429–430.

Pineda RG, Foss J, Richards L, Pane CA. Breastfeeding changes for VLBW infants in the NICU following staff education. *Neonatal Netw.* 2009;28(5):311–319.

Pinelli J, Atkinson SA, Saigal S. Randomized trial of breastfeeding support in very low-birth-weight infants. *Arch Pediatr Adolesc Med.* 2001;155(5):548–553.

Pinelli J, Symington A. Non-nutritive sucking for promoting physiologic stability and nutrition in preterm infants. *Cochrane Database Syst Rev.* 2005;3:CD001071. doi: 10.1002/14651858.CD001071.pub2.

Polberger S, Lonnerdal B. Simple and rapid macronutrient analysis of human milk for individualized fortification: basis for improved nutritional management of very-low-birth-weight infants. *J Pediatr Gastroenterol Nutr.* 1993;17:283–290.

Preyde M, Ardal F. Effectiveness of a parent "buddy" program for mothers of very preterm infants in a neonatal intensive care unit. *CMAJ.* 2003;168(8):969–973.

Prime DK, Garbin CP, Hartmann PE, Kent JC. Simultaneous breast expression in breastfeeding women is more efficacious than sequential breast expression. *Breastfeed Med.* 2012;7(6):442–447. doi: 10.1089/bfm.2011.0139.

Qi Y, Zhang Y, Fein S, et al. Maternal and breast pump factors associated with breast pump problems and injuries. *J Hum Lact.* 2014;30(1):62–72; quiz 110–112. doi: 10.1177/0890334413507499.

Quan R, Yang C, Rubinstein S. Effects of microwave radiation on anti-infective factors in human milk. *Pediatrics.* 1992;89(4 Pt 1):667–669.

Quan R, Yang C, Rubinstein S. The effect of nutritional additives on anti-infective factors in human milk. *Clin Pediatr (Phila).* 1994;33(6):325–328.

Raimbault C, Saliba E, Porter RH. The effect of the odour of mother's milk on breastfeeding behaviour of premature neonates. *Acta Paediatr.* 2007;96(3):368–371.

Ramasethu J, Jeyaseelan L, Kirubakaran CP. Weight gain in exclusively breastfed preterm infants. *J Trop Pediatr.* 1993;39(3):152–159.

Rassin DK, Gaull GE, Järvenpää AL, Räihä NC. Feeding the low-birth-weight infant: II. Effects of taurine and cholesterol supplementation on amino acids and cholesterol. *Pediatrics.* 1983;71:179–186.

Reyna BA, Pickler RH, Thompson A. A descriptive study of mothers' experiences feeding their preterm infants after discharge. *Adv Neonatal Care.* 2006;6(6):333–340.

Rocha NM, Martinez FE, Jorge SM. Cup or bottle for preterm infants: effects on oxygen saturation, weight gain, and breastfeeding. *J Hum Lact.* 2002;18(2):132–138.

Rochow N, Fusch G, Choi A, et al. Target fortification of breast milk with fat, protein, and carbohydrates for preterm infants. *J Pediatr.* 2013;163(4):1001–1007. doi: 10.1016/j.jpeds.2013.04.052.

Rodriguez NA, Meier PP, Groer MW, et al. A pilot study to determine the safety and feasibility of oropharyngeal administration of own mother's colostrum to extremely low-birth-weight infants. *Adv Neonatal Care.* 2010;10(4):206–212. doi: 10.1097/ANC.0b013e3181e94133.

Rodriguez NA, Miracle DJ, Meier PP. Sharing the science on human milk feedings with mothers of very-low-birth-weight infants. *J Obstet Gynecol Neonatal Nurs.* 2005; 34(1):109–119.

Ross ES, Browne JV. Developmental progression of feeding skills: an approach to supporting feeding in preterm infants. *Semin Neonatol.* 2002;7(6):469–475.

Rossman B, Kratovil AL, Greene MM, et al. "I have faith in my milk": the meaning of milk for mothers of very low birth weight infants hospitalized in the neonatal intensive care unit. *J Hum Lact.* 2013;29(3):359–365. doi: 10.1177/0890334413484552.

Saarela T, Kokkonen J, Koivisto M. Macronutrient and energy contents of human milk fractions during the first six months of lactation. *Acta Paediatr.* 2005;94(9): 1176–1181.

Sameroff A. Nonnutritive sucking in newborns under visual and auditory stimulation. *Child Dev.* 1967;38(2): 443–452.

Sangild P, Petersen YM, Schmidt M, et al. Preterm birth affects the intestinal response to parenteral and enteral nutrition in newborn pigs. *J Nutr.* 2002;132(9): 2673–2681.

Sankaran K, Papageorgiou A, Ninan A, Sankaran R. A randomized, controlled evaluation of two commercially available human breast milk fortifiers in healthy preterm neonates. *J Am Diet Assoc.* 1996;96(11): 1145–1149.

Santiago MS, Codipilly CN, Potak DC, Schanler RJ. Effect of human milk fortifiers on bacterial growth in human milk. *J Perinatol.* 2005;25(10):647–649.

Scanlon KS, Alexander MP, Serdula MK, et al. Assessment of infant feeding: the validity of measuring milk intake. *Nutr Rev.* 2002;60(8):235–251.

Schanler RJ. The role of human milk fortification for premature infants. *Clin Perinatol.* 1998;25(3):645–657.

Schanler RJ. The use of human milk for premature infants. *Pediatr Clin North Am.* 2001;48(1):207–219.

Schanler RJ. CMV acquisition in premature infants fed human milk: reason to worry? *J Perinatol.* 2005;25(5): 297–298.

Schanler RJ. Outcomes of human milk fed preterm infants. *Semin Perinatol.* 2011;35:29–33.

Schanler RJ, Atkinson SA. Effects of nutrients in human milk on the recipient premature infant. *J Mammary Gland Biol Neoplasia.* 1999;4(3):297–307.

Schanler RJ, Hurst NM, Lau C. The use of human milk and breastfeeding in premature infants. *Clin Perinatol.* 1999;26(2):379–398.

Schanler RJ, Shulman RJ, Lau C. Feeding strategies for premature infants: beneficial outcomes of feeding fortified human milk versus preterm formula. *Pediatrics.* 1999; 103(6 Pt 1):1150–1157.

Scheel CE, Schanler RJ, Lau C. Does the choice of bottle nipple affect the oral feeding performance of very-low-birthweight (VLBW) infants? *Acta Paediatr.* 2005; 94(9):1266-72.

Schmolzer G, Urlesberger B, Haim M, et al. Multi-modal approach to prophylaxis of necrotizing enterocolitis: clinical report and review of literature. *Pediatr Surg Int.* 2006;22(7):573–580.

Shaker CS, Woida AM. An evidence-based approach to nipple feeding in a level III NICU: nurse autonomy, developmental care, and teamwork. *Neonatal Netw.* 2007;26(2):77–83.

Sharland M, Khare M, Bedford-Russell A. Prevention of postnatal cytomegalovirus infection in preterm infants. *Arch Dis Child Fetal Neonatal Ed.* 2002;86(2):F140.

Shin H, White-Traut R. The conceptual structure of transition to motherhood in the neonatal intensive care unit. *J Adv Nurs.* 2007;58(1):90–98.

Shoji H, Koletzko B. Oxidative stress and antioxidant protection in the perinatal period. *Curr Opin Clin Nutr Metab Care.* 2007;10(3):324–328.

Shulman RJ, Schanler RJ, Lau C, et al. Early feeding, antenatal glucocorticoids, and human milk decrease intestinal permeability in preterm infants. *Pediatr Res.* 1998a;44(4):519–523.

Shulman RJ, Schanler RJ, Lau C, et al. Early feeding, feeding tolerance, and lactase activity in preterm infants. *J Pediatr.* 1998b;133(5):645–649.

Sidell EP, Froman RD. A national survey of neonatal intersive-care units: criteria used to determine readiness for oral feedings. *J Obstet Gynecol Neonatal Nurs.* 1994, 23:783–789.

Simmer K, Metcalf R, Daniels L. The use of breastmilk in a neonatal unit and its relationship to protein and energy intake and growth. *J Paediatr Child Health.* 1997; 33(1):55–60.

Simpson C, Schanler RJ, Lau C. Early introduction of oral feeding in preterm infants. *Pediatrics.* 2002;110(3): 517–522.

Singhal A, Cole TJ, Fewtrell M, Lucas A. Breastmilk feeding and lipoprotein profile in adolescents born preterm: follow-up of a prospective randomised study. *Lancet.* 2004;363(9421):1571–1578.

Sisk PM, Lovelady CA, Dillard RG, Gruber KJ. Lactation counseling for mothers of very low birth weight infants: effect on maternal anxiety and infant intake of human milk. *Pediatrics.* 2006;117(1):e67–e75.

Slusher T, Hampton R, Bode-Thomas F, et al. Promoting the exclusive feeding of own mother's milk through the use of hindmilk and increased maternal milk volume for hospitalized, low birth weight infants (< 1800 grams) in Nigeria: a feasibility study. *J Hum Lact.* 2003;19(2):191–198.

Spatz DL. Ten steps for promoting and protecting breastfeeding in vulnerable populations. *J Perinat Neonatal Nurs.* 2004;18(4):412–423.

Spatz DL. Report of a staff program to promote and support breastfeeding in the care of vulnerable infants at a children's hospital. *J Perinat Educ.* 2005;14(1): 30–38.

Spatz DL. Roles and responsibilities of health professions: focus on nursing. Breastfeed Med. 2010;5:243–244. doi: 10.1089/bfm.2010.0036.

Stocks RJ, Davies DP, Allen F, Sewell D. Loss of breastmilk nutrients during tube feeding. Arch Dis Child. 1985; 60:164–166.

Sullivan S, Schanler RJ, Kim JH, et al. An exclusively human milk-based diet is associated with a lower rate of necrotizing enterocolitis than a diet of human milk and bovine milk-based products. *J Pediatr.* 2010;156(4): 562–567.e1. doi: 10.1016/j.jpeds.2009.10.040. Epub December 29, 2009.

Sweet L. Breastfeeding a preterm infant and the objectification of breastmilk. *Breastfeed Rev.* 2006;14(1):5–13.

Sweet L, Darbyshire P. Fathers and breast feeding very-low-birthweight preterm babies. *Midwifery.* 2009;25(5): 540–553. doi: 10.1016/j.midw.2007.09.001.

Taylor SN, Basile LA, Ebeling M, Wagner CL. Intestinal permeability in preterm infants by feeding type: mother›s milk versus formula. *Breastfeed Med.* 2009;4(1):11–15. doi: 10.1089/bfm.2008.0114.

Telang S, Berseth CL, Ferguson PW, et al. Fortifying fresh human milk with commercial powdered human milk fortifiers does not affect bacterial growth during 6 hours at room temperature. *J Am Diet Assoc.* 2005; 105(10):1567–1572.

Thompson N, Pickler RH, Munro C, Shotwell J. Contamination in expressed breast milk following breast cleansing. *J Hum Lact.* 1997;13(2):127–130.

Tornhage CJ, Serenius F, Uvnäs-Moberg K, Lindberg T. Plasma somatostatin and cholecystokinin levels in preterm infants during kangaroo care with and without nasogastric tube-feeding. *J Pediatr Endocrinol Metab.* 1998;11(5):645–651.

Tornhage CJ, Stuge E, Lindberg T, Serenius F. First week kangaroo care in sick very preterm infants. *Acta Paediatr.* 1999;88(12):1402–1404.

Torres AG, Ney JG, Meneses F, Trugo NM. Polyunsaturated fatty acids and conjugated linoleic acid isomers in breast milk are associated with plasma non-esterified and erythrocyte membrane fatty acid composition in lactating women. *Br J Nutr.* 2006;95(3):517–524.

Uauy R, Birch E, Birch D, Peirano P. Visual and brain function measurements in studies of n-3 fatty acid requirements of infants. *J Pediatr.* 1992;120(4 pt2): S168–S180.

Uauy R, Hoffman DR. Essential fat requirements of preterm infants. *Am J Clin Nutr.* 2000;71(1 suppl):245S–250S.

Ustundag B, Yilmaz E, Dogan Y, et al. Levels of cytokines (IL-1beta, IL-2, IL-6, IL-8, TNF-alpha) and trace elements (Zn, Cu) in breast milk from mothers of preterm and term infants. *Mediators Inflamm.* 2005;(6):331–336.

Uvnas-Moberg K. Physiological and endocrine effects of social contact. *Ann N Y Acad Sci.* 1997;807:146–163.

Uvnas-Moberg K. Oxytocin may mediate the benefits of positive social interaction and emotions. *Psychoneuroendocrinology.* 1998;23(8):819–835.

Valentine CJ, Hurst NM, Schanler RJ. Hindmilk improves weight gain in low-birth-weight infants fed human milk. *J Pediatr Gastroenterol Nutr.* 1994;18(4):474–477.

van den Berg A, van Elburg RM, Teerlink T, et al. A randomized controlled trial of enteral glutamine supplementation in very low birth weight infants: plasma amino acid concentrations. *J Pediatr Gastroenterol Nutr.* 2005;41(1):66–71.

van der Strate BW, Harmsen MC, Schäfer P, et al. Viral load in breast milk correlates with transmission of human cytomegalovirus to preterm neonates, but lactoferrin concentrations do not. *Clin Diagn Lab Immunol.* 2001;8(4):818–821.

Vohr BR, Poindexter BB, Dusick AM, et al. Beneficial effects of breast milk in the neonatal intensive care unit on the developmental outcome of extremely low birth weight infants at 18 months of age. *Pediatrics.* 2006;118(1):e115–e123.

Vohr BR, Poindexter BB, Dusick AM, et al. Persistent beneficial effects of breast milk ingested in the neonatal intensive care unit on outcomes of extremely low birth weight infants at 30 months of age. *Pediatrics.* 2007;120(4):e953–e959.

Walker M. Test weighing and other estimates of breastmilk intake. *J Hum Lact.* 1995;11(2):91–92.

Wang B, McVeagh P, Petocz P, Brand-Miller J. Brain ganglioside and glycoprotein sialic acid in breastfed compared with formula-fed infants. *Am J Clin Nutr.* 2003;78(5):1024–1029.

Ward PP, Paz E, Conneely OM. Multifunctional roles of lactoferrin: a critical overview. *Cell Mol Life Sci.* 2005;62(22):2540–2548.

Waterland RA, Berkowitz RI, Stunkard AJ, Stallings VA. Calibrated-orifice nipples for measurement of infant nutritive sucking. *J Pediatr.* 1998;132(3 Pt 1): 523–526.

Wauben IP, Atkinson SA, Grad TL, et al. Moderate nutrient supplementation of mother's milk for preterm infants supports adequate bone mass and short-term growth: a randomized, controlled trial. *Am J Clin Nutr.* 1998;67(3):465–472.

Wauben IP, Atkinson SA, Shah JK, et al. Growth and body composition of preterm infants: influence of nutrient fortification of mother's milk in hospital and breastfeeding post-hospital discharge. *Acta Paediatr.* 1998; 87(7):780–785.

Wheeler JL, Johnson M, Collie L, et al. Promoting breastfeeding in the neonatal intensive care unit. *Breastfeed Rev.* 1999;7:15–18.

Whitelaw A, Liestol K. Mortality and growth of low birth weight infants on the kangaroo mother program in Bogota, Colombia. *Pediatrics.* 1994;94(6 Pt 1): 931–932.

Williamson MT, Murti PK. Effects of storage, time, temperature, and composition of containers on biologic components of human milk. *J Hum Lact.* 1996;12(1):31–35.

Woltil HA, van Beusekom CM, Siemensma AD, et al. Erythrocyte and plasma cholesterol ester long-chain polyunsaturated fatty acids of low-birth-weight babies fed preterm formula with and without ribonucleotides: comparison with human milk. *Am J Clin Nutr.* 1995;62(5):943–949.

Woodward DR, Rees B, Boon JA. Human milk fat content: within-feed variation. *Early Hum Dev.* 1989;19(1): 39–46.

Wooldridge J, Hall WA. Posthospitalization breastfeeding patterns of moderately preterm infants. *J Perinat Neonatal Nurs.* 2003;17(1):50–64.

Xiao X, Xiong A, Chen X, et al. Epidermal growth factor concentrations in human milk, cow's milk and cow's milk-based infant formulas. *Chin Med J (Engl).* 2002; 115(3):451–454.

Yasuda A, Kimura H, Hayakawa M, et al. Evaluation of cytomegalovirus infections transmitted via breast milk in preterm infants with a real-time polymerase chain reaction assay. *Pediatrics.* 2003;111(6 Pt 1):1333–1336.

Zachariassen G, Faerk J, Grytter C, et al. Nutrient enrichment of mother's milk and growth of very preterm infants after hospital discharge. *Pediatrics.* 2011;127(4): e995–e1003. doi: 10.1542/peds.2010-0723. Epub March 14, 2011.

Zarban A, Taheri G, Chankandia T, et al. Antioxidant and radical scavenging activity of human colostrum, transitional and mature milk. *J Clin Biochem Nutr.* 2009;45: 150–154.

The Preterm Infant Breastfeeding Behavior Scale (PIBBS)

The PIBBS is used to describe the infant's behavior, as defined by the scale. It does not assess the infant's breastfeeding behavior capacity in a way that can be quantified by a total score.

Scale Items	Maturational Steps	Score
Rooting	Did not root	0
	Showed some rooting behavior	1
	Showed obvious rooting behavior	2
Areolar grasp (How much of the breast was inside the baby's mouth?)	None, the mouth only touched the nipple	0
	Part of the nipple	1
	The whole nipple, not the areola	2
	The nipple and some of the areola	3
Latched-on and fixed to the breast (scored on a continuous scale)	Did not latch on at all so the mother felt it	0
	Latched on for 5 minutes or less	1
	Latched on for 6–10 minutes	2
	Latched on for 11–15 minutes or more	3
Sucking	No sucking or licking	0
	Licking and tasting, but no sucking	1
	Single sucks, occasional short sucking bursts (2–9 sucks)	2
	Repeated short sucking bursts, occasional long bursts (>10 sucks)	3
	Repeated (2 or more) long sucking bursts	4
Longest sucking burst (in consecutive sucks, scored on a continuous scale)	1–5	1
	6–10	2
	11–15	3
	16–20	4
	21–25	5
	26–30 or more	6
Swallowing	Swallowing was not noticed	0
	Occasional swallowing was noticed	1
	Repeated swallowing was noticed	2

Definition of Terms

1. Rooting: Some rooting (mouth opening, tongue extension, hand-to-mouth movements) and obvious rooting (simultaneous mouth opening and head turning). Examples of suggestions to mothers for stimulation of rooting are touching the infant's lips with the nipple and expressing some milk on the lips.

2. Areolar grasp: Part of the nipple, whole nipple, or nipple and part of the areola. The mother can facilitate this by encouraging the infant to continue rooting until he shows a wide open mouth, by shaping her breast into a form that fits the infant's mouth, and then letting the infant latch-on and pulling him close to her body; in order for successful latching-on to take place the mother should sit in an upright position; with proper support for her back, arms, and feet; and with a pillow under the infant that supports a comfortable position in front of the breast.

3. Duration of latching-on: Momentarily, less than a minute, or several minutes. The infant is assisted in staying fixed at the breast by adjustment of the mother's and infant's position and of the areolar grasp.

4. Sucking: occasional sucks, short or long (10 consecutive sucks or more) sucking bursts, occasional or repeated bursts. The mother can encourage sucking by talking to the infant and by gently depressing the breast tissue in front of the infant's mouth, which makes the nipple touch the hard palate.

5. The longest sucking burst: Maximum number of consecutive sucks, a measure of sucking maturity.

6. Swallowing: Occasional or repeated. When swallowing is noticed, the mother can be asked to commence test weighing (if this is included in the unit policy), and the milk given by alternative methods can be reduced.

Source: Nyqvist KH, Ewald U, Sjoden PO. Supporting a preterm infant's behaviour during breastfeeding: a case report. *J Hum Lact.* 1996;12(3):221–228. Reprinted with permission.

Chapter 14

Donor Milk Banking

Frances Jones

Introduction

Donor human milk banks recruit and screen mothers who have excess milk beyond what their own baby needs or are willing to express for the milk bank. In addition, bereaved mothers may donate to milk banks, reporting that this is helpful in their grieving process (Wellborn, 2012). The banks then collect, process, screen, store, and distribute the donated milk to specific individuals for whom human milk is prescribed by a licensed healthcare provider (Human Milk Banking Association of North America [HMBANA], 2013). Pasteurized human donor milk (PHDM) and donor milk banks should not be confused with handling and storage of a mother's own milk for her own infant.

This chapter describes donor human milk banking and discusses issues surrounding clinical uses of donor human milk, including safety and availability. Included as well is a history of donor human milk banking and milk-banking procedures. Information on informal milk sharing, particularly the increased interest in sharing human milk via the Internet, is also discussed. Research regarding donor milk is described, and selected case studies are presented to illustrate the benefits of donor milk for a range of conditions in infants.

Use of Donor Milk

The World Health Organization (WHO, 2003, 2011), the American Academy of Pediatrics (Eidelman & Schanler, 2012), and the Canadian Pediatric Society (Kim & Unger, 2010) all mention donor milk in their recent infant feeding statements as an alternative when a mother's own milk is not available. For premature or sick infants, the preponderance of evidence indicates that *not* providing human milk presents a risk to the infant (Arslanoglu et al., 2010; Lucas & Morley, 1994; Lucas et al., 1989, 1990, 1992, 1994; Stuebe, 2009). In some neonatal intensive care units (NICUs), use of pasteurized donor milk in the absence of mother's own is the standard of care (Kim & Unger, 2010).

More and more healthcare providers as well as parents and insurers are finding this a compelling argument to support the investment necessary to make PHDM available to every needy infant (Carroll & Herrmann, 2012; Mackenzie, 2013). Article 24 of the Convention on the Rights of the Child (United Nations, 1990) recognizes the right of every child to "the enjoyment of the highest attainable standard of health and to facilities for the treatment of illness and rehabilitation to health." For healthcare providers, the question becomes one of offering the highest standard of care to all infants regardless of the individual mother's ability to provide milk.

Medical Indications

Recognizing the importance of mothers' own milk for their babies, donor milk banks provide human milk not to replace mothers' own milk, but rather to complement mothers' efforts to provide human milk particularly when there is an infant with a medical need (Baack et al., 2012; Giuliani et al., 2012; Ley et al., 2011; Montjaux-Regis et al., 2012; Vieira et al., 2011) (see Figure 14-1). In the hospital setting, PHDM may be used to supplement a mother's own milk or for babies whose mothers are not yet fully lactating; most often, however, it is used for high-risk and premature and ill infants.

The use of donor milk is growing in North American healthcare facilities. In maternity hospitals providing advanced care, 11.5% used donor milk in 2007, but that percentage had increased to 22% by 2011. Most of the increase in use occurred in the NICUs of these hospitals: 25.1% of NICUs used PHDM in 2007 versus 45.2 % in 2011 (Perrine & Scanopn, 2013). The use of PHDM in hospital NICUs may potentially affect the rate of exclusive breastfeeding. An Italian study of 83 NICUs found that centers with milk banks and access to pasteurized donor milk had significantly higher rates of exclusive breastfeeding at discharge than centers that did not have a milk bank or use donor milk (Arslanoglu et al., 2013). In contrast, an American study examining two level 3 NUCUs found that the provision of donor milk reduced formula-feeding rates but did not influence breastfeeding rates (Delfosse et al., 2013). Further research is needed to elucidate the reasons for the different results from these two studies.

Donor milk is used therapeutically for older infants as well. Documented uses include the following:

- In infants who are otherwise healthy but not thriving on human milk substitutes (HMBANA, 2013)
- To decrease feeding intolerance (Edwards & Spatz, 2012)

Figure 14-1 DIAGNOSIS CODES FOR DONOR MILK ORDERS PLACED TO HMBANA BANKS IN 2012.

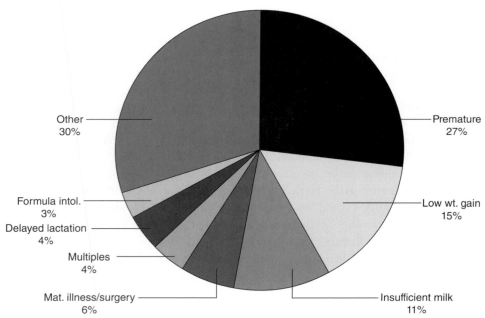

Source: Data from Human Milk Banking Association of North America 2012 Annual Report.

- In infants with short-gut syndrome or post surgery for necrotizing enterocolitis (Olieman et al., 2010)
- As a source of immunoglobulin A (IgA) for an IgA-deficient infant who is not being breastfed or an older child or adult suffering from IgA deficiency (Merhav et al., 1995; Tully, 1990)
- Post surgery, including children undergoing cardiac surgery who develop chylothorax and receive fat-free donor milk (Chan & Lechtenberg, 2007) (see the Box 14-4 case study later in this chapter)
- In children with kidney problems or congenital malformations such as cleft palate, and as part of the treatment for severe gastrointestinal infections (HMBANA, 2013)

Recent research demonstrated that 18 HIV-exposed uninfected infants fed human donor milk and followed for 18 months had normal growth of the thymus and contracted fewer infections than other healthy infants. Those babies receiving human milk (either donor or mother's own) had fewer infections than those fed formula, suggesting that the human donor milk provided to this vulnerable population offered benefits for their maturing immune systems (Jeppesen et al., 2013) (see Table 14-1).

Nonmedical Indications

In the United States and Canada, PHDM is also occasionally used for infants with no specific medical need—for example, babies who are adopted or babies of mothers with mastectomies or those requiring medication incompatible with breastfeeding. However, when there is no identified medical need for human milk, the processing fee is not covered by health insurance or the healthcare system; that is, patients and families are responsible for the expense. Milk can be dispensed for these babies only

Table 14-1 INFANT DIAGNOSES FOR WHICH DONOR MILK HAS BEEN ORDERED FROM HMBANA MEMBER BANKS

Categories	Common Medical Reasons for Ordering Pasteurized Human Donor Milk
<ul><li>Prematurity/late preterm<ul><li>◄ Mother is often pumping but may have difficulty establishing a supply or have more than one infant.</li></ul></li><li>Full-term infant with a medical problem<ul><li>◄ Some infant problems make breastfeeding difficult, such as cleft palate, Pierre Robin syndrome, low muscle tone, or cardiac anomaly. Many of these mothers are pumping but are having problems with their milk supply.</li></ul></li><li>Higher-risk infant with mother with a medical problem<ul><li>◄ Mother is being treated for cancer or other illness, has had a mastectomy, has died during childbirth, or has some other condition incompatible with breastfeeding; and her baby is premature, late preterm, or at risk for allergies or other conditions increased by lack of human milk.</li></ul></li></ul>	<ul><li>High risk for necrotizing enterocolitis (NEC) (premature/preterm)</li><li>Formula allergy or other feeding intolerance</li><li>Postsurgical nutrition (e.g., cardiac, kidney, bowel [post NEC])</li><li>Severe gastrointestinal infections</li><li>Metabolic disorders</li><li>Respiratory illness</li><li>Hypoglycemia</li><li>Hyperbilirubinemia</li><li>Poor growth/failure to thrive</li><li>Congenital anomalies and syndromes</li></ul>

Reproduced from Human Milk Banking Association of North America 2012 Annual Report. Used with permission.

when there is sufficient milk available to provide for recipients with a medical need first (HMBANA, 2013). In a few hospitals in North America, donor milk is offered when any breastfed baby has medical need of supplementation (see the Box 14-2 case study later in this chapter).

History of Donor Milk Banking

Until the 1900s, mothers primarily breastfed their children (Jefferson, 1954). When a mother was unavailable or had insufficient milk, families used wet nurses (women who nursed children to whom they were not biologically related) or sought donated human milk from friends, relatives, or strangers. Women who wet-nursed or provided donor milk were verbally screened for diseases and healthy lifestyles. In addition, the health of their children was assessed. These early practices formed the foundation for modern milk banking.

Prior to the late 1800s, attempts to replace human milk with other substances often proved fatal. By the late 1880s, with the advances in science and increased understanding of food composition, a number of companies, including Nestlé, sold artificial feeding products throughout Europe, Australia, and the Americas (Apple, 1986; Wood, 1955). By the beginning of the 1900s, improved sanitation, greater understanding of infant nutrition, and availability of refrigeration resulted in increased success using artificial feeding products made from modified animal milk (Baker, 1914; Blackman, 1977; Jefferson, 1954). As the marketing increased, the support for artificial feeding increased, although as one physician stated, "It is difficult to overcome a prejudice in favor of breast milk" (Tow, 1934).

Between 1900 and 1950, a cultural shift occurred. Artificial feeding replaced breastfeeding as the "norm" in North America and many other developed countries. This shift resulted from changes in physicians' and women's roles, increased belief in science, and aggressive marketing of artificial feeding products. During the first half of the 1900s, mothering came under the purview of physicians, reflecting the idea that mothers needed direction from physicians, who were almost exclusively male. In addition, increasing numbers of women began working outside the home, a condition that made breastfeeding difficult.

Science held a privileged status in society during this era, and physicians emphasized the close relationship between science and medicine (McHaffie, 1927). The specialty of pediatrics, first established in the early 1900s, included directions for infant feeding as part of the pediatrician's job. Proprietary companies realized the value of a partnership with the medical community. In the 1930s, the American Medical Association (AMA) published specific advertising guidelines for infant foods stating that physicians should provide direction to every mother on infant feeding (Apple, 1980). These guidelines restricted manufacturers from publishing instructions on artificial feeding products. Mothers were directed to visit their physicians, who provided instruction sheets supplied by manufacturers of human milk substitutes. When they adhered to these guidelines, the companies were awarded the AMA seal of approval for their products, allowed to advertise in the *Journal of the American Medical Association* (*JAMA*), and permitted to have displays at AMA conferences. These arrangements proved to be financially advantageous to both parties. Companies sold greater amounts of their products, and physicians had more patient visits. This relationship between health professionals and proprietary companies contributed to the shift of infant feeding from the domestic sphere, in which women helped other women, to the scientific, medical world, and from breastfeeding to artificial feeding.

Almost 90 years later, this relationship persists, with product marketing becoming more pervasive through funding of journals, newsletters, conferences, meetings, research, websites, gifts, and travel for medical professionals and allied health providers (Brady, 2012; Wright & Waterston, 2006). Common marketing themes of best nutrition, physician endorsement, and pseudoscience have remained constant throughout more than 100-plus years of marketing of artificial feeding.

During this period, modern milk banking was born. The technical advances that made artificial feeding products possible also made milk banking possible. In 1909, the first milk bank was established in Vienna, Austria. In 1910, two more milk banks were established: one in Boston, Massachusetts, and one in Germany. Interest in milk banking grew as premature infants of earlier gestational ages and infants with more complex illnesses survived owing to advances in health care.

The Boston Milk Bank provided education and support to a number of institutions, resulting in the establishment of milk banks in both Canada and the United States (Barret & Hiscox, 1939). The publicity surrounding the births of the premature Dionne quintuplets in northern Ontario also gave milk banking a boost, as the quintuplets received frozen donor milk shipped by train from Toronto and parts of the northeastern United States (Breton, 1978).

By the 1940s, the American Academy of Pediatrics (AAP) had developed guidelines for donor milk banking. By the early 1980s, there were about 30 milk banks in the United States and about 23 such facilities in Canada. Donor milk was dispensed either raw or pasteurized, depending on the preference of the milk bank. Use was primarily for infants in medical need, particularly those who were premature or ill. The Human Milk Banking Association of North America was founded in 1985 with the goal of standardizing donor milk banking operations (HMBANA, 2013).

In the mid-1980s, potential transmission of two viruses through human milk raised concerns. Cytomegalovirus (CMV) in human milk was recognized to have potentially serious neurological consequences for preterm infants (Rawls et al., 1984; Yeager et al., 1983), and human immunodeficiency virus (HIV), the cause of acquired immune deficiency syndrome (AIDS), was identified as being transmissible in human milk. Many milk banks closed as the concerns over possible spread of disease decreased the amount of milk ordered. To address the concerns about potential pathogen transmission, requirements for screening of donors, including serum screening, and heat processing of all donor milk were suggested as the appropriate standard. Many more banks closed because they had no funding to support this additional processing. At the same time, the development and marketing of specialty formulas, particularly for preterm infants, convinced many practitioners that human milk was replaceable. By the late 1990s, the number of donor milk banks in North America reached an all-time low (Jones, 2003).

However, the pendulum quickly swung back as ever smaller and younger-gestational-age infants survived as the result of ongoing medical advances and research increased on appropriate nutrition for preterm infants. This research led to increased awareness of the many benefits of human milk and, in turn, a resurgence of interest in donor milk banking. In North America, the number of human milk banks and the size of some of the banks began to increase dramatically by the early 2000s (see Figure 14-2 and Table 14-2). The number of HMBANA donor milk banks has increased steadily in the 21st century, with 13 banks in operation in 2013 and 7 more banks in development (see Figure 14-3). It has been estimated that to serve the NICUs in the United States, 8 million ounces of PHDM is needed (Rivera, 2007). Currently, the American HMBANA banks dispense about one-fourth of this amount, demonstrating a need for more donors and facilities to process the required milk.

Donor Milk Today

Today, donor milk banking is expanding globally. More than 500 nonprofit milk banks operate around the world in Africa, Asia, Australia, Central America, North America, South America, and Europe (Technical Advisory Group on Milk Banking Meeting [TAG], 2012). Both Russia and China are working on establishing milk banks but do not as yet have a formal system of milk banking.

Globally, Brazil leads the world in number of donor milk banks, with more than 200 such milk banks found in Brazilian hospitals (Almeida & Dorea, 2006; Ortiz, 2012). Donor milk banking is integrated into the promotion, protection, and support of breastfeeding nationally. Brazil has national

Figure 14-2 IN 2013 THERE WERE 11 NON-PROFIT MILK BANKS IN THE UNITED STATES AND 2 IN CANADA.

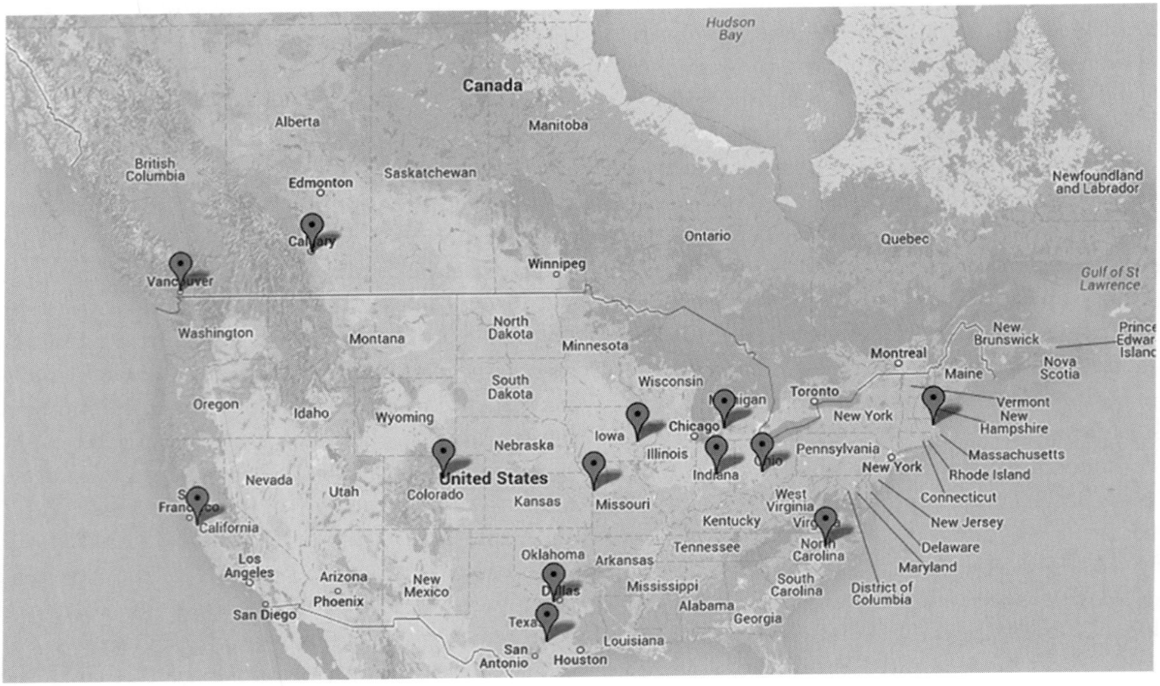

Source: Data from Human Milk Banking Association of North America

milk banking standards, a National Human Milk Bank Network, national breastfeeding promotion, and donor milk banking conferences (RedeBlh, 2013).

Brazil provides a creative model, particularly for countries with limited resources. In this country, there is active support of donor milk banking at the federal, state, and local levels. A national reference milk bank at FIOCRUZ University in Rio de Janeiro acts as the liaison between the milk banks and the Ministry of Health (Gutiérrez & de Almeida, 1998). It provides mandatory, standardized training for all milk bank personnel across the country and monitors all of the milk banks by reviewing bacteriologic screening of milk prior to and after pasteurization. The Internet facilitates communication within the Brazilian system. Each milk bank

is located in a hospital and provides breastfeeding support and education as well as the traditional work of milk banks—that is, donor recruitment and milk screening and processing (Ortiz, 2012).

Further integrating breastfeeding into the healthcare system, as part of their Emergency Medical Technician (EMT) training, fire fighters receive 40 hours of breastfeeding education and clinical training, including time spent in a donor milk bank. In some states, fire fighters collect milk from donors daily, since few Brazilian homes have large refrigerators or freezers to accommodate storing the milk for any length of time at home. As EMTs, they also provide breastfeeding advice. Interestingly, letter carriers for the postal service are trained to promote and support breastfeeding as well. Both of these groups of government employees are well

Figure 14-3 In 2013 There Were Six Developing Banks in the United States and One in Canada. These bank are receiving guidance from HMBANA. Once they successfully complete all necessary steps, they will become distributing banks and fully fledged HMBANA members.

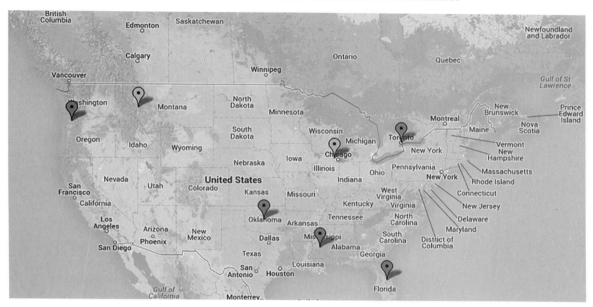

Source: Data from Human Milk Banking Association of North America

Table 14-2 Current Member Banks in the Human Milk Banking Association of North America

Canada	United States
Alberta	**California**
Calgary Mothers' Milk Bank	Mothers' Milk Bank
103-10333 Southport Rd. S.W.	751 South Bascom Ave.
Calgary, Alberta T2W 3X6	San Jose, CA 95128
Phone: 403-475-6455	Phone: 408-998-4550
Fax: 888-334-4372	Toll free: 877-375-6645
www.calgarymothersmilkbank.ca	Fax: 408-297-9208
	http://mothersmilk.org
	mothersmilkbank@hhs.co.santa-clara.ca.us

(continues)

Table 14-2 CURRENT MEMBER BANKS IN THE HUMAN MILK BANKING ASSOCIATION OF NORTH AMERICA (*CONTINUED*)

British Columbia

BC Women's Milk Bank
C & W Lactation Service
1U 50- 4450 Oak St.
Vancouver, BC V6H 3N1
Phone: 604-875-2282
Fax: 604-875-2871
www.bcwomens.ca
Fjones@cw.bc.ca

Colorado

Mothers' Milk Bank
Presbyterian/St. Luke's Medical Center and Rocky Mountain Hospital for Children
1719 E, 19th Ave.
Denver, CO 80218
Phone: 303-869-1888
www.milkbankcolorado.org
Laraine.Lockhart-Borman@healthonecares.com

Indiana

Indiana Mothers' Milk Bank, Inc.
4755 Kingsway Dr., Suite 120
Indianapolis, IN 46205
Phone: 317-536-1670
Fax: 317-536-1676
www.immb.org
info@immb.org

Iowa

Mother's Milk Bank of Iowa Department of Food and Nutrition Services University of Iowa Hospitals and Clinics
University of Iowa at Liberty Square
119 2nd St., Suite 400
Coralville, IA 52241
Phone: 319-384-9929
Toll free: 877-891-5347
Fax: 319-384-9933
www.uichildrens.org/mothers-milk-bank
jean-drulis@uiowa.edu

Michigan

Bronson Mothers' Milk Bank
601 John St., Suite N 1300
Kalamazoo, MI 49007
Phone: 269-341-6146
Fax: 269-341-8365
www.bronsonhealth.com
Duffc@bronsonhg.org

Missouri

Heart of America Mothers' Milk Bank at Saint Luke's Hospital
4401 Wornail Rd.
Kansas City, MO 64111
Phone: 816-932-4888
kcmilkbank@saint-lukes.org

New England

Mothers' Milk Bank of New England
PO Box 60-0091
Newtonville, MA 02460 or
225 Nevada St., Room 201
Newtonville, MA 02460
Phone: 617-527-6263
Fax: 617-527-1005
www.milkbankne.org
info@milkbankne.org

North Carolina

WakeMed Mothers' Milk Bank and Lactation Center
3000 New Bern Ave.
Raleigh, NC 27610
Phone: 919-350-8599
Fax: 919-3590-8923
www.wakemed.org
Suevans@wakemed.org

Ohio

OhioHealth Mothers' Milk Bank
4850 E. Main St.
Columbus, OH 43213
Phone: 614-566-0630
Fax: 614-566-0637
www.ohiohealth.com
ffeehan@ohiohealth.com

Texas

Mothers' Milk Bank at Austin
2911 Medical Arts St., Suite 12
Austin, TX 78705
Phone: 512-494-0800
Toll free: 877-813-6455
Fax: 512-494-0880
www.milkbank.org
info@milkbank.org

Mothers' Milk Bank of North Texas

600 Magnolia Ave.
Ft Worth, TX 76104
Phone: 817-810-0071
Toll free: 866-810-0071
Fax: 817-810-0087
www.texasmilkbank.org
info@TexasMilkBank.org

Note: Two additional banks were expected to be fully operational HMBANA banks before the end of 2013. Check the HMBANA website at www.hmbana.org for the most recent updates.

Data from Human Milk Banking Association of North America.

represented at national breastfeeding meetings, with several hundred members attending such conferences. Brazil also has an annual national donor milk day to honor milk bank donors. Well-known local celebrities are featured on posters breastfeeding their children and supporting donor milk banking. In 2012, to increase global awareness of milk banking, Brazilian milk bank representatives requested that all milk banks celebrate International Donors Day on May 19 each year (De Almeida, 2012).

Brazil has been reaching out to other countries, particularly in South and Central America, to export its model of milk banking, which fits well with limited-resource countries. The Brazilian and Ibero-American Network of Human Milk Banks was established to promote this model, with 23 countries involved in Latin America, the Caribbean, and Africa, as well as Spain and Portugal in Europe (Ortiz, 2012).

Countries where Muslim religious beliefs predominate provide challenges for milk banks. However, a new bank is opening in Izmir, Turkey. Here milk will be screened and tested, but not pooled. Recipient babies will receive milk from only one donor, and the donor mother and recipient mother will meet as "milk kinship," which means there can be no marriages between these families (Arslanoglu, 2012; El-Khuffash & Unger, 2012; Shaikh & Ahmed, 2006).

In recent years, increased demand for donor human milk has led to the establishment of additional regional organizations, including those in South America and Europe. In October 2010, the European Milk Banking Association was founded; at the time of this text's writing, it had 25 country members, with 186 milk banks in operation and 13 banks in development. South Africa established the Human Milk Banking Association of South Africa (HMBASA) in 2009.

These regional groups and individual country organizations have come together under the umbrella of the International Milk Banking Initiative (IMBI) founded by HMBANA and the United Kingdom Association of Milk Banks (UKAMB) for cooperation, collaboration, education, and research. In addition, in 2012 the international nonprofit organization Program for Appropriate Technology in Health (PATH) received funding from the Bill and Melinda Gates Foundation to develop milk banking technology particularly for resource-poor areas in India and Africa (TAG, 2012). PATH has a mandate to "transform global health through innovation" (PATH, 2013). Its website (www.path.org) provides further information on the organization's progress in expanding milk banking.

Safety

Donor milk banks worldwide have an enviable track record of product safety. There has never been a recorded case of a patient becoming seriously ill from donor milk received from a recognized milk bank anywhere in the world. Table 14-3 compares the safety of donor milk from banks following HMBANA or similar guidelines to the safety of human milk substitutes for preterm infants. Despite this outstanding record, some neonatologists still express concerns about the safety of donor milk (Miracle et al., 2011). As a result of ongoing education and dissemination of current research, however, more donor milk is being used in healthcare systems.

Availability

As with all donor tissue, use of PHDM requires a prescribing healthcare provider's order. Nonprofit donor milk banks provide milk almost exclusively for patients with a medical need. Access may be restricted by availability of donor milk. To ensure that they can provide milk to vulnerable, high-risk infants, milk banks rely on a well-informed public and healthcare system to identify and screen an adequate number of donors. When supplies are limited, high-risk infants may be vulnerable to increased mortality and morbidity.

In most countries, PHDM is available only in an inpatient setting. However, in North America, donor milk is frequently dispensed to patients at home. The HMBANA 2012 annual report indicated that 28% of milk distributed by member facilities went to outpatients. These patients may be able to remain at home only because the human milk provides needed therapeutic properties. Access to PHDM may be restricted when healthcare providers or families of patients are

Table 14-3 THE SAFETY OF DONOR HUMAN MILK COMPARED TO HUMAN MILK SUBSTITUTES (FORMULA)

Donor Human Milk

Screening procedures for donors and banking procedures in North America were developed with input from the Centers for Disease Control (CDC), American Academy of Pediatrics (AAP), and U.S. Food and Drug Administration (FDA) (HMBANA, 2013) and similar governmental bodies around the world (Gutiérrez & de Almeida, 1998).

Banking procedures are reviewed and updated regularly based on current research (HMBANA, 2013; Gutiérrez & de Almeida, 1998).

Human milk is designed to meet the needs of human infants (Schanler, 2007; Steube, 2009).

There has never been a recall for tainted or inadequate formulation of the milk.

There is no documented morbidity or mortality attributed to donor milk from a recognized donor milk bank following standard screening and processing procedures.

Human Milk Substitutes

Standards developed by Codex Alimentarius (Codex Alimentarius, 2007), an international commission created by the World Health Organization (WHO) and the Food and Agriculture Organization of the United Nations (UN) are the standards used by the U.S. Food and Drug Administration (FDA).

Modifications of infant formulas, even for the preterm infant, are registered with the FDA but do not require clinical trials or other testing for approval (FDA, 2006).

"Formula" is bovine milk or soy extract modified to approximate human milk as closely as possible (Codex Alimentarius, 2007).

There are constant recalls of formula for contamination and incorrect formulation (Codex Alimentarius, 2007; USFDA, 2006; Walker, 2013).

There are regular reports documenting evidence of morbidity and mortality due to contaminated or incorrectly formulated "formula" (Codex Alimentarius, 2007; FDA, 2006; Walker, 2013).

Data from Lucas et al., 1978.

unaware of the availability of pasteurized milk and/or there are inadequate donations made to the nonprofit banks.

The expense of screening donors, processing and dispensing the milk, and record keeping require milk banks to charge for their services. Many healthcare systems and insurance companies pass this processing fee on to the patient. Therefore, cost can be a barrier, as the processing fee in 2013 typically amounted to $5–6 per ounce (30 mL) plus the expense of overnight shipping. Many HMBANA banks have a process whereby they provide charitable care particularly in cases of medical need.

Milk Banking Procedures

In 1985 when HMBANA was established, one of its primary goals included supporting the creation of

new banks and developing standards for screening of donors and processing of their milk (HMBANA, 2013). *Guidelines for Establishment and Operation of a Donor Human Milk Bank* (available from HMBANA at www.hmbana.org) is updated annually, or more often if needed. Each member bank follows the mandatory guidelines as a minimum standard. These guidelines have been used as the basis for milk bank guidelines in countries around the world.

Donor Screening

Detailed donor screening involves verbal, written, and serum screening. In some developing countries, serum screening is not done, but all milk is pasteurized, thereby destroying both viruses and bacteria. When a prospective donor contacts the milk bank, a general conversation covers the requirements for donation, type of screening done, and storage requirements for donor milk. If the donor wishes to proceed, the initial screening questionnaire is completed by phone or in person (or in some cases on the Internet). The mother then receives a more detailed set of forms asking about health and lifestyle issues as well as consent to contact the mother's and baby's healthcare provider(s). Generally, healthy lactating women who meet requirements for blood donation and are not taking contraindicated medications are acceptable donors. Once the milk bank receives and reviews these forms, the mother is contacted to complete the process. The mother's primary healthcare provider is asked specific questions that focus on the health and suitability of the mother as a donor. The healthcare provider for the donor's child is also contacted to confirm that milk donation will not have an adverse effect on the child. Once the healthcare provider forms are received and reviewed, the mother's blood is screened for HIV types 0, 1, and 2; human T-lymphoma virus (HTLV); hepatitis B; hepatitis C; and syphilis (HMBANA, 2013). A retrospective review of 1091 potential milk bank donors underlined the importance of blood screening, as it identified an incidence of 3.3% positive results on screening serology for syphilis, hepatitis, HTLV, or HIV (Cohen, 2010).

After the mother's blood screening results are received and reviewed, the mother is contacted about arrangements for getting her milk to the milk bank. Although a mother can continue breastfeeding her own baby, a donor is temporarily disqualified for a period following consumption of certain medications or alcohol, and during certain short-term medical conditions.

Storage and Handling of Milk

The fundamental principles of good hand hygiene and using clean equipment are emphasized to each donor. All prospective donors receive information about correct cleaning of breast pump equipment. Donors mark each container of milk with their name and/or identification number and the time and date of expression. The milk is stored frozen in an appropriate freezer (one that is cold enough to keep ice cream hard) at home until there is enough accumulated to justify shipping the milk to the milk bank.

Processing of Milk

Once donor screening is complete, the frozen milk may be delivered to the milk bank. The frozen milk may be delivered to the milk bank directly (see Figure 14-4) or shipped via overnight express (see Figure 14-5). In some cases, the milk is sent to a depot of a particular milk bank and then shipped to the bank. All banks provide instructions for overnight shipping and nearly all provide shipping containers and pay shipping expenses.

Figure 14-4 DONOR BRINGS MILK TO THE MOTHERS' MILK BANK AT WAKEMED, RALIEGH, NORTH CAROLINA. MOTHERS WHO LIVE IN THE AREA BRING THEIR MILK TO THE BANK, AND MOTHERS FROM FARTHER AWAY SHIP THEIR MILK BY OVERNIGHT EXPRESS.

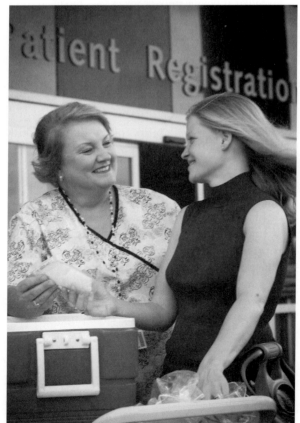

Figure 14-5 A Volunteer at the WakeMed Mothers' Milk Bank Unpacking a Shipment of Frozen Milk.

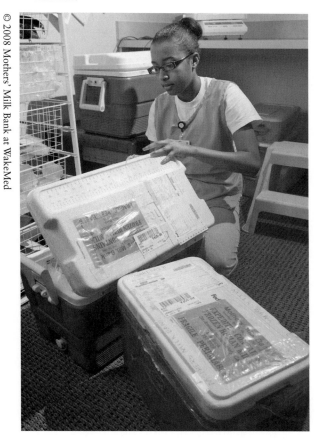

Milk banks store raw milk from screened donors in designated freezers. Prior to processing, the milk is thawed by placing it in a refrigerator overnight or by carefully monitoring it at room temperature for a few hours. Some banks analyze milk for protein or total calories and pool it to optimize either caloric or protein content for specific recipients—a practice called targeted pooling. Other banks pool milk based on time of expression and appearance (i.e., amount of fat that has risen to the top). Milk expressed by mothers whose babies were born at or before 36 weeks' gestation is pooled separately for the 4 weeks after birth and referred to as "premie" milk. This milk is distributed to hospitals for premature infants because of research indicating that it has a higher protein and mineral content, thereby improving growth in this population. Before pasteurization was implemented, in North America thawed milk was pooled (usually four to six donors), poured into individual bottles, and capped. In the United Kingdom and a number of other countries, there is no pooling due to the theoretical risk of Creutzfeldt-Jakob disease (CJD) (*NICE Guidelines*, 2010).

Pasteurization

In North American banks, pasteurization is done using a shaking water bath (see Figure 14-6) or a human milk pasteurizer (see Figure 14-7). Both methods effectively achieve Holder pasteurization. This type of pasteurization process rapidly heats and agitates the milk, holding the temperature of the milk at 62.5°C for 30 minutes. The milk is then rapidly cooled in chilled water or an ice slurry. The bottles are dried and labeled with batch number, date, and name of the milk bank (see Figure 14-8). In a few developed countries with a very low incidence of HIV, such as Germany and Norway, donor milk is still screened and dispensed raw in some situations (Grovslien & Gronn, 2009).

Figure 14-6 A Shaking Water Bath Set Up to Pasteurize Donor Milk. Note the temperature probe in a test bottle with the electronic reader on the counter.

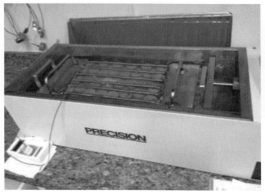

Figure 14-7 A MILK TECHNICIAN AT BC WOMEN'S MILK BANK CLOSING THE LID ON THE HUMAN MILK PASTEURIZER. NOTE THE TEMPERATURE PROBE IN A SAMPLE BOTTLE (USED FOR THIS PURPOSE) AND THE DATA LOGGER IS HELD IN HER HAND WHILE SHE CLOSES THE LID. ONCE PASTEURIZATION IS COMPLETE THE DATA WILL BE DOWNLOADED ONTO THE COMPUTER AND PROCESSING DATA FOR THE BATCH WILL BE CHECKED FOR APPROPRIATE PROCESSING TEMPERATURES.

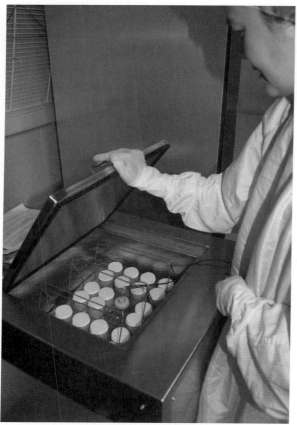

Figure 14-8 BOTTLES OF PASTEURIZED MILK FROM THE BC WOMEN'S MILK BANK. THE BOTTLE LABEL INCLUDES WHERE THE MILK WAS PROCESSED AS WELL AS THE EXPIRATION DATE (BASED ON WHEN THE MILK WAS EXPRESSED) AND THE BATCH NUMBER. SOME BANKS ALSO INCLUDE CALORIES AND PROTEIN ON THEIR BOTTLE LABELS.

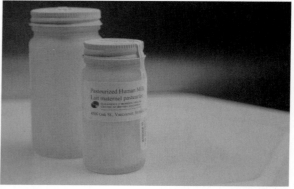

Screening Milk

Once the pasteurization is complete, a random sample bottle of milk is tested in a certified laboratory to ensure that there is no bacterial growth. Milk is not dispensed until negative test results are received, which usually takes about 48 hours (see Figure 14-9). If very low contamination is reported, the milk is retested to assure that the results are not a laboratory error. The milk is discarded if bacterial growth is still found.

Storage of Milk in the Milk Bank

Milk is stored frozen in separate freezers depending on whether it is raw or processed. The freezers are monitored and equipped with alarms to ensure that the temperature stays at −20°C or colder (see Figure 14-10).

Figure 14-9 STAFF AT WAKEMED MOTHERS' MILK BANK PACKING MILK FOR SHIPPING TO A RECIPIENT. MILK IS PACKED IN COOLERS WITH DRY ICE AND SHIPPED OVERNIGHT EXPRESS FROM MILK BANKS TO RECIPIENTS ANYWHERE IN THE COUNTRY IN BOTH UNITED STATES AND CANADA.

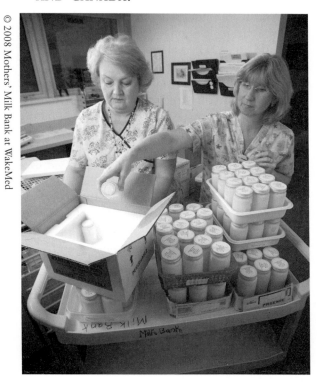

© 2008 Mothers' Milk Bank at WakeMed

Figure 14-10 FROZEN PROCESSED MILK READY FRO DISTRIBUTION AT THE SAN JOSE MILK BANK.

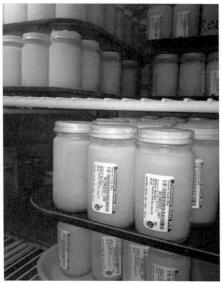

© 2013 Mothers' Milk Bank at San Jose

Recalls

Although a recall has never been necessary in an HMBANA member bank, the *Guidelines* require that every bank complete a mock recall every 3 years to ensure its recall process is workable. Currently, HMBANA requires each member bank to complete an annual accreditation process by peer-review site visits or review by an informed third party such as a health department official (HMBANA, 2013).

Informed Decision Making

Fully informed consent for selecting feeding options for infants in healthcare settings includes information on the availability of donor milk in situations where the mother cannot provide her own (Eidelman & Schanler, 2012; WHO, 2003). The evidence that human milk is the most appropriate form of nutrition and immunologic protection for preterm and fullterm infants and that not

Records

Milk bank records are carefully maintained and kept in secure areas. All banks use computer and/or written records to document all stages of screening, processing, dispensing, and contact with both donors and recipients. All milk banks are required to keep records for at least 10 years or until all recipients of the milk reach 21 years of age.

breastfeeding or providing human milk puts the infant at risk is becoming more compelling each year (Eidelman & Schanler, 2012; Stuebe, 2009).

Wet-Nursing, Informal Sharing, and Sale of Milk

In addition to obtaining PHDM from a milk bank, some mothers are increasingly seeking out milk from informal milk-sharing sources. A realistic understanding of the potential risks associated with this practice is necessary to make informed decisions.

Human milk carries a low risk of disease transmission, even in a donor situation. A study of 1091 potential donors to a HMBANA milk bank found that 3.3% of the donors tested positive on serological screening testing, including for syphilis (6), hepatitis B (17), hepatitis C (3), HTLV (6), and HIV (4) (Cohen et al., 2010). Moreover, human milk is not sterile and contains normal skin flora as well as pathogenic organisms (de Oliveira et al., 2009; Landers & Updegrove, 2010) and, like any other food, needs to be handled and stored appropriately to avoid contamination. It is an excellent growth medium for bacteria if heavily contaminated or if left at room temperature too long.

Wet-nursing, the first form of milk sharing, is the practice of breastfeeding someone else's child for hire. Wet-nursing has occurred throughout human history (Stevens et al., 2009) and continues today (Thorley, 2009). An increased demand for human milk in developed countries resulted in a resurgence of wet-nursing as reported in the popular press. This service is similar to having a nanny. There may be risks for the wet nurse (donor mother) and her child as well as the recipient child. For the donor mother, if the recipient child were to become ill, she needs to consider what, if any, her legal liability would be. For the recipient child, disease transmission risk (HIV, HTLV, possibly hepatitis B, and other viruses) is low, but it is still present.

Milk may also be contaminated if it is not handled appropriately. Direct purchase from a donor mother creates another potential risk—namely, that the milk may be altered to increase volume. Some milk sharers offer their milk via the Internet

because they have not passed the milk bank screening (Gribble, 2013). With informal milk sharing, there is no easy way for recipients to check whether they are receiving safe milk.

Risks for the donor's own child include the potential for inadequate milk intake and exposure to illness. Lactating breasts usually increase the volume of milk produced to meet the demand placed on them, however, and the woman's immune system will be developing antibodies to protect against any bacteria, viruses, or parasites to which she is exposed. In a hospital setting, if the mother wishes to have someone else provide milk for or breastfeed her child, it is essential to document all relevant information in the infant's and mother's charts.

Around 2005, the establishment of increasing numbers of Internet milk-sharing groups resulted in a dramatic increase in informal milk sharing over the Internet. The accuracy of the information provided on these milk-sharing sites varies widely, and the number of sites has increased over the last few years. Whereas some of these sites mention the importance of informed choice, safe handling, and sharing milk responsibility, they do not screen donors or handle or process milk. Unlike formal milk banks, where both donors and milk are screened and processed, informal milk sharing leaves the responsibility for "screening" up to families. In situations where the donor is well known to the recipient (a close friend or family member), the risk is probably fairly low. However, in situations where the donor and the recipient are strangers who connect over the Internet, it is impossible to define the risk. A number of sources, including the U.S. Food and Drug Administration (FDA, 2010) and Health Canada (2006, 2010), have expressed concern about the risks associated with milk sharing, including the possible spread of disease and potential for contamination of the milk.

Three well-known Internet sites promote milk sharing but do not condone the selling of human milk. *Milk Share*, established in 2004, permits donors or prospective recipients to connect for an initial $20 fee. *Eats on Feets*, established in 2010 (see http://www.eatsonfeets.org/), and *Human Milk 4 Human Babies* (http://hm4hb.net/) facilitate donors and recipients in making connections. In contrast, the website *Only the Breast*, set up in 2009, permits the buying, selling, or sharing of human milk (http://www.onlythebreast.com/). In 2013, the Internet group known as the Mother's Milk Coop appeared, describing itself as "nursing mothers (who) want to shape the future of milk banking," although the site offers sophisticated screening including blood tests (http://www.mothersmilk.coop/).

The novel use of the Internet to share human milk appears to fascinate the media. Recently several stories in lay journals and newspapers have focused on stranger-to-stranger donors and recipients. Unfortunately, the media seem to miss the important story—namely, why so many women are seeking "second best" donor milk rather than feeding their own children (Block, 2010).

In North American milk banks, several layers of donor screening, pasteurization, and a final bacterial screen of milk must be navigated before the milk is released. Each bank has well-trained donor screening personnel with access to expert advisors and current tissue banking resources. Some milk-sharing Internet groups suggest using screening criteria such as HMBANA published criteria. Unauthorized use of HMBANA screening forms and application of blood testing guidelines to assess donor suitability do not guarantee safe milk, however.

For healthcare providers, such as physicians, nurses, midwives, and International Board Certified Lactation Consultants (IBCLCs), to actively involve themselves in an informal exchange of milk raises both ethical and liability questions. The role of the healthcare provider in this type of situation is to provide information to enable the mother to make her own informed choice.

Currently, in Canada and the United States there are no federal laws to regulate the sale of human milk. However, Health Canada and the FDA are monitoring the sale of milk over the Internet. Health Canada (2006, 2010) has released a cautionary bulletin regarding this practice. A few U.S. states, including California, Maryland, New York, and Texas, have health facility regulations or laws covering donor milk banking—both collecting donor milk and dispensing it—that include adherence to HMBANA's guidelines. It is important for IBCLCs to be aware of any regulations or laws applicable where they practice.

For-Profit and Not-for-Profit Milk Banking

When women donate their milk, it is important that they clearly understand how it will be used and whether anyone will profit financially from their donation. There is one for-profit milk bank in California, which pays collection sites by the ounce for collecting milk and sells the processed milk to hospitals for a profit. Italy also has a for-profit bank (www.mommilk.eu).

In the case of HMBANA member banks, donors sign a consent form acknowledging that they will not be paid for their milk or their efforts, and that any of their milk not usable for infants may go to research on donor milk (HMBANA, 2013). Recipients are charged a processing fee (similar to that charged by other tissue banks) to partially cover the expense of screening, processing, and testing the milk; this fee is not payment for the milk itself.

Ethical questions arise with a for-profit milk banking model. In this scenario, milk becomes a commodity used to generate income for investors. Whether the for-profit bank is contacting women directly or through collection sites that are paid for the milk they collect, there is greater potential for the donor mother to feel pressured to provide a specific volume of milk regardless of her own infant's needs. Providing PHDM is less financially beneficial than producing specialty products such as human milk fortifiers made from human milk. Whereas 100% human milk fortifier has a strong appeal to breastfeeding supporters, its production presents an ethical question—produce PHDM for as many children as possible or reduce the available supply by producing a human milk fortifier (Miracle et al., 2011)?

Research Findings on Donor Milk

In 1992, Lucas and colleagues published the results of a multicenter study involving NICUs in the United Kingdom. This study found that infants fed at least some human milk in the first month of life (mother's own or donor, all by gavage) had higher IQs at 7.5–8 years old, even when controlling for psychosocial influences. Interestingly, given that this study was done in the late 1980s, at least some of the donor milk was "drip milk," or milk collected in breast shells while women breastfed their own children on the opposite breast. Even though drip milk has since been shown to have a very low fat content, the babies who received it had good long-term outcomes. Follow-up studies of this multicenter NICU cohort in the United Kingdom showed that as they reached adolescence, the children who were fed human milk (either mother's own or donor milk) had lower cholesterol and better high-density lipoprotein (HDL) to low-density lipoprotein (LDL) ratios than those children fed preterm formula (Singhal et al., 2004).

A meta-analysis of four randomized controlled trials compared the use of donor milk to human milk substitutes (formula) in terms of the incidence of necrotizing enterocolitis (NEC), a devastating bowel disease that is frequently fatal for preterm infants. Results showed the protective effect of donor human milk (McGuire & Anthony, 2003). Although none of the individual studies in this meta-analysis showed a significant risk associated with formula use, aggregating the numbers from the smaller, individual studies revealed that infants who were fed donor milk when the mother's own milk was not available were four times less likely to develop confirmed NEC. A subsequent systematic review and meta-analysis of seven studies, including five randomized controlled trials, comparing donor milk with formula found donor milk reduced the risk of NEC (Quigley et al., 2007). This Cochrane review evaluating five randomized controlled trials demonstrated a significant increased risk of NEC in preterm and low-birth-weight infants exposed to formula. In addition, the donor milk group had fewer episodes of feeding intolerance and diarrhea compared to the formula group (Boyd et al., 2007).

In contrast, Schanler et al. (2005) reported that donor milk "offered little observed short-term advantage over [preterm formula] for feeding extremely premature infants." However, the authors were careful to qualify that the parameters they measured were short-term, and as Wight pointed out (2005), this study showed a significantly lower incidence of chronic lung disease as well as a trend toward fewer days on a ventilator among the babies fed mother's own and donor milk compared to those fed preterm formula.

In addition, in an attempt to reduce NEC rates, donor milk has been used to create human milk fortifiers to replace the use of bovine-based products. Sullivan (2010) demonstrated a reduced rate of NEC with the provision of an exclusively human milk diet including fortifiers made from human milk. NEC levels in this study dropped significantly, matching the level achieved in many NICUs that use bovine fortifiers and demonstrate high breastfeeding/human milk feeding rates. Notably, of the 18 studies' authors, only one did not receive financial remuneration from the fortifier company. Embleton et al. (2013) noted that infants in this study who received bovine fortifiers also received bovine milk–based formula when insufficient mother's milk was available. Thus it is not clear whether the decrease in NEC rates resulted from use of human milk fortifier or the human milk that the other group received instead of formula.

Research over the last few years highlights the importance of "priming" the immune system appropriately through early exposure to human milk to ensure effective immunity to infection and decrease the risk of immune disorders later in life. Human milk components such as oligosaccharides and long-chain polyunsaturated fatty acids, which are not affected by pasteurization and are therefore present in donor milk, contribute to development of a healthy immune system and are not found in formula (Bertina et al., 2008; Gottrand, 2008; Kuntz et al., 2008; Marks et al., 2013; Puthia et al., 2013). A U.S. study in a large neonatal unit showed better feeding tolerance and decreased infections when using fortified mother's own milk. In addition, there was more rapid achievement of full feeds with no untoward effects related to slower weight gain, because the feedings were better tolerated (Schanler et al., 1999). Many clinicians who regularly use donor milk find the same results among babies fed donor milk.

Finally, Wight (2001) estimated that because of the reductions in length of stay, NEC incidence, and sepsis incidence, there is a relative savings of approximately $11 to the hospital or healthcare plan for each $1 spent to buy donor milk from a nonprofit bank. As far as total costs of donor milk are concerned, Carroll and Herrmann (2013) found that in a U.S. NICU, with babies weighing less than 1500 g or less than 33 weeks' gestation, most mothers were unable to provide all the milk needed. The cost of providing donor milk, either partially or exclusively, to this group ranged from $27 to $590 per day. A second study calculated the cost savings of providing a 100% human milk–based diet (including fortifiers made from human donor milk) versus mother's milk with bovine fortifier for extremely premature infants (Ganapathy et al., 2012). The authors found a shorter expected NICU length of stay and smaller total hospital costs due in part to the reduced rate of NEC associated with this practice. As discussed earlier, Embleton et al. (2013) question the reliability of the evidence used to support the current claims of effectiveness of human milk–based fortifiers. To date, no studies have compared the cost of the increased risk for high-risk infants denied PHDM due to lack of availability with the cost savings from using a 100% human milk diet. Another approach to examine the costs associated with use of donor milk is to compare the costs of providing 100 mL of the mother's own milk versus PHDM or commercial formula. The lowest institutional cost to feed very low-birth-weight infants in the NICU is realized with provision of the mother's own milk (Jegier et al., 2013).

Several published case reports describe the use of donor milk for treatment of a variety of conditions or to provide immunologic support and appropriate nutrition to full-term infants and older children (Tully et al., 2004) as well as some adults. Donor milk has been used as adjunct to other therapies in infants with chronic renal failure (Anderson & Arnold, 1993), metabolic disorders (Arnold, 1995), IgA deficiency, and allergy (Tully, 1990).

Although specific research has not been published, milk banks report many cases of feeding intolerance and allergy that have been treated with donor milk, including infants who have failed to thrive on anything but human milk. Donor milk is typically a treatment of last resort in these cases, both because of the expense and because it is not a commonly used therapy, so fewer clinicians have experience with it.

Some adult conditions respond to human milk, including hemorrhagic conjunctivitis (Centers for Disease Control and Prevention, 1982), IgA deficiency in liver transplant recipients (Merhav et al., 1995), and gastrointestinal problems such as severe reflux (Wiggins & Arnold, 1998). Research from the University of Lund in Sweden first published in 1995 found that human milk contains a unique protein, multimeric alpha-lactalbumin, that induces apoptosis (programmed cell death) in certain cancer cells (Gustafsson et al., 2005; Hakansson et al., 1995). The research group also discovered that alpha-lactalbumin-oleic acid isolated from human milk is successful as a topical treatment for skin papillomas resistant to traditional treatment (Gustafsson et al., 2004). Further work has been reported using a rat model to investigate the use of HAMLET (human alpha-lactalbumin made lethal to tumor cells), extracted from human milk, as a very specific treatment for human glioblastomas (brain tumors) (Gustafsson et al., 2005). Research focusing on the structure and function of HAMLET continues, with the goal of developing clinical applications (Noteborn, 2009). Evidence from mouse and human trials has shown that HAMLET may potentially have value in the future treatment of a number of cancers (Mossberg et al., 2009; Pettersson-Kastberg et al., 2009). Rough et al. (2009) published results from adult patients' point of view on use of human milk for cancer therapy. Most patients reported improved quality-of-life measures in the physical, psychological, and spiritual domains (McGuire, 2012).

Some of the newer research on donor milk has focused on the effects of pasteurization. Although some factors such as erythropoietin and interleukin are decreased following pasteurization, many other beneficial components such as oligosaccharides are unaffected by this process (Bertina et al., 2008; Untalan et al., 2009).

Selected Case Studies

The vast majority of individual infants receiving donor milk are premature infants, and in many countries, including Brazil and the United Kingdom, they are the only recipients of donor milk. In contrast, in North America, donor milk has also been used in many other situations. Boxes 14-1 to 14-5 illustrate cases in which donor milk was used in situations that are common in many hospitals and communities.

A TRIBUTE TO MARY ROSE TULLY

Sadly, Mary Rose Tully, my coauthor on the previous edition of this chapter, died of pancreatic cancer in January 2010. Mary Rose was one of the founders of the Human Milk Banking Association of North America and worked tirelessly to support nonprofit milk banking as well as breastfeeding women for many decades. From 2001 until her death, she was the Director of Lactation Services at Women's & Children's Hospitals, University of North Carolina (UNC) Healthcare, Chapel Hill; Adjunct Associate Professor, School of Public Health, University of North Carolina; and a faculty member in the Center for Infant & Young Child Feeding & Care at UNC. Her wonderful sense of humor and dedication to the fields of lactation and breastfeeding are greatly missed.

SUMMARY

Donor milk banking and the use of donor human milk in clinical situations is one significant strategy in the promotion, protection, and support of breastfeeding. The use of banked donor milk is a strong endorsement of the incomparable and irreplaceable nature of human milk. The first choice is always the mother's own milk except in very unusual circumstances. The 2002 WHO Global Strategy for Infant and Young Child Feeding (2003) states:

> For those few health situations where infants cannot, or should not, be breastfed, the choice of the best alternative—expressed breast milk from an infant's own mother, breast milk from a healthy wet nurse or a human-milk bank, or a breast milk substitute fed with a cup, which is a safer method that a feeding bottle and teat—depends on individual circumstances. (Section 18: [40])

BOX 14-1 BABY B CASE STUDY

Baby B was born at 28 weeks, 6 days, by emergency C-section due to fetal distress after her mother's membranes ruptured. Her mother, Marina, has Crohn's disease and developed hypertension and pre-eclampsia during pregnancy. Baby B was Marina's second baby. Her first baby was born at term by vaginal birth.

Marina described the breastfeeding as not going well, as she had little milk and gave up within the first week to completely formula-feed her baby. She was very emotional about her "failure" with her first baby. Baby B weighed 710 grams (1 pound, 9 ounces), with intrauterine growth restriction (IUGR) and was admitted to the NICU. Within 6 hours of birth, Marina learned how to hand-express her breastmilk and, within the first 24 hours, she began using her hands while pumping to maximize milk production. She was able to express a few drops of clear colostrum and was very excited. The doctors started her baby on trophic feeds within the first 24 hours using mother's expressed milk and pasteurized donor milk. Having Crohn's disease and a baby at high risk for NEC, Marina was concerned about the development of her baby's gut and was pleased that pasteurized human milk was available in the NICU for her fragile baby.

Source: BC Women's Milk Bank. Used with permission.

Box 14-2 Baby M Case Study

Baby M was born at 23:30, weighing 4252 grams (9 pounds, 6 ounces), by vaginal birth to a mother with gestational diabetes. Baby M was placed on her mother's abdomen at delivery, dried off, and placed skin-to-skin on her mother's chest. First breastfeeding took place at 30 minutes after birth. Her mother has large breasts and short nipples, and Baby M sucked on and off for about 10 minutes but did not latch well. Her mother was taught hand expression and expressed a few drops of colostrum onto a spoon and was shown how to give it to her baby. Her mother was reassured that this amount is normal and would increase over the next few days. Baby M fell asleep skin-to-skin for transfer to the postpartum area.

On admission to postpartum, the Baby M was hypoglycemic with a blood sugar of 2.0 mmol/L at 2 hours of age and needed additional milk to increase the blood sugar. Her mother could not latch the baby or express any more colostrum. Supplemental feeding options were reviewed and informed consent given to feed the baby 5 cc of pasteurized donor milk by spoon. A retest of the baby's blood sugar after an hour indicated the blood sugar level was 2.2 mmol/L. Another 5 cc of donor milk by spoon was given, and an hour later the blood glucose check indicated 2.6 mmol/L (normal range).

The mother was taught feeding cues, to keep her baby skin-to-skin, and to attempt breastfeeding on demand. Baby M's mother attempted breastfeeding about every 3 hours followed by hand expression and giving her baby her expressed colostrum by spoon until at about 24 hours, with the help of her primary nurse, and the baby began to latch and feed effectively.

Source: BC Women's Milk Bank. Used with permission.

Box 14-3 Baby L Case Study

Baby L, a healthy term breastfeeding infant with above-average weight gain, started out doing well. At 2 weeks of age, his mother had to discontinue breastfeeding for medical reasons and began feeding formula. Within 7 days of formula introduction, Baby L experienced significant weight loss. He began experiencing severe symptoms of reflux: excessive crying, frequent vomiting, refusing to feed, arching and crying when feeding was attempted, and blood in stools. He also developed a rash on his trunk. Additionally, his mother noticed a significant increase in mucus production, watery red eyes, and excessive coughing. Baby L was hospitalized for respiratory symptoms, feeding intolerance, and weight loss at 4 weeks of age. Several feeding trials with multiple formulas were attempted and failed to improve his symptoms.

At the recommendation of the pediatric gastroenterologist, Baby L was started on pasteurized donor milk. Within 5 days, his symptoms were greatly improved. At 2 weeks after donor human milk feedings started, all symptoms were gone.

At approximately 4 months of age, a feeding trial was attempting using a hypoallergenic formula. Within 24 hours, an eczema-type rash appeared on Baby L's trunk and mucus production increased. He experienced severe wheezing that prompted an emergency room visit. His oxygen saturation was low upon admission. He was diagnosed with severe allergies.

At 8 months old, Baby L remained on donor human milk with no return of symptoms and above-average weight gain.

Source: 2013 Mothers' Milk Bank of North Texas.

BOX 14-4 BABY K CASE STUDY

Baby K was born at 41 weeks' gestation and weighed 2892 grams (6 pounds, 6 ounces). Born with a ventricular septal defect (VSD), an atrial septal defect (ASD), and an aortal coarctation, she underwent heart surgery at 6 days of age. The surgeon nicked a lymph node and the baby developed chylothorax, a condition that is incompatible with feedings that contain fat. Baby K did not tolerate Portagen formula. The milk bank provided nonfat donor human milk, which was initially given via gastric nasal tube, and then orally. Baby K started on 40 mL per feeding and her family was able to take her home a week sooner than expected. The number of calories per day was not an issue at this point, as getting any nutrition was the critical challenge. Donor milk was the only medical choice for this fragile child, as it helped to prevent infections and helped in her recovery from surgery.

Note: To provide low-fat donor milk, the milk bank uses a process that involves refrigerating the frozen milk for at least 12 hours and removing the low-fat whey via tubing and syringe. This low-fat milk is placed in a new container and provided for feeding. To produce even lower-fat milk, the removed whey can be centrifuged and the aspiration process repeated.

Source: 2013 Mothers' Milk Bank Denver Colorado.

BOX 14-5 BABY P CASE STUDY

Baby girl P was born at 35 weeks' gestation due to placental insufficiency. She spent 5 days in the NICU, during which time her mother was breastfeeding and expressing milk for her. At 2 weeks postpartum, her mother's supply was still only at half what Baby P needed, and she began to exhibit signs of feeding intolerance whenever formula was used. Treatment for reflux did not alleviate the symptoms (discomfort and difficulty with stooling). She was tried on six different formulas. She was then referred to a pediatric gastroenterologist, who recommended even more formulas to try.

Based on the parents' observation that when she was fed strictly her mother's milk, Baby P was comfortable and happy, the parents went to the Internet seeking donor milk. They found the HMBANA website and contacted their nearest milk bank. After discussions with the baby's physicians, donor milk was prescribed and her symptoms began to subside quickly. After 3 weeks, the physician wanted to try two more hypoallergenic formulas. Baby P's symptoms returned with each of them. She had difficulty with stooling and stopped gaining weight well. She was put back on donor milk and began thriving and gaining weight well. Her mother observed that milk from donors on dairy-free diets seemed to agree with her the most. Milk from a pool of three donors on dairy-free diets was tried. Baby P's symptoms increased, so the milk bank created pools from each donor separately. One donor's milk gave her the most relief from symptoms. The milk bank contacted that donor with a request to increase her volume, if possible. She did for several weeks. During this time, Baby P's mother developed mastitis and her milk supply diminished completely, so starting at 5 months Baby P was exclusively on donor milk and thriving even when she did not get exclusively dairy-free milk.

This case is unusual because targeting of a specific donor to the recipient is rarely done, but is possible in situations such as this one, where the baby is not thriving.

Used with permission of WakeMed Health & Hospitals Milk Bank.

KEY CONCEPTS

- Donor human milk banks recruit and screen donors, and collect, process, screen, and distribute donated milk to meet the needs of individuals for whom donor milk is prescribed by a licensed healthcare provider.
- Donating milk can be therapeutic for a bereaved mother and provision of information enables mothers to make informed decisions about this option.
- The screening process is based on blood and tissue donor screening, with additional criteria unique to human milk.
- Donor milk is provided in situations where the mother's own milk is insufficient or unavailable and there is a medical need for human milk.
- Effective support of breastfeeding is important but use of donor milk, when the mother's own milk is not available, ensures the highest standard of care particularly for ill and high-risk infants.
- The first known donor milk bank was established in Vienna in 1909.
- The first known milk bank in North America was established in 1910 in Boston, Massachusetts.
- By the 1940s, the American Academy of Pediatrics had developed guidelines for donor milk banking.
- During the 1970s and early 1980s, there was a proliferation of formal and informal hospital and community-based donor milk banks.
- The Human Milk Banking Association of North America (HMBANA) was founded in 1985 with a goal of standardizing milk banking operations.
- In the mid-1980s, with the awareness of CMV and HIV combined with the development and promotion of specialty preterm formulas, many donor milk banks closed.
- Currently donor milk banking is growing globally as research indicates that human milk—mother's own or donor—is optimal for infants.
- Pasteurized human milk from screened donors has a stronger safety record than products that are used to replace it.

- One of the primary barriers to use of donor milk is the lack of awareness and education among healthcare providers.
- For healthcare professionals to involve themselves in an informal exchange of human milk raises both ethical and liability questions. Although informal sharing usually carries a low risk, screening of potential donors needs to be completed by personnel trained to complete milk bank screening. Over the last 10 years, there has been an upswing in milk sharing due to the use of the Internet and increased awareness of the value of human milk. Unfortunately, effective support for breastfeeding has not enjoyed the same response.
- HMBANA member banks in North America, as well as most donor milk banks everywhere else in the world, are nonprofit organizations, which ensures that the safest product is available at the lowest possible cost.

INTERNET RESOURCES

American Academy of Pediatrics statement on breastfeeding and human milk: http://pediatrics.aappublications.org/content/early/2012/02/22/peds.2011-3552

Breastfeeding Committee of Canada (BCC): www.breastfeedingcanada.ca

CDC breastfeeding resources: www.cdc.gov/breastfeeding

European Milk Banking Association: http://www.europeanmilkbanking.com/

Human Milk Banking Association of North America: www.hmbana.org

Journal of Human Lactation: http://jhl.sagepub.com/archive

United Kingdom Association for Milk Banking: www.ukamb.org

United States Breastfeeding Committee: www.usbreastfeeding.org

REFERENCES

Almeida SG, Dorea JG. Quality control of banked milk in Brasilia, Brazil. *J Hum Lact.* 2006;22:335–339.

Anderson A, Arnold LD. Use of donor breast milk in the nutrition management of chronic renal failure: three case histories. *J Hum Lact.* 1993;9:263–264.

Apple RD. "To be used only under the direction of a physician": commercial infant feeding and medical practice, 1870–1940. *Bull Hist Med.* 1980;54:402–417.

Apple RD. "Advertised by our loving friends": the infant formula industry and the creation of new pharmaceutical markets, 1870–1910. *J Hist Med Allied Sci.* 1986;41:3–23.

Arnold LD. Use of donor milk in the treatment of metabolic disorders: glycolytic pathway defects. *J Hum Lact.* 1995;11:51–53.

Arslanoglu S. *Establishing the first HMB in Turkey.* Presentation given at the HMBANA Conference "Embracing Human Milk in the 21st Century: Practice, Research and Results." Las Vegas, NV, April 23–24, 2012.

Arslanoglu S, Ziegler EE, Moro GE. Donor human milk in preterm infant feeding: evidence and recommendations. *J Perinatal Med.* 2010;38:347–351.

Arslanoglu S, Moro GE, Bellù R, et al. Presence of human milk bank associated with elevated rate of exclusive breastfeeding in VLBW infants. *J Perinatal Med.* 2013;41:129–131.

Baack ML, Norris AW, Yao J, Colaizy T. Long chain polyunsaturated fatty acid levels in US donor human milk: meeting the needs of premature infants? *J Perinatol.* 2012;32:598–603.

Baker J. The infants' milk stations: their relation to the pediatric clinics and to private physician. *Arch Pediatr.* 1914;31:165–170.

Barret C, Hiscox I. The collection and preservation of breast milk. *Can Nurs.* 1939;1:15–18.

Bertina E, Coppa GV, Giuliani F, et al. Effects of Holder pasteurization on human milk oligosaccharides. *Int J Immunopathol Pharmacol.* 2008;21:381–385.

Blackman J. Lessons from history of maternal care and childbirth. *Midwives Chron Nurs Notes.* 1977;3:46–49.

Block J. Move over milk banks: Facebook and milk sharing. 2010. Available at: http://www.time.com/time/health /article/0,8599,2032363,00.html. Accessed May 20, 2013.

Boyd CA, Quigley MA, Brocklehurst P. Donor breast milk versus formula for preterm infants: systematic review and meta analysis. *Arch Dis Child Fetal Neonatal Ed.* 2007;92:F169–F175.

Brady JP. Marketing breast milk substitutes: problems and perils throughout the world. *Arch Dis Child.* 2012;97:529–532.

Breton P. *The Dionne years.* New York, NY: WW Norton; 1978.

Carroll K, Herrmann K. Introducing donor human milk to the NICU: lessons for Australia. *Breastfeed Rev.* 2012;20:19–26.

Carroll K, Herrmann KR. The cost of using donor human milk in the NICU to achieve exclusively human milk feeding through 32 weeks of postmenstrual age. *Breastfeed Med.* 2013;8:286–290.

Centers for Disease Control and Prevention. *Morbidity and Mortality Weekly Report (MMWR).* Acute hemorrhagic conjunctivitis—American Samoa. *MMWR.* 1982;3:1.

Chan GM, Lechtenberg E. The use of fat-free human milk in infants with chylous pleural effusion. *J Perinatol.* 2007;27:434–436.

Codex Alimentarius. *Standard for infant formula and formulas for special medical purposes intended for infants.* Geneva, Switzerland: World Health Organization; 2007.

Cohen R. Retrospective review of serological testing of potential human milk donors. *Arch Dis Child Fetal Neonatal Ed.* 2010;95:F118–F120.

De Almeida JAG. *The Iberoamerican program of human milk banks: creating a world day of human milk donation. Donor breastmilk: in support of breastfeeding.* Lisbon, Spain: EMBA International Congress; October 5–6, 2012.

Delfosse NM, Ward L, Lagomarcino AJ, et al. Donor human milk largely replaces formula-feeding of preterm infants in two urban hospitals. *J Perinatol.* 2013;33:446–451.

de Oliveira PR, Yamamoto AY, de Souza CB, et al. Hepatitis B viral markers in banked human milk before and after Holder pasteurization. *J Clin Virol.* 2009;45:281–284.

Edwards TM, Spatz D. Making the case for using donor human milk in vulnerable infants. *Adv Neonatal Care.* 2012;12:273–278.

Eidelman AI, Schanler R. Breastfeeding and the use of human milk. Section on Breastfeeding. *Pediatrics.* 2012;129:e827–e841.

El-Khuffash A, Unger S. The concept of milk kinship in Islam: issues raised when offering preterm infants of Muslim families donor human milk. *J Hum Lact.* 2012;28:125–127.

Embleton N, King C, Jarvis C, et al. Effectiveness of human milk-based fortifiers for preventing necrotizing enterocolitis in preterm infants: case not proven. *Breastfeed Med.* 2013;8:421.

Food and Drug Administration (FDA). *Frequently asked questions about FDA's regulation of infant formula.* College Park, MD: FDA; 2006.

Food and Drug Administration (FDA). Use of donor human milk. 2010. Available at: http://www.fda.gov/Science Research/SpecialTopics/PediatricTherapeuticsResearch /ucm235203.htm. Accessed May 20, 2013.

Ganapathy V, Hay JW, Kim JH. Costs of necrotizing enterocolitis and cost-effectiveness of exclusively human milk-based products in feeding extremely premature infants. *Breastfeed Med.* 2012;7:29–37.

Giuliani F, Prandi G, Coscia A, et al. Donor human milk versus mother's own milk in preterm VLBWIs: a case control study. *J Biol Regul Homeost Agent.* 2012;26(3 suppl):19–24.

Gottrand F. Long-chained polyunsaturated fatty acids influence the immune system of infants. *J Nutr.* 2008;138:1807S–1812S.

Gribble KD. Peer-to-peer milk donors' and recipients' experiences and perceptions of donor milk banks. *JOGNN.* 2013;42:451–461.

Grovslien AH, Gronn M. Donor milk banking and breastfeeding in Norway. *J Hum Lact.* 2009;25:206–210.

Gustafsson L, Leijonhufvud I, Aronsson A, et al. Treatment of skin papillomas with topical alpha-lactalbumin-oleic acid. *N Engl J Med.* 2004;350:2663–2672.

Gustafsson L, Hallgren O, Mossberg AK, et al. HAMLET kills tumor cells by apoptosis: structure, cellular mechanisms, and therapy. *J Nutr.* 2005;135:1299–1303.

Gutiérrez D, de Almeida JA. Human milk banks in Brazil. *J Hum Lact.* 1998;14:333–335.

Hakansson A, Zhivotovsky B, Orrenius S, et al. Apoptosis induced by a human milk protein. *Proc Natl Acad Sci USA.* 1995;92:8064–8068.

Health Canada. *Information update: Health Canada raises concerns about sale and distribution of human milk.* Ottawa, Canada: Health Canada; 2006.

Health Canada. Health Canada raises concerns about the use of unprocessed human milk. 2010. Available at: http://www.hc-sc.gc.ca/ahc-asc/media/advisories-avis/_2010/2010_202-eng.php. Accessed April 24, 2014.

Human Milk Banking Association of North America (HMBANA). *Guidelines for the establishment and operation of a donor human milk bank.* Raleigh, NC: HMBANA; 2013.

Jefferson DL. Child feeding in the United States in the nineteenth century. *J Am Diet Assoc.* 1954;30:335–344.

Jegier BJ. The institutional cost of acquiring 100 mL of human milk for very low birth weight infants in the neonatal intensive care unit, 2013. *J Hum Lact.* 2013;29:390–399.

Jeppesen DI, Ersbøll AK, Hoppe TU, et al. Normal thymic size and low rate of infections in human donor milk fed HIV-exposed uninfected infants from birth to 18 months of age. *Int J Pediatr.* Epub April 30, 2013. doi: 10.1155/2013/373790.

Jones F. History of North American donor milk banking: one hundred years of progress. *J Hum Lact.* 2003;19:313–318.

Jones F. *Best practice for expressing, storing and handling human milk in hospitals, homes and child care settings.* Fort Worth, TX: HMBANA; 2011.

Kim, J, Unger S. Position statement: human milk banking. Canadian Pediatric Society. *Paediatr Child Health.* 2010;15:595–598.

Kuntz S, Rudloff S, Kunz C. Oligosaccharides from human milk influence growth-related characteristics of intestinally transformed and non-transformed intestinal cells. *Br J Nutr.* 2008;99:462–471.

Landers S, Updegrove K. Bacteriologic screening of donor human milk before and after Holder pasteurization. *Breastfeed Med.* 2010;5:117–121.

Ley SH, Hanley AJ, Stone D, O'Connor DL. Effects of pasteurization on adiponectin and insulin concentrations in donor human milk. *Pediatr Res.* 2011;70:278–281.

Lucas A, Morley R. Does early nutrition in infants born before term programme later blood pressure? *BMJ.* 1994;309:304–308.

Lucas A, Morley R, Cole TJ, et al. Early diet in preterm babies and developmental status in infancy. *Arch Dis Child.* 1989;64:1570–1578.

Lucas A, Brooke OG, Morley R, et al. Early diet of preterm infants and development of allergic or atopic disease: randomised prospective study. *BMJ.* 1990;300:837–840.

Lucas A, Morley R, Cole TJ, et al. Breast milk and subsequent intelligence quotient in children born preterm. *Lancet.* 1992;339:261–264.

Lucas A, Morley R, Cole TJ, Gore SM. A randomised multicentre study of human milk versus formula and later development in preterm infants. *Arch Dis Child Fetal Neonatal Ed.* 1994;70:F141–F146.

Mackenzie C. Mothers' knowledge of and attitudes toward human milk banking in South Australia: a qualitative study. *J Hum Lact.* 2013;29:222–229.

Marks LR, Clementi EA, Hakansson AP. Sensitization of *Staphylococcus aureus* to methicillin and other antibiotics *in vitro* and *in vivo* in the presence of HAMLET. *PLoS One.* 2013;8(5):e63158.

McGuire E. Ruth goes home: an adult's use of human milk. *Breastfeed Rev.* 2012;20:44–48.

McGuire W, Anthony MY. Donor human milk versus formula for preventing necrotising enterocolitis in preterm infants: systematic review. *Arch Dis Child Fetal Neonatal Ed.* 2003;88:F11–F14.

McHaffie LP. The artificial feeding of young babies. *Can Nurs.* 1927;23:635–664.

Merhav HJ, Wright HI, Mieles LA, Van Thiel DH. Treatment of IgA deficiency in liver transplant recipients with human breast milk. *Transpl Int.* 1995;8:327–329.

Miracle DJ, Szucs KA, Torke AM, Helft PR. Contemporary ethical issues in human milk-banking in the United States. *Pediatrics.* 2011;128:1186–1191.

Montjaux-Regis N, Cristini C, Arnaud C, et al. Improved growth of preterm infants receiving mother's own raw milk compared with pasteurized donor milk. *Acta Paediatr.* 2012;100:1548–1554.

Mossberg AK, Wullt B, Gustafsson L, et al. Bladder cancers respond to intravesical instillation of HAMLET. *Int J Cancer.* 2007;121:1352–1359.

NICE guidelines: donor breast milk banks: the operation of donor breast milk bank services. CG93. United Kingdom: National Institute for health and care Excellence; 2010. Available at: http://pathways.nice.org.uk/pathways/donor-breast-milk-banks/donor-breast-milk-banks-overview.

Noteborn MH. Proteins selectively killing tumor cells. *Eur J Pharmacol.* 2009;625:165–173.

Olieman JF, Penning C, Ijsselstijn H, et al. Enteral nutrition in children with short-bowel syndrome: current evidence and recommendations for the clinician. *J Am Diet Assoc.* 2010;110:420–426.

Ortiz F. Breast milk banks. From Brazil to the world. Inter Press Service News Agency; 2012. Available at: http://www.ipsnews.net/2012/09/breast-milk-banks-from-brazil-to-the-world/PATH. Accessed April 14, 2013.

Program for Appropriate Technology in Health (PATH). Driving transformative innovation to save lives 2013. Available at: www.path.org. Accessed April 23, 2014.

Perrine CG, Scanopn KS. Prevalence of use of human milk in US advanced care neonatal units. *Pediatrics.* 2013;131:1066–1071.

Pettersson-Kastberg J, Mossberg AK, Trulsson M, et al. Alpha-lactalbumin, engineered to be nonnative and inactive, kills tumor cells when in complex with oleic acid: a new biological function resulting from partial unfolding. *J Mol Biol.* 2009;394:994.

Puthia M, Storm P, Nadeem A, et al. Prevention and treatment of colon cancer by peroral administration of HAMLET (human a-lactalbumin made lethal to tumour cells). *Gut.* 2013. Available at: http://gut.bmj .com/content/early/2013/01/23/gutjnl-2012-303715 .full. Accessed June 20, 2013.

Quigley MA, Henderson G, Anthony MY, McGuire W. Formula milk versus donor breast milk for feeding preterm, low birth weight infants. *Cochrane Database Syst Rev.* 2007;4:CD002971.

Rawls WE, Wong CL, Blajchman M, et al. Neonatal cytomegalovirus infections: the relative role of neonatal blood transfusion and maternal exposure. *Clin Invest Med.* 1984;7:13–19.

RedeBlh: Brazil Milk Bank website. 2013. Available at: http://www.redeblh.fiocruz.br/cgi/cgilua.exe/sys/start .htm?tpl=homeRed. Accessed May 10, 2013.

Rivera A. *Growth issues for preterm infants fed donor milk.* Human Milk for Human Infants: Evidence & Application, HMBANA Conference. Fort Worth, TX, November 8, 2007.

Rough SM, Sakamoto P, Fee CH, Hollenbeck CB. Qualitative analysis of cancer patients' experiences using donated human milk. *J Hum Lact.* 2009;25:211–229.

Schanler RJ. Evaluation of the evidence to support current recommendations to meet the needs of premature infants: the role of human milk. *Am J Clin Nutr.* 2007;85:625S–628S.

Schanler RJ, Shulman RJ, Lau C. Feeding strategies for premature infants: beneficial outcomes of feeding fortified human milk versus preterm formula. *Pediatrics.* 1999;103:1150–1157.

Schanler RJ, Lau C, Hurst NM, Smith EO. Randomized trial of donor human milk versus preterm formula as substitutes for mothers' own milk in the feeding of extremely premature infants. *Pediatrics.* 2005;116:400–406.

Shaikh U, Ahmed O. Islam and infant feeding. *Breastfeed Med.* 2006;1:164–167.

Singhal A, Cole TJ, Fewtrell M, Lucas A. Breast milk feeding and lipoprotein profile in adolescents born preterm: follow-up of a prospective randomised study. *Lancet.* 2004;363:1571–1578.

Steube A. The risks of not breastfeeding. *Rev Obstet Gynecol.* 2009;2:222–231.

Stevens EE, Patrick TE, Pickler R. A history of infant feeding. *J Perinatal Ed.* 2009;18(2):32–39.

Stuebe A. The risks of not breastfeeding for mothers and infants. *Rev Obstet Gynecol.* 2009 Fall;2(4):222–231.

Sullivan S. An exclusively human milk–based diet is associated with a lower rate of necrotizing enterocolitis than a diet of human milk and bovine-based products. *J Pediatr.* 2010;156:562–567.

Technical Advisory Group (TAG) on Milk Banking Meeting. Seattle, WA: PATH; November 2012.

Thorley V. Mothers' experiences of sharing breastfeeding or breastmilk co-feeding in Australia 1978–2008. *Breastfeed Rev.* 2009;17:9–18.

Tow A. Simplified infant feeding: a four hour feeding schedule. *Arch Pediatr.* 1934;51:49–50.

Tully MR. Banked human milk in the treatment of IgA deficiency and allergy symptoms. *J Hum Lact.* 1990;6:75.

Tully MR, Lockhart-Borman L, Updegrove K. Stories of success: the use of donor milk is increasing in North America. *J Hum Lact.* 2004;20:75–77.

United Nations. UN Convention on the Rights of the Child. 1990. Available at: http://www.ohchr.org/EN /ProfessionalInterest/Pages/CRC.aspx. Accessed July 9, 2013.

Untalan PB, Keeney SE, Palkowetz KH, et al. Heat susceptibility of interleukin-10 and other cytokines in donor human milk. *Breastfeed Med.* 2009;4:137–144.

Vandenberg LN, et al. Human exposures to bisphenol A: mismatches between data and assumptions. *Rev Environ Health.* 2013;28(1):37–58.

Vieira AA, Soares FV, Pimenta HP, et al. Analysis of the influence of pasteurization, freezing/thawing and offer processes on human milk's macronutrient concentrations. *Early Hum Dev.* 2011;7:577–580.

Walker M. Recalls of infant feeding products. 2013. NABA. Available at: http://www.naba-breastfeeding. org/images/Formula%20Recalls-W.pdf. Accessed July 31, 2013.

Wellborn J. *Lactation support for the bereaved mother: a toolkit— information for healthcare providers.* Fort Worth, TX: HMBANA; 2012.

Wiggins PK, Arnold LD. Clinical case history: donor milk use for severe gastroesophageal reflux in an adult. *J Hum Lact.* 1998;14:157–159.

Wight NE. Donor human milk for preterm infants. *J Perinatol.* 2001;21:249–254.

Wight NE. Donor milk: down but not out. *Pediatrics.* 2005;116:1610.

Wood AL. The history of artificial feeding of infants. *J Am Diet Assoc.* 1955;31:474–482.

World Health Organization (WHO). *Guidelines on optimal feeding of low birth-weight infants in low- and middle-income countries.* Geneva, Switzerland: WHO; 2011.

World Health Organization (WHO). *Global strategy for infant and young child feeding.* Geneva, Switzerland: WHO; 2003.

Wright CM, Waterston AJ. Relationships between paediatricians and infant formula milk companies. *Arch Dis Child.* 2006;91:383–385.

Yeager AS, Palumbo PE, Malachowski N, et al. Sequelae of maternally derived cytomegalovirus infections in premature infants. *J Pediatr.* 1983;102:918–922.

Expressing, Storing, and Handling Human Milk

Human milk is a living tissue. As such, it has many properties that both preserve its integrity and protect the infant. However, it is important to recognize that each step in the collection and storage process may affect the final product. Expression, collection, and storage recommendations may vary somewhat depending on the health of the child or infant, whether premature, full-term, healthy, or ill. Recommendations will also depend on where the milk will be stored and fed, whether in the home, hospital, or child care setting.

To preserve the composition of the milk and maximize the benefit to the infant, freshly expressed milk should be used whenever possible (Edwards & Spatz, 2012; Auslanangu et al., 2010, Montjaux-Regis et al., 2011). Providing optimal nutrition is important. As long as human milk has been expressed and stored in a manner that renders the product bacteriologically safe, human milk is far superior to any replacement product except in extremely unusual circumstances. There is limited research on the precise effect of storage on human milk and none to show that at a specific time or temperature the milk spoils. In the case of a preterm or ill infant, use of fresh milk is always optimal, and milk that has been refrigerated and not been used within 48 hours probably should be frozen to better preserve the immunologic properties. However, freezing decreases the activity of the digestive enzymes in the milk.

Issues to consider that may affect the immunological function, caloric content, and nutritional value of the milk include the following:

- Careful hand washing and appropriate cleaning of pump parts
- Determining the most appropriate type of expression/pump for the mother's situation and baby's condition
- Type of storage container
- Clean (sterile is not necessary)
- Glass or hard plastic containers are preferred for preserving immunologic function of the milk. Note: Scientific concerns have been raised regarding storage or heating of any food in polycarbonate plastics (hard, clear plastics) because they can release bisphenol A, an endocrine disruptor, into the milk or other food (Vandenberg et al., 2013).
- Polyethylene bags increase the risk of spillage from tears in the bag, and research has shown that fats tend to stick to the plastic (Jones, 2011).

Human milk that has been refrigerated retains its antibacterial activity for several days, and data show that bacterial counts in refrigerated expressed milk gradually decrease over time (Jones, 2011). However, enzymatic activity continues during refrigeration and is significantly slowed by freezing, so the recommendation to freeze preterm infants' milk that has not been used within 48 hours is at least partially based on slowing enzyme activity. Shortterm storage for healthy full-term infants or young children who receive most of their nutrition through direct breastfeeding presents a wider range of options when compared to storage for premature or otherwise compromised infants. Optimal handling and storage is far more critical when infants are premature or otherwise compromised and may have implications for nutrient supplementation. When infants are receiving all of their nutrition from expressed milk, every effort must be made to maximize the nutritional and immunologic value of the milk. For example, Buss et al. found that loss of vitamin C is significant during storage (Buss et al., 2001); therefore, babies primarily fed expressed, stored milk require vitamin C supplementation. Even when storage and handling of milk is optimal,

premature infants may need additional fortification of their human milk feedings given their individual nutritional needs.

In addition to optimal handling and storage, it is important that each baby receive his or her own mother's milk. Many facilities require two staff members to check the label on the milk container prior to feeding it to the infant to minimize the risk of error. When an infant receives another mother's milk in error, the most commonly expressed concern is disease transmission. Although the chances of this are minimal, followup should include an apology to both mothers that the error occurred, blood testing of the unintended donor (or confirmation that it has been done recently), and counseling and reassurance for both the mother whose milk was misappropriated and the parents of the baby given the wrong milk (Jones & Tully, 2006).

Section
Four

Beyond Postpartum

CHAPTER 15   Women's Health & Breastfeeding

CHAPTER 16   Maternal Employment & Breastfeeding

CHAPTER 17   Child Health

CHAPTER 18   The Ill Child: Breastfeeding Implications

CHAPTER 19   Infant Assessment

The reproductive phase of a woman's life span can potentially last up to 40 years although actual childbearing years are fewer. Most women are healthy during their childbearing years, and it is rare that a mother's health is detrimental to her ability to lactate. Nonetheless, some mothers encounter health issues, acute or chronic, many of which can be treated or resolved in a manner that preserves breastfeeding. Major concerns for the breastfeeding woman include her child's health, her employment outside the home, and concerns relating to her fertility and resumption of sexual activity after the birth of her infant. Infant assessment provides the baseline for assisting both the healthy and the ill breastfeeding child.

Chapter 15

Women's Health and Breastfeeding

Barbara Morrison
Karen Wambach

Pregnancy, birth, and breastfeeding make up important phases of a woman's life during her reproductive years. However, because most women are healthy during this period, it is also a time for health promotion both for the mother and for her family (Fielding & Gilchick, 2011; Zell, 2011). Habits changed and established during the reproductive years can affect each family member for the rest of their life. While women's health care is worthy of a book in and of itself, in this chapter we discuss the impact of a number of health issues on breastfeeding, from initial recovery after birth, to birth spacing and interconception care, to the influence of acute and chronic illnesses. Areas for health promotion are highlighted (Fahey & Shenassa, 2013). Although lactation consultants usually do not see the more serious health concerns described in this chapter, they need a working knowledge of these conditions so as to plan care based on the wishes and needs of the breastfeeding mother who has a health problem.

Postpartum Health and Care

Because of the cyclical nature of menstruation, pregnancy, birth, and breastfeeding, it is difficult to know where to start the discussion of issues of women's health during the reproductive years. Given that this text and chapter focus on breastfeeding and the impact of women's health on breastfeeding, and vice versa, we will begin with the immediate postpartum period when breastfeeding is initiated. Indeed, the primary focus of care in the first days and weeks after birth is the establishment of breastfeeding. This time is significant because of the neurohormonal changes accompanying birth that not only initiate and stimulate contractions, but also influence women's instinctive emotional, physical, social, and behavioral responses during the transition to motherhood (Dixon et al., 2013; Saltzman & Maestripieri, 2011):

- High levels of oxytocin resulting from labor and pushing promote calm and connectedness (Uvnas-Moberg, 2003) as well as milk letdown and involution.
- Falling levels of progesterone after delivery of the placenta allow for increasing levels of prolactin (Djiane & Durand, 1977).
- High levels of prolactin lead to the up-regulation of prolactin receptors so that milk production can occur (Kim et al., 1997).
- Release of oxytocin reduces stress and anxiety, improves social memory, and increases generosity toward and trust in others (Bell et al., 2014; Carter, 2014; Uvnas-Moberg et al., 2005).
- The endogenous opioids—that is, oxytocin and norepinephrine—contribute to a sense of comfort and security for mother and infant (Nelson & Panksepp, 1998).
- Release of oxytocin and prolactin promotes maternal behaviors (Feldman et al., 2011; Grattan et al., 2001).

Table 15-1 ACTION INDUCED OR STIMULATED BY ELEVATED LEVELS OF OXYTOCIN AND RELATED HORMONES DURING THE POSTPARTUM

Maternal Characteristics	Interaction Characteristics	Physiological Characteristics
Connection	Well-being	Decreased cortisol levels
Relaxation	Friendliness	Relaxation of muscles
Calm	Closeness	Decreased cardiovascular activity
Contentment	Trust	Activation of vagal, parasympathetic nervous system
Happy	Loyalty	Suppression of HPA axis
Peaceful	Giving	Suppression of SAM system
Warm	Receiving	Low, healthy, balanced level pulse rate and blood pressure
Open	Love	Stimulation of growth and restorative processes
Generous	Unity	Promotion of digestion and storing of nutrients
Empathetic	Positive social interaction	Related to sense well-being and relaxation
Reduced arousal	Stimulates maternal interactions	Participates in metabolic prerequisites for milk production—stimulating glucagon release and mobilization of glucose
	Stimulates attachment between mother & child	Reduced levels of anxiety
		More social activity

Note: HPA: hypothalamic-pituitary-adrenocortical axis; SAM: sympatho-adreno-medullary regulatory processes

- Elevated prolactin levels suppress sexual drive and fertility (Lyons & Broberger, 2014).

See Table 15-1 for additional ways that oxytocin affects both mother and infant.

With an appreciation for what is happening physiologically, care providers can create a postpartum environment promoting prolonged periods of skin-to-skin holding, frequent breastfeeding, rest, support with breastfeeding and infant care, and decreased stressors such as numerous interruptions so the hormonal milieu remains optimal for lactogenesis and attachment (Bick et al., 2012; Morrison & Ludington-Hoe, 2012; Wray, 2006a). Unfortunately, postpartum care has become known as the "Cinderella" (Wray, 2006a) of perinatal care, causing mothers to express their frustrations and desires as follows:

- "Constant interruptions from visitors, doctors, cleaners, paper sellers, bounty people, etc. I just wanted some sleep" (Wray, 2006b, p. 250).
- "They [breastfeeding sessions] were good, but it was hard having visitors; probably would

have done it [breastfeeding] more. Tried to squeeze it in when visitors left" (Morrison et al., 2006, p. 713).
- "I do like the two-hour quiet, no visitors, one until three. I think that's a really important thing" (Beake et al., 2010, p. 4).
- "I have been impressed by the number of hours, the amount of bedside time that the staff working here are able to provide rather than just saying, 'I will come and spend a few minutes trying to help you.' . . . People have been prepared to come and spend an hour full stop helping you" (Beake et al., 2010, p. 5).
- "I got the impression that because I chose to bottle-feed, feeding help and advice was overlooked" (Wray, 2006b, p. 252).

In our hurry to get back to "normal," we have forgotten that important physiological, psychological, and social work is being done as mothers and newborns adjust to life together outside the womb (Clements, 2009). It is incumbent upon healthcare providers to provide an environment and support in ways that enhance the processes occurring within and between the mother–newborn dyad. Indeed, Bick and colleagues (2012) reported that after multiple revisions to in-hospital postpartum care and processes to improve breastfeeding and maternal health (Box 15-1), more mothers initiated breastfeeding and breastfed at any point or exclusively for a longer duration, they had fewer common morbidities while hospitalized, and they expressed greater satisfaction with their own care. Similar breastfeeding and satisfaction

results have been reported in the United States for hospitals achieving the Baby-Friendly Hospital designation (DiFrisco et al., 2011; Taylor et al., 2012).

Numerous health benefits accrue for mothers who exit early postpartum care confident in their breastfeeding abilities and who breastfeed, preferably exclusively, for an extended period of time. The neurohormonal adaptations occurring during lactation influence reproduction, sexuality, and both the short- and long-term health benefits and risk reductions for mothers and infants.

BOX 15-1 CHANGES MADE IN ONE MATERNITY UNIT IN AN ENGLISH HOSPITAL TO IMPROVE BREASTFEEDING AND MATERNAL HEALTH OUTCOMES

- Revision of care processes informed by continuous quality improvement methodology
  - ◀ Set goals
  - ◀ Support breastfeeding initiation and duration
  - ◀ Enhance women's postnatal recovery through evidence-based practices and mothers' desires for care and preparation for discharge
- Diagnose the current situation
  - ◀ Interviews with wide range of stakeholders to elicit perceptions of barriers and facilitators to effective in-patient postpartum care
  - ◀ Process mapping of the "journey" mothers travel through postpartum care to identify restrictions in the system following various modes of birth
  - ◀ Identifying where revisions to care were necessary and possible
- Change in documentation of care to comply with the *Clinical Negligence Scheme for Trusts* (CNST) maternity clinical risk management standards
- Pilot and implement documentation to enhance support for breastfeeding and to identify maternal physical and psychological heath needs in a timely manner
  - ◀ Symptom checklist to prompt early identification and management of common maternal morbidities such as breastfeeding issues, backache, urinary problems, or pain
  - ◀ Signs and symptoms checklist for early identification of potentially severe morbidities such as upper genital tract infections or elevated blood pressure, with referral as indicated
- Longer stays in delivery suite (2 to 3 hours) after vaginal births to facilitate skin-to-skin contact and early breastfeeding initiation
- Transfer of responsibility for care of women identified as high risk to midwife immediately after birth
- Postpartum discharge preparation beginning in the delivery suite
- Multiple education methods for parents including demonstrations of infant care and revised postnatal information booklet with translation into languages commonly spoken by mothers
- Numerous workshops for staff to discuss revisions to care systems and processes, to explain new documentation and to provide opportunity for discussion of concerns

Source: Data from Bick et al., 2012.

Lactation, Fertility, Sexuality, and Contraception

Fertility, sexuality, and contraception are interrelated aspects of reproduction, and breastfeeding affects each, making the reproductive aspects of women's lives more complex during lactation than during the nonlactating state (Figure 15-1). Although breastfeeding clearly has a fertility-reducing effect on the nursing mother, the nature of this effect is not fully understood. In general, the infant's suckling initiates a cycle of neuroendocrine events that results in the inhibition of ovulation. One consequence of this inhibition is the creation of a hypoestrogenic state in the woman. Similar to what occurs with menopause, the hypoestrogenic state of lactating women may cause a dry, sometimes atrophic, vaginal mucosa, possibly resulting in pain upon intercourse. Because of this and other circumstances, many breastfeeding women have sexual intercourse infrequently and, therefore, are at reduced risk of pregnancy. Emotions related to motherhood, such as intense (albeit normal) involvement with the infant, and feelings of undesirability on the part of a mother who has not recovered her prepregnancy body, may affect her sexual behavior as well. Fear of subsequent pregnancy may also play a role in coital behavior, thereby influencing risk of pregnancy. As some contraceptives may relieve the vaginal symptoms of hypoestrogenicity as well as lessen the fear of pregnancy, coital frequency may also be related to family planning choice. These are but a few examples of the interrelationships among fertility, sexuality, contraception, and lactation. It is fitting that they should be explored together.

Fertility

The Demographic Impact of Breastfeeding

The natural birth-spacing effect of breastfeeding has been recognized for many years. In the past few decades, demographers have been able to quantify, in various ways, the degree of contraceptive protection

Figure 15-1 The Interrelationships Among Fertility, Contraception, and Lactation. (A) In the absence of a family planning intention, the phenomena of reproduction and sexual behavior (fertility and sexuality) are related in the most simple and direct manner. (B) When a family planning method is used for spacing or limiting pregnancies, it clearly affects fertility, and sometimes also sexual behavior (e.g., coitus-dependent methods). (C) Lactation can have independent effects on fertility, sexual behavior, and contraceptive decisions and patterns of use.

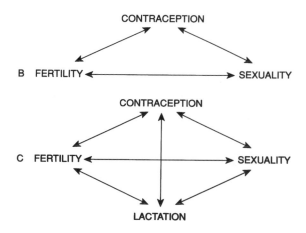

that results from breastfeeding. In populations without access to modern methods of family planning, birth spacing is the major determinant of total fertility (the total number of children a woman will bear), and the birth interval depends for the most part on breastfeeding (Bongaarts & Menken, 1983; Bongaarts & Potter, 1983). Demographers describe the fertility-suppressing effect of breastfeeding as the extent to which contraceptive prevalence would need to increase to offset a projected decline in breastfeeding and its concomitant decrease in natural contraceptive protection (Bongaarts & Potter, 1983). For example, in countries where contraceptive prevalence is low and breastfeeding prevalence is high, modest declines in breastfeeding duration would require the tripling or better of other contraceptive use to prevent an increase in the existing, already high fertility in the country (Thapa et al., 1988). In more developed countries where breastfeeding practices have profoundly decreased, such as the United States and the United Kingdom, the contraceptive effects of breastfeeding are demographically insignificant and the prevalence of contraceptive use is high.

Menstrual Cycle

During the normal menstrual cycle in the nonlactating woman, the hypothalamus secretes gonadotropin-releasing hormone (GnRH) in a pulsatile fashion, which in turn triggers a pulsatile release of luteinizing hormone (LH) from the anterior pituitary. LH pulses play a major role in follicular growth and estrogen secretion. In the first days of the menstrual cycle, the growing ovarian follicles produce increasing amounts of estrogen, which in turn appear to increase the frequency of LH pulses. When estrogens reach a critical level, a surge of LH occurs, which is followed by ovulation in about 17 hours. After ovulation, a corpus luteum is formed that produces estrogens and progesterone, and GnRH and LH secretion declines.

By about 4 weeks postpartum, plasma levels of LH return to a normal level in nonbreastfeeding women, and cyclicity begins anew, although the first few cycles are not always normal. In lactating women, LH levels remain lower than normal and, more importantly, pulsation is not normal. In exclusively breastfeeding women, baseline levels of LH remain lower than normal even in the presence of follicular development. Presumably, suckling interferes with the normal secretion of GnRH by the hypothalamus, in turn disrupting normal pulsatile LH secretion (Figure 15-2). Thus, normal follicular development does not ensue. Small amounts of estrogen are secreted but they are insufficient to cause an LH surge and ovulation. An experiment to test this presumption involved the administration of pulsatile GnRH to breastfeeding women, after which follicular development, ovulation, and luteinization were observed (Labbok, 2007; McNeilly, 2001a, 2001b).

Increased levels of prolactin are clearly associated with breastfeeding patterns. It has been postulated that prolactin has inhibitory effects on gonadotropin secretion and/or ovarian function. Nevertheless, the role of prolactin remains uncertain: some lactating women show normal ovulatory cycles despite high levels of prolactin (Diaz et al., 1995), and pulsatile GnRH infusion can induce follicular development and ovulation in hyperprolactinemic breastfeeding women (Glasier et al., 1986). Possibly, the decline in suckling causes both the decrease in prolactin and the improvement in LH pulsation, while the relationship between prolactin and hypothalamic inhibition is only coincidental (McNeilly, 2001a, 2001b). The complexity of the return of fertility for lactating women is appreciated, as is the irony that the baby is in charge of it all.

Lactational Amenorrhea

The period of lactational amenorrhea rather than the period of breastfeeding is considered the phase of natural infertility (Aryal, 2007; Short et al., 1991). The duration of lactational amenorrhea depends on numerous factors; however, if a mother exclusively breastfeeds for the first 6 months postpartum, lactational amenorrhea is 98% effective as a method of contraception. This effectiveness rate is similar to the effectiveness of reversible methods of fertility regulation such as pills or intrauterine devices (IUDs). Obviously, a small proportion of women experience their first normal postpartum ovulation and conceive during the period of lactational amenorrhea. Therefore, investigators posit that a woman will have no more than one ovulation during amenorrhea. If she

Figure 15-2 PHYSIOLOGICAL MECHANISMS INVOLVED IN LACTATIONAL INFERTILITY.

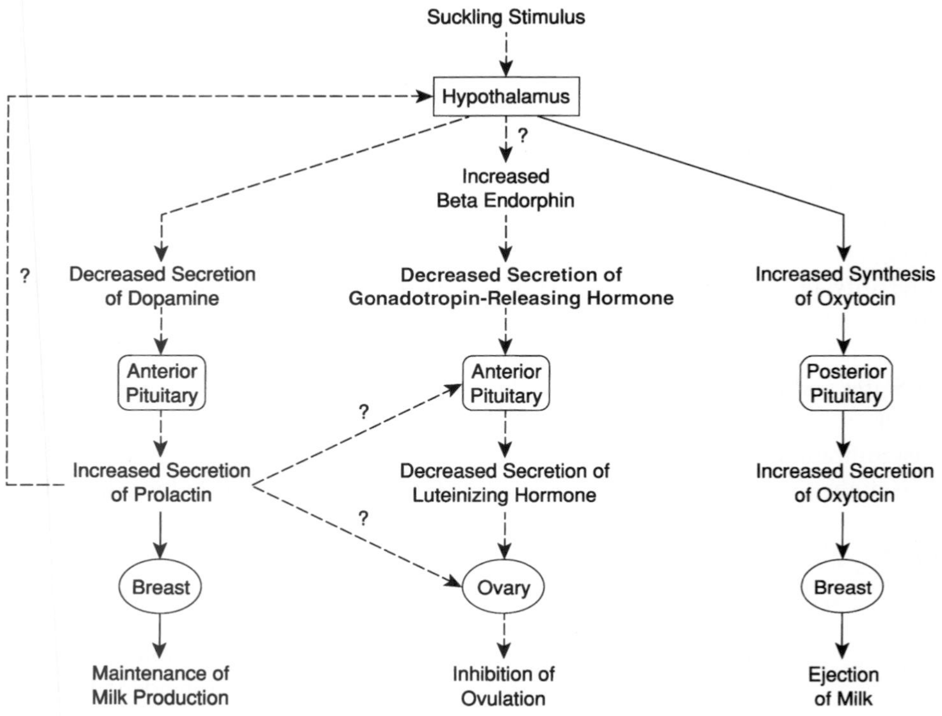

Source: Adapted from Short, 1984.

does ovulate during amenorrhea, the event will usually occur shortly (0 to 3 weeks) before the first postpartum menses.

The duration of lactational amenorrhea and the concomitant return of ovulation and menses are highly variable among different populations around the world (Garcia & Mella, 2013). For example, in urban populations, first menses will occur before the sixth month postpartum for as many as 30% of exclusively breastfeeding mothers (McNeilly et al., 1994; Tracer, 1996). Some women repeatedly experience "inadequate" menstrual cycles—that is, cycles in which too little progesterone is produced to sustain a fertilized ovum after the end of lactational amenorrhea. Indeed, some women who wish to conceive are unable to do so until after the breastfeeding child has been totally weaned, as even token breastfeeding may provide enough inhibitory stimuli to prevent ovulation or to allow adequate progesterone production. Generally, the earlier in the postpartum period that a woman experiences her first menses, the less likely it is that this first bleeding episode will be preceded by ovulation (Howie et al., 1981, 1982; Perez et al., 1972). The earlier in the postpartum period that the first ovulation occurs, the less likely it is to be characterized by a luteal phase of adequate duration and progesterone production (McNeilly et al., 1982).

The Suckling Stimulus

The infant's suckling is the stimulus that controls the negative feedback inhibition of the normal cycling of the hypothalamic–pituitary–ovarian axis, but accurate measurement or quantification of the suckling stimulus has proved difficult. In general, researchers have relied on measures such as the frequency of breastfeeding episodes, the duration of each episode, total minutes of suckling, and intervals between suckling episodes, as well as each of these measures classified by day and by night. All of these approaches have led to development of indices of how often suckling occurred. However, recent work by Geddes and colleagues (Geddes et al., 2008, 2012; Sakalidis et al., 2013) using ultrasound to visualize tongue movement and pressure sensors to measure intra-oral vacuum has provided descriptions of suckling characteristics. Use of ultrasound and other new technologies hold promise for better understanding the role of infant suckling in lactational amenorrhea (Geddes, 2009).

While suckling is recognized as the stimulus that controls the negative feedback inhibition of fertility and reproduction, researchers from around the world have demonstrated that the relative frequency of breastfeeds or the breastfeeds as a proportion of all feeds is the best correlate of the risk of ovulation during breastfeeding. Women whose first ovulation occurs before 6 months postpartum have a significantly lower percentage of breastfeeds to total feeds in the first 6 months (84%) compared to women whose first ovulation occurs later (88%) (Eslami et al., 1990; Gray et al., 1990). Although the difference in breastfeeds as a proportion of all feeds is statistically significant (84% versus 88%), this difference is clinically insignificant; thus this factor cannot be used in practice as a sign of impending fertility. Other studies have shown that women do not ovulate if they breastfed their baby at least 6 times in 24 hours for a total of at least 65 minutes (Andersen & Schioler, 1982; McNeilly et al., 1983, 1985). Such frequency and duration of breastfeeding appear effective in maintaining levels of prolactin consistent with those observed during anovulation (Delvoye et al., 1977). However, subsequent prospective studies on the return of ovulation during lactation found no such minimum value of breastfeeding frequency that could be relied upon to suppress ovarian activity; some women may ovulate despite up to 15 breastfeeding episodes per day (Elias et al., 1986; Israngkura et al., 1989; Rivera et al., 1988; Shaaban et al., 1990).

The wide range of minimal feeding frequency required to prevent ovulation may be due to measurement differences across studies and mothers' definitions of a breastfeed. For example, for some women, a breastfeed is a highly ritualized affair that takes some time to accomplish. It involves changing the baby's diaper, preparing a beverage for the mother to consume during the feed, taking the phone off the hook, settling into a particular rocking chair, suckling for 20 minutes or so, and putting the baby (who may have slipped off to sleep) back into the crib. These breastfeeds occur, for example, five to six times a day and one to two times per night, perhaps with the baby nursing in the parents' bed. By contrast, other women may identify their baby's cue to feed before the first whimper. Such a mother may breastfeed for 3 to 4 minutes until the baby regains serenity, as often as 15 to 20 times day and night. Given these different definitions of a "breastfeed," it is not surprising that a "magic number" of breastfeeds that will keep all women ovulation free has not been identified.

Nevertheless, when studying a large number of women, frequent breastfeeding remains an important correlate of lactational infertility (Jones, 1988, 1989) depending on which other variables are measured and controlled. Thus, while it is difficult to generalize across mother–baby pairs the total number of minutes of suckling needed for the mother to remain anovulatory, many investigators hypothesize that since frequent suckling produces higher milk yields than occasional suckling, mothers who breastfeed more frequently will also feed for a longer total duration; that is, the more milk there is, the longer it will take for the baby to obtain it. Howie et al. (1981) found this relationship to be so strong that frequency and duration could be substituted one for the other. Like every other aspect of breastfeeding (and fertility), this generalization needs to be tempered by recognition of normal individual variations. For example, the need of a given baby to suckle for comfort may affect both breastfeeding frequency and duration. Some babies are efficient sucklers and obtain milk quickly, whereas others are more methodical and unhurried, just as children and adults vary in their speed of food consumption at the dinner table.

Another correlate of the duration of lactational infertility is actually a measure of not breastfeeding. The interval between breastfeedings is an inverse expression of both frequency and duration: the number of intervals will be high if the frequency is high, and the length of the average interval will be low if the duration or the frequency of breastfeeds is high. Measuring average intervals between feedings yields no new information or advantage over measuring frequency and duration of feedings. However, the longest interval between feedings reflects a different characteristic from all others mentioned thus far.

Recognizing that the duration of lactational infertility is strongly influenced by infant feeding patterns, the World Health Organization (WHO) conducted a prospective study of more than 4000 breastfeeding women in seven countries to learn whether the duration of lactational infertility could be predicted (WHO, 1998b, 1998c). Eighty-three variables were available for analysis: 32 were infant feeding variables and 51 were other characteristics of the mother and infant. Many measures of the suckling stimulus (such as breastfeeding frequency, duration, and intervals between feeds) were tested. As should be expected, not all of the 32 breastfeeding (or infant feeding) factors were significant predictors of the duration of lactational amenorrhea because these factors are often interrelated, or simply slightly different ways of defining the same variable. After controlling for center-related differences across the five developing country and two developed country settings, 10 factors were found, in a multivariate analysis, to be significantly related to the duration of amenorrhea; 7 of the 10 were infant feeding characteristics (Box 15-2). Whether the infant was breastfeeding versus totally weaned was, not surprisingly, a highly significant predictor of lactational amenorrhea. The total duration of breastfeeding per 24 hours and the interval between birth and the first breastfeed were also significant determinants of the duration of amenorrhea. Several significant factors were related to supplementation, such as the time until regular supplementation commenced and the percentage of all feeds that were breastfeeds.

BOX 15-2 FACTORS RELATED TO DURATION OF AMENORRHEA

Nonfeeding Variables

1. (High) number of live births = longer amenorrhea***
2. (High) maternal body mass index at 6 to 8 weeks postpartum = shorter amenorrhea***
3. (High) percentage follow-up visits in which infant was ill = longer amenorrhea***

Feeding Variables

4. (Long) time from delivery to first breastfeed = shorter amenorrhea**
5. (Yes) regular supplementation with any food or drink = shorter amenorrhea**
6. (High) total 24-hour duration of breastfeeding = longer amenorrhea*
7. (High) percentage of feeds constituted by breastmilk = longer amenorrhea***
8. (High) frequency of water/noncaloric supplements = longer amenorrhea***
9. (Yes) weaned = shorter amenorrhea***
10. (Yes) supplements compose 50% of feeds = shorter amenorrhea**

* $p < 0.05$
** $p < 0.01$
*** $p < 0.001$

Source: Adapted from World Health Organization, 1998a, 1998b.

The WHO Multinational Study of Breastfeeding and Lactational Amenorrhea clearly demonstrated a profound effect of suckling on the duration of amenorrhea. It also suggested that, among a large number of ways of defining the suckling stimulus, the simple presence of breastfeeding and the 24-hour duration of breastfeeding were the breastfeeding factors most closely associated with the duration of amenorrhea. Had the study not measured the suckling stimulus in these particular ways, some other quantification of the suckling stimulus—such as the frequency of breastfeeding or the longest interval between suckling episodes—would have proved to be statistically significant.

Supplemental Feeding

The role that supplementation plays in the return of fertility is anything but straightforward. A prevailing assumption is that anything that decreases the child's suckling behavior or the need to suckle will be a secondary cause of the recovery of fertility. Supplementation may have the effect of decreasing hunger, thirst, and possibly the emotional need for comfort, thereby reducing suckling at the breast.

The pioneering work of the Medical Research Council in Edinburgh found this to be the case (Howie et al., 1981). In a sample of Scottish women, the initiation of supplements to the infant occurred very shortly before the first ovulation. Supplementation was thought to be causally related to the recovery of ovulation because of the close temporal relationship between the two events. By contrast, in studies conducted in developing countries, instances have been observed in which supplements are introduced to the baby without any impact on the underlying maternal ovarian hormone profile (Figure 15-3). In such cases, the supplements usually consist of gradual additions to the baby's diet; like the maternal ovarian hormone levels, the breastfeeding behaviors remain essentially unchanged. A study of well-nourished Australian women who breastfed for an extended period of time also did not find supplementation to be associated with returning fertility (Lewis et al., 1991), presumably because the introduction of supplements was gradual and their quantities were small. By contrast, in the Scottish studies, a supplement generally consisted of a milk substitute that was given as a replacement for a breastfeed, so that the suckling stimulus was decreased.

Supplementation has also been shown to have an effect on the duration of lactational amenorrhea independent of breastfeeding frequency and duration (Benitez et al., 1992; Jones, 1989). It is possible that supplementation might change some of the more elusive characteristics of breastfeeding, such as suckling strength, rather than just frequency and duration. As seen in Box 15-2, five of the seven significant infant feeding variables that predicted the return of menses in the large WHO study were actually measures of supplementation (WHO, 1998b). The effect of supplementation on the return of fertility is likely to be a function of the degree to which weaning foods replace the suckling stimulus. Additionally, the strength and the nature of the relationship between infant feeding characteristics (such as breastfeeding frequency and time until supplementation) and the return of fertility change with the duration of lactation. For example, if the duration of lactation is short, supplementation is probably more strongly associated with the return of fertility than if lactation extends over a long period.

The Repetitive Nature of the Recovery of Fertility

A significant association exists between the duration of lactational infertility after one pregnancy and the duration in the same woman after her next pregnancy (Kennedy, 1993). This relationship has been confirmed in several large prospective studies. For example, Ford (1992) reported that in sample of 418 Bangladeshi women followed through the course of breastfeeding two consecutive babies, the length of amenorrhea while breastfeeding the first child had significant predictive value for the subsequent length of amenorrhea. In addition, in the WHO Multinational Study of Breastfeeding and Lactational Amenorrhea (WHO, 1998b), the duration of lactational amenorrhea after the previous pregnancy was recorded at the time of admission. This single predictor was so highly significant and explained so much of the variance in the duration

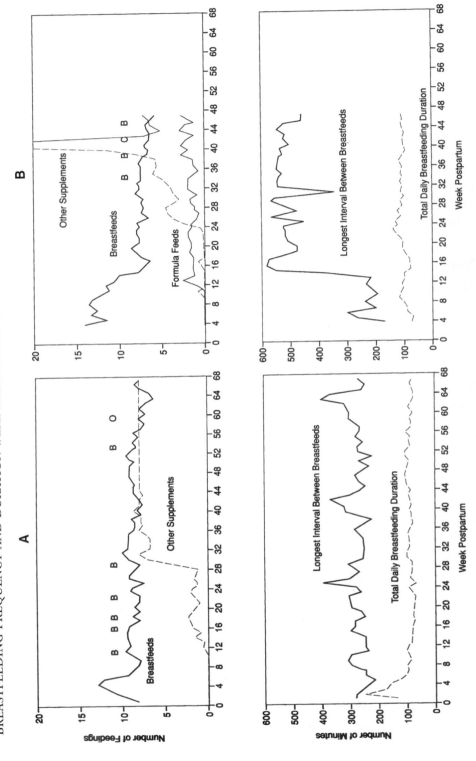

Figure 15-3 THE EFFECT OF SUPPLEMENTATION ON BREASTFEEDING. (A) IN ONE EXAMPLE, THE INTRODUCTION OF SUPPLEMENTS AT POSTPARTUM WEEK 28 HAD NO EFFECT ON BREASTFEEDING FREQUENCY, DURATION, OR THE INTERVAL BETWEEN FEEDINGS. (B) IN ANOTHER EXAMPLE, THE INTRODUCTION OF SUPPLEMENTS AT ABOUT WEEK 9 COINCIDED WITH A DECREASE IN BREASTFEEDING FREQUENCY AND AN INCREASE IN THE LONGEST INTERVAL BETWEEN BREASTFEEDS. OVULATION WAS STILL POSTPONED FOR ABOUT 10 MONTHS, PROBABLY BECAUSE BREASTFEEDING FREQUENCY AND DURATION WERE HIGH ENOUGH.

Source: Data from Rivera R, Kennedy KI, Ortiz E, et al. Breastfeeding and the return to ovulation in Durango, Mexico. Fertil Steril. 1988;49:780–787.

of lactational amenorrhea in the prospective study that no other factor in a multivariate analysis was significantly associated with the duration of lactational amenorrhea.

If a woman is to experience the same duration of infertility (or of amenorrhea) while breastfeeding two consecutive babies, the breastfeeding behavior must presumably be essentially similar in both cases. In turn, the amount of neurosensory stimulation received by the mother through suckling would be approximately the same, eliciting roughly the same fertility-repressing effect in the woman. We can suppose that this is likely to happen in many cases because several factors would be almost the same in both breastfeeding couplets:

- The organism of the mother is the same; that is, her basic physiology is essentially the same unless a long interval between births causes age-related changes in organismic responses to reproductive hormones.
- A mother's orientation to infant feeding, and her ideas and habits about breastfeeding, probably remain constant across the two experiences. However, if a mother's pattern of breastfeeding changes markedly, the length of recovery of fertility will also differ.
- Two infants with markedly different needs and personalities could potentially cause different effects on the mother's return to fertility.

If the duration of the previous period of lactational amenorrhea is known, this information may be useful in making a decision about when to start postpartum contraception. Additionally, information about the average duration of lactational amenorrhea may inform community programs as to the most effective approaches to postpartum contraception (Weiss, 1993).

The Bellagio Consensus

By 1988, researchers on five continents had completed prospective studies of the changes in ovarian hormones in breastfeeding women. Many of these researchers gathered in Bellagio, Italy, to determine whether their findings about women with vastly different patterns of breastfeeding behavior could be synthesized into a statement about how breastfeeding might predict women's recovery of fertility (Box 15-3). The basis for the Bellagio consensus statement was a collection of published and unpublished studies of the pregnancy rates (3 studies in two countries), as well as data on the probability of a recognizable pregnancy from prospective studies on the recovery of ovulation during lactation (10 studies in seven countries). Among these studies, the highest pregnancy rate reported in fully breastfeeding amenorrheic women during the first 6 months postpartum was lower than 2% (Family Health International, 1988; Kennedy et al., 1989).

The Bellagio Consensus states that bleeding in the first 56 days postpartum can be ignored. This claim has been confirmed by several prospective studies of postpartum bleeding. For 477 experienced breastfeeding mothers in the Philippines, postpartum bleeding lasted a median of 27 days and did not vary by age, parity, breastfeeding frequency, or level of supplementation. Additionally, more than

---

BOX 15-3 THE BELLAGIO CONSENSUS

Lactational amenorrhea should be regarded as a potential family planning method in all maternal and child health programs in developing and developed countries.

Postpartum women should be offered a choice of using breastfeeding as a means of family planning, either to help achieve optimal birth spacing of at least 2 years, or as a way of delaying the introduction of other contraceptives. They should be informed of how to maximize the antifertility effects of breastfeeding to prevent pregnancy.

Breastfeeding provides more than 98 percent protection from pregnancy during the first 6 months postpartum if the mother is "fully" or nearly fully breastfeeding and has not experienced vaginal bleeding after the 56th day postpartum.

one-fourth of these mothers experienced a subsequent bleeding episode beginning not later than postpartum day 56. Only 10 mothers may have had their first cyclic menses before day 56, but none of them became pregnant (although not all were sexually active at this point) (Visness et al., 1997). In another prospective study of 72 fully breastfeeding mothers in developed countries, nearly half of them experienced some bleeding or spotting between the sixth and eighth weeks postpartum. Despite ovarian follicular development in 7 of the 72 cases, none of the mothers ovulated in the first 8 weeks postpartum. Finally, findings from the WHO Multinational Study of Breastfeeding regarding the return of menses are consistent with the advice to ignore bleeding prior to postpartum day 56 (WHO, 1999a).

The Bellagio Consensus is important because it reflects principles that are believed to be applicable across cultures. Yet this aspect of the consensus is also one of its weaknesses: when making generalizations that apply to a range of breastfeeding patterns and practices, some possible situations cannot be accommodated. For example, in societies in which a child is breastfed for 2 years or more, or among mothers in industrialized countries who choose to breastfeed for these longer periods, lactational amenorrhea alone may be a viable marker of returning fertility. Cognizant of this fact, Kennedy, Rivera, and McNeilly (1989, p. 485) issued a cautionary note:

> Guidelines specific to a particular country or population for using breastfeeding as a postpartum family-planning method can be developed based on this consensus. Local infant feeding practices, the average duration of amenorrhea, and the ongoing changes in women's status and health practices should be considered in adapting these general guidelines.

The consensus is also important because it represents the framework for the actual use of lactational amenorrhea as a method of contraception. Guidelines on how to integrate the lactational amenorrhea method (LAM) into family planning and breastfeeding support programs have been developed based on the Bellagio Consensus (Labbok et al., 1994).

During the 8 years after the Bellagio Consensus, a new body of research was undertaken to test the consensus prospectively. Four clinical trials of the contraceptive efficacy of LAM were conducted in Chile (Perez et al., 1992), in Pakistan (Kazi et al., 1995), in the Philippines (Ramos et al., 1996), and on a multinational scale (Labbok et al., 1997). These studies observed women who chose to use LAM as their postpartum contraceptive method and were taught and actually used the method. The researchers found cumulative 6-month life-table rates of pregnancy during correct use of the method of 1.0%, 0.5%, 1.5%, and 0.6%, respectively. Additionally, secondary data analyses conducted on the data sets used for the original consensus showed that the protection from pregnancy under the LAM conditions can outlast the parameters set in the Bellagio Consensus (Rojnik et al., 1995; Short et al., 1991; Weiss, 1993). The largest secondary analysis was from the WHO Multinational Study of Breastfeeding and the Return of Menses, where the findings on pregnancy during lactation also upheld the claims made in the Bellagio Consensus (WHO, 1999a). On the basis of these studies and unpublished research from a variety of sources, scientists who reconvened at Bellagio in 1995 were able to conclude "the Bellagio Consensus has clearly been confirmed" (Kennedy et al., 1996). Having accumulated data and experience from prospective clinical trials, the group at "Bellagio II" was able to draw conclusions about the modification of LAM on a local level (see Box 15-3).

Questions continue to be asked about the mechanisms underlying lactational amenorrhea. Energy balance has been explored in relationship to nutritional intake (McNeilly, 2001a; Valeggia & Ellison, 2009) and work (Garcia & Mella, 2013; Valdes et al., 2000). However, the role of nutrition and work/exercise in the suppression of fertility during lactation is complex, making it difficult to confirm any correlations. Energy allocation models even allow consideration of the effects of social, political, and cultural practices on fertility regulation (Daglas & Antoniou, 2012). Energy balance can also impact hormone release as a response to stressor and nonnoxious stimuli.

Perhaps the greatest unspoken question at this time has to do with the healthfulness of 6 months of exclusive breastfeeding and maternal ability to exclusively breastfeed for at least 6 months. A meta-analysis done in the early part of the 21st century compared health outcomes with 4 versus 6 months of exclusive breastfeeding (Kramer & Kakuma, 2002). The authors of the analysis proposed a dose effect and, therefore, suggested that longer duration of exclusive breastfeeding provides greater benefit to mothers and infants (Kramer & Kakuma, 2012).

In the years since the original meta-analysis, numerous organizations—including the Academy of Breastfeeding Medicine (ABM), the American Academy of Pediatrics (AAP), the American Dietetic Association (ADA), the Centers for Disease Control and Prevention (CDC), and WHO—have developed position papers and guidelines promoting at least 6 months of exclusive breastfeeding with continued exclusive breastfeeding as complementary foods are introduced (ABM, 2008; AAP, 2012; ADA, 2009), The International Lactation Consultant Association publishes *Clinical Guidelines for the Establishment of Exclusive Breastfeeding* (ILCA, 2014).

Postpartum Well-Being and Sexual Health

Postpartum well-being and sexual health are complex and influenced by physical, hormonal, social, cultural, and emotional changes accompanying the transition to parenthood (Leeman & Rogers, 2012). While sexual health encompasses much more than sexual expression, the discussion in this section is based on two assumptions:

- A stable union between a breastfeeding woman and her male partner is presupposed simply for convenience. Nevertheless, the majority of lactating mothers are heterosexual, and there is little, if any, research focusing on the sexuality of breastfeeding single and lesbian women. It is likely that much of the following discussion will apply to all women.
- Libido or sexual desire is the main driving force or motivation for sexual expression (although

the desire to please one's partner is also recognized as a motivation). It is recognized that many women have intercourse against their will or without sexual desire, but the role of breastfeeding in coercive or indifferent sexual relationships is not considered here.

Libido

At least five categories of factors may influence sexual drive or desire during lactation:

- Common situational factors unrelated to breastfeeding
- Libido-inhibiting influences related to parturition
- Libido-inhibiting influences of lactation
- Libido-enhancing factors related to pregnancy, birth, and lactation
- Lactation factors related to the breastfeeding woman's partner

Common Situational Factors Unrelated to Breastfeeding

Many preexisting factors that either facilitated or inhibited sexual arousal before pregnancy or birth remain a part of a woman's living experience, family routine, or personal preference after birth (Yee et al., 2013). Preexisting factors that inhibit libido—such as the chronic illness of one of the partners, fear of pregnancy, or lack of privacy—persist and are unrelated to breastfeeding. If a couple has a dysfunctional or unsatisfying sexual rapport, it is no more likely to be spontaneously remedied by lactation than a faltering marriage is to be "saved" by adding a child to the family chemistry.

Conversely, there is no reason to assume that individualized stimuli per se, such as a preferred cologne, a special song, or candlelight, should lose their excitatory effects because a baby joins the family. Opportunity to attend to the old stimuli, however, is another matter. Some of the preexisting sexual stimuli or circumstances associated with sexual opportunity may be decreased due to having a young baby in the home. For example, the couple may find that they now lack time alone and that they endure constant interruptions—especially, it seems, at night. The quiet evening at home may seem gone forever.

Libido-Inhibiting Influences Related to Parturition

Physical recovery from vaginal delivery takes approximately 6 weeks, albeit with some variation across women. Postpartum abstinence or perineal rest is recommended during this time period to allow for healing and to prevent infection. Indeed, postpartum abstinence is sensible until the mother decides she has sufficient physical comfort to resume sexual activity.

Tenderness from the episiotomy, tears, and vulvo-vaginal or perineal stress following vaginal delivery usually lasts for several months. Although the mother's stitches may have dissolved and the perineum healed, she may still experience discomfort during intercourse. Indeed, results of multiple studies over the past three to four decades (Abraham et al., 1990; Barrett, Pendry, et al., 2000; Grudzinskas & Atkinson, 1984; Yee et al., 2013) suggest that many mothers resume intercourse within the first 3 months and that 40% to 50% of them report experiencing dyspareunia (pain upon intercourse). By 6 months postpartum, reports of dyspareunia decrease by half, but mothers report achieving comfort during intercourse from 1 month to more than 12 months post birth. Mode of birth and presence of an episiotomy are not significant predictors of either the resumption of sexual activity or the rating of sexual function (Abraham et al., 1990; Yee et al., 2013). After the initial distressing event, many mothers refrain from further coitus (Grudzinskas & Atkinson, 1984). Indeed, the anticipation of pain during intercourse may cause mothers to avoid sexual suggestion. A clear understanding of feelings and ongoing communication may help the couple to defer intercourse until some future time and to express their love and caring in other ways.

Another source of pain during intercourse may stem from the precipitous decline in ovarian steroid levels soon after birth. This decline leads to a state of hypoestrogenemia. Especially among breastfeeding women, the period of hypoestrogenemia can endure for the entire lactation course. As in menopause, lactation-related hypoestrogenemia can cause the vaginal epithelium to be very thin and to secrete little fluid during arousal. In such a case, dryness and pain are experienced during intercourse, and vaginal tears are possible. Although dyspareunia declines greatly by the sixth postpartum month, breastfeeding is one of the few predictors of prolonged discomfort or pain, probably due to vaginal dryness (Barrett, Pendry, et al., 2000). Atrophy of the vaginal mucosa can be relieved quickly and easily by the use of inert, water-based lubricants.

The drastic hormonal changes postpartum can also be associated with noticeable mood changes. The immediate effect is usually temporary and probably overlaps with the period of postpartum abstinence. In some women, postpartum depression can follow delivery immediately or occur after a few days or weeks. Although the etiology of postpartum depression is not well understood, it probably has both endogenous and exogenous sources. Some women experience emotional vulnerability when their progesterone levels are low, as happens during the postpartum period. (By way of analogy, the symptoms of premenstrual syndrome in the nonpregnant woman are often relieved by progesterone administration.) The overwhelming needs of the new baby plus other familial and extra familial responsibilities are more than enough to make a normal person weary. Thus the role of exogenous sources in development of postpartum depression should not be underestimated. Depression is commonly characterized by a lack of sexual drive, and postpartum depression is no exception.

Even if the mother does not experience postpartum depression, she will probably be spending most of her emotional energy caring for and bonding with her newborn. This process is sometimes likened to a love affair in which infatuation with one's beloved is like an obsession. It is difficult to refrain from thinking about and doing things for the object of one's affection. Between mother and infant, this bonding serves exceedingly important functions by creating an enduring parental talent and commitment in the mother and a sense of trust and security in the infant.

However, this process can preclude opportunity and emotional availability for the partner.

One mother described these feelings during lactation:

> When you are home and you touch, hold, hug, and nurse all day, you're not so interested in it when your husband walks through the door. But then his day has been all talk all day and no touch, and he's ready. It creates a problem. (Riordan, 1983)

Psychological factors unrelated to hormones or to attachment can also be strong inhibitors of libido. Fear of pregnancy can be an important inhibitor of sexual drive. If the new baby was unplanned—and especially if a contraceptive failure occurred—sexual inhibition could understandably be great. Parents of a firstborn child sometimes have trouble synthesizing the roles of lover and mother or father, because the parental role was previously understood subconsciously to be asexual. Colic or minor or major problems with the infant can decrease sexual interest in either partner, and if a mother who has no previous parenting experience faces a difficult parenting challenge, she may be even less emotionally available to her partner. Preexisting marital difficulties may manifest themselves in an exclusive emphasis on the child and neglect of the adult love relationship. One mother suggested that the factors contributing to a decrease in the frequency of sexual relations were not very complex or deeply rooted and were probably unrelated to any particular psychological construct. She declared simply, "Our priorities changed! When you have kids, there are lots of other things to do, and your values change."

Libido-Inhibiting Influences of Lactation

Libido is thought to be elevated during the middle of the menstrual cycle in normal, nonlactating women. The midcycle is the period during which peaks in follicle-stimulating hormone, luteinizing hormone, and estrogen are observed. Accordingly, libido in the breastfeeding woman may be linked to one or more of these substances.

A study of parturients in New South Wales showed that breastfeeding duration longer than 5 months was associated with longer duration of discomfort during intercourse as well as longer periods of lactational amenorrhea (Abraham et al., 1990). This finding supports an association between the hormonal milieu during breastfeeding and sexual activity. It is recognized that mothers who bottle-feed their babies tend to resume coitus earlier and to have intercourse more frequently than breastfeeding mothers, which similarly supports a hormone–libido association (Meston & Frohlich, 2000).

Another hormone that can influence libido and is present in high levels during breastfeeding is prolactin. Nonbreastfeeding women and men with abnormally high levels of prolactin frequently complain of decreased sexual interest; if given bromocriptine (a dopamine agonist that lowers prolactin levels), their sexual desire returns. A few studies have identified a similar phenomenon in breastfeeding mothers who report decreased sexual desire during breastfeeding as compared to prepregnancy levels of sexual desire (Meston & Frohlich, 2000). During the initiation of breastfeeding, prolactin levels are excessively high to facilitate the up-regulation of prolactin receptors. Elevated prolactin levels have also been associated with mood disturbances such as anxiety and depression, which can cause decreased sexual desire as well. More research is needed to fully understand the interaction between prolactin and sexual desire and behavior, especially in breastfeeding mothers.

As if the emotional demands of parenthood are not enough, breastfeeding adds another dimension of complexity. Exhaustion may be the most pervasive inhibitor of sexual desire. A London study of primiparous women conducted by Robson, Brant, and Kumar (1981) reported that 25% of mothers indicated tiredness reduced their libido and enjoyment of sex. Of course, the nonbreastfeeding woman with a new infant is also vulnerable to exhaustion, especially if she has other small children to care for. Breastfeeding women, however, may be more vulnerable to this effect if frequent night feeding disturbs their sleep and because of the extra energy needed to make breastmilk. If the breastfeeding infant sleeps in the parents' bed, this practice may afford the mother a better night's sleep. Conversely, the presence of the infant could inhibit sexual expression, in which case the couple could choose another site for lovemaking.

Finally, some fathers or partners may feel that they are in competition with the baby, not only for the breastfeeding mother's attention but also for her breasts. The woman's breasts are often an important aspect of eroticism for the couple. If either or both partners feel that the breasts are off-limits for sexual play because the woman is producing milk, then the couple's sexual expression may be negatively affected. Even if the couple feels no taboo about the woman's breasts, there may be a dislike of milk leakage and a fear of eliciting it. The breasts may be tender, and the new mother may be tired of having her breasts "handled." Conversely, there is little harm in breast stimulation and even suckling by the woman's partner, especially after the baby has had his fill. The partner may actually help to prevent or relieve engorgement by periodically stimulating milk secretion or ejection.

Libido-Enhancing Factors Related to Pregnancy, Birth, and Lactation

Especially in the context of a planned pregnancy, the birth can be a positive and fulfilling experience, and many couples express this mutual happiness in lovemaking. Childbirth is a major life event. When it occurs under emotionally and physically healthy conditions, sexual expression can be particularly joyful and rewarding. In contrast to the possible inhibitors mentioned earlier, pregnancy, childbirth, and breastfeeding can have the effect of magnifying an appreciation of the womanliness of the mother by her partner. For example, to some men and women, the shape or fullness of the lactating breasts is particularly arousing. The breastfeeding woman may feel more interested in sexual relations after a few months postpartum because of the interaction of some of the factors mentioned previously. Her perineum is less tender, she may be experiencing some ovarian activity, she no longer has the body shape of a pregnant woman, and she feels more normal. One mother described it this way:

> To me, sex is best of all during the later breastfeeding period because (1) I feel physically better than at any other time, (2) [there is] no fear of pregnancy and no contraceptives [are] needed because for me breastfeeding is a 100% effective contraceptive for at least 1 year after the birth of a baby, and (3) there is something about nursing a little baby that gives you an "all's right with the world" kind of feeling. I feel so happy and loving toward my whole family, husband, and other children as well as the baby. Sex just seems to be a nice, natural expression of this good feeling. (Kenny, 1973, p. 225)

Human sexual expression can be a creative activity in addition to being procreative. It is obviously a personal endeavor for the lovers both as individuals and as a couple. For this reason, some potentially inhibiting factors may actually be arousing factors that add to the likelihood that the couple will have sexual intercourse. For example, one couple may make love more frequently in times of stress, while another couple may experience a paucity of emotional reserve for lovemaking under the same circumstances. The former pattern may be quite functional because orgasm helps to release tension and promotes relaxation and a feeling of well-being, thereby providing one or both partners with more psychic energy with which to cope with the causes of stress. For some couples, pregnancy itself often stimulates erotic responses. As a consequence, to some people, having given birth and becoming nonpregnant again may be less sexually stimulating than being "great with child."

Because each person and each couple are unique, any discussion of sexuality during lactation must be couched in generalities, recognizing that individual expression varies widely. Unfortunately, very few women talk to their healthcare professional about their sexual health. It seems possible that many couples could have better sexual satisfaction if they were equipped with a few simple facts and some lubricant.

Factors Related to the Breastfeeding Woman's Partner

The possibility of role conflict has already been mentioned and serves as a reminder that men also experience psychological adjustments to accommodate the major life event of birth. No doubt the experience is most profound the first time that a man becomes a father. While fathers are often assumed to be ever ready, willing, and wanting sex, this is an overgeneralization, possibly reflecting the relative lack of a cycle in the male capacity to fertilize. Fathers are subject to libidinal influences in everyday life, and, analogous to the female perspective discussed at the beginning of this section, these facilitators and inhibitors do not disappear with the birth of a child or during the lactation course of a partner. When the father has witnessed his pregnant partner's metamorphosis into lactating mother, this transformation may affect his perception of her as a sex partner, either because of her body's obvious changes or because of the meaning he ascribes to her maternity. Motherhood or lactation may make her more or less sexually appealing to him.

Fear of hurting his partner during vaginal intercourse may inhibit male sexual expression. A man may feel guilty for desiring his breastfeeding partner if he perceives that she has "more important" maternal matters. Identifying and talking about their sexual feelings, desires, and inhibitions, while earnestly caring for the welfare of each other, can help the couple through this sometimes awkward period.

Sexual Behavior During Lactation

To measure a level of sexual functioning or behavior in breastfeeding women, studies of lactational amenorrhea have examined other variables, including resumption of postpartum intercourse and coital frequency. While first intercourse and coital frequency are relatively easy variables to quantify, they do not yield a complete understanding of sexual practices during lactation. Unfortunately, little qualitative information about sexual behavior during lactation is reported in the scientific literature.

Information on the timing of initiation of sexual intercourse for lactating women may be gleaned from studies conducted around the world. Outcomes of these studies indicate that 50% to 80% of breastfeeding women resume intercourse by 6 to 8 weeks postpartum. Some mothers initiate coitus as early as 3 to 4 weeks after birth (Barrett, Pendry, et al., 2000; Udry & Deang, 1993). Data on frequency of sexual intercourse have been obtained both prospectively and retrospectively.

To provide a context for interpretation of coital frequency during lactation, 91 normally cycling, non-pregnant, non-lactating North Carolina women who were married or cohabitating participated a retrospective and prospective study of frequency of sexual intercourse. First, the women reported from memory their "usual" weekly frequency of sexual intercourse. Then they recorded each morning, for 1 to 3 months, whether they had intercourse during the previous 24 hours. The women reported a significantly higher frequency of coitus for the period prior to the first interview (2.5 times per week) compared with their later prospective recordings (1.7 times per week)—an average of 0.8 episode per week. This overestimate occurred uniformly in subgroups of women and was thought to be caused by the women's tendency to report a frequency that would exist in the absence of travel, illness, menses, and other influencing factors. The prospective data showed trends toward decreased coital frequency with increasing age, education, income, and duration of relationship. Also, women who were currently using an intrauterine device or who had undergone a tubal ligation had intercourse twice as often (2.0 times per week) as women with "no" contraceptive use (1.1 times per week) (Hornsby & Wilcox, 1989).

Studies of coital frequency among lactating women show variance from less than once every other week to 4 to 6 times per week during the first 6 months postpartum (Udry, 1993; Visness & Kennedy, 1997). A number of factors have been found to explain this variability but there is no consistency among studies. For example, age, education, and the number of living children appear to be unrelated to coital frequency. In contrast, maternal age is related in two ways: younger women report an increase in frequency with time postpartum, and their overall frequency is greater than that reported by older women (Udry & Deang, 1993; Visness & Kennedy, 1997). Other factors, such as fear of pregnancy, may be stronger correlates of sexual behavior, as may psychological factors such as perceived locus of control (the perception that one is in control of one's life and fate rather than the victim of forces outside oneself).

Does breastfeeding affect the resumption of sexual activity or coital frequency? When comparing breastfeeding and nonbreastfeeding mothers, breastfeeding mothers show lower coital frequencies (Islam & Khan, 1993; Udry, 1993). Breastfeeding women also have a lower preferred frequency of intercourse; delay the resumption of coitus for a longer period; have a greater reduction in sexual interest and enjoyment compared with prepregnancy levels; experience more pain during intercourse; and are slightly more depressed at 3 months postpartum (Alder & Bancroft, 1988; Barrett, Pendry, et al., 2000). All of these differences disappear by 6 months postpartum, except for dyspareunia. By contrast, earlier research by Masters and Johnson (1966) and by Kenny (1973) reported a more prompt return of sexual desire, plus a return to higher levels of sexual functioning, among breastfeeding women than among bottle-feeders. These studies were conducted during a time and at locations in which breastfeeding was not popular. It is unknown whether women who were less sexually inhibited were the ones who breastfed. Another group of studies report that breastfeeding does not appear to influence resumption of coitus, coital frequency, and other indices of sexuality (Grudzinskas & Atkinson, 1984; Knodel & Chayovan, 1991; Robson et al., 1981)

What do these conflicting results mean? Does breastfeeding stifle sexual experience, accelerate it, or neither? Conflicting results can be due to differences in research methodology or to cultural norms. Additional psychological, behavioral, and biological hypotheses are needed. Can breastfeeding have either an inhibiting or a stimulating effect? Perhaps breastfeeding is a swing factor, sometimes enhancing sexual feelings and sometimes acting as the obstacle to their expression.

Whether breastfeeding enhances, inhibits, or does not influence sexual desire or sexual behavior, it is clear that large numbers of women are sexually active before the traditional time of the postpartum check-up (i.e., 6 weeks postpartum). For lactation consultants, awareness of the issues related to return of sexual desire and initiation of intercourse may come up as a topic of conversation. Knowledge of the great variability in sexual behavior will aid the practitioner in addressing this topic, especially since lactation consultants are likely to see mothers in the early days and weeks after birth. One could also argue that the initial postpartum follow-up visit should take place earlier. Mothers need support and encouragement as they establish breastfeeding, especially given that exclusive breastfeeding for 6 months is the expectation. Additionally, new mothers should always have access to care in the event of unexpected pain, vaginal discharge, or other physical concerns or reinforcement of anticipatory guidance to prevent and resolve these types of problems. Lastly, making informed decisions about family planning for the future requires education closer to the time the contraception is actually needed. Given that the majority of women have some sexual discomfort or concerns postpartum, health professionals should initiate discussion of sexual issues—actual or potential—and contraception in a timely manner, meaning before sexual activity is resumed.

Women's Health Across the Childbearing Years

Family planning and reproductive health, while frequently considered the primary foci of health care for women of childbearing age, represent only a fraction of women's health concerns. Certainly, during pregnancy and birth, there is intensive use of healthcare services to assure health and safety of mother and fetus/infant. In contrast, postpartum health care is limited, and few national statistics exist on healthcare utilization and health problems encountered by mothers during the first postpartum year (Cheng et al., 2006). Besides physical concerns of involution of the reproductive system and return to non-pregnant physiology, the postpartum period is distinguished by psychosocial adaptations such as adjusting to the parenting role, changing family relationships, and alterations in self-perception and body image (Fahey & Shenassa, 2013). These transitions, along with physical recovery and the work of caring for an infant, are not completed by the 6-week check-up, which traditionally is considered the end of perinatal care. Instead, mothers are at heightened vulnerability to stressors and health concerns, both physical and psychological, for at least the first full year after giving birth (Fahey & Shenassa, 2013). Many of these concerns may influence breastfeeding exclusivity and duration as well as the mother's ability to care for her infant.

Stress and Stressors

Stress has long been associated with health, illness, and disease. Indeed, a large body of evidence supports the notion that stress—especially chronic environmental and psychosocial stress—is a significant contributor to physiological dysregulation, poor mental health, poor physical health, chronic diseases, and shortened life span (Beckie, 2012). A recent national study in the United States demonstrated just how much stress individuals are experiencing (National Public Radio [NPR], Robert Wood Johnson Foundation, & Harvard School of Public Health, 2014). Approximately half of the respondents indicated they had experienced a major stressful event within the past year, and during the month prior to completing the survey 26% of the respondents reported having a "great deal" of stress, 37% experienced "some stress," 23% reported "not very much" stress, and 14% indicated they had "no stress at all" (p. 3). Common stressors included too many responsibilities, health, finances (especially for those with annual incomes of less than $20,000), and parenting.

Stress, and responses to it, stem from individuals' perceptions of the safety or threat level in their environment. In a process known as neuroception, neural circuits interpret situations and persons as safe or unsafe, friendly or hostile, isolating or integrating, caring or indifferent, or, ultimately, life threatening (Porges, 2007). The nervous system stimuli are converted into neural, electrical, chemical, and biological signals that are responsible for the physical, emotional, and mental experiences of stress and their interpretation into behavioral responses (Zender & Olshansky, 2012). Thus stress can be defined as the activation of neuroendocrine system, sympathetic and autonomic nervous systems, and immunological and metabolic systems when seeking to adapt to environmental challenges (McEwen, 2012).

Of course, not all stress is negative. Short-term, resolvable stress stimulates and actually strengthens physiological health and adaptive responses (Zender & Olshansky, 2012). Positive stress can lead to a sense of mastery, control, and accomplishment when challenges end with satisfying outcomes. Such resolution leads to the development of high self-esteem and enhanced ability to cope with future challenges and stressors (McEwen, 2007). In many situations, stress may be interpreted as tolerable, especially if mediators such as social support, knowledge, and financial stability are present and coping abilities are adequate (McEwen, 2005).

Distress or negative and toxic stress occurs when environmental and psychological demands exceed an individual's ability to cope. The transition from stress to distress is determined by the quantity, chronicity, and intensity of stressors, as well as their resolvability, in relationship to individuals' capacity to cope (Zender & Olshansky, 2012). For example, stress or stressors tolerable to one person can be exacerbated by chaos, abuse, neglect, and poor social and emotional support, thereby becoming distress for another person. Women of childbearing age experience stress from major life events but perhaps more so from the pressures and conflicts of daily life. For many women, the accumulation and chronicity of such stress alters their physiological systems, producing a chronic stress burden (McEwen, 2012). In an attempt to ease this stress burden, brain circuits are remodeled to adjust the balance among anxiety, mood control, memory, and decision making (Karatsoreos & McEwen, 2013). If the chronic stress burden continues, the changes to the brain and body—although initially adaptive—can become maladaptive, leading to altered health behaviors; problems with diet, physical activity, sleep, and substance use; and disease, both mental and physical (McEwen, 2013).

While the most studied reaction to stress is the "fight or flight" response, another model of stress reactivity has been proposed by Taylor (2002, 2006) and others (Turton & Campbell, 2005). Based in evolutionary theory, Taylor's model suggests that women, and especially mothers, react to stress by "tending and befriending." Because mothers are unable to fight or flee because of their responsibilities to offspring, the "tending" response favors both mother and child survival. "Tending" in threatening situations includes quieting and caring for offspring while blending into the environment. "Befriending" involves seeking or providing social support and sharing the burdens of child rearing and protection. In times of stress, women will talk to friends, share problems, ask for directions when lost, or "clear the air" as they discuss concerns with others (Taylor, 2002).

The neural circuitry of "tend and befriend" appears to be regulated by the hormone oxytocin as well as endogenous opioid peptides, prolactin, vasopressin, dopamine, and many others (Taylor, 2002; Uvnas-Moberg, 2003). Besides stimulating labor and milk letdown, oxytocin is the hormone of affiliation. The high levels of oxytocin observed immediately after birth promote an otherworldly calm and an intense, visceral connection with the newborn (Uvnas-Moberg et al., 2005). Beyond birth, the somatosensory stimulation of breastfeeding and associated skin-to-skin contact and dyadic interactions maintain the elevated levels of oxytocin. For mothers, the elevated oxytocin reduces the fight-or-flight neuroendocrine responses to stress (inhibits release of cortisol), lessens anxiety, induces calm and even mild sedation, enhances sociability, and triggers the initiation of mothering (Uvnas-Moberg & Petersson, 2005).

A critical aspect of mothering is nurturance, without which the human species would not survive (Taylor, 2002). Nurturing significantly influences the architecture of the nervous (including the brain) and endocrine systems for both mother and infant, and is especially critical during infants' first two to three years of life. Stimulated by maternal social presence and the senses (smell, sound, taste, and especially touch, movement, and ingestive behaviors), the developing neuroendocrine structures provide infants with increasing abilities to regulate their physiological state responses in a rapidly and dramatically changing environment (Rincon-Cortes & Sullivan, 2014). As the neural structures become more sophisticated, they provide the framework for stress management across the life span (Porges & Furman, 2011). Feldman and colleagues (2010) demonstrated the significance of nurturance, consisting of maternal social presence and touch, on stress reactivity using two still-face (mother and infant start in free play; mother ceases interaction for a specified period and then reunites with infant in play) paradigms: still face alone or still face with maternal touch. The results of their study demonstrate how maternal touch during moments of simulated maternal deprivation (still face) decreases the infant's physiological stress response. Additionally, the magnitude of the stress response is reduced in both the autonomic nervous system (vagal tone) and the hypothalamic–pituitary–adrenal axis (cortisol reactivity), suggesting touch provides multidimensional responses to stress.

Indeed, nurturance/touch as a sensitive, synchronized component of mother–infant communication and ongoing maternal (or other committed caregiver) involvement influences the organizing of infants' physiological systems (e.g., state regulation, emotional control), thereby positively influencing the functioning of the developing child's stress-management systems. By contrast, intrusive, missynchronous maternal or parental touch and communication lead to physiological and behavioral dysregulation (Bystrova et al., 2009) and less advantageous reactions to stress. In summary, communication and tactile patterns experienced within the context of early mother–infant interactions affect neuroendocrine and, ultimately, epigenetic expression, thereby influencing mothers' and infants' capacities to manage stress not only in the immediate moment of interaction but also during their lifetime and across generations (McEwen, 2003).

This brief discussion of stress and the formation of stress response and reactivity is intended to help breastfeeding practitioners anticipate maternal concerns related to stress and the impact of stress on breastfeeding initiation, continuation, and exclusivity. Just as breastfeeding and skin-to-skin contact have an anxiolytic effect, so stress—especially chronic social stress—can impair breastfeeding and mothering behaviors secondary to remodeling of the neuroendocrine system as an adaptation to the chronic stress (Murgatroyd & Nephew, 2012). Lactation consultants and other lactation practitioners have the opportunity to reverse some of the impact of chronic social stress by taking the following steps:

1. Acknowledging mothers' many responsibilities and daily worries.
2. Providing mothers with the opportunity to talk about their current stress. Specifically, practitioners should ask what is bothering new mothers or causing stress (do not assume you know).
3. Supporting mothers in problem solving. (Listen: Mothers frequently know the answer to their problems, but just need an audience to voice it.)
4. Affirming positive parenting actions.
5. Providing breastfeeding support. (The first five actions all lead to the release of oxytocin.)
6. Encouraging breastfeeding as much as mother is able (the best thing mother can do for infant intelligence and social development).
7. Encouraging kangaroo care (skin-to-skin holding) and holding/carrying of the infant (extremely important actions in ongoing neuroendocrine development).

As mothers feel valued, important to their infant, and recognized for their expertise in relation to their infant, they will reap the benefits of elevated levels of oxytocin, attenuated (lessened) stress, and readjustment of their stress reactivity set point. Additionally, as they develop their mothering abilities, their infants will garner lifelong advantages such as independence, greater cognitive abilities, lowered reactivity to stress, and an ability to confidently take risks.

Immediate Postpartum Concerns

Primary concerns or stressors starting immediately after birth include breastfeeding initiation, newborn care, maternal–infant bonding and attachment, pain, bleeding, and infection prevention. Breastfeeding initiation is covered in another chapter, and bonding and attachment are addressed briefly in the discussion of stress.

Pain

Pain during the postpartum can come from multiple sources (Table 15-2). Regardless of its location, pain and discomfort are likely to interfere with breastfeeding initiation and infant care, possibly undermining mother's confidence and development of maternal identity (Eshkevari et al., 2013; Karlstrom et al., 2007). Mothers' experiences of pain vary. During pregnancy, sensitivity to pain may be heightened due to elevated levels of estrogen stimulating peripheral and central pain mechanisms. Once the placenta is delivered, the estrogen level declines precipitously, reducing pain sensitivity. Additionally, oxytocin is known to blunt peripheral nerve hypersensitivity. Thus the elevated levels of oxytocin during labor, birth, and breastfeeding may lead to decreased pain sensations and to fewer reports of chronic pain during the postpartum period (Gutierrez et al., 2013). Oxytocin also stimulates endogenous opioid production, which modulates pain as well as elevates mood.

Multiple theories of pain have been developed over the ages (Moayedi & Davis, 2013). An early pain theory, known as the specificity theory, proposed dedicated pathways for pain and other somatosensory modalities. According to this model, with distinct receptors and associated sensory fibers, stimuli are transported to the spinal cord and on to the brain for interpretation. High- or low-threshold stimuli provide signals for intensity of pain. The intensity theory postulates that pain, rather than consisting of signals transported along distinct pathways, is an emotion or

Table 15-2 LOCATION, PHYSIOLOGICAL CAUSES AND NONPHARMACOLOGIC MANAGEMENT OF POSTPARTUM DISCOMFORTS

Location of Discomfort	Causes of Discomfort	Nonpharmacologic Management

• Tissue trauma	• Extensive tissue damage
	• Release of inflammatory peptides, lipids, and mediators
	• Release of histamine and neurotransmitters
	• Inflammatory mediators stimulate activation of primary afferent nociceptors (pain) and transmission of impulses to spinal cord.
		• Nociceptive impulses can be inhibited at spinal cord level by stimulating release of descending modulatory neurotransmitters serotonin and endogenous opioids
		  ▼ Music (Good, 1996)
		  ▼ Meditation
		  ▼ Relaxation (Good, 1996)
		  ▼ Guided imagery
		  ▼ Holding infant skin-to-skin (Handlin et al., 2009)
		  ▼ Social support
		  ▼ Choice of words

▼ Perineal pain
  o Microtrauma due to tissue stretching
  o Episiotomy
  o Lacerations
  o Peri-uretheral tears
	• See above	• Ice/cold pack to perineum first 24–28 hours (East et al., 2012)
		  ▼ 30 minutes on (continuous), 30–60 minutes off
		  ▼ Minimizes perineal edema and inflammation
		  ▼ Decreases local circulation through local vasoconstriction
		  ▼ May reduce possible hematoma formation
		• Warm compresses (starting after 48 hours, warmth earlier will increase edema and pain)
		  ▼ Relaxes and loosens tissues
		  ▼ Increases blood flow to area helping to promote circulation & healing (Eshkevari et al., 2013)
		• Topical products including anesthetic sprays are not any better than placebo for relieving perineal discomfort (Hedayati et al., 2005)

▼ Cesarean incision	• See above	• Potent analgesic initially (Good & Moore, 1996)
		• Comfort measures—measures beyond pain medication to assure mother's comfort (Kolcaba et al., 2006)
		  ▼ Early ambulation
		  ▼ Shower first postoperative day
		  ▼ Splinting with pillow or blanket when coughing and turning
		  ▼ Abdominal binder
		  ▼ Heating pad or warm compresses after 48 hours

• Uterine involution → cramping	• Contracting of the myometrium after birth as uterus returns to pre-pregnant size ▼ Discomfort and cramping pain ▼ Contractions increase with release of oxytocin during breastfeeding ▼ Contractions increase with distended bladder ▼ More severe in women who have had previous childbirth experience ▼ Administration of utero-tonic medications	• Education regarding possibilities of uterine contractions with breast-feeding • Empty bladder • Heating pads, warm packs, ice packs—depending on mother's personal and cultural preferences (anecdotal evidence) • Mild analgesic 20–30 minutes before feeding
• Hemorrhoids	• Venous distention and engorgement of the anal canal • Exacerbated by prolonged pushing/straining during second stage • Contributing factors ▼ Constipation ▼ Genetics ▼ Lack of pelvic floor muscle support • Tend to decrease in size with improved circulation after delivery	• Increased dietary fiber and fluids • Chilled witch hazel compresses (or witch hazel saturated paper towels) • Warm sitz baths (tub soak) • Topical local anesthetics • Hydrocortisone-containing cream or suppository for severe itching (Eshkevari et al., 2013) • High fiber laxatives (Alonso-Coello et al., 2005) • Stool softner (Colace) • Interventions to treat hemorrhoids during pregnancy and postpartum have not been adequately evaluated (Quijano & Abalos, 2005)
• Flatulence (gas pains)	• Postoperative ileus or inhibited gastrointestinal motility (van Bree et al., 2012) ▼ Inhibition of motility associated with anesthetics and opioid analgesics ▼ Handling of intestine during surgery activates inhibitory neuronal reflexes → intestinal edema due to excessive intravascular fluid loading • Decreased motility due to relaxin and other hormones of pregnancy	• Periparturm and perioperative fluid management • Early ambulation • Early feeding/eating • Gum chewing (Purkayastha et al., 2008) • Rocking in a rocking chair

(continues)

Table 15-2 LOCATION, PHYSIOLOGICAL CAUSES AND NONPHARMACOLOGIC MANAGEMENT OF POSTPARTUM DISCOMFORTS *(CONTINUED)*

Location of Discomfort	Causes of Discomfort	Nonpharmacologic Management
• Breast discomforts ▼ Nipple pain and trauma	• Pain sensation on frictional and suction lesions • Incorrect latch 　▼ Tugging on tip of nipple 　▼ Latch broken inaccurately 　▼ Flat nipples 　▼ Overweight/obese with pendulous breasts • Physical trauma 　▼ Cracked 　▼ Sore 　▼ Bleeding 　▼ Edematous 　▼ Erythemic 　▼ Blistered 　▼ Fissures 　▼ Eschar • Care practices associated with higher incidence nipple soreness (Morland-Schultz & Hill, 2005) 　▼ Use of pacifier 　▼ Use of feeding bottle 　▼ Early breastfeeding in upright/sitting position 　▼ Many hands helping with attachment • Nipple pain generally resolves within 7 days	• Prenatal education—breastfeeding positioning and attachment technique (Grade A recommendation, The Joanna Briggs Institute, 2009) • Laid-back positioning with newborn self attaching (Colson et al., 2008) • Early postpartum education (Grade B recommendation, Cadwell et al., 2004) 　▼ Positioning of infant and attachment 　▼ Assessment and correction of latch 　▼ Infant suck strength and pattern • Warm water compress (Grade B) 　▼ Lanolin or vitamin A ointments with heat (superior properties in relief of pain) • Breast shell and ointment or expressed breastmilk/colostrum for frictional pain • Antenatal nipple preparation (use with caution due to risk of uterine contractions, Grade C) • Prevention and treatment methods neither confirmed or supported (The Joanna Briggs Institute, 2009) 　▼ Keep nipples clean and dry 　▼ Breast shells 　▼ Breast shields 　▼ Aerosol spray 　▼ Hydrogel dressing 　▼ Modified lanoline or vitamin A 　▼ Collagenase or dexpanthenol ointment

▼ Engorgement

- Breast fullness secondary to lactogenesis II
  ▼ Insufficient milk removal
  ▼ Milk stasis
  ▼ Edema
  ▼ Inflammation

- Skin-to-skin holding as much as possible from birth through lactogenesis
- Frequent breastfeeding as lead by baby
- Manual expression or pumping (ABM Protocol Committee, 2009)
- Cold compress or gel pack—decreases blood flow through tissues, decreasing inflammation & pain (Mangesi & Dowswell, 2010)
- Warm compresses or shower before feeding to soften tissue and allow infant to latch on.
- *Gua-Sha* (scraping therapy)—using Chinese principles of 12 meridians and collaterals to remove blood and metabolic waste congesting surface tissues and muscles thus promoting normal circulation and metabolic processes (Chiu, 2010)
- Relief for Sabbath-observant Jewish women
  ▼ Frequent breastfeeding
  ▼ Manual expression with different hand than usual
  ▼ Express less than 17 ml at a time
  ▼ Have a non-Jewish person turn on electric breast pump if no other manner for milk expression.
  ▼ Waste or alter milk so it is unusable—hand express into open sink
  ▼ Hot water bottle with water heated before the Sabbath
  ▼ Breast massage without cream or oil
  ▼ Bag of ice or frozen vegetables applied to breast after feeding (Chertok, 1999)

sensory system that responds to stimuli that are stronger than "usual" (Moayedi & Davis, 2013).

The conceptualization of pain was revolutionized in 1965 when Melzack and Wall introduced the gate control theory (as cited in Moayedi & Davis, 2013). Building on physiological evidence corroborating the more simplistic theories of pain, Melzack and Wall recognized that activation of two types of neuron fibers, pain and touch, causes them to send signals to the dorsal horn of the spinal cord. In the dorsal horn, these signals converge and impulses are transmitted to the sensory forebrain (Mendell, 2014). Within the spinal neurons, signals are modulated; activity from large neural fibers (touch) closes the "gate" inhibiting impulse transmission, while small fiber (pain) activity opens the gate (Trout, 2004). The descending spinal control pathways also influence the inhibition effects of the gate. The experience of pain, both sensory and affective, occurs when small fiber activity exceeds the inhibition abilities of the spinal cord, thereby leading to opening of the gate and allowing transmission of impulses to the forebrain, where they are interpreted (Mendell, 2014).

With further investigation, Melzack recognized that the gate control theory did not fully explain experiences of pain (Trout, 2004); in turn, he developed the neuromatrix theory of pain (Melzack, 2005). This theory postulates that pain is multidimensional, having both parallel and cyclic processing loops in the brain. Melzack (1999) describes the neuromatrix as a "network, whose spatial distribution and synaptic links are initially determined genetically and are later sculpted by sensory inputs. . . . Thalamocortical and limbic-cortical loops that comprise the neuromatrix, diverge to permit parallel processing in different components of the neuromatrix and converge to permit interactions between the output products of processing" (p. 86). Repeated cyclical processing and syntheses of nerve impulses create a characteristic pattern, a so-called neurosignature—each individual. The output patterns form the "body–self neuromatrix," which is composed of sensory, affective, and cognitive neuromodules that produce the multiple

dimensions of pain experiences and the concurrent homeostatic and behavioral responses (Box 15-4). Thus, when managing pain, all of these dimensions need to be assessed (Table 15-3) and taken into consideration when planning pharmacologic and nonpharmacologic pain management interventions (Good & Moore, 1996) so mothers are fully mindful while providing newborn care.

Postpartum Hemorrhage and Dysfunctional Uterine Bleeding

Normal uterine bleeding (lochia) following birth ceases in approximately 3 to 5 weeks. The median duration of lochial flow for breastfeeding women is 27 days (Visness, Kennedy, & Ramos, 1997). Nearly half of women who fully breastfeed experience some vaginal bleeding or spotting between 6 and 8 weeks postpartum (Visness, Kennedy, & Ramos, 1997). Abnormal bleeding can inhibit breastmilk synthesis. Willis and Livingstone's (1995) description of 10 cases of insufficient milk following severe postpartum hemorrhage has been substantiated by more recent research (Thompson et al., 2010). In the early weeks postpartum, excessive bleeding may be caused by placental fragments retained in the uterus.

Bleeding caused by a relaxed uterus occurs less often in mothers providing skin-to-skin contact and breastfeeding (Saxton et al., 2013), because the oxytocin released by the suckling infant causes the uterus to contract during each suckling episode. Later bleeding may result from miscarriage or the irregular onset of hormonal function. Treatment includes hormonal therapy or nonsteroidal anti-inflammatory drugs (NSAIDs). If bleeding is excessive, prolonged, or unexplained, curettage of the uterine lining may be necessary.

Nonpharmacologic interventions for excessive postpartum bleeding include emptying the mother's bladder, placing the baby in skin-to-skin contact, and breastfeeding. If these interventions are unsuccessful, the physician usually orders intravenous oxytocin. If the uterus fails to respond to the oxytocin,

Box 15-4 Input and Output Factors Contributing to Patterns of Activity Generated by the Sensory, Affective, and Cognitive Neuromodules of the Body–Self Neuromatrix, Which Produces the Multiple Dimensions of the Pain Experience, and Homeostatic and Behavioral Responses as Described by Melzack (1999, 2001, 2005)

Body–Self Neuromatrix	
Inputs to Body–Self Neuromatrix	**Outputs from Body–Self Neuromatrix**

Cognitive-evaluative-related brain areas

- Tonic input from brain
  - ◄ Memories of past experiences
  - ◄ Cultural learning
  - ◄ Personality variables
- Phasic input from brain
  - ◄ Attention
  - ◄ Expectation
  - ◄ Meaning
  - ◄ Anxiety
  - ◄ Depression

Sensory-discriminative signaling systems

- Phasic cutaneous sensory input
- Tonic somatic input
  - ◄ Trigger points
  - ◄ Deformities
- Visceral inputs
- Visual, auditory, vestibular, and other sensory input
- Musculoskeletal inputs
- Intrinsic neural inhibitory modulation

Motivational-affective-related brain areas

- Hypothalamic–pituitary–adrenal system
- Noradrenalin–sympathetic system
- Immune system
  - ◄ Cytokines
- Oxytocin system
  - ◄ Endogenous opioids
- Limbic system

Pain perception

- Cognitive-evaluative dimension
- Sensory-discriminative dimension
- Motivational-affective dimension

Action programs

- Involuntary action patterns
- Voluntary action patterns
- Social communication
- Coping strategies

Stress-regulation programs

- Endocrine system
  - ◄ Coritsol level
  - ◄ Norepinephrine levels
  - ◄ Oxytocin levels
  - ◄ Endorphin levels
- Immune system activity
  - ◄ Cytokine levels
- Autonomic system activity
- Homeostatic/stress responses
- Behavioral responses

→	Time	→	Time	→	Time	→

Adapted from Melzack R, 1999; 2001; 2005.

Table 15-3 Dimensions of Pain as Delineated in the McGill Pain Questionnaire

Measurement	Dimension	Descriptors
Pain location	Sensory	On a drawing of the human body, patient identifies area of body that are painful. Number of pain sites is summed.
Pain intensity	Sensory	0 = no pain 3 = distressing 1 = mild 4 = horrible 2 = discomforting 5 = excruciating

Pain quality:
What does your pain feel like?
	Sensory	• *Continuous Pain* ◂ Splitting pain
		  ◂ Throbbing pain ◂ Electric-shock pain
		  ◂ Cramping pain ◂ Piercing
		  ◂ Gnawing pain • *Predominantly Neuropathic Pain*
		  ◂ Aching pain ◂ Hot—burning pain
		  ◂ Heavy pain ◂ Cold—freezing pain
		  ◂ Tender ◂ Pain caused by light touch
		  ◂ Sharp ◂ Itching
		• *Intermittent Pain* ◂ Tingling/pins and needles
		  ◂ Shooting pain ◂ Numbness
		  ◂ Stabbing pain
		  ◂ Sharp pain
		Rate intensity of each type of pain, add number of types of pain and intensity scores.

	Affective	• Tiring/exhausting • Depression • Sickening • Anxiety • Fear/Fearful • Tension • Punishing/cruel • Autonomic properties Rate intensity of each affective description, add number of affective descriptions and intensity scores.
	Cognitive	• Overall appraisal of pain • Qualities/evaluative words
Pain pattern: How does your pain change with time?	Sensory	• Continuous • Intermittent • Steady • Brief • Constant • Momentary • Rhythmic • Transient • Periodic
Alleviating and aggravating Factors	Behavioral	• What kinds of things decrease your pain? • What kinds of things increase your pain?

Sources: Dworkin et al., 2009; Ngamkham et al., 2012.

then methylergonovine maleate (Methergine), a derivative of an ergot alkaloid, is given. Unlike with crude ergot preparations, no adverse effects have been reported following the use of methylergonovine by nursing mothers. Prostaglandin may also be given. None of these medications suppresses lactation.

Anxiety almost always accompanies excessive bleeding. Interventions should focus on relieving the mother's anxiety and assisting in determining the cause of the bleeding while maintaining breastfeeding. Additionally, skin-to-skin contact with her baby and social support may have an anxiolytic effect on the mother secondary to the increase in oxytocin stimulated by these activities. The mother should be referred to a physician for an immediate appointment or, if the bleeding is especially severe and a physician is not available, she should be taken to the hospital emergency room. Because leaving her alone simply increases her fear, someone should stay with her until she can be medically evaluated. A dilation and curettage (D&C), if required, can usually be performed in an outpatient setting, which reduces the likelihood and duration of mother–infant separation.

Fatigue

Fatigue is frequently a stressor for new mothers as they adjust to their infants' around-the-clock schedules (Wambach, 1998). Mothers should be encouraged to rest as frequently as they can, seek help (especially with household chores), and if at all possible delay returning to work for at least 12 weeks post birth. Unaddressed fatigue can lead to more serious physical and mental health issues as well as early discontinuation of breastfeeding.

Re-lactation and Induced Lactation

Re-lactation and induced lactation are very similar processes and considerations. Re-lactation is the process of restimulating lactation days, weeks, or months after lactation initially ended. Induced lactation is the process of stimulating lactation when a woman has not had the benefit of the hormones of pregnancy and has never lactated or has not lactated in the recent past.

In developing countries, re-lactation is routinely initiated as part of the rehydration therapy that is offered to ill and seriously malnourished infants and young children. For these children, nutritional difficulties generally start after weaning from the breast and introduction of bottle-feedings and frequently are accompanied by diarrhea. In rehydration centers, the mothers receive additional foods and the babies are put to breast frequently and for long periods. Complementary foods are provided only after suckling. The mothers live at the center with other mothers receiving the same assistance. They become a mutual support system along with the staff (more oxytocin), who strongly support the importance of reestablishing breastfeeding. In nearly all cases, the mothers re-lactate fully, and the babies' health status is improved.

In developed countries, the purpose of re-lactation is to enable breastfeeding after an untimely weaning, or to initiate breastfeeding delayed by neonatal or maternal illness or prematurity (de Aquino & Osorio, 2009). Re-lactation is also an option for a mother who bottle-feeds at first but has a change of mind or discovers her infant cannot tolerate infant formula.

Induced lactation, sometimes called adoptive lactation, is undertaken by adoptive parents who want their child to have the benefits of breastfeeding (Denton, 2010). For the adoptive family, induced lactation is one means of overcoming the attachment and bonding problems experienced by many adopted infants. Adopted neonates and infants are particularly vulnerable to stress and excessive stress reactivity, so breastfeeding and skin-to-skin holding, as much as possible, can recreate the habitat they missed in the first few days after birth and change the course of development within their nervous, endocrine, immunologic, and other body systems. In some cultures, breastfeeding a child other than a birth child is a way of turning the relationship into that of a mother and her own child (Saari & Yusof, 2014). Establishing the "blood relationship" makes the child a member of the family with all the same rights and responsibilities. Whatever the motivation is to induce lactation and to breastfeed an adopted child, the experience may also help ease mothers' and parents' disappointment at not experiencing their own pregnancy and birth as well as build their confidence in becoming a mother and parent (Denton, 2010).

Inducing lactation or re-lactating requires a lot of motivation and commitment (Denton, 2010). Inducing lactation generally begins 6 months before the expected arrival of the infant (see the protocol for inducing lactation in Box 15-5). The mother-to-be starts by taking a combined oral contraceptive continuously to simulate pregnancy and stimulate breast development through proliferation of ducts and growth of the mammary epithelium. She also begins taking domperidone, a dopamine agonist (raises prolactin levels), to enhance milk production. When she begins to pump her breasts according to the protocol, she can begin taking an herbal galactogogue (Table 15-4). The galactogogue stimulates an increase in prolactin as preparation for the nursing phase or breast stimulation (Saari & Yusof, 2014). Re-lactating mothers may also use a galactogogue, but these agents are not necessary in all cases.

At this point, inducing lactation and re-lactating become the same process. All mothers inducing lactation will begin stimulating the breasts by pumping or suckling an infant. Just as for the mother who just gave birth and is breastfeeding, frequency of breast emptying and time spent stimulating the breast are important components for developing a good breastmilk supply. Emptying the breasts should occur every 2 to 3 hours during the day and once or twice at night, for a total of 8 to 12 breast emptyings per 24 hours. The duration of each episode should be 20 to 30 minutes. If milk is expressed, it can be saved for later use.

Re-lactation is generally easier to accomplish than induced lactation, especially if the interval between the end of the pregnancy or the last day of previous breastfeeding (or pumping) is short. A milk supply can be reestablished with sufficient, regular stimulation. For many mothers, a supplemental nurser is invaluable to establishing the milk supply (see the *Breast Pumps and Other Technologies* chapter).

For example, when attempting to re-lactate, an Italian mother used a supplemental nurser about one to three times a day because the cleaning and preparation of the device seemed complicated. "But after 2 weeks of regular use, a drop of milk started coming out from her breast after the feedings, and the stools of her baby had a 'yogurtlike' smell. She became very enthusiastic and started using the supplemental nurser at each feeding (five to six times a day)" (Smedberg, 2007, p. 26).

Whether the woman is inducing lactation or re-lactating, her breastmilk supply may not always meet the baby's demand for nutrition. The supplemental nurser allows all the advantages of breastfeeding while assuring the baby gets enough to eat. After the milk supply is established, ongoing production or galactopoiesis depends on supply and demand (autocrine system) through the emptying of the breasts by breastfeeding or pumping (see the *Anatomy and Physiology of Lactation* chapter for a review of hormonal mechanisms).

Given that breastfeeding is a dyadic activity, it is important to consider the infant's role in the process. The age of the infant at the time breastfeeding is attempted can make a critical difference in its success. With a newborn or a baby younger than 1 month, the usual experience is that the baby will, with little encouragement, root at and accept the breast, especially if given time in kangaroo (skin-to-skin) care and allowed to move to the breast at his own pace (baby-led feeding). Similarly, the younger the baby, the greater the likelihood he will be willing to suckle, particularly within the first 3 months of life. If the baby has previously breastfed, the chances of success are even greater. Older infants may not be willing to accept or may outright reject the breast, particularly if they have never been to breast. Between 3 and 6 months of age, individual infants may be more or less willing breastfeed; after 6 months, however, most babies cannot be convinced that the breast will provide either nutrition or nurturing. Other considerations influencing successful breastfeeding include the baby's suckling style, the frequency with which he is put to breast, the strength of his suckling, and the duration of each suckling episode.

BOX 15-5 INDUCED LACTATION PROTOCOL

Regular Protocol: Approximately 6 Months to Prepare Before Baby Arrives

- *Six months before baby is expected*: Start combination progesterone–estrogen birth control pills equivalent to Ortho 1/35 (1 mg norethindrone + 0.035 mg ethinyl estradiol) to stimulate breast development (must contain at least 1 mg of progesterone [2 to 3 mg is better] and no more than 0.035 mg of estrogen). Take continuously (without stopping, only active pills, no sugar pills). Also take 10 mg domperidone 4 times per day for 1 week. Then increase the dosage to 20 mg 4 times per day. *Note*: For women over the age of 35 or are unable to use the estrogen–progesterone combination birth control pill, replace it with EITHER Provera 2.5 OR prometrium 100 mg.
- *Five months before baby is expected:* Continue to take the birth control pill and domperidone 20 mg 4 times per day.
- *Four months before baby is expected:* Take an "active" birth control pill each day and maintain the domperidone dosage of 20 mg 4 times per day.
- *Six weeks before baby is expected:* Stop the combination progesterone–estrogen pill. There will be vaginal bleeding. Continue the domperidone at maximum dosage of 20 mg 4 times daily.
- Begin expressing milk, preferably using an electric pump with a double setup for pumping both breasts. Pump every 3 hours and once during the night. Pump for 5–7 minutes on the low or medium setting; massage, stroke, shake; and pump for 5–7 more minutes. Encourage the mother if at first very little (or no) milk is expressed. Freeze any pumped milk. Once pumping has started, the mother can take herbs considered to be galactogogues.
- Put the baby to breast immediately after arrival. Use a supplementer with breastmilk, donor human milk, or formula (last choice) to ensure that the baby receives sufficient nutriment for hydration and growth.
- The amount of daily infant milk intake varies according to the weight and age of the baby. A baby who is over 7 pounds (3.7 kg) and over 1 week old should be receiving at least 600 ml/day.
- Continue taking the domperidone 20 mg 4 times daily until satisfactory milk supply is achieved. The dosage can be slowly dropped to see if the milk volume can be maintained with a lower dose.

Accelerated Protocol: Where There Is Little Time to Prepare

- Start combination oral progesterone–estrogen birth control pills to stimulate breast development. Take continuously (without stopping for 1 week a month).
- Start taking domperidone 20 mg 4 times daily at the same time as the combination oral contraceptive pills.
- If significant breast changes occur within 30 days, stop taking the birth control pill while continuing to take domperidone.
- Begin pumping breasts and continue domperidone (see Regular Protocol above).

Adapted from Newman and Goldfarb: The Newman Goldfarb Protocols for induced lactation, http://www.asklenore.info/breastfeeding /induced_lactation/regular_protocol.shtml

Table 15-4 PHARMACOLOGIC AND HERBAL GALACTOGOGUES: ADVERSE EFFECTS, ACTIONS, AND ADDITIONAL COMMENTS

	Adverse Effects	Actions and Comments
Synthetic Galactogogues		
Dopamine Antagonists	Block dopamine receptors in the CNS, inducing increase of prolactin synthesis in lactotropic cells of the anterior pituitary (Tabares et al., 2014).	
Metoclopramide	Crosses blood–brain barrier Anxiety Dystonia Depression Gastrointestinal disturbances Insomnia Sedation Suicidal ideation Risk of tardive dyskinesia Tremor/seizures Infants: Intestinal discomfort	Metoclopramide concentrations in human milk are similar to therapeutic concentration in adults and can be detected in breastfeeding infants. Clearance in infants is prolonged, possibly resulting in excessive serum concentrations and risk of conditions associated with overdose (Sachs & AAP Committee on Drugs, 2013).
Domperidone	Minimally crosses blood–brain barrier With IV use: • Arrhythmia • Cardiac arrest • Sudden death Oral administration in children and infants: QT-wave prolongation	• In June 2004, the FDA issued a warning regarding breastfeeding women's use of domperidone because of safety concerns. • Not an approved product in the United States. • Outside the United States, oral formulations are labeled as *not* recommended for use during lactation (Sachs & AAP Committee on Drugs, 2013). • No data suggest use of oral domperidone by breastfeeding mothers produces similar negative effects (Osadchy et al., 2012).
Chlorpromazine (CNS tranquilizer)	Adverse effects in development of CNS (short- and long-term use) • Mothers: Extrapyramidal symptoms • Infants: Lethargy May induce changes in neonate CNS development by causing alterations in the undeveloped brain	• May induce lobulo-aveolar growth and initiation of milk secretion. • Increases milk production and weight gain in women with hypogalactia (Tabares et al., 2014).

Table 15-4 PHARMACOLOGIC AND HERBAL GALACTOGOGUES: ADVERSE EFFECTS, ACTIONS, AND ADDITIONAL COMMENTS (*CONTINUED*)

	Adverse Effects	Actions and Comments
Sulpiride	Acute dystonic reactions Endocrine disruption Extrapyramidal symptoms Fatigue Headache Lethargy Sedation Tremor Weight gain	• Increase in prolactin levels and milk secretion.
Oxytocin	No reported adverse effects in women or infants with appropriate dosing	• Induces milk ejection in cases of dysfunctional ejection reflex. • Subsequent milk removal removes the feedback inhibitor of lactation (FIL) inducing milk production. • Indicated in cases of agalactia or hypogalactia secondary to dysfunction of the milk-ejection reflex related to stress and premature birth. • May help with treatment of mastitis by inducing letdown and breast emptying (Tabares et al., 2014).
Thyrotropin-releasing hormone (TRH)	Mothers: • Iatrogenic hyperthyroidism • Brief episodes of sweating Infants: No side effects	• Synthesized in the hypothalamus, THR stimulates secretion of thyroid-stimulating hormone and prolactin by the anterior pituitary. • Oral TRH elevates prolactin blood concentrations. • Effective in induction of lactation in mothers with agalactia 10–150 days after birth. • Effects as a galactogogue vary (Tabares et al., 2014).
Herbal Galactogogues		
Herbal supplements	Pharmacokinetics and pharmacodynamics of active ingredients in galactogogue plants are not well characterized. More rigorous research (well-designed, well-conducted clinical trials) is needed to determine the mechanism of action and to establish therapeutic ranges, dosages, and side effects. Standardization of material and preparations to ensure efficacy, safety, and composition is also needed (Sachs & AAP Committee on Drugs, 2013; Tabares et al., 2014).	

(continues)

Table 15-4 PHARMACOLOGIC AND HERBAL GALACTOGOGUES: ADVERSE EFFECTS, ACTIONS, AND ADDITIONAL COMMENTS (*CONTINUED*)

	Adverse Effects	Actions and Comments
Fenugreek (*Trigonella foenum graecum*)	• Contains coumarin, which may interact with NSAIDs, possibly causing bleeding or increased bruising • Diarrhea • Dyspnea, wheezing, rhinitis • Hypoglycemia • Nausea, diarrhea, flatulence • Fainting • Facial edema • Possible uterine stimulant • If allergic to chickpeas or other Fabaceae family plants such as soybeans or peanuts, may be allergic to fenugreek (Zapantis et al., 2012) • Maple-syrup odor to urine and sweat • May interfere with absorption of oral medications • Infants: Maple-syrup odor in infants	• Efficacy to facilitate lactation has not been established. Study results have been equivocal (Reeder et al., 2013), although more studies are supporting fenugreek as a galactogogue that induces significant increase in milk production and shortens neonatal weight recovery (Sakka et al., 2014; Turkyilmaz et al., 2011). • Fenugreek seed seems to have a mastogenic effect, stimulating growth of mammary glands and enhancing sweat production (mammary glands are modified sweat glands). • Appears to stimulate endogenous hormones secretion (estrogen), thereby elevating prolactin.
Fennel (*Foeniculum vulgare*)	• Atopic dermatitis • Photosensitivity • Good source of calcium, magnesium, and iron	Appears to have an estrogenic effect, leading to increased milk production and higher milk fat content (Tabares et al., 2014).
Anise (*Pimpinella anisum*)	Not known	Strong estrogenic activity from main oil constituents: trans-anethole and estragole (Tabares et al., 2014).
Shatavari (*Asparagus racemosus*)	• Runny nose • Itchy conjunctivitis • Contact dermatitis • Throat tightening and cough during preparation • Diuretic-like effects	• Phytoestrogenic properties lead to increased milk secretion; there is a gradual decrease in milk secretion when the drug is withdrawn (Gupta & Shaw, 2011; Sharma & Bhatnagar, 2011). • Elevation of prolactin levels.
Milk thistle (*Silybum marianum*)	• Well tolerated when administered orally • Gastrointestinal disturbances: Nausea, flatulence, diarrhea • If allergic to other members of Asteraceae/Compositae plant family (e.g., ragweed, marigolds, daisies), may exhibit allergic reactions to milk thistle derivatives	• Estrogenic effect with promising lactogenic properties. • Increased milk production.

Table 15-4 Pharmacologic and Herbal Galactogogues: Adverse Effects, Actions, and Additional Comments (*continued*)

	Adverse Effects	Actions and Comments
Torbangun, Spanish thyme, Indian borage (*Coleus amboinicus lour*)	• May cause hypoglycemia and stimulate the thyroid gland • Theoretically capable of increasing risk of bleeding • Potential abortifacient effects: Do not use in pregnant women (Zapantis et al., 2012)	Proliferation of secretory mammary cells (Mortel & Mehta, 2013).

Note: AAP = American Academy of Pediatrics; CNS = central nervous system; FDA = Food and Drug Administration.

Numerous signs and symptoms will indicate that the induction of lactation or re-lactation has been at least partially successful. Many mothers often report mild to moderate changes in menstrual cycling, some breast changes (including a feeling of fullness, a change in breast shape, and occasional leaking of milk), and other indicators of increasing milk production, especially when breastfeeding occurs very frequently. Another obvious indication of an increasing supply of breastmilk is the change in infant stooling: less stool odor, a softening of the stool so that it more closely resembles the nearly liquid breastmilk stool, and a resultant lightening of the color from dark brown to mustard yellow. Because these stool changes usually occur gradually, the healthcare worker assisting the adoptive mother needs to remind her that they are an indication of an increase in the proportion of human milk versus artificial formula that the baby is receiving. In a few instances, mothers have reported a cessation of menstrual bleeding, although such a response is rare; it probably reflects a highly responsive mother and a baby whose suckling pattern is both vigorous and frequent. One mother laughingly reported, "If *your* baby sucked like a vacuum cleaner, you'd get milk in a week, too!" Often mothers find that as breastfeedings increase in frequency and volume, the amount of necessary supplemental fluid declines.

Keeping priorities clear from the outset can provide the mother–infant dyad with a unique relationship built on the special closeness that characterizes the breastfeeding experience. The clinician who assists a family with re-lactation or induced lactation is in a position to observe how mother and baby must truly work together to enjoy that which cannot be duplicated with any other method of feeding. However, placing emphasis only on the mother's milk supply as evidence of success can increase the woman's anxiety and, in turn, inhibit her milk production and milk-ejection reflex. Thus the clinician needs to weigh carefully—with plenty of discussion with the mother—both the benefits and the more problematic elements of induced lactation and re-lactation. Breastfeeding is a two-person activity; failure to keep this point continuously in mind in assisting the mother to re-lactate or induce lactation is likely to result in disappointment and a sense of failure that is avoidable. Realistic expectations are especially important with re-lactation. Even if the mother never produces a single drop of milk, the closeness and intimacy that mother and baby derive from this special relationship cannot be underestimated (Davis, 2001).

Galactogogues

Galactogogues—especially herbal galactogogues—have been used across the millennia to enhance lactation (refer to Table 15-4). Unfortunately, there is a paucity of research determining the efficacy and mechanism of action of these agents and establishing therapeutic ranges, dosage, and side effects for a majority of the galactogogues and, therefore, for the use of exogenous hormones and galactogogues as preparation for induced lactation or re-lactation. Additionally, standardization of material and preparations to ensure the efficacy, safety, and composition of herbal galactogogues is also needed (Sachs & AAP Committee on Drugs, 2013; Tabares et al., 2014). As interest in and demand for adequate breast-milk supply and ability to breastfeed at-risk infants (e.g., preterm, low-birth-weight, sick, and adopted infants) grow, more research will be done to assure the safety and efficacy of galactogogues. Indeed, just in the past 6 to 8 years, more randomized clinical trials focusing on the safety and efficacy of domperidone for breastfeeding dyads have been completed (Wan et al., 2008).

Other Measures to Initiate and Enhance Lactation

Even if galactogogues are not used, initiation and enhancing lactation can be accomplished by employing the following measures:

- Lots of kangaroo care or skin-to-skin time
- Consultation with a lactation specialist, especially someone who is knowledgeable about induced lactation and re-lactation
- Use of proper breastfeeding technique
- Activities that will increase the release of oxytocin:
  - ◄ Touch
  - ◄ Social support
  - ◄ Emotional support (maximize)
  - ◄ Massages
  - ◄ Warm bath or shower
- Frequent breastfeeding or pumping
- Prolonging the duration of pumping
- Increasing frequency of milk expression
- Looking at a picture of the infant while pumping
- Having a piece of infant's clothing to smell while pumping or expressing milk

Most of all, the healthcare provider should be as supportive as possible with mothers, helping them to focus on the good and pleasant aspects of the experience rather than the unmet goals and expectation.

Acute Illnesses and Infections

Immunizations are the primary intervention for preventing communicable diseases. The immunization efforts undertaken in the United States over the years have prevented millions of cases of serious, communicable diseases and represent one of the country's top public health achievements. Widespread immunization efforts have led to eradication of smallpox worldwide and greatly limited cases of numerous other deadly diseases (National Foundation for Infectious Diseases [NFID], 2014). While some controversy has arisen regarding this issue, pregnancy is an important time to promote vaccinations, as this activity is a four-for-one healthcare intervention. Specifically, bringing expectant mothers' vaccinations up-to-date (1) protects the mother, (2) improves her chance of having a healthy birth, (3) provides passive antibody protection for the infant during the first few months after birth when his immunologic status is low, and (4) models health promotion habits for the mother to continue while raising her child. The risk to the mother and developing fetus is minimal from any inactivated vaccine, and the benefits of vaccinating pregnant women usually outweigh the potential risk, especially when the likelihood of disease exposure is high and the infection poses a risk to mother or her developing child (American College of Obstetrics and Gynecology [ACOG], Committee on Obstetric Practice, 2013). The immunization schedule for women of reproductive age appears in Table 15-5. Guidelines for immunizations during pregnancy and breastfeeding as well as current vaccine recommendations can be found at www.cdc.gov/vaccines.

Acute illnesses such as colds, upper respiratory tract infections, and gastroenteritis are not contraindications for breastfeeding. For most infections, the key descriptor is *self-limiting*. Usually, such infections are not life threatening; furthermore, the infected mother provides antibody protection to her infant through continued breastfeeding, thereby decreasing her baby's exposure or modifying the illness. Interruption of breastfeeding renders infants more susceptible to the maternal illness, exposes them unnecessarily

Table 15-5 IMMUNIZATIONS AND PREGNANCY

Vaccine	Before Pregnancy	During Pregnancy	After Pregnancy	Type of Vaccine
Hepatitis A	Yes, if indicated	Yes, if indicated	Yes, if indicated	Inactivated
Hepatitis B	Yes, if indicated	Yes, if indicated	Yes, if indicated	Inactivated
Human papillomavirus (HPV)	Yes, if indicated, through 26 years of age	No, under study	Yes, if indicated, through 26 years of age	Inactivated
Influenza IIV	Yes	Yes	Yes	Inactivated
Influenza LAIV	Yes, if less than 50 years of age and healthy; avoid conception for 4 weeks	No	Yes, if less than 50 years of age and healthy; avoid conception for 4 weeks	Live
MMR	Yes, if indicated, avoid conception for 4 weeks	No	Yes, if indicated, give immediately postpartum if susceptible to rubella	Live
Meningococcal: • polysaccharide • conjugate	If indicated	If indicated	If indicated	Inactivated
Pneumococcal Polysaccharide	If indicated	If indicated	If indicated	Inactivated
Tdap	Yes, if indicated	Yes, vaccinate during each pregnancy ideally between 27 and 36 weeks' gestation	Yes, immediately postpartum, if not received previously	Toxoid/ inactivated
Tetanus/ Diphtheria Td	Yes, if indicated	Yes, if indicated, Tdap preferred	Yes, if indicated	Toxoid
Varicella	Yes, if indicated, avoid conception for 4 weeks	No	Yes, if indicated, give immediately postpartum if susceptible	Live

Source: Reproduced from Centers for Disease Control and Prevention, "Immunization & Pregnancy"

to the hazards of formula, and removes an important source of comfort. Continued breastfeeding and skin-to-skin contact also reduce maternal stress, thereby expediting the mother's healing.

Postpartum infections expose the breastfeeding dyad to potential delayed breastfeeding, prolonged hospital stay, and possible separation. Urinary tract infections (UTI) are the most common problem in mothers seen by primary care providers. Frequency of UTIs secondary to catheterization during labor or surgery has decreased with implementation of a policy in which catheters are removed within 24 hours. *Escherichia coli* is the most common pathogen associated with UTIs. Breastfeeding women with a UTI are treated with antibiotics, prompting some concern related to the safety of taking a medication while breastfeeding. Self-treatment is also suggested: drinking at least six to eight glasses of water each day, drinking cranberry juice, avoiding caffeine, and urinating frequently and immediately after sexual intercourse.

Antibiotics are commonly used to treat postpartum infections. These medications usually pose no danger to the infant; thus antibiotic therapy is not justification to interrupt or cease breastfeeding (see the *Drug Therapy and Breastfeeding* chapter). In addition to UTIs, other postpartum infections treated with antibiotics include mastitis (see the *Breast-Related Problems* chapter for a detailed discussion), puerperal infections (puerperal fever), and wound infections from cesarean incisions and episiotomies.

Group B *Streptococcus* (GBS) is the leading cause of neonatal sepsis and a common cause of neonatal morbidity and mortality. In approximately 10% to 40% of pregnant women, GBS (a normal body flora) colonizes their gastrointestinal and genitourinary systems, but without symptoms (Nasri et al., 2013; Plumb & Clayton, 2013). To try to prevent early onset (within the first 6 days) of neonatal sepsis, expectant mothers in the United States are routinely screened for GBS infection between 35 and 37 weeks' gestation (Money et al., 2013). In the United Kingdom, guidelines for prevention of early onset of disease is built on risk-based management (Homer et al., 2014). Both management approaches achieve similar outcomes.

Approximately 1 in every 100 to 200 infants who carry GBS develops signs and symptoms of GBS bacterial infection. Factors increasing the risk of neonatal sepsis for affected babies include preterm and low birth weight, prolonged labor, prolonged rupture of membranes (more than 12 hours), severe changes in fetal heart rate during the first stage of labor, and gestational diabetes (Ohlsson & Shah, 2014). In the United States, women with positive GBS cultures are given antibiotics intravenously during labor; while this antibiotic prophylaxis appears to rapidly reduce GBS bacteria levels, there is no conclusive evidence supporting the routine use of antibiotics (Ohlsson & Shah, 2014). Additionally, very few women who are GBS positive give birth to infants infected with GBS, and prophylactic antibiotics can have a variety of harmful effects—for example, severe maternal allergic reactions, increase in drug-resistant

organisms, exposure of newborns to resistant bacteria, and postpartum maternal and neonatal yeast infections (Ohlsson & Shah, 2014).

Besides reducing GBS bacteria levels, antibiotics wipe out healthy bacterial flora, diminishing protection from pathogenic invaders and support for the immune system. When they experience a loss of normal flora from such treatment, infants are not colonized with beneficial bacteria as they pass through the vagina, thereby compromising healthy immune system development and increasing the potential for development of allergies (Donnelly, 2014). In addition, deliberately creating insufficient normal flora increases the incidence of antibiotic-resistant infections, such as *E. coli*, which are more difficult to treat and, in turn, more lethal. One final consideration in judging the efficacy of routine prophylactic antibiotic therapy for GBS is the finding that among 10,000 mother–fetal dyads, such treatment saved the lives of just *three* full-term newborns (Donnelly, 2014).

Some concern has arisen that GBS can be passed to infants through breastmilk. Indeed, several case reports in the literature describe breastmilk as being the source of late-onset or recurrent GBS infections (Jones & Steele, 2012; Wang et al., 2007). In rare cases, GBS may persistently colonize infants' mucous membranes, influencing the pathogenesis of recurrent GBS infection. Cultures of samples taken from women with maternal mastitis may also be revealed as GBS. Nevertheless, the rarity of GBS in breastmilk was demonstrated by Burianova and colleagues (2013). They compared the breastmilk of mothers colonized with GBS before delivery and noncolonized mothers during the first week after term birth. Of the 243 samples, only two (0.82%) breastmilk cultures were GBS positive and both samples were from GBS-negative mothers.

Early introduction of formula and human milk fortifiers may make infants more susceptible to infection. Certain human milk fortifiers reduce the antibacterial properties of preterm breastmilk by the addition of iron. When iron is added to breastmilk either directly or by a fortifier containing iron, it may saturate lactoferrin, thereby decreasing its antibacterial action (Chan, 2003).

When an infant in the special care nursery receiving mother's milk becomes clinically ill, the following steps should occur (Byrne et al., 2006):

- Review with the mother proper hygiene for milk expression at home and in the hospital.
- If signs of infection occur in an infant and/or a mother, culture the mother's milk and withhold it while providing banked milk until cultures are negative for potential pathogens.
- Observe mothers of these infants in the special care nursery closely for signs of mastitis (especially if the GBS status of the mother is unknown or positive).

Questions may arise about the transfer of the antibiotic into mothers' milk and the effect on the baby. None of the antibiotics commonly used (penicillin, ampicillin, or—if penicillin allergic—clindamycin or erythromycin) are contraindicated in pregnant or nursing mothers. In fact, antibiotics to prevent GBS are directly given to infants.

Methicillin-Resistant Staphylococcus aureus

Staphylococcus aureus has long been recognized as a common pathogen. Unfortunately, with the frequent use of antibiotics, *S. aureus* strains have become resistant to many of the frequently prescribed antibiotics. Of special concern is methicillin-resistant *S. aureus* (MRSA), a virulent bacterium commonly found in hospitals and now in the community (Kriebs, 2008). Community-associated MRSA frequently presents as soft-tissue or wound infections, while healthcare-associated MRSA tends to be a more systemic infection.

Numerous individuals are carriers of *S. aureus*, with the nares being the most common site of colonization, although the vagina and other body surfaces may be colonized as well. Carrier status is transient, so treatment is not recommended. Indeed, Dr. Ruth Lawrence, an honored breastfeeding expert,

suggested the following breastfeeding guidelines when mother is colonized with MRSA:

> An infant who is term and otherwise well and home should continue breastfeeding. If still hospitalized, term, and healthy, mother and infant can be isolated together [and breastfeeding can continue]. If mother is sick [and] if baby is positive, then breastfeed, but treat both. The main reason not to breastfeed would be an infant in the neonatal intensive care unit and premature/sick when the milk might be the only contact between them. (Quoted in Kriebs, 2008, p. 249)

If mothers have an actively infected lesion on the breast, mastitis, abscess, or surgical incision drainage, then breastfeeding/breastmilk should be withheld from the baby while the mother undergoes 24 hours of appropriate antibiotic therapy. Mothers should pump and dump during this time. Additionally, infants must be observed closely for any signs of infection, including conjunctivitis or skin lesions.

The number of cases of mastitis testing positive for MRSA is increasing (Reddy et al., 2007), but it is difficult to readily trace the transmission pathway. Case studies have reported MRSA transmission to newborns through breastmilk even though mothers did not have any signs or symptoms of mastitis or other infection (Behari et al., 2004; Kawada et al., 2003). In a case-controlled study of 100 breastfeeding mothers with mastitis and 99 breastfeeding mothers without mastitis, Amir, Garland, and Lumley (2006) reported no difference in the number of mothers with *S. aureus* nasal colonization between breastfeeding mothers with mastitis and the control mothers. Conversely, significantly more infants of mothers with mastitis were nasal carriers of *S. aureus* than were control infants.

Even though mother and baby may be infected with the identical organism, it is nearly impossible to know if the infant acquired the organism in the nursery and then transferred it to the mother, or whether the mother was the initial reservoir and the baby was the secondary target. When this issue was looked at in another way by Schanler et al. (2011), milk cultures (collected prospectively) were not predictive of subsequent infection in neonates less than 30 weeks' gestation. The authors of this study concluded that routine milk cultures do not provide sufficient data to be useful in clinical management of preterm infants.

Nurses can take several important actions to decrease a newborn's risk of MRSA infection. The fetus is in a germ-free state while in the womb but becomes exposed to bacteria flora while passing through the birth canal. As a defense against MRSA infection, it is important to populate the newborn's skin and orifices, nose, and mouth with nontoxic bacterial species. Immediately placing the infant in skin-to-skin contact with the mother after birth will transfer maternal *Staphylococcus epidermis* bacteria to which mother has developed antibodies and immunoglobulins; this protection is then reinforced with early and frequent breastfeeding. The more skin-to-skin contact newborns have with their parents, the less likely MRSA will settle in and on them—in essence, "first come, first stay" (Kitajima, 2003). Additionally, continued skin-to-skin contact and breastfeeding calm and decrease stress for all newborns, thereby providing further protection from MRSA, GBS, and other infections (see the discussion on inflammation in the mental health section). Box 15-6 summarizes guidelines and techniques to decrease the risk of transmission of MRSA and other nosocomial infections.

For both MRSA and Group B *Streptococcus*, it is difficult to eradicate the carrier state (nasal, oral, anogenital), so the end point of treatment for shedding of these organisms is uncertain. Decision-making goals should include not only the "medical" care of the mother and the infant, but also the considerable benefits to the infant from receiving the mother's milk and skin-to-skin care. Mothers need ongoing support of breastfeeding or pumping of breastmilk so that the infant may receive the maximal benefit of breastmilk for up to a year or longer.

In summary, MRSA infections are minimized with the following measures:

- Mothers hold and nurse their babies immediately after birth, starting while still in the delivery room

- The newborn rooms-in, with mother and baby staying in close proximity
- Both mother and baby receive minimal interventions by healthcare providers

Tuberculosis

Approximately one-third of tuberculosis (TB) cases in the United States occur in people between 25 and 44 years of age (CDC, 2011). Tuberculosis in women in their childbearing years can reflect other coexisting influences, such as HIV/AIDS (Loto & Awowole, 2012), drug abuse associated with conditions of urban poverty (Burr et al., 2014), and the influx of immigrants from areas of the world where there is a high prevalence of tuberculosis (CDC, 2013). Women with tuberculosis who are being treated appropriately with anti-tuberculosis drugs at the time of giving birth may and should breastfeed (CDC, 2011; WHO, 1998a). Separation of the mother from her infant is rarely justified unless the tuberculosis is discovered at birth and the mother is considered contagious. In that case the dyad is separated for two weeks, and mother should begin pumping immediately. Breastfeeding should then continue while the mother continues her medication regimen (AAP, 2012).

A latent TB infection (LTBI) during pregnancy is usually treated with a 9-month course of daily or twice weekly isoniazid (INH) (CDC, 2011). Women taking INH should also take pyridoxine (vitamin B_6) supplementation. When active TB is diagnosed during pregnancy the woman should be treated as soon as it is suspected with isoniazid (INH), rifampin (RIF), and ethambutol (EMB) daily for 2 months, followed by INH and RIF daily, or twice weekly for 7 months, for a total of 9 months (CDC, 2011). The risk of drug toxicity to an infant breastfed by a mother taking anti-tuberculosis medication is minimal. A breastfeeding newborn might receive 6% to 20% of the therapeutic dose of isoniazid and 1% to 11% of other drugs, such as rifampin, ethambutol, and streptomycin (Snider & Powell, 1984). Moreover, infants exposed to tuberculosis are themselves treated with a therapeutic dose of isoniazid.

BOX 15-6 GUIDELINES AND TECHNIQUES FOR DECREASING RISK OF TRANSMISSION OF MRSA AND OTHER NOSOCOMIAL INFECTIONS

- Facilitate skin-to-skin contact and breastfeeding as soon as possible after delivery. At a minimum the newborn's mouth should be placed on mother's nipple to receive the bacterium on the mother's skin as well as to enhance milk flow.
- Promote the growth of bifido bacteria in the baby's intestines by immediate feeding of breastmilk.
- Encourage frequent skin-to-skin holding.
- Have mother and baby room-in as well as place the beds side by side. This will reduce the likelihood of horizontal infection from other caregivers.
- Teach mother good latching techniques to prevent nipple damage.
- Have staff wash their hands with disinfectant soap or hand-hygiene gels immediately before and after contact with the newborn or mother (foam in, foam out).
- Use gloves (non-latex) when handling newborns.
- Use gown and mask when needed to avoid contamination of clothes or splash/droplet exposure.
- Disinfect baby scales, BP cuffs, stethoscopes, breast pumps and other items handled by staff.
- Screen and treat MRSA carrier staff.
- Educate mothers about the following:
  - ◄ Frequent hand washing with warm soapy water or antibacterial gel/foam
  - ◄ Keeping open lesions covered with a bandage
  - ◄ Disposal of soiled bandages or materials that have touched an infected wound in separate bags
  - ◄ Warning signs of MRSA breast infections
- Educate families about the following:
  - ◄ Risks of intrafamilial spread of skin infections
  - ◄ Hand washing
  - ◄ Not sharing personal items, such as razors, sports equipment, bed linens, and towels
  - ◄ Continue skin-to-skin holding and breastfeeding

The 1998 policy of the Global Program for Vaccines and Immunization states, "Infants in situations where they are at risk of TB infection should be immunized with BCG (Bacillus Calmette-Guérin) as soon after birth as possible" (WHO, 1998a). Thus, women who have moved to the United States from countries where TB is endemic and have been vaccinated with BCG will probably have a positive purified protein derivative (PPD) test. PPD, which consists of an intradermal injection on the forearm, is a screening test for TB. If it is positive, the injection site will appear as a reddened induration. There is no reliable way to tell if a positive PPD is from BCG vaccination or infection (Lake, 2001), and a mother with this result will need to be followed up with more testing.

If a breastfeeding mother becomes acutely ill with TB, breastfeeding may have to be interrupted. The mother's breasts should not be allowed to become engorged; a staff member should arrange for the mother to express her milk so that the woman's breasts remain comfortable.

Headaches

Migraine headaches—hormonally sensitive headaches of an episodic nature—tend to lessen through the course of pregnancy and menopause

(Sances et al., 2003; Silberstein, 1993). Postpartum headaches can be caused by oral contraceptives or by having epidural or spinal anesthesia during childbirth, but they can also occur for no apparent reason. Breastfeeding delays the postpartum recurrence of migraine headaches.

Some women have a brief but intense headache when they have an orgasm. It is thought that the rise in blood pressure and heart rate during sexual activity are similar to the physiological process that produces migraine.

Thorley (2000) identified two types of lactational headaches:

- Type 1 occurs on the first letdown during a feed and is linked to the surge of oxytocin from the letdown.
- Type 2 is triggered by overfullness of the breast and is relieved by breastfeeding or pumping.

In addition to oxytocin surge at letdown and breast overfullness, trigger factors for headaches in lactating women include the baby sleeping through the night (Thorley, 1997) and breastfeeding twins (Wall, 1992). A family history of lactational headaches that disappear with weaning can also be a factor (Walker, 1999).

Rest and ice packs should be tried before resorting to medications. Propranolol (Inderal), sumatriptan succinate (Imitrex), and NSAIDs—the standard drugs used for migraine headaches—are all listed as being compatible with breastfeeding. Ergotamine alkaloids (Cafergot, DHE-45) are contraindicated in breastfeeding mothers owing to their suppression of prolactin (Hale, 1999).

Chronic Illnesses

Asthma

Between 3.7% and 8.7% of pregnant women have active asthma that may improve, worsen, or remain unchanged during pregnancy (Mihălțan et al., 2014). Women with a family history of asthma should be encouraged to breastfeed exclusively because of the long-term protective effect of breastfeeding on asthma (Dogaru et al., 2014) (also see the *Biological Specificity of Breastmilk* chapter).

The main concern for the breastfeeding mother is the effect of medications taken to control her asthma. Asthma therapy should be continued during lactation and generally does not have to be altered. The two central classes of antiasthmatic medications are corticosteroids and bronchodilators, including beta agonists (albuterol, terbutaline, and metaproterenol). Beta agonists are used to treat acute exacerbations and to prevent exercise-induced asthma. Most antiasthma medications are administered by metered-dose inhalers, which avoid systemic side effects of the medication by delivering the drug directly to the lungs. Metered aerosol inhalers deliver a given amount of a drug, and the likelihood of overdose is small. Halogenated corticosteroids given by inhalation provide selective topical effects that lessen the amount of corticosteroids transferred into breastmilk (see the *Drug Therapy and Breastfeeding* chapter for more information). Theophylline (Theo-Dur, Slo-BID, Slo-phyllin) is used less frequently now. Although the infant receives only a small percentage (less than 10%) of the maternal dose (Ellsworth, 1994), this drug may occasionally cause infant irritability and insomnia.

Smoking

Women who smoke are less likely to breastfeed and are likely to breastfeed for a shorter period of time than nonsmokers (Amir & Donath, 2002; Giglia et al., 2006; Horta et al., 1997; Liu et al., 2006). They are also less likely to breastfeed exclusively for 6 months (Brown et al., 2013). The fat content of breastmilk of smoking mothers is lower than that of nonsmokers and contains nicotine. The milk of mothers exposed to secondhand smoke also contains smaller concentrations of the lipids that are essential for infant growth (Baheiraei et al., 2014), and mothers who are exposed to secondhand smoke breastfeed for a shorter time than those who are not exposed to such smoke (Horta et al., 1997). The mother who smokes also exposes her infant to secondhand smoke that raises inhaled carbon monoxide to unsafe levels, aggravates allergies, and increases the child's risk of developing respiratory illnesses (Horta et al., 1997). Maternal cigarette smoking is associated with respiratory illnesses, tremors, and muscular rigidity (Vagnarelli, 2006).

The breastfeeding smoker is also at greater risk for breast abscess (Bundred et al., 1992) and breast periductal inflammation (Furlong et al., 1994). Among women with Crohn's disease, smoking resumption in the postpartum period is associated with relapses of this chronic disease (prevalence odds ratio [POR], 1.85; 95% confidence interval [CI], 0.62–5.54) (Julsgaard et al., 2014). Thus there are several reasons related to maternal and infant health to support efforts at smoking cessation during pregnancy and in the postpartum period during lactation.

In one case report, a heavy-smoking lactating mother delivered a baby who had spontaneous tremors, fluctuations of muscular rigidity, and opisthotonus at 48 hours of life (Vagnarelli, 2006). The symptoms could be controlled by swaddling or wrapping the baby in a blanket. The absence of any other etiology generated a suspicion of exposure to heavy tobacco smoke and potential neonatal nicotine withdrawal syndrome. This diagnosis was supported by extremely high concentration of hair nicotine and cotinine in the infant's and mother's hair. The presence of nicotine and cotinine in breastmilk confirmed that the mother did not quit smoking after delivery, despite her reports that she had. The breastfed infant continued to have three to four crises of tremor and muscular rigidity for a month.

Despite the damning evidence about the detrimental effects of smoking, Amir and Donath (2002) maintain that the reasons smokers breastfeed less often and for a shorter period are psychological, not physiological. Their study shows that some women who want to smoke and to breastfeed can and do breastfeed for a long duration of time, debunking a myth about the consistent negative physiological effect on lactation.

The ongoing concern about smoking and breastfeeding begs the question: When we insist that women do not smoke and breastfeed, do we invite the possibility that some mothers will give up breastfeeding rather than stop smoking? Mothers are highly motivated to give the best care to their babies. Given this motivation, there is a need to develop specific programs for smoking cessation. Until these programs are developed, mothers who continue to smoke should be encouraged to breastfeed.

Alterations in Endocrine and Metabolic Functioning

Anything that affects control of the endocrine system can also affect the production of breastmilk. The following discussion of diabetes mellitus, thyroid problems, and pituitary dysfunction explains common and uncommon conditions that may affect the breastfeeding mother's milk supply. Any woman with symptoms that suggest she might have an altered metabolic functioning should be referred to a physician for further evaluation and treatment.

Diabetes

Diabetes is a chronic disease of impaired carbohydrate metabolism caused by insufficient insulin or the inefficient use of insulin. Pregnant women with diabetes mellitus can be classified into two main categories: (1) women who have prepregnancy diabetes (type 1 [T1DM] or type 2 [T2DM]) and (2) women who develop gestational diabetes (GDM). Type 1 diabetes is a serious disease in which insulin is not being produced as a result of autoimmunity directed at the beta cells of the pancreas (Type 1A) or destruction of the beta cells without evidence of autoimmune processes (Type 1B). Type 2 diabetes, which is characterized by an impaired response to insulin and β-cell dysfunction, used to be seen infrequently in pregnancy because the diagnosis was usually made after the reproductive years. Type 2 diabetes is much more common in pregnant women today, however, and is often part of a metabolic syndrome along with hypertension, obesity, dyslipidemia, and polycystic ovarian syndrome (PCOS) (Joham et al., 2014).

Gestational Diabetes

Gestational diabetes—a glucose intolerance that occurs in as many as 9% of all pregnancies in the United States—manifests itself only during pregnancy (DeSisto et al., 2014). Gestational diabetes is far more common now than it was a decade ago because more women (and men) are obese today. Gestational diabetes is detected in the same ways as other forms of diabetes and during pregnancy is often diagnosed during routine glucose tolerance testing. Most women with gestational diabetes will revert to normal glucose metabolism in the postpartum period. However, it is now well documented that many women who had GDM will later develop T2DM. In fact, a meta-analysis of 20 retrospective and prospective cohort studies showed that the risk of developing T2DM later in life was 7 times higher in women with GDM than in women without GDM (Bellamy et al., 2009).

Breastfeeding should be encouraged among mothers with GDM because evidence also indicates that lactation improves glucose metabolism in the early postpartum period in these women (Gunderson et al., 2014; Much et al., 2014). Nevertheless, additional prospective, well-designed studies are necessary to more fully support the contention that lactation protects women with GDM from future T2DM (Gunderson et al., 2014). Healthcare providers' encouragement of the breastfeeding choice on a prenatal basis is essential because there is greater likelihood that women with GDM will not initiate breastfeeding (Finkelstein et al., 2013).

Lactation consultant/specialist support is also essential for women with GDM because of their risk for delayed onset of lactogenesis II (Matias et al., 2014; Nommsen-Rivers et al., 2010). In the largest study to date of early lactation outcomes in women with GDM, Matias and colleagues (2014) found that among 883 participants in the Study of Women, Infant Feeding, and Type 2 Diabetes After GDM Pregnancy (SWIFT study), one-third of women with recent GDM experienced delayed onset of lactogenesis. Maternal obesity, insulin treatment, and suboptimal in-hospital breastfeeding were key risk factors for such a delay.

Early breastfeeding support for women with GDM and these risk factors is certainly indicated to ensure successful lactation. In-hospital support and education to facilitate early skin-to-skin contact, frequent breastfeeding, rooming-in, and careful monitoring of infant intake, output, and glucose levels as needed are warranted. Finally, women with a history of gestational diabetes should be screened with a fasting plasma glucose at 6 weeks postpartum and annually thereafter (Taylor et al., 2005).

Type 1 Diabetes

With improvement in the monitoring and control of maternal blood sugar, women with type 1 diabetes (T1DM) who have well-controlled glucose levels can usually look forward to a safe and relatively healthy pregnancy and birth. It is commonplace today for a woman with diabetes to experience a normal delivery and for the infant to remain with the mother from birth and to breastfeed without the need for special care. The current use of subcutaneous insulin infusion pumps and multiple daily insulin doses has decreased the erratic glucose levels once seen, resulting in fewer perinatal complications. During pregnancy, the mother's blood glucose levels should be maintained below 130 mg/dL as much as possible. During labor and delivery, and for some time after delivery, blood glucose levels are closely monitored.

According to one recent U.S. study, rates of breastfeeding among women with type 1 diabetes are lower than those among the general childbearing population (Cordero et al., 2014). Of 392 mothers with pregestational diabetes in this study, 159 (41%) initiated breastfeeding. A regression model showed that the strongest predictor of initiation was the intention to breastfeed, followed by higher education (odds ratio [OR], 1.91; 95% CI, 1.18–3.10). Conversely, women who did not breastfeed were more likely to be African American, smokers, or those whose infants were admitted to the NICU. In this study, 45% of the 251 white women and 27% of 97 African American women initiated breastfeeding. At the time of discharge from the hospital, 29 infants (13%) were exclusively breastfed, 53 (23%) were breastfed with formula supplementation, and the remaining 144 (64%) were taking formula exclusively. These findings may not be representative of all diabetic women in the United States, but they certainly do suggest that prenatal education and counseling related to the benefits of breastfeeding are needed.

The woman with type 1 diabetes not only can, but should, be encouraged to breastfeed her infant. Colostrum helps to stabilize the infant's blood sugar. Although breastfeeding should begin as soon after birth as possible, this is usually not the case. Infants of mothers with diabetes are occasionally placed in the special care unit after delivery (Cordero et al., 2014). If breastfeeding is delayed, the mother should be encouraged to begin expressing or pumping her milk as soon as she feels able.

Lactating women with type 1 diabetes have a delay of about one day in lactogenesis II, or "coming in" of their milk (Arthur et al., 1994; Bitman et al., 1989; Hartmann & Cregan, 2001; Miyake et al., 1989; Murtaugh et al., 1998). These mothers and their neonates need additional attention and care to establish lactation. In addition to early, frequent feedings, pumping to stimulate the milk supply is advised. It may be necessary to supplement the neonate during the first 2 to 3 days after birth due to hypoglycemia (Cordero et al., 2014). According to the Academy of Breastfeeding Medicine's Protocol Committee (2009), expressed human milk is the first choice for supplementing the newborn, followed by pasteurized donor human milk, and lastly protein hydrolysate formulas. The ABM protocol for blood glucose monitoring and treatment of hypoglycemia should also be followed because the infant of the diabetic mother is at increased risk for hypoglycemia (Wight et al., 2014).

During the immediate postnatal period, sudden but normal hormonal changes may cause marked fluctuations in maternal blood glucose levels. Maternal hypoglycemia can be expected to occur immediately post birth, with this condition lasting 5 to 7 hours after delivery. In addition, lactose excretion in the urine drops to a low level 2 to 5 days after birth, but then rises rapidly. These sudden metabolic shifts of erratic blood glucose levels and an increase in insulin reaction require close monitoring. Juggling the feeding schedule of the infant and the amount of milk taken at each feeding are factors to be considered in maintaining good diabetic balance. Nighttime feedings present special challenges to the breastfeeding mother with diabetes. The mother should be encouraged to test her glucose levels during the night. She may need an additional snack at night.

Lactose is reabsorbed from the breast and is normally excreted in the urine; therefore, nurses and mothers should be aware that in testing the urine after delivery, the presence of lactose might result in a false-positive result if copper-reducing urine testing (Clinitest) is used. For this reason, testing with Testape or Diastix, which measure only glucose, is preferred. Once she is physiologically stable, the woman with type 1 diabetes can return to treatment with subcutaneous injection insulin or to injection via a portable infusion pump.

Blood glucose meters are reliable means of testing blood glucose by the mother at home. By keeping a daily record of blood glucose levels, the mother can self-monitor day-to-day changes. Once the blood glucose level stabilizes, it is generally lower during lactation. For example, early research by Ferris et al. (1988, 1993) compared 30 mothers with type 1 diabetes with 30 controls and found that fasting plasma glucose levels in mothers during the exclusive breastfeeding period were significantly lower than were the glucose levels of the women with type 1 diabetes who had stopped breastfeeding or who had never breastfed, even in the face of markedly higher caloric intake by the breastfeeding mothers.

Women with type 1 diabetes usually take insulin by injection. Insulin, a large peptide that does not pass into breastmilk, is not a problem medication with breastfeeding.

In addition to providing the known physiological advantages of breastfeeding for the infant, breastfeeding helps to fulfill the mother's need to feel normal in spite of her diabetic condition. An advantage of working with these women is their keen awareness of their body functions and the importance of diet. They are more knowledgeable than the average woman about physiology and are quick to notice changes that may forewarn of problems. These mothers are likely to need prolonged professional and peer support as they continue to breastfeed over time—a recommendation supported by Swedish researchers in a recent study. With the aim of identifying needs to develop supportive activities, Berg (2012) explored breastfeeding attitudes and the impact of breastfeeding on the daily life of mothers with type 1 diabetes compared with mothers without diabetes. Compared to the reference group, mothers with diabetes did not differ significantly in their rating of how breastfeeding impacted their daily lives at 2 and 6 months (i.e., very much or quite a lot). However, the mothers with diabetes remained more affected by disruptions in daily life and felt more worried about their health both at 2 and 6 months after childbirth.

Mothers with diabetes may be more susceptible to mastitis, especially if their blood glucose level is not well controlled (Ferris et al., 1988; Gagne et al., 1992). Any infection will quickly raise the level of blood glucose. Self-care teaching should emphasize recognizing early symptoms of mastitis and seeking prompt treatment while continuing to breastfeed. Mothers with diabetes are also at risk for candidiasis if blood glucose levels are elevated. Preventing this problem involves careful control of blood glucose, drying the nipple after breastfeeding, and being aware of the early symptoms.

Once lactation is established, most women who have diabetes report that their breastfeeding experiences are no different from those of mothers without diabetes. Notably, the mother with diabetes needs additional calories while breastfeeding. As her child begins to wean, the mother will again need to make alterations in her diet and insulin intake to compensate for a decrease in milk production. If weaning is gradual, fewer problems and adjustments arise.

Type 2 Diabetes

Like women with GDM and T1DM, women with type 2 diabetes (T2DM) are less likely to initiate breastfeeding, according to some researchers (Taylor et al., 2005). However, the benefits of breastfeeding for maternal and infant health should be emphasized in prenatal and early postpartum teaching and support. Mothers with T2DM and their infants have physical and emotional issues similar to those of mothers with T1DM and their infants, although the former group's glucose control may not be as volatile in the early postpartum period.

Diabetes therapy during and after pregnancy and during lactation often consists of metformin. There is no evidence of long-term impact on the offspring

of women who used metformin during pregnancy, but more evidence is required (Simmons, 2010).

Thyroid Disease

The thyroid gland controls the body's metabolism and promotes normal growth and development of the central nervous system and brain. It produces three hormones: thyrosine/thyroxine (T_4), triiodothyronine (T_3), and calcitonin. Iodine combines with thyroglobulin, a protein substance found in the follicles of the thyroid, to produce T_4 and T_3. T_4 can be produced only in the thyroid gland. In contrast, only 20% of T_3 is manufactured in the thyroid; the remainder is produced by the removal of one iodine atom from T_4 outside the thyroid (Speller et al., 2012). T_3 and T_4 are chemically similar and are known as the thyroid hormones.

T_3 and T_3 production is regulated by a feedback mechanism involving the hypothalamus and the anterior pituitary. Thyrotropin-releasing hormone (TRH), produced in the hypothalamus, stimulates the production of thyroid-stimulating hormone (TSH) by the pituitary, while thyroid hormones themselves inhibit the production of TSH. Thus, TSH levels rise in response to low T_3 or T_4 levels (hypothyroidism) and stimulate the thyroid to produce more hormone, whereas high levels of T_3 or T_4 (hyperthyroidism) inhibit production of TSH, slowing T_3 and T_4 production.

The physiologic changes of pregnancy influence the thyroid quite profoundly. The size of the thyroid increases by approximately 10% due to a 20% to 40% increase in production of thyroid hormones; this change supports maternal needs and fetal development of the brain. The maternal iodine requirement is also increased during pregnancy, and iodine stores should be replete at conception with an iodine intake of more than 150 g per day (De Groot et al., 2012). Thyroid screening tests are pregnancy trimester specific, with overall decreases in TSH, increases in thyroxin-binding globulin, and lower T_4 and higher T_3 concentrations being apparent (Carney et al., 2014; De Groot et al., 2012).

Postpartum thyroid dysfunction is fairly common and includes hypothyroidism, hyperthyroidism, and postpartum thyroiditis (PPT). Some thyroid disease is considered an immune-mediated dysfunction (e.g., PPT and Graves's disease). Breastfeeding women who develop disorders of the thyroid gland can be treated and continue to breastfeed in most cases.

Hypothyroidism

Maintaining full-term pregnancy is rare in untreated women who suffer from hypothyroidism; therefore, most breastfeeding women with a history of hypothyroidism are on replacement therapy. For the untreated breastfeeding woman, hypothyroidism can result in a reduced milk supply. Other symptoms in the mother are thyroid swelling or nodules (goiter), cold intolerance, dry skin, thinning hair, poor appetite, extreme fatigue, and depression. When the thyroid deficiency is not known, these problems are often attributed to postpartum hormonal changes and changes in lifestyle (notably, constant care of the baby) and remain undiagnosed—at least for a time. When the infant of one mother suddenly and completely weaned, the mother, who subsequently received a diagnosis of hypothyroidism, reported that she "never experienced any fullness in the breast—it was as though I'd dried up overnight." (personal communication). In another case, hypothyroidism developed in a preterm infant whose initial screening thyroid function test results were normal at 2 weeks of life. The infant's mother was packing her cesarean incision with iodine-soaked gauze, resulting in a markedly increased breastmilk iodine concentration. Treatment with oral L-thyroxine normalized the infant's thyroid function tests (Smith et al., 2006).

These maternal complaints, which are sometimes coupled with the infant's failure to gain weight satisfactorily on breastmilk alone, should alert the healthcare provider, nurse, or lactation consultant to the possibility of thyroid deficiency and to the reality that the mother needs further medical diagnostic evaluation. If replacement therapy of thyroid extract with synthetic T_4 (thyroxine, sodium levothyroxine, or Synthroid) or other thyroid preparation is adequate, the relief of the symptoms and an increase in the milk supply can be quite dramatic. The daily replacement dose of thyroid extract is 0.25 to 1.12 mg of sodium levothyroxine or an equivalent dose of another thyroid preparation. Women whose replacement therapy was established before pregnancy should be reevaluated after the baby's birth to determine whether adjustment is necessary; in most cases, the thyroid replacement dose is cut back to the prepregnancy dose (De Groot et al., 2012).

Hyperthyroidism

An excess of thyroid hormone is characterized by loss of weight (despite an increased appetite), nervousness, sweating, heat intolerance, muscle weakness, decreased exercise tolerance, frequent bowel movements, heart palpitations, a rapid pulse at rest, and hypertension (Carney et al., 2014). Hyperthyroidism in the year following birth occurs in approximately 9% of women (Goldstein, 2013). Graves's disease accounts for nearly 95% of hyperthyroidism in pregnancy (Carney et al., 2014), but is less common postpartum, accounting for only 0.2% of such cases (De Groot et al., 2012).

The ability to lactate does not appear to be affected with hyperthyroidism, although the mother's nervousness may complicate her ability to cope with the daily caregiving of her infant. However, in a recent case study, Goldstein (2013) reported on a new case of Graves's disease in a mother with lactation failure in her first and second pregnancies.

Generally, laboratory diagnosis of hyperthyroidism can be established by values from just two laboratory tests: serum TSH and serum free T_4 index. When evaluation of the thyroid using a radioactive substance is deemed essential, technetium-99m pertechnetate is the preferred agent (Stagnaro-Green et al., 2011). Treatment of hyperthyroidism consists of antithyroid medications such as methimazole or propylthiouracil, both of which are safe during lactation (Carney et al., 2014). (See also the *Drug Therapy and Breastfeeding* chapter.)

Postpartum Thyroiditis

Postpartum thyroiditis (PPT) is thought to be an autoimmune disorder. Women with a history of type 1 diabetes, thyroglobulin or thyroperoxidase autoantibodies, Graves's disease, or viral hepatitis are at increased risk of developing PPT. Asymptomatic women should be screened at 3 and 6 months postpartum using serum TSH measurement (Carney et al., 2014; De Groot et al., 2012).

Postpartum thyroiditis is the most common form of postpartum thyroid dysfunction, affecting approximately 7% of women in the first year post childbirth. At this time, there is not enough evidence to recommend universal screening (De Groot et al., 2012). PPT may present as hyperthyroidism (32%) or hypothyroidism (43%), or begin with hyperthyroidism and progress to hypothyroidism (25%) (Carney et al., 2014). Women who have experienced PPT are at risk for permanent hypothyroidism within 5 to 10 years after giving birth and should be screened annually (Carney et al., 2014; De Groot et al., 2012).

The symptoms of PPT—fatigue, depression, and anxiety—may go unrecognized in the postpartum period. Treatment depends on presenting symptoms and laboratory findings. Women with a hypothyroid condition who are breastfeeding should be treated with levothyroxine (De Groot et al., 2012). The hyperthyroid phase of PPT is caused by autoimmune destruction of the thyroid and leads to release of stored thyroid hormone; thus antithyroid medication is not useful for this condition. Beta blockers may be used to treat symptoms in these women. However, differentiation of the hyperthyroid phase of PPT from Graves's disease is important because Graves's disease requires antithyroid therapy. Radioactive iodine uptake testing is generally required for this purpose and necessitates a temporary interruption in breastfeeding. The radioiodine uptake is elevated or normal in Graves's disease and low in PPT. Due to their shorter half-life, ^{123}I or technetium scans are preferred to ^{131}I scans in women who are breastfeeding. Nursing can resume several days after an ^{123}I or technetium scan (Stagnaro-Green et al., 2011).

Pituitary Dysfunction

Severe postpartum hemorrhage and hypotension may result in the pituitary gland's failure to produce gonadotropins, which leads to a condition known as *panhypopituitarism* or *Sheehan's syndrome*. Along with

lactation failure, the affected woman experiences loss of pubic and axillary hair, intolerance to cold, breast and vaginal tissue atrophy, low blood pressure, secondary hypothyroidism, and adrenal failure, all of which manifest over years (Dökmetaş et al., 2006; Sert et al., 2003). Milder cases of pituitary disruption may occur, with less severe symptoms and delay in milk synthesis. DeCoopman's (1993) report that lactation continued following pituitary resection suggests that the role of the pituitary gland may be temporary in the early establishment of lactation rather than an essential requirement throughout its course.

Prolactinomas (prolactin-secreting adenomas) are the most common pituitary tumors, occurring at a rate of 30 to 50 cases per 100,000 population; 80% to 90% of these tumors occur among women, giving a rate of approximately 1 case per 1200 women (Domingue et al., 2014). These adenomas stimulate the secretion of prolactin and lead to secondary galactorrhea, amenorrhea, and infertility.

Dopamine agonists such as bromocriptine (BRC) and cabergoline (CAB) are the mainstay of treatment for prolactinomas; they reduce tumor size (and compression on the optic chiasm), normalize prolactin levels, and restore fertility in women who wish to conceive (Glezer & Bronstein, 2014; Wang et al., 2012). A recent review indicated that cabergoline was more effective than bromocriptine in reducing resistant prolactin levels and restoring fertility (Wang et al., 2012). Nevertheless, BRC remains the drug of choice for induction of pregnancy due to its shorter half-life and concerns for fetal development in the first trimester. BRC is discontinued as soon as pregnancy is confirmed. According to the Endocrine Society Guidelines, only women who experience symptomatic tumor growth during pregnancy are allowed to continue BRC, or CAB in those who cannot tolerate BRC (Glezer & Bronstein, 2014).

Women with prolactinomas may breastfeed without restriction. Evidence suggests that the number of pregnancies per woman and duration of lactation do not impact the remission rate (Dominigue et al., 2014). Auriemma et al. (2013) evaluated 143 pregnancies in 91 women with hyperprolactinemia and observed that treatment with CAB had to be restarted within 6 months after lactation in 29 women, while 68% remained normoprolactinemic up to 60 months after giving birth. There was no difference in serum prolactin levels among women who breastfed for less than 2 months versus those who nursed 2 to 6 months. The authors concluded that nursing does not influence hyperprolactinemia recurrence.

Cystic Fibrosis

Cystic fibrosis (CF) is a hereditary autosomal recessive genetic disorder of infants, children, and adults. Prevalence of CF is highest in North America, where the disease affects 1 in 3000 Caucasians of Northern European descent. Lower prevalence of CF is observed in other groups—Latino-Americans, 1:10,000; African Americans, 1:15,000. The disorder is uncommon in Africa and Asia, where prevalence ranges from 1:35,000 to 1:350,000 (Antunovic et al., 2013).

In CF, a single gene defect (CF transmembrane regulator gene [CFTR]) on chromosome 7 affects the apical membrane of epithelial cells that line the airways, biliary tree, intestines, vas deferens, female reproductive tract, sweat ducts, and pancreatic ducts. The disorder is associated with widespread dysfunction of the exocrine glands and is marked by chronic pulmonary infection, obstruction of the pancreatic ducts, and pancreatic enzyme deficiency.

In the past, children with CF rarely lived to adulthood. In more recent years, early and ongoing sophisticated treatment regimens have substantially increased the life span of those with CF; more than 40% of CF patients are now older than 18 years of age (Antunovic et al., 2013). Although women with cystic fibrosis may have reduced fertility secondary to CFTR effects on ovulatory function, uterine fluid composition, and cervical mucus (Ahmad et al., 2013), pregnancy does occur (Tonelli & Aitken, 2007). With adequate pulmonary and nutritional management and status monitoring, including management of diabetes (which is fairly prevalent in CF), women with CF can successfully complete pregnancy (McMullen et al., 2006).

There is limited evidence on the prevalence of breastfeeding among mothers with CF. In a study of pregnancy morbidity and outcomes in 22 Swedish and Norwegian women with CF, 26 of 33 babies (79%) were breastfed and all stopped breastfeeding before 3 months of age (Ødegaard et al., 2002). Mothers who delivered preterm infants were significantly less likely to breastfeed their babies (50% versus 88% of term infants; $p < 0.05$). In CF clinics in Toronto, Canada, pregnancy and fetal outcomes were identified in 49 women with CF who gave birth to 74 babies between 1968 and 1993 (Gilljam et al., 2000). Breastfeeding information was available for 43 pregnancies in 29 women and indicated approximately 50% breastfed one or all of their children; about half breastfed for 1 to 3 months, and the remainder for longer than 4 months.

Early case studies have provided descriptions of the breastfeeding experiences of mothers with CF and their infants' outcomes. Shiffman et al. (1989) reported breastfeeding duration of two women was 1 to 2 months, during which time the babies grew at appropriate rates. In both cases, the concentrations of milk sugar, electrolytes, sodium, potassium, and chloride were within normal limits. At the same time, concentrations of milk proteins, fat, and immunoglobulin A (IgA) appeared to decrease during periods of pulmonary exacerbations. Michel and Mueller (1994) reported on five cases in which infants maintained adequate growth, including one who exclusively breastfed for 6 months. Welch and colleagues (1981) described a 20-year-old woman with CF whose early breastfeeding course was normal and whose baby grew appropriately through the first 10 weeks postpartum. Thereafter, the mother continued to lose weight and her respiratory status began to worsen. She began antibiotic therapy and stopped breastfeeding. In another case, a breastfeeding mother with CF in Italy had to receive intravenous antibiotic treatment with tobramycin; the drug was not detected in her breastmilk, and lactation continued (Festini et al., 2006). Another case report documented the normal growth of an infant through 6 weeks of exclusive breastfeeding by a 24-year-old mother with CF. These authors concluded that breastfeeding is an "acceptable option" for women with the disease, as long as the maternal diet is closely monitored and vitamin and caloric supplementation is offered when necessary (Golembeski & Emergy, 1989).

Mothers with CF should be encouraged to breastfeed. Concern about the mother's own health status while breastfeeding and caring for a young infant warrants close monitoring of her pulmonary and nutrition needs. Considerations do not include the quality of the mother's milk. Although there are some differences in lipid composition, the breastmilk of mothers with CF contains nutrients sufficient to supply the energy needs of the nursing infant (Edenborough et al., 2008). In addition, breastfeeding conveys immunological advantages to the nursing infant. Because individuals with CF are chronic carriers of bacterial pathogens (such as *Staphylococcus aureus* and *Pseudomonas*), breastmilk lymphocytes, sensitized to the bacterial pathogens carried by the mother, will protect the infant against these infections.

Polycystic Ovarian Syndrome

Polycystic ovarian syndrome (PCOS) is a common endocrine disorder in women that is characterized by abnormal ovulation, clinical or laboratory indices of increased androgen levels, and polycystic ovaries. The prevalence of PCOS is anywhere from 6% to 8% (Carmina & Aziz, 2006). Originally called Stein-Leventhal syndrome, PCOS features clinical manifestations including amenorrhea or irregular menses, hirsutism (unusual hair growth), persistent acne, androgen-dependent alopecia, abdominal obesity, hypertension, and infertility. Unusual breast development has also been noted. A classic radiographic study of breast tissue identified frequent aberrations that included hypoplasia and large breasts filled primarily with fatty tissue (Balcar et al., 1972). Tissue samples from another study demonstrated abnormalities of the glandular parenchyma (Fonseca, 1985). Clinical observations by lactation consultants have cited tubular-shaped breasts with a large space between them and large-diameter nipples in women with PCOS (Wilson-Clay & Hoover, 2013).

Marasco (2005) hypothesized a connection between insufficient milk supply and PCOS. It was thought that the high levels of androgens associated with PCOS interfere with the hormones necessary for full lactation, and subsequent research has supported this hypothesis. Vanky et al. (2008) reported that in comparison to matched controls ($n = 99$), women with PCOS ($n = 36$) breastfed less at 1 month postpartum; dehydroepiandrosterone sulfate (DHEAS) levels among those women at 32 and 36 weeks' gestation were negatively associated with breastfeeding at 1 and 3 months after birth. A randomized clinical trial ($n = 186$), Carlsen and colleagues (2010) likewise found support for a negative association between mid-pregnancy androgen levels and breastfeeding at 3 and 6 months in mothers without PCOS.

Vanky and colleagues (2012), in follow-up to a randomized trial, investigated breast size change and the impact of metformin during pregnancy on breastfeeding in women with PCOS. Metformin is the drug of choice for treatment of PCOS. It improves the endocrinopathy associated with PCOS, facilitates conception, appears to reduce first-trimester miscarriage and gestational diabetes, does not appear to cause birth defects, and appears to be safe in the first 6 months of infancy (Glueck et al., 2006; Glueck & Wang, 2007; Hale & Rowe, 2014). Vanky et al. (2012) found no differences in the duration of exclusive or partial breastfeeding between mothers with PCOS who were treated with metformin and a group of placebo-treated women. The duration of both exclusive and partial breastfeeding correlated positively with breast size change in pregnancy. The basal metabolic index (BMI) was negatively associated with breastfeeding duration. Late-pregnancy androgens had no effect on breast size changes or duration of breastfeeding. In closer examination, women who had no change in breast size during pregnancy were found to have higher blood pressure, were more obese, and had higher fasting insulin and triglyceride levels early in pregnancy compared to those women with breast changes, suggesting metabolic disturbance in the women without breast changes. Among those women who had stopped breastfeeding at 3 months, the majority gave insufficient or no milk supply as the reason for weaning.

Marasco, Marmet, and Shell (2000) described three additional cases of breastfeeding women with PCOS who had insufficient milk supply. While working with a mother who is experiencing a delay with her milk coming in, it is wise to ask questions about menstrual problems, infertility, miscarriages, and ovarian cysts. Marasco (2005, p. 28) cautions healthcare professionals:

> When primary lactation failure is evident, great sensitivity is needed in guiding the mother through the process of deciding how she wants to proceed. Remember that she is facing a complex situation that does not offer a guarantee of full results and that she may even have come to us hesitantly, afraid of "fanaticism" that ignores the emotions and realities of her situation. Anything that feels like subtle pressure can heap more guilt upon her, resulting in anger and resentment.

More research is needed to evaluate the effects of metformin use during lactation. Although safety for the nursing infant has been supported (Glueck et al., 2006; Glueck & Wang, 2007; Hale & Rowe, 2014) and this treatment is therapeutic for the patient with PCOS who has taken metformin throughout pregnancy, little is known about metformin's effects, if any, on breastfeeding outcomes.

Gestational Ovarian Theca Lutein Cysts

Theca lutein cysts are an unusual condition in which, during pregnancy, both ovaries are enlarged by multiple cysts that produce a high level of testosterone. Several weeks postpartum, the cysts resolve and the testosterone level returns to normal. Women with this condition usually have delayed lactogenesis II. After testosterone drops (to approximately 300 ng/dL), milk production begins, and the mother is able to breastfeed (Hoover et al., 2002).

If the testosterone level is high, an ultrasound should be ordered to determine whether ovarian cysts are present. If cysts are found on ultrasound, documenting their resolution supports the diagnosis and also rules out the possibility of malignancy. Betzold, Hoover, and Snyder (2004) described four cases of women with gestational ovarian theca lutein cysts. Three of the four women were eventually able to supply 100% of their infants' caloric requirements through breastfeeding.

Mood Disorders During Lactation

Pregnancy, birth, and the postpartum period are a time of emotional and psychosocial challenges and adjustments, a time of healing and growth, and, one hopes, a time of confidence building and empowerment. However, they are also a time when anxiety and depression can become overwhelming, having devastating, long-lasting effects on the mother, infant, and family (Ystrom, 2012). Conversely, hormonal and physiological changes accompanying birth and lactation create an adaptive physiologic state that can be protective against mood disorders (Donaldson-Myles, 2011). This physiologic state is designed to protect the mother–infant dyad from extraneous, bothersome environmental stimuli and to promote calm, nurturing, and optimal functioning of immune and metabolic systems while blunting reactivity to stress (Groer, 2005; also see the discussion of stress in this chapter).

Peripartum Depression

Peripartum depression, formerly known as postpartum depression (PPD), comprises a spectrum of disorders that occur during pregnancy and postpartum, and can last through the first 12 months after birth. The label "peripartum" for this form of depression acknowledges that as many as 50% of mood disorders begin during the third trimester of pregnancy (American Psychological Association, 2013). The incidence of peripartum depression is estimated to range from 5.5% to 33.1%, and each year more than 400,000 infants are born to mothers who are or will become depressed (McDonagh et al., 2014). Peripartum depression is the leading cause of disability in women, being responsible for $30 billion to $50 billion in lost productivity and direct medical costs each year in the United States (ACOG, 2010).

Commonly described as a triad of mood disorders, peripartum depression encompasses a variety of syndromes ranging from mild depression and anxiety, including hopelessness, desolation, agitation, and fatigue, to severe forms of emotional disorders such as major depression and psychosis (Zauderer & Davis, 2012).

- *Baby "blues" (maternity blues, postpartum blues):* A common mild transient affective syndrome experienced by 70% to 80% of women following birth. Characteristic symptoms include emotional lability with mood swings possible several times a day, weeping, anxiety, fatigue, insomnia, irritability, mood elevation, and cognitive difficulties such as poor attention, distractibility, and poor short-term memory (Quintero et al., 2014). Depression and sadness are generally not typical symptoms of the baby blues. Generally, the onset of this condition occurs during the first few days after delivery, with increasing intensity and then spontaneous resolution being observed after 7 to 10 days. The baby blues is more common in women having their first child.

- *Peripartum depression:* An episode of mild to moderate depression occurring shortly (within 4 to 6 weeks) after childbirth. If a mother has a depressive episode after one pregnancy, her risk of recurrence with subsequent pregnancies is as high as 50% to 62%. Symptoms of PPD are similar to those observed with major depression: tearfulness, emotional lability and irritability, despondency, feelings of inadequacy or guilt related to parenting abilities, thoughts of harming self or baby, sadness, reduced or increased appetite, insomnia or hypersomnia, feelings of helplessness and hopelessness, anxiety, and despair (Quintero et al., 2014). When they have severe depression, mothers may reject their baby. Because every new mother experiences at least some of these symptoms, they may be wrongly interpreted as baby blues. Peripartum depression lasts at least 2 weeks but usually longer. Typically depression begins during the third trimester of pregnancy or after delivery; however, it can also occur after weaning (Sharma & Corpse, 2008).

- *Postpartum psychosis:* Although it remains rare (1 to 2 cases per 1000 births), psychosis is the most severe of the peripartum disorders (Quintero et al., 2014). Mothers with a personal or family history of mood disorders, especially bipolar disorder type 1, are at significantly greater risk. Other risk factors include primiparity, cesarean birth, and discontinuation of mood stabilizers including lithium. Peripartum psychosis typically begins 2 to 4 weeks postpartum, with acute delusional symptoms being combined with confusion and mood manifestations. The primary difference between perinatal psychosis and other perinatal psychiatric disorders is the presence of psychotic symptoms or disturbances in perception of reality such as delusions, hallucination, thought disorganization, irrational ideas, feelings of failure, self-accusatory thoughts, and, sometimes, threats to commit suicide. Women with postpartum psychosis are a danger to themselves and to their children and should *never* be left alone.

New mothers with high levels of life stress and few supportive relationships (especially in regard to a husband or partner) more frequently suffer from peripartum depression. There is no consistent evidence that the mother's age, the number of children she has, or complications during the pregnancy and birth are associated with the appearance of depression.

For many years, research focused on the impact of depression—especially untreated depression—on breastfeeding duration (Dennis & McQueen, 2009; Henderson et al., 2003; Nishioka et al., 2011) and infant social development, in the form of insecure attachment, behavioral problems, impaired cognitive function, increased risk of abuse and neglect, and childhood psychiatric symptoms and diagnosis (Freeman, 2012). Numerous researchers have compared depressive symptomatology between breastfeeding mothers and bottle-feeding mothers. They report that breastfeeding mothers have less depression (Tashakori et al., 2012). Also, the longer mothers breastfeed, the lower their risk for and severity of PPD (Akman et al., 2008). These findings have led to a reversal of the research question to "What is the impact of breastfeeding on postpartum depression?" (Donaldson-Myles, 2011; Hahn-Holbrook et al., 2013). When the question is asked in this manner, the findings indicate that mothers with lower Edinburgh Postnatal Depression Scale (EPDS) and State-Trait Anxiety scores and higher levels of oxytocin during breastfeeding have a more positive affect—that is, they are happier, have more positive moods, report more positive events, and perceive less stress (Groer, 2005; Stuebe et al., 2013).

Hahn-Holbrook and colleagues (2013) reported outcomes supporting both views of the interaction between breastfeeding and depression: women who had depressive symptomatology prenatally weaned their infants 2.3 months earlier than women without such symptomatology (depressive symptomatology → early weaning). However, women without prenatal depressive symptoms who were more fully breastfeeding (closer to exclusive breastfeeding) at 3 months had declines in depressive symptoms for up to 2 years (↑ breastfeeding at 3 months → ↓ depression symptoms over 2 years), illustrating the protective effect of breastfeeding on depression and mood alterations (Groer et al., 2002; Hahn-Holbrook et al., 2013).

To explain the cause of postpartum depression, a psychoneuroimmunology (PNI) framework has been suggested. Recent research has confirmed that rather than inflammation independently being *a* risk factor for depression along with stress, sleep disturbance, pain, psychological trauma, and a history of depression or trauma, it is *the* risk factor undergirding the other five factors and explaining depression in general (Kendall-Tackett, 2007). Additionally, the inflammation process provides a perspective on the mechanisms by which previously identified psychosocial, behavioral, and physical factors increase the risk for depression. In particular, physical and psychological stressors trigger the inflammatory response system. Expectant mothers are especially vulnerable to inflammation starting during the third trimester of pregnancy, as inflammation levels rise significantly during this period and are exacerbated by common experiences of the last trimester and new motherhood (e.g., sleep disturbance, pain, psychological stress and trauma, and history of depression or trauma). Therefore, it is important to identify known physical and psychological risk factors or causes of depression and to be proactive in addressing inflammation and depression risk factors so as to increase expectant mothers' resilience to other stressors. (For a more complete discussion, see Kendall-Tackett, 2007.)

When Beck first proposed a substantive theory of postpartum depression in 1993, she shared reflections of mothers who had suffered from PPD. These women reported loss of control as a basic social and psychological problem in PPD. One mother confided, "I had absolutely no control, and that was the scariest thing because I always had control." Another woman said of her feelings, "I just couldn't get out of the pain. It's like you hurt so bad, and you don't want to be that way, and yet you lost all control of everything" (Beck, 1993). When their depression started, these mothers felt trapped with no foreseeable escape. "One night I had my first severe panic attack. I felt like everything was closing in on me. Something just snapped in me, and there was no going back." Mothers described this period as "going to the gates of hell and back" and "your worst possible nightmare." As the mothers regained control, gradually the number of "good days" increased, but they mourned the lost time they would not be able to recapture with their infants. When the mothers recovered, they talked about how their symptoms just eventually faded away. "When I was sick, I didn't want my baby. I didn't love my husband. I didn't want to work. I hated everything. When I got better, it all melted away" (Beck, 1993). Because of the devastating effects of mood disorders and with new understanding of the processes of PPD, prevention is the primary intervention.

Prevention and Treatment

Perinatal mood disorders are preventable or at least the severity can be decreased by (1) reducing maternal stress and (2) reducing maternal inflammation (Kendall-Tackett, 2007). Nature has its own way of meeting both of these goals, thereby attenuating the risk of postpartum depression: *breastfeeding*. The neuroendocrinology of breastfeeding mothers—especially the release of oxytocin and prolactin—induces calm, has amnesic effects, encourages a positive mood, and decreases maternal reactivity to stressors (Donaldson-Myles, 2012; Groer et al., 2002; Uvnas-Moberg, 1998a, 1998b). Prolactin and oxytocin down-regulate hypothalamic–pituitary–adrenal axis functioning. Specifically, high prolactin levels buffer stress responses by opposing the effects of cortisol, and oxytocin moderates the effects of adrenocorticotropic hormone (ACTH) and cortisol (Donaldson-Myles, 2012). With down-regulation of the stress response, energy is conserved and directed toward milk production and nurturing behaviors (Groer & Davis, 2006). Additionally, exclusive breastfeeding increases maternal immune competence, thereby decreasing the harmful effects of stress (Groer & Morgan, 2007). Thus, when breastfeeding is going well, stress is lowered and activation of the maternal inflammatory response system is avoided, which in turn lowers the mother's risk of depression (Kendall-Tackett, 2007). Breastfeeding also protects infants of depressed mothers by reducing their stress through mechanisms similar to those occurring in mothers.

Numerous other therapies and interventions can help reduce stress in ways similar to breastfeeding. Specifically, the following measures stimulate the release of oxytocin, which then activates the endogenous opioid system, elevating mood.

- Kangaroo care (KC). The ventral surfaces of both mother and infant are particularly sensitive to touch, so KC effortlessly stimulates the release of oxytocin. Continuous KC is associated with continuous pulsatile release of oxytocin, maintaining reduced reactivity to stress and strengthening the bond between mother and baby. Besides the immunological protection achieved by reducing stress, KC provides direct immunological effects. Several different types of wraps are available to facilitate hands-free KC.
- Social support. Social support is a key protective factor, whereas a primary risk factor for peripartum mood disorders is lack of social support. Because of changes in social structure, the support of extended family or the "village" is no longer available for most mothers. Especially in Western cultures, the nuclear family has become the functioning social unit. Therefore, it is important to find other means of constructing social support by building strong, trusting relationships (Deligiannidis & Freeman, 2014; Zauderer & Davis, 2012):
  - Significant other
  - Friendships
  - Continuity of care with midwife or other healthcare provider who is respectful and provides true family-centered care
  - Group prenatal care—encourages the development of social interactions that mothers and fathers interpret as supportive (Arnold et al., 2014; Risisky et al., 2013), leading to similar or improved perinatal and breastfeeding outcomes when compared to women receiving individualized care (Tanner-Smith et al., 2013, 2014)
  - Counseling, psychotherapy, and cognitive behavioral therapies (Guille et al., 2013)
  - Support group (e.g., La Leche League, church group, play group)—decreases sense of isolation
- Education/obtaining knowledge of PPD:
  - Education about the spectrum of perinatal mood disorders to foster appropriate understanding and coping strategies for emotional fluctuations of pregnancy and postpartum
  - Bibliotherapy—reading about others' experiences lets the mother know she is not alone and increases understanding (Zauderer & Davis, 2012)
  - Lullaby therapy—soothing; mothers learn to recognize their infant's cues to the music as well as their own feelings (Zauderer & Davis, 2012)
- Exercise.
- Bright light therapy.
- Massage.
- Acupuncture.

For many mothers, these therapies are adjuvants to supplements (Table 15-6) or pharmacologic

Table 15-6 ACTIONS OF NATURAL SUPPLEMENTS IN DECREASING SEVERITY OR PREVENTING PERIPARTUM MOOD DISORDERS

Supplement	Action
Omega-3 fatty acids	Powerful anti-inflammatories, lowering pro-inflammatory cytokines thereby improving mood by decreasing inflammation.
S-adenosyl methionine	May affect depression positively because it is needed for biosynthesis of serotonin and dopamine (neurotransmitter synthesis). May effect anti-oxidative, anti-inflammatory and neuroprotective processes with biological roles in depression. Found in the body naturally.
St. John's Wort (*hypericum perforatum L.*)	Anti-inflammatory. Helpful in reducing mild to moderate anxiety and depression by inhibiting nerve cells in the brain from reabsorbing serotonin, or by decreasing levels of a protein involved in the body's immune system functioning.
Kava (*Piper methysticum*)	Considered to be a natural tranquilizer. Works by enhancing GABA, a neurotransmitter.
Valerian (*Valeriana officinalis*)	Has anxiolytic effects shown to be effective for mild to moderate anxiety and insomnia, without the drowsiness and side effects of benzodiazepines. Works by increasing the usage of GABA in the body.
B vitamins	Increases tolerance for stress, may decrease anxiety.
Vitamin C	Enhances immune system, which can be depleted of vitamin C during stress.
Folic acid	Coenzyme or co-substrate involved in neurotransmitter metabolism avoiding activation of inflammatory response system. Depression has been found in women who are deficient in folic acid. Associated with better response to antidepressants when taken as a supplement.
Vitamin D (Sun or bright light therapy)	Coenzyme in neurotransmitter metabolism avoiding activation of inflammatory response system. To prevent or treat depression, especially in the winter months.

GABA – γ-aminobutyric acid

Data from Deligiannidis & Freeman, 2014; Kendall-Tackett, 2007; Zauderer & Davis, 2012.

medications. Both supplements and antidepressants decrease inflammation, but many women prefer the natural supplements so as to avoid possible side effects from antidepressant medications. Certainly, antidepressants are the most aggressive line of defense. If the mood disorder is severe enough or not amenable to other treatments, however, antidepressants are the intervention of choice to minimize the significant, negative consequences to infant, mother, and family (Guille et al., 2013). Evidence for the efficacy and safety of antipsychotic and antidepressant agents during pregnancy and breastfeeding is limited due to the small sample sizes and sparse controlled trials and, therefore, inadequate to allow well-informed decisions about treatment (Galbally et al., 2014; McDonagh et al., 2014). Newer, non-tricyclic compounds such as selective serotonin-reuptake inhibitors (SSRIs) produce very low or undetectable plasma concentrations in nursing infants and, therefore, continuation of breastfeeding during treatment should be encouraged (Berle & Spigset, 2011). (See also the *Drug Therapy and Breastfeeding* chapter.)

Peripartum depression has been a concern for decades due to the negative consequences for maternal and infant development. It is incumbent on healthcare providers to provide education regarding peripartum mood disorders and to routinely screen for them during pregnancy and postpartum (ACOG, 2010). Healthcare providers serving pediatric patients are encourage to screen mothers for PPD at least at the 1- and 4-month well-child visits (Myers et al., 2013; Sheeder et al., 2009). Screening includes a thorough personal and family history and psychological assessment upon admission to care, making note of significant risk factors for depression (Scottish Intercollegiate Guidelines Network [SIGN], 2012). As pregnancy progresses, mothers should be asked about depressive or affective symptoms at each encounter. If a mother is at high risk for mental illness, a plan for psychiatric management and referral to a psychiatric specialist should be developed. For lactation consultants, peer counselors, and other breastfeeding support personnel, referral to a healthcare provider or facility should be initiated if mood disorders are suspected or if there is a threat of harm to mother, infant, or other family members. Because peripartum mood disorders negatively affect the whole family and the community, it is our obligation to routinely screen new mothers so they can be treated in a timely manner.

Autoimmune Diseases

Inflammatory Bowel Disease

Inflammatory bowel disease (IBD) is a chronic autoimmune process of unknown origin. The predominant hypothesis for its etiology suggests that genetically susceptible individuals develop an aberrant response to luminal bacteria (Yarur & Kane, 2013). IBD primarily affects the gastrointestinal (GI) tract and has two major forms: ulcerative colitis (UC), which involves the colon (ulcerative proctitis, proctosigmoiditis, left-sided colitis, pancolitis, and fulminant colitis), and Crohn's disease (CD), which can occur in any part of the GI tract but mainly affects the ileum and the colon.

IBD is characterized by periods of active disease and remission. Symptoms of UC depend on the location of the inflammation and range from rectal bleeding and pain, to bloody diarrhea, abdominal cramps and pain, and inability to move the bowels, to weight loss and fatigue. Symptoms of CD include bleeding, diarrhea, nausea, weight loss, abdominal pain, fatigue, and fever. Management of IBD has progressed to include a multidisciplinary team approach including gastroenterologists, surgeons, and registered dietitians. Drug therapy for IBD can include sulfasalazine, mesalamine (acute phase), corticosteroids, antibiotics, and immunosuppressive drugs.

Rates of IBD have increased over time, according to a systematic review of prevalence and incidence studies (Molodecky et al., 2012). The highest incidence rates of IBD occur in the Westernized nations of Northern Europe, Canada, and Australia (Molodecky et al., 2012). Similarly, the prevalence of IBD is highest in Europe and Canada. There appears to be no sex differentiation of occurrence of IBD.

IBD occurs most frequently between 20 and 40 years of age, meaning that it disproportionately affects reproductive-age individuals (Molodecky et al., 2012). There is some evidence of decreased fertility in persons with IBD, in both sexes, and especially among those with more severe forms of IBD who have had surgery (Yarur & Kane, 2013). Pregnancy outcomes for women with IBD compared to controls without IBD indicate higher rates of prematurity, low birth weight, and cesarean births. When disease activity is controlled, there is less evidence of these effects, except for low birth weight and cesarean birth (Yarur & Kane, 2013). In the past, pregnancy was discouraged in women with IBD. Even today, women with CD are encouraged to postpone pregnancy until they experience remission of their disease (Cury & Moss, 2014). During pregnancy, monitoring and managing nutritional status are important. In pregnant women with small-bowel CD, folic acid, vitamin D, and vitamin B_{12} may all need to be supplemented. Based on observational data, most drug treatments are safe in pregnancy and lactation, including 5-aminosalicylic acid, thiopurines, anti-tumor necrosis factor, and anti-integrins. Methotrexate should be avoided due to its teratogenicity (Cury & Moss, 2014).

Work in other autoimmune disorders has found that breastfeeding may be associated with an increased risk for developing postpartum disease relapse; however, in a study of 122 women attending an IBD center in Chicago, breastfeeding did not appear to make any difference in disease activity for either Crohn's disease or ulcerative colitis, after adjusting for cessation of medications. Approximately half of the women attending the center did not breastfeed, and only 29% of those women with CD breastfed their infants. The low percentage of those breastfeeding mainly reflected concern about the effects of maternal medications on the breast-feeding infant (Kane & Lemieux, 2005).

In more recent studies in North America and Europe that enrolled larger samples and tallied greater percentages of breastfeeding initiation and duration, relapse of CD was either reduced or no different in breastfeeding versus nonbreastfeeding women (Julsgaard et al., 2014; Manosa et al., 2013; Moffatt et al., 2009). Furthermore, in one study women overall had greater adherence to their medications (Julsgaard et al., 2014). Thus breastfeeding should be encouraged in women with IBD as well as adherence to the medical regimen and not smoking.

Systemic Lupus Erythematosus

Systemic lupus erythematosus (SLE), an autoimmune disease that is multisystemic in nature, primarily affects women of childbearing age (Tsokas, 2011); therefore, lactation consultants are often called upon to care for women with this problem. In the United States, members of ethnic minority groups (African, Hispanic, or Asian origin), as compared with members of other racial or ethnic groups, tend to have an increased prevalence of SLE and greater involvement of vital organs. The 10-year survival rate for this disease is approximately 70% (Tsokas, 2011).

The clinical presentations of lupus are remarkably diverse and include headaches, arthritic symptoms of joint, redness and swelling, and a butterfly rash on the cheeks and nose. Raynaud's phenomenon (RP) is present in 18% to 46% of cases (Pavlov-Dolijanovic et al., 2013). Fatigue is a major symptom, and the diagnosis of chronic fatigue syndrome and fibromyalgia may also be made concomitantly. The American Society of Rheumatology (Tan et al., 1982) has established 11 criteria associated with the disease, with 4 needed for formal diagnosis of SLE (Table 15-7).

Women with lupus have higher rates of miscarriage and infant prematurity. Nevertheless, women who have good management of their condition prior to pregnancy, thus entering pregnancy in a stable remission period, and who continue their medications experience few flares of a mild nature

Table 15-7 AMERICAN COLLEGE OF RHEUMATOLOGY CRITERIA FOR THE DIAGNOSIS OF SYSTEMIC LUPUS ERYTHEMATOSUS

Criterion	Description
Malar rash	A rash on the cheeks and nose, often in the shape of a butterfly
Discoid rash	A rash that appears as red, raised, disk-shaped patches
Photosensitivity	A reaction to sunlight that causes a rash to appear or get worse
Oral ulcers	Sores in the mouth
Arthritis	Joint pain and swelling of two or more joints
Serositis	Inflammation of the lining around the lungs (pleuritis) or inflammation of the lining around the heart that causes chest pain, which is worse with deep breathing (pericarditis)
Kidney disorder	Persistent protein or cellular casts in the urine
Neurologic disorder	Seizures or psychosis
Blood disorder	Anemia (low red blood cell count), leukopenia (low white blood cell count), lymphopenia (low level of specific white blood cells), or thrombocytopenia (low platelet count)
Immunologic disorder	Positive test for anti-double-stranded DNA, anti-Sm, or antiphospholipid antibodies
Abnormal antinuclear antibodies	Positive antinuclear–antibody test

Source: Data from Tan EM, Cohen AS, Fries JF, et al. The 1982 revised criteria for the classification of systemic lupus erythematosus. *Arthritis Rheum.* 1982;25:1271–1277.

and are well managed with a temporary increase in prednisone dose (Andreoli et al., 2012). Lupus may be exaggerated after delivery, so close observation for lupus flares is needed.

Breastfeeding is feasible for most women with SLE. Treatment of the pregnant and lactating woman is tailored to the individual and her symptomatology. The main concern is the safety of medications that can enter the milk. Table 15-8 provides information about the medications commonly used in SLE, including whether they are allowed during lactation.

The lactation consultant working with the woman who has SLE should be aware of the plan of care for the mother as prescribed by her healthcare team. Lactation care should be tailored to the individual woman, just as with any other mother. Special considerations may include the following:

- Joint pain and swelling may impact holding the infant during feeding.
  - ◄ Assist with positioning that promotes ease and comfort.
  - ◄ Use of breastfeeding pillows may be helpful.
  - ◄ Laid-back nursing may be useful and facilitate infant-led nursing.

- ◄ A baby sling may offer support and lessen stress on the shoulders.
- Raynaud's phenomenon, which may be triggered by cold or emotional stress, is caused by vasospasm of the small vessels of the fingers, toes, nose, chin, and, in the breastfeeding mother, the nipples, causing pain and blanching before, during, and after the feeding. The vasospasm results in blanching, cyanosis, and reactive hyperemia (Pavlov-Dolijanovic et al., 2013).
  - ◄ Ensure warmth of the mother overall and of her breasts during feedings with comfortable warm clothing and room temperature.
  - ◄ Warm compresses to the breast may relieve spasms and promote comfort.
  - ◄ Avoid vasoconstrictive agents such as caffeine and nicotine.
  - ◄ Nifedipine, a calcium-channel blocker, is sometimes used to treat RP and was reported to be effective in 10 of 15 (67%) of breastfeeding mothers with RP in one study (Barrett et al., 2013). (Also see the *Breast-Related Problems* chapter.)

Table 15-8 MEDICATIONS FOR SLE AND LACTATION

Drug	Allowed During lactation?
Prednisone	Allowed
Non-steroidal anti-inflammatory (NSAIDs)	Allowed
Azathioprine	Allowed
Cyclosporine	Allowed
Tacrolimus	Allowed
Sulphasalazine	Allowed if healthy full-term baby
Methotrexate	Avoid
Cyclophosphamide	Avoid
Mycophenolate mofetil	Avoid
Warfarin/acenocoumarol	Allowed
Low molecular weight heparin (e.g., enoxaparin)	Allowed
Intravenous immunoglobulin	Allowed
Rituximab	Avoid (no information)
Belimumab	Avoid (no information)

Multiple Sclerosis

Multiple sclerosis (MS) is a progressive degenerative neurological disorder that is characterized by such symptoms as weakness, fatigue, incoordination, paralysis, and speech and visual disturbances. It affects twice as many women as men, and the diagnosis usually is made during the reproductive years (ages 20 to 40). This condition is known for its unpredictability and the variability of its prognosis and symptoms; it is an immune-mediated or an autoimmune disorder in which the myelin sheath covering the nerves is attacked by the person's own immune system. There are four disease courses in MS: relapsing–remitting MS (RRMS; the most common), primary progressive MS (PPMS), secondary progressive MS (SPMS), and progressive relapsing MS (PRMS). Each disease course can be mild, moderate, or severe.

There is no cure for multiple sclerosis, but treatments can help speed recovery from attacks, modify the disease course, and manage symptoms. Corticosteroids and plasma exchange transfusions are used to manage attacks. Immune-modulating therapies (IMTs), also known as disease-modifying therapies (DMTs), are the mainstay for ongoing treatment of MS and are prescribed soon after diagnosis. DMTs include the parenterally administered beta interferons (1A and 1B), glatiramer acetate, natalizumab, and mitoxantrone, plus the oral preparations of dimethyl fumarate, fingolimoda, and teriflunomide. The safety of DMTs in pregnancy and breastfeeding is not well established, although more evidence is becoming available based on case reports, prospective cohort studies, pregnancy registries, and safety databases maintained by manufacturers (Cree, 2013). In most cases, DMTs are discontinued prior to conception or at the time of pregnancy diagnosis; avoidance of these agents continues through the postpartum period if the mother breastfeeds her infant. At this time, only glatiramer acetate is thought to be relatively safe for use in women who have to remain on DMTs during pregnancy (Cree, 2013). However, interferon has been thought to be safe from the lactation perspective because of its large molecular weight, which means that transfer of this drug into breastmilk is limited. Its lactation risk category is moderately safe—L3 (Hale & Rowe, 2014).

In the woman with MS, the decision to bear a child is complex (Prunty et al., 2008), and healthcare providers are challenged to provide accurate information about the risk of relapse during pregnancy and postpartum and the overall impact on the progression of MS following pregnancy and lactation (Wundes et al., 2014). Most experts believe pregnancy is safe for women with MS. Studies consistently report remission of symptoms during pregnancy, followed by substantially increased exacerbations or relapses in the postpartum period, especially in the first 3 months (Confavreux et al., 1998; Hellwig et al., 2012; Vukusic et al., 2004; Worthington et al., 1994). The presence of an immunosuppressive factor in the maternal serum during the pregnancy may be protective; the subsequent drop in serum hormonal levels after birth may provoke exacerbations.

There is mixed evidence regarding the impact of breastfeeding on postpartum exacerbations of MS. Overall, however, it appears that exclusive breastfeeding is protective against postpartum relapse. In a California prospective case-controlled study of 39 pregnant women with MS and 29 age- and parity-matched pregnant controls, Langer-Gould (2009) found that 69% of those with MS breastfed compared with 96% of the controls. Breastfeeding women in the MS group were more likely to begin daily formula feedings within the first 2 months compared to controls. The primary reason for not breastfeeding or starting early formula feedings was to take medications for MS. Women who did not breastfeed or who started regular supplemental feedings within 2 months postpartum had a higher risk of relapses in the year after giving birth and had earlier relapses compared to those who exclusively breastfed (unadjusted hazard ratio [HR], 5.0; 95% CI, 1.7–14.2; $P = 0.003$). Exclusive breastfeeding in the first 2 months was also protective against relapses in the subgroup of 22 women who had used immunomodulatory agents (IMAs) prior to pregnancy (possibly reflecting a more serious disease prepregnancy).

In a prospective Finish study of 61 mothers with MS, 55 (91%) initiated breastfeeding and 32 (52.5%) continued to breastfeed for 6 or more months; 1 mother started interferon treatment at 2 weeks postpartum while breastfeeding for 5 months (Airas et al., 2010). In this sample, breastfeeding was less frequent in mothers with active prepregnancy disease and duration of breastfeeding was shorter. The researchers found significantly higher rates of prepregnancy relapse among mothers who breastfed for less than 2 months compared with mothers who nursed for greater than 2 months. They also found no significant differences in the rate of postpartum relapse frequency between the group that breastfed for more than 2 months and the group that breastfed for less than 2 months. From this study, it appears that women with more serious disease before and after pregnancy are more likely to choose not to breastfeed.

Newer evidence on this topic comes from a larger sample of German women with MS, some of whom were exposed to either interferon-beta (IFNβ) or glatiramer acetate (GLAT) in the first trimester of pregnancy. Hellwig et al. (2012) followed 335 pregnancies of women with MS to evaluate exposure to DMTs during pregnancy and to further determine whether exclusive breastfeeding by these mothers influenced postpartum relapse rate. They identified 78 pregnancies exposed to IFNβ preparations, 41 with GLAT exposure, and 216 pregnancies without DMT exposure at any time in pregnancy. The study was partly prospective and partly retrospective. The annualized relapse rate (ARR) decreased continuously during pregnancy across all groups and was not significantly different between groups. In nonexposed mothers, the pattern of a decreased relapse rate during pregnancy was typical of what is generally seen, with this rate decreasing steadily and then increasing drastically in the first 3 months postpartum ($p < 0.001$). In IFNβ- or GLAT-exposed women, however, this typical pattern was not as obvious. In total, 170 women exclusively breastfed in the first 3 months after giving birth. Exclusive breastfeeding was associated with a reduced postpartum relapse rate as compared with nonexclusively breastfeeding or nonbreastfeeding women with MS ($p < 0.0001$).

In the year before pregnancy, the relapse rates had been similar throughout all groups. Thus prepregnancy disease activity did not appear to influence breastfeeding choice in these women, and exclusive breastfeeding was protective against relapse rates.

Additional study is needed to make more definitive statements regarding the impact of breastfeeding on relapse risk in the postpartum period. In the meantime, new mothers with MS must be given information based on the evidence (conflicting as it is) and make the choice that is right for them. Certainly, the advantages of breastfeeding to the infant must be conveyed to the mother as well. In fact, breastfeeding for more than 4 months may be protective against MS in later life, at least according to a recent German case control study (Conradi et al., 2013).

For the mother with MS who chooses to breastfeed, support is needed. These mothers, especially, need support of all kinds, including help with household work and child care. Furthermore, the concern the disabled woman has for her children and the consequences of living with a disability in a socially isolating and stigmatizing environment may lead to depression (Harrison & Stuifbergen, 2002).

Rheumatoid Arthritis

Rheumatoid arthritis (RA) is a chronic inflammatory disease thought to be caused by a genetically influenced autoimmune response. Symptoms include pain and swelling of the joints, pain on movement, and fatigue.

RA symptoms usually go into remission during pregnancy and then relapse postpartum. According to a recent review (Akasbi et al., 2014), retrospective studies indicate that approximately 75% to 90% of patients with RA improve during pregnancy, while prospective studies indicate approximately 65% of patients improve. Women who become pregnant while they have stable or low disease activity realize fewer beneficial effects of pregnancy, but their disease remains mainly stable. By comparison, patients with high disease activity at conception benefit the most from pregnancy. Flares after pregnancy occur in 39% to 62% of patients, according to prospective studies. New-onset RA has been reported to be

3–5 times more frequent within the first 6 months after delivery cited in the review by Akasbi et al. (2014). The problem is greater for breastfeeding women, probably owing to their hyperprolactinemic state; prolactin has been shown to act as an immunostimulator (Brennan & Silman, 1994; Hampl & Papa, 2001). The most severe symptoms occur after a first pregnancy; symptoms are less severe following subsequent pregnancies (Barrett, Brennan, et al., 2000). In contrast to these studies that described lactation as a predictor of RA in the postpartum period, it has been suggested that women who lactate, especially those who do so for more than 13 months, are at lower risk of developing RA in later life (Nommsen-Rivers, 2005; Pikwer et al., 2009).

NSAIDs are used as first-line therapy to decrease pain and inflammation of the joints in RA (Akasbi et al., 2014). Other drugs considered safe for use during lactation include sulfasalazine, a combination of an aspirin-like anti-inflammatory component and a sulfur antibiotic-like component, which is used to treat RA as a disease-modifying drug. Antimalarial agents are compatible with breastfeeding except for premature babies aged younger than 1 month. Corticosteroids are safe during breastfeeding, but if the dose is more than 40 mg/day, breastfeeding should be postponed 4 hours after the mother takes the drug. All anti-tumor necrosis factor-alpha (anti-TNF-α) agents are compatible with lactation.

Methotrexate therapy, which is used for severe cases of RA, is contraindicated with breastfeeding, according to the American Academy of Pediatrics (see the *Drug Therapy and Breastfeeding* chapter). Hale and Rowe (2014) recommended that women who must use methotrexate pump and discard their milk for a minimum of 4 days.

There has been little research into the breastfeeding experiences of women with RA, and most of the existing studies are now quite old. However, the evidence is useful for supporting breastfeeding women with RA. One study described women with RA often feeling overwhelmed with fatigue both during pregnancy and postpartum (Carty et al., 1986). Although these mothers need additional rest, they also need to continue range-of-motion exercises to promote flexibility and reduce stiffness. Periodic rest periods and the wearing of removable braces or splints to support joints will help to reduce fatigue as well (Carty et al., 1986).

Physically Challenged Mothers

Increasing numbers of women who are physically impaired are choosing to become pregnant and to breastfeed. For these women, breastfeeding is more than the giving of good nutrition: it helps to normalize this aspect of their life experience. Breastfeeding builds the mother's confidence and self-esteem by proving that her body is capable of nourishing her baby even though she may be able to do little else quite as easily. Using the mother's knowledge of her health problem and the breastfeeding specialist's expertise in breastfeeding can lead to some ingenious solutions to any difficulties experienced during this process (Minami, 2000).

Spinal Cord Injury

In a study of women who had spinal cord injury, 67 percent reported having sexual intercourse after injury (Jackson & Wadley, 1999). As a rule, the lower the injury, the less loss of function (Cesario, 2002). A woman with a spinal cord injury should be able to breastfeed her baby if her injury is below the sixth cervical vertebra (C6) (Craig, 1990; Halbert, 1998). Oxytocin-triggered milk ejection is reduced if the injury is between T4 and T6, the point of origin for the nerves that innervate the breast and nipples (see the *Anatomy and Physiology of Lactation* chapter). If she can breastfeed, chances are that the mother has function of her upper extremities and can position the baby for breastfeeding and perform other baby care activities, but she may need help.

Cowley (2005) reported three cases in which women with spinal cord injury successfully breastfed their babies. Two of these amazing women maintained their milk supply through relaxation and mental imaging.

Conversely, a recent case study described a 33-year-old woman with a C4 AIS D tetraplegia (based on the American Spinal Injury Association

Impairment Scale [AIS]) (Liu & Krassioukov, 2013). After giving birth and commencing breastfeeding, she experienced hypogalactia of the right breast. This woman experienced Brown-Séquard-plus syndrome (BSPS), which is defined as an incomplete spinal cord injury (SCI) syndrome with ipsilateral weakness and contralateral loss of both pinprick and temperature sensation. In this case, her injury also impacted the descending spinal autonomic pathways needed for lactation on her right side. Although she attempted several interventions to improve the lactation amount, she was not able to increase milk production on the right side and she eventually began formula feeding. It is unfortunate that a lactation consultant or other knowledgeable specialist did not encourage the mother to continue to feed from the left side; perhaps her milk supply would have compensated for the lack of production in the right breast. The authors noted that the International Standards to document remaining Autonomic Functions after SCI (ISAFSCI) were developed in 2009 but do not include lactation function. They also noted that further attention is needed by SCI specialists relative to childbearing women's needs in the postpartum period.

Breastfeeding and Physical Challenges

In some disorders involving impaired mobility, especially those that are immunologically mediated (e.g., RA, MS, and myasthenia gravis), pregnancy may bring a period of remission followed by postpartum relapse. Often, women suffering from such a disease feel so good during their pregnancy that they take it for granted that their condition has improved. When the condition worsens after birth, it is doubly difficult because additional energy is now required to care for a new baby.

Physically challenged parents are adaptive and even ingenious in devising ways to carry out basic baby care activities. A case study (Thomson, 1995) of a mother with a congenital below-elbow limb absence describes how the mother positioned her baby at the breast: "Using her right hand, she held her breast between her thumb and fingers in the same plane as the baby's mouth, when closed. She then placed her breast in the baby's mouth by leaning forward. This mother had her older daughter help her to attach for about 4 months. After this, the baby was able to 'hop on' by herself."

The lesson for the nurse and lactation consultant assisting mothers with disabilities is simple: creativity counts. Often the mother with a disability knows better than anyone else how important flexible thinking is in solving a problem or overcoming a problem that may seem to be unsolvable. Ask for the mother's help in thinking through the situation. Together, a solution may be found.

For example, 3 years before her baby's birth, one mother suffered a debilitating stroke, one outcome of which was substantial loss of arm and hand control and strength. She and her lactation consultant experimented with a variety of slings that the mother could put on with one hand and wear to keep her baby close to her. This was especially important when the mother had to move the baby from one room to another or out of the house: She was fearful when she could not hang onto a handrail when going down stairs, for example. After practicing with several different positions, the mother identified alternative ways to present the breast to the baby that were both comfortable and required a minimum of movement by the mother. By the time the baby was 3 months old, he had learned to help his mother by scooting up to the breast himself when placed on the bed next to her.

Good parenting occurs even when a mother is severely disabled. Generally, these mothers find that breastfeeding is more convenient than bottle-feeding. Breastfeeding also renders caring for the infant simpler, because there is nothing to measure, prepare, pour, or sterilize. Yet friends and relatives may react negatively, concerned that the mother should not breastfeed due to her limited energy or abilities. These mothers need compassionate support and guidance, even more so than women with normal mobility. Suggestions for the physically disabled mother and her family on breastfeeding and baby care are listed in Box 15-7.

Because the physically challenged mother is usually under continuing medical care and has so

Box 15-7 Baby Care Guidelines for Physically Disabled Breastfeeding Mothers

- Mothers with some upper-body strength who are confined to a wheelchair can use a harness or a wide belt with a long strip of Velcro to lift and retrieve a crawling baby from the floor.
- One or two special "feeding nests" for breastfeeding that are easily accessible and comfortable for the mother can be set up. Group together a crib or other sleeping place for the infant, diaper-changing supplies, and a comfortable place to breastfeed.
- If the baby is small, he can be laid diagonally across the mother's knees on a pillow to breastfeed. Put other pillows under the mother's arms for support. Elevate the mother's feet on a footrest to keep the infant secure during the feeding.
- A mother who cannot elevate her feet can rest her forearm holding the infant on a pillow placed across her knees. This arrangement ensures that if the infant rolls, he will roll toward the mother.
- Changing tables and cribs can be adapted so that they are accessible to a wheelchair, and the room can be arranged so that moving about is minimized. A low-sided pram or baby stroller makes it easier to slide the baby out onto the mother's lap without requiring much lifting.
- A baby sling allows the mother's arms to be free while ensuring that the baby is safe and supported during breastfeeding. This is also helpful when the mother has unilateral weakness or paralysis (e.g., as from a stroke).
- A bell tied to the baby's shoes keeps track of where the mobile child is.
- A toddler will quickly learn to climb on his mother's knee for a ride and to sit still while the chair is moving.
- The baby can be given extra cuddling such as touching at night in bed if there are barriers to physical contact during the day.
- A baby clothed in overalls with crossed straps can be picked up fairly easily.
- The mother's use of a nursing bra that opens in the front instead of the back, one with an easy-to-fasten clip or Velcro that can be handled with one hand, will facilitate breastfeeding. The usual clip for opening and closing the bra flap can be replaced with Velcro. Some all-elastic bras are easily pulled down to allow the baby to breastfeed.
- Maternity clothes can be altered to incorporate Velcro openings or large ring zippers. Antique buttonhooks are helpful to manipulate the small buttons found on many garments.
- The mother should plan rest periods during the day and should sit to work whenever possible.
- The mother can sleep with the infant or have the father or someone else bring the baby to her to nurse during the night.
- Use of an intercom system that picks up the sound of the baby crying is helpful. If the mother is deaf, the sound can be transformed into flashing light signals.
- If the mother cannot lift both the baby and herself, she might care for her baby on the floor (preferably carpeted), feeding, changing, and playing with him. This enables her to roll the baby to her, instead of lifting him, when he needs attention. A beanbag will provide support for breastfeeding.

many needs, the healthcare professional working with the disabled breastfeeding mother may find her role expanding to that of a case manager; the professional may coordinate medical, family, and community support and services. If the mother has someone to help her with the physical tasks, diplomatically arrange for that person to take over the household jobs and care of older children and let the mother take care of her baby. Many of these mothers are already on medications, and their physicians should be consulted about the safety of taking specific medications while breastfeeding. Most medications are compatible with breastfeeding (see the *Drug Therapy and Breastfeeding* chapter), especially with short-term use. If the physician recommends weaning, the healthcare provider should research the drug using up-to-date references and, if necessary, act as an advocate for the mother in her desire to continue to breastfeed.

For peer support, set up group sessions that include any woman who has a disability and has given birth in the last 5 years. The purpose of these sessions is to provide information about coping with the demands placed on physically challenged women by pregnancy, birthing, and early infant care, and to allow the more experienced women to serve as mother-to-mother role models for those women having a first child.

Nurses and healthcare professionals can learn a great deal from the mother who has developed extraordinary survival skills to work around inconveniences. For example, one mother has no left hand and lower arm, yet she tends to breastfeed her baby on her left side, propping her baby against her upper-left arm so that her right hand is free. This mother also needs a battery- or electric-powered pump—not a hand-operated device—to express her milk.

For mothers who are blind and cannot rely on visual cues, breastfeeding is a way to communicate with their infant nonvisually through touch, smell, sound, and even intuitive sensitivity (Martin, 1992).

Until recently, limited information was available regarding breastfeeding (and all other aspects of childbearing) among women with disabilities.

Unfortunately, society's general view remains that women with a physical disability are not capable of having or caring for a child. Even now, only a few resources for these families exist. Two such resources are La Leche League International and the Australian Breastfeeding Association. Both organizations have developed educational materials, including audiocassette tapes and Braille material, for the physically challenged mother who is breastfeeding. These organizations will also refer the mother to another woman who has had a similar experience. Finally, additional information on assisting women with physical and other disabilities can be found in the *Core Curriculum for Lactation Consultant Practice*, in Chapter 32, "Breastfeeding Mothers with Disabilities" (Siebenaler & Rogers, 2013).

Epilepsy (Seizure Disorders)

Epilepsy and seizure disorders are classified into two major groups: partial and generalized. Partial or focal seizures begin in a specific area of the brain and produce symptoms ranging from simple repetitive movements to more complex abnormal movements and bizarre behavior. Generalized seizures have no specific point of origin in the brain. The most common type is a major motor seizure, formerly called grand mal epilepsy.

All women with epilepsy should be encouraged to breastfeed their babies. Seizure disorders can be so well controlled by medications that seizures are rarely a problem for the lactating mother. However, nurses and lactation consultants need to know about the effect of the medication on the breastfed infant. The physician will prescribe antiseizure medications on the basis of diagnosis of the seizure and its pattern of occurrence, and on the tolerance and response of the mother to the prescribed drug.

The advantages of breastfeeding outweigh the risks of infant exposure to antiepileptic drugs (AEDs) (Pennell et al., 2007). The concentrations of AEDs secreted in breastmilk are generally low and not usually harmful. AEDs for seizure disorders include levetiracetam (Keppra), phenytoin

(Dilantin), carbamazepine (Tegretol), primidone (Mysoline), and phenobarbital. Phenobarbital taken in higher-than-average amounts (50–100 mg two or three times daily), however, may cause drowsiness in infants or mothers; primidone may also cause sedation in the infant. The estimated maximal dose of carbamazepine that the breastfed baby would consume in breastmilk is 3% to 5% of the weight-adjusted maternal dose, an amount similar to other drugs, such as phenytoin and valproic acid.

Evidence related to AED exposure in utero is now available, although studies on this topic have produced conflicting results. In an attempt to evaluate the pooled evidence related to in utero exposure versus nonexposure, Banach and colleagues (2010) conducted a meta-analysis of 7 studies involving 239 exposed children of mothers with epilepsy, 58 nonexposed children of mothers with epilepsy, and 436 nonexposed children of mothers without epilepsy. Outcomes included developmental cognitive outcomes. The findings indicated that exposure to valproic acid during pregnancy was associated with significantly reduced intelligence in children whose mothers were treated for epilepsy. Exposure to carbamazepine in pregnancy was not associated with reduced IQ in children, although one measure of IQ was lower in the subanalysis. The authors recommended that clinicians inform families of the potential cognitive adverse effects of valproic acid.

The meta-analysis just described did not look at postnatal exposure via breastfeeding. Evidence to support the importance of breastfeeding for children of mothers taking antiepileptic drugs (AED) is now available, although further study of these agents is warranted. Meador and colleagues (2014) conducted a prospective study of American and British children of epileptic mothers on monotherapy (i.e., carbamazepine, lamotrigine, phenytoin, or valproate), called the Neurodevelopmental Effects of Antiepileptic Drugs [NEAD] Study. In total, 42.9% of children were breastfed a mean of 7.2 months. Breastfeeding rates and duration did not differ across drug groups. At age 3 years, there was no significant difference between breastfed versus nonbreastfed children in intelligence test scores (IQ). However, at 6 years of age, children who were breastfed scored 4 points higher on IQ testing and had better verbal skills (also 4 points higher). Of note, lower IQ was found among those children who were exposed to valproic acid via breastmilk, similar to previous research on intrauterine exposure. Like Banach et al. (2010), these authors caution that mothers should not take valproic acid during pregnancy or lactation.

In the unusual case in which the mother has seizures, breastfeeding is in no way contraindicated. Dropping or harming the infant during a seizure is no more probable during breastfeeding than it is during bottle-feeding. Usually, a prodromal warning (aura) alerts the mother of an impending seizure, and she is able to take safety precautions to protect her infant (Box 15-8).

BOX 15-8 GUIDELINES FOR A BREASTFEEDING MOTHER WITH A SEIZURE DISORDER

1. On each level of the house, make sure there is a playpen in which to quickly place the baby when a seizure seems imminent.
2. Pad the arms of the rocker or chair where the mother usually breastfeeds with extra pillows and cushions.
3. Place guardrails padded with pillows around the mother's bed if she customarily takes her infant to bed to breastfeed.
4. Attach to the baby and to the stroller or baby carrier tags stating that the mother has a seizure disorder, along with other pertinent information, whenever she is away from home.

Surgery

Surgery of any kind is a stressful experience. Surgery that is scheduled when the mother is breastfeeding and caring for a small child or infant raises the possibility of separation from the baby and the inability to care for him. The mother who enters the hospital in advance of a surgical procedure may have sufficient time to make plans. If she knows on which unit she will be housed, she can learn the visitation policy for that floor in that hospital (whether her baby and other minor children will be allowed to visit her) and determine how long she will be in the hospital, whether a fully automatic breast pump will be available, and what the staff's knowledge and experience with breastfeeding mothers is.

Getting in touch with a lactation consultant in the hospital ensures that someone knowledgeable is aware of the mother's concerns about preserving lactation and the breastfeeding relationship. This person may be able to arrange for a breast pump to use in advance of the surgery (and immediately thereafter if needed). Guidelines for helping the breastfeeding mother who undergoes surgery are summarized in Box 15-9.

Generally, surgery is likely to result in a temporary reduction in a woman's milk supply as measured by expressing breastmilk. However, once the mother is fully awake, she may feel uncomfortably full. If the surgery involved the breast, pumping should begin as soon as possible to avoid putting further pressure on the operative site from engorgement and to relieve the mother's discomfort. A mother who donated her kidney to her sister, for example, continued to breastfeed and pump while in the hospital.

If the staff has limited experience in assisting breastfeeding women, a referral should be made to the in-hospital lactation consultant so that she can provide care for the mother. Most hospitals allow a breastfeeding infant to stay with the mother after the surgery if another adult is present to take care of the infant. If this is not possible, the baby can be brought to the hospital to be breastfed.

During her hospitalization, the mother may be receiving one or more medications. If she must be separated from her baby, she needs to determine whether she will express and discard her milk or send it home with a family member to be given to the baby. Once the mother is at home, how her baby will react to her depends on several factors, including the length of time the mother was absent, the means by which the baby was fed in her absence, and the baby's age at the time of the separation.

Finally, on the healthcare provider side, the surgeon(s) who will be involved with the breastfeeding mother must be knowledgeable about

---

BOX 15-9 SURGERY AND THE BREASTFEEDING MOTHER: GUIDELINES FOR CARE

- Encourage the mother to plan for help at home after surgery to allow time to recuperate.
- Use an outpatient surgical facility rather than an inpatient facility.
- Arrange for breastfeeding of the baby immediately before the surgery.
- Assist the mother in breastfeeding as soon as she awakes from anesthesia.
- Make rooming-in arrangements for the breastfeeding child if an inpatient facility is required. (Most hospitals require that another adult be present to care for the baby.)
- Express and freeze a supply of breastmilk before the surgery (if needed).
- Aid the mother in conditioning the baby to cup-feedings before surgery if it is determined that temporary supplementary feedings will be necessary.
- Encourage the mother to take postoperative analgesia to alleviate pain. (The infant will receive only a small dose through breastmilk.)
- Show the mother how to "splint" the surgical area with pillows if abdominal surgery is performed. Cover the incision area with dressings.

breastfeeding considerations, including the pharmacokinetics of drugs in the maternal system, the possible adverse effects to the infant, and ways to minimize drug exposure to the infant. Resources for physicians include *Medications and Mothers' Milk* by Thomas Hale and Hilary Rowe (2014) and the Drugs and Lactation Database (LactMed) on the U.S. National Library of Medicine TOXNET website (http://toxnet.nlm.nih.gov). The LactMed resource is a peer-reviewed and fully referenced database of drugs to which breastfeeding mothers may be exposed. Mothers should be open in their communication with their surgeon about their breastfeeding and their desire to protect their infant and themselves as much as possible. Such a partnership is important to all involved.

Transplants

Recipients of solid-organ transplants are usually advised against breastfeeding because of the questionable safety of immunosuppressant agents. Limited data suggest that infant exposure to tacrolimus via breastmilk is low. A case report described a 29-year-old woman who was exclusively breastfeeding her healthy 3-month-old infant while on tacrolimus plus other drugs relevant to her transplant. The baby ingested approximately 0.5% of the maternal dose (weight adjusted). Thus maternal tacrolimus therapy may be compatible with breastfeeding (Gardiner & Begg, 2006).

Donating Blood

Is it a good idea for a breastfeeding woman to donate blood? It depends on the circumstances. For example, it would not be a good idea for a mother to give blood soon after childbirth. The American Red Cross says that lactating women may donate blood if they wish to do so, but the organization suggests waiting at least 6 weeks after an uncomplicated term delivery or cesarean birth. If a blood transfusion was necessary during delivery, the mother should wait for 12 months. If a breastfeeding mother does give blood, she should eat especially well, stay hydrated, and avoid lifting her baby or heavy items with the arm used to donate the blood (La Leche League International, 2001). Recipients of smallpox vaccine should not donate blood for 21 days or until the scab has separated.

The Impact of Maternal Illness and Hospitalization

Hospitalization of a mother is a traumatic experience for all members of the family. A mother faced with the prospect of separation from her infant, whether brief or prolonged, is a mother in crisis. For the breastfeeding woman and her infant, it is essential that ongoing, intimate, and regular contact be maintained. Today, a mother with an acute illness is more likely to be treated as an outpatient than to be hospitalized. As a result, separation because of hospitalization is not as frequent a barrier to breastfeeding as it was in past decades.

If the mother is hospitalized, the baby should be allowed to room-in with the mother or at least be brought to her for breastfeeding at frequent intervals. Nurses and lactation consultants can be advocates for changing polices and for relaxing hospital restrictions that create an unnecessary additional hardship for families.

A mother who is acutely or chronically ill may find that the decisions about her health care and advice regarding breastfeeding are divided among her obstetrician, the baby's pediatrician, and the medical specialist or surgeon. Additional healthcare professionals such as a dietitian, nurse practitioner, or physician's assistant may be involved as well. Even when all parties agree that breastfeeding is desirable, childbirth may be riskier for the mother and infant, and they are more likely to be separated postpartum. Although it is possible to establish breastfeeding after an initial separation, doing so can be more difficult, especially if the separation lasts more than a few days (Coates & Riordan, 1992). Moreover, when an illness is associated with a reduced milk supply, the mother is further traumatized when she is lectured about breastfeeding more often and about "supply and demand" when the care provider does not first assess the total picture and the possibility that the woman is already breastfeeding frequently.

Chronic illnesses present a somewhat different potential dilemma for the breastfeeding mother and the clinician assisting her. Not surprisingly, women with disabilities are likely to be depressed. They also worry about their children more than other mothers (Harrison & Stuifbergen, 2002). In some cases, the nature of the chronic illness and its effect on the mother's functioning may interfere to a greater or lesser extent with her ability to breast-feed. In other cases, creative alternatives to "usual" solutions are all that are needed to give the mother the opportunity to experience the same infant feed-ing as do those mothers who do not have a chronic illness. Additionally, drug therapy, particularly because it is likely to be long term, may pose risks to the breastfeeding infant that are not an issue if the mother has an acute, self-limiting illness. Thus the clinician needs to look beyond the illness itself and examine how the condition is being managed and what the mother wants to do, given complete information relating to the risks and benefits of breastfeeding to herself and to her baby in light of her chronic illness. In many cases, the therapy of choice need not be changed because it poses no dan-gers for the suckling infant.

Care must be taken to accurately interpret the mother's desire to begin or to continue breastfeed-ing when faced with uncommon difficulties or situations. Occasionally, when an illness or a breast-feeding problem occurs, health professionals may be asked to give permission to wean to a woman who no longer wants to continue breastfeeding. Even if there is no reason to wean, a relatively minor dif-ficulty can occasionally present a mother with a socially acceptable "out" from a situation that she finds emotionally uncomfortable or finds inconve-nient for her lifestyle. The comment—namely, that the physician, lactation consultant, or nurse "told me to wean" because of a problem—may partially reflect the mother's own desires. Avoiding judg-mental responses and encouraging her to air con-flicting feelings may enable the mother to place her breastfeeding experience in context, so that she can focus on the positive aspects of her experience rather than on its more problematic elements.

ACKNOWLEDGMENT

This chapter is a compilation of topics from two chapters from previous editions of the book, those dealing with women's health and fertility, sexuality, and contraception. Dr. Jan Riordan was the origi-nal author of the *Women's Health* chapter, while Dr. Kathleen Kennedy authored the *Fertility, Sexual-ity, and Contraception* chapter. In our revision of the chapter, we have maintained the principal content but revised the evidence undergirding the prin-ciples as necessary. We acknowledge and laud the work of these two experts as we carry on their work.

SUMMARY

This chapter reviewed health and reproductive conditions that relate to the lactating mother and suggested interventions that facilitate the lacta-tion process. Admittedly, this discussion does not include the full range of acute or chronic disease that the health professional will encounter in prac-tice. Likewise, it does not fully cover reproductive issues such as fertility, sexuality, and contraception. To find information on these conditions that the mother may develop or face while she is lactating, we recommend reviewing public health, gyneco-logical, and medical–surgical texts for physicians and nurses that more thoroughly discuss the condi-tions described here and others not addressed.

KEY CONCEPTS

- The immediate postpartum period is marked by the neurohormonal changes accompany-ing birth that not only initiate and stimu-late contractions, but also influence women's instinctive emotional, physical, social, and behavioral responses during the transition to motherhood.
- Care providers who have knowledge and appreciation for the physiologic changes of

postpartum can create an environment in which prolonged periods of skin-to-skin holding, frequent breastfeeding, rest, support with breastfeeding and infant care, and decreased stressors to facilitate the optimal hormonal milieu for lactogenesis and attachment.

- The child's suckling initiates a cycle of neuroendocrinologic events that result in the inhibition of ovulation.
- Anything that decreases the child's suckling behavior or the need to suckle will be a secondary cause of the recovery of fertility. Supplementation may have the effect of decreasing hunger, thirst, and possibly the emotional need for comfort, thereby reducing suckling at the breast.
- A significant association exists between the duration of lactational infertility after one pregnancy and the duration in the same woman after her next pregnancy.
- Breastfeeding provides more than 98% protection from pregnancy during the first 6 months postpartum if the mother is "fully" or nearly fully breastfeeding and has not experienced vaginal bleeding after the 56th day postpartum.
- Once menstruation has resumed, fertility is returning or already has returned. Menses is an absolute indication of the need for another contraceptive method if continued protection is desired.
- The tenderness from episiotomy or vulvovaginal or perineal stress following vaginal delivery usually lasts for several months and can cause pain or discomfort during intercourse.
- Postpartum women produce low levels of estrogen which can endure for the entire lactation course. As a result the vaginal epithelium is very thin and secretes little fluid during sexual arousal. The use of inert, water-based lubricants can facilitate comfort during sexual intercourse.
- Most women experience change in their sexual practices after delivery. The frequency of sex is often lower, although some women report better quality in their sex lives.

- Very few women talk to their healthcare professional about their sexual health.
- Mothers are at heightened vulnerability to stressors and health concerns, both physical and psychological, for at least the first full year after giving birth.
- The postpartum period is often marked by negative and positive stress. Breastfeeding and skin-to-skin contact have an anxiolytic effect.
- Chronic social stress can impair breastfeeding and mothering behaviors secondary to remodeling of the neuroendocrine system as an adaptation to the chronic stress.
- Primary concerns or stressors starting immediately after birth include breastfeeding initiation, newborn care, maternal–infant bonding and attachment, pain, bleeding, and infection prevention.
- Pain management includes assessment of multiple dimensions that need consideration when planning pharmacologic and nonpharmacologic pain management interventions.
- Excessive postpartum bleeding can be controlled by pharmacologic agents and non-pharmacologic management, including breastfeeding. Anxiety often accompanies excessive bleeding, and skin-to-skin contact with the newborn can reduce it.
- Induced lactation involves taking hormones to mimic pregnancy and stimulate production of breastmilk. The protocol for induction typically begins with an oral combination of hormones (progesterone/estrogen) in addition to domperidone or Reglan, regular pumping of the breasts, and finally suckling by the infant.
- Herbal galactogogues are taken to increase breastmilk supply, although little scientific evidence supports their effectiveness and safety.
- Immunizations are important to the health of the mother and her child and are encouraged during pregnancy and lactation.
- Women with tuberculosis who have been treated appropriately for 2 or more weeks (and who are otherwise considered to be

noncontagious) may and should breastfeed. If the mother is acutely ill with TB, breastfeeding may have to be interrupted.

- U.S. women are routinely screened for Group B *Streptococcus* (GBS), a leading cause of neonatal sepsis. Those at risk for GBS infection are given antibiotics intravenously during labor and can breastfeed.

- Skin-to-skin contact and breastfeeding right after birth help prevent MRSA infection in newborns.

- Breastfeeding may delay return of migraine headaches. Two types of lactational headaches can occur. Type I occurs with the first letdown during a feed and is linked to the surge of oxytocin from the letdown. Type 2 is triggered by overfullness of the breast and is relieved by breastfeeding or pumping.

- Women with a family history of asthma should be encouraged to breastfeed exclusively because of the long-term protective effect of breastfeeding on asthma. Asthma medications are generally compatible with breastfeeding.

- Women with type 1 diabetes should be encouraged to breastfeed their infants. If breastfeeding is delayed, the mother should be encouraged to begin expressing or pumping her milk as soon as she feels able.

- Lactating women with type 1 diabetes have a delay of about 1 day in lactogenesis II.

- For the untreated breastfeeding woman, hypothyroidism can result in a reduced milk supply. If replacement therapy (0.25–1.12 mg of sodium levothyroxine or equivalent doses of other thyroid preparation) is adequate, relief of the symptoms and increase in the milk supply can be dramatic.

- Mothers with cystic fibrosis can breastfeed. The breastmilk of these mothers contains nutrients sufficient to supply the energy needs of the nursing infant despite some differences in lipid composition. The mother's diet should be closely monitored to avoid excessive weight loss.

- Polycystic ovarian syndrome can interfere with the production of hormones necessary for full lactation and lead to high levels of testosterone.

- Theca lutein cysts—a condition where ovaries are enlarged by multiple cysts that produce a high level of testosterone—usually delay lactogenesis. Several weeks postpartum, the cysts will resolve and the testosterone level return to normal.

- Women who suffer from severe peripartum depression should be supported, closely monitored, and medicated. First-choice medications for breastfeeding women with severe depression are sertraline (Zoloft) and paroxetine (Paxil). Sertraline has the least drug-interaction potential.

- Women with autoimmune conditions should be encouraged to breastfeed. Rheumatoid arthritis and systemic lupus erythematosus symptoms usually go into remission during pregnancy and then a relapse occurs postpartum. Women with lupus sometimes have a reduced milk supply.

- Physically challenged mothers should be supported to breastfeed, tailoring care and support to the individual problems.

- In the case in which a mother has seizures, breastfeeding is in no way contraindicated. Dropping or harming the infant during a seizure is no more probable during breastfeeding than during bottle-feeding. With a few exceptions, antiepileptic drugs do not constitute a contraindication for breastfeeding, although the infant should be monitored for idiosyncratic reactions.

- Hospitalization of a mother is a traumatic experience given the prospect of separation from her infant, whether brief or prolonged. For the breastfeeding woman and her infant, it is essential that ongoing, intimate, and regular contact be maintained. The health care team should provide individualized and compassionate care to the mother and support continued lactation.

INTERNET RESOURCES

Centers for Disease Control and Prevention, information on breastfeeding and infections and other conditions: http://www.cdc.gov /breastfeeding/disease/index.htm

Cystic Fibrosis Foundation: http://www.cff.org/

Protocols for induced lactation: A Guide for Maximizing Breastmilk Production: http:// www.asklenore.info/breastfeeding/induced _lactation/gn_protocols.html

Information on domperidone from Dr. Jack Newman: http://www.breastfeedinginc.ca/

Office on Women's Health: http://www .womenshealth.gov/

Multiple Sclerosis Foundation: http://www .msfocus.org/

Polycystic Ovarian Syndrome Association: http://www.pcosupport.org/

Postpartum Support International online support network for PPD: http://www .postpartum.net

REFERENCES

Abraham S, Child A, Ferry J, et al. Recovery after childbirth: a preliminary prospective study. *Med J Aust.* 1990;152: 9–12.

Academy of Breastfeeding Medicine (ABM) Board of Directors. ABM statements: position on breastfeeding. *Breastfeed Med.* 2008;3(4):267–270. doi: 10.1089/ bfm.2008.9988.

Academy of Breastfeeding Medicine (ABM) Protocol Committee. ABM clinical protocol #3: hospital guidelines for the use of supplementary feedings in the healthy term breastfed neonate, revised 2009. *Breastfeed Med.* 2009;4(3):175–182. doi: 10.1089/bfm.2009.9991.

Ahmad AL, Ahmed A, Patrizio P. Cystic fibrosis and fertility. *Curr Opin Obstet Gynecol.* 2013;25(3):167–172. doi: 10.1097/GCO.0b013e32835f1745.

Airas L, Jalkanen A, Alanen A, et al. Breast-feeding, postpartum and prepregnancy disease activity in multiple sclerosis. *Neurology.* 2010;75(5):474–476. doi: 10.1212/ WNL.0b013e3181eb5860.

Akasbi N, Abourazzak FE, Harzy T. Management of pregnancy in patients with rheumatoid arthritis. *OA Musculoskeletal Med.* 2014;2(1):3.

Akman I, Kuscu MK, Yurdakul Z, et al. Breastfeeding duration and postpartum psychological adjustment: role of maternal attachment styles. *J Paediatr Child Health.* 2008;44:369–373. doi: 10.1111/j.1440-1754.2008. 01336.x.

Alder E, Bancroft J. The relationship between breastfeeding persistence, sexuality, and mood in postpartum women. *Psychol Med.* 1988;18:389–396.

Alonso-Coello P, Guyatt GH, Heels-Ansdell D, et al. Laxatives for the treatment of hemorrhoids. *Cochrane Database Syst Rev.* 2005;4:CD004649. doi: 10.1002/ 14651858.CD004649.pub2.

American Academy of Pediatrics (AAP), Section on Breastfeeding. Breastfeeding and the use of human milk. *Pediatrics.* 2012;129:e827. doi: 10.1542/peds.2011-3552.

American College of Obstetricians and Gynecologists (ACOG), Committee on Obstetrical Practice. Committee opinion no. 453: screening for depression during and after pregnancy. *Obstet Gynecol.* 2010;115: 394–395. (Reaffirmed 2012.)

American College of Obstetricians and Gynecologists (ACOG), Committee on Obstetrical Practice. Committee opinion no. 558: Integrating vaccinations into practice. *Obstet Gynecol.* 2013;121:898–903.

American Dietetic Association (ADA). Position of the American Dietetic Association: promoting and supporting breastfeeding. *J Am Diet Assoc.* 2009;109(11): 1926–1942. doi: 10.1016/j.jada.2009.09.018.

American Psychiatric Association. (2013). Diagnostic and statistical manual of mental disorders (5th ed.). Arlington, VA: American Psychiatric Publishing.

Amir LH, Donath SM. Does maternal smoking have a negative physiological effect on breastfeeding? The epidemiological evidence. *Birth.* 2002;29:112–123.

Amir LH, Garland SM, Lumley J. A case-control study of mastitis: Nasal carriage of *Staphylococcus aureus*. *BMC Family Pract.* 2006;7:57. doi: 10.1186/1471-2296-7-57.

Andersen AN, Schioler V. Influence of breastfeeding pattern on pituitary–ovarian axis of women in an industrialized community. *Am J Obstet Gynecol.* 1982;143:673–677.

Andreoli L, Fredi M, Nalli C, et al. Pregnancy implications for systemic lupus erythematosus and the antiphospholipid syndrome. *J Autoimmun.* 2012;38(2–3): J197–J208. doi: 10.1016/j.jaut.2011.11.010.

Antunovic SS, Lukac M, Vujovic D. Longitudinal cystic fibrosis care. *Clin Pharmacol Ther.* 2013;93(1):86–97. doi: 10.1038/clpt.2012.183.

Arnold J, Morgan A, Morrison B. Paternal perceptions of and satisfaction with group prenatal care in Botswana. *Online J Cultural Competence Nurs Healthcare.* 2014;4(2): 17–26. doi: 10.9730/ojccnh.org/v4n2a2.

Arthur PG, Kent JC, Hartman PE. Metabolites of lactose synthesis in milk from diabetic and nondiabetic women during lactogenesis II. *J Pediatr Gastroenterol Nutr.* 1994;19:100–108.

Aryal TR. Differentials of post-partum amenorrhea: a survival analysis. *J Nepal Med Assoc.* 2007;46(166):66–73.

Auriemma RS, Perone Y, Di Sarno A, et al. Results of a single-center observational 10-year survey study on recurrence of hyperprolactinemia after pregnancy and lactation. *J Clin Endocrinol Metab.* 2013;98(1):372–379. doi: 10.1210/jc.2012-3039.

Baheiraei A, Shamsi A, Khaghani S, et al. The effects of maternal passive smoking on maternal milk lipid. *Acta Med Iran.* 2014;52(4):280–285.

Balcar V, Silinkova-Malkova E, Matys Z. Soft tissue radiography of the female breast and pelvic peritoneum in the Stein-Leventhal syndrome. *Acta Radiol Diag.* 1972;12:353–362.

Banach R, Boskovic R, Einarson T, Koren G. Long-term developmental outcome of children of women with epilepsy, unexposed or exposed prenatally to antiepileptic drugs: a meta-analysis of cohort studies. *Drug Saf.* 2010;33(1):73–79. doi: 10.2165/11317640-000000000-00000.

Barrett G, Pendry E, Peacock J, et al. Women's sexual health after childbirth. *BJOG.* 2000;107(2):186–195.

Barrett JH, Brennan P, Fiddler M, Silman A. Breast-feeding and postpartum relapse in women with rheumatoid and inflammatory arthritis. *Arthritis.* 2000;43:1010–1015.

Barrett ME, Heller MM, Stone HF, Murase JE. Raynaud phenomenon of the nipple in breastfeeding mothers: an underdiagnosed cause of nipple pain. *JAMA Dermatol.* 2013;149(3):300–306.

Beake S, Rose V, Bick D, et al., A qualitative study of the experiences and expectations of women receiving in-patient postnatal care in one English maternity unit. *BMC Pregnancy Childbirth.* 2010;10:article 70. http://www.biomedcentral.com/1471-2393/10/70.

Beck CT. Teetering on the edge: a substantive theory of postpartum depression. *Nurs Res.* 1993;42:42–48.

Beckie TM. A systematic review of allostatic load, health, and health disparities. *Biol Res Nurs.* 2012;14(4):311–346. doi: 10.1177/1099800412455688.

Behari P, Englund J, Alcasid G, et al. Transmission of methicillin-resistant *Staphylococcus aureus* to preterm infants through breastmilk. *Infect Control Hosp Epidemiol.* 2004;25:778–780.

Bell AF, Erickson EN, Carter CS. Beyond labor: the role of natural and synthetic oxytocin in the transition to motherhood. *J Midwifery Women's Health.* 2014;00:1–9. doi:10.1111/jmwh.12101.

Bellamy L, Casas JP, Hingorani AD, Williams D. Type 2 diabetes mellitus after gestational diabetes: a systematic review and meta-analysis. *Lancet.* 2009;373(9677):1773–1779. doi: 10.1016/S0140-6736(09)60731-5.

Benitez I, de la Cruz J, Suplido A, et al. Extending lactational amenorrhea in Manila: a successful breast-feeding education program. *J Biosoc Sci.* 1992;24:211–231.

Berg M, Erlandsson L, Sparud-Lundin C. Breastfeeding and its impact on daily life in women with type 1 diabetes during the first six months after childbirth: a prospective cohort study. *International Breastfeeding Journal.* 2012;7:20. Available at: http://www.internationalbreastfeedingjournal.com/content/7/1/20

Berle JO, Spigset O. Antidepressant use during breastfeeding. *Curr Women's Health Rev.* 2011;7:28–34.

Betzold CM, Hoover KL, Snyder CL. Delayed lactogenesis 11: a comparison of four cases. *J Midwifery Women's Health.* 2004;49:133–137.

Bick D, Murrelis T, Weavers A, et al. Revising acute care systems and processes to improve breastfeeding and maternal postnatal health: a pre and post intervention study in on English maternity unit. *BMC Pregnancy Childbirth.* 2012;12:article 41. Available at: http://www.biomedcentral.com/1471-2393/12/41.

Bitman J, Hamosh M, Hamosh P, et al. Milk composition and volume during the onset of lactation in a diabetic mother. *Am J Clin Nutr.* 1989;50:1364–1369.

Bongaarts J, Menken J. *Determinants of fertility in developing countries.* New York, NY: Academic Press; 1983.

Bongaarts J, Potter RG. *Fertility, biology and behavior.* New York, NY: Academic Press; 1983.

Brennan P, Silman A. Breast-feeding and the onset of rheumatoid arthritis. *Arthritis Rheum.* 1994;37:808–813.

Brown CR, Dodds L, Attenborough R, et al. Rates and determinants of exclusive breastfeeding in first 6 months among women in Nova Scotia: a population-based cohort study. *CMAJ Open.* 2013;1(1):E9–E17. doi: 10.9778/cmajo.20120011. eCollection 2013.

Bundred NJ, Dover MS, Coley S, Morrison JM. Breast abscesses and cigarette smoking. *Br J Surg.* 1992;79:548–559.

Burianova I, Paulova M, Cermak P, Janota J. Group B *Streptococcus* colonization of breast milk of Group B *Streptococcus* positive mothers. *J Hum Lact.* 2013;29:586–590. doi: 10.1177/0890334413479448.

Burr CK, Storm DS, Hoyt MJ, et al.Integrating health and prevention services in syringe access programs: a strategy to address unmet needs in a high-risk population. *Public Health Rep.* 2014;129 Suppl 1:26-32.

Byrne PA, Miller C, Justus K. Neonatal Group B streptococcal infection related to breast milk. *Breastfeeding Medicine.* 2006;1(4):263–270.

Bystrova K, Ivanova V, Edhborg M, et al. Early contact versus separation: effects on mother–infant interaction one year later. *Birth.* 2009;36(2):97–109.

Cadwell K, Turner-Maffei C, Blair A, et al. Pain reduction and treatment of sore nipples in nursing mothers. *J Perinatal Education.* 2004;13(1):29–35.

Carlsen SM, Jacobsen G, Vanky E. Mid-pregnancy androgen levels are negatively associated with breastfeeding. *Acta Obstet Gynecol Scand.* 2010;89(1):87–94. doi: 10.3109/00016340903318006.

Carmina E, Aziz R. Diagnosis, phenotype, and prevalence of polycystic ovary syndrome. *Fertil Steril.* 2006;86(suppl 1):S7–8.

Carney LA, Quinlan JD, West JM. Thyroid disease in pregnancy. *Am Fam Physician.* 2014;89(4):273–278.

Carter CS. Oxytocin pathways and the evolution of human behavior. *Annu Rev Psychol.* 2014;65:10.1–10.23. doi: 10.1146/annurev-psych-010213-115110.

Carty E, Conine TA, Wood-Johnson F. Rheumatoid arthritis and pregnancy: helping women to meet their needs. *Midwives Chron.* 1986;99:254–257.

Centers for Disease Control and Prevention (CDC). TB elimination: tuberculosis and pregnancy. 2011a. Available at: http://www.cdc.gov/tb/topic/populations/pregnancy/default.htm.

Centers for Disease Control (CDC). *Reported tuberculosis in the United States, 2012.* Atlanta, GA: U.S. Department of Health and Human Services, CDC; October 2013.

Cesario SK. Spinal cord injuries: nurses can help affected women and their families achieve pregnancy and birth. *AWHONN Lifelines.* 2002;6:225–232.

Chan GM. Effects of powdered human milk fortifiers on the antibacterial actions of human milk. *J Perinatol.* 2003;23:620–623.

Cheng C-Y, Fowles ER, Walker LO. Postpartum maternal health care in the United States: a critical review. *J Perinatal Educ.* 2006;15(3):34–42. doi: 10.1624/105812406X1.

Chertok I. Relief of breast engorgement for the Sabbath-observant Jewish woman. *JOGNN.* 1999;28:356–369.

Chiu J-Y. Effects of *Gua-Sha* therapy on breast engorgement: a randomized controlled trial. *J Nurs Res.* 2010;18(1): 1–8.

Clements M. Breastfeeding, the mother in charge. *UN Chron.* 2009;46(1/2):24–27.

Coates MM, Riordan J. Breastfeeding during maternal or infant illness. *Clin Iss Perin Wom Health Nurs.* 1992;3(4): 683–694.

Colson SD, Meek JH, Hawdon JM. Optimal positions for the release of primitive neonatal reflexes stimulating breastfeeding. *Early Hum Develop.* 2008;84:441–449. doi: 10.1016/j.earlhumdev.2007.12.003.

Confavreux C, Hutchinson M, Hours MM, et al. Rate of pregnancy-related relapse in multiple sclerosis. Pregnancy in Multiple Sclerosis Group. *N Engl J Med.* 1998;339:285–291.

Conradi S, Malzahn U, Paul F, et al. Breastfeeding is associated with lower risk for multiple sclerosis. *Mult Scler.* 2013;19(5):553–448. doi: 10.1177/1352458512459683.

Cordero L, Thung S, Landon MB, Nankervis CA. Breastfeeding initiation in women with pregestational diabetes mellitus. *Clinical Pediatrics.* 2014; 53(1): 18–25.

Cowley KC. Psychogenic and pharmacologic induction of the let-down reflex can facilitate breastfeeding by tetraplegic women: a report of 3 cases. *Arch Phys Med Rehabil.* 2005;86:1261–1264.

Craig D. The adaptation to pregnancy of spinal cord injured women. *Rehab Nurs.* 1990;15:6–9.

Cree BA. Update on reproductive safety of current and emerging disease-modifying therapies for multiple sclerosis. *Mult Scler.* 2013;19(7):835–843. doi: 10.1177/1352458512471880.

Cury DB, Moss AC. Treatment of Crohn's disease in pregnant women: drug and multidisciplinary approaches. *World J Gastroenterol.* 2014;20(27):8790–8795.

Daglas M, Antoniou E. Cultural views and practices related to breastfeeding. *Health Sci J.* 2012:6(2):353–361.

Davis M. Breastfeeding my adopted baby. *New Beginnings.* May–June 2001:48.

de Aquino RR, Osorio MM. Relactation, translactation, and breast-orogastric tube as transition methods in feeding preterm babies. *J Hum Lact.* 2009;25(4):420–426. doi: 10.1177/0890334409341472.

DeCoopman J. Breastfeeding after pituitary resection: support for a theory of autocrine control of milk supply? *J Hum Lact.* 1993;9:35–40.

De Groot L, Abalovich M, Alexander EK, et al. Management of thyroid dysfunction during pregnancy and postpartum: an Endocrine Society clinical practice guideline. *J Clin Endocrinol Metab.* 2012;97(8):2543–2565. doi: 10.1210/jc.2011-2803.

Deligiannidis KM, Freeman MP. Complementary and alternative medicine therapies for perinatal depression. *Best Pract Res Clin Obstet Gynaecol,* 2014;28(1):85–95. doi: 10.1016/j.bpobgyn.2013.08.007.

Delvoye P, Demaegd M, Delogne-Desnoeck J. The influence of the frequency of nursing and of previous lactation experience on serum prolactin in lactating mothers. *J Biosoc Sci.* 1977; 9:447–451.

Dennis C-L, McQueen K. The relationship between infant-feeding outcomes and postpartum depression: a qualitative systematic review. *Pediatrics.* 2009;123:e736. doi: 10.1542/peds.2008-1629.

Denton Y. Induced lactation in the nulliparous adoptive mother. *Br J Midwifery.* 2010;18(2):84–87.

DeSisto CL, Kim SY, Sharma AJ. Prevalence estimates of gestational diabetes mellitus in the United States, Pregnancy Risk Assessment Monitoring System (PRAMS), 2007–2010. *Prev Chronic Dis.* 2014;11:130415. doi: http://dx.doi.org/10.5888/pcd11.130415.

Diaz S, Seron-Ferre M, Croxatto HB, Veldhuis J. Neuroendocrine mechanisms of lactational infertility in women. *Biol Res.* 1995;28:155–163.

DiFrisco E, Goodman KE, Budin WC, et al. Factors associated with exclusive breastfeeding 2 to 4 weeks following discharge from a large, urban, academic medical center striving for Baby-Friendly designation. *J Perinatal Educ.* 2011;20(1):28–35. doi: 10.1891/1058-1243.20.1.28.

Dixon L, Skinner J, Foureur M. The emotional and hormonal pathways of labour and birth: integrating mind, body and behavior. *N Z Coll Midwives J.* 2013;48:15–23.

http://dx.doi.org/10.12784/nzcomjnl48.2013.3 .15-23.

Djiane J, Durand P. Prolactin–progesterone antagonism in self-regulation of prolactin in the mammary gland. *Nature.* 1977;266(14):641–643.

Dogaru CM, Nyffenegger D, Pescatore AM, et al. Breastfeeding and childhood asthma: systematic review and meta-analysis. *Am J Epidemiol.* 2014;179(10):1153–1167. doi: 10.1093/aje/kwu072.

Dökmetaş HS, Kilicli F, Korkmaz S, Yonem O. Characteristic features of 20 patients with Sheehan's syndrome. *Gynecol Endocrinol.* 2006;22(5):279–283.

Domingue ME, Devuyst F, Alexopoulou O, et al. Outcome of prolactinoma after pregnancy and lactation: a study on 73 patients. *Clin Endocrinol (Oxf).* 2014;80(5): 642–648. doi: 10.1111/cen.12370.

Donaldson-Myles F. Postnatal depression and infant feeding: A review of the evidence. British Journal of Midwifery, 2011;19(10):619-624.

Donaldson-Myles F. Can hormones in breastfeeding protect against postnatal depression? *Br J Midwifery.* 2012; 20(2):88–93.

Donnelly L. Group b strep: A holistic approach. *Midwifery Today.* 2014;109:9–22.

Dworkin RH, Turk DC, Revicki DA, et al. Development and initial validation of an expanded and revised version of the Short-Form McGill Pain Questionnaire (SF-MPQ-2). *Pain.* 2009;144:35–42. doi: 10.1016/j.pain.2009.02.007.

East CE, Begg L, Henshall NE, et al. Local cooling for relieving pain from trauma sustained during childbirth. *Cochrane Database Syt Rev.* 2012;5:CD006304. doi: 10.1002/14651858.CD006304.pub3.

Edenborough FP, Borgo G, Knoop C, et al. Guidelines for the management of pregnancy in women with cystic fibrosis. *J Cystic Fibrosis.* 2008;7(S1):S2–S32.

Elias MF, Teas J, Johnston J, Bora C. Nursing practices and lactational amenorrhea. *J Biosoc Sci.* 1986;18:1–10.

Ellsworth A. Pharmacotherapy of asthma while breastfeeding. *J Hum Lact.* 1994;10:39–41.

Eshkevari L, Trout KK, Damore J. Management of postpartum pain. *J Midwifery Women's Health.* 2013;58: 622–631. doi: 10.1111/jmwh.12129.

Eslami SS, Gray RH, Apelo R, Ramos R. The reliability of menses to indicate the return of ovulation in breastfeeding women in Manila, the Philippines. *Stud Fam Plann.* 1990;21:243–250.

Fahey JO, Shenassa E. Understanding and meeting the needs of women in the postpartum period: the Perinatal Maternal Health Promotion Model. *J Midwifery Women's Health.* 2013;58:613–621. doi: 10.1111/jmwh.12139.

Family Health International. Breastfeeding as a family planning method. *Lancet.* 1988;2:(8621):1204–1205.

Feldman R, Gordon I, Zagoory-Sharon O. Maternal and paternal plasma, salivary, and urinary oxytocin and parent–infant synchrony: considering stress and affiliation components of human bonding. *Devel Sci.* 2011;14(4):752–761. doi: 10.1111/j.1467-7687.2010.01021.x.

Feldman R, Singer M, Zagoory O. Touch attenuates infants' physiological reactivity to stress. *Devel Sci.* 2010;13(2): 271–278. doi: 10.1111/j.1467-7687.2009.00890.x.

Ferris AM, Dalidowitz CK, Ingardia CM, et al. Lactation outcome in insulin-dependent diabetic women. *J Am Diet Assoc.* 1988;88:317–322.

Ferris AM, Neubauer SH, Bendel RB, et al. Perinatal lactation protocol and outcome in mothers with and without insulin-dependent diabetes mellitus. *Am J Clin Nutr.* 1993;58:43–48.

Festini F, Ciuti R, Taccetti G, et al. Breast-feeding in a woman with cystic fibrosis undergoing antibiotic intravenous treatment. *J Matern Fetal Neonatal Med.* 2006; 19:375–376.

Fielding JE, Gilchick RA. Positioning for prevention from day 1 (and before). *Breastfeed Med.* 2011;6(5):249–255. doi: 10.1089/bfm.2011.0059.

Finkelstein SA, Keely E, Feig DS, et al. Breastfeeding in women with diabetes: lower rates despite greater rewards. A population-based study. *Diab Med.* 2013;30:1094–1101.

Fonseca AM. Histologic and histometric aspects of the breast in polycystic ovary syndrome. *Arch Gynecol.* 1985;237: 380–381.

Ford K. Correlation between subsequent lengths of postpartum amenorrhea in a prospective study of breastfeeding women in rural Bangladesh. *J Biosoc Sci.* 1992; 24:89–95.

Freeman MP. Postpartum depression, breastfeeding, and other postdelivery concerns. *Nurs Pract Wom Health.* 2012. Available at: http://www.npwh.org/files/11-06L(1).pdf.

Furlong AJ, al-Nakib L, Knox WF, et al. Periductal inflammation and cigarette smoke. *J Am Coll Surg.* 1994;179: 417–420.

Gagne MG, Leff EW, Jefferis SC. The breast-feeding experience of women with type I diabetes. *Health Care Wom Int.* 1992;13:249–260.

Galbally M, Snellen M, Power J. Antipsychotic drugs in pregnancy: a review of their maternal and fetal effects. *Therap Adv Drug Safety.* 2014. E-pub ahead of print. doi: 10.1177/2042098614522682.

Garcia PV, Mella C. Analysis of factors involved in lactational amenorrhea, *J Biosafety Health Educ.* 2013;1(4). doi: 10.4172/2332-0893.1000109.

Gardiner SJ, Begg EJ. Breastfeeding during tacrolimus therapy. *Obstet Gynecol.* 2006;107(2):453–455.

Geddes DT. The use of ultrasound to identify milk ejection in women: tips and pitfalls. *Int Breastfeed J.* 2009;4: article 5. doi: 10.1186/1746-4358-4-5.

Geddes DT, Kent JC, Miloulas LR, Hartmann PE. Tongue movement and intra-oral vacuum in breastfeeding infants. *Early Hum Devel.* 2008;84(7):471–477. doi: 10.1016/j.earlhumdev.2007.12.008.

Geddes DT, Sakalidis VS, Hepworth AR, et al. Tongue movement and intra-oral vacuum of term infants during breastfeeding and feeding from an experimental teat that released milk under vacuum only. *Early Hum Devel.* 2012;88(6):443–449. doi: 10.1016/j.earlhumdev.2011.10.012.

Giglia R, Binns CW, Alfonso H. Maternal cigarette smoking and breastfeeding duration. *Acta Paediatr.* 2006;95:1370–1374.

Gilljam M, Antoniou M, Shin J,et al. Pregnancy in cystic fibrosis: fetal and maternal outcome. *Chest.* 2000;118:85–91.

Glasier A, McNeilly AS, Baird DT. Induction of ovarian activity by pulsatile infusion of LHRH in women with lactational amenorrhea. *Clin Endocrinol.* 1986;24:243–252.

Glezer A, Bronstein MD. Prolactinomas, cabergoline, and pregnancy. *Endocrine.* July 2, 2014. E-pub ahead of print.

Glueck CJ, Salehi M, Sieve L, Wang P. Growth, motor, and social development in breast- and formula-fed infants of metformin-treated women with polycystic ovary syndrome. *J Pediatr.* 2006;148(5):628–632.

Glueck CJ, Wang P. Metformin before and during pregnancy and lactation in polycystic ovary syndrome. *Expert Opin Drug Saf.* 2007;6(2):191–198.

Goldstein AL. New-onset Graves' disease in the postpartum period. *J Midwifery Women's Health.* 2013;58(2):211–214. doi: 10.1111/jmwh.12016.

Golembeski DJ, Emergy MG. Lipid composition of milk from mothers with cystic fibrosis (letter). *Pediatrics.* 1989;31(suppl):631–632.

Good M. Effects of relaxation and music on postoperative pain: a review. *J Adv Nurs.* 1996;24:905–914.

Good M, Moore SM. Clinical practice guidelines as a new source of middle-range theory: focus on acute pain. *Nurs Outlook.* 1996;44:74–79.

Grattan DR, Pi XJ, Andrews AB, et al. Prolactin receptors in the brain during pregnancy and lactation: Implications for behavior. *Hormones Behav.* 2001;40:115–124. doi: 10.1006/hbeh.2001.1698.

Gray RH, Campbell OM, Apelo R, et al. Risk of ovulation during lactation. *Lancet.* 1990;335:25–29.

Groer M. Differences between exclusive breastfeeders, formula-feeders, and controls: a study of stress, mood, and endocrine variables. *Biol Res Nurs.* 2005;7:106–117. doi: 10.1177/1099800405280936.

Groer M, Davis MW. Cytokines, infections, stress, and dysphoric moods in breastfeeders and formula feeders. *JOGNN.* 2006;35:599–607. doi: 10.1111/j.1552-6909.2006.00083.x.

Groer M, Davis MW, Hemphill J. Postpartum stress: current concepts and the possible protective role of breastfeeding. *JOGNN.* 2002;31:411–417.

Groer M, Morgan K. Immune, health and endocrine characteristics of depressed postpartum mothers. *Psychoneuroendocrinology.* 2007;32:133–139.

Grudzinskas JG, Atkinson L. Sexual function during the puerperium. *Arch Sex Behav.* 1984;13:85–91.

Guille C, Newman R, Fryml LD, et al. Management of postpartum depression. *J Midwifery Women's Health.* 2013;58:643–653. doi: 10.1111/jmwh.12104.

Gunderson EP. Impact of Breastfeeding on Maternal Metabolism: Implications for Women with Gestational Diabetes. *Curr Diab Rep.* 2014; 14:460. doi: 10.1007/s11892-013-0460-2.

Gupta M, Shaw B. A double-blind randomized clinical trial for evaluation of galactogogue activity of *Asparagus racemosus* wild. *Iran J Pharmaceut Res.* 2011;10(1):167–172.

Gutierrez S, Liu B, Hayashida K, et al. Reversal of peripheral nerve injury–induced hypersensitivity in the postpartum period: role of spinal oxytocin. *Anesthesiology.* 2013;118:152–159.

Hahn-Holbrook J, Haselton MG, Schetter CD, Glynn LM. Does breastfeeding offer protection against maternal depressive symptomatology? A prospective study from pregnancy to 2 years after birth. *Arch Women's Ment Health.* 2013;16:411–422. doi: 10.1007/s00737-013-0348-9.

Halbert L. Breastfeeding in women with a compromised nervous system. *J Hum Lact.* 1998;14:327–331.

Hale T. *Clinical Therapy in Breastfeeding Patients.* TX: Pharmasoft Medical Publishing; 1999.

Hale T, Rowe H. *Medications and mothers' milk,* 16th ed. Amarillo, TX: Pharmasoft Medical Publishing; 2014.

Hampl J, Papa D. Breastfeeding-related onset, flare, and relapse of rheumatoid arthritis. *Nutrition Reviews.* 2001;59(8):264–268

Handlin L, Jonas W, Petersson M, et al. Effects of sucking and skin-to-skin contact on maternal ACTH and cortisol levels during the second day postpartum: influence of epidural analgesia and oxytocin in the perinatal period. *Breastfeed Med.* 2009;4(4):207–220. doi: 10.1089.bfm.2009.0001.

Harrison T, Stuifbergen A. Disability, social support, and concern for children: depression in mothers with multiple sclerosis. *JOGNN.* 2002;31:444–453.

Hartmann P, Cregan M. Lactogenesis and the effects of insulin-dependent diabetes mellitus and prematurity. *J Nutr.* 2001;131:3016S–3020S.

Hedayati H, Parsons J, Crowther CA. Topically applied anaesthetics for treating perineal pain after childbirth. *Cochrane Database Syst Rev.* 2005;2:CD004223. doi: 10.1002/14651858.CD004223.pub2.

Hellwig K, Haghikia A, Rockhoff M, Gold R. Multiple sclerosis and pregnancy: experience from a nationwide database in Germany. *Ther Adv Neurol Disord.* 2012;5(5):247–253. doi: 10.1177/1756285612453192.

Henderson JJ, Evans SF, Straton JAY, et al. Impact of postnatal depression on breastfeeding duration. *Birth.* 2003;30(3):175–180.

Homer CS, Scarf V, Catling C, Davis D. Culture-based versus risk-based screening for the prevention of group B streptococcal disease in newborns: a review of national guidelines. *Women Birth*. 2014;27(1):46–51. doi: 10.1016/j.wombi.2013.09.006.

Hoover K, Barbalinardo L, Pia Platia M. Delayed lactogenesis II secondary to gestational ovarian theca lutein cysts in two normal singleton pregnancies. *J Hum Lact*. 2002; 18:264–268.

Hornsby PP, Wilcox AJ. Validity of questionnaire information on frequency of coitus. *Am J Epidemiol*. 1989;130: 94–99.

Horta BL, Victora CG, Menezes AM, Barros FC. Environmental tobacco smoke and breastfeeding duration. *Am J Epidemiol*. 1997;146:128–133.

Howie PW, McNeilly AS, Houston MJ, et al. Effect of supplementary food on suckling patterns and ovarian activity during lactation. *Br Med J*. 1981;283:757–759.

Howie PW, McNeilly AS, Houston MJ, et al. Fertility after childbirth: postpartum ovulation and menstruation in bottle and breastfeeding mothers. *Clin Endocrinol*. 1982;17:323–332.

International Lactation Consultant Association (ILCA). *Clinical guidelines for the establishment of exclusive breastfeeding*. Raleigh, NC: ILCA; March 2014.

Islam MM, Khan HTA. Pattern of coital frequency in rural Bangladesh. *J Fam Welfare*. 1993;39:38–43.

Israngkura B, Kennedy KI, Leelapatana B, Cohen HS. Breastfeeding and return to ovulation in Bangkok. *Int J Gynaecol Obstet*. 1989;30:335–342.

Jackson AB, Wadley V. A multicenter study of women's self-reported reproductive health after spinal cord injury. *Arch Phys Med Rehabil*. 1999;80:1420–1428.

Joanna Briggs Institute. Clinical updates 128: the management of nipple pain and/or trauma associated with breastfeeding. *Austral Nurs J*. 2009;17(2):32–35.

Joham AE, Ranasinha S, Zoungas S, et al. Gestational diabetes and type 2 diabetes in reproductive-aged women with polycystic ovary syndrome. *J Clin Endocrinol Metab*. 2014;99(3):E447–E452. doi: 10.1210/jc.2013-2007.

Jones RE. A hazards model analysis of breastfeeding variables and maternal age on return to menses postpartum in rural Indonesian women. *Hum Biol*. 1988;60:853–871.

Jones RE. Breastfeeding and postpartum amenorrhea in Indonesia. *J Biosoc Sci*. 1989;21:83–100.

Jones S, Steele RW. Recurrent Group B bacteremia. *Clin Pediatr*. 2012;51(9):884–887. doi: 10.1177/0009922811409203.

Julsgaard M, Nørgaard M, Hvas CL, et al. Self-reported adherence to medical treatment, breastfeeding behaviour, and disease activity during the postpartum period in women with Crohn's disease. *Scand J Gastroenterol*. 2014; 49(8):958–966. doi: 10.3109/00365521.2014.920913.

Kane S, Lemieux N. The role of breastfeeding in postpartum disease activity in women with inflammatory bowel disease. *Am J Gastroenterol*. 2005;100:102–105.

Karatsoreos IN, McEwen BS. Resilience and vulnerability: a neurobiological perspective. *F1000 Prime Reports*. 2013;5:13. doi: 10.12703/P5-13.

Karlstrom A, Engström-Olofsson R, Norbergh KG, et al. Postoperative pain after cesarean birth affects breastfeeding and infant care. *JOGNN*. 2007;36:430–440. doi: 10.1111/J.1552-6909.2007.00160.x.

Kawanda M, Okuzumi K, Hitomi S, Sugishita C. Transmission of *Staphylococcus aureus* between health, lactating mothers and their infants by breastfeeding. *J Hum Lact*. 2003;19:411–417. doi: 10.1177/0890334403257799.

Kazi A, Kennedy KI, Visness CM, Khan T. Effectiveness of the lactational amenorrhea method in Pakistan. *Fertil Steril*. 1995;64:717–723.

Kendall-Tackett K. A new paradigm for depression in new mothers: the central role of inflammation and how breastfeeding and anti-inflammatory treatments protect maternal mental health. *Int Breastfeed J*. 2007;2:6. doi: 10.1186/1746-4358-2-6.

Kennedy KI. Fertility, sexuality and contraception during lactation. In: Riordan J, Auerbach K, eds. *Breastfeeding and human milk*. Sudbury, MA: Jones and Bartlett; 1993:435–437.

Kennedy KI, Labbok MH, Van Look PFA. Consensus statement—lactational amenonorrhea method for family planning. *Int J Gynecol Obstet*. 1996;54:55–57.

Kennedy KI, Rivera R, McNeilly AS. Consensus statement on the use of breastfeeding as a family planning method. *Contraception*. 1989;39:477–496.

Kenny JA. Sexuality of pregnant and breastfeeding women. *Arch Sex Behav*. 1973;2:215–229.

Kim JY, Mizoguchi Y, Yamaguchi H, et al. (1997). Removal of milk by suckling acutely increases the prolactin receptor gene expression in the lactating mouse mammary Kjos gland. *Molecul Cell Endocrinol*. 1997;131: 31–38.

Kitajima H. Prevention of methicillin-resistant *Staphylococcus aureus* infections in neonates. *Pediatr Int*. 2003;45: 238–245.

Knodel J, Chayovan N. Coital activity among married Thai women. In: *Demographic and Health Surveys World Conference proceedings, Vol. 2*. Columbia, MD: IRD/Macro International; 1991.

Kolcaba K, Tilton C, Drouin, C. Comfort theory: a unifying framework to enhance the practice environment. *JONA*. 2006;36(11):538–544.

Kramer MS, Kakuma R. *The optimal duration of exclusive breastfeeding: a systematic review*. Geneva, Switzerland: World Health Organization; 2002: WHO/FCH/CAH/01.23. Available at: http://whqlibdoc.who.int/hq/2001/WHO_NHD_01.08.pdf.

Kramer MS, Kakuma R. Optimal duration of exclusive breastfeeding. *Cochrane Database Syst Rev*. 2012;8: CD003517. doi: 10.1002/14651858.CD003517. pub2.

Kriebs JM. Methicillin-resistant *Staphylococcus aureus* infections in the obstetric setting. *J Midwifery Women's Health.* 2008;53:247–250. doi:10.IOI6/j.jmwh.2008.02.001.

Labbok M. Breastfeeding, birth spacing, and family planning. In: Hale TW, Hartmann PE. *Hale & Hartmann's textbook of human lactation.* Amarillo, TX: Hale Publishing; 2007:305–318.

Labbok MH, Hight-Laukaran V, Peterson AE, et al. I. Multicenter study of the lactational amenorrhea method (LAM): duration and implications for clinical guidance. *Contraception.* 1997;55:327–336.

Labbok MH, Perez A, Valdes V, et al. *Guidelines: breastfeeding, family planning and the lactational amenorrhea method— LAM.* Washington, DC: Institute for Reproductive Health; 1994.

Lake MF. Tuberculosis in pregnancy. *AWHONN Lifelines.* 2001;5:35–41.

La Leche League International. Question from breastfeeding mothers: should lactating women donate blood? *New Beginnings.* 2001;18(4):227.

Langer-Gould A, Huang SM, Gupta R, et al. Exclusive breastfeeding and the risk of postpartum relapses in women with multiple sclerosis. *Arch Neurol.* 2009;66(8): 958–963. doi: 10.1001/archneurol.2009.132.

Leeman LM, Rogers RG. Sex after childbirth: postpartum sexual function. *Obstet Gynecol.* 2012;119:647–655. doi: 10.1097/AOG.0b013e3182479611.

Lewis PR, Brown JB, Renfree MB, Short RV. The resumption of ovulation and menstruation in a well-nourished population of women breastfeeding for an extended period of time. *Fertil Steril.* 1991;55:529–536.

Liu J, Rosenberg KD, Sandoval AP. Breastfeeding duration and perinatal cigarette smoking in a population-based cohort. *Am J Public Health.* 2006;96:309–314.

Liu N, Krassioukov AV. Postpartum hypogalactia in a woman with Brown-Séquard-plus syndrome: a case report. *Spinal Cord.* 2013;51(10):794–796. doi: 10.1038/sc.2013.51.

Loto OM, Awowole I. Tuberculosis in pregnancy: a review. *J Pregnancy.* 2012;2012:379271. doi: 10.1155/2012/379271.

Lyons DJ, Broberger C. Tidal waves: network mechanisms in the neuroendocrine control of prolactin release. *Frontiers Neuroendocrinol.* 2014. E-pub ahead of print. doi: 10.1016/j.yfrne.2014.02.001.

Mangesi L, Dowswell T. Treatments for breast engorgement during lactation. *Cochrane Database Syst Rev.* 2010;9: CD006946. doi: 10.1002/14651858.CD006946.pub2.

Manosa M, Navarro-Llavat M, Marin L, et al. Fecundity, pregnancy outcomes, and breastfeeding in patients with inflammatory bowel disease: a large cohort survey. *Scand J Gastroenterol.* 2013;48:427–432.

Marasco L. Polycystic ovary syndrome. *Leaven,* April–May 2005:7–29.

Marasco L, Marmet C, Shell M. Polycystic ovary syndrome: a connection to insufficient milk supply? *J Hum Lact.* 2000;15:143–148.

Martin DC. LLL and the mother who is blind. *Leaven.* 1992; 28(5):67–68.

Masters WH, Johnson VE. *Human sexual response.* Boston, MA: Little, Brown; 1966.

Matias SL, Dewey KG, Quesenberry CP Jr, Gunderson EP. Maternal prepregnancy obesity and insulin treatment during pregnancy are independently associated with delayed lactogenesis in women with recent gestational diabetes mellitus. *Am J Clin Nutr.* 2014;99(1): 115–121. doi: 10.3945/ajcn.113.073049.

McDonagh M, Matthews A, Phillipi C, et al. *Antidepressant treatment of depression during pregnancy and the postpartum period.* Evidence Report/Technology Assessment No. 216. (Prepared by the Pacific Northwest Evidence-based Practice Center under Contract No. 290-2007-10057-I.) AHRQ Publication No. 14-E003-EF. Rockville, MD: Agency for Healthcare Research and Quality; July 2014. Available at: http://www .effectivehealthcare.ahrq.gov/reports/final.cfm.

McEwen BS. Early life influences on life-long patterns of behaviour and health. *Mental Retard Devel Disabil Res Rev.* 2003;9:149–154. doi: 10.1002/mrdd.10074.

McEwen B. Stressed or stressed out: what is the difference? *J Psychiatry Neurosci.* 2005;30:315–318.

McEwen B. Physiology and neurobiology of stress and adaptation: central role of the brain. *Physiol Rev.,* 2007;87:873. doi: 10.1152/physrev.00041.2006.

McEwen B. Brain on stress: how the social environment gets under the skin. *PNAS.* 2012;109(suppl 2): 17180–17185. Available at: http://www.pnas.org/cgi /doi/10.1073/pnas.1121254109.

McEwen B. The brain on stress: toward an integrative approach to brain, body, and behavior. *Persp Psychol Sci.* 2013;8(6):673–675. doi: 10.1177/1745691613506907.

McMullen AH, Pasta DJ, Frederick PD, et al. Impact of pregnancy on women with cystic fibrosis. *Chest.* 2006; 129(3):706–711.

McNeilly AS. Lactational control of reproduction. *Reprod Fertil Dev.* 2001a;13:583–590.

McNeilly AS. Neuroendocrine changes and fertility in breastfeeding women. *Prog Brain Res.* 2001b;113: 207–214.

McNeilly AS, Glasier A, Howie PW. Endocrine control of lactational infertility-I. In: Dobbing J, ed. *Maternal nutrition and lactational infertility.* New York, NY: Raven Press; 1985:1–16.

McNeilly AS, Glasier AF, Howie PW, et al. Fertility after childbirth: pregnancy associated with breastfeeding. *Clin Endocrinol.* 1983;18:167–173.

McNeilly AS, Howie PW, Houston MJ, et al. Fertility after childbirth: adequacy of postpartum luteal phases. *Clin Endocrinol.* 1982;17:609–615.

McNeilly AS, Tay CCK, Glasier A. Physiological mechanisms underlying lactational amenorrhea. *Ann N Y Acad Sci,* 1994;709:145–155. doi: 10.1111/j.1749-6632.1994. tb30394.x.

Meador KJ, Baker GA, Browning N, et al. Breastfeeding in children of women taking antiepileptic drugs: cognitive outcomes at age 6 years. *JAMA Pediatr.* 2014; 168(8):729–736. doi: 10.1001/jamapediatrics. 2014.118.

Melzack R. From the gate to the neuromatrix. *Pain.* 1999; suppl 6:S121–S126.

Melzack R. Pain and the neuromatrix in the brain. *J Dental Educ.* 2001;65(12):1378–1382.

Melzack R. Evolution of the neuromatrix theory of pain. The Prithvi Raj Lecture: presented at the Third World Congress of World Institute of Pain, Barcelona 2004. *Pain Pract.* 2005;5(20):85–94.

Mendell LM. Constructing and deconstructing the gate theory of pain. *Pain.* 2014;155:210–216. doi: 10.1016/j.pain. 2013.12.010.

Meston CM, Frohlich PF. The neurobiology of sexual function. *Arch Gen Psychiatry.* 2000;57:1012–1030.

Michel SH, Mueller DH. Impact of lactation on women with cystic fibrosis and their infants: a review of five cases. *J Am Diet Assoc.* 1994;94:159–155.

Mihălţan FD, Antoniu SA, Ulmeanu R. Asthma and pregnancy: therapeutic challenges. *Arch Gynecol Obstet.* July 18, 2014. E-pub ahead of print.

Minami J. Helping mothers with chronic illness. *Leaven.* 2000;36:5–6.

Miyake A, Tahara M, Koike K, Tanizawa O. Decrease in neonatal suckled milk volume in diabetic women. *Eur J Obstet Gynecol Reprod Biol.* 1989;33:49–53.

Moayedi M, Davis KD. Theories of pain: from specificity to gate control. *J Neurophysiol.* 2013;109:5–12. doi: 10.1152/jn.00457.2012.

Moffatt DC, Ilnyckyj A, Bernstein CN. A population-based study of breastfeeding in inflammatory bowel disease: initiation, duration, and effect on disease in the postpartum period. *Am J Gastroenterol* 2009;104: 2517–2523.

Molodecky NA, Soon IS, Rabi DM, et al. Increasing incidence and prevalence of the inflammatory bowel diseases with time, based on systematic review. *Gastroenterology.* 2012;142(1):46–54.

Money D, Allen VM; Society of Obstetrician and Gynaecologists of Canada.The prevention of early-onset neonatal group B streptococcal disease. *J Obstet Gynaecol Can.* 2013;35(10):939–951.

Morland-Schultz K, Hill P. Prevention of and therapies for nipple pain: a systematic review. *JOGNN.* 2005;34: 428–437. doi: 10.1177/0884217505276056.

Morrison B, Ludington-Hoe SM. Interruptions to breastfeeding dyads in an LDRP unit. *Am J Matern Child Nurs.* 2012;37(1):36–41. doi: 10.1097/ NMC.0b013e31823851d5.

Morrison B, Ludington-Hoe SM, Anderson GC. Interruptions to breastfeeding dyads on postpartum day 1 in a university hospital. *JOGNN.* 2006;35:709–716. doi: 10.1111/J.1552-6909.2006.00095.x.

Mortel M, Mehta SD. Systematic review of the efficacy of herbal galactogogues. *J Hum Lact.* 2013;29(2): 154–162. doi: 10.1177/0890334413477243.

Much D, Beyerlein A, Roßbauer M, et al. Beneficial effects of breastfeeding in women with gestational diabetes mellitus. *Molecular Metabolism.* 2014; 3: 284–292.

Murgatroyd CA, Nephew BC. Effects of early life social stress on maternal behavior and neuroendocrinology. *Psychoneuroendocrinology.* 2012;38(2):219–228. doi:10.1016/ j.psyneuen.2012.05.020.

Murtaugh MA, Ferris AM, Capacchione CM, Reece EA. Energy intake and glycemia in lactating women with type 1 diabetes. *J Am Diet Assoc.* 1998;98:642–652.

Myers ER, Aubuchon-Endsley N, Bastian LA, et al. *Efficacy and safety of screening for postpartum depression.* Comparative Effectiveness Review 106. (Prepared by the Duke Evidence-based Practice Center under Contract No. 290-2007-10066-I.) AHRQ Publication No. 13-EHC064-EF. Rockville, MD: Agency for Healthcare Research and Quality; April 2013. Available at: http://www.effectivehealthcare.ahrq.gov/reports/final .cfm.

Nasri K, Chehrei A, Manavi MS. Evaluation of vaginal group B streptococcal culture results after digital vaginal examination and its pattern of antibiotic resistance in pregnant women. *Iran J Reprod Med.* 2013;11(12): 999–1004.

National Foundation for Infectious Diseases. Call to action. Improving vaccination rates in pregnant women: Timely intervention – lasting benefits. Bethesda, MD: author; 2014.

National Public Radio (NPR), Robert Wood Johnson Foundation, Harvard School of Public Health. The burden of stress in America. July 2014. Available at: http://media .npr.org/documents/2014/july/npr_rwfj_harvard_stress _poll.pdf.

Nelson EE, Panksepp J. Brain substrates of infant–mother attachment: contributions of opioids, oxytocin, and norepinephrine. *Neurosci Biobehav Rev.* 1998;22(3): 437–452.

Ngamkham S, Vincent C, Finnegan L, et al. The McGill Pain Questionnaire as a multidimensional measure in people with cancer: an integrative review. *Pain Manag Nurs.* 2012;13(1):27–51. doi: 10.1016/j.pmn.2010.12.003.

Nishioka E, Haruna M, Ita E, et al. Prospective study of the relationship between breastfeeding and postpartum depressive symptoms appearing at 1–5 months after delivery. *J Affective Disorders.* 2011;133:553–559.

Nommsen-Rivers L. Evidence of a dose–response relationship between duration of lactation and future risk of rheumatoid arthritis. *J Hum Lact.* 2005;21:213–214.

Nommsen-Rivers LA, Chantry CJ, Dewey KG. Early breastfeeding outcomes in gestational diabetic primiparas delivering term infants. *FASEB J.* 2010;24:91.4 (meeting abstract).

Ødegaard I, Stray-Pedersen B, Hallberg K, et al. Maternal and fetal morbidity in pregnancies of Norwegian and

Swedish women with cystic fibrosis. *Acta Obstet Gynecol Scand.* 2002;81:698–705.

Ohlsson A, Shah VS. Intrapartum antibiotics for known maternal Group B streptococcal colonization. Cochrane Database Syst Rev. 2014 Jun 10;6:CD007467. doi: 10.1002/14651858.CD007467.pub4.

Osadchy A, Moretti ME, Koren G. Effect of domperidone on insufficient lactation in puerperal women: a systematic review and meta-analysis of randomized controlled trials. *Obstet Gynecol Int.* 2012;article 642893. doi: 10.1155/2012/642893.

Pavlov-Dolijanovic S, Damjanov NS, Vujasinovic Stupar NZ, et al. Is there a difference in systemic lupus erythematosus with and without Raynaud's phenomenon? *Rheumatol Int.* 2013;33(4):859–865. doi: 10.1007/s00296-012-2449-6.

Pennell PB, Gidal BE, Sabers A, et al. Pharmacology of antiepileptic drugs during pregnancy and lactation. *Epilepsy Behav.* 2007;11(3):263–269.

Perez A, Labbok MH, Queenan JT. Clinical study of the lactational amenorrhoea method for family planning. *Lancet.* 1992;339:968–970.

Perez A, Vela P, Masnick GS, Potter RG. First ovulation after childbirth: the effect of breastfeeding. *Am J Obstet Gynecol.* 1972;114:1014–1047.

Pikwer M, Bergström U, Nilsson JA, et al. Breast feeding, but not use of oral contraceptives, is associated with a reduced risk of rheumatoid arthritis. *Ann Rheum Dis.* 2009;68(4):526–530. doi: 10.1136/ard.2007.084707.

Plumb J, Clayton G. Group B streptococcus infection: risk and prevention. *Pract Midwife.* 2013;16(7):27–30.

Porges SW. The polyvagal perspective. *Biol Psychol.* 2007; 74(2):116–143.

Porges SW, Furman SA. Early development of the autonomic nervous system provides a neural platform for social behaviour: a polyvagal perspective. *Infant Child Devel.* 2011;20:106–118. doi: 10.1002/icd.688.

Prunty M, Sharpe L, Butow P, Fulcher G. The motherhood choice: themes arising in the decision-making process for women with multiple sclerosis. *Mult Scler.* 2008; 14(5):701-4. doi: 10.1177/1352458507086103.

Purkayastha S, Tilney HS, Darzi AW, et al. Meta-analysis of randomized studies evaluating chewing gum to enhance postoperative recovery following colectomy. *Arch Surg.* 2008;143:788–493.

Quijano CE, Abalos E. Conservative management of symptomatic and/or complicated haemorrhoids in pregnancy and the puerperium. *Cochrane Database Syst Rev.* 2005;3:CD004077. doi: 10.1002/14651858.CD004077.pub2.

Quintero J, Fernandez-Rojo S, Chapela E, et al. Postpartum emotional psychopathological outcomes. *J Gen Pract.* 2014;2:162. doi: 10.4172/2329-9126.1000162.

Ramos R, Kennedy K, Visness C. Effectiveness of lactational amenorrhea in prevention of pregnancy in Manila, the Philippines: non-comparative prospective trial. *Br Med J.* 1996;313:909–912.

Reddy P, Qi C, Zembower T, et al. Postpartum mastitis and community-acquired methicillin-resistant *Staphylococcus aureus. Emerg Infect Dis* [serial on the Internet]. 2007. Available at: http://wwwnc.cdc.gov/eid/article/13/2/06-0989. doi: 10.3201/eid1302.060989.

Reeder C, LeGrand A, O'Connor-Von SK. The effect of fenugreek on milk production and prolactin levels in mothers of preterm infants. *Clin Lact.* 2013;4(4):159–165. doi: 10.1891/2158-0782.4.4.159.

Rincon-Cortes M, Sullivan R. Early life trauma and attachment: immediate and enduring effects on neurobehavioral and stress axis development. *Frontiers Endocrinol.* 2014;5:article 33. doi: 10.3389/fendo.2014.00033/.

Riordan J. *A practical guide to breastfeeding.* St. Louis, MO: Mosby; 1983.

Risisky D, Asghar SM, Chaffee M, DeGennaro N. Women's perceptions using the CenteringPregnancy model of group prenatal care. *J Perinatal Educ.* 2013;22(3):136–144. doi: 10.1891/1058-1243.22.3.136.

Rivera R, Kennedy KI, Ortiz E, et al. Breastfeeding and the return to ovulation in Durango, Mexico. *Fertil Steril.* 1988;49:780–787.

Robson KM, Brant HA, Kumar R. Maternal sexuality during first pregnancy and after childbirth. *Br J Obstet Gynaecol.* 1981;88:882–889.

Rojnik B, Kosmelj K, Andolsek-Jeras L. Initiation of contraception postpartum. *Contraception.* 1995;51:75–81.

Saari Z, Yusof FM. Induced lactation by adoptive mothers: a case study. *Jurnal Teknologi.* 2014;68(1):123–132.

Sachs HC, American Academy of Pediatrics (AAP) Committee on Drugs. The transfer of drugs and therapeutics into human breast milk: an update on selected topics. *Pediatrics.* 2013;132:e796. doi: 10.1542/peds.2013-1985.

Sakalidis VS, Williams TM, Garbin CP, et al. Ultrasound imaging of infant suckling dynamics during the establishment of lactation. *J Hum Lact.* 2013;29(2):205–213. doi: 10.1177/0890334412452933.

Sakka AE, Salama, M, Salama, K. The effect of fenugreek herbal tea and palm dates on breast milk production and infant weight. *J Pediatr Sci.* 2014;6:e202.

Saltzman W, Maestripieri D. The neuroendocrinology of primate maternal behavior. *Prog Neuropsychopharmacol Biol Psychiatry.* 2011;35(5):1192–1204. doi: 10.1016/j.pnpbp.2010.09.017.

Sances G, Granella F, Nappi RE, et al. Course of migraine during pregnancy and postpartum: a prospective study. *Cephalalgia.* 2003;23:197–205.

Saxton A, Fahy K, Skinner V, Hastie C. Effects of immediate skin-to-skin contact on breastfeeding after birth on postpartum (PPH) rates: a cohort study. *Women Birth.* 2013;26:S16–S17.

Schanler RJ, Fraley JK, Lau C, et al. Breastmilk cultures and infection in extremely premature infants. *J Perinatol.* 2011;31(5):335–8. doi: 10.1038/jp.2011.13.

Scottish Intercollegiate Guidelines Network (SIGN). *Management of perinatal mood disorders: a national clinical guideline.* Edinburgh, UK: SIGN; 2012.

Sert M, Tetiker T, Kirim S, Kocak M. Clinical report of 28 patients with Sheehan's syndrome. *Endocr J.* 2003; 50(3):297–301.

Shaaban MM, Kennedy KI, Sayed GH, et al. The recovery of fertility during breastfeeding in Assiut, Egypt. *J Biosoc Sci.* 1990;22:19–32.

Sharma K, Bhatnagar M. *Asparagus racemosus* (Shatavari): a versatile female tonic. *Int J Pharmaceut Biol Arch.* 2011; 2(3):855–863.

Sharma V, Corpse CS. Case study revisiting the association between breastfeeding and postpartum depression. *J Hum Lact.* 2008;24:77–79.

Sheeder J, Kabir K, Stafford B. Screening for postpartum depression at well-child visits: is once enough during the first 6 months of life? *Pediatrics.* 2009;123(6): e982–e988. doi: 10.1542/peds.2008-1160.

Shiffman ML, Seale TW, Flux M, et al. Breast-milk composition in women with cystic fibrosis: report of two cases and a review of the literature. *Am J Clin Nutr.* 1989;49: 612–617.

Short RV, Lewis PR, Renfree MB, Shaw G. Contraceptive effects of extended lactational amenorrhea: beyond the Bellagio consensus. *Lancet.* 1991;337:715–717.

Siebenaler N, Rogers J. Breastfeeding mothers with disabilities. In: Mannel R, Martens PJ, Walker M, eds. *Core curriculum for lactation consultant practice*, 3rd ed. Burlington, MA: Jones & Bartlett; 2013:603–620.

Silberstein SD. Headaches and women: treatment of the pregnant and lactating migraneur. *Headache.* 1993;33: 533–540.

Simmons D. Metformin treatment for Type 2 diabetes in pregnancy? *Best Practice & Research Clinical Endocrinology & Metabolism.* 2010;24:625–634.

Smedberg C. Relactation after breast cancer: a case study. *Leaven.* April–May–June 2007. Available at: http://www .lalecheleague.org/llleaderweb/lv/lvaprmayjun07p26 .html.

Smith VC, Svoren BM, Wolfsdorf JI. Hypothyroidism in a breast-fed preterm infant resulting from maternal topical iodine exposure. *J Pediatr.* 2006;149:566–567.

Snider DF, Powell KE. Should women taking antituberculosis drugs breastfeed? *Arch Intern Med.* 1984;144:589–590.

Speller E, Boddribb W, McEntyre E. Breastfeeding and thyroid disease: a literature review. *Breastfeed Rev.* 2012; 20(2):41–47.

Stagnaro-Green A, Abalovich M, Alexander E, et al. Guidelines of the American Thyroid Association for the diagnosis and management of thyroid disease during pregnancy and postpartum. *Thyroid.* 2011;21(10): 1081–1125. doi: 10.1089/thy.2011.0087.

Stuebe AM, Grewen K, Meltzer-Brody S. Association between maternal mood and oxytocin response to breastfeeding. *J Women's Health (Larchmt).* 2013;22(4):352–361. doi: 10.1089/jwh.2012.3768.

Tabares FP, Jaramillo JVB, Ruiz-Cortés ZT. Pharmacological Overview of Galactogogues. Veterinary Medicine International. 2014, Article ID 602894, 20 pages. doi: 10.1155/2014/602894

Tan EM, Cohen AS, Fries JF, et al. The 1982 revised criteria for the classification of systemic lupus erythematosus. *Arthritis Rheum.* 1982;25:1271–1277.

Tanner-Smith EE, Steinka-Fry KT, Lipsey MW. Effects of CenteringPregnancy group prenatal care on breastfeeding outcomes. *J Midwifery Women's Health.* 2013;58: 389–395. doi: 10.1111/jmwh.12008.

Tanner-Smith EE, Steinka-Fry KT, Lipsey MW. The effects of CenteringPregnancy group prenatal care on gestational age, birth weight, and fetal demise. *Matern Child Health J.* 2014;18:801–809.

Tashakori A, Behbahani AZ, Irani RD. Comparison of prevalence of postpartum depression symptoms between breastfeeding mothers and non-breastfeeding mothers. *Iran J Psychiatry.* 2012;7(2):61–65. doi: 10.1007/ s10995-013-1304-z.

Taylor EC, Nickel NC, Labbock MH. Implementing the ten steps for successful breastfeeding in hospitals serving low-wealth patients. *Am J Public Health.* 2012;102(12): 2262–2268. doi: 10.2105/AJPH.2012.300769.

Taylor JS, Kacmar JE, Nothnagle M, Lawrence RA. A systematic review of the literature associating breastfeeding with type 2 diabetes and gestational diabetes. *J Am Coll Nutr.* 2005;24:320–326.

Taylor SE. *The tending instinct: How nurturing is essential to who we are and how we live.* New York, NY: Times Books; 2002.

Taylor SE. Tend and befriend: behavioral bases of affiliation under stress. *Curr Direct Psychol Sci.* 2006;15(6): 273–277.

Thapa S, Short RV, Potts M. Breastfeeding, birth spacing and their effects on child survival. *Nature.* 1988;335(6192): 679–682.

Thomson VM. Breastfeeding and mothering one-handed. *J Hum Lact.* 1995;11:211–215.

Thompson JF, Heal LJ, Roberts CL, Elwood DA. Women's breastfeeding experience following a significant postpartum haemorrhage: a multicentre cohort study. *Int Breastfeed J.* 2010;5:5.

Thorley V. *Lactation and headaches.* Presented at Breastfeeding: The Natural Advantage Conference; Sydney, Australia; October 1997.

Thorley V. Headaches in breastfeeding women. *Birth Issues.* 2000;9(3):85–88.

Tonelli MR, Aitken ML. Pregnancy in cystic fibrosis. *Curr Opin Pulm Med.* 2007;13(6):537–540.

Tracer DP. Lactation, nutrition and postpartum amenorrhea in lowland Papua New Guinea, *Hum Biol.* 1996;68(2): 277–292. Available at: http://www.jstor.org/stable /41465472.

Trout KK. The neuromatrix theory of pain: implications for selected nonpharmacologic methods of pain relief for labor. *J Midwifery Women's Health.* 2004;49:482–488. doi: 10.1016/j.jmwh.2004.07.009.

Tsokos GC. Systemic lupus erythematosus. *N Engl J Med.* 2011;365(22):2110–2121. doi: 10.1056/NEJM-ra1100359.

Turkyilmaz E, Hirfanoglu IM, Turan O, et al. The effect of galactogogue herbal tea on breast milk production and short-term catchup of birth weight in the first week of life. *J Altern Complement Med.* 2011;17(2): 139–142.

Turton S, Campbell C. Tend and befriend versus fight or flight: gender differences in behavioral response to stress among university students. *J Appl Biobehav Res.* 2005;10(4):209–232.

Udry JR. Coitus as demographic behaviour. In: Gray R, ed. *Biomedical and demographic determinants of reproduction.* Oxford, UK: Clarendon Press; 1993:85–97.

Udry JR, Deang L. Determinants of coitus after childbirth. *J Biosoc Sci.* 1993;25:117–125.

Uvnas-Moberg K. Antistress pattern induced by oxytocin. *News Physiol Sci.* 1998a;13:22–26.

Uvnas-Moberg K. Oxytocin may mediate the benefits of positive social interaction and emotions. *Psychoneuroendocrinology.* 1998b;23(8):819–835.

Uvnas-Moberg K. *The oxytocin factor: tapping the hormone of calm, love and healing.* Cambridge, MA: Da Capo Press; 2003.

Uvnas-Moberg K, Arn I, Magnusson D. The psychobiology of emotion: the role of the oxytocinergic system. *Int J Behav Med.* 2005;12(2):59–65.

Uvnas-Moberg K, Petersson M. Oxytocin, a mediator of anti-stress, well-being, social interaction, growth and healing. *Z Psychosom Med Psychother.* 2005;51(1): 57–80.

Vagnarelli F. TDM grand rounds: neonatal nicotine withdrawal syndrome in an infant prenatally and postnatally exposed to heavy cigarette smoke. *Ther Drug Monit.* 2006;28(5):585–588.

Valdes V, Labbok MH, Pugin E, Perez A. The efficacy of the lactational amenorrhea method (LAM) among working women. *Contraception.* 2000;62:217–219.

Valeggia C, Ellison PT. Interactions between metabolic and reproductive functions in the resumption of postpartum fecundity. *Am J Hum Biol.* 2009;21(4):559–566. doi: 10.1002/ajhb.20907.

van Bree SHW, Nemethova A, Cailotto C, et al. New therapeutic strategies for postoperative ileus. *Nat Rev Gastroenterol Hepatol.* 2012;9:675–683. doi: 10.1038/nrgastro.2012.134.

Vanky E, Isaksen H, Moen MH, Carlsen SM. Breastfeeding in polycystic ovary syndrome. *Acta Obstet Gynecol Scand.* 2008;87:531–535. doi: 10.1080/00016340802007676.

Vanky E, Nordskar JJ, Leithe H, et al. Breast size increment during pregnancy and breastfeeding in mothers with polycystic ovary syndrome: a follow-up study of a randomised controlled trial on metformin versus placebo. *BJOG.* 2012;119(11):1403–1409. doi: 10.1111/j.1471-0528.2012.03449.x.

Visness CM, Kennedy KI. The frequency of coitus during breastfeeding. *Birth.* 1997;24(4):253–257.

Visness CM, Kennedy KI, Gross BA, et al. Fertility of fully breastfeeding women in the early postpartum period. *Obstet Gynecol.* 1997;89:164–167.

Visness CM, Kennedy KI, Ramos R. The duration and character of postpartum bleeding among breastfeeding women. *Obstet Gynecol.* 1997;89:159–163.

Vukusic S, Hutchinson M, Hours M, et al. Pregnancy and multiple sclerosis (the PRIMS study): clinical predictors of post-partum relapse. *Brain.* 2004;127(pt 6): 1353–1360.

Walker J. Lactational headaches. *Nurs Mothers Assoc Australia Talkabout.* 1999;39(1):12–13.

Wall VR. Breastfeeding and migraine headaches. *J Hum Lact.* 1992;8:209–212.

Wambach K. Fatigue in breastfeeding primiparae over the first nine weeks post partum. *J Hum Lact.* 1998;14: 219–230.

Wan EW, Davey K, Page-Sharp M, et al. Dose-effect study of domperidone as a galactagogue in preterm mothers with insufficient milk supply, and its transfer into milk. *Br J Clin Pharmacol.* 2008;66(2):283-9. doi: 10.1111/j.1365-2125.2008.03207.x.

Wang AT, Mullan RJ, Lane MA, et al. Treatment of hyperprolactinemia: a systematic review and meta-analysis. *Syst Rev.* 2012;1:33. doi: 10.1186/2046-4053-1-33.

Wang L, Chen CT, Liu WH, Wang YH. Recurrent neonatal Group B streptococcal disease associated with infected breast milk. *Clin Pediatr.* 2007;46:547–549.

Weiss P. The contraceptive potential of breastfeeding in Bangladesh. *Stud Fam Plann.* 1993;22:294–307.

Welch MJ, Phelps DL, Osher AB. Breast-feeding by a mother with cystic fibrosis. *Pediatrics.* 1981;67:664–666.

Wight N, Marinelli KA; Academy of Breastfeeding Medicine. ABM clinical protocol #1: guidelines for blood glucose monitoring and treatment of hypoglycemia in term and late-preterm neonates, revised 2014. *Breastfeed Med.* 2014;9(4):173–179. doi: 10.1089/bfm.2014. 9986.

Willis CE, Livingstone V. Infant insufficient milk syndrome associated with maternal postpartum hemorrhage. *J Hum Lact.* 1995;11:123–126.

Wilson-Clay B, Hoover K. *The breastfeeding atlas,* 5th ed. Manchaka, TX: LactNews Press; 2013.

World Health Organization (WHO). Breastfeeding and maternal tuberculosis. *WHO Division of Child Health and Development.* 1998a;23:1–3.

World Health Organization (WHO). The WHO multinational study of breastfeeding and lactational amenorrhea: I. Description of infant feeding patterns and the return of menses. *Fertil Steril.* 1998b;70:448–460.

World Health Organization (WHO). The WHO multinational study of breastfeeding and lactational amenorrhea: II. Factors associated with the length of amenorrhea. *Fertil Steril.* 1998c;70:461–471.

World Health Organization (WHO). The WHO multinational study of breastfeeding and lactational amenorrhea: III. Pregnancy during breastfeeding. *Fertil Steril.* 1999a; 72(3):431–440.

World Health Organization (WHO). The WHO multinational study of breastfeeding and lactational amenorrhea: IV. Postpartum bleeding and lochia in breastfeeding women. *Fertil Steril.* 1999b;72(3):441–447.

Worthington J, Jones R, Crawford M, Forti A.. Pregnancy and multiple sclerosis: a 3-year prospective study. *J Neurol.* 1994;241:228–233.

Wray J. Postnatal care: is it based on ritual or a purpose? A reflective account. *Br J Midwifery.* 2006a;14(9): 520–526.

Wray J. Seeking to explore what matters to women about postnatal care, *Br J Midwifery.* 2006b;4(5):248–254.

Wundes A, Pebdani RN, Amtmann D. What do healthcare providers advise women with multiple sclerosis regarding pregnancy? *Mult Scler Int.* 2014;2014:819216. doi: 10.1155/2014/819216.

Yarur A, Kane SV. Update on pregnancy and breastfeeding in the era of biologics. *Dig Liver Dis.* 2013;45(10): 787–794. doi: 10.1016/j.dld.2013.02.001.

Yee LM, Kaimal AJ, Nakagawa S, et al. Predictors of postpartum sexual activity and function in a diverse population of women. *J Midwifery Women's Health.* 2013;58: 654–661. doi:10.1111/jmwh.12068.

Ystrom E. Breastfeeding cessation and symptoms of anxiety and depression: a longitudinal cohort study. *BMC Pregnancy and Childbirth.* 2012;12:36. http://www .biomedcentral.com/1471-2393/12/36.

Zapantis A, Steinberg JG, Schilit L. Use of herbals as galactogogues. *Pharmacy Practice.* 2012;25(2):222–231. doi: 10.1177/0897190011431636.

Zauderer C, Davis W. Treating postpartum depression and anxiety naturally. *Holist Nurs Pract.* 2012;26(4): 203–209.

Zell BL. Breastfeeding as a community health imperative. *Breastfeed Med.* 2011;6(5):303–304. doi: 10.1089/ bfm.2011.0090.

Zender R, Olshansky E. Biology of caring: researching the healing effects of stress response regulation through relational engagement. *Biol Res Nurs.* 2012;14(4): 419–430. doi: 10.1177/1099800412450505.

Maternal Employment and Breastfeeding

Wilaiporn Rojjanasrirat
Karen Wambach

Introduction

A large proportion of childbearing age women work outside the home in the United States and other industrialized countries of the world (International Labour Organization [ILO], 2012; U.S. Bureau of Labor Statistics, 2013). The decision to return to work soon after childbirth presents significant challenges for women who wish to continue breastfeeding. Women who continue to breastfeed when they return to work often face difficulties, especially if their worksite lacks a supportive environment and their schedules lack flexibility. Coupled with an increasing focus on prolonging exclusive breastfeeding to 6 months and overall breastfeeding to 1 year or beyond, the challenges of combining breastfeeding and work outside the home become very apparent. In fact, the impact of work on breastfeeding is a public health and global health issue (Calnen, 2007; United States Breastfeeding Committee, 2011).

This chapter focuses on breastfeeding and working women, as well as the influence of maternal employment on breastfeeding practice and duration. Strategies to manage the continuation of breastfeeding and employment at the individual, workplace, community, national, and international levels are described.

Historical Perspective and Statistics on Maternal Employment

Historically, women have always worked, either paid or unpaid. The focus of this chapter is on paid work outside the home in combination with breastfeeding. Maternal employment in the United States and other industrialized nations has increased rapidly over the past few decades. Based on data from the U.S. Bureau of Labor Statistics (2013), between 1975 and 2000, the proportion of U.S. working women with children younger than 18 years of age increased from 47.4% to 72.9%. Furthermore, the proportion of first-time mothers employed on a full-time basis increased from 40% in 1961–1965 to 56% in 2006–2008 (U.S. Bureau of Labor Statistics, 2009). The number of women participating in the labor market in the United States varies with the age of the youngest child, marital status, and race. Rates of employment are highest among married women with young children. In 2011, the workforce participation rate for mothers with infants younger than 1 year was 55.8% (U.S. Bureau of Labor Statistics, 2013). Globally, approximately 1.3 billion women participated in the workforce in 2012, representing

39.9% of the total workforce of 3.3 billion people (ILO, 2011).

Many factors contribute to the increasing participation of women and mothers in the workforce. The majority of women work to earn money needed to support their families (Christrup, 2001; Hawkins et al., 2007; Smith et al., 2001). During the last 40 years, many families have come to depend on a second income (Laughlin, 2011). Maternal age and educational attainment in relation to childbearing have also changed over time, with women first pursuing their education and subsequently obtaining employment, and only then having children. The proportion of women aged 25 to 64 who participate in the labor force with a college degree increased threefold from 1970 to 2010, and the mean maternal age for first-time mothers increased 3.6 years from 21.4 years in 1970 to 25.0 years in 2007 (Laughlin, 2011; Matthews & Hamilton, 2009). Also reflective of women's educational attainment, women accounted for more than 52% of all people employed in management and professional occupations, financial industry, education, and health services in 2010. Women's earnings as a proportion of men's earnings have improved over time. Women working full time earned 81% of what men did in 2010, compared with only 62% in 1979 (U.S. Department of Labor, 2011). Not surprisingly, women report career development and personal enjoyment as major reasons for returning to work after childbirth, in addition to finances, self-fulfillment, workplace policy, work motivation, and family or baby motivation (Killien, 1998; Nichols & Roux, 2004).

As women's and mothers' participation in the workforce has increased over time, the conditions influencing women as they bear children have evolved. For example, legislative, judicial, and regulatory changes related to maternal employment were enacted in the 1970s and 1980s that affected policy on employee pregnancy, birth, and childcare support. The Pregnancy Discrimination Act, enacted in 1978, covered hiring and firing policies for pregnant women and women following childbirth (Spain & Bianchi, 1996).

Conditions in the home often present challenges for working mothers. Working mothers usually play multiple roles and share domestic responsibilities such as household chores; thus, they juggle to maintain a balance between work and family. Many women report that neither their employers nor public policy adequately recognizes or supports women's family responsibilities (Killien, 2005; Killien et al., 2001). Studies have revealed that postpartum mothers experience many resiliency challenges such as role overload, family stress, maternal–infant separation anxiety, and financial and psychosocial issues when they return to work (Cooklin et al., 2012; Nichols & Roux, 2004).

As more women work outside the home, potential conflicts arise between breastfeeding, which demands a woman's unique ability to meet her baby's needs, and her efforts to balance the demands of work and family.

The Effect of Work on Breastfeeding

The National Immunization Survey (NIS) indicates that the prevalence of breastfeeding initiation and duration through 6 months and 1 year of age in the United States has risen substantially, to 76.9%, 47.2%, and 25.5%, respectively (Centers for Disease Control and Prevention [CDC], 2012). Although breastfeeding initiation rates in the United States have been rising over the past decade, the rates at 6 and 12 months are still far below the *Healthy People 2020* goals. The prevalence of continued exclusive breastfeeding for the birth years 2009 to 2011 at 3 and 6 months were 36% and 16.3%, respectively (CDC, 2012).

The increasing number of women with infants younger than 1 year of age entering the workforce each year has serious implications, as many women will choose to combine breastfeeding and employment. Some empirical evidence suggests that employment has a negative impact on women's decision to initiate breastfeeding, especially among those women who plan to return to work in the first few to 12 weeks postpartum (Fein & Roe, 1998;

Lindberg, 1996; Mandal et al., 2010; Mirkovic et al., 2014; Ogbuano et al., 2011; Roe et al., 1999), while other evidence suggests no impact on breastfeeding initiation (Kimbro, 2006; Noble & ALSPAC Study Team, 2001; Ong et al., 2005; Ryan et al., 2006). Studies conducted outside the United States on maternal employment status and breastfeeding also indicate that full-time employed women in non-U.S. countries are less likely to initiate breastfeeding than mothers who are not employed (Chen et al., 2006; Chuang et al., 2010; Hawkins et al., 2007).

For many women both inside and outside the United States, the workplace seems to be incompatible with long breastfeeding duration. In a longitudinal study known as Infant Feeding Practice Study II, Mandal and colleagues (2010) analyzed the relationships among mothers' work status, initiation, and breastfeeding duration. Women working fewer than 35 hours per week were more likely than full-time workers to initiate breastfeeding. Furthermore, working more than 34 hours per week was associated with significantly shorter breastfeeding duration. Numerous studies indicate that full-time working mothers are less likely to breastfeed at 6 months compared to those who work part time or are unemployed (Arthur et al., 2003; Chuang et al., 2010; Kimbro, 2006; Roe et al., 1999; Ryan et al., 2002). Ryan et al., (2006) reported that 65.5% and 26.1% of women who worked full time were breastfeeding their infants at hospital discharge and at 6 months, respectively, compared to 64.8% and 35% of those women who did not work. Note that while initiation rates were similar in both groups, the continuation rates were measurably different. Some studies have suggested that the longer women delayed their return to work, the lower the negative effect of employment on their breastfeeding experience (Arthur et al., 2003; Chuang et al., 2010; Mandal et al., 2010; Ogbuanu et al., 2011; Skafida, 2012). Most international studies, particularly those conducted in developing countries, report that working negatively affects breastfeeding (Aikawa et al., 2012; Chen et al., 2006; Cooklin et al., 2008; Ong et al., 2005).

The intensity of breastfeeding has also been associated with duration of breastfeeding. Working mothers who exclusively breastfeed (no formula supplementation) are more likely to continue breastfeeding longer than those who partially breastfeed (Aikawa et al., 2012; Ong et al., 2005). In addition, when a mother is satisfied and views breastfeeding as a special time with the baby that she does not want to give up, she is more likely to breastfeed longer (Rojjanasrirat, 2004).

Type of occupation is also associated with duration of breastfeeding. Women who are classified as professional, administrative, or managerial have a longer duration of breastfeeding than do women in lower-skill occupations such as clerical and service jobs (Piper & Parks, 1996; Visness & Kennedy, 1997; Whaley et al., 2002). In contrast, Kimbro (2006) reported that women in service occupations and administrative positions wean earlier than other women. In general, there is a need for more research to test interventions and set policies that support breastfeeding among women in service jobs as well as among those who do shift work.

Facilitators and Barriers to Breastfeeding in the Workplace

A number of barriers to breastfeeding in the workplace have been identified (Johnston & Esposito, 2007; Mills, 2009; Skafida, 2012). Significant factors and reasons for early weaning among working mothers include insufficient milk supply, lack of knowledge regarding management of breastfeeding in the workplace, lack of time to pump, and work facilities that are not conducive to breastfeeding (Arthur et al., 2003; Bar-Yam, 1998; Chuang et al., 2010; Ong et al., 2005; Roe et al., 1999; Rojjanasrirat, 2004; Scott et al., 2006). Arthur et al. (2003) examined the breastfeeding decisions and experiences of female physicians related to employment. They reported that the three major factors contributing to complete discontinuation of breastfeeding are returning to work (45%), diminishing milk supply (31%), and lack of time to pump (18%).

Factors enhancing or facilitating the continuation of breastfeeding in the workplace include on-site child care, long maternity leave, flexible work schedules, availability of a lactation room, types of breast pumps, and a supportive environment (family-friendly employers) (Arthur et al., 2003; Fein et al., 2008; Hawkins et al., 2007; Ortiz et al., 2004; Stevens & Janke, 2003; Witters-Green, 2003). Feeding the infant directly at the breast during the workday is the most effective strategy for combining employment and breastfeeding, according to one team of researchers (Fein et al., 2008). Sattari et al. (2013), in their study of 130 female U.S. physicians, found a discrepancy between mothers' breastfeeding duration goals and their actual breastfeeding duration (i.e., a shorter duration then intended), with longer duration of breastfeeding being related to not having to make up missed calls/work that occurred as a result of pregnancy or maternity leave, longer length of maternity leave, sufficient time at work for milk expression, and perceived level of support for breastfeeding efforts at work from colleagues, program directors, or division/section chiefs.

Consideration of these barriers and facilitators when planning for combining work and breastfeeding can enhance success in ongoing breastfeeding. We turn now to strategies to manage breastfeeding and work, beginning with the individual woman's efforts and then moving to a discussion of the other key players in the quest to support breastfeeding among employed woman.

Individual Strategies to Manage Breastfeeding and Work

Prenatal Planning and Preparation

Just as pregnancy is a time of planning that focuses on caring for and feeding a baby, so pregnancy is the best time to plan for one's return to employment. Some women have already thought about a plan, often before they ever become pregnant. Preconception planning, as advocated by Johnston and Esposito (2007) in their review of the literature on barriers and facilitators for breastfeeding among working mothers, may be suggested by healthcare providers through the use of posters, videos, and pamphlets, as well as referral to lactation consultants; such measures may enhance attitudes and commitment to continued breastfeeding after returning to work. Preconception and prenatal planning allow women to sort out and debunk existing myths about breastfeeding, especially those saying that combining breastfeeding and employment is difficult and not worth the effort. Thus the healthcare worker who has contact with the employed pregnant woman does her a great service simply by asking how she plans to combine breastfeeding and returning to work. In some cases, the mother's reply to such a question will identify fallacies that need to be corrected and areas in which information needs to be shared.

For mothers who are ambivalent or undecided about continued breastfeeding after returning to work, healthcare workers can share information on the benefits of continued breastfeeding in general and in combination with employment, including the following advantages:

- Optimal infant health, growth, and development
- Fewer work absences due to infant illness, lower expenses for infant health care, and increased employee morale (Cohen et al., 1995; Ortiz et al., 2004)
- Lower expenses for infant nutrition
- Less energy and time spent in purchasing, storing, and preparing formula
- Feeling more connected and bonded to the baby during the workday when pumping or feelings of enhanced motherliness (Rojjanas-rirat, 2004; Stevens & Janke, 2003)
- Periodic lactation breaks that restore the mother's perspective
- The opportunity to restore feelings of closeness while nursing the baby when back together (Stevens & Janke, 2003)

The healthcare worker should begin by encouraging the pregnant woman, especially the first-time breastfeeding mother, to learn as much as she can about breastfeeding so she can be sure to get off to a smooth start when breastfeeding after returning to work. This includes learning about infant feeding patterns, breast pump alternatives, milk expression and storage, and maintaining the optimal milk supply (Angeletti, 2009; Biagoli, 2003; Fein et al., 2008; Mills, 2009). Numerous resources including books, pamphlets, and websites may also provide the woman with helpful information (see the Internet resources and other sources of information listed at the end of this chapter).

The woman should also talk with women who have already combined breastfeeding and employment to obtain practical tips. Individual breastfeeding counseling is an important strategy for care providers such as nurses or lactation consultants to identify specific needs, establish rapport through active listening, acknowledge specific concerns or myths, and encourage the woman with consistent information. In a qualitative study among low-income working women, Rojjanasrirat and Sousa (2010) found that some women anticipated multiple challenges and felt uncertain regarding the decision to continue breastfeeding after returning to work. Prenatal breastfeeding classes, especially those with an emphasis on planning for return to work while breastfeeding, can be very helpful and can boost a mother's knowledge and confidence about breastfeeding.

The healthcare provider can help the mother begin planning for breastfeeding when she returns to work. The timing of the return to work should be decided before the baby arrives and in most cases is planned in consultation with the woman's family and her employer. The constraints of official maternity leave and family financial needs often determine the timing. However, the longer that a mother can stay at home after birth the better, as demonstrated by research showing a detrimental effect of shorter maternity leave on breastfeeding duration (Arthur et al., 2003; Chuang et al., 2010; Mandal et al., 2010; Ogbuanu et al., 2011; Skafida, 2012).

The employed pregnant woman should seek support from her employer and determine if there is a breastfeeding policy. As part of this effort, she should verify, as required by Section 7(r) of the Fair Labor Standards Act (FSLA)—Break Time for Nursing Mothers Provision (U.S. Department of Labor, 2010), that there is a private space in which to express her milk (note that this regulation applies to businesses with more than 50 employees). Although not required by the FLSA, she should also ask about facilities to store her expressed milk (see Figure 16-1). An open discussion with the employer about the economic benefits of continued breastfeeding after returning to work can help women gain support. For example, the woman should include in the conversation the benefits of increased productivity, reduced absenteeism, and lower healthcare costs due to long-term breastfeeding (Cohen et al., 1995). Further discussion of worksite considerations appears later in this chapter.

The healthcare provider should discuss different work options and the woman's specific plans or goals for breastfeeding while employed. Will she work full time or part time? Research indicates that women who work part time breastfeed longer (Haider et al., 2003; Hawkins et al., 2007; Mandal et al., 2010; Ogbuanu et al., 2011; Ryan et al., 2006). Therefore, encouraging the woman to work less, if financially possible, is recommended.

Figure 16-1 EXPRESSING BREASTMILK IN THE WORKPLACE.

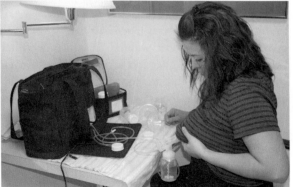

Courtesy of Wilaiporn Rojjanasrirat

Working at Home

Working at home is an option for some mothers, particularly where connecting to the job electronically, via computer modems, the Internet, and fax machines is possible. Telecommuting offers an opportunity for parents who previously worked elsewhere to continue employment while remaining at home with an infant or young child (Bettinelli, 2012). It not only enables the new mother to resume an organized way of life, but also teaches her that a less structured day that recognizes the baby's needs has its own rewards. However, even these workers will likely need to go into the workplace periodically to attend meetings and to share their work with others in face-to-face encounters. Therefore, when preparing to engage in telecommuting, mothers may wish to make part-time/flexible childcare arrangements to allow for times when separation from the baby is necessary.

Job Sharing

Yet another employment option is job sharing. According to the U.S. Department of Labor, job sharing occurs when "two (or more) workers share the duties of one full-time job, each working part-time, or two or more workers who have unrelated part-time assignments share the same budget line" (http://www.dol.gov/compliance/topics/wages -other.htm, para. 1). Advantages to the employer may include greater productivity, greater worker satisfaction, and lower turnover. One study of two community-based private practice physician groups with 13 years of job sharing (Vanek & Vanek, 2001) found that job sharers perceived their situation as successful and most wanted to continue. They had significantly higher job satisfaction than their counterparts who did not job share. The flexibility of job sharing may be appropriate for an employee who wishes to maintain work skills while avoiding stress and burnout, which may occur with having young children.

In another description of job sharing, two University of Tennessee pharmacy faculty members described a major job-sharing benefit for the employer as retention of experienced employees who together offer a wider range of skills than a single employee (Rogers & Finks, 2009). The benefits to the workers, as employees, included balanced work and family lives and maintenance of their knowledge and skills by remaining in the workforce.

Another study ($n = 2775$ male and female exempt and non-exempt employees) conducted by the American Business Collaboration (ABC, 2007) found that flexibility in jobs was exceptionally important. Among those workers who engaged in job sharing, 96% reported having the flexibility they needed; among those who telecommuted (worked from home), 86% reported having the flexibility they needed. In addition, 85% to 90% of women in this survey assigned high importance to workplace flexibility as a factor in their work satisfaction. Work–life balance and flexibility of work schedule were found to be secondary in importance to only salary, job security, and benefits in determining job satisfaction. In fact, exempt women ranked work–life balance and flexibility higher than benefits and almost even with job security.

Although these literature descriptions did not address breastfeeding specifically, their implications for working breastfeeding mothers are certainly apparent.

The Childcare Dilemma

Another area that the healthcare provider should inquire about is childcare decisions. Whether to use a daycare facility, where such care will be provided, when the baby will be enrolled and for how many hours and days, and the effects of such care on both the child and his parents are issues that figure in decision making during the prenatal or early postpartum period. In some cases, the father may take on such care, particularly when the parents' work hours differ or when the father's work is flexible and he can rearrange his schedule to accommodate his partner's job situation. In other families, however, the mother may not have a partner who is available, or she may be a single parent. Other relatives may not be potential caregivers because of geographical distance, disinclination to provide such assistance, physical or psychological incapacity, and many other reasons. Regardless of the ultimate decision of who will care for the baby, the daycare dilemma is a significant issue for all working mothers and families.

The substantial growth in the number of mothers going back to work has increased the demand for child care. In 2011, 12.5 million (61%) of the 20.4 million U.S. children younger than 5 years of age were in some form of childcare arrangement. Across various types of childcare arrangements, the preschoolers of employed mothers spent an average of 36 hours per week in child care, versus 21 hours for children of non-employed mothers (Laughlin & U.S. Census Bureau, 2013). Furthermore, attendance at daycare programs increases children's exposure to potentially infectious agents and, therefore, increases their risk of contracting an infectious disease (Gordon et al., 2007). Studies have shown an increased incidence of upper respiratory infections and diarrhea associated with center-based childcare attendance. Thus it is even more important for mothers to continue to breastfeed as long as possible to protect their infants from infectious illness if they will be cared for in a daycare center.

Pertinent to childcare provider choice and continued breastfeeding after return to work are the following questions: Has a childcare provider been chosen or is there on-site day care in the workplace? Is the childcare provider supportive of continued breastfeeding after returning to work? Is the childcare provider knowledgeable about breastfeeding and human milk qualities (e.g., milk appearance, rapid digestibility)? Is the childcare provider familiar with how to store and warm human milk? In addition, the mother needs to ask how babies are fed at the daycare center—specifically, are they given a bottle to hold while lying alone in a crib or on a pad on the floor, or are they held? Angeletti (2009) speaks to the importance of educating mothers on which knowledge childcare providers should have related to breastfeeding—for example, allowing for paced feedings similar to breastfeeding, watching for feeding cues such as lip smacking or rooting instead of feeding on a rigid schedule, and allowing infants to pace themselves by pausing intermittently and deciding when the feeding is finished to more closely resemble a breastfeeding session.

In 2011, the American Academy of Pediatrics (AAP) and the American Public Health Association (APHA) published the third edition of *Caring for Our Children: National Health and Safety Performance Standards: Guidelines for Early Care and Education Programs*. Within this comprehensive set of health and safety national guidelines for early care and education programs (ECE), including those in personal homes, are guidelines on how to accommodate breastfeeding mothers and infants. The guidelines include the following points: (1) allowing the mother to feed her baby on-site; (2) having a breastfeeding policy that is posted and communicated; (3) following procedures for storing and handling breastmilk, and feeding breastfed infants; and (4) training staff in the policies and procedures. Another strategy recommended by *The CDC Guide to Strategies to Support Breastfeeding Mothers and Babies* (CDC, 2013) encourages the implementation of the AAP/APHA ECE guidelines and provides evidence from the Infant Feeding Practices Study II (IFPS II) that showed a significant association between support from childcare providers and breastfeeding at 6 months. Thus the healthcare provider should make the mother or mother-to-be aware of such guidelines and encourage her to query prospective childcare providers about their policies/procedures for supporting breastfeeding mothers and their children.

Other examples of formal efforts by state or national organizations to promote childcare support of breastfeeding mothers and infants include the Rhode Island Department of Health's *Tips for Childcare Providers* on preparing and storing breastmilk, and the Australian Breastfeeding Association's *Caregiver's Guide to the Breastfed Baby*. In addition, information sources such as La Leche League International's pamphlet entitled, *The Balancing Act* address issues that many employed mothers face while breastfeeding and include tips on how to prepare the childcare provider for the breastfeeding infant. All of these and other resources are listed in the list of Internet resources at the end of this chapter. Finally, additional alternatives to infant day care such as longer paid maternity leave need to be developed and supported by the government.

An alternative is a system that enables—perhaps even encourages—parents to remain with their infants during the first few months of life. Sweden and Norway are two of the leading countries in terms of advocating for parental leave (ILO, 2010). In Sweden, if an employee has been working for an employer for the previous 6 months, or not less than 12 months in the previous 2 years, the parent is entitled to parental leave until the child reaches 18 months. Paid benefits include 80% of earnings up to 390 days and then a flat rate for the last 90 days (total of 480 days) if the parent was insurable for 240 consecutive days prior to birth. If the parents do not meet this requirement, they receive the flat benefit during the entire leave period. In Norway, an employee is entitled to parental leave during the child's first year of life. Paid parental leave consists of 46 weeks at 100% of wages or 56 weeks at 80% of wages. Of this time, 10 weeks are reserved for the father. To be eligible for this benefit, the parent must have been employed and earning a pensionable income for at least 6 of the last 10 months prior to using this benefit.

Special Issues Related to Returning to Work

The day on which a mother returns to work, even when she has prepared for it throughout her time at home after the baby's birth, is often characterized by the emotional and physical tugs she feels. Rarely is this day one in which she is as productive as she was prior to the baby's birth. Informing the mother that her first day back is likely to be emotionally trying and less productive is prudent anticipatory guidance.

The timing of return to work—particularly if it is full-time employment—will influence the specific problems that the breastfeeding mother encounters and the length of time that she may have to deal with them. Breastfeeding problems typical of the early postpartum include the following:

- Concern about an inadequate or fluctuating milk supply
- Engorgement
- Leaking
- Baby's need for frequent feedings
- Baby's frequently changing feeding patterns, including appetite spurts and nighttime nursing

The helping professional should inform the mother that each of these difficulties will resolve over time and that the longer she is home with the baby, the less likely it is that any of these issues will prove insurmountable. None of these issues will be a major obstacle after the baby is older than 4 months; pointing this fact out may encourage the mother to see that these difficulties need not reduce breastfeeding duration when she returns to work very soon after her baby's birth. This information may also assist her in making decisions about the length of her leave from work, if she has an opportunity to extend it beyond the usual 4 to 6 weeks. Extended maternity leaves have been demonstrated to increase breastfeeding duration after returning to work (Arthur et al., 2003; Mandal et al., 2010; Ogbuanu et al., 2011).

Helping the mother to maintain realistic expectations about her first days on the job will enable her to see that most of the problems that she encounters will not be specific to breastfeeding (Thompson & Bell, 1997), but rather will be specific to the working woman with a family. How she plans to breastfeed can make a difference. For example, women who practiced exclusive breastfeeding in the first postpartum month and whose postpartum behaviors were consistent with their prenatal intention to fully or partially breastfeed are more likely to breastfeed longer than 6 months after returning to work (Meedya et al., 2010; Piper & Parks, 1996; Thulier & Mercer, 2009). Furthermore, among American women employed by the Special Supplemental Nutrition Program for Women, Infants, and Children (WIC), four variables predicted breastfeeding duration: intent to exclusively breastfeed, delayed introduction of infant formula, attendance at breastfeeding support groups, and availability of work-site breast pumps (Whaley et al., 2002). Ways in which breastfeeding can be continued after the mother returns to work include the following:

- Hand-expressing breastmilk
- Breast pumping
- Having the baby brought to the mother during meal breaks
- Substituting formula for those feedings that occur during the mother's workday

Maintaining an Adequate Milk Supply

Maintaining an adequate milk supply is an issue for many women after they return to work (Arthur et al., 2003; Chezem et al., 1997; Lewallen et al., 2006; Rojjanasrirat, 2004; Slusser et al., 2004) and can even be a concern prior to returning to work (Rojjanasrirat & Sousa, 2010). Women who return to employment and discontinue breastfeeding before they had planned may develop negative feelings such as guilt, sadness, and depression (Chezem, et al., 1997; Rojjanasrirat, 2004; Yimyam & Morrow, 1999). Women who regularly express breastmilk breastfeed for longer durations than those who do not express milk regularly (Slusser et al., 2004; Win et al., 2006). Other factors that influence the frequency and the amount of time expressing breastmilk include the mother's age, supplementation, skills and efficiency at breastmilk expression, and type of breast pump.

In a study conducted in a large company with on-site lactation support, mothers of 3- and 6-month-old infants expressed breastmilk at work approximately two to three times each day. Most spent less than 1 hour per day in an employment environment supportive of breastfeeding (Slusser et al., 2004). The appropriate use of breast pumps may be a means to maintain milk supply and help mothers to achieve 6 months of exclusive breastfeeding. If mothers notice their supply dropping after returning to work, they should increase their pumping during the workday and increase feedings at the breast during the evening, night, and early morning. Childcare providers should be informed not to feed the infant in the hour preceding the mother's return from work so that she may feed the infant at the breast soon after arrival at the center or upon arrival at home.

Hand Expression and Pumping

Prior to the mother's return to work, the lactation consultant or other healthcare worker who is counseling the mother will want to discuss the need to express milk when she is away from her baby. Decisions must be made regarding how much breastmilk the mother desires for her baby's diet: all breastmilk or a combination of breastmilk and commercial formula. This decision and the baby's age upon the mother's return to work will determine the need and frequency for milk expression, either by hand or by pump (Angeletti, 2009).

Based on their now-classic research, Auerbach and Guss (1984) suggested that 7 to 10 days before the mother returns to work is a good time for her to begin practicing expression and pumping and to begin stockpiling milk. Other authors suggest that 2 weeks is needed to become proficient at pumping and to start building a supply of milk, once the mother's milk supply is established (Bocar, 1997; Neifert, 2000; Wyatt, 2002). In Rojjanasrirat's (2004) descriptive study of breastfeeding experiences of working mothers, women reported that part of their strategic plan for managing breastfeeding and work included beginning to pump a "few weeks" before returning to work or pumping "early" to store their milk and adjust to "the whole process" (p. 225).

Mothers also must decide if they will use a bottle or other device such as a cup to feed expressed milk to the baby. In either case, practice with the new method should commence prior to mother's return to work. However, it is recommended that bottles not be introduced before mother's milk is well established (when the child reaches 3–4 weeks of age) (Biagoli, 2003; Neifert, 2000).

As a general rule, the earlier in the postpartum period the mother returns to full-time work, the more frequently she will need to express or pump her breasts. The major reasons for expressing milk at work are to give the baby human milk feedings in the mother's absence and to maintain the mother's milk supply. The mother is also protecting her baby from infections and allergies by continued feeding of her breastmilk. In addition, the mother who is comfortable as a result of pumping is a more efficient worker. Lastly, painful engorgement contributes to embarrassing leaking, an increased risk of mastitis from milk stasis (Fetherston, 1998; Hager & Barton, 1996; Iatrakis et al., 2013; Potter, 2005; Thompsen et al., 1984), and reduction of the milk supply from overfull distended breasts and its sequelae (e.g., feedback inhibition of lactation [FIL]) (Peaker & Wilde, 1996).

When the mother begins expressing milk, she may be dismayed that she obtains so little (sometimes barely enough to cover the bottom of a small 4 oz bottle). However, each time she expresses, she will probably obtain more milk. Just as she had to learn to breastfeed, so her body needs to learn to respond to the stimulation of hand expression or breast pumping to trigger the milk-ejection reflex. Mothers should expect no more than half an ounce with the first several pumping or expression sessions.

During practice sessions, the mother should express or pump in the morning, when she is more likely to feel rested and when she may have more residual milk volume, rather than later in the afternoon or evening. Usually two practice sessions, timed about 1 hour after two consecutive morning feedings, are sufficient to develop her milk-expression skills. Mothers who feel particularly full late in the evening have also found that expressing breastmilk at this time helps to build up a sizable stockpile of milk. Remind the mother that the milk she obtains in this way is "excess," not an indication of the amount of milk the baby obtains. Furthermore, milk is still present in the breasts after breastfeeding, regardless of the rate at which the baby is growing (Daly & Hartmann, 1995).

Frequency of pumping or expression in the workplace depends on how old the baby is and how long mother is away from the baby. Earlier return to work generally necessitates more frequent expression, ideally as frequently as the baby eats, but at least every 3 hours. A later return to work (i.e., after 3 months) may allow the mother to stretch out the time between pumping sessions, but she should not go longer than 4 hours, especially in the days early after returning to work. Generally, mothers should plan to pump at least three times during an 8-hour workday for at least 20 minutes if using a double pump. As the mother becomes adept at expressing or pumping and as her baby gets older, she may find that she can reduce the duration of each expression period or the number of pumping sessions to two and then to one per day. Slusser et al. (2004) found there were significant differences ($p < 0.05$) in pumping frequency between women with 3-month-old children and those with 6-month-old children, with mothers pumping an average of 2.2 (SD = 0.8) times per day and 1.9 (SD = 0.6) times per day, respectively. The majority of women pumped less than 1 hour per day at each time period; however, there were significantly more women at 6 months than 3 months pumping less than 1 hour ($p < 0.05$). In evaluating a lactation program in an academic medical center, Wambach et al. (2014) found that breastfeeding staff, students, and faculty ($n = 27$) used the lactation rooms 1 to 5 days per week (mean = 4.04, SD = 1.692) and expressed their milk 1 to 3 times per day, with a mean of 2.09 (SD = 0.996).

When babies are cared for near the workplace, mothers may use their lunch time to go to the baby for a relaxed midday nursing session, or sometimes they can have the baby brought to them. In either case, breastfeeding stimulates the breasts more effectively than do either the best electric pumps or the accomplished mother who hand-expresses her milk. Furthermore, both parties enjoy their time together; the baby is nourished and nurtured at the breast, and the mother may also grab a quick sandwich at the babysitter's house or childcare center. In contrast, some mothers may travel periodically for their work; in such a case, they will need to pump during the time away, store their milk appropriately, and transfer it home at the end of the trip. In the United States, the transport of human milk in containers containing greater than 3 ounces is permitted in carry-ons on airplanes according to the Transportation Security Administration rules (see the list of Internet resources at the end of the chapter).

Although hand expression is an option, most women choose to use a mechanical pump of some kind (automated or non-automated). The mother will need to rent or purchase this equipment. Many mothers actually purchase a pump prior to giving birth—a good way to avoid making decisions about the best pump for them during the very busy time following birth and leading up to returning to work. The questions in Box 16-1 are a useful guide for the mother who is planning to pump her breasts.

There is a pump that is best suited for each mother's needs. Considerations in choosing a pump include the age of the infant (amount of milk needed); how long and how frequently the dyad will be separated; which facilities are available (i.e., electrical access); how easily the pump can be cleaned; and how comfortable, costly, and convenient the pump is (Angeletti, 2009; Biagoli, 2003; Biancuzzo, 1999). An important consideration when selecting a breast pump is that it must be easy to clean. If the user cannot be assured that cleaning is possible at home or work, with or without a dishwasher, the pump should not be purchased.

The pump should be easy and comfortable to use. Comfort depends on the closeness of fit of the pump flange on the mother's breast, the angle of "pull" for cylinder-style pumps, and other factors. The angle of the flange varies from one pump to another, as do the shape, size, and degree of fullness of each mother's breasts. Optimally, the mother should experiment with several pumps before purchasing one. The next best alternative is for her to talk with other mothers who are successfully pumping and compare the efficiency and reported comfort of different pumps, keeping in mind that what works for one person may not work for another. The healthcare worker who assists the mother should be familiar with the many types of pumps available and the criteria for choosing the pump that best fits the mother's needs. Additionally, pump instructions should be reviewed to determine whether the pictures demonstrating use of the equipment are accurate. Mothers can also be referred to the U.S. Food and Drug Administration, which regulates breast pumps in the United States, to read its guidelines for choosing and using a breast pump (http://www.fda.gov/MedicalDevices/ProductsandMedicalProcedures/HomeHealthandConsumer/ConsumerProducts/BreastPumps/default.htm).

Efficiency and effectiveness of the pump are factors of importance and need to be gauged based on whether the mother is comfortable with the pump during its use, whether her breasts feel softer after using the pump, and whether, over time, the amount of milk she obtains tends to increase. Double pumping is generally more effective and efficient (Figure 16-2). Prime et al. (2012) compared the efficiency and effectiveness of simultaneous pumping of both breasts (SIM) versus sequential pumping (SEQ) in 31 Australian breastfeeding women. These researchers found SIM yielded more milk ejections ($p < 0.001$) and greater amounts of milk at 2, 5, and 10 minutes ($p < 0.01$) and removed a greater total amount of milk ($p < 0.01$) and percentage of available milk ($p < 0.05$) than SEQ expression. After SIM expression, the cream content of both

Figure 16-2 DOUBLE PUMP SET-UP WITH BLUE ICE FOR CHILLING EXPRESSED MILK IN THE WORKPLACE.

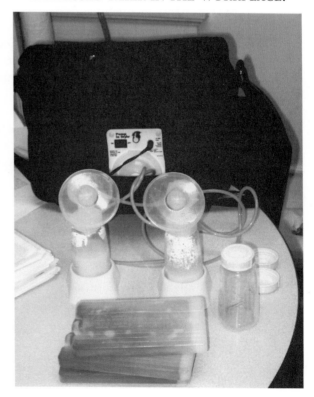

BOX 16-1 QUESTIONS TO ASK A MOTHER WHO IS PLANNING TO USE A BREAST PUMP

1. Is there a pump available for expressing her milk in the workplace?
2. What is the experience of other women who have used the breast pump in the workplace?
3. Is an automated or nonautomated pump needed based on frequency of use?
   - For occasional use (once a week)—hand expression or nonautomated pump (suck/release totally regulated by mother)
     - ◀ Cylinder pumps
     - ◀ Trigger or handle pumps
   - For part-time (once a day) or dependent (frequent pumping)—automated pump
     - ◀ 20 cycles per minute
     - ◀ Partially or fully automated
   - Battery-operated or battery-electric
     - ◀ 21–40 cycles per minute
     - ◀ Partially or fully automated
     - ◀ Compression component with some
   - Electric
     - ◀ 40–78 cycles per minute
     - ◀ Fully automated
     - ◀ Bilateral pumping possible
     - ◀ Most effective in mimicking infant sucking
4. Is the pump easy to clean? Are washable parts dishwasher safe?
5. Is the pump easy to assemble, disassemble, and use?
6. Is the pump physically comfortable to use?
7. Is the pump effective in obtaining milk quickly? Can the suck/release mechanism be adjusted easily? Is the pump self-cycling? Is the suction adequate?
8. Are the instructions accompanying the pump understandable, accurate, and easy to follow?
9. What is the cost (initial investment and daily, weekly, or monthly rental fee) of using the pump?
10. Are extra or replacement parts available without having to purchase a new kit?
11. Are both single and double pumping options available if desired?
12. What have other mothers reported about using specific equipment?
13. What size and weight is the pump?
14. How much noise does it make?
15. Can standard bottles be used to collect the milk?
16. Does the mother feel emotionally and psychologically comfortable pumping her milk? If she does not, has she considered expressing her milk by hand or breastfeeding without expressing her milk for the periods when she is separated from her baby?

Source: Adapted from Angeletti (2009); Biagoli (2003); Biancuzzo (1999); Bocar (1997).

the overall (8.3% [$p < 0.05$]) and post-expression (12.6% [$p < 0.001$]) milk was greater.

When the mother begins offering solid foods to her baby, feedings become less frequent or shorter; at that time, the amount obtained by pumping usually declines. If the foregoing efficiency criteria are met, however, the pump can still be considered efficient. See the *Breast Pumps and Other Technology* chapter for an in-depth discussion of breast pumps.

Human Milk Storage

Human milk is a dynamic substance that kills bacteria. This bactericidal ability is highest in the first several hours after expression, even when the breastmilk is not refrigerated (Ogundele, 2000), and some investigators have reported that colony counts remain low in such milk for at least 48 hours

(Hamosh et al., 1996). For this reason, when women use careful hand washing and clean containers in which their own fresh milk is stored for less than 6 to 8 hours prior to refrigeration, they are not endangering their healthy babies (see Box 16-2). Mothers who prefer to refrigerate their milk should do so in a clean, capped glass or plastic container and use the milk within 8 days after it has been refrigerated (Pardou et al., 1994). Polyethylene bags designed for milk collection and storage are also appropriate; however, there can be fat loss in these bags and spillage and tearing of the bags may be issues as well (Jones, 2011).

If a mother plans to use the milk before 8 days, it should be refrigerated rather than frozen, as suggested by Pardou et al. (1994), who found that antimicrobial properties were better preserved with refrigeration rather than freezing. Longer storage

---

BOX 16-2 GENERAL GUIDELINES FOR STORING HUMAN MILK

- Always use a clean container.
- Standard glass or plastic baby bottles (preferably bisphenol A [BPA] free), clean food storage containers with tight-fitting solid lids, and disposable feeding bottle liners.
- Label each container with date and time of the earliest contribution to the container, particularly if "layering" different expressions into the same container. Include baby's name for daycare center storage.
- Store milk in the approximate quantities that the baby is likely to need for one feeding.
- If refrigerated within 4 to 6 hours, store in a clean, tightly capped container for the unrefrigerated interim period (60–85°F or 16–29°C) (Jones, 2011).
- Milk may be stored in an insulated cooler bag with ice packs for 24 hours (39°F or 4°C).
- If refrigerated, use within 4–8 days. Store milk in the back of the main body of the refrigerator, where the temperature is the coolest (39°F or 4°C). Consider storing in a separate bin or box for convenience and protection of bags, if used (Jones, 2011).
- Milk can be stored in a normal refrigerator with other food items. The U.S. Occupational Safety and Health Administration and CDC say human milk does not require special handling or storage in a separate container.
- If frozen in a freezer maintained at −4°F or −20°C, use within 12 months (Jones, 2011).*
- Discard any remaining milk that was not used at the feeding for which it was thawed and warmed.
- Use thawed milk within 24 hours.
- Match the "age" of the milk as closely as possible to the baby's age in order to optimize the degree of fit between the baby's needs and the properties of the milk.

*Shake while thawing to remix the creamy portion that separates during storage.

equates to greater loss of vitamin C in the milk, as found by Buss et al. (2001), who recommended using milk stored in the refrigerator within 24 hours or milk stored in a freezer within 1 month. Milk stored in the freezer compartment of a refrigerator (top, bottom, or side models) should be placed as far away from the door as possible; most mothers use frozen milk within 1 month of the date when it was expressed, but if temperatures inside the freezer are maintained at $-4°F$ $(-20°C)$, it can be kept for 3 months. If a deep-freezer, again maintained at $-4°F$ $(-20°C)$ is used to store the milk, it can be used up to 12 months after the date of expression (Jones, 2011). The mother should be reminded that human milk is a substance that is matched to the baby's age: milk obtained when the baby was 3 months old will not as completely meet that same baby's needs when he is 6 months old. Therefore she should label the milk with the date expressed and use the milk that was expressed first.

If the mother finds that her milk changes in odor or consistency after storage, or if the baby begins to refuse it, the mother may need to reduce the storage time and freeze rather than refrigerate it to avoid possible adverse reactions. Once the milk has been frozen, it should be thawed either (1) quickly in a container of warm water (98°F [37°C]) or (2) slowly at room temperature, monitored, and refrigerated before thawed completely (Jones, 2011). Milk should not be heated very quickly on a stove or in a microwave oven. Although some research (Carbonare et al., 1996; Ovesen et al., 1996) suggests that microwave heating does not negatively impact immunoglobulins (IgA) and nutrients (vitamins B1 and E, linoleic and linolenic acids), microwave heating nearly always results in uneven distribution of the heat. This can go unnoticed because the container rarely feels as warm as the center portion of the fluid; thus the milk can be too hot in some spots and substantially cooler in others. Even water-warmed milk should be mixed well and tested on the inside of the caregiver's wrist before offering it to the baby. For feeding the term or older infant, the temperature of feedings can be at room temperature, body temperature, or straight from the refrigerator (Jones, 2011). Mixing should be

done not only for heat distribution, but also to ensure that the creamy portion of the milk is redistributed.

The fat content of milk is altered with refrigeration as well as when the milk is frozen and then thawed for reuse (Pardou et al., 1994). Loss of fat can be minimized when the container is shaken gently before offering its contents to the baby, and single-serving amounts should be stored to prevent wastage. When giving thawed milk, the unused portion should be discarded to prevent bacterial colonization. Mothers should be told not to refreeze thawed milk. However, small amounts of fresh milk can be added to frozen milk. It is recommended that the fresh milk be refrigerated before being added to the frozen milk.

Fatigue and Loss of Sleep

Sleep deprivation is a fact of life for nearly all parents of very young infants. For women who return to work following childbirth, loss of sleep and fatigue become bigger concerns, and may be compounded in the breastfeeding mother. Evidence from research into infant and maternal sleep, as well as maternal fatigue, is mixed, but illustrative of potential problems that employed and non-employed breastfeeding mothers may experience. First, a recent large study in Asia ($n = 10,321$) indicated that 6-month-old breastfed infants had less consolidated sleep and more frequent and longer nighttime awakenings than non-breastfed infants, but that maternal nursing behaviors moderated that relationship (i.e., nursing at the start of nighttime and during nighttime to put the infant to sleep) (Ramamurthy et al., 2012). However maternal employment status was not addressed in the study. Another study of infant sleep in Australia ($n = 4500$) found that after adjustment for covariates including maternal employment, mothers reported infants who were breastfed at 6 months were 66% more likely to wake during the night and 72% more likely to report difficulty sleeping alone, compared to non-breastfed infants (Galbally et al., 2013).

The relationships between breastfeeding and perceived fatigue have been supported in some studies

(McGovern et al., 2006; Pugh & Milligan, 1993; Wambach, 1998), whereas other studies have suggested that perceived fatigue is not dependent on types of feeding (Callahan et al., 2006). Wambach (1998) examined fatigue levels among first-time breastfeeding mothers over the first 9 weeks postpartum, finding levels were moderate during the first 3 weeks postpartum and then decreased to mild levels at 6 and 9 weeks. It was also demonstrated that women experiencing greater difficulty in combining working and breastfeeding had greater fatigue. A prospective study of 817 working mothers at 5 weeks postpartum revealed that breastfeeding mothers experienced significantly more fatigue than women not breastfeeding (McGovern et al., 2006). Finally, more recently, Radtke Demirci et al. (2012) conducted a secondary analysis of data from the 2004 Sleep in America Poll that included 77 dyads of mothers and infants aged 6 to 11 months. The analysis revealed no difference in sleep duration between breastfeeding mothers and formula-feeding mothers. Breastfed mothers were awoken more frequently by their infant, but there was no statistically significant difference in the amount of time for which the mothers were awake at night or experienced daytime sleepiness.

Knowing that fatigue and sleep disturbances may affect breastfeeding, and vice versa, can guide healthcare providers and lactation consultants in helping mothers who plan to return to work to manage their own and their infants' sleep patterns. Many employed breastfeeding mothers who work during the day find that their babies' sleep patterns change after their return to work. Instead of taking short naps during the day and sleeping longer at night, the baby begins to sleep for very long periods during the day and remains awake later into the evening. Called "reverse-cycle breastfeeding," this coping behavior enables the baby to tolerate many hours away from his mother. Often, the baby's waking time with his mother may alternate between short breastfeeding episodes and simply nestling in her arms. Such behavior need not mean that the mother loses still more sleep. In fact, what better built-in "excuse" than breastfeeding does a mother have for

lying down when she gets home? Sleep-saving techniques that families have found work well include any one of a variety of co-sleeping arrangements:

- Keeping the baby's cradle or crib in the parents' room
- Creating an extension on the parents' bed
- Placing a spare mattress on the floor of the baby's room for late-night cuddling and nursing away from other family members (McKenna et al., 1997)

Workplace Strategies to Support Breastfeeding and Work

Support for breastfeeding in the workplace requires four essential elements: time, space, person, and policy (Bar-Yam, 1998; Dunn et al., 2004; Ortiz et al., 2004). These elements are included in the definition of support for breastfeeding in the workplace in *The CDC Guide to Strategies to Support Breastfeeding Mothers and Babies* (CDC, 2013). The CDC describes such support as "several types of employee benefits and services," including "developing corporate policies to support breastfeeding women; providing designated private space for breastfeeding or expressing milk; allowing flexible scheduling to support milk expression during work; giving mothers options for returning to work, such as teleworking, part-time work, and extended maternity leave; providing on-site or near-site child care; providing high-quality breast pumps; and offering professional lactation management services and support" (p. 23).

These four essential elements are considered important strategies to assist women in their workplace to continue breastfeeding successfully.

- *Time.* Working mothers need flexible time to express breastmilk, clean the breast pump, and store breastmilk during the working hours. Examples of flexible time include providing appropriate break time for breastfeeding or pumping daily and traveling time between the workplace and the nursing mothers' room (NMR) or child care. The frequency and amount of time it takes to pump depend on the baby's age and the type and quality of the pump (Slusser et al., 2004).

- *Space.* A private area or facility is needed where mothers can be comfortable expressing breastmilk. More and more companies in the United States and around the world are providing their employees with nursing mothers' rooms (Dunn et al., 2004; Ortiz et al., 2004; Smith et al., 2013; Witters-Green, 2003). The nursing mothers' room should be clean and have electrical outlets, a sink to wash hands, a comfortable chair, and a refrigerator to store breastmilk.

- *Person.* Persons such as an employer, office manager, supervisor, or human resources director have important roles as gatekeepers in facilitating and supporting the needs of the working mothers who desire to maintain breastfeeding while they are employed. Understanding colleagues also contribute to the success of combining breastfeeding and work (Bar-Yam, 1998; Libbus & Bullock, 2002; Rojjanasrirat, 2004; Sattari et al., 2013; Witters-Green, 2003). Key personnel such as managers, supervisors, and human resources personnel should also be educated and made aware of the need to support and respect the needs of breastfeeding working mothers.

- *Policy.* Breastfeeding policy is another workplace strategy that provides women with the opportunity to breastfeed while working. A written policy should enable working women to maintain lactation while separated from their infants with adequate accommodation for breastfeeding (Dozier & McKee, 2011; Dunn et al., 2004). For instance, a supportive environment allows mothers to breastfeed or express breastmilk in a reasonable break time and to have a choice of part-time employment, job sharing, and/or an extended maternity leave.

Other sources of support for the working mother may include the spouse, significant others, friends, and healthcare providers. Table 16-1 presents an assessment checklist that healthcare providers can use when discussing returning to work with their breastfeeding patients.

Legislation and public policies can contribute significantly to women successfully sustaining breastfeeding while working. In the United States, the Patient Protection and Affordable Care Act was signed into law on March 23, 2010, and included Section 4207, which amends the Fair Labor Standards Act to require employers to provide reasonable break time and space for breastfeeding mothers to express breastmilk in the workplace for a child aged up to 1 year (U.S. Department of Labor, 2010). This law states that employers with more than 50 employees must provide a private space other than a bathroom for the breastfeeding mothers' use. The FLSA makes it illegal for an employer to discriminate against an employee for filing a complaint regarding an employer's failure to comply with this provision (Murtagh & Moulton, 2011). As noted previously, employers with fewer than 50 employees are exempt from the FLSA break time requirement if compliance with the provision would impose an undue hardship. Employers must document such hardship through a written application for exemption to the U.S. Department of Labor.

Lactation Programs in Work Sites

The establishment of a lactation support program in the workplace is an important strategy to reduce barriers to breastfeeding among working mothers, enhance breastfeeding success, and promote positive health outcomes for both mother and the baby (Balkam et al., 2011; Chow et al., 2011; Click, 2006; Eldridge & Croker, 2005; Mills, 2009; Smith et al., 2013). In addition, economic and employer benefits related to supporting breastfeeding in the workplace include significant healthcare cost savings associated with fewer child illnesses, increased employee morale, and decreased employee absenteeism (Cohen et al., 1995). The Business Case for Breastfeeding is a national initiative that was created in 2008 by the U.S. Department of Health and Human Services to increase workplace lactation support (U.S. Department of Health and Human Services, 2010). The program is

---

Table 16-1 ASSESSMENT CHECKLIST FOR COMBINING WORK AND BREASTFEEDING

Type of Work

What is your work setting? (office, factory, on the road)

Do you have your own office?

Do you keep your own schedule/control your own time?

Does your job involve travel?

Are most of your colleagues women?

Space

Is there a facility or private breastfeeding/pumping area in the workplace?

Can you use the same space every day?

Does the room have a sink, chair, electrical outlets?

Are breast pumps available there?

Is the nursing/pumping area near your work space?

Is there a refrigerator to store your milk?

If there is no designated space, where will you pump?

Time

How old will baby be upon your return to work?

Do you plan to express milk/breastfeed when you return to work?

Will you have time to pump?

Will you use an electric or manual pump? Is there a double pump?

Is the pump easy to clean with each use?

Can a break be taken reliably at the same time every day?

If there is on-site or near-site day care, can you go there to nurse the baby?

Support

Does your supervisor need to be informed or consulted?

Does your supervisor feel supportive about your breastfeeding plan?

Are there other colleagues breastfeeding or planning to breastfeed at work?

Are there mothers at work who have done so in the past?

Does your partner feel supportive of your plan to nurse and work?

Do daycare providers recognize the importance of breastfeeding?

Do they know how to handle breastmilk?

Will an on-site or near-site provider call the mother to nurse, if you request?

Work Allies

Who can help you find the time and space to pump or breastfeed?

Who is responsible for signing up spare offices/rooms?

Did you discuss the breastfeeding issue with your supervisor?

What is his/her response or concerns about breast-feeding at the workplace?

Are there any policies in the workplace regarding nursing mothers?

Are there any policies regarding flexibility for new mothers returning to work?

Do you have any of the following programs at your workplace?

    Earned time

    Flex time

    Compressed work week

    Telecommuting

    Part time

    Job sharing

    Phase back

    On-site or near-site day care

Do you plan to take advantage of one or more of them?

Who is the person you need to contact to arrange one or more of these programs?

    Supervisor(s)

    Human resources officer

    Benefits officer

    Employee relations officer

Source: Adapted from Bar-Yam (1998).

designed for employers, employees, healthcare professionals, and those involved in supporting breastfeeding employees at work by educating employers about the value of supporting breastfeeding mothers. The initiative offers a comprehensive, multifaceted approach including the curriculum "Implementing the Business Case for Breastfeeding in Your Community," which was provided to state breastfeeding coalitions in 30 states and 6 cities. The list of the 32 states that currently participate in the Business Case for Breastfeeding initiatives can be found on this website: http://www.usbreastfeeding.org /Employment/WorkplaceSupport/tabid/105 /Default.aspx. Very recently the U.S. Department of Health and Human Services, Office on Women's Health developed additional online searchable resources based on the Business Case for Breastfeeding for employers to tap into when creating workplace support for breastfeeding employees. The *Supporting Nursing Moms at Work: Employer Solutions* (2014) can be used by breastfeeding coalitions, WIC agencies, and other community partners to assist local employers and their employees with worksite lactation support (see http://www.womenshealth. gov/breastfeeding/employer-solutions/index.php).

The recently released U.S. *Healthy People 2020* goals for breastfeeding initiation and duration now also include recommendations to increase the proportion of workplace lactation support programs from the baseline 25% to 38% (see http://www .healthypeople.gov/2020/topicsobjectives2020 /default.aspx). The enforcement of the Fair Labor Standard Act, previously mentioned, coupled with other events may increase the likelihood of the availability of workplace lactation support programs for breastfeeding mothers in the United States. According to a Society for Human Resource Management (SHRM) report, 6% of employers in 2012 provided lactation support programs, including education and consultation; 43% of the SHRM survey respondents reported that their employers offered flexible break time (SHRM, 2012).

Generally, components of the lactation support program include a room for milk expression, pump purchase or rental service, on-site classes, lactation telephone support, support group, and staff

Figure 16-3 Space for Expressing Mother's Milk in a College Setting.

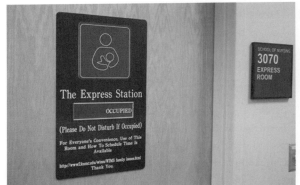

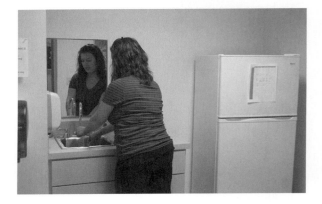

(Balkam et al., 2011; Click, 2006; Marinelli et al., 2013). Most milk-expression rooms are equipped with a sink with running water, an electrical outlet, a comfortable chair, a table, and a refrigerator (Figure 16-3).

Studies of on-site lactation programs are limited (Balkam et al., 2011; Cohen & Mrtek, 1994; Ortiz et al., 2004; Slusser et al., 2004; Smith et al., 2013). Results indicate that working women who are provided with access to a pumping facility and flexible time are more likely to continue breastfeeding until their children reach 6 months or 1 year of age (Cohen & Mrtek, 1994; Dodgson & Duckett, 1997; Ortiz et al., 2004) or to breastfeed exclusively at 6 months (Smith et al., 2013). Cohen and Mrtek (1994) reported that in two settings where lactation programs were in place, 75% of women who returned to work and were still breastfeeding continued to do so for 6 months or longer. In addition, Cohen et al. (1995) found that increased duration of breastfeeding led to low incidence of child illnesses. These findings translated into far fewer employee absences related to infant illness and, therefore, less lost time to the company. In a cross-sectional survey, Balkam et al. (2011) evaluated the effects of components of a workplace lactation program on breastfeeding duration among 128 women employed in the public sector. The findings demonstrated that the number of workplace lactation program services women received was positively related to exclusive breastfeeding at 6 months of infant age. Finally, a recent mixed-method workplace study in Australia examined employee perspectives on barriers to and facilitators of combining employment and breastfeeding, including employment arrangements and workplace factors linked with exclusive breastfeeding at 6 months (Smith et al., 2013). Key findings included that more workplace support was related to more exclusive breastfeeding at 6 months. Furthermore, employees who had exclusively breastfed for 6 months were likely to take fewer days off to care for sick babies and to have fewer hospitalizations for their babies.

Although reports of work-site programs and their effectiveness are impressive and promising, none of them has used an experimental design; that is, they lack a control group. Randomized controlled trials are needed to establish the effectiveness of workplace interventions to support the continuation and intensity of breastfeeding (Abdulwadud & Snow, 2012). In addition, little is known about the experiences of women who work in lower-skilled and service jobs, which account for a relatively large segment of working women in the United States. Barriers to continued breastfeeding after returning to work are likely much higher for these women, many of whom are disadvantaged or members of an ethnic minority. Some preliminary findings (Rojjanasrirat et al., 2010) indicated that women in low-income WIC populations who attempted to combine breastfeeding and work faced multiple challenges. Using focus group interviews, the

17 WIC women in that study perceived barriers to breastfeeding in terms of the difficult nature of their job (e.g., waitress, sales clerk, cashier, teacher); time issues such as no break time, too busy, or no flexible time allowed; support issues such as lack of support from coworkers and feeling intimidated by male coworkers; lack of privacy; lack of space or a facility to pump; and childcare issues such as high cost and low levels of trust in childcare providers. In the Fragile Families and Child Wellbeing study, among a sample of 4900 mostly low-income, unmarried U.S. mothers, Kimbro (2006) reported that within 1 month after returning to work, a mother had 32% higher odds of discontinuing breastfeeding than a mother who did not start working during that time. Furthermore, 50% and 75% of the mothers discontinued breastfeeding by 3 months and 6 months, respectively. The challenges to continued breastfeeding appear to be greater among low-wage workers. Further research is needed to determine how women in low-wage jobs manage to combine breastfeeding and work. A recently developed reliable and valid measure of mothers' perceptions of workplace breastfeeding support could be used in such research (Bai et al., 2008).

The Employer's Perspective

Employers can provide a supportive work environment for women to succeed at combining breastfeeding and employment. Workplace breastfeeding support in the United States depends primarily on the initiative taken by individual employers, as the enforcement provisions of the FSLA legislation are limited to large employers/businesses. Employers' knowledge regarding benefits of breastfeeding and needs of working mothers for continued breastfeeding has been found to vary among studies (Bridges et al., 1997; Brown et al., 2001; Chow et al., 2011; Dunn et al., 2004; Libbus & Bullock, 2002). Studies indicate that employers lack knowledge regarding short- and long-term benefits of breastfeeding and see very little value for their business in supporting breastfeeding in the work environment (Bridges et al., 1997; Dunn et al., 2004; Libbus & Bullock, 2002). Other research has demonstrated that employers that have been exposed to or had experiences working with employees who previously breastfed tended to be more positive in their support of breastfeeding in the workplace (Bridges et al, 1997; Libbus & Bullock, 2002; Witters-Green, 2003).

Dunn and colleagues (2004) examined breastfeeding policies and practices among 157 Colorado businesses. They reported that available benefits and services conducive to breastfeeding were mostly found in large companies (more than 500 employees) and included 3 months' maternity leave, flex time, job sharing, part-time options, refrigerators for breastmilk storage, and break time for pumping milk or feeding the infant. They also found that only 3% to 7.5% of the study participants had a written policy regarding workplace breastfeeding support. Despite the evidence of long-term benefits of on-site lactation support that accrued to employers (Cohen et al., 1995; Ortiz et al., 2004), most were not aware of the benefits of breastfeeding such as decreased employee turnover, improved morale, decreased employee absenteeism, and increased recruitment ability (Dunn et al., 2004). Brown, Poag, and Kasprzycki (2001) conducted a qualitative study of employers' knowledge, attitudes, and practices in providing breastfeeding support for lactating employees using two focus groups of human resources personnel from large employers and small employers. Participants reported that allowing employees time to breastfeed or express their milk would have an adverse effect on other employees' morale.

As noted previously, intervention research and randomized clinical trials related to supporting breastfeeding in the workplace are nonexistent at this time. However, researchers have now developed two measures of employer and manager attitudes and intentions to provide workplace breastfeeding support: the Employer Support for Breastfeeding Questionnaire (ESBQ) (Rojjanasrirat et al., 2010) and the Manager's Attitude Toward Breastfeeding Support Questionnaire (Chow et al., 2012). Both theory-based measures were developed and tested using rigorous instrument development and psychometric principles, and were assessed as reliable and valid. These measures could be used to measure, evaluate, and compare employers' attitudes and intentions to support breastfeeding in the workplace. Targeted strategies to develop or improve support by educating employers about supporting breastfeeding mothers could then be implemented and further evaluated with the measures. These targeted strategies could be augmented with the toolkit from the Business Case for Breastfeeding or the Breastfeeding Friendly Workplace program to provide information about the financial benefits for employers and strategies to implement a workplace lactation support (Marinelli et al., 2013).

Community Strategies to Support Breastfeeding and Work

Healthcare Providers and Lactation Consultants

Throughout this chapter, we have discussed how the healthcare professional and lactation specialist can assist the breastfeeding mother who works away from home. Physicians, nurses, midwives, lactation consultants, and other healthcare providers play an important role in promoting breastfeeding. Every healthcare encounter should be used to inform and support the mother who plans to combine, or is currently combining, breastfeeding and employment. In the prenatal period, efforts to assist the pregnant woman to plan her return to work include information sharing and prenatal breastfeeding classes. Referral to a community or health plan-affiliated lactation consultant during the prenatal period can facilitate establishment of a therapeutic relationship that will promote successful breastfeeding and preparation for return to work. The lactation consultant can provide the mother with assistance related to milk expression, maintaining her milk supply once she has returned to work, and other issues that may arise related to continued breastfeeding.

Breastfeeding Support Groups

La Leche League International (LLLI) is a notable community resource for breastfeeding women who return to work. LLLI provides information on combining breastfeeding and employment through its pamphlets and books, as well as on its website. LLLI Mother-to-Mother Forums, including one specifically for mothers working outside the home and one for pumping/milk expression issues, are online discussions where mothers can log into and ask for support. These forums include postings on balancing work, breastfeeding, and the home; pumping issues; family matters; issues regarding rights to pump at work; and time demands. For those who prefer face-to-face contact, support can also be gained at LLLI local group meetings.

Internet resources for the healthcare provider and breastfeeding mothers are listed at the end of this chapter. Healthcare providers should be aware of the variation in quality of breastfeeding information on the Web and evaluate websites prior to recommending them to their patients. Dornan and Oermann (2006) conducted a descriptive study to evaluate the quality of 30 websites on breastfeeding for patient education on the top three Internet search engines. These researchers used the Health Information Technology Institute's criteria for evaluating health information on the Internet (credibility, content, disclosure, links, design, interactivity, caveats, and readability) and eight criteria from the American Academy of Pediatrics Policy Statement on Breastfeeding for evaluating the websites. The top five quality websites at that time were offered by La Leche League International; ProMOM, Inc.; Breastfeeding Basics; American Academy of Pediatrics; and MedlinePlus, all of which contained accurate information regarding breastfeeding and employment.

Another community resource regarding breastfeeding in general, and in relation to breastfeeding and employment in the United States, is the Special Supplemental Nutrition Program for Women, Infants, and Children (WIC). A notable effort, "Loving Support Makes Breastfeeding Work," was the result of a cooperative agreement between the U.S. Department of Agriculture's Food and Nutrition Service (FNS) and Best Start Social Marketing, Inc. "Loving Support" is national in scope and implemented at the state agency level. The goals of this campaign are fourfold: (1) encourage WIC participants to initiate and continue breastfeeding; (2) increase referrals to WIC for breastfeeding

support; (3) increase general public acceptance and support of breastfeeding; and (4) provide technical assistance to WIC state and local agency professionals in breastfeeding promotion, including provision of promotional materials. Promotional materials pertinent to breastfeeding employment include a pamphlet and poster entitled "Busy Moms: Breastfeeding Works Around My Schedule."

National and Global Strategies in Promoting and Supporting Breastfeeding

Legislative Support and Public Advocacy

The United States lags behind several developed countries in legislative and federal policy regarding protection of families, mothers, and breastfeeding. However, in 2010, the Patient Protection and Affordable Care Act was signed into law; it includes Section 4207, which offers protection for working mothers who continue breastfeeding after returning to the workplace (see http://www.gpo.gov/fdsys/pkg/BILLS-111hr3590enr/pdf/BILLS-111hr3590enr.pdf). The amendment requires employers to provide reasonable space and break time for working mothers to express breastmilk. This protection of breastfeeding may increase the likelihood of longer breastfeeding duration and exclusivity. However, the law mandates only larger companies (50 or more employees) to comply with its dictates. Employers with fewer than 50 employees are exempt from the provision (Murtagh & Moulton, 2011).

The enactment of the Family Medical Leave Act (FMLA) in 1993 provided for employees to take up to 12 weeks of unpaid leave during a 1-year period for various family and medical reasons, including childbirth or adoption. This legislation supports mothers who can afford to take unpaid leave beyond the traditional 6-week maternity leave so that they can establish breastfeeding solidly before returning to work. However, *paid* maternity leave is not mandated in the United States (Calnen, 2007). In surveys conducted by Abt Associates for the U.S. Department of Labor in 2012, only 17%

of workplaces reported that they were covered by FMLA and only 59% of employees were eligible for the FMLA protections (U.S. Department of Labor, 2012). Notably, low-income, less-educated, and ethnic minority women are less likely to be covered by or eligible for FMLA benefits (Galtry, 2003; Hen & Waldfogel, 2003). Even when covered and eligible, many employees cannot afford to take unpaid time off. Thus, although FMLA is a significant step forward in protection of maternity and breastfeeding rights, it is by no means universal or socially equitable because it rules out benefits for those mothers who are economically and socially vulnerable and, therefore, less likely to initiate and continue breastfeeding for long durations.

Most countries provide maternity protection law in some forms. Paid maternity leave, another form of maternity protection, is mandated in several countries in the world. Whereas most European countries provide the longest paid maternity leave, many Asian and Middle Eastern countries as well as the United States are in the lower bracket in terms of paid maternity leave, designated as 12 weeks or less (World Alliance for Breastfeeding Action [WABA], 2011). WABA reported that approximately 68% of countries in the world now mandate breastfeeding breaks, some of which are paid for.

Policy and legislation to promote, support, and protect breastfeeding in the United States, and specifically regarding breastfeeding and employment, are progressing, with steady and encouraging adoption of pertinent initiatives over the last 14 years. In 2000, the U.S. Department of Health and Human Services published *HHS Blueprint for Action on Breastfeeding*. This document introduced an action plan for breastfeeding based on education, training, awareness, support, and research. In January 2011, the release of the *Surgeon General's Call to Action to Support Breastfeeding* by the U.S. Department of Health and Human Services brought maternal employment and breastfeeding to the forefront as an important public health issue. Specific actions and strategies to support breastfeeding mothers and infants based on the evidence were outlined in this document. Actions related to breastfeeding and employment include the following foci:

- Action 13: Work toward establishing paid maternity leave for all employed mothers.
- Action 14: Ensure that employers establish and maintain comprehensive, high-quality lactation support programs for their employees.
- Action 15: Expand the use of programs in the workplace that allow lactating mothers to have direct access to their babies.
- Action 16: Ensure that all childcare providers accommodate the needs of breastfeeding mothers and infants.

The U.S. Department of Health and Human Services' website lists several documents and resources in support of *The Surgeon General's Call to Action to Support Breastfeeding*, including resources for employers (see http://www.surgeongeneral.gov/library/calls/breastfeeding/calltoactiontosupport breastfeeding.pdf).

Unlike the federal government, several states in the United States have enacted breastfeeding legislation, many have pending legislation on this topic, and many are revising their existing legislation. Currently, 45 states, the District of Columbia, and the Virgin Islands have laws that specifically allow women to breastfeed in any public or private location. As of 2011, a total of 24 states, the District of Columbia, and Puerto Rico had enacted 28 statutes containing a total of 51 provisions relevant to breastfeeding in the workplace. Of 51 provisions, 21 were related to break times or milk expression (National Conference of State Legislation, 2010). For additional information, readers are encouraged to visit La Leche League's and the United States Breastfeeding Committee's websites to learn more about breastfeeding legislation (see the Internet resources listed at the end of this chapter). In addition, readers may access state and federal legislative websites to follow legislation through the process of becoming law (e.g., Thomas Legislative Information can be found at http://thomas.loc.gov/). In a study using the 2009 National Immunization Survey analyzing breastfeeding duration using multiple levels of the social–ecological model, breastfeeding at 6 months was associated with being from a state that had a worksite breastfeeding statute in place. However, the state worksite breastfeeding statute alone did not directly affect breastfeeding duration when controlling for year enacted and other state characteristics such as years since founding of state breastfeeding coalition and breastfeeding-supportive hospital practices (Dozier & McKee, 2011).

Advocacy efforts regarding breastfeeding and employment globally and nationally are abundant. The United States Breastfeeding Committee (USBC) is an overarching group formed to coordinate breastfeeding advocacy activities in the United States (see the list of Internet resources at the end of the chapter). The committee is composed of representatives from health professional associations, breastfeeding support organizations, relevant government departments, and nongovernmental organizations. Approximately 50 member organizations make up the committee, including such notables as the American Academy of Pediatrics; International Lactation Consultant Association; Association of Women's Health, Obstetric, and Neonatal Nurses; the Centers for Disease Control and Prevention; and Wellstart International. Regional representatives from local and state breastfeeding coalitions are also voting members of the USBC. Many of these members have published position papers or established advocacy programs relative to promoting and supporting breastfeeding in relationship to employment. For example, a current initiative by the USBC at the time of this edition was an effort to gain support for a change in the federal law that requires employers to provide nursing mothers who are hourly wage-earners ("non-exempt" employees) with reasonable break time and a private, non-bathroom location to express breastmilk for 1 year after the child's birth. Currently, U.S. law protecting breastfeeding does not cover "exempt" or salaried employees. The Supporting Working Moms Act, therefore, would ensure a fair and uniform national policy by extending the existing federal provision to cover approximately 12 million "exempt" executive, administrative, and professional employees.

In conclusion, strides are being made in the United States, but there is much yet to do in the overall area of protecting and promoting family and maternal interests. In other countries of the world, breastfeeding advocacy groups are also prevalent and endorse support and protection of the working mother in her right to breastfeed (see the list of Internet sources). The efforts of the International Labour Organization to support breastfeeding women in the workplace are especially notable.

International Labour Organization

The International Labour Organization is an agency of the United Nations that focuses on labor standards, policies, and programs. Among the primary goals of the ILO are to protect the maternity health needs of women workers and their babies and to promote the retention of women in the workforce throughout their childbearing years. The ILO is composed of representatives of governments, workers, and employers. This UN agency sets international labor standards through conventions and recommendations. Upon ratification of an ILO convention, its articles are binding on member states through a regulatory mechanism that influences national law and practice.

The ILO has issued three conventions related to maternity protection for working women. In 1919, convention 3 recognized the need to give women workers maternity leave and breastfeeding breaks. In 1952, maternity leave was increased to 12 weeks in convention 103. The latest ILO Maternity Protection Convention 2000 (convention 183) provides for at least 14 weeks of paid maternity leave and the right to one or more breastfeeding breaks daily (see the Internet resources list). The convention also allows for a reduction of working hours for breastfeeding mothers, which gives added flexibility in settings where short breaks are not feasible.

The widened scope of convention 183 affects all employed women. Provisions relating specifically to breastfeeding women are health protection at the workplace; paid maternity leave of not less than 14 weeks; 6 weeks of compulsory leave after childbirth; cash benefits at no less than two-thirds of previous earnings; and nondiscrimination and employment protection in relation to pregnancy and breastfeeding.

The convention also emphasizes that maternity protection is a social responsibility and that the burden of costs should thus be shared by all of society. Recommendation 191 (ILO, 2000), which accompanies convention 183, further encourages an extension of maternity leave to at least 18 weeks and the adaptation of the frequency and length of nursing breaks to the particular needs of mothers and babies. It also promotes the establishment of adequate hygienic facilities at or near the workplace for nursing mothers.

Breastfeeding advocates can make use of several areas within ILO standards where the needs of breastfeeding women are addressed. When national or workplace policies are being created or updated, the ILO works to ensure that, for example, breastfeeding breaks are sufficient in number and frequency and that minimum requirements for a hygienic facility for breastfeeding or expression of milk are met. "Flexibility" is the key word. In light of the recommendation of exclusive breastfeeding for 6 months, maternity leave should be long enough to enable working women to meet this goal.

Improvements in maternity protection measures for working women can be best achieved by working together with trade unions and other social partners. The ILO conducted a study focusing on how countries' provisions conformed to the ILO's maternity protection conventions 183 and 191 among 167 ILO members. The results indicated that globally, 30% of the member states fully met the requirements of convention 183 on all three aspects: "maternity leave for at least 14 weeks at a rate of at least two-thirds of previous earnings, paid by public or social security funds, and practice where the employer is not solely responsible for payment" (ILO, 2012, p. IX). Although paternity leave is not included in the ILO standards, 49 countries provided some types of parental leaves that fathers can use during and after the birth of a child.

Clinical Implications

When providing information about breastfeeding and employment, the lactation consultant or other healthcare provider is wise to sprinkle such information throughout several discussions of breastfeeding, maintaining a matter-of-fact attitude and establishing a positive expectation that this combination of roles is possible. The lactation consultant should discuss breastfeeding with the mother well in advance of her return to work (Johnston & Esposito, 2007; Mills, 2009; Rojjanasrirat et al., 2010; Stewart-Glenn, 2008). The mother should be encouraged to identify her breastfeeding goals early in pregnancy and be aware of several breastfeeding options available based on the individual work circumstances (see Box 16-3). The combined breastfeeding and work assessment checklist presented earlier in Table 16-1 may be used to assess the important work-related elements so the appropriate planning can be done to support the mother's breastfeeding goal.

The role overload often experienced by the full-time employed mother necessitates that she learn how to organize her time for maximum efficiency. In breastfeeding, she has found an ideal combination for meeting the physical and psychological needs of her young child. In returning to work, she need not feel that she must shorten the period of lactation that she had planned. Some mothers who return to work may choose to breastfeed exclusively, whereas some may elect to breastfeed partially and supplement with artificial milk. It is crucial that mothers understand clearly the consequences of each option. Mothers who choose to return to work early and desire to breastfeed exclusively may anticipate pumping frequently to maintain their milk supply.

Other mothers may choose not to express their milk at all. These women will need to know that expressing for comfort, at least during the first week or two, may be necessary if they are to avoid unpredictable, potentially embarrassing leak spots while their body is adjusting to the lack of breast stimulation during the workday. These mothers also must

Box 16-3 Decisions the Employed Breastfeeding Mother Must Make

When to Return to Work

- Work intensity: Women must determine the status or intensity of their employment whether they choose to work part-time or full-time, or to not return to work after childbirth.
- Breastfeeding goals: Breastfeeding goals can be determined by considering factors such as length of maternity leave, breastfeeding intensity (exclusive or partial breastfeeding), work intensity, work circumstances, and amount of support available.

How Long to Breastfeed

- The decision regarding how long to breastfeed depends on a mother's breastfeeding goals and if weaning would occur due to mother-led reasons or baby-led reasons.

How Often to Pump

- The frequency of milk expression or pumping when a mother returns to work depends on the age of the baby and the duration of separation time between the mother and her child.
- The older the baby, the less frequent is the time needed to pump each day. Generally, mothers should express at least twice within 8 to 10 hours of work to maintain milk supply.

How Much Supplementation to Use

- How much supplementation or breastmilk substitute is used depends on breastfeeding intensity. For mothers who plan to breastfeed exclusively, they should avoid supplementation to prevent decreased milk production.
- Breastmilk substitutes are used for missed breastfeeding when mothers choose to breastfeed partially. The disadvantage of this option is that the mother's milk supply will decline as the baby receives more supplementation.

Child-Care Decisions

- Decisions on using child care services depend on several factors, such as issues of trust, convenience, and finances.
- The options for child care include the following: in the baby's own home, in a neighbor's or friend's home, in the home of someone who provides daycare services, or in a daycare center.

be informed that milk stasis resulting from infrequent emptying of the breast could lead to diminishing milk supply, plugged/blocked ducts, and mastitis.

Some new mothers will choose to return to work as soon as possible, often because they are financially unable to do otherwise; other women will make every effort to delay returning to work. The type of job that the woman has, the degree of involvement of coworkers and supervisors, her relationship with them, her seniority, and a wide array of other factors will influence these decisions. The healthcare worker can provide information about maternal employment and breastfeeding, but only the mother can implement the final plan.

The lactation consultant can share with the mother how other women have coped with similar situations and should answer her questions based on research evidence whenever possible. Babies do know when a mother is not available and adapt to her absence by altering sleep patterns. Changes in wakeful and sleepy periods are typical in families in which the mother works at times when the baby has previously been awake a great deal. Increased breastfeeding frequency when the mother is home (reverse-cycle nursing) is a common reaction, particularly in very young babies who breastfeed often. Such a pattern needs to be pointed out to the childcare provider; the mother should ask that the provider not wake the baby for feedings. Instead, the provider should let the baby indicate when he wants to be fed during the day. These reverse-cycle nursing episodes do not always increase during the mother's nighttime sleeping hours; rather, they tend to occur more frequently during the early daytime hours when she is preparing to leave for work and during the evening hours after she has returned home. Many mothers find that setting the alarm an hour earlier than they plan to be up reminds them to offer the baby the breast before heading for the shower or the kitchen to start the day. If she is encouraged to see this as the baby's touching and social time, the mother is more likely to view such behavior as a sign of the baby's attachment to her.

No "magic bullet" will resolve daycare issues. Unlike other countries, in which government subsidies enable many mothers to stay home for a substantial period following the birth of their babies, the United States has no federal policy supporting paid maternity leave. At the same time, increasing numbers of families make economic choices that mandate a two-worker household. In addition, daycare workers, often because they are so poorly paid, represent a workforce that has a high turnover, inadequate training, and lack of job commitment.

Summary

The role of the healthcare worker is to inform the working mother that she is not alone and that other women have in most cases faced what she is likely to encounter. In some cases, mothers have found partial solutions; in other cases, their solutions have enabled them, and will enable others, to proceed with breastfeeding with minimal interruption. Whatever the mother's individual situation, the person providing information needs to do so from a perspective of what has worked for others, recognizing that each mother's situation has unique strengths and pitfalls.

In settings in which institutionalized day care is well organized and carefully supervised, many families' concerns can be set aside. In other daycare situations, the increased illness rates and other issues related to meeting the infant's and child's many needs warrant considerable concern. At-home care is both more expensive and more difficult to obtain; in addition, it provides no guarantee that some of the problems that have surfaced in group settings, including child neglect or abuse, will not occur.

The length of time that a child breastfeeds (even if it is 2 years) represents a very small amount of the total time that the child will live in the parents' home. The length of the mother's employment is likely to last far longer than her child's infancy. The longer the mother is home during the baby's early weeks and months, the shorter the time that breastfeeding is most likely to be negatively affected by that employment.

Key Concepts

- Currently 55.8% of married women return to the labor force while their children are younger than 1 year of age.
- More women choose to breastfeed, and many will continue to breastfeed after they return to work.
- Research indicates that returning to work does not affect breastfeeding initiation but does adversely affect duration of breastfeeding.
- Working full time versus part time affects breastfeeding duration negatively.

- The sooner a mother returns to work, typically the shorter the duration of breastfeeding.
- The longer a mother stays at home before returning to work, typically the longer the breastfeeding duration.
- Level of job skill is associated with combining breastfeeding and employment: combined breastfeeding and employment increase as job skills increase.
- Prenatal planning is important to women who choose to combine breastfeeding and employment. Key to planning is learning about breastfeeding and combining it with employment, decisions regarding work options and timing of the return to work, assessing workplace support of breastfeeding, and childcare decisions.
- Four elements have been identified as enhancers of breastfeeding in the workplace: time, space, person, and policy.
- Benefits of combined breastfeeding and employment to employers include decreased absenteeism owing to decreased infant illness, which translates into decreased healthcare costs and increased worker productivity.
- Evidence indicates that lactation support programs in the workplace reduce healthcare costs, absenteeism, and infant illness while increasing breastfeeding duration.
- Breastfeeding problems may depend on the age of the infant and the timing of the return to work.
- Common concerns for women who breastfeed and work outside the home include loss of sleep, fatigue, maintaining an adequate milk supply, and daycare issues.
- Decisions regarding exclusive or partial breastfeeding upon returning to work and the baby's age will determine the need and frequency of milk expression.
- Several factors must be considered when choosing a breast pump, including cleanliness, ease of use, comfort, efficiency, and cost.
- Human milk storage guidelines exist to promote safety and are based on research evidence.

- Community resources for the breastfeeding employed woman include healthcare providers, lactation consultants, La Leche League International, breastfeeding support groups, and online information and support.
- Legislative support and public advocacy are increasing to promote and protect women's rights to breastfeed after returning to work.
- The International Labour Organization has been instrumental in protecting maternal rights, including breastfeeding in the workplace, since 1919.

INTERNET RESOURCES

Breastfeeding Position Papers and Professional Organization Information on Breastfeeding and Return to Work

Academy of Breastfeeding Medicine: http://www.bfmed.org /Media/Files/Documents/pdf/Statements/ABM _position_on_mothersinworkplace_2013.pdf

American Academy of Family Physicians: http://www.aafp .org/about/policies/all/breastfeeding-support.html

American Academy of Pediatrics: http://www2.aap.org /breastfeeding/sectionOnBreastfeeding.html

http://www.aafp.org/afp/2003/1201/p2215.html

International Lactation Consultant Association: http://www .ilca.org/files/resources/ilca_publications /BreasfeedingandWorkPP.pdf

United States Breastfeeding Committee: www.usbreast feeding.org

Breast Pump Information

Breastfeeding and pumping: http://kidshealth.org/parent /pregnancy_newborn/breastfeed/breastfeed_pump .html

Travelers' health: http://wwwnc.cdc.gov/travel/yellowbook /2014/chapter-7-international-travel-infants-children /travel-and-breastfeeding

U.S. Food and Drug Association, breast pump information for consumers: http://www.fda.gov/MedicalDevices /ProductsandMedicalProcedures/HomeHealthhand Consumer/ConsumerProducts/BreastPumps /ucm061944.htm

Work and breastfeeding. www.workandpump.com

Breastfeeding Advocacy, Consumer Information, and Discussion Forums

Innate Motherhood: http://www.internetmom.org /Breastfeeding.html

Medline Plus breastfeeding information for the consumer: http://www.nlm.nih.gov/medlineplus/breastfeeding .html

Mother-to-Mother Forum for Working and Breastfeeding Mothers: http://forums.llli.org/index.php

Transportation Security Administration: http://www.tsa.gov /traveling-formula-breast-milk-and-juice

Breastfeeding Promotion and Support

Centers for Disease Control and Prevention, The CDC Guide to Strategies to Support Breastfeeding Mothers and Babies: http://www.cdc.gov/breastfeeding/resources /guide.htm

La Leche League International: http://www.llli.org

National Women's Health Information Center: http://www .womenshealth.gov/breastfeeding/

U.S. Department of Agriculture National Breastfeeding Loving Support campaign: http://www.nal.usda.gov /wicworks/Learning_Center/loving_support.html

Breastfeeding and Child Care

Australian Breastfeeding Association Breastfeeding Workplace Accreditation Program: https://www.breastfeeding.asn .au/bfinfo/caregivers.html

Rhode Island Department of Health, Tips for childcare providers: http://www.health.ri.gov/breastfeeding/for /childcareproviders/

U.S. Department of Agriculture: http://fnic.nal.usda.gov /lifecycle-nutrition/breastfeeding

U.S. Department of Health and Human Services, Maternal and Child Health Bureau (MCHB): http://www.mchb .hrsa.gov

Other Non-U.S. National Initiatives and Resources

Breastfeeding Committee of Canada: http://www.breastfeeding canada.ca

International Confederation of Free Trade Unions: http:// www.ituc-csi.org/spip.php?page=recherche&recherche =breastfeeding+in+the+workplace

International Labour Organization: http://www.ilo.org /global/about-the-ilo/newsroom/comment-analysis /WCMS_218710/lang--en/index.htm

Public Services International (PSI): http://www.world-psi.org /en/breastfeeding-work-also-good-employers

REFERENCES

Abdulwadud OA, Snow ME. Interventions in the workplace to support breastfeeding for women in employment. *Cochrane Database Syst Rev.* 2012;10:CD006177.

Aikawa T, Pavadhgul P, Chongsuwat R, et al. Maternal return to paid work and breastfeeding practices in Bangkok, Thailand. *Asia Pac J Public Health.* 2012; doi: 10.1177/1010539511419647.

American Academy of Pediatrics (AAP), American Public Health Association (APHA), National Resource Center for Health and Safety in Child Care and Early Education. *Caring for our children: national health and safety performance standards. Guidelines for early care and education programs.* Elk Grove Village, IL: American Academy of Pediatrics; Washington, DC: American Public Health Association; 2011.

American Business Collaboration (ABC). *The new career paradigm: flexibility briefing.* 2007. http://www.shrm.org /Publications/HRNews/documents/ABC_NCP _Flexibility_Briefing.pdf.

Angeletti MA. Breastfeeding mothers returning to work: possibilities for information, anticipatory guidance and support from US health care professionals. *J Hum Lact.* 2009;25:226–232.

Arthur CR, Saenz RB, Replogle WH. The employment-related breastfeeding decisions of physician mothers. *J MS Med Assoc.* 2003;44:383–387.

Auerbach KG, Guss E. Maternal employment and breastfeeding: a study of 567 women's experiences. *Am J Dis Child.* 1984;138:958–960.

Bai Y, Peng J, Fly AD. Validation of a short questionnaire to assess mothers' perception of workplace breastfeeding support. *J Am Diet Assoc.* 2008;108:1221–1225.

Balkam JA, Cadwell K, Fein SB. Effect of components of a workplace lactation program on breastfeeding duration among employees of a public-sector employer. *Matern Child Health J.* 2011;15:677–683.

Bar-Yam NB. Workplace lactation support, part 1: a return to work breastfeeding assessment tool. *J Hum Lact.* 1998;14:249–254.

Bettinelli M. Breastfeeding policies and breastfeeding support programs in the mother's workplace. *J Matern Fetal Neonatal Med.* 2012;25(suppl 4):81–82. doi: 10.3109/14767058.2012.715033.

Biagoli F. Returning to work while breastfeeding. *Am Fam Phys.* 2003;68:2199–2206.

Biancuzzo M. Selecting pumps for breastfeeding mothers. *JOGNN.* 1999;28:417–426.

Bocar D. Combining breastfeeding and employment: increasing success. *J Perinat Neonat Nurs.* 1997;11:23–43.

Bridges CB, Frank DI, Curtin J. Employer attitudes toward breastfeeding in the workplace. *J Hum Lact.* 1997;13:215–219.

Brown CA, Poag S, Kasprzycki C. Exploring large employers' and small employers' knowledge, attitudes, and practices on breastfeeding support in the workplace. *J Hum Lact.* 2001;17:39–46.

Buss IH, McGill F, Darlow BA, Winterbourn CC. Vitamin C is reduced in human milk after storage. *Acta Paediatr.* 2001;90:813–815.

Callahan S, Sejourne N, Denis A. Fatigue and breastfeeding: an inevitable partnership? *J Hum Lact.* 2006;22: 182–187.

Calnen G. Paid maternity leave and its impact on breast-feeding in the United States: an historic, economic, political and social perspective. *Breastfeed Med.* 2007;2:34–43.

Carbonare SB, Palmeira P, Silva ML, Carneiro-Sampaio MM. Effect of microwave radiation, pasteurization and lyophilization on the ability of human milk to inhibit *Escherichia coli* adherence to Hep-2 cells. *J Diarrhoeal Dis Res.* 1996;14:90–94.

Centers for Disease Control and Prevention (CDC). Breastfeeding report card—United States. 2012. Available at: http://www.cdc.gov/breastfeeding/pdf/2012Breast feedingReportCard.pdf.

Centers for Disease Control and Prevention (CDC). *The CDC guide to strategies to support breastfeeding mothers and babies.* Atlanta, GA: U.S. Department of Health and Human Services; 2013.

Chen YC, Wu YC, Chie WC. Effects of work-related factors on the breastfeeding behavior of working mothers in a Taiwanese semiconductor manufacturer: a cross-sectional survey. *BMC Public Health.* 2006;6:160.

Chezem J, Montgomery P, Fortman T. Maternal feelings after cessation of breastfeeding: influence of factors related to employment and duration. *J Perinat Neonat Nurs.* 1997;11:61–70.

Chow T, Smithey Fulmer I, Olson BH. Perspectives of managers toward workplace breastfeeding support in the state of Michigan. *J Hum Lact.* 2011;27:138–146.

Chow T, Wolfe EW, Olson B. Development, content validity, and piloting of an instrument designed to measure managers' attitude toward workplace breastfeeding support. *J Acad Nutr Diet.* 2012;112:1042–1047.

Christrup SM. Breastfeeding in the American workplace. *J Gender Soc Pol Law.* 2001;9:472–503.

Chuang CH, Chang PJ, Chen YC, et al. Maternal return to work and breastfeeding: a population-based cohort study. *Int J Nurs Stud.* 2010;47:461–474.

Click ER. Developing a worksite lactation program. *MCN.* 2006;31:313–317.

Cohen R, Mrtek MB. The impact of two corporate lactation programs on the incidence and duration of breast-feeding by employed mothers. *Am J Health Prom.* 1994;8:436–441.

Cohen R, Mrtek MB, Mrtek RG. Comparison of maternal absenteeism and infant illness rates among breast-feeding and formula-feeding women in two corporations. *Am J Health Prom.* 1995;10:148–153.

Cooklin AR, Donath SM, Amir LH. Maternal employment and breastfeeding: results from the longitudinal study of Australian children. *Acta Paediatr.* 2008;97:620–623.

Cooklin AR, Rowe HJ, Fisher JR. Paid parental leave supports breastfeeding and mother–infant relationship: a prospective investigation of maternal postpartum employment. *Aust N Z J Public Health.* 2012;36:249–256.

Daly SEJ, Hartmann PE. Infant demand and milk supply: the short-term control of milk synthesis in lactating women. *J Hum Lact.* 1995;11:27–37.

Dodgson JE, Duckett L. Breastfeeding in the workplace: building a support program for nursing mothers. *AAOHN J.* 1997;45:290–298.

Dornan BA, Oermann MH. Breastfeeding websites for patient education. *MCN.* 2006;31:18–23.

Dozier AM, McKee KS. State breastfeeding worksite statutes…breastfeeding rates… and… *Breastfeed Med.* 2011;6:319–324.

Dunn BF, Zavela KJ, Cline AD, Cost PA. Breastfeeding practices in Colorado businesses. *J Hum Lact.* 2004;20:170–177.

Eldridge S, Croker A. Breastfeeding friendly workplace accreditation: creating supportive workplaces for breastfeeding women. *Breastfeed Rev.* 2005;13:17–22.

Fein SB, Mandal B, Roe BE. Success of strategies for combining employment and breastfeeding. *Pediatrics.* 2008;122:S56–S62.

Fein SB, Roe B. The effect of work status on initiation and duration of breastfeeding. *Am J Pub Health.* 1998;88:1042–1046.

Fetherston C. Risk factors for lactation mastitis. *J Hum Lact.* 1998;14:109.

Galbally M, Lewis AJ, McEgan K, et al. Breastfeeding and infant sleep patterns: an Australian population study. *J Paediatr Child Health.* 2013;49:E147–E152.

Galtry J. The impact on breastfeeding of labour market policy and practice in Ireland, Sweden, and the USA. *Soc Sci Med.* 2003;57:167–177.

Gordon RA, Kaestner R. Korenman S. The effects of maternal employment on child injuries and infectious disease. *Demography.* 2007;44:307–333.

Hager WD, Barton JR. Treatment of sporadic acute puerperal mastitis. *Infect Dis Obstet Gynecol.* 1996;4:97–101.

Haider SJ, Jacknowitz A, Schoeni RF. Welfare work requirements and child well-being: evidence from the effects on breast-feeding. *Demography.* 2003;40:479–497.

Hamosh M, Ellis LA, Pollock DR, et al. Breastfeeding and the working mother: effect of time and temperature of short-term storage on proteolysis, lipolysis, and bacterial growth in milk. *Pediatrics.* 1996;97:492–498.

Hawkins SS, Griffiths LJ, Dezateux C, et al., Millennium Cohort Study Child Health Group. Maternal employment and breast-feeding initiation: findings from the Millennium Cohort Study. *Paediatr Perinat Epidemiol.* 2007;21:242–247.

Hen W, Waldfogel, J. Parental leave: the impact of recent legislation on parents' leave taking. *Demography.* 2003;40(4):191–200.

Iatrakis G, Zervoudis S, Ceausu I, et al. Clinical features and treatment of lactational mastitis: the experience from a binational study. *Clin Exp Obstet Gynecol.* 2013;40(2):275–276.

International Labour Organization (ILO). R191 Maternity Protection Recommendation 2000. Available at: http://www.ilo.org/public/english/employment/skills/hrdr/instr/r_191.htm.

International Labour Organization (ILO). Maternity at work: a review of national legislation. 2nd ed. 2010. Available at: http://www.ilo.org/wcmsp5/groups/public/---dgreports/---dcomm/---publ/documents/publication/wcms_124442.pdf.

International Labour Organization (ILO). Economically active population, estimates and projections. 6th ed. [database]. 2011. Available at: http://laborsta.ilo.org/applv8/data/EAPEP/eapep_E.html.

International Labour Organization (ILO). Global employment trends for women 2012 (brief). December 2012. Available at: http://www.ilo.org/trends.

Johnston M, Esposito N. Barriers and facilitators for breastfeeding among working women in the United States. *JOGNN*. 2007;36:9–20.

Jones F. *Best practice for expressing, storing and handling human milk in hospital, homes, and child care settings.* Fort Worth, TX: Human Milk Banking Association of North America; 2011.

Killien MG. Postpartum return to work: mothering stress, anxiety, and gratification. *Can J Nurs Res.* 1998;30:53–66.

Killien MG. The role of social support in facilitating postpartum women's return to employment. *JOGNN*. 2005;34:639–646.

Killien M, Habermann B, Jarrett M. Influence of employment characteristics on postpartum mothers' health. *Women's Work, Health, and Quality of Life.* 2001;33:63–81.

Kimbro RT. On-the-job moms: work and breastfeeding initiation and duration for a sample of low-income women. *Matern Child Health J.* 2006;10:19–26.

Laughlin L. Maternity leave and employment patterns of first-time mothers: 1961–2008. 2011. Available at: http://www.census.gov/prod/2011pubs/p70-128.pdf. Accessed February 16, 2013.

Laughlin L, U.S. Census Bureau. Who's minding the kids? Child care arrangements. Spring 2013. Available at: http://www.census.gov/prod/2013pubs/p70-135.pdf.

Lewallen LP, Dick MJ, Flowers J, et al. Breastfeeding support and early cessation. *J Obstet Gynecol Neonatal Nurs.* 2006;35(2):166–172.

Libbus MK, Bullock FC. Breastfeeding and employment: an assessment of employer attitudes. *J Hum Lact.* 2002;18:247–251.

Lindberg LD. Women's decisions about breastfeeding and maternal employment. *J Marr Fam.* 1996;58:239–251.

Mandal B, Roe BE, Fein SB. The differential effects of full-time and part-time work status on breastfeeding. *Health Policy.* 2010;97:79–86.

Marinelli KA, Moren K, Taylor JS, Academy of Breastfeeding Medicine. Breastfeeding support for mothers in work-place employment or educational settings: summary statement. *Breastfeed Med.* 2013;8:137–142.

Matthews JT, Hamilton BE. *Delayed childbearing: more women are having their first child later in life.* NCHS Data Brief, no. 21. Hyattsville, MD: National Center for Health Statistics; 2009.

McGovern P, Dowd B, Gjerdingen D, et al. Postpartum health of employed mothers 5 weeks after childbirth. *Ann Fam Med.* 2006;4:159–167.

McKenna J, Mosho S, Richard C. Bedsharing promoted breastfeeding. *Pediatrics.* 1997;100:214–219.

Meedya S, Fahy K, Kable A. Factors that positively influence breastfeeding duration to 6 months: a literature review. *Women Birth.* 2010;23:35–45. doi: 10:1016/j.wombi.2010.02.002.

Mills SP. Workplace lactation programs: a critical element for breastfeeding mothers' success. *AAOHN.* 2009;57:227–231.

Mirkovic KR, Perrine CG, Scanlon KS, Grummer-Strawn LM. In the United States, a mother's plans for infant feeding are associated with plans for employment. *J Hum Lact.* 2014;30:291–297.

Murtagh L, Moulton, AD. Working mothers, breastfeeding, and the law. *Am J Public Health.* 2011;101:217–223.

National Conference of State Legislation. Breastfeeding laws, 2010. Available at: http://www.ncsl.org/issues-research/health/breastfeeding-state-laws.aspx.

Neifert M. Supporting breastfeeding mothers as they return to work. *Am Acad Pediatr Newsl.* 2000. Available at: http://www.aap.org/healthtopics/breastfeeding.cfm. Accessed October 10, 2007.

Nichols MR, Roux GM. Maternal perspectives on postpartum return to the workplace. *JOGNN.* 2004;33:463–471.

Noble S, ALSPAC Study Team. Maternal employment and the initiation of breastfeeding. *Acta Paediatr.* 2001;90:423–428.

Ogbuanu C, Glover S, Probst J, et al. The effect of maternity leave length and time of return to work on breastfeeding. *Pediatrics.* 2011;127:1414–1427.

Ogundele MO. Techniques for the storage of human breastmilk: implications for antimicrobial functions and safety of stored milk. *Eur J Pediatr.* 2000;159:793–797.

Ong G, Yap M, Li FL, Choo TB. Impact of working status on breastfeeding in Singapore. *Eur J Pub Health,* 2005;15:434–430.

Ortiz J, McGilligan K, Kelly P. Duration of breast milk expression among working mothers enrolled in an employer-sponsored lactation program. *Pediatr Nurs.* 2004;30:111–119.

Ovesen L, Jakobsen J, Leth T, Reinholdt J. The effect of microwave heating on vitamins B1 and E, and linoleic and linolenic acids, and immuno-globulins in human milk. *Int J Food Sci Nutr.* 1996;47:427–436.

Pardou A, Serruys E, Mascart-Lemone F, et al. Human milk banking: influence of storage processes and of bacterial contamination on some milk constituents. *Biol Neonate.* 1994;65:302–309.

Peaker M, Wilde CJ. Feedback control of secretion from milk. *J Mammary Gland Biol Neoplasia.* 1996;1:307–314.

Piper S, Parks PL. Predicting the duration of lactation: evidence from a national survey. *Birth.* 1996;23:7–12.

Potter B. Women's experiences of managing mastitis. *Comm Pract.* 2005;78:209–212.

Prime DK, Garbin CP, Hartmann PE, Kent JC. Simultaneous breast expression in breastfeeding women is more efficacious than sequential breast expression. *Breastfeed Med.* 2012;7:442–447.

Pugh L, Milligan R. A framework for the study of childbearing fatigue. *Adv Nurs Sci.* 1993;15:60–70.

Radtke Demirci J, Braxter BJ, Chasens ER. Breastfeeding and short sleep duration in mothers and 6–11 month-old infants. *Infant Behav Dev.* 2012;35:884–886.

Ramamurthy MB, Sekartini R, Ruangdaraganon N, et al. Effect of current breastfeeding on sleep patterns in infants from Asia-Pacific region. *J Paediatr Child Health.* 2012;48:669–674.

Roe B, Whittington LA, Fein SB, Teisl MF. Is there competition between breast-feeding and maternal employment? *Demography.* 1999;36:157–171.

Rogers KC, Finks FW. Job sharing for women pharmacists in academia. *Am J Pharmaceut Educ.* 2009;73 (7, Article 135):1–5.

Rojjanasrirat W. Working women's breastfeeding experiences. *MCN.* 2004;29:222–227.

Rojjanasrirat W, Sousa V. Perceptions of breastfeeding and planned return to work or school among low-income pregnant women in the USA. *J Clin Nurs.* 2010;19:2014–2022.

Rojjanasrirat W, Wambach KA, Sousa VD, Gajewski B. Psychometric evaluation of the Employer Support for Breastfeeding Questionnaire (ESBQ). *J Hum Lact.* 2010;26(3):286–296.

Ryan AS, Zhou W, Acosta A. Breastfeeding continues to increase into the new millennium. *Pediatrics.* 2002;110:1103–1109.

Ryan AS, Zhou W, Arensberg MB. The effect of employment status on breastfeeding in the United States. *Women's Health Iss.* 2006;16:243–251.

Sattari M, Serwint JR, Neal D, et al. Work-place predictors of duration of breastfeeding among female physicians. *J Pediatr.* 2013;163:1612–1617.

Scott JA, Binns CW, Oddy WH, Graham KI. Predictors of breastfeeding duration: evidence from a cohort study. *Pediatrics.* 2006;117:646–655.

Skafida V. Juggling work and motherhood: the impact of employment and maternity leave on breastfeeding duration: a survival analysis on Growing Up in Scotland data. *Matern Child Health J.* 2012;16:519–527.

Slusser WM, Lange L, Dickson V, et al. Breast milk expression in the workplace: a look at frequency and time. *J Hum Lact.* 2004;20:164–169.

Smith JP, McIntyre E, Craig L, et al. Workplace support, breastfeeding and health. *Family Matters.* 2013;93:58–73. Available at: http://www.aifs.gov.au/institute/pubs/fm2013/fm93/fm93f.html.

Smith K, Downs B, O'Connell M. *Maternity leave and employment patterns: 1961–1995, Current Population Reports,* Washington, DC: U.S. Census Bureau; 2001.

Society for Human Resource Management (SHRM). Employee benefits: the employee benefits landscape in a recovering economy. 2012. Available at: http://www.shrm.org/Research/SurveyFindings/Articles/Documents/2012_EmpBenefits_Report.pdf

Spain D, Bianchi S. *Balancing act: motherhood, marriage, and employment among American women.* New York, NY: Russell Sage Foundation; 1996.

Stevens KV, Janke J. Breastfeeding experiences of active duty military women. *Mil Med.* 2003;168:380–384.

Stewart-Glenn J. Knowledge, perceptions, and attitudes of managers, coworkers, and employed breastfeeding mothers. *AAOHN J.* 2008;56:423–431.

Thompsen AC, Espersen T, Maigaard S. Course and treatment of milk stasis, noninfectious inflammation of the breast, and infectious mastitis in nursing women. *Am J Obstet Gynecol.* 1984;149:492–495.

Thompson PE, Bell P. Breast-feeding in the workplace: how to succeed. *Iss Comp Pediatr Nurs.* 1997;20:1–9.

Thulier D, Mercer J. Variables associated with breastfeeding duration. *J Obstet Gynecol Neonatal Nurs.* 2009;38:259–268. doi: 10.1111/j.1552-6909.2009.01021.x.

United States Breastfeeding Committee. *Statement on lactation accommodations in the workplace* [position paper]. Washington, DC: United States Breastfeeding Committee; 2011.

U.S. Bureau of Labor Statistics. Women in the labor force: a databook (Report 1018). 2009. Available at: http://www.bls.gov/cps/wlf-databook2009.htm.

U.S. Bureau of Labor Statistics. Women in the labor force: a databook (Report 1040). 2013. Available at: http://www.bls.gov/cps/wlf-databook-2012.pdf.

U.S. Department of Health and Human Services. *HHS blueprint for action on breastfeeding.* Washington, DC: U.S. Department of Health and Human Services, Office on Women's Health; 2000.

U.S. Department of Health and Human Services. Business case for breastfeeding. 2010. Available at: http://www.womenshealth.gov/breastfeeding/government-in-action/business-case-for-breastfeeding/index.cfm.

U.S. Department of Health and Human Services, Office on Women's Health. Supporting Nursing moms at work: employer solutions. 2014. Available at: http://www.womenshealth.gov/breastfeeding/employer-solutions/index.php.

U.S. Department of Labor. Wage and hour division. 2010. Available at: http://www.dol.gov/whd/nursingmothers/Sec7rFLSA_btnm.htm.

U.S. Department of Labor. Women in the labor force: a databook (Report 1034). 2011. Available at: http://www.bls.gov/cps/wlf-databook2011.htm.

U.S. Department of Labor. Family and medical leave in 2012: executive summary by Abt Associates Inc. Washington, DC. 2012. Available at: http://www.dol.gov/asp/evaluation/fmla/FMLA-2012-Executive-Summary.pdf.

Vanek EP, Vanek JA. Job sharing as an employment alternative in group medical practice. *Med Group Manage J.* 2001;48:24–40.

Visness CM, Kennedy KI. Maternal employment and breastfeeding: findings from the 1988 National Maternal and Infant Health Survey. *Am J Public Health.* 1997;87: 945–950.

Wambach K. Maternal fatigue in breastfeeding primiparae during the first nine weeks postpartum. *J Hum Lact.* 1998;14:219–229.

Wambach K, Prusia, V, Britt C, Murray L. Supporting breastfeeding: evaluation of the University of Kansas Medical Center Express Stations. International Lactation Consultant Association Conference, Phoenix, AZ., July 25, 2014.

Whaley SE, Meehan K, Lange L, et al. Predictors of breastfeeding duration for employees of the Special Supplemental Nutrition Program for Women, Infants, and Children (WIC). *J Am Diet Assoc.* 2002;102:1290–1293.

Win NN, Binns CW, Zhao Y, et al. Breastfeeding duration in mothers who express breast milk: a cohort study. *Int Breastfeed J.* 2006;1:28.

Witters-Green R. Increasing breastfeeding rates in working mothers. *Fam Sys Health.* 2003;21:415–434.

World Alliance for Breastfeeding Action (WABA). Status of maternity protection by country. Available at: http://www.waba.org.my/whatwedo/womenandwork/pdf/mpchart2011a.pdf.

Wyatt SN. Challenges of the working breastfeeding mother: workplace solutions. *AAOHN J.* 2002;50:61–66.

Yimyam S, Morrow M. Breastfeeding practices among employed Thai women in Chiangmai. *J Hum Lact.* 1999; 15:225–232.

Chapter 17

Child Health

Heather Baker

This chapter reviews child health issues, beginning with the fundamentals of normal growth and development of infants and children, and then reviewing the prominent theories of child development. The discussion then focuses on the rich textures of mother–infant social interaction. Woven from the sophisticated sensory abilities of the newborn, they create a lifelong bond. Next, questions about such children's health issues as immunization, vitamin D, oral and dental health, and obesity are answered. The chapter concludes with the practical considerations of introducing solids and a discussion of weaning.

Developmental Outcomes and Infant Feeding

Before addressing specific elements of growth and development, it is useful to consider studies that compare developmental outcomes between breastfed and bottle-fed babies. A number of studies suggest that breastfeeding has a long-term benefit on cognitive and intellectual development in childhood, extending to young adulthood (Table 17-1).

These findings raise questions: Which elements of breastfeeding play a role in promoting development and intelligence? Is it the nutritional or immunological aspects of breastmilk, or are there environmental and emotional interactions connected with breastfeeding that cannot be controlled? Which

systems can support successful breastfeeding? Lucas et al. (1992) controlled for maternal interaction by studying preterm infants who received their mothers' milk via tube feedings, and compared them with children who got formula or children whose mothers intended to provide them with breastmilk but did not. Because all the infants were fed only by tube, the effects of breastmilk per se were separate from the normally intertwined effect of intimate maternal contact. The IQ scores of the children fed human milk were, on average, 8.5 points higher than those of the children not fed human milk. Nisbett et al. (2012), in a comprehensive review, reported that breastfeeding, and longer duration of breastfeeding, may increase IQ by as much as 6 to 8 points, although other confounding factors, such as genetic, social class, and the mother's IQ, may not have been considered in all studies.

Several breastmilk components have been suggested to explain the advantages realized by breastfed children, most prominently the presence of longer-chain polyunsaturated fatty acids, particularly arachidonic acid (AA) and docosahexaenoic acid (DHA), in human milk. These fatty acids are essential nutrients for infants, because they are present in structural lipids in brain and nervous tissue (Drobetz et al., 2012; Farquharson et al., 1992). Differences in visual performance between breastfed and formula-fed full-term infants, for example, are thought to result from the provision

Table 17-1 STUDIES ON BREASTFEEDING AND CHILDREN'S INTELLIGENCE, DEVELOPMENT, AND MOTOR SKILLS

Source

Singhal et al., 2007 (United States)

Method

Two hundred sixty-two children aged 4 to 6 years; breastfeeding benefits on dietary intake of docosahexaenoic acid (DHA). Children assigned either DHA or arachidonic acid ($n = 94$) or control formula ($n = 90$) for 6 months. Random dot E test and Sonksen-Silver acuity system used to assess visual responses.

Findings

Breastfed children had significantly greater likelihood of foveal stereoscopic vision maturation and stereoacuity ($P = 0.001$), independent of partial confounding ($P = 0.005$). Stereoacuity did not differ significantly between children who received DHA supplemented or control formula. Results suggest factors other than DHA in breastmilk account for benefits.

Source

Julvez et al., 2007 (Norway)

Method

Behavioral areas as related to long-term breastfeeding were assessed on 4 year olds, from Menorca ($n = 420$) and Spain ($n = 79$).

Children assessed for neuropsychological function (McCarthy test), attention-hyperactivity behavior (ADHA Criteria of DSM-IV) and social behavior (California Preschool Competence Scale).

Findings

Long-term breastfeeding (< 12 and 20 weeks) associated with fewer attention and hyperactivity symptoms and improvement in neuropsychological and sociobehavioral outcomes.

Outcomes remained significant when included as covariates in the regression models.

Source

Martin et al., 2007 (United Kingdom)

Method

Cohort study with a 60 year follow-up of 1414 participants from England and Scotland, assessing breastfeeding with social class mobility.

Findings

Participants who breastfed were 41% more likely to move up social class in adulthood ($P = 0.007$) than bottle-fed infants. Longer breastfeeding duration associated with upward mobility.

Source

Eickmann et al., 2007 (Brazil)

Method

One hundred ninety-one infants from low-income population, tested at 12 months, using Bayley Scales of Infant Development II. Controlled for covariates.

Table 17-1 Studies on Breastfeeding and Children's Intelligence, Development and Motor Skills (*continued*)

Findings

Full breastfeeding at 1 month associated with small but significant benefits in mental development (+3.0 points, $P = 0.02$).

No association with breastfeeding longer than 1 month or benefits in motor development.

Source

Vohr et al., 2006 (United States)

Method

1035 extremely low-birth-weight infants assessed at 18 months, corrected age with three tests: Bayley Mental and Development Indexes and Behavioral Rating Scale.

Findings

Infants with highest ingestion of breastmilk in NICU scored higher on Bayley tests than infants with lower or no breastmilk intake. For each 10 ml/kg/day breastmilk increase, score points increased: development by 0.53, psychomotor by 0.63, behavioral by 0.82. A five-point (1/2 SD) increase in IQ suggests long-term benefits of breastfeeding for extremely low-birth-weight infants.

Source

Hart et al., 2006 (United States)

Method

Effect of natural docosahexaenoic acid (DHA) levels in breastmilk on neurobehavioral outcomes in newborn infants. Breastmilk from $n = 20$ mothers collected 9 days postpartum. Tested with Brazelton Neonatal Behavioral Assessment Scale (NBAS).

Findings

Pearson correlations revealed positive association between DHA concentrations in breastmilk and infant scores on NBAS. State cluster scores suggest breastmilk DHA beneficial to neonatal neurobehavioral functioning.

Source

Sacker et al., 2006 (United Kingdom)

Method

Cohort study of 14,660 term singleton infants who weighed > 2500 g at birth.

Findings

Infants never breastfed 50% more likely to have gross motor coordination delays than infants who had been breastfed exclusively for 4 months and 40% more likely to have fine motor delays than infants who were breastfed for a prolonged period.

(Continues)

Table 17-1 Studies on Breastfeeding and Children's Intelligence, Development and Motor Skills (*continued*)

Source

Slykerman et al., 2005 (New Zealand)

Method

550 European children, half small for gestational age (SGA), and half appropriate for gestational age (AGA). IQ assessed at 3.5 years, using Stanford Binet Intelligence Scale, breastfeeding duration assessed by maternal interviews.

Findings

SGA children breastfed longer than 12 months had adjusted IQ scores 6.0 points higher ($P = 0.06$) than nonbreastfed infants. Breastfeeding not significantly related to IQ scores for the total SGA and AGA sample.

Source

Daniels et al., 2005 (Philippines)

Method

Normal birth weight (NBW, $n = 1790$) and low-birth-weight (LBW, $n = 189 < 2500$ g) infants, born close to term, in Philippines, 1983–1984. Cognitive ability assessed at ages 8.5 and 11.5 years with Nonverbal Intelligence Test.

Findings

Scores at 8.5 years higher for infants breastfed longer (12 to < 18 months versus < 6 months): NBW (1.6 points), and LBW (9.8 points). Findings indicate importance of both predominant and long-term partial breastfeeding in LBW infants born close to term.

Source

Rao et al., 2002 (Norway, Sweden)

Method

529 full-term small for gestational age (SGA) and normal weight Norwegian and Swedish infants followed up to 5 years. Norwegian Weschler Intelligence-Revised and Raven Progressive Matrices used to measure IQ.

Findings

Total IQ increased linearly with duration of exclusive breastfeeding for durations over 12 weeks giving an 11-point advantage in total IQ for SGA children exclusively breastfed for 24 weeks compared to those exclusively breastfed for 12 weeks.

Source

Wigg et al., 1998 (Australia)

Method

Cognitive assessments on 375 children at 2, 4, 7, and 11 to 13 years. Bayley Mental Development and Wechsler Full-Scale IQ.

Findings

Small, nonsignificant effect of breastfeeding on scores. Breastfed children had higher scores on Bayley Mental Development at ages 2 and 4, and higher IQ at ages 7 and 11.

Table 17-1 STUDIES ON BREASTFEEDING AND CHILDREN'S INTELLIGENCE, DEVELOPMENT AND MOTOR SKILLS (*CONTINUED*)

Source

Johnson et al., 1996 (United States)

Method

204 children measured at age 3. Stanford-Binet, Hollingshead Index of Social Status used; controlled for socioeconomic status, mother's intelligence, smoking, gender, and birth order.

Findings

Initiation of breastfeeding predicted scores on intelligence tests at age 3. Breastfeeding associated with 4.6 higher mean in intelligence.

Source

Floury et al., 1995 (United Kingdom)

Method

592 first-born infants; Bayley Scales of Infant Development used.

Findings

Higher mental development (3.7–5.7 points) significantly related to breastfeeding at 2 weeks after discharge after control for social and demographic factors. No differences for psychomotor development or behavior.

Source

Temboury et al., 1994 (Spain)

Method

364 healthy infants measured between 18 and 29 months of age. Bayley Scales of Infant Development used; controlled for maternal and infant variables.

Findings

Low results on the Index of Mental Development associated with bottle-fed infants, lower-middle and lower social class, mother education, temper tantrums, and having siblings.

Source

Rogan & Gladen, 1993 (United States)

Method

855 newborns; Bayley Scales of Infant Development and McCarthy Scale used; prospective case control.

Findings

Statistically significant but small increases in scores among breastfed children on cognitive skills, not motor skills. Slightly higher English grades on report cards after adjusting for confounding variables.

(Continues)

Table 17-1 STUDIES ON BREASTFEEDING AND CHILDREN'S INTELLIGENCE, DEVELOPMENT AND MOTOR SKILLS (*CONTINUED*)

Source

Lucas et al., 1992 (United Kingdom)

Method

926 low-birth-weight infants tube-fed with human milk or formula. Measured at 8.5 years of age; Weschler Intelligence Scale for Children used.

Findings

Children used; randomized trial of feeding mode; controlled for maternal contact, social class, education.

Dose-response relationship between proportion of breastmilk and IQ. Breastfed children scored 8.3 points higher.

Source

Morley et al., 1988 (United Kingdom)

Method

771 low-birth-weight infants; Bayley Mental Scale and Developmental Profile 11 used; measured at 18 months postterm; randomized controlled trial of feeding mode.

Findings

Breastfed children had significant 4.3-point advantage on the Bayley Mental Developmental Index over the children who received only formula. ($P < 0.005$).

---

of AA and DHA in breastmilk. Randomized trials have demonstrated improved visual and mental development in infants receiving a formula supplemented with DHA (Birch et al., 2000; Singhal et al., 2007; Wagner & Rosenkrantz, 2012; Wang & Brand-Miller, 2003). Another possible reason for enhanced cognitive function of breastfed children is the high concentration of sialic acid in breastmilk. Maturation of the brain is associated with total sialic concentration. Breastfed infants have higher brain sialic acid levels than do formula-fed infants because human milk is a rich source of sialic acid containing oligosaccharides, while formula contains very little of this component (Wang & Brand-Miller, 2003).

Development of the nervous system also depends on the amount, quality, and timing of sensory stimulation of the developing infant. Several components of the breastfeeding relationship have been suggested as enhancers of infant stimulation, such as the skin-to-skin contact (SSC) involved in breastfeeding. Infant suckling also releases prolactin and oxytocin in the mother, which are thought to contribute to mothering behavior.

Oxytocin and Breastfeeding

Abundant research demonstrates that oxytocin plays a significant role in maternal–child relationships and growth and development of children, in particular attachment, bonding, trust, and socialization. The influence of oxytocin, a neuropeptide, has been studied extensively in humans and animals, by means of observation of behaviors and responses to trust games and human faces, intranasal administration of oxytocin, serum sampling, and magnetic resonance imaging (MRI) of the neural system. Lactation, sensory stimulation, infant suckling, touching, mother–infant socialization, and even related sights, sounds, or smells associated with the mother–infant relationship stimulate the release of oxytocin, which is sometimes referred to as the "anti-stress hormone," or the "love" hormone (Winberg,

2005). There appears to be a complex interaction of multiple neuroendocrine systems involved, with oxytocin playing the major role in stress reduction, prosocial behavior, bonding, and the development of trust. Oxytocin is associated with numerous anti-stress responses: lowering of blood pressure and cortisol levels, as well as increased relaxation, calming, sedation, blood flow and warmth over the mammary glands and nipples, digestion, healing, and stimulation of growth (Strathearn, Fonagy, et al., 2009; Uvnas-Moberg, 1997).

In relationship to trust, Riedl and Javor (2012) summarize significant interactions as follows. Oxytocin (OXT), dopamine (DOP), serotonin (SER), and estrogen (EST) are associated with approach behavior and trust. Cortisol (COR), arginine vasopressin (AVP), and testosterone (TES) are more strongly associated with avoidance behavior and distrust. Levels of DOP, a neurotransmitter associated with reward processing and promotion of maternal behavior, have been shown to be enhanced by OXT; collectively, these relationships are referred to as the oxytocinergic and dopaminergic system (Strathearn, 2011). The interaction of OXT release and touch is associated with increased levels of SER, a neurotransmitter with multiple functions, including roles in calmness, positive mood, and decreased stress activity. Depression is known to be a result of SER deficiency. EST, a hormone, facilitates the uptake of OXT. COR, a hormone secreted by the adrenal cortex, is associated with stress and the "fight-or-flight" response. Stress-induced COR elevation has been shown to impair social memory. Chronic stress is associated with inflammatory and other negative health factors, and can be considered "toxic" and injurious over time to organ systems, including brain regions associated with regulating attention and memory (Nisbett et al., 2012). AVP, a neuropeptide, has been associated with behaviors such as aggression, territoriality, and enhanced stress responsiveness, and may also be associated with distrust. TES, a hormone, is associated with competition and dominance, and may be associated with reduced personal trust and sociality, although this relationship remains less clearly defined.

Growth and Development

Physical Growth

Infant and child growth is affected by genetic makeup, general health, and nutrition. Infants and children vary in their tempo of growth and development, which tends to be marked by spurts of growth separated by plateaus. Still, there are universal patterns of growth for all children. These universal patterns include cephalocaudal growth (growth that proceeds from head to foot), proximodistal growth (growth that occurs from the center outward), and general-to-specific movements. The infant's head accounts for about one-fourth of the infant's length at birth and illustrates cephalocaudal direction of growth. Maturation of motor skills also follows the cephalocaudal pattern: an infant masters control of his head before he masters arm and trunk control, which is followed by leg control (Figure 17-1).

Proximodistal and general-to-specific development are illustrated by the sequence of muscle control: infants control large muscles before they control small muscles. For example, the child is able to wave "bye-bye" before he is able to grasp with his whole hand and before he is able to hold a small object with his thumb and forefinger (pincer grasp). Some evidence indicates that breastfeeding has a beneficial effect on neurological development in children.

Weight and Length

Change, rather than stability, is the hallmark of infancy; weight increases faster in infancy than at any other time of life. The average neonate weighs about 3000 to 4000 g (6.5–8.5 lb). Because full-term infants are born with excess fluid, they lose 5% to 10% of their birth weight following birth and then stabilize within a few days. Generally speaking, infants double their birth weight by about 5 months of age, triple it by 1 year of age, and quadruple it by 2 years of age.

As discussed earlier in this text, weight patterns of formula-fed infants differ from those of infants who are fed exclusively at the breast. Their

Figure 17-1 PHYSICAL DEVELOPMENT, BIRTH TO 56 WEEKS.

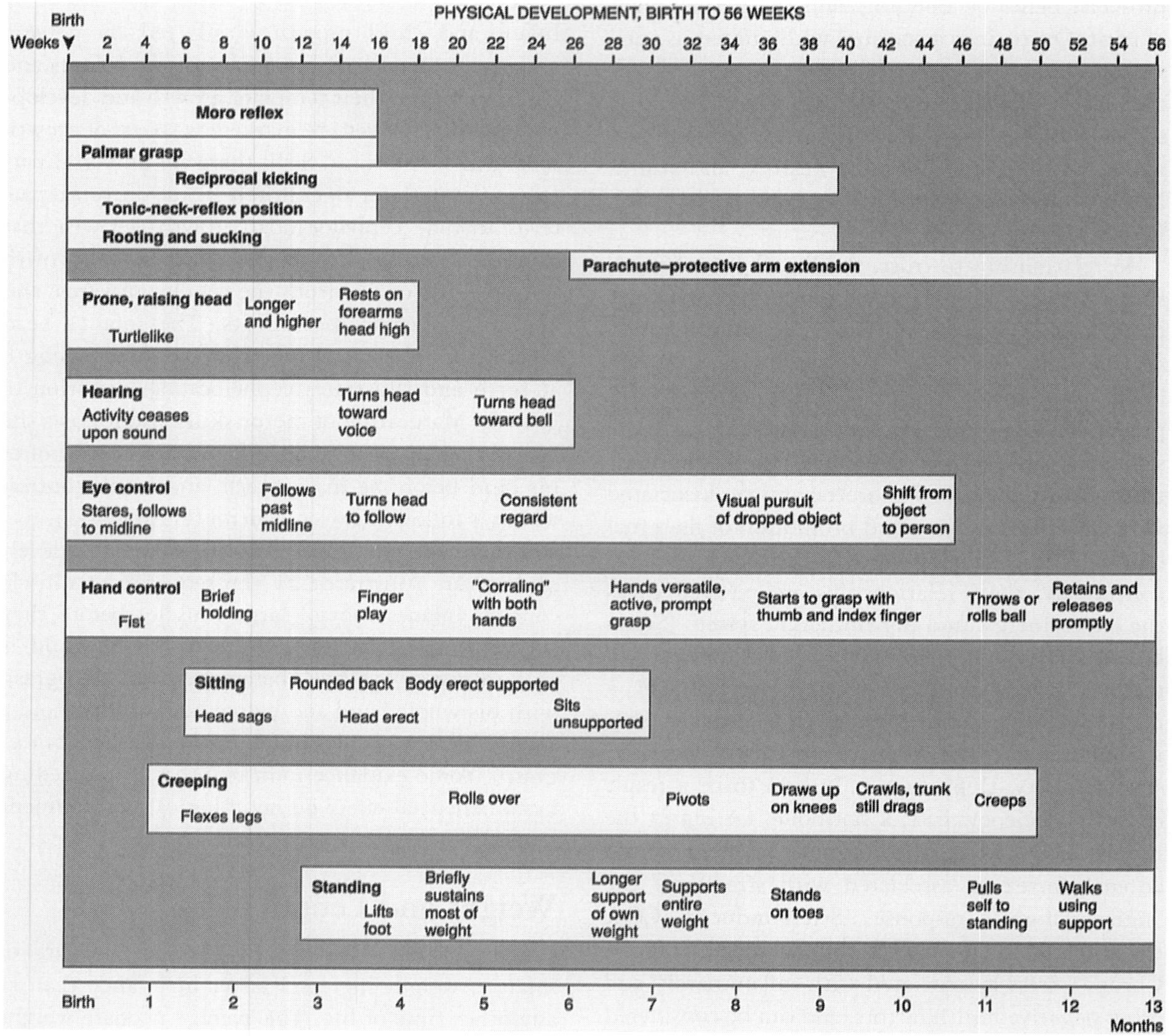

weights are similar for the first few months, but at 3 to 4 months, formula-fed infants begin to weigh more than do their breastfed counterparts. This appears to hold cross-culturally: formula-fed Japanese babies 6 to 8 months old weigh significantly more (135 g) than do those breastfed (Yoneyama et al., 1994). North American breastfed babies gain an average of 35 g (approximately 1 oz) per day at 1 month and 19 g (0.6 oz) per day at

4 months, whereas formula-fed infants gain an average of 34.4 g per day at 1 month and 23 g per day at 4 months. Despite their slightly slower weight gain, breastfed infants at 4 months have more body fat (Butte et al., 1995).

Length at birth is about 50 to 53 cm (20–21 in) and, on average, male infants tend to be 5 oz heavier and 0.5 inch longer than females. A baby grows about 1 inch each month for the first 6 months and about 0.5 inch per month for the next 6 months. By the infant's first birthday, his length has increased by 50%. Length and head-circumference growth are similar for both breastfed and formula-fed infants (Butte et al., 1990). The weight of the baby's brain increases most rapidly during infancy as nerve cells enlarge, become longer and branched, and gain myelin sheathing. By 18 months of age, the infant's brain is 75% of its adult weight. If the infant becomes malnourished, the first growth factor to be affected is weight. Only when malnourishment is severe and long-standing are the infant's length or head circumference compromised.

In 2006, the World Health Organization (WHO) released new International Child Growth Standards for birth to age 5, based on research begun in 1997 on more than 8000 children in six countries: Brazil, Ghana, India, Norway, Oman, and the United States. The new growth charts are based on infants who were exclusively breastfed for 6 months, with the addition of complementary foods after 6 months in addition to continuing breastfeeding. In 2007, WHO released new growth standards for children from 5 to 19 years of age. A detailed description of WHO standards and growth charts can be found online at http://www.who.int/childgrowth /standards/en/ and http://www.who.int/growthref /en/.

Senses

Neonates and young infants have remarkably well-developed sensory capabilities. At birth, infants' auditory nerve tracts have sufficient myelin sheathing to allow them to hear well; they can differentiate various tastes and smells. This ability to selectively respond through their senses enhances infants' early attempts to locate and attach to the nipple and to distinguish between the child's own mother and other individuals.

Within several days after birth, breastfeeding infants respond preferentially to breast or axillary odors from their mother. In striking contrast, bottle-feeders display no evidence of recognizing axillary odors from their mothers. While feeding at the breast, the neonate's nostrils are in close proximity with the mother's bare skin, which provides the opportunity to become familiar with her characteristic odor (Makin & Porter, 1989). When nipple searching was observed in 30 newborns after one of the mother's breasts had been washed and dried to partially eliminate the natural odor, 22 infants selected the unwashed breast. Maternal breast odor elicited mouthing, suggesting that olfactory discrimination helps prepare the infant's brain to expect food, and to initiate breastfeeding. Additionally, when breast odor is present without allowing access to the breast, infants may display heightened arousal (Winberg, 2005).

As early as 2 months before birth, hearing develops in the womb. The fetus is already responding both to internal sounds from the mother and to noises outside the mother. Some young infants, for instance, appear to recognize their mother's favorite soap opera when it comes on television. Neonates discriminate between differences in pitch and can detect the direction of the source of sound. Loud, low sounds are likely to disturb and alarm the infant, whereas soft, high-pitched sounds have a calming effect; therefore, the higher-range tones of the female voice tend to quiet and focus the baby's attention. When one baby starts crying in a nursery, others will do the same. Newborns respond to sound by differentiating the caregiver's voice from that of strangers. They also sense heat, cold, pressure, and pain.

The neonate's vision is less developed because retinal structures and the optic nerve are not yet complete. A neonate focuses mainly on large objects close to his face and sees best at a range of 8 to 12 inches, with 9 inches as the optimum—just about the distance between the baby's face and the mother's face while the baby is being held at the breast level. Neonates are able to follow and track a moving object with their eyes and prefer moving objects to stationary ones.

Babies seem to have an innate visual preference. They prefer more complex stimuli, such as the human face, to a plain surface and will look at a face longer than at other visual patterns. All infants have dark, smoky eyes at birth. Their lids are puffy, and the tear ducts do not function. Eye muscles may occasionally drift to a crossed position, referred to as intermittent strabismus.

The sense of touch seems well developed in infants. For example, when testing vision or hearing, it is important not to stimulate them with touch, as they will respond to the touch—an outcome that may potentially confuse testing results. Sensory stimulation, grooming, licking, and stroking have been studied in the animal kingdom, demonstrating that the amount of time devoted to social grooming in primates exceeds the requirements for cleaning. Grooming is associated with an increase in OXT levels, calming, growth, and social bonding (Dunbar, 2010; Uvnas-Moberg, 1998). The positive effects of sensory stimulation have been demonstrated in infants, especially skin-to-skin contact with preterm infants. In humans, as in mammals, the provision of touch during moments of maternal unavailability reduces infants' physiologic reactivity to stress, as measured by cortisol levels (Feldman et al., 1999). In older children, a daily 5- to 10-minute massage in 4- to 5-year-olds children with aggression and deviant behavior at daycare centers yielded a significant reduction in aggression scores (von Knorring et al., 2008).

As children grow older, sensory deprivation has been associated with developmental delay and attachment disorders. In adults, sensory stimulation, such as massage, is known to improve health and work performance, and to significantly reduce blood pressure, anxiety, and job stress (Ardiel & Rankin, 2010).

Reflexes

The fragile appearance of neonates belies the sophistication of their reflexes, which are designed to enhance survival. Reflexes protect the infant and give the central nervous system and brain time to mature and to begin to govern coordinated behaviors.

Rooting, suckling, swallowing, and gag reflexes are directly applicable to breastfeeding. The rooting reflex initiates the act of suckling milk from the mother's breast and is considered vital to life.

The suck–swallow reflex is presumably developed at 34 weeks' gestation. Synchronized coordination of suckling and swallowing with breathing appears to be achieved consistently by infants of more than 37 weeks' postconception age (Bu'Loc et al., 1990), but many low-birth-weight infants can suckle at the breast. By 3 to 4 months after birth, the rooting reflex begins to diminish. Earlier in this text, we described the infant's oral and suckling capabilities as the cockpit of the nervous system. The presence of rooting, sucking, swallowing, and gag reflexes are barometers that indicate an intact, functioning central nervous system.

Levels of Arousal and Sleep

Young infant behavior can be described by several levels of arousal states (Burns et al., 2013, pp. 256–261; Gill et al., 1988; Prechtl & Beintema, 1975). The Anderson Behavioral State Scale (Gill et al., 1988) lists 15 categories, with states ranging from very quiet sleep to hard crying (Box 17-1). The infant's most complex interaction with his environment is made in the quiet awake state; at this time, the neonate fixates on and follows objects and turns his head toward any sound. It is an excellent time for breastfeeding. The neonate becomes more alert when he senses a new stimulus; if it is repeated, the infant responds less or habituates to the stimulus (Als & Brazelton, 1981). This decrement in response allows the neonate to control his behavioral state. Overactive infants are said to lack this ability to habituate (respond less to repeated stimuli).

Sleep is important to brain organization. Quality and duration of sleep are increasingly being recognized as an essential aspect of health promotion and chronic disease prevention. Chronic sleep disruption in childhood is linked with daytime sleepiness, attention problems, and poor academic performance, and has also been associated with chronic disease, such as diabetes, cardiovascular disease, obesity, depression, attention-deficit/hyperactivity disorder (ADHD), and oppositional symptoms (Cortese et al., 2006; Shur-Fen Gau, 2006;

BOX 17-1 ANDERSON BEHAVIORAL STATE SCALE: BEHAVIORAL STATES

Sleep
Very quiet sleep
Quiet sleep
Restless sleep
Very restless sleep
Quiet awake
Awake
Drowsy
Alert inactivity
Restless
Restless awake
Very restless awake
Fussing
Crying
Hard crying

Source: Data from Gill NE et al. Effect of nonnutritive sucking on behavioral state in preterm infants before feeding. *Nurs Res.* 1988;37:347–350.

Taheri, 2006). Promoting healthy sleep patterns, or good "sleep hygiene," begins in young infants. Circadian rhythms (i.e., the sleep–awake cycles) are regulated by light and dark as well as by the secretion of melatonin, a hormone that promotes sleep. Light suppresses melatonin and darkness promotes melatonin release.

There are two basic alternating sleep cycles: nonrapid eye movement (NREM), or restorative deep, quiet sleep (QS); and rapid eye movement (REM), or active sleep (AS), when the brain is active and dreaming and arousals occur (National Sleep Foundation, 2013). Sleep cycles are initially irregular, with more REM arousal sleep occurring in newborns, but mature into a regular sleep–wake cycle by age 3 to 6 months. Using a consistent daily routine is helpful in establishing sleep–wake cycles. Infants may need a variety of movement, sound, or touch to calm them. Putting the infant to bed while still awake but drowsy may facilitate self-soothing, or self-regulation behavior for going to sleep.

Although infants differ in the number of hours of sleep, each baby gets as much sleep as he needs.

Newborns sleep an average of 16.5 hours per day, with an average range of 12 to 18 hours; some sleep a total of about 10 hours, whereas others sleep up to 23 hours. Generally, infants fuss and cry before falling asleep.

The sleeping pattern of breastfed infants differs from that of formula-fed infants. Breastfed infants wake more often during the night and have shortened sleep patterns (Mosko et al., 1996, 1997). The expression "He sleeps just like a baby" simply is not true during the first few months of life for any infant. The typical pattern is one of frequent, short periods of sleep interrupted by crying and fussing. This normal sleep and arousal pattern occurs night and day, and is not a sleep disorder.

Both emotional and physical closeness can facilitate sleep. In a study of 45 families, the emotional quality of parenting during bedtimes was assessed by means of questionnaires, sleep diaries, direct observation of parent–child interactions, and video monitoring of infant sleep, at ages 1, 3, 6, 12, and 24 months. Results suggest that whatever bedtime practices parents decide to use, the effect of maternal/parent emotional availability and calming at bedtime may be as important, if not more important, than bedtime practices in predicating infant sleep quality (Teti et al., 2010). Another study, comparing 28 relatively healthy preterm infants with control groups, suggests that SSC promotes more mature sleep organization, which may lead to improved brain maturation and positive neurodevelopment. A 2- to 3-hour session, comparing SSC or incubator care between feedings, demonstrated by EEG recordings and sleep observations that the SCC group showed a more mature sleep organization than the control group, with decreased arousals, REM sleep, and indeterminate sleep, and with increased quiet sleep or NREM sleep (Ludington-Hoe et al., 2006).

The American Academy of Pediatrics (AAP, 2011b) has updated recommendations for safe sleeping as well as for avoidance of suffocation and entrapment related to sudden infant death syndrome (SIDS) and other sleep-related disorders in two publications. These recommendations are extensive, but basically include supine positioning; use of a firm sleep surface; breastfeeding; room-sharing without bed-sharing; routine immunization; consideration of a pacifier (after breastfeeding is well established); avoidance of soft or loose bedding and overheating; and avoidance of exposure to tobacco smoke, alcohol, and illicit drugs. During the first year of life, infants should be placed on their back for sleeping; when they can roll from supine to prone position and from prone to supine position, they can be allowed to remain in whichever sleep position they assume. Sleeping in car seats or other sitting devices is not recommended. When cloth carriers or slings are used, ensure that the infant's head and face are visible, and the nose and mouth are clear of obstructions. AAP recommends that infants be brought to bed for feeding, comforting, and bonding, but then returned to the crib when the parent is ready for sleep. Infant beds should meet safety standards, and bed slats should be 2 ⅜ inches apart. Bumper pads, portable bed rails, or wedges on adult beds or couches to prevent infants from falling off are not recommended.

Theories of Development

Nature Versus Nurture

Which is more important in a child's development: nature (genes, heredity) or nurture (environment)? At one end of the spectrum, how a child develops is thought to be determined at conception; at the other end, development is seen as a product of the environment. Although we can demonstrate that breastfeeding appears to optimize development, the issue is still complex. For example, are the overall parenting patterns of a woman who chooses to breastfeed different from those of a woman who chooses to bottle-feed? We cannot say that any one aspect of child development is determined exclusively by either nature or nurture; clearly, each plays a role. The extent of influences from nature versus nurture differ among developmental theorists. How these two issues interact are addressed in two classic theories about child development.

Erikson's Psychosocial Theory

Eric Erikson (1963, 1968) identified stages of development that center on conflicts. These conflicts are central issues of crucial importance to the personality at each stage of life. Characteristics of the first two stages (infant and toddler) of Erikson's theory are shown in Table 17-2. Each stage requires resolution of its particular conflict, and each stage widens the social radius of the infant's influence.

The first conflict is trust versus mistrust. According to Erikson, the first year is when confidence in having one's needs met and feeling physically safe results in the infant's either trusting or mistrusting his environment.

Once trust, as opposed to mistrust, is established, the toddler moves into the next stage, in which autonomy must be mastered over shame and doubt. By then (18 months to 3 years of age), the child walks, runs, and expresses himself verbally, eagerly exploring his exciting new world but still needing reassurance and returning to his mother for "emotional refueling." If an infant is lovingly fed and his biological needs are cared for, he develops

Table 17-2 THEORIES OF DEVELOPMENT

Theorist	Infant	Toddler
Erikson (psychosexual)	Trust versus mistrust (birth–1 year)	Autonomy versus shame and doubt (1–3 year)
	Requires basic needs (food, comfort, warmth) to be met	Increasing independence in eating, dressing, toileting, and bathing
	Learns to trust self (and environment)	Father becomes important
		Limits (firm and consistent) lead to security
	Mutual giving and getting between self and caregivers	Acquires "will"; feeling of self control, bias for self-esteem
	Mistrust results if needs not met consistently or inadequately	
Piaget (cognitive)	Sensorimotor (birth–2 years); uses senses, motor skills, reflexes to explore	Excessive criticism and expectation of perfection leads to shame and doubt about ability to control self and world
	Object permanence	Proconceptual (2–7 years)
	Trial and error	Self-centered; other-centeredness begins
	"Insight" problem solving	Perception from own point of view
	Able to think before acting (18–24 months)	Use of symbols, especially language
		Literal interpretation of works and action
		Judges thing for outcome, consequence to self
		Transductive reasoning

Source: Data from Erikson, 1963; Piaget & Inhelder, 1969.

a sense of trust in the world. Being left hungry or crying for long periods results in a sense of mistrust of the world. Breastfeeding for nourishment becomes breastfeeding for reassurance and comfort in this stage. The process of individuation—a realization that he is a separate individual—unfolds gradually as the child begins to assert control over his life.

Piaget's Cognitive Theory

Jean Piaget (1952) identified the major periods through which humans pass in the course of intellectual maturation. The first is the sensorimotor stage, in which an infant's knowledge of the world comes primarily through his sensory experiences and motor activities. Its main features are presented in Table 17-3.

As infants experience sensory and motor activities, they construct schemas (concepts or models) for dealing with information and experiences. These schemas are put into play through complementary processes of assimilation and accommodation. Assimilation refers to the process of absorbing new information from the environment and using current structures to deal with the information. Accommodation refers to the process by which the infant alters his behavior and adjusts existing schemas to the requirements of objects or events to integrate new learning with old (and thus adapt to his ever-expanding environments). For example, if a child is breastfed, and a pacifier is given to him, the pacifier nipple may be sufficiently different so that the old sucking patterns do not work well. When this happens, disequilibrium occurs, and the child must restructure the existing view of suckling so that it fits with the new information or experience (accommodation). Through these processes, schemas are developed and refined.

Table 17-3 CHARACTERISTICS OF INFANTS' THINKING: SENSORIMOTOR STATE

Major Task

Conquest of Object

Throughout this stage, infants are unable to think. Intelligence proceeds from directly acting, as a whole, on the environment to more goal-directed attending to and action on particular objects to make specific events occur. All the senses and motor skills are actively used to define and interpret objects and events.

Perception

- *Birth–3 months:* View of world and self undifferentiated; unconscious of self.
- *4–6 months:* View of world centered around body; self-centered.
- *After 6 months:* View of world as centered around objects.
- *6–12 months:* Self seen as separated from objects.
- *12–18 months:* Objects seen to have constancy and permanence.
- *18–24 months:* Represents spatial relationships between objects and between objects and self (e.g., knows smaller things fit inside larger things).

Thought

- *Birth–3 months:* Not present. Uses inborn reflexes and senses.
- *4–6 months:* Questions presence of thought. Uses combination of reflexes and senses purposively. Develops habits.
- *6–12 months:* Knows objects by how he or she uses them. Knows objects have constant size before knows objects have same form; serially acts out two previously separate behaviors in goal-directed sequences.
- *12–24 months:* Object permanence stimulates purposive, intentional use of behaviors to find hidden objects and to cause event via trial and error—problem solve via "insight": can now see effect when given the cause (e.g., knows where train will come out when it goes into tunnel). Symbolism and memory begin—uses deferred imitation to discover new ways of acting (e.g., when "pretends" sleep means "know" symbolic sleeping).

Reasoning

- *Birth–6 months:* Not present.
- *6–24 months:* Syncretism (1) perceives "whole"—impression without analysis of parts or synthesis of relations, (2) lacks systematic exploratory behavior until end of state, (3) begins to connect series of ideas into a confused whole.

Language

- *Birth–3 months:* Undifferentiated cry. Use of different intensities, patterns, and pitches of cry for different feelings (e.g., pain, hunger, fatigue).
- *6–8 weeks:* Cooing: contented and happy sounds.
- *3–6 months:* Babbling: repeated various sounds for sensation of pleasure. Laughing: when happy or excited.
- *6–12 months:* Spontaneous vocalization: imperfect imitation. Echolalia: conscious imitation of sounds.
- *12–18 months:* Expressive jargon: use of information, rhythms, and pauses to imitate sentence sounds.
  Holophrases: use of one word to convey meaning.
  Gestures: substitute for or add meaning to speech.
- *18–24 months:* Telegraphic speech: use of noun and verb to convey many meanings.

Table 17-3 CHARACTERISTICS OF INFANTS' THINKING: SENSORIMOTOR STATE (CONTINUED)

Play

- *Birth–6 months:* Exercise play: repetition of actions and sounds for pleasure (e.g., rolling over, babbling).
- *6–12 months:* Exploratory play: pleasure from causing effect and reconfirming skill (e.g., "peek-a-boo," "drop and retrieve," "pat-a-cake").
- *12–24 months:* Deferred imitation: imitates previously observed actions (not reasons for or purposes of actions) from memory (e.g., pretends to be "Daddy" and goes through getting dressed, shaving, then walks outside, and gets in the "car").

Source: Data from Servonsky J., Opas S. Nursing Management of Children. Boston, Mass: Jones & Bartlett; 1997:22.

The concept of object permanence is a feature of the sensorimotor period. Piaget (1952) suggested that the infant younger than 6 to 9 months of age lacks the ability to engage in mental representation of the unseen. For instance, when an object such as a toy is out of sight, it ceases to exist, and the infant does not search for it. With the ability for mental representation, the infant realizes that an object or person continues to exist when out of sight, and he searches for a hidden object. It is now quite certain that person permanency precedes object permanency; an infant does recognize his mother, father, or caretaker long before 8 months and experiences loss or anxiety when an all-important person is not present. Later, as the child broadens the ability to recognize a separate existence from his mother, he begins to tolerate brief periods of separation from different caretakers. The ability roughly coincides with diminishing separation anxiety and with Erikson's establishment of trust progressing to the beginnings of autonomy.

Social Development

As infants grow, their periods of waking and socializing lengthen. By 2 to 8 weeks of age, a baby smiles spontaneously to pleasurable stimuli, particularly at human faces. Babies coo and babble to their parents and other fascinated adults who coo and babble back. By 3 months, the infant is interested in his environment and playfully reaches out to grasp objects, including breasts, nipples, noses, and hair. By 6 months of age, the infant reaches out to be picked up, squeals with pleasure at recognition of his mother, and enjoys games such as peek-a-boo.

Language and Communication

Because infants hear well from birth, they are able to discriminate between different intonations and between vowels and consonants. This ability to understand the spoken word is called passive, or receptive, language. The ability to produce meaningful utterances is called expressive language. The speech center in the brain borders on the areas of the motor cortex that control both mouth–tongue movement and hand movement. This proximity explains why we tend to express ourselves with both our hands and our mouths. Infants likewise use many gestures in association with sounds and expressive language. Children consistently acquire language communication in a definable sequence (Figure 17-2):

- Crying—from birth; different rhythms signifying emotions and needs (hunger, anger, pain)
- Cooing and gooing—starting after birth; a wide variety of meaningless speech sounds
- Babbling—3 to 12 months ("mama-mama," "dada-dada")
- Holophrasing—12 months; one-word sentences

Figure 17-2 ADAPTIVE-SOCIAL DEVELOPMENT, BIRTH TO 56 WEEKS.

ADAPTIVE - SOCIAL DEVELOPMENT, BIRTH TO 56 WEEKS

Birth
Weeks ▼ 2 4 6 8 10 12 14 16 18 20 22 24 26 28 30 32 34 36 38 40 42 44 46 48 50 52 54 56

Crying
Tearless hunger cry — Differentiable — May stop when mother appears — Crying reduced — Cries easily — Vocalizes "m-m-m" while crying; Rapid changes from tears to smiles — Increased frustration cry

Language
Infant mews — Babbles, coos — Blows bubbles — Coos; carries on "conversation" — "Talks" to toys or self — "Da-da" "ma-ma" (not meaningful) — Adjusts to "where is the ..." and "bye-bye" — Waves bye-bye — Adjusts to simple commands — Responds to "where is the shoe?" by looking for shoe

Smile
Responds to social stimulation by smiling — Laughs aloud, initiates social contact by smile — Smiles at mirror image

Socializing
Enjoys cuddling and motion — Responds to presence of people — Visually pursues moving person — Knows mother; stares at strangers — Shows interest in father and sibling — Fear of strangers; affection for family group appears — Waves hands — Increasing imitation — May release object on request — Actively solicits attention — Offers object to mother or acquaintance

Feeding
Extrusion reflex disappears — Some ability to wait for food — Easy to feed; pats breast — Mouthing of nipple largely disappears

Interst in self
Puts everything in mouth, plays contentedly alone — Reaches for mirror image — Smiles at mirror image — Approaches mirror image socially, even vocalizes

Birth 1 2 3 4 5 6 7 8 9 10 11 12 13
Months

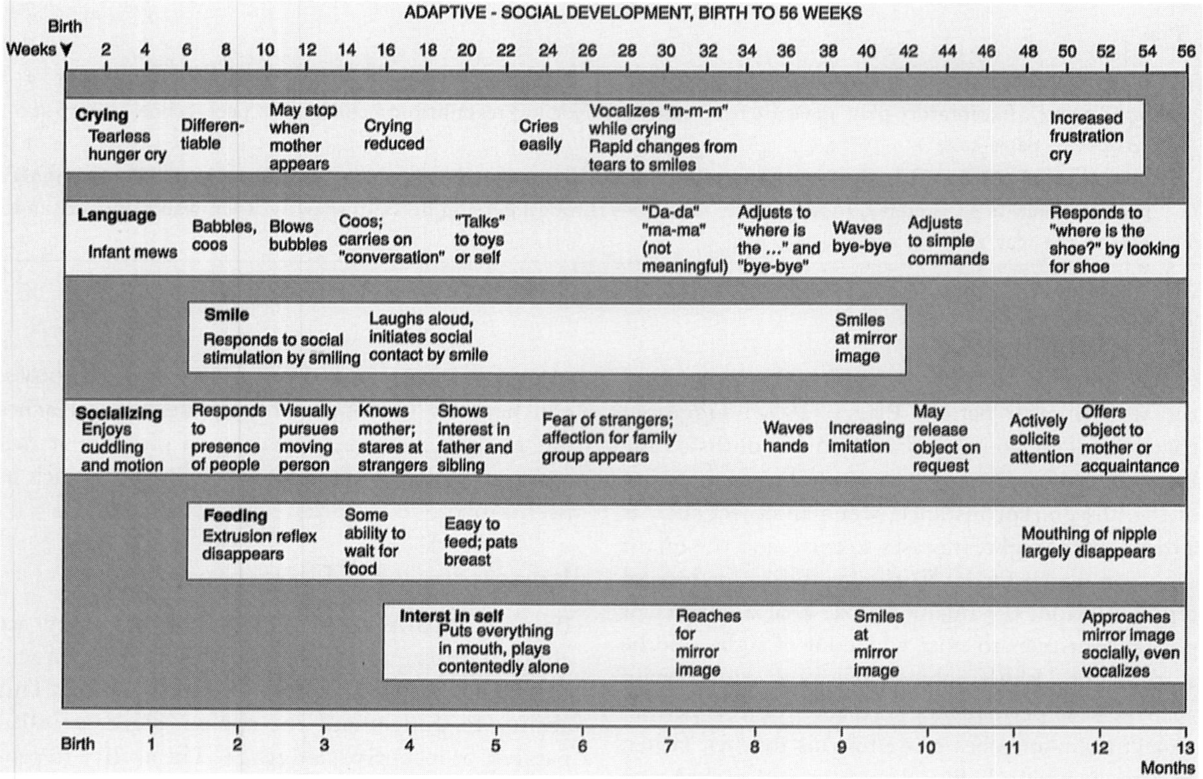

- Telegraphic speech—18 months; subject–verb–object
- Complete sentences—2 years

The duration of a baby's crying during the early months of life typically increases until about 6 weeks of age, followed by a gradual decrease until 4 months of age. Infants cry more and are more wakeful during the late afternoon and evening. If the infant is carried during fussy periods, crying and fussing decrease, but the number of feedings and the duration of his sleep do not change (McKenna et al., 1997).

Mothers and babies interact with each other using a variety of communications that are visual, vocal, tactile, and postural. Babies coo, goo, and babble whenever they are alert and content. These sounds change from week to week and are elicited by the smiling faces of adults, by voices, or by touch. Any mother who has breastfed knows that feeding at the breast is a prime time for her baby to communicate actively with coos, babbling, and speech sounds as he looks into the eyes of his mother (Figure 17-3). These exquisite sensory interchanges further strengthen the bond between mother and baby.

Epstein (1993) videotaped breastfeeding mothers and their babies during feedings to investigate maternal–infant interactions. These videos were later observed and analyzed. The interactions between the mothers and infants were elaborate and complex, with each breastfeeding dyad interacting with its own individual style. All of the mothers

Figure 17-3 MUTUAL CAREGIVING PROMOTES THE MATERNAL ROLE-TAKING PROCESS.

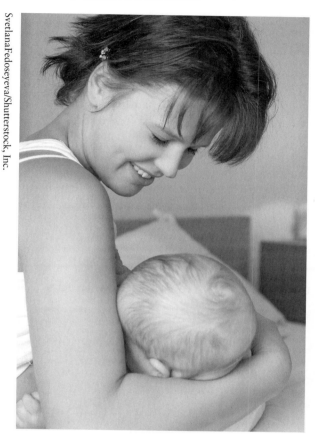

SvetlanaFedoseyeva/Shutterstock, Inc.

Mothers speak to their infants in a universal dialogue that instinctively uses exaggerated upbeat tones and facial gestures to talk to babies. Mothers use slowly rising crescendo and decrescendo allowing the baby time to process each short vocal package before the next communication arrives. How a mother talks to her baby is more important than what she says.

This sing-song quality of the mother's speech is tailored to the baby's listening abilities. Smiling, grasping, and talking all play important roles in the attachment process (i.e., the reciprocal development of an affectional tie between the mother or caregiver and the baby) (Pridham & Chang, 1992). During these interactions, the mother not only gives care to her infant but the newborn also gives care back to his mother. For this reason, Anderson (1977) called the mother and infant "mutual caregivers" (p. 53):

> As the mother holds her infant to her breast, assumes the en face position, and talks to her newborn, her eyes are the optimal distance away and her head, mouth, and eyes move slowly and within a closely circumscribed range. Her newborn will also be sending stimuli, such as changes in facial expression, vocalizations, and eye-to-eye contact. This mother's response to such stimuli is immediate.

In a review of the theoretical framework for studying factors that affect the maternal role, Mercer (1981) emphasized the role of the infant in his mother's maternal role-taking process. The newborn's ability to see, hear, and track the human face shows socialization capabilities at birth that allow the infant to be an active partner with the mother in the attachment process. Each new infant presents a challenge to maternal adaptation, and previous experience with infants makes little difference to becoming the parent of a new child. Moreover, the transition process of being mother to a new infant is different in the second and third months from the process in the first month (Pridham & Chang, 1992). Breastfeeding plays an important role in a mother's feelings of competence. Indeed, Tarkka (2003) reported that breastfeeding was a main predictor

and babies looked at their partners' bodies, not just at their faces, during the breastfeeding session. All of the mothers had happy and affectionate expressions on their faces as they watched their babies, yet the amount of time they maintained the positive expression differed between mothers. Certain babies in the study even smiled and laughed with their mother's nipples in their mouths. Babies and mothers were observed vocalizing to one another. In some dyads, intricate vocal interactions occurred. Babies made sounds that their mothers initiated, which resulted in the babies continuing to make sounds and the mothers continuing to imitate them. In all of these cases, the sounds that the babies made seemed to be expressions of pleasure.

of a woman's competence as a mother. Competence was measured as the ability to make independent childcare decisions, to find pleasure in parenthood, and to meet the demands of being a parent.

The infant uses play as a part of the communication process. During the earliest (sensorimotor) stage of life, infants begin with exercise play, such as repeating newly learned actions for pleasure. Stick out your tongue at a young infant, and he will stick out his tongue at you. Next, infants play to explore their skills, crawling backward down the stairs, for example, or pushing a finger into the mother's mouth while breastfeeding and then squealing with glee when she pretends to bite the finger (Figure 17-4). The older baby's playful activities as he breastfeeds are a part of communication and attachment with his mother. Deferred imitation play begins at around 18 months of age, when toddlers begin to imitate the behavior and language they see and hear. For example, little girls, who are already adopting the gender role of their mothers, will very seriously and readily "nurse" their dolls at their breasts (Figure 17-5).

Attachment and Bonding

This exquisite dance of reciprocal reinforcement in the mother–infant dyad leads to the mother's "taking in" her maternal role, cementing the mother–infant bond. Early theorists paved the way for understanding the processes of bonding and attachment. Konrad Lorenz (1935) noted the behavior and imitation of the mother animal by the young, which is necessary for survival, and labeled it imprinting. It is believed that attachment and bonding are the human equivalent of imprinting.

Figure 17-4 DEVELOPING MOTOR SKILLS BY EXPLORING THE ENVIRONMENT.

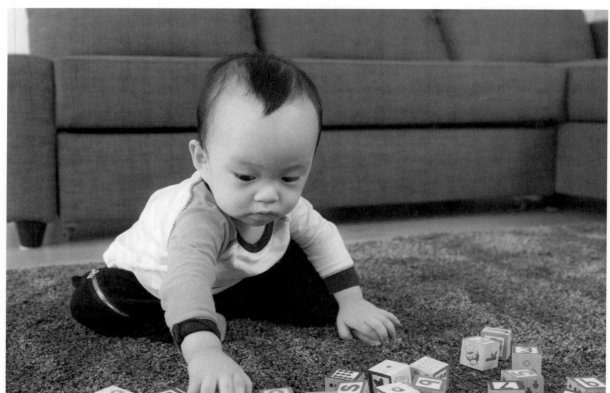

leungchopan/ShutterStock, Inc.

Figure 17-5 A CHILD "NURSING" A DOLL.

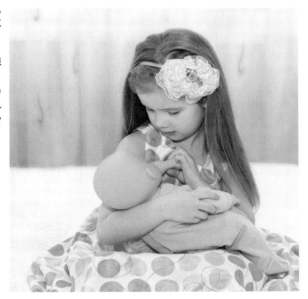

Svitlana-ua/ShutterStock, Inc.

Bowlby's seminal paper (1958), which introduced the principles of attachment theory, emphasized the importance of an infant's developing a primary attachment to a caring, responsible adult. Later, Harlow and Harlow (1965) demonstrated the importance of contact comfort for the attachment and emotional well-being of the newborn rhesus monkey. When presented with "surrogate" mothers—one formed out of unpadded chicken wire and equipped with milk-filled bottles, the other made out of padded terry cloth but without bottles—the baby monkeys spent much more time with the warm, cloth-covered mothers, going only briefly to the bottles for food.

Mothers who room-in with their infants after birth touch their infants' face and head more often than do mothers who have minimal contact with their newborn (Prodromidis et al., 1995). Rubin (1967) showed a progressive attachment that results from touching: a mother first explores her newborn's extremities with her fingertips, rapidly moves to the baby's arms and legs, and finally caresses the trunk with the palm of her hand. A conceptual model for the maternal–infant bonding might well be like the weaving of a tapestry. Rubin (p. 240) described bonding as follows:

> Not a cord, nor a bond, nor a welding job, rather a large creative work, framed between the child and the mother's own significant social world, systematically and progressively developed for durability against time and stress to form the substance of her own personal identity and the fabric of her relationship with this particular child.

Ainsworth et al. (1978) studied brief infant separation from mothers in a laboratory situation to measure the degree of attachment. Mothers defined by the researchers as "securely attached" to their infants were most sensitive to their baby's needs, whereas mothers identified as "insecurely attached" to their infants were less emotionally expressive, felt more aversion to close body contact with the babies, and were more frequently irritated, resentful, and angry. A multitude of circumstances affect the mother–child relationship, which begins before the child is born; even though the baby is unseen, the mother imagines or fantasizes about her child.

Strathearn, Fonagy, et al. (2009) studied the neuroendocrine basis of human mother–infant attachment with 30 first-time mothers, using adult attachment interviews, temperament and behavioral questionnaires, maternal–infant social interaction and "en face" infant cues, functional MRI scanning, and serum levels of OXT, free COR, epinephrine, and norepinephrine to test whether differences in attachment were related to brain reward and peripheral OXT response to infant cues. These studies were conducted in four phases: (1) prenatal attachment patterns, (2) videotaping and OXT sampling at 7 months, (3) MRI scanning at 11 months, and (4) assessment of child development at 14 months. On viewing their own infants' smiling and crying faces, mothers with secure attachment showed greater peripheral OXT response and activation of DOP-associated circuits and brain reward regions. Insecure or dismissing mothers showed distancing in response to their own infant's sad faces, and increased brain activation in regions associated with feelings of unfairness, pain, and disgust. These results suggest that insecure mothers may interpret their own infant's face as representing an omitted reward, which may lead to avoidance or rejection of negative infant cues. This information may also help to better understand attachment patterns across generations and determine how secure maternal attachment may facilitate developmental advantages for children.

These early parent–child attachments form the foundation for trust. Impaired trust, attachment, and bonding heralds a negative psychosocial outcome, and may be associated with child neglect, a prevalent and increasing form of child abuse/maltreatment. Neglected children are more likely to develop a non-organic failure to thrive; show a progressive decline in cognitive functioning over time, more delayed language development, and less competent social and academic functioning; and are at increased risk for developing childhood aggression (Strathearn, 2011; Tomlinson & Landman, 2007). When Strathearn Mamun, et al. (2009) investigated whether breastfeeding was protective against maternally perpetrated maltreatment, they concluded that breastfeeding, among other factors, may help protect against maternally perpetrated child neglect (omission of appropriate child care). In their study, a total of 7223 Australian mother–infant dyads were monitored prospectively over 15 years. Maternal maltreatment increased as breastfeeding duration decreased. After adjusting for confounding, the odds ratio for nonbreastfed infants was 2.6 times higher than for breastfed infants. Other risk factors were observed as well. Cultural risk factors included limited social support, young maternal age, unplanned pregnancy, low education unemployment, and poverty. Parent-related risk factors included anxiety and depression. Child-related risk factors included prematurity.

Biological systems identified as contributing to maternal caregiving behavior focus on OXT and DOP, as these substances affect reward pathways in response to social cues. In a mother with insecure attachment, which may be associated with emotional neglect, Strathearn (2011) noted reduced brain activation of the DOP reward system in response to infant face cues, and decreased peripheral OXT response to mother–infant contact.

Research to test whether the administration of intranasal OXT could reverse some of these neurological differences is ongoing. OXT release during lactation appears to exert long-term anxiolytic and bonding effects through changes in specific brain regions. This information may contribute to efforts geared toward decreasing maternal neglect (Strathearn, 2011; Uvnas-Moberg, 1997).

The mother's perceptions of the "dream child" and, subsequently, her relationship with that child will not only be influenced by her self-concept but also by her total life experience. Her culture, social relationship, economic status, and state of health can all add to or detract from her relationship with her unborn child. If she experiences social isolation and economic deprivation during her pregnancy, her emotional reserves will be lowered. If she experiences physical discomfort and ill health, her physical stamina may be depleted. Thus the support she receives during pregnancy and from her total environment will affect her acceptance and readiness for mothering.

The infant's birth forces the mother to compare her real-life baby with her dreams, fantasies, and expectations. If reality and expectations are congruent, attachment begins soon after birth; if they are divergent, the mother must first work through the loss of the "dream child" and strive to fall in love with this stranger who bears little resemblance to the child of her fantasies.

Klaus and Kennell (1975) moved the concept of attachment one step further by popularizing the existence of a sensitive period for attachment shortly after birth. Barring excessive medication of the mother during delivery, a newborn will normally be in an alert state for at least 1 hour following birth. During this period, the mother will spend a significant amount of time gazing en face (face to face) into her infant's eyes, touching, and stroking. The neonate is born in a state of readiness for this human interaction. The infant's remarkable perceptual and sensory abilities (hearing, seeing, smelling, and tasting) at birth facilitate the attachment process. As attachment becomes established, the newborn is observed to move his arms and legs in rhythm to the cadences of the mother's voice, in a synchronous pattern that may be the foundation for later speech (Condon & Sander, 1974). Such interaction is known as entrainment, and its effects carry over into later life (Figure 17-6).

An active partner in the attachment process, the infant initiates about half of the parent–infant interaction. Through predictable and clear-cut transmission of cues or nonverbal signals, neonates are capable of producing the desired behavior in the parent and selectively reinforcing parent behavior. In many ways, the infant is as competent as the parents, and perhaps even more so than young, inexperienced parents.

The baby's cry is an impossible-to-ignore cue for attention, and his mother responds by picking up, feeding, or carrying him. The perceptive mother is attuned to her baby's cues and reacts to them appropriately. If he coos and smiles, she reacts happily to his pleasure. The infant's contentment or irritability signal the mother to increase or decrease stimulation. If parents are aware of these cues as a method of communication for their infant, they respond

---

Figure 17-6 COMPONENTS OF ATTACHMENT.

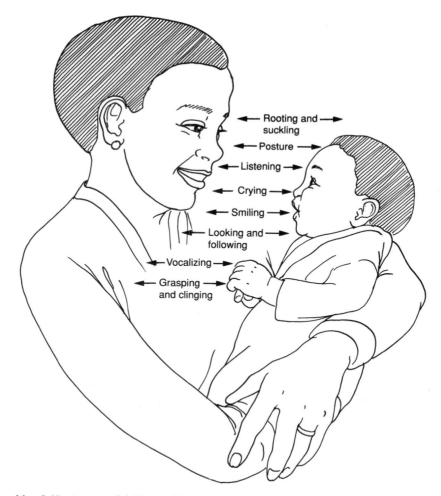

Source: Adapted from Mott S. *Nursing care of children and families.* Boston: Addison-Wesley; 1993:206.

by viewing their infants as individuals. Informing mothers about the behavioral characteristics of their babies is an effective means of enhancing the interaction between mothers and their infants (Anderson, 1981; Strathearn, 2011).

Breastfeeding, with its frequent touching, holding, and eye-to-eye contact, offers enhanced opportunities for attachment and responding to infant cues. Certainly, the frequency of subjective verbal responses by mothers who state that they "feel closer" to the breastfed child merits serious consideration. Through breastfeeding, the infant may exert more control—for example, the decision to end the feeding is a shared decision between the mother and baby when the mother "reads" and responds to her baby's behaviors. In bottle-feeding, in contrast, the mother is chiefly responsible for ending the feeding.

Maternal bonding consists of two global aspects: the first is related to preoccupations with infant safety, the second concerns developing a selective and unique bond with the baby. Even mothers of normal healthy babies experience thoughts and worries. Initial separation increases these preoccupations (Feldman et al., 1999).

Increasingly scientists are recognizing the role of developing self-regulatory skills as important to developing higher-level intellectual functioning. In a study of 267 mother–child dyads, cognitive development, self-regulation, and delay of gratification were measured in children age 5 to 7 years, with the use of cognitive testing and "gummy bear" rewards. The study showed better cognitive development, increased ability to delay self-gratification as the child's age increased, and duration of breastfeeding were significant predictors of self-regulation and delay of gratification in children, even after other variables were controlled (Drobetz et al., 2012). The authors further pointed out that duration of breastfeeding may be protective against obesity and ADHD, as both of these conditions are associated with self-regulatory deficits. Nisbett et al. (2012) described self-regulatory behaviors, or self-discipline, in older children as being able to wait in line, controlling desire to call out in class, and persevering at tasks that may be boring or difficult.

The common practices today of rooming-in and mother–baby care in maternity care were the result of many studies of maternal–infant attachment and bonding in the 1970s that demonstrated that mother–baby contact was associated with stronger attachment. Mother–infant touching, skin-to-skin contact, and kangaroo mother care (KMC) increase the incidence and duration of exclusive or nearly exclusive breastfeeding and strengthen mother–infant bonding, both in healthy term infants and in preterm and very preterm infants, who are at increased risk for long-term ill health problems and infections. In low-birth-weight infants, KMC has been found to reduce mortality, morbidity, length of hospital stay, and financial costs; and to increase infant growth, breastfeeding, and mother–infant attachment (Anderson et al., 2003; Conde-Agudelo et al., 2011; Flacking et al., 2011).

Numerous published reports relating to the safety, efficacy, and feasibility of kangaroo care have associated it with both immediate and long-term effects (Anderson, Moore, et al., 2003). In a survey of U.S. neonatal intensive care units, about 80% were found to practice some form of kangaroo care in their units (Engler et al., 2002). Kangaroo care is now commonly practiced in neonatal care units both in the United States and worldwide. Case Western Reserve University nurse researchers Gene Cranston Anderson (Anderson et al., 2001; Anderson, Chiu, et al. 2003b) and Susan Ludington-Hoe (Ludington-Hoe & Swinth 1996; Ludington-Hoe et al., 2000) have led clinical research teams that study kangaroo care.

The intervention of skin-to-skin contact may be critical for mothers, especially those who have low-birth-weight babies or are otherwise unable to take their infants home. By promoting skin-to-skin touching, kangaroo care builds the components of bonding and even has been shown to increase the volume of breastmilk production (Hurst et al., 1997). The positive encounter of SSC provides a bonding experience that helps to offset the mother's experience of loss, thereby avoiding bonding failure (Anderson et al., 2003).

Although immediate postpartum mother–child contact is desirable, it is no longer considered critical. Almost all parents are attached to their babies, even if they experience marked disruption of the early parent–child contact, which most healthy mothers and babies now take for granted. For example, Hedberg-Nyqvist and Ewald (1997) found that Swedish infants who were separated from their mothers on the first day because they were ill or because of a complicated delivery breastfed for as many months as did those who had immediate contact with their mothers. Parents should be assured that not having the opportunity to interact and bond with their baby soon after birth will not cause irreparable damage to their child.

The 1991 WHO/UNICEF Baby-Friendly Hospital Initiative (BFHI) and "Ten Steps to Successful Breastfeeding" (also discussed in the *Tides in Breastfeeding Practice* chapter) have been adopted in many countries, and have national support from the U.S. Surgeon General's Call to Action and the Centers for Disease Control and Prevention for facilitating breastfeeding practices. The BFHI emphasizes rooming-in, breastfeeding within 1 hour of birth, and exclusive breastfeeding on demand. Studies show that mothers who breastfeed within the first hour of birth are significantly more likely to be exclusively breastfeeding 2 to 4 weeks after delivery (DiFrisco et al., 2011). In the United States, The Joint Commission has expanded performance requirements for accredited hospitals to include the perinatal measurement set, including exclusive breastmilk feeding in the hospital, becoming mandatory for hospitals with 1100 or more births per year, effective January 1, 2014 (Joint Commission Release, 2012).

A large study by DelBono and Rabe (2012), based on the U.K. Millennium Cohort, showed that in hospitals that participated in the UNICEF BFHI, breastfeeding initiation rates increased by as much as 15%, and rates of exclusive breastfeeding at 4 and 8 weeks increased by 8% to 9%, compared to nonparticipating hospitals. This study found significant positive effects of breastfeeding on cognitive outcomes throughout childhood as well as improvement in child emotional development and maternal mental health.

A non-SSC variation of KMC involving the use of baby carriers was studied by Pisacane et al. (2012). In this investigation, mothers used comfortable baby carriers with their newborns for at least 1 hour per day during the first month of life. Breastfeeding rates were similar in both the intervention and control groups at hospital discharge, but higher at the 2- and 5-month follow-ups for the intervention group that used the baby carriers. These results suggest that the use of simple baby carriers in healthy term infants during the first month of life may be associated with increased breastfeeding.

Temperament

Researchers have studied the temperament of the infant and how it influences parenting. The longitudinal work of Thomas and Chess (1977) suggested that every child exhibits a particular temperament from birth and that (1) infants have individual characteristics even as newborns, (2) these characteristics differentiate infants one from another, and (3) they remain constant over time. Categories of response that influence a child's temperament include activity level, regularity of body functions, adaptability, response to new situations, sensory threshold, intensity of reaction, quality of mood, distractibility, and attention span and persistence. These characteristics were rated for three temperaments: the easy child, the difficult child, and the slow-to-warm-up child. These characteristic temperament styles are profiled in Table 17-4.

Sears (1987) reduced these three temperament characteristics to two categories—that is, high-need and low-need babies—and popularized the concept for parents to understand and use. High-need babies are fussy, seem to breastfeed "all the time," and cry if put down; low-need babies are content and cuddly and do not need constant carrying or attention.

Two questionnaires or tools used for assessing the temperament of an infant or child are the Infant Temperament Questionnaire (ITQ) for infants 4 to 12 months of age (Carey & McDevitt, 1978) and the Toddler Temperament Scale for children 1 to 3 years of age (Hegvik et al., 1982). The ITQ scores identify a child's temperamental style; the results

Table 17-4 CHARACTERISTICS OF TEMPERAMENT STYLES IN CHILDREN

Factor	Easy Child	Slow-to-Warm-Up Child	Difficult Child
Activity level—amount of physical activity during sleep, feeding, play, dressing	High	Medium	Low
Regularity—of body functions in sleep, hunger, bowel movements	Fairly regular	Variable	Fairly irregular
Adaptability to change in routine—ease or difficulty to adapt with which initial response can be modified in socially desirable way	Generally adaptable	Variable	Generally slow
Response to new situations—initial reaction to new stimuli, foods, people, places, toys, or procedures	Approach	Variable	Withdrawal
Level of sensory threshold— amount of external stimulation, such as sounds necessary to or changes in food or people, produce a response	High threshold (much stimulation needed)	Medium threshold	Low threshold (little stimulation needed)
Intensity of response—energy content of responses regardless of their quality	Generally intense	Variable	Generally mild
Positive or negative mood—energy content of responses regardless of their quality	Generally positive	Variable	Generally negative
Distractibility—effectiveness of external stimuli (sounds, toys, people) in interfering with ongoing behavior	Easily distractible	Variable	Nondistractible
Persistence and attention span—duration of maintaining specific activities with or without external obstacles	Persistent	Variable	Nonpersistent
Percentage of all children	40%	15%	10%

Source: Data from Carey (1978); Servonsky & Opas (1987, p. 180).

may be used as an opportunity for making parents aware of their child's temperament and for suggesting appropriate parenting skills.

More recently, the Infant Toddler Temperament Tool (IT3; http://www.ecmhc.org/temperament/) was developed by the Center for Early Childhood Mental Health Consultation at Georgetown University, as part of work funded by the Office of Head Start. The IT3 allows parents of infants and toddlers to recognize and explore their own temperament traits and those of the child. The tool results support parents in understanding how adult and child similarities and differences in temperament traits may affect relationships.

Stranger Distress

As the infant grows older, the significance of his major caregiver is recognized and, during the second half of the first year of life, another developmental phenomenon appears: stranger distress. The infant who up to that time has been curious about everything in his environment, including strangers, suddenly frowns and cries and may even attempt physical escape when a stranger approaches. Stranger distress appears quite suddenly as early as 6 months but more commonly at 8 months. It is more pronounced when the mother or primary caretaker is not present. As a consequence, exposure to a variety of strangers is disruptive to an infant at this age. Although stranger distress occurs at about the same period of development as that of separation anxiety, it is a separate phenomenon.

Separation Anxiety

As the mother or father leaves the room, anxious eyes follow. Almost instantly, the child's face is contorted by rage; he cries loudly and may throw himself wildly about, kicking and screaming. No action brings solace at this point. This behavior is the first phase of separation anxiety, a phenomenon that emerges toward the middle of the first year of life, peaks from 13 to 20 months, and decreases after the second birthday. Separation anxiety, according to psychoanalytic theory, is the painful effect of anxiety engendered by the threat of actual separation from a loved one. Bowlby (1973) and Robertson (1958) delineated three phases of separation anxiety in young children: (1) protest, (2) despair, and (3) denial.

Protest

In an angry and yearning attempt to recover his mother or primary caregiver, the child violently cries and throws himself about, kicking and screaming. He is angry with the world and with his mother for leaving him. He feels that she must be angry with him as well, because she left him. The protest phase can last from a few hours to several days, depending on the energy of the child, his age, his relationship with his mother, and the quality of the new environment.

Despair

Gradually, the child moves into quiet grieving and mourning as he begins to accept his fate. He shows little interest in his environment but suffers intensely; his expression is one of great sadness. Regressive behavior, such as thumb sucking, occurs as the child turns inward for solace.

Detachment or Denial

The child develops a defense mechanism to deal with his loss by detaching himself from the importance of his mother's love. He gradually begins to interact with others, approaching anyone and even appearing cheerful. This stage is often misinterpreted as adapting or "settling in." Actually, he is coping with his loss by indiscriminately attaching to caretakers. When he is reunited with his mother at this point, he may appear uninterested and may not seem to recognize her.

Clinical Implications

Deviations from normal patterns of attachment signal that a problem may be present; hence assessing the infant's or child's growth and developmental level—and being able to apply a working knowledge of developmental patterns—is as important as knowing the specifics of a child's health problem. If a baby is being examined, for example, the close proximity of his mother helps to reduce stranger distress. Although clothing that appears "friendly" (nonwhite) helps to ameliorate the baby's distress, by no means does it prevent his crying and avoidance behavior as the examiner approaches him, especially for the first time.

How can healthcare workers who are strangers to the child minimize this fear? First, take advantage of his attachment to his mother by relating to the mother first in the presence of the child. During this interaction with his mother, the child is carefully observing her response to and acceptance of the "stranger" and will take cues from her. Even body position is important; turning slightly sideways away from the child to avoid en face contact while talking with the mother is less threatening to the child. Spitz (1946) demonstrated in one of his films that when a stranger approaches with his back to the child, the child becomes curious and will even reach out after a bit and tug at the stranger. Using a soft, low voice rather than a loud or high-pitched tone is more pleasing to the child and facilitates his acceptance of this new person in his life.

Nursing and medicine have made great progress in recognizing and applying development theories in practice. Because a comprehensive listing and discussion of developmental assessment and screening tools is not within the scope of this text, we refer the reader to the many excellent references that discuss child development in detail. In addition, we remind the reader of the use of assessment tools, such as the Bayley Scales of Infant Development, Denver Development Screening Test, Denver Prescreening Developmental Questionnaire (PDQ II), Ages and Stages Questionnaires (ASQ-3), Modified Checklist for Autism in Toddlers (M-CHAT), and Brazelton Neonatal Behavior Assessment Scale.

Breastfeeding, in addition to providing maternal and child health benefits, is important in establishing healthy mother–infant attachments and trust. Clinical support of breastfeeding may be an important educational or training process for helping new mothers for secure bonds with their new infants.

Immunizations

Immunizations have greatly reduced the incidence of childhood diseases worldwide. Many infections that contributed to high infant mortality in the past can now be prevented through a series of immunizations. Additionally, a number of combination vaccines that reduce the number of injections required are available and generally preferred over separate injections of equivalent component vaccines. The exact timing of the immunizations is not as important as the fact that the child eventually receives the complete immunization series. The United States Recommended Childhood Immunization Schedules are approved and published annually by the Advisory Committee on Immunization Practices (ACIP) of the Centers for Disease Control and Prevention (CDC), the American Academy of Pediatrics (AAP), and the American Academy of Family Physicians (AAFP). The recommended and catch-up schedules are available on the CDC website (CDC, 2013a; http://www.cdc.gov/vaccines/schedules). The CDC also offers healthcare organizations a Web-based "content syndication" program that consistently displays and updates current immunization information on a subscribing organization's website. Other countries may follow a similar schedules or recommendations of the World Health Organization (http://www.who.int). Information on breastfeeding and vaccines is available on the Internet from LactMed (http://toxnet.nlm.nih.gov).

Vaccines are designed to stimulate the antigen–antibody immune response, for the purpose of providing protection for future exposures to specific disease antigens, and are made primarily from bacteria or viruses. Whole organisms (live, attenuated or killed), modified proteins, polysaccharide sugars, or DNA technologies are used to prepare vaccines. Immunization may be active or passive. Active immunization involves administration of vaccines to stimulate the immune response, whereas passive immunity involves protective administration of exogenous antibodies, such as immunoglobulins (IGs).

Several types of vaccines are available:

- Live, attenuated vaccines contain weakened organisms (primarily viruses), such as measles–mumps–rubella (MMR) or varicella (VAR). Live viruses induce long-lasting immunity, but many are associated with contraindications, precautions, or adverse reactions.
- Inactivated vaccines are made from whole, killed organisms, and include the majority of recommended vaccines. Killed vaccines are noninfectious, usually induce shorter periods of protection, and may require multiple doses and booster injections.
- Toxoid vaccines are made from weakened toxins (poisons) from bacteria that cause disease through toxins, such as the tetanus toxoid.
- Subunit vaccines include only essential parts or antigens instead of whole organisms, such as the pertussis component of DTaP. They are less likely to cause side effects.
- Conjugate vaccines combine bacterial outer-coat polysaccharides from one organism with specific proteins from a different organism to enhance the immune response, such the *Haemophilus influenzae* type b (Hib) vaccine used for infants and young children.
- Recombinant vaccines are made with genetically engineered DNA technology, by inserting DNA from one species into another to produce vaccines, such as the two hepatitis B recombinant vaccines licensed in the United States.

Guidelines, precautions, and contraindications for vaccine administration are available from the CDC, manufacturers' inserts, the Immunization Action Coalition's *Needle Tips* (http://www.immunize.org), and the current AAP *Red Book* (Pickering et al., 2012).

Recommendations for immunizing young children are the same for breastfed children as for nonbreastfeeding children. With rare exceptions, inactivated and live vaccines do not affect the safety of breastmilk, and breastfeeding does not limit the immune response to most routine vaccines for infants or toddlers (Farren & McEwen, 2004). Data suggest that breastfeeding enhances infant immune responses to vaccines and decreases side effects such as fever, and that maternal antibodies in breastmilk do not significantly interfere with the infant's immune responses. Rotavirus (RV) is one exception being studied. Although breastfeeding protects infants against gastroenteritis caused by rotavirus, breastfeeding may reduce the infant's immune response to the vaccine, as compared to nonbreastfeeding infants (LactMed, 2013; Sachs & Committee on Drugs, 2013).

Most vaccines are administered parenterally, making them one of the most painful procedures performed in childhood. They are given either intramuscularly (IM) or subcutaneously (SC). Techniques for reducing pain during immunizations include breastfeeding, skin-to-skin contact, maternal holding during immunizations, putting sucrose on the tongue or pacifier, applying pressure to the injection site before vaccination, and having children blow a pinwheel or bubbles during the procedure (Burns et al., 2013; Efe & Ozer, 2007; Tansky & Lindberg, 2010).

Hepatitis B Vaccine (Given IM)

In the United States, the recommended age for beginning primary immunization of infants is at birth, with the hepatitis B (HepB) inactivated viral vaccine being administered prior to hospital discharge, given to all newborns who weigh at least 2000 g (4.4 lb). Infants weighing less than 2000 g and whose mothers are negative for the hepatitis surface antigen (HbsAg negative) should receive the first dose either within 1 month after birth or before discharge. Only monovalent HepB vaccine can be used for the birth dose. The HepB series can be completed with two doses of single-antigen vaccine (ages 1–2 and 6–18 months), or up to three doses of combination vaccine (ages 2, 4, 6, and 12–15 months). Infants born to HbsAg-positive mothers should receive the first HepB dose plus hepatitis immune globulin (HBIG) 0.5 mL IM within 12 hours after birth, at separate sites. If the mother's HbsAg status is unknown, the first HepB dose should is given within 12 hours of birth, regardless of weight. Then, if the mother is found to be HbsAg positive, the newborn should receive HBIG no later than 7 days after birth. For infants weighing less than 2000 g, HBIG is given in addition to HepB within 12 hours of birth.

Rotavirus Vaccine (Given Orally)

A series of RV (live virus) vaccinations are recommended for all infants, as early as 6 weeks to a final dose no later than 8 months of age. The series should not be started after 14 weeks, 6 days of age. Currently two RV vaccines are available: RV-1 (Rotarix) is administered in a two-dose series at 2 and 4 months, and RV-5 (RotaTequ) is administered in a three-dose series at 2, 4, and 6 months. The original RV (RotaShield) vaccine, which was introduced in 1999, was removed from the market due to associated intussusception. A low incidence of intussusception is associated with current RV vaccination; however, the CDC reports that the benefit of vaccination outweighs this low risk, and it continues to recommend RV vaccine to prevent rotavirus disease, a worldwide leading cause of gastroenteritis and death in young children.

Diphtheria, Tetanus Toxoids, and Acellular Pertussis Inactivated Bacterial Vaccines (Given IM)

The combined diphtheria/tetanus toxoid/acellular pertussis (DTaP) vaccine is given only to children younger than the age of 7 years. Acellular pertussis (Tdap) and tetanus toxoid (Td) vaccines are given to those 7 years of age and older. Td is given for 10-year tetanus boosters and wound management.

The primary schedule for administering the DTaP vaccine consists of a five-dose series, given at 2, 4, 6, and 12–18 months and 4–6 years. A one-dose DTaP vaccine is given to adolescents at 11–12 years, with Td boosters every 10 years. In the United States, the acellular (weakened) pertussis vaccine has replaced the older (whole-cell) pertussis (DPT) vaccine because it produces fewer side effects.

In October 2012, the ACIP recommended administration of a dose of Tdap to pregnant women for each pregnancy, ideally between 27 and 36 weeks' gestation, regardless of any prior history of receiving Tdap. If Tdap is not given during pregnancy, it should be administered immediately postpartum. Since 2005, the ACIP has recommended protection, or "cocooning" of infants from pertussis (whooping cough) by Tdap vaccination of those who come in close contact with them, at least 2 weeks prior to contact. Young infants have the highest incidence of hospitalizations and deaths due to pertussis, and they are not fully protected from this infection until their third dose of DTaP vaccine is given at 6 months of age. There is evidence of transplacental transfer of maternal pertussis antibodies from mother to infant, which may provide protection against pertussis early in life (CDC, 2013a).

Haemophilus influenzae *Type b* Vaccine (Given IM)

Before the introduction of the Hib vaccine in 1987, *H. influenzae* type b bacteria accounted for several serious infectious diseases—such as pneumonia, bacteremia, meningitis, epiglottitis, septic arthritis, cellulitis, otitis media, and purulent pericarditis, among others—in young children, with children aged 6 to 18 months being at the highest risk. Administration of the Hib vaccine has reduced the incidence of Hib disease by 99% (Burns et al., 2013, p.436). Hib inactivated bacterial conjugated vaccine may be given in a four-dose series (2, 4, 6, and 12–15 months) or a three-dose series (2, 4, and 12–15 months), depending on the specific vaccine product used. A combination Hib-HepB vaccine is also available. Hib is not routinely recommended for children age 5 years and older, except for those with high-risk immunocompromising conditions.

Pneumococcal Inactivated Bacterial Vaccines (Given IM and IM/SC)

Two pneumococcal virus (PCV) vaccines are currently available in the United States: PCV13 and PPSV23. The 13-valent PCV13 pneumococcal conjugate (diphtheria protein carrier) vaccine (given IM), introduced in 2010, replaced the original 7-valent PCV7 vaccine for the primary four-dose series of immunization against pneumococcal infections, given at 2, 4, 6, and 12–15 months. For children aged 14 through 59 months who received the PCV7 series, one dose of PCV13 is recommended. Children with incomplete vaccinations should complete their series with PCV13. PCV13 is not routinely recommended for healthy children age 5 years and older, except for those with specific high-risk medical conditions. Previous anaphylaxis to PCV or any diphtheria toxoid–containing vaccine is a contraindication. The 23-valent PPSV23 polysaccharide vaccine (given IM or SC) may be given to children 2 years and older with medical conditions that place them at high risk for pneumococcal disease.

Polio Vaccines (Given IM or SC in the United States, or Orally in Some Countries)

Two types of vaccines protect against polio: inactivated viral polio vaccine (IPV) and live viral oral polio vaccine (OPV). Prior to 2000, OPV was used for immunization against polio. IPV, given by IM or SC injection, has since replaced OPV in the United States, for the purpose of reducing the risk of vaccine-associated paralytic polio associated with OPV. However, OPV is still used in many parts of the world, and breastfed infants are successfully immunized if they are given OPV. U.S. children follow a four-dose schedule for IPV, with the vaccine being given at 2, 4, and 6–18 months and 4–6 years.

Influenza Vaccine (Given IM or Intranasally)

There are two basic types of influenza vaccine: inactivated (viral) influenza vaccine (IIV), given

IM, and live, attenuated (viral) influenza vaccine (LAIV), given intranasally. Influenza vaccines are reformulated for the flu season each year, and annual vaccination of all children, beginning at 6 months of age, is recommended. For most healthy, non-pregnant persons age 2 through 49 years, either LAIV or IIV may be used; otherwise, IIV is recommended. Two doses of IIV, spaced 4 weeks apart, are recommended for children age 6 months through 8 years who are first-time vaccinees or who meet specific guidance criteria.

Measles–Mumps–Rubella and Varicella Vaccines (Given SC)

There are two MMR live, attenuated viral vaccines: MMR (M-M-R II), a trivalent vaccine including measles, mumps, and rubella, and MMRV, a quadrivalent vaccine including measles, mumps, rubella, and varicella (chickenpox). Varicella single-antigen live, attenuated viral vaccine (VAR) is also available. The vaccine for all four diseases is recommended to be administered on a two-dose schedule, given at ages 12–15 months and 4–6 years. The following combinations can be administered: MMR plus VAR (given at separate sites) or the MMRV combination vaccine. The CDC recommends that MMR plus VAR be used for the first dose given to the 12- to 47-month age group. This recommendation is based on studies indicating an increased risk for febrile seizures following the first dose of MMRV, as compared to either the first dose of MMR plus VAR, or the second dose of MMRV (CDC, 2013c). MMR may temporarily suppress tuberculin activity. If tuberculin testing is needed, the tuberculosis (TB) skin test should be given before or on the same day as MMR, or else 4–6 weeks following MMR (Immunization Action Coalition [IAC], 2013).

Hepatitis A Inactivated Viral Vaccine (Given IM)

Hepatitis A (HepA) immunization is recommended as a two-dose series, spaced 6 to 18 months apart, in all children aged 12 to 23 months. Vaccination of previously unvaccinated children age 2 years and older and certain high-risk groups is recommended, using a two-dose series, spaced 6 to 18 months apart.

Human Papillomavirus Inactivated Viral Vaccine (Given IM)

Two human papillomavirus (HPV) vaccines are available: HPV4 and HPV2. A three-dose series, given at 0, 1–2, and 6 months to all adolescents aged 11 to 12 years is recommended (although the series may be given as early as age 9 years). Either HPV4 or HPV2 may be administered to females through 26 years, and only HPV4 to males through age 21 years.

Meningococcal Inactivated Bacterial Vaccines (Given IM)

Three types of meningococcal virus (MCV) vaccines for children are available: two meningococcal conjugate quadrivalent vaccines (Menactra [MCV4-D] and Menveo [MCV4-CRM]), plus Hib-MenCY, a bivalent meningococcal-*Haemophilus influenzae* type b conjugate vaccine, licensed in 2012. Menactra is recommended as a two-dose schedule given to children at ages 11–12 years and 16 years. Children with high-risk conditions may receive meningococcal vaccines in combinations, beginning at the following minimal ages: Menactra at 9 months or older, Menveo at 2 years or older, and Hib-MenCY at 6 weeks or older, following a four-dose schedule at 2, 4, 6, and 12–15 months). A polysaccharide vaccine, Menomune (MPSV4), given SC, is preferred for older adults.

Questions about risks of vaccination have been raised by concerned citizens and advocacy groups. In response, the U.S. Congress created the Vaccine Adverse Event Reporting System (VAERS), a national surveillance system administered by the Food and Drug Administration (FDA) and the CDC. VAERS maintains a database of reports of adverse events following vaccinations. More information on reporting adverse cases to VAERS can be found on the CDC website (www.cdc.gov /vaccines).

The public has shown considerable concern regarding the issue of childhood vaccines and the risk for autism spectrum disorder (ASD). These concerns have been focused on certain vaccines, such as MMR; vaccine ingredients, such as thimerosal (mercury); and the number of vaccines and vaccine antigens recommended in the childhood immunization schedule, including the number of vaccines given in a single day and the total antigens given in the first 2 years. Although the number of recommended vaccines has increased, the number of specific antigens in the vaccines has decreased, due to changes in vaccine preparations. A large CDC study, published in 2013, showed neither the number of antigens received in one day nor the total antigens received in the first 2 years of life is related to the development of autism (DeStefano, 2013; DeStefano et al., 2013). Previous reliable studies have not shown a positive association between specific vaccines (e.g., MMR) or ingredients (e.g., thimerosal) and autism. Thimerosal was taken out of childhood vaccines in 2001. Autism rates have continued to increase, and studies to determine the etiology of autism continue.

Vitamin D and Rickets

Vitamin deficiencies are rare in exclusively breastfed infants, except when the maternal diet is deficient. Maternal supplementation and dietary improvement are preferable to offering foods to infants younger than 4 to 6 months of age. Overall, human milk provides the vitamins and minerals needed by healthy full-term infants, except in special situations. Preterm infants represent a different situation and need supplementation if birth weight is less than 1500 g (very low birth weight [VLBW]). For preterm infants between 1500 and 2500 g, the need for supplementation is individualized. Fat-soluble vitamins in human milk are only minimally affected by what the mother eats, but are toxic if overdosed. Conversely, the maternal diet does affect the level of water-soluble vitamins in breastmilk.

Selected cases of common vitamin and mineral deficiencies are discussed in this section of the text. For example, mothers who are on a strict vegan diet may need supplements of vitamin B_{12}.

After a number of published studies showed high bioavailability of iron in human milk and indicated that breastfed infants have normal iron levels, the recommendation for breastfed infants to receive iron supplements was lifted. Preterm infants are at risk for iron deficiency due to reduced stores of iron at birth, and should be given supplemental iron. Additionally, maternal conditions, such as smoking, hypertension with uterine growth restriction, diabetes, or anemia can result in reduced fetal iron stores (Baker & Greer, 2010).

Vitamin D plays a role in immune function, and has been the subject of controversy and increasing research. Deficiency of vitamin D is recognized as highly prevalent in the United States and worldwide, affecting 30% to 50% of the general population (Lavie et al., 2011). Human milk does not normally contain adequate vitamin D to prevent vitamin D deficiency states and rickets. Rickets is the most severe form of vitamin D deficiency in children, with a peak incidence in infants between 3 and 18 months of age. This condition presents with skeletal deformities, osteopenia, growth failure, and predisposition to respiratory infections. There are also concerns for older children and adults raised by vitamin D deficiency. Most notably, vitamin D deficiency is associated with immune deficiency; allergy and asthma; autoimmune disease; increased rates of cancers; cardiovascular disease and hypertension; psychiatric disease; and type 1 diabetes, metabolic syndrome, and type 2 diabetes (Harris et al., 2013; Lavie et al., 2011; Malone & Kessenich, 2008; Wagner & Greer, 2008). Vitamin D deficiency is prevalent in overweight and obese children, especially in severely obese and minority children (Turner et al., 2013).

Sources for producing vitamin D include sunlight exposure, foods such as fatty fish and fortified cereals or milk, and dietary supplements. Lifestyle changes in the United States have reduced sun exposure significantly, resulting from more time spent indoors and use of sunscreen or other barriers to avoid sun exposure and subsequent risk of skin cancer. Northern latitudes, clouds, pollution, and cultural practices that keep women covered also reduce sun exposure. Dark skin pigmentation blocks more sunlight, increasing the risk of vitamin D deficiency in dark-skinned individuals. Vitamin D status is measured by serum concentrations of 25-hydroyvitamin D, 25(OH)D, reported in units of nanomoles per liter (nmol/L) or nanograms per milliliter (ng/mL): 1 nmol/L = 0.4 ng/mL. The Institute of Medicine (IOM) lists the following serum 25(OH)D concentrations as related to health status:

- Deficiency: < 30 nmol/L (< 12 ng/mL)
- Inadequate, at risk: 30–50 nmol/L (12–20 ng/mL)
- Adequate: ≥ 50 nmol/L (≥ 20 ng/mL)
- Potential toxicity: > 125 nmol/L (> 50 ng/mL)

For optimal health, 25(OH)D levels greater than 30 ng/mL are recommended (National Institutes of Health [NIH], 2011; Pramyothin & Holick, 2012).

The American Academy of Pediatrics' 2008 clinical report supports the AAP guidelines for limiting sun exposure and keeping infants younger than 6 months out of direct sunlight. The report also recommends vitamin D supplementation of 400 international units per day (400 IU/day), comparable to 1 teaspoon of cod liver oil, for all breast-fed infants, for children and adolescents beginning in the first few days of life, and for children who receive less than 1000 mL of vitamin D–fortified milk per day (Wagner & Greer, 2008). Another recent report suggests limiting cow milk intake to 500 mL (2 cups) per day to avoid iron deficiency, yet still maintain sufficient vitamin D levels (Maguire et al., 2012). Infant formulas in the United States and Canada are supplemented with vitamin D, but may not be able to compensate for low maternal gestational stores. The Institute of Medicine's Recommended Dietary Allowances (RDAs) for vitamin D are higher for children older than 1 year and adults, ranging between 600 IU/day and 800 IU/day, with an upper tolerable amount of 4000 IU/day (NIH, 2011). Ongoing research indicates that many experts lean toward even higher amounts of vitamin D supplementation. In Canada, the recommended infant dose is 800 IU/day during winter, and other guidelines suggest the need to individualize dosing according to risk factors for deficiency, such as dark skin pigment or reduced sunlight conditions (Madhusmitam et al., 2008).

Infants of mothers with vitamin D deficiency are born with low stores of this vitamin—a condition associated with high risk for respiratory infections in infants and potential for chronic illnesses later in life (Kaludjerovic & Vieth, 2010; Maxwell et al., 2012). Vitamin D supplementation to pregnant women, as high as 2000 to 4000 IU/day, is effective in replenishing maternal stores of vitamin D, as measured by 25(OH)D maternal serum levels and infant cord blood levels at birth (Dawodu et al., 2013). Supplementing lactating mothers with high doses of vitamin D—as high as 6400 IU/day—is effective in raising vitamin D levels in breastmilk (Wagner & Greer, 2008). However, direct supplementation to the infant rather than through breastmilk remains recommended practice. More research is needed to evaluate the long-term effects of maternal high dosing to elevate breastmilk levels of vitamin D, as well as identifying and supplementing pregnant women who are at risk for vitamin D deficiency.

Dental Health and Orofacial Development

The first primary (deciduous) teeth to erupt are the lower central incisors, which appear at about 6 to 8 months of age. By 2.5 years of age, children have a full set of primary teeth that will be replaced by permanent teeth. Although breastfeeding helps to protect the teeth, healthy dental practices should not be neglected because the child is breastfeeding.

Dental health begins with good oral care, which promotes healthy baby teeth and prevents decayed and abscessed teeth that cause pain and suffering in children. As soon as new teeth erupt, they should be cleaned daily with soft cloths and toothbrushes, and inspected by parents for discoloration or white spots that indicate early caries. The American Academy of Pediatric Dentistry (AAPD, 2012a) recommends that, based on risk factors, children visit the dentist as early as 6 months of age, 6 months after the first tooth erupts, and no later than 12 months of age.

Fluoride in water supplies is effective in preventing dental caries, and is supported by the AAPD, the American Dental Association (ADA), and the AAP. The U.S. Department of Health and Human Services (USDHHS) recommends 0.7 mg of fluoride per liter of water, or 0.7 part per million (ppm), for fluoridation of community water supplies; this recommendation replaces or lowers the earlier recommendations of 0.7 to 1.2 ppm (CDC, 2013b; USDHHS, 2011), in an effort to balance the optimal level for preventing tooth decay with minimization of the incidence of fluorosis, a complication of excessive, cumulative systemic fluoride that can result in white spots, staining, or pitting of tooth enamel. Dental fluorosis can develop in child 8 years and younger, during enamel development of permanent teeth. Children who drink fluoride-deficient water are at risk for caries and can benefit from fluoride supplements. However, it is important to assess community fluoridation levels and to base fluoride supplement dosages on the recommended dietary fluoride supplementation schedule (AAPD, 2012b; CDC, 2001). Fluoride supplementation is not recommended for infants younger than 6 months of age, and nonfluoridated water sources may need to be considered for reconstituting powdered formula if the water supply is fluoridated (Markowitz, 2012).

Professional fluoride applications that are effective in reducing tooth decay include oral fluorides in the form of tablets, lozenges, or drops; fluoride gels or foam; and fluoride sealants or varnishes. Fluoride mouth rinses, recommended by a healthcare provider, may be used if the child is able to spit and not swallow the rinse. Xylitol—used as a sweetener, and available in chewing gum, syrup, and other products—has been shown to reduce caries (Burns et al., 2013, pp. 795–797; Hall & Hall, 2013). Brushing the teeth twice daily with fluoride toothpaste, applied as a thin film or pea-sized amount on the toothbrush, is protective in reducing tooth decay, and is recommended for children 2 years and older. Fluoride toothpaste may be recommended for children younger than 2 years who have risk factors for caries.

Risk factors leading to caries and poor dental health include a mother or primary care provider with active tooth decay, low socioeconomic status, nutritional deficiencies, special healthcare needs, poor oral hygiene and lack of dental care, sweetened pacifiers, putting babies to bed with a bottle, fruit juices, sodas, sweetened foods, "sippy" cups, iron deficiency, lead exposure, and tobacco smoke.

Nursing-bottle caries is a term applied to progressive dental caries aggravated by sucking on a bottle while sleeping and is associated with a high count of lactobacilli in dental plaque (Smith & Moffatt, 1998). *Streptococcus mutans* is a major factor in this plaque biofilm on teeth. Decay usually starts with the maxillary (upper) incisors and spares the mandibular (lower) incisors.

Several studies suggest that human milk is protective against caries and that breastfed children have less dental decay than do those who are fed otherwise. Immune factors in human milk, such as secretory immunoglobulin A and G (IgA and IgG), are protective, and lactoferrin in breastmilk has a bactericidal effect (Al-Dashti et al., 1994; Altshuler, 2006; Oulis et al., 1999; Weerheijm et al., 1998). Other probable reasons for this include the mechanical differences between breastfeeding and bottle-feeding. Drawn deep into the child's mouth, the human nipple rests at the junction of the hard and soft palates during breastfeeding, posterior to the child's teeth. A suckle is automatically followed by a swallow, thus preventing the teeth from being bathed in pooled milk. In contrast, the milk from a bottle flows out spontaneously with only the slightest pressure into the anterior part of the mouth, permitting stagnation of the milk on and around the teeth.

Brazilian children who were premature and did not breastfeed were at higher risk for developmental enamel defects of primary teeth and tooth decay (Lunardelli & Peres, 2006). A few studies have reported a condition similar to nursing-bottle caries that occurred in breastfed children, especially those who breastfed for 2 to 3 years and spent long, uninterrupted periods at the breast. Although these cases represent a small percentage of young children who breastfeed, nursing caries are associated with the practice of breastfeeding at night "at will" after 6 months of age (Al-Dashti et al., 1994; Matee et al., 1994). A study of 629 Iowa children, aged birth to 4 years (Spitz et al., 2006), suggests that maternal reports of child temperament may be early indicators of risk factors for caries. Children reported as having "easy" temperaments were more likely to be breastfed throughout the night, while children perceived as "difficult" were more likely to be bottle-fed to sleep. As the number of breastfeeding toddlers increases, however, it is reasonable to expect that some of them will develop dental disease, especially after the introduction of solids that often contain sugar.

A lack of methodological consistency in studies on dental caries in breastfed children makes it difficult to draw conclusions. For example, none of the studies reported the dietary habits of the remainder of the children's diet. If a child ingests a sugar-rich food and then breastfeeds, the lips are pressed against the teeth, thus restricting flow of saliva and facilitating caries development (Bowen et al., 1997). As a result, when Valaitis et al. (2000) reviewed 151 articles on caries and breastfeeding, they were unable to come to a conclusion. Erickson (1999) conducted a unique in vitro study on caries development and human milk. She found that when children's teeth were exposed to human milk as the only carbohydrate source, caries did not occur. By comparison, when breastmilk was supplemented with 10% sucrose, caries development was rapid.

Dental caries are also thought to be an inherited trait; therefore, children who experience such tooth decay probably represent a group who are more susceptible, and prolonged nocturnal exposure to human milk becomes a risk factor. It could be argued that some breastfed children develop caries not because they were breastfed, but in spite of it. The susceptibility of the child's teeth to decay cannot be clinically predicted, and caries may be extensive before they become evident.

Orofacial development is a health issue in which breastfeeding has a measurable impact (Palmer, 1998). The orofacial development of a child is affected by feeding methods, swallowing patterns, and finger sucking (Sanger & Bystrom, 1982). The mechanisms by which bottle-feeding might contribute to the development of malocclusion include a forward thrusting of the tongue, which in turn leads to underdevelopment of the masseter and buccinator muscles, abnormal swallowing patterns, and increased prevalence of nonnutritive sucking. A study of preschool children in Puerto Rico (Lopez Del Valle et al., 2006) revealed that breastfeeding helped prevent malocclusions, such as space deficiency, open bites and cross-bites, and decreased thumb sucking and pacifier use. In Brazil, children ages 3 years to 6 years were studied for the relationship between breastfeeding, nasal breathing, and deleterious oral habits (Trawitzki et al., 2005). The breastfeeding time period was longer among nasal breathers. Mouth-breathing children were breastfed for shorter time periods and had statistically significant deleterious oral habits, such as suction (P = 0.004) and biting habits (P = 0.0002).

Solid Foods

Every breastfed infant reaches a point when breastmilk alone no longer fulfills his nutritional needs. If breastfeeding is continued exclusively, the baby will eventually become malnourished. How long exclusive breastfeeding can satisfy the nutrient needs of babies is a crucial public health issue, especially in areas with an unsafe water supply and poor sanitation, where early supplements are likely to be associated with infections.

Introducing Solid Foods

Solid foods are not necessary, nor are they recommended, before a baby is 4 to 6 months of age. Developmental cues for introducing solid foods to the infant are the fading of his tongue-extrusion reflex, eruption of teeth, the ability to sit, and purposeful movement of the baby's hands and fingers, all of which normally occur during the middle months of the first year of life. Most infants will at first actively resist the advances of even the most enterprising parent in attempts to spoon-feed them during the early months of life. Before 6 months of age, a baby has a tongue-extrusion reflex and is unable to push food to the back of his mouth. In the full-term baby, the prenatal storage of iron acquired during the last trimester of pregnancy gradually begins to diminish by 4 to 5 months of age, and external sources of iron are needed (Pisacane et al., 1995).

Early introduction of solids is still a common practice in the United States, even though the

American Academy of Pediatrics' Committee on Nutrition has consistently held that no nutritional advantage results from the introduction of supplemental foods prior to 4 to 6 months of age. A study of mothers in Kentucky found that by 1 month of age, 12% of mothers reported that their infant had received solid food and cereal added to the bottle. Fruit juices were given to one-fifth of the study infants by 1 to 2 months of age (Barton, 2001).

Despite official recommendations and a concerted effort to teach parents to delay solids, many infants still receive solid foods during their first few months of life. The first solid food is usually iron-fortified rice cereal, the least allergic first food. Some parents wrongly believe or have been told that feeding solids to the baby will help him sleep through the night. However, feeding infants solids prior to bedtime is not related to evening sleep patterns; according to well-controlled studies, babies who receive solids before bedtime have the same sleep patterns as do babies who are not given solids (Keane et al., 1988; Macknin et al., 1989).

Energy-intake patterns between breastfed and formula-fed infants discussed earlier in this text indicate that breastfed infants maintain energy-intake levels below those of formula-fed infants. These patterns persist even after solid foods are introduced. If breastfeeding infants are given solids at from 3 to 6 months, their milk intakes decline significantly; the energy from solids generally replaces that from breastmilk. Although the infant breastfeeds fewer times during the day, the frequency of night feedings remains the same (Heinig et al., 1993). This is not true for formula-fed infants, who continue to take about the same amount of formula when early solids are given.

In industrialized countries, infants fed solids early appear to have about the same incidence of illness as do infants who are fed solids later. In developing countries, however, the risk of diarrhea is such that the risks of introducing solids before 6 months outweigh any potential benefits.

Choosing the Diet

The U.S. Department of Agriculture developed MyPlate, a useful tool for educating families about a healthful diet. Information about this tool is available at http://www.choosemyplate.gov. MyPlate illustrates healthy meal portions, and emphasizes recommended portions of grains, fruits, vegetables, beans, peas, lean meats, fish, and poultry. A Mediterranean diet has long been considered to be a healthy diet, as it is rich in fruits, vegetables, whole grains, fish, nuts, and olive oil (as the main source of dietary fat).

If solids are started after 6 months of age, the sequence of food introduction is not critical. If solids are introduced earlier, the following order is suggested: cereals, yellow vegetables, fruits, meats, and (last) legumes. For cereal that requires mixing with a liquid, breastmilk (rather than cow milk) avoids any potential allergic reaction.

Infants need additional water when solids are started because of their added osmolar load. Historically, fruit juice was recommended by pediatricians as a source of vitamin C and water. Because fruit juice tastes sweet, children readily accept it. Although fruit juice has some benefits such as the vitamins and in some cases calcium that it contains, it also has potential detrimental effects (AAP, 2001). Children can become addicted to consuming fruit juices and other sugar-sweetened beverages at the expense of eating other foods, especially healthy, fresh foods. It has been recommended that honey not be given to infants younger than 1 year of age because there is a highly unlikely, but possible, chance of contracting botulism from this food (Lawrence & Lawrence, 2005).

A basic rule is to feed the infant foods in as close to a natural state as possible: pieces of raw, peeled apples; slices of banana; toasted whole-wheat bread; orange sections; and a chicken leg with the skin removed are all good choices. They can be picked up and held and are tasty, nutritious, and satisfying to chew. Feeding small amounts at first, followed by gradually increased amounts (along with continued breastfeeding), avoids constipation. Parents should be prepared for changes in consistency, odor, and frequency of stool when solids are begun. Generally, all foods eaten by the family can be given to the infant in a consistency that he can handle. The beginning eater enjoys foods of all kinds and relishes the tactile pleasures of squeezing, smearing, and crushing his food—an activity he should be allowed with impunity because it is also a learning experience. General guidelines for initiating solid foods are found in Table 17-5.

Breastfed babies are exposed to a variety of flavors of whatever is transmitted in their mothers' breastmilk (Mennella, 1995). As a result, it seems likely that they would be more accepting of novel flavors in solid foods than are formula-fed infants who are not so exposed. Likewise, flavors from the mother's diet during pregnancy are transmitted to amniotic fluids and swallowed by the fetus. Consequently, food flavors eaten by women during pregnancy are experienced by infants before their first exposure to solid foods (Mennella et al., 2001). To test this assumption, Sullivan and Birch (1994) compared acceptance of vegetables by 4- to 6-month-old infants. These infants were randomly assigned to be fed one vegetable on 10 occasions for 10 days. The researchers found that breastfeeding infants ate more vegetables than did formula-fed infants. Thus breastmilk may facilitate the acceptance of solid foods during the important transition from suckling to feeding solids. Babies who are given cereal were more accepting of it if this food was mixed with mother's milk rather than water (Mennella & Beauchamp, 1997). In situations in which families are unable to provide high-quality solids, continued breastfeeding beyond 1 year of age is also recommended to enhance linear growth in toddlers (Marquis et al., 1997).

Foods prepared at home are not only more wholesome and nutritious but cost less than do commercially prepared baby foods. Carrots and applesauce, for example, cost about half the store price when prepared at home, and blended beef and chicken provide more nutrients by weight than do their commercial counterparts, chiefly because

---

Table 17-5 INTRODUCING SOLID FOODS INTO A BREASTFED INFANT'S DIET

When to Introduce	Approximate Total Daily Intake of Solids*	Description of Food and Hints Giving Them
6–7 months if infant is breastfed	*Dry cereal:* Start with 1/2 tsp (dry measurement); gradually increase to 2–3 tb. *Vegetables:* Start with 1 tsp; gradually increase to 2 tb. *Fruit:* Start with 1 tsp; gradually increase to 2 tb. Divide food among 4 feedings per day (if possible).	*Cereal:* Offer iron-enriched baby cereal. Begin with single grains. Mix cereal with an equal amount of breastmilk. *Vegetables:* Try a mild-tasting vegetable first (carrots, squash, peas, green beans). Stronger-flavored vegetables (spinach, sweet potatoes) may be tried after infant accepts some mild-tasting ones. *Fruits:* Mashed ripe banana and unsweetened, cooked, bland fruits (apples, peaches, pears) are usually well-liked. Apple juice and grape juice (unsweetened) may be introduced. Initially, dilute juice with an equal amount of water. Introduce one new food at a time and offer it several times before trying another new food. Give a new food once daily for a day or two; increase to twice daily as the infant begins to enjoy the food. Watch for signs of intolerance. Include some foods that are good sources of vitamin C (other than orange juice).

(Continues)

Table 17-5 INTRODUCING SOLID FOODS INTO A BREASTFED INFANT'S DIET (*CONTINUED*)

6–7 months if infant is breastfed	*Meat:* Start with 1 tsp and gradually increase to 2 tb. Divide food among 4 feedings per day (if possible). *Dry cereal:* Gradually increase up to 4 tb. *Fruits and vegetables:* Gradually increase up to 3 tb of each.	*Meat:* Offer pureed or milled poultry (chicken or turkey) followed by lean meat (veal, beef); lamb has a stronger flavor and may not be as well-liked initially. Liver is a good source of iron; it may be accepted at the beginning of a meal with a familiar vegetable. Continue introducing new cereals, fruits, and vegetables as the infant indicates he is ready to accept them, but always one at a time; introduce legumes last.
7–9 months if infant is breastfed	*Dry cereal:* Up to 1/2 cup. *Fruits and vegetables:* Up to 1/4 to 1/2 cup of each. *Meats:* Up to 3 tb. Divide food among 4 feedings per day (if possible).	Soft table foods may be introduced—for example, mashed potatoes and squash and small pieces of soft, peeled fruits. Toasted whole grain or enriched bread may be added when the infant begins chewing.
8–12 months if infant is breastfed	*Dry cereal:* Up to 1/2 cup. *Bread:* About 1 slice. *Fruits and vegetables:* Up to 1/2 cup of each. Divide food among 4 feedings per day (if possible).	If introduction of solids is delayed until now, it is not necessary to use strained fruits and vegetables. Continue using iron-fortified baby cereals. Table foods cut into small pieces may be added gradually. Start with foods that do not require too much chewing (cooked, cut green beans and carrots, noodles, ground meats, tuna fish, soft cheese, plain yogurt). If fish is offered, check closely to be sure there are no bones in the serving. Mashed, cooked egg yolk and orange juice may be added at about 9 months of age. Sometimes offer peanut butter or thoroughly cooked dried peas and beans in place of meat.

* Some infants do not need or want these amounts of food; some may need a little more food.

they contain less water. With the aid of an electric blender, food mill, or grinder, preparing baby food is easily accomplished. The foods should be selected from high-quality fresh or frozen fruits, vegetables, or meats, with special attention to hygienic preparation and storage. For convenience, small individualized portions can be stored safely in the refrigerator or freezer for reasonable periods. A list of foods that can be quickly and easily prepared appears in Box 17-2.

Some parents prefer to buy commercial baby food rather than to make their own. In addition to being expensive, commercial baby foods are generally produced by pulverizing fruit, grain, vegetable, and meat ingredients with water and adding filler ingredients such as colorings, additives, and preservatives (Randle, 1999).

For families on vegan diets, their infants may need supplements of vitamin B_{12} when dairy products and eggs are excluded from the diet. Older infants may need zinc supplements and reliable sources of iron and vitamin D as well as vitamin B_{12}. Timing of solid-food introduction is similar to that recommended for nonvegetarians. Tofu, dried beans, and meat analogs are introduced as protein sources around the middle of the first year (Mangels & Messina, 2001).

Choosing Feeding Location

The best place to feed a baby is at the family table at mealtime, in a high chair or on someone's knee. Young children love to be considered one of the family and to sit at the same height as the rest of the family. Even before the infant is ready to take solids, he enjoys being nearby during meals and can "join in" by chewing on such food as a bread crust or a banana.

Delaying Solid Foods

Current recommendations American Public Health Association, 2007; 2013; (American Academy of Pediatrics, 2012; World Health Organization, 2014) include exclusive breastfeeding for the first 6 months of life, with continued breastfeeding for at least the first 1 to 2 years, and introduction of complementary foods between at 6 months of age. Some evidence suggests that breastfeeding for at least

4 months prevents or delays occurrence of atopic dermatitis, cow milk allergy and food allergy, allergic rhinitis, asthma, and wheezing in early childhood. There is no convincing evidence for delaying introduction of complementary foods or highly allergic foods beyond 4 to 6 months of age (Greer et al., 2008).

Food allergy (FA) is increasing worldwide and in the United States, with peanuts recognized as the most common allergen, followed by milk and shellfish. New recommendations from the American Academy of Allergy, Asthma and Immunology (AAAA) state that infants can safely tolerate highly allergenic foods, such as cow milk, egg, peanuts and tree nuts, soy, wheat, fish, and shellfish, when they are as young as 4 months. Egg yolk, which is high in protein and iron, is considered hypoallergenic, and egg white is considered more allergenic. Recent studies indicate that it may be beneficial to introduce egg at an early age, in smaller amounts, either cooked or in baked goods. Early introduction of highly allergenic foods after complementary foods have been initiated might actually prevent development of allergies to these foods. Most pediatric guidelines suggest introducing foods at a rate no faster than one new food every 3 to 5 days; highly allergenic foods should be introduced at home, so that children can be monitored for adverse

---

BOX 17-2 QUICK, EASY-TO-PREPARE INFANT FOODS

- Yogurt (low-fat)
- Fresh fruit: cut-up apples, pears, oranges, bananas, grapes, or any fruit in season
- Cheese, cut into chewable pieces
- Toast of whole grain bread, cut into strips
- Chicken: leg, wing, or cut-up pieces
- Egg: soft-boiled; hard-boiled as finger food
- Vegetables: mashed; whole (e.g., peas); in strips or pieces as finger food
- Crackers: whole grain; cheese spread
- Custard
- Cottage cheese
- Dried fruit: apples, dates, figs, prunes (pitted)
- Liver: sauteed and cut into strips
- Tuna: drained; with grated cheese

reactions. Special consideration is recommended for children already diagnosed with allergic conditions or at especially high risk for developing allergy (i.e., those with at least one first-degree relative, parent, or sibling with allergic disease). Studies suggest that partial whey hydrolysate formulas have a preventive effect on atopic disease and cow milk protein allergy (Azad et al., 2013; Fleischer et al., 2013; Ismail et al., 2012; Syed et al., 2013).

FA is currently regarded as a complex dysfunction of the normal immune tolerance mechanisms. All foods are recognized by the gut as foreign antigens, and allergic individuals demonstrate immune responses to these antigens. Tolerance is believed to suppress this response in nonallergic individuals. FA develops in two stages: sensitization to allergens, followed by elicitation of immunoglobulin E (IgE) and inflammatory response after allergen reexposure. Levels of IgE, associated with allergy, rise in direct time sequence to the introduction of solid foods, and can also be verified by positive allergy tests later in life.

Before the age of 6 months, the infant's intestine lacks the necessary digestive enzymes to completely digest complex proteins and starches down to amino acids and simple sugars. At the same time, the infant's intestinal mucosa is permeable to some intact proteins and starches. Alterations in the intestinal microflora have been linked to the development of allergic disease. The "hygiene hypothesis" suggests that changes in the pattern of intestinal colonization during infancy, such as reduced microbial diversity in early life, decreased exposure to infectious agents, and use of antibiotics in childhood, are important factors in developing FA. Studies have shown that a more diverse intestinal microflora in the first week of life is associated with a reduced risk of subsequent eczema in infants at risk of allergic disease (Ismail et al., 2012). Infants with eczema at 12 months of age had reduced intestinal microbial diversity from as early as the first week of life, compared to high-risk infants who did not develop eczema in infancy. Early-life exposure to pets or siblings may also influence the diversity and composition of gut microbiota, offering some protection against allergic disease (Azad et al.,

2013). The use of probiotic live organisms to balance gut microflora is being investigated.

Treatment of allergic disease consists of avoidance of the offending allergen, delivery of epinephrine in the case of accidental ingestions, and symptom management. No effective cure is currently available.

Obesity

Childhood obesity, a complex and growing problem throughout the world, is most commonly measured by the 2000 CDC body mass index (BMI)-for-age-growth charts for children 2 to 18 years of age. Overweight is defined as a BMI at or above the 85th percentile to the 95th percentile; obesity is defined as a BMI at or above the 95th percentile or a BMI of 30—whichever is lower; and extreme obesity is defined as a BMI above 30. Comparison BMI ranges for adults are as follows: underweight (less than 18.5), normal (18.5–24.9), overweight (25–29.9), and obese (30 or greater) (Barlow, 2007). WHO growth standards are recommended in weight–length ratio charts for children younger than age 2 years.

Approximately 21% to 24% of U.S. children are overweight, and 16% to 18% are obese (Schwarz, 2012). According to WHO, worldwide obesity has doubled since 1980. The National Health and Nutrition Examination Survey (NHANES) data indicate that obesity prevalence in the United States was relatively stable between 1960 and 1980, but more than doubled from 1980 to 2006. The 2009–2010 data indicate no change, or a leveling off of childhood obesity prevalence at 16.9%. Data from the Pediatric Surveillance System (PedNSS), collected by the CDC from 2003 through 2010 as part of a national study of low-income preschool-aged children, showed, for the first time, a decline in obesity and extreme obesity among low-income preschool children (CDC, 2012; Ogden, 2012). Significant ethnic differences have been documented, with higher rates of overweight and obesity being observed in non-Hispanic black, Mexican American, Native American, Alaskan Native, and Pacific Islander populations (Matheson & Robinson, 2008).

Obesity in childhood increases the risk for obesity as an adult. Obesity is associated with significant long-term health problems (AAP, 2012; Barlow, 2007; Bruney, 2011; Burns et al., 2013, pp. 174–179; Schwartz, 2012), such as the following:

- Endocrine and cardiovascular disorders: metabolic syndrome, insulin resistance, acanthosis nigricans of the skin associated with hyperinsulinemia, hypertension, hyperlipidemia, abdominal obesity, type 1 and type 2 diabetes mellitus, polycystic ovary syndrome, gynecomastia, accelerated growth and bone maturation
- Respiratory disorders: obstructive sleep apnea, asthma, exercise intolerance, reactive airway, obesity hypoventilation
- Gastrointestinal disorders: fatty liver disease, gallstones and cholecystitis, gastroesophageal reflux
- Orthopedic disorders: excessive bowing of legs, slipped femoral epiphysis, increased risk for fractures and musculoskeletal discomfort
- Psychosocial disorders: depression, eating disorders, social isolation, peer problems and lower self-esteem

Childhood obesity involves complex interactions between genetic predisposition, metabolism, environment, and human behavior. Family history of obesity, having obese parents, excessive maternal weight gain during pregnancy, and rapid weight gain during early infancy place children at increased risk for obesity (Hediger et al., 2001; Ludwig et al., 2013; Maffeis, 1999). Specific obesity-associated genes and metabolic influences are currently being studied. Hormones, such as insulin and leptin, influence appetite satiety and fat distribution. Intake of high-fructose corn syrup and other high-glycemic foods, decreased physical activity, and chronic stress can all lead to the hyperinsulinemia, resulting in insulin and leptin resistance. Bruney (2011) reported on two studies that showed changes in intestinal microflora of infants preceding development of overweight; these studies raised questions regarding the benefits of probiotic supplementation as well as advocated judicious antibiotic

prescribing. Vitamin D deficiency has also been associated with obesity in children and adolescents (Bruney, 2011; Turner et al., 2013).

Environmental and behavioral factors affecting the risk of obesity include dietary habits, physical activity, cultural differences, effects of media advertising, family stressors, and low socioeconomic status. Consumption of sugar-sweetened beverages, increased serving sizes and snack foods, sedentary lifestyles, increased television viewing or other screen time, fewer physical education classes, and less physical outside play time are some examples of these factors. The American Academy of Pediatrics recommends that parents limit total noneducational screen time to no more than 2 hours per day, avoid screen exposure for infants younger than 2 years of age, and keep televisions out of children's bedrooms (AAP, 2011a). The AAP also recommends encouraging children and adolescents to be physically active for at least 60 minutes per day in unstructured and fun activities they enjoy.

Early diet plays a role in obesity. Are breastfeeding children, then, less likely to become obese? Many large studies have shown that breastfed babies are less likely than bottle-fed infants to become obese (Armstrong & Reilly, 2002; Arnez & von Kries, 2005; Bergmann et al., 2003; Kramer, 1981; Singhal & Lanigen, 2006; Toschke et al., 2002). Other research has shown no or an insignificant relationship between breastfeeding and later obesity (Butte, 2001; Dewey, 2003; Li et al., 2003), and some studies found that breastfed children were more likely to become fat (Agras et al., 1990; Kersey et al., 2005). The literature is contradictory in part because many studies are characterized by small sample sizes, missing data, lack of adequate control for confounding factors (e.g., the mother's nutritional awareness, exercise patterns), and methodological problems (e.g., operational definitions of obesity, the distinction between a "breastfed" infant versus a "bottle-fed" infant, and the timing of feedings). Moreover, differences in exercise patterns of children were typically not included in studies as a confounding factor.

A review of breastfeeding and pediatric overweight research summarizes significant findings

(CDC, Division of Nutrition and Physical Activity, 2007). Breastfeeding appears to be protective against obesity, and this effect may persist into the teenage and adult years. Exclusive breastfeeding appears to have a stronger effect than combined breastfeeding and formula-feeding, and longer duration of breastfeeding reduces the odds of becoming overweight. Several biological associations may also reduce the risk for overweight. Breastfed infants self-regulate their milk intake according to their caloric needs, are more likely to actively suckle and respond to internal hunger and satiety cues, and, at the same time, control their mother's milk production. This early programming of self-regulation may affect later weight gain. In contrast, the satiated bottle-fed baby is more likely to be passive in the feeding process and be encouraged to empty the bottle and not develop control over food intake.

Studies by Li et al. (2010, 2012) compared weight gain by both milk type (formula versus breastmilk) and feeding mode (breast versus bottle). Infants who were fed by bottle (either formula or expressed breastmilk) gained more weight, regardless of the type of milk, than infants who fed at the breast.

Leptin—the hormone that regulates appetite and satiety—is present in breastmilk but not in formula, and may be protective against risk for overweight in breastfed infants. A large meta-analysis showed that formula-fed infants had higher plasma insulin concentrations, a more prolonged insulin response, and higher protein intake (stimulates insulin secretion), which may influence deposition of fat and create a significant positive relationship between high protein intake early in life and increased risk of obesity later in life (Arnez & von Kries, 2005). A large study review (Owen et al., 2006) concluded that breastfeeding in infancy is associated with lower blood glucose in infancy, along with marginally lower insulin concentrations and reduced risk of type 2 diabetes mellitus later in life.

Childhood obesity is a multifaceted disease and a public health issue. Breastfeeding, along with genetic, racial, socioeconomic, and behavioral factors, affects later obesity and the risks of developing cardiovascular disease, hypertension, metabolic syndrome, and diabetes mellitus. Other dietary factors, such as early introduction of sweet drink consumption when infants are developing taste preferences, can lead to excessive sugar intake and the long-term consequences of type 2 diabetes mellitus, low nutrition, low calcium intake, low bone density, dental caries, and some behavior issues (Saalfield & Jackson-Allen, 2006).

Prevention of childhood overweight and obesity begins with optimal maternity care practices and holistic prevention and treatment strategies. Initial treatment for obesity ideally consists of lifestyle changes including diet, exercise, and behavioral modification. The National Association of Pediatric Nurse Practitioners (NAPNAP) has developed the *Healthy Eating and Activity Together* (HEAT) clinical practice guideline, which offers culturally appropriate interventions intended to enhance the family's ability to achieve the ideal balance between nutrition and physical activity to support optimal growth and wellness (http://www.napnap.org). Treatment of obesity involves changes by the whole family, and barriers may need to be overcome. For example, the research results reported by De La et al. (2009) indicate that the majority of parents of overweight children tend to underestimate their child's weight.

A limited number of medications are available to treat older children and adolescents with obesity. Bariatric surgery is available for morbidly obese adolescents, and the two procedures most commonly used for this indication are laparoscope adjustable gastric banding and gastric bypass surgery (Woo, 2009).

Long-Term Breastfeeding

Long-term breastfeeding is considered "comfort nursing"—a form of nurturance and a special bonding rather than nourishment. Nutritional benefits are considered secondary at this point in the child's development. The conceptual difference is that breastfeeding is considered as a "process" rather than a "product" (Van Esterik, 1985). Do older breastfeeding children receive sufficient food to grow? Nutrition in long-term breastfeeders in the United

States appeared to be adequate in one study. When daily food intake of these children was measured, their nonbreast intake of complementary foods met RDA energy requirements (Buckley, 2001).

Weaning

In the United States, weaning usually takes place during the first year of life. Women who breastfeed longer than this have difficulty with acceptance by relatives, peers, and health professionals (Page-Goertz, 2002). If "baby-led weaning" is practiced, weaning usually takes place between the child's second and fourth birthdays (Sugarman & Kendall-Tackett, 1995). To counteract social pressures for early weaning, women with breastfeeding toddlers find peer support from one another, sometimes changing their circle of friends.

In a study by Wrigley and Hutchinson (1990) of 12 mothers who practiced long-term breastfeeding, one mother reported that her obstetrician told her anyone who breastfed an infant past 6 months of age was "perverted." Another said that her father thought she was "strange." Many healthcare workers who wholeheartedly support breastfeeding and would never advocate taking a security blanket away from a baby reel in horror when a mother breastfeeds a walking child. Page-Goertz (2002) advises, "To avoid embarrassing moments at the mall due to the toddler's increasing language skills, parents may want to teach their child a code word for breastfeeding. Examples are 'pillow' and 'nums.' This can prevent a child from yelling 'BOOBY, mom—now!'"

Ideally, the time for weaning is a joint decision in which both the mother and the baby reach a state of readiness to begin weaning around the same time; however, this is not always the case. The child may be ready before his mother; more often, the mother is ready before her child. In a unique study of weaning times of 36 primates, anthropologist Dettwyler (1995) determined what would be a natural duration of breastfeeding in modern humans. Her evidence suggests that 2.5 years is the minimum duration of time for breastfeeding, and that 4 or 5 years, or longer, is within the normal range for humans.

Sometimes, the decision is made to wean quickly. Although the literature offers considerable advice about gradual weaning, there is little information for the anxious mother in a situation in which weaning must be rapid and will necessarily be traumatic. The following nondrug therapies may make deliberate weaning easier and at the same time avert plugged ducts or mastitis:

- Shower and allow the warm water to run over the breasts, or soak the breasts by lying down in the tub.
- Use a breast pump or manual expression to relieve breast fullness.
- Wear a supportive, comfortable bra.
- Observe for signs of plugged ducts or a breast infection.
- Expect to feel very emotional during this time and seek support from people who will listen sympathetically.
- Give the baby extra cuddling and holding.

It may take several days before the mother finds it is no longer necessary to express breastmilk for comfort. As described earlier in this text, an Australian method for reducing engorged breasts is to wear cool raw cabbage leaves in the bra. Doing so has been reported to quickly relieve engorgement.

Implications for Practice

Care providers assume responsibility for educating families in optimal infant-feeding practices and for providing rationales and support when they are needed. The introduction of foods other than breastmilk is culturally influenced and common worldwide. Some mothers encourage their babies to eat as much as possible, believing that a plump baby represents the picture of health. Competition among mothers can also lead to the early introduction of baby foods. Mothers who feel pressure to give their babies solids may misinterpret the baby's cries as hunger, when the baby merely needs stimulation by holding and interacting. Education is a powerful tool for teaching healthy food practices.

It is not unusual for children, usually from about 2 years of age, to become very fussy about food and to refuse to eat certain items; they may especially dislike vegetables. Children will go through periods of eating very little for a period from as short as a week to as long as a few months; then they gradually start eating more again. The mother should be reassured that "this too shall pass" and that her child will start eating again. Meanwhile, she should make the food the child does like easily available and neither force the child to eat nor mask his natural appetite by offering sugary foods.

Choices about weaning should be based on the mother's own wishes rather than on the expectations of others and call for active listening to her feelings. If the mother enjoys breastfeeding but feels pressure to wean, pointing out the advantages of continued breastfeeding and the cultural differences in weaning practices may be all the reinforcement she needs. Conversely, if she expresses resentment each time her baby breastfeeds and is impatient for each feeding to end, she is entitled to know options for safe and comfortable weaning techniques. Some women report that after weaning their baby, they experienced improvement in mood and sexuality and felt less fatigue (Forster et al., 1994).

ACKNOWLEDGMENT

Jan Riordan, a pioneer in the world of breastfeeding, was the original author of this chapter. I was honored when she invited me to be her co-author beginning with the third edition. For this fifth edition, as solo author, a number of changes in organizing and updating the material were made, but the content honors Dr. Riordan's initial work, in particular regarding the psychosocial concerns.

SUMMARY

Imperative to assisting a breastfeeding family is recognition and knowledge of a wide array of areas of child health. Taking the holistic view, breastfeeding is but one aspect of the child's overall health and welfare. This chapter has offered readers basic information derived from research findings and clinical experiences. Teaching parents and incorporating research findings into the daily lives of families are the linchpins of effective practice.

KEY CONCEPTS

- Worldwide studies indicate that breastfed infants are more likely to have higher intellectual ability and cognitive development compared with those who were not breastfed.
- Universal child growth patterns include cephalocaudal and proximodistal growth.
- Generally, both breastfed and bottle-fed infants double their birth weight by the middle of the first year of life and triple it by 1 year. Breastfeeding infants weigh slightly more than their formula-fed counterparts for the first 3 to 4 months.
- The infant's brain grows rapidly during infancy.
- Neonates are born with well-developed sensory abilities of hearing, smell, touch, and taste. Their visual preference is for human faces and moving objects.
- Sleep is irregular in early infancy but matures into more regular sleep–wake cycles by age 3 to 6 months.
- Theories about early developmental stages include (1) trust versus mistrust and autonomy versus shame and doubt (Erickson), and (2) sensorimotor, assimilation, and accommodation (Piaget).
- Breastfed infants tend to be more wakeful, cry more often during the late afternoon and evening, and wake more frequently during the night.
- Attachment and bonding are facilitated by kangaroo mother care, skin-to-skin contact, and breastfeeding, resulting in a series of physical contact and sensory interactions between mother and baby as "mutual caregivers." The role of oxytocin release associated with breastfeeding and mother–infant bonding is being extensively studied.
- Stranger distress and separation anxiety, which occur during the second half of the first year of life, are normal phenomena where the child fears strangers and being apart from the primary caretaker.

- Developmentally speaking, the ability to tolerate solids offers no evidence that their early introduction is advantageous. In fact, the practice may initiate a chain of disadvantages that include allergies and obesity.
- Recommendations for immunizations are usually the same for breastfed children as for nonbreastfed children.
- The increased incidence of vitamin D deficiency, which is associated with potential systemic health problems and rickets, has led to recommendations for vitamin D supplementation of all infants, children, and adolescents
- Breastfeeding infants generally have fewer dental caries. Reported cases of dental caries are usually associated with nighttime feedings, genetic predisposition, and dietary sugar.
- Solids foods are not necessary before 4 to 6 months of age. Developmental cues for introducing solid foods are fading of the child's tongue-extrusion reflex, the eruption of teeth, the ability to sit, and purposeful movement of the baby's hands and fingers, all of which normally occur during the middle months of the first year of life. Full-term babies have storage of iron that begins to diminish by 4 to 5 months of age.
- Total solid-food elimination for the first 4 to 6 months of life, in addition to exclusive breastmilk feeding, appears to reduce atopic disease in children who are at hereditary risk. Delaying the introduction of solid foods beyond this period does not appear to have a significant protective effect on the development of atopic disease.
- Breastfeeding appears to have a protective effect against later obesity, but it appears to be weaker than genetic, racial, socioeconomic, dietary, and behavioral factors.
- Co-sleeping facilitates breastfeeding. Safe co-sleeping includes bedding that fits tightly to the mattress, no soft pillows or space between the bed and the wall, and placing the baby on his back or side. The American Academy of Pediatrics recommends room-sharing without bed-sharing.
- Ideally weaning takes place when both the mother and the baby reach a state of readiness around the same time. Cross-culturally, weaning takes place around 2.5 years of age.

INTERNET RESOURCES

Academy of General Dentistry: http://www.agd.org

Alberta Health Services: http://www.albertahealthservices.ca/default.asp

American Academy of Pediatric Dentistry: http://www.aapd.org

American Academy of Pediatrics (AAP): http://www.aap.org

American Dental Association: http://www.ada.org

Bright Futures at American Academy of Pediatrics: A national resource for child health promotion: http://www.brightfutures.org

Centers for Disease Control and Prevention: http://www.cdc.gov

Healthy Steps: Focus on first 3 years of life: http://www.healthysteps.org

Immunization Action Coalition: http://www.immunize.org/

National Association of Pediatric Nurse Practitioners (NAPNAP): Information resource for child health promotion special initiatives: http://www.napnap.org

- KySS: Keep your children/yourself Safe and Secure (mental health)
- HEAT: Healthy Eating and Activity Together (childhood obesity)

Sleep Foundation: http://www.sleepfoundation.org/

UNICEF: http://www.unicef.org/

World Health Organization: http://www.who.int/en

REFERENCES

Agras WS, Kraemer HC, Berkowitz RI, Hammer LD. Influence of early feeding style on adiposity at 6 years of age. *J Pediatr.* 1990;116:805–811.

Ainsworth MDS, Blehar M, Waters E, Wall S. *Patterns of attachment: a Psychological Study of the Strange Situation.* Hillsdale, NJ: Lawrence Erlbaum; 1978.

Al-Dashti AA, Williams SA, Curzon MEJ. Breast feeding, bottle feeding and dental caries in Kuwait, a country with low-fluoride levels in the water supply. *Community Dent Health.* 1994;12:42–47.

Als H, Brazelton TB. A new model of assessing the behavioral organization in preterm and full-term infants. *J Am Acad Child Psychol.* 1981;20:239.

Altshuler A. Early childhood caries: new knowledge has implications for breastfeeding families. *Leaven.* April–May–June 2006;27–31.

American Academy of Pediatric Dentistry (AAPD). Reference manual, oral health policies: policy on the dental home. 2012a;34(6):24–25. Available at: http://www.mychildrensteeth.org/policies/. Accessed April 29, 2012.

American Academy of Pediatric Dentistry (AAPD). Reference manual, oral health policies: policy on use of fluoride. 2012b;34(6):43–44. Available at: http://www.mychildrensteeth.org/policies/. Accessed April 29, 2012.

American Academy of Pediatrics (AAP). The use and misuse of fruit juice in pediatrics. *Pediatrics.* 2001;107:1210–1213.

American Academy of Pediatrics (AAP). Children, adolescents, obesity, and the media. *Council on Communications and Media.* 2011a;128(1):201–208.

American Academy of Pediatrics (AAP). SIDS and other sleep-related infant deaths: expansion of recommendations for a safe infant sleeping environment. Task Force on Sudden Infant Death Syndrome. *Pediatrics.* 2011b;128:1030; originally published October 17, 2011; doi: 10.1542/peds.2011–2284. *Pediatrics.* 2011;128;e1341; originally published online October 17, 2011; doi: 10.1542/peds.2011–2285.

American Academy of Pediatrics (AAP). Breastfeeding and the use of human milk. Section on Breastfeeding. *Pediatrics.* 2012;29(3):e827–e841.

American Public Health Association. Policy No. 200714. A call to action to support breastfeeding: a fundamental public health issue. 2007. Available at: http://www.apha.org/advocacy/policy/policysearch/default.htm?id=1360. Accessed April 2, 2014.

American Public Health Association. Policy No. 20132. An update to a call to action to support breastfeeding: a fundamental public health issue. 2013. Available at: http://www.apha.org/advocacy/policy/policysearch/default.htm?id=1448. Accessed April 2, 2014.

Anderson GC. The mother and her newborn: mutual caregivers. *JOGNN.* 1977;6:50–55.

Anderson GC. Enhancing reciprocity between mother and neonate. *Nurs Res.* 1981;30:89–93.

Anderson GC, Chiu SH, Dombrowski MA, et al. Mother–newborn contact in a randomized trial of kangaroo (skin-to-skin) care. *JOGNN.* 2003;32:604–611.

Anderson GC, Dombrowski MA, Swinth JY. Kangaroo care: not just for stable preemies anymore. *Reflect Nurs Leadership.* 2001;27:32–34.

Anderson GC, Moore E, Hepworth J, Bergman N. Early skin-to-skin contact for mothers and their healthy newborn infants (Cochrane review). In: *The Cochrane library.* Oxford, UK: Update Software; Issue 2, 2003.

Anderson GC, et al. Skin-to-skin for breastfeeding difficulties postbirth. In: Field T, ed. *Advances in touch.* New Brunswick, NJ: Johnson & Johnson; 2003.

Ardiel EL, Rankin CH. The importance of touch in development. *Paediatr Child Health.* 2010;15(3):153–156.

Armstrong J, Reilly JJ. Breastfeeding and lowering the risk of childhood obesity. *Lancet.* 2002;359:2003–2004.

Arnez F, von Kries R. Protective effect of breast-feeding against obesity in childhood. *Adv Exp Med Biol.* 2005;569:40–48.

Azad M, Konya T, Maughan H, et al. Infant gut microbiota and hygiene hypothesis of allergic disease: impact of household pets and siblings on microbiota composition and diversity. *Allergy Asthma Immunol.* 2013;9:15. Available at: http://www.aacijournal.com/content/9/1/15. Accessed August 30, 2013.

Baker D, Greer F. American Academy of Pediatrics, Committee on Nutrition. Diagnosis and prevention of iron deficiency and iron-deficiency anemia in infants and young children (0–3 years of age). *Pediatrics.* 2010;126(5):1040–1050.

Barlow S. Expert committee recommendations regarding the prevention, reference assessment, and treatment of child and adolescent overweight and obesity: summary report. *Pediatrics.* 2007;120(suppl 4):S164–S192.

Barton SJ. Infant feeding practices of low-income rural mothers. *MCN.* 2001;26:93–98.

Bergmann KE, Bergmann RL, Von Kries R, et al. Early determinants of childhood overweight and adiposity in a birth cohort study: role of breastfeeding. *Int J Obesity.* 2003;27:162–172.

Birch EE, Garfield S, Hoffman DR, et al. A randomized controlled trial of early dietary supply of long-chain polyunsaturated fatty acids and mental development in term infants. *Dev Med Child Neurol.* 2000;41:174–181.

Bowen WH, Pearson SK, Rosalen PL, et al. Assessing the carcinogenic potential of some infant formulas, milk and sugar solution. *JADA.* 1997;128:865–871.

Bowlby J. The nature of the child's tie to his mother. *Int J Psychoanal.* 1958;39:350–372.

Bowlby J. *Attachment and loss: separation,* Vol. 2. New York: Basic Books; 1973.

Bruney T. Childhood obesity: effects of micronutrients, supplements, genetics and oxidative stress. *J Nurs Pract.* 2011;7(8):647–652.

Buckley KM. Long-term breastfeeding: nourishment or nurturance? *J Hum Lact.* 2001;17:304–312.

Bu'Loc F, Woolridge MW, Baum JD. Development of coordination of sucking, swallowing and breathing:

ultrasound study of term and preterm infants. *Dev Med Child Neurol.* 1990;32:669–678.

Burns CE, Dunn AM, Brady MA, et al., eds. *Pediatric Primary care,* 5th ed. St Louis: Saunders; 2013.

Butte NF. The role of breastfeeding in obesity. In: Schanler R, ed. Breastfeeding 2000, part 1. *Pediatr Clin North Am.* 2001;48:189–198.

Butte NF, Smith EO, Garza C. Energy utilization of breast-fed and formula-fed infants. *Am J Clin Nutr.* 1990;51: 350–358.

Butte NF, Wong WW, Fiorotto M, et al. Influence of early feeding mode on body composition of infants. *Bio Neonate.* 1995;67:414–424.

Carey WB, McDevitt SC. Revision of the infant temperament questionnaire. *Pediatrics.* 1978;61:735–739.

Centers for Disease Control and Prevention (CDC). Recommendations for using fluoride to prevent and control dental caries in the United States. *MMWR.* 2001;50(No. RR-14);8. Available at: http://www.cdc.gov/mmwr/PDF/rr/rr5014.pdf. Accessed July 15, 2013.

Centers for Disease Control and Prevention (CDC). Division of Nutrition and Physical Activity. Research to practice series no. 4: does breastfeeding reduce the risk of pediatric overweight? Atlanta: Centers for Disease Control and Prevention; 2007.

Centers for Disease Control and Prevention (CDC). Trends in the prevalence of extreme obesity among US preschool children living in low-income families, 1998–2010. *JAMA.* 2012;308(24):2563–2565.

Centers for Disease Control and Prevention (CDC). Advisory Committee on Immunization Practices (ACIP) recommended immunization schedules for persons aged 0 through 18 years and adults aged 19 years and older—United States, 2013. *MMWR.* 2013a;62(1):1–19.

Centers for Disease Control and Prevention (CDC). Community water fluoridation: frequently asked questions. Updated July 10, 2013b. Available at: http://www.cdc.gov/fluoridation/faqs/. Accessed August 30, 2013.

Centers for Disease Control and Prevention (CDC). Prevention of measles, rubella, congenital rubella syndrome and mumps. *MMWR.* 2013c:62(4):7–8, 14–15.

Conde-Agudelo A, Belizán JM, Diaz-Rossello J. Kangaroo mother care to reduce morbidity in low birthweight infants (Cochrane review). The Cochrane Collaboration. *Cochrane Library.* 2011;3. Available at: http://www.thecochranelibrary.com. Accessed April 2, 2014.

Condon WS, Sander LW. Neonate movement is synchronized with adult speech: interaction participation and language acquisition. *Science.* 1974;183:99.

Cortese S, Konofal E, Yateman N, et al. Sleep and alertness in children with attention-deficit/hyperactivity disorder: a systematic review of the literature. *Sleep.* 2006;29(4):504–511.

Daniels MC, Adair LS. Breast-Feeding influences cognitive development in Filipino children. J Nutr. 2005;135:2589–2595.

Dawodu A, Saadi H, Vekdache G, et al. Randomized controlled trial (RCT) of vitamin D supplementation in pregnancy in a population with endemic vitamin D deficiency. *J Clin Endocrinol Metab.* 2013;98(6); 2337–2346.

De La O, Jordan KC, Ortiz K, et al. Do parents accurately perceive their child's weight status? *J Pediatr Health Care.* 2009;23(4):216–221.

DelBono E, Rabe B. *Breastfeeding and child cognitive outcomes: evidence from a hospital-based breastfeeding support policy.* 2012. No. 2012-29. Funded by ESRC under grant RES-062-1693.

DeStefano F. Vaccines and autism: CDC study says no connection. Centers for Disease Control. *Medscape from WebMD.* Accessed April 18, 2013.

DeStefano F, Price CS, Weintraub ES. Increasing exposure to antibody-stimulating proteins and polysaccharides in vaccines is not associated with risk of autism. *J Pediatr.* 2013;163(2):561–567.

Dettwyler KA. A time to wean. In: Stuart-Macadam P, Dettwyler KA, eds. *Breastfeeding: biocultural perspectives.* New York: Aldine de Gruyter; 1995:39–73.

Dewey KG. Is breastfeeding protective against child obesity? *J Hum Lact.* 2003;19:9–18.

DiFrisco E, Goodman KE, Holmes B. Factors associated with exclusive breastfeeding 2 to 4 weeks following discharge from a large, urban, academic medical center striving for baby-friendly designation. *J Perinatal Educ.* 2011;20(1):28–35.

Drobetz R, Maercker A, Spieß CK, et al. A household study of self-regulation in children: internal links and maternal antecedents. *Swiss J Psychol.* 2012;71(4):215–226.

Dunbar RIM. The social role of touch in humans and primates: behavioural function and neurobiological mechanisms. *Neurosci Biobehav Rev.* 2010;34:260–268.

Efe E, Ozer ZC. The use of breast-feeding for pain relief during neonatal immunization injections. *Appl Nurs Res.* 2007;20:10–16.

Eickmann SH de Lira PI, Lima Mde C, et al. Breast feeding and mental and motor development at 12 months in a low-income population in northeast Brazil. *Paediatr Perinat Epidemiol.* 2007;21:129–137.

Engler AJ, Ludington-Hoe SM, Cusson RM, et al. Kangaroo care: national survey of practice, knowledge, barriers and perceptions. *MCN.* 2002;27:146–152.

Epstein K. The interactions between breastfeeding mothers and their babies during the breastfeeding session. *Early Child Dev Care.* 1993;87:93–104.

Erickson PR. Investigation of the role of human breastmilk in caries development. *Pediatr Dentistry.* 1999;21:86–90.

Erikson EH. *Childhood and society,* 2nd ed. New York: Norton; 1963.

Erikson EH. *Identity, youth and crisis.* New York: Norton; 1968.

Farquharson J, Cockburn F, Patrick WA, et al. Infant cerebral cortex phospholipid fatty-acid composition and diet. *Lancet.* 1992;340:810–813.

Farren E, McEwen M. The basics of pediatric immunizations. *Newborn Infant Nurs Rev.* 2004:4(1):5-14.

Feldman R, Weller A, Leckman JF, et al. The nature of the mother's tie to her infant: maternal bonding under conditions of proximity, separation, and potential loss. *J Child Psychol Psychiatry.* 1999.40:929–939.

Flacking R, Ewald U, Wallin L. Positive effect of kangaroo mother care on long-term breastfeeding in very preterm infants. *JOGNN.* 2011;40:190–197. doi: 1111/j.1552-6909.2011.01266.x.

Fleischer D, Spergel JM, Assa'ad AH, Pongracic JA. Primary prevention of allergic disease through nutritional interventions. *J Allergy Clin Immunol Pract.* 2013;1(1):29–36.

Floury CV, Leech AM, Blackhall A. Infant feeding and mental and motor development at 18 months of age in first-born singletons. *Int J Epidemiol.* 1995;24(3 suppl 1):S21–S26.

Forster C, Abraham S, Taylor A, Llewellyn-Jones D. Psychological and sexual changes after the cessation of breastfeeding. *Obstet Gynecol.* 1994;84:872–876.

Gill NE, Behnke M, Conlon M, et al. Effect of nonnutritive sucking on behavioral state in preterm infants before feeding. *Nurs Res.* 1988;37:347–350.

Greer FR, Sicherer SH, Burks AW; American Academy of Pediatrics Committee on Nutrition. Effects of early nutritional interventions on the development of a topical disease in infants and children: the role of maternal dietary restriction, breastfeeding, timing of introduction of complementary foods, and hydrolyzed formulas. *Pediatrics.* 2008;121:183–191.

Hall M, Hall R. Preventive dental services. *Primary Care Clin Rev.* 2013;23(3):42–50.

Harlow HF, Harlow M. The affectional systems. In: Schrier A, Harlow H, Stollnitz F, eds. *Behavior of nonhuman primates,* Vol. 2. New York: Academic; 1965:287–334.

Harris HW, Jaiswal P, Holmes V, Weisler RH. Vitamin D deficiency and psychiatric illness. *Curr Psychiatry.* 2013;12(4);19–25.

Hart SL, Boylan LM, Carroll SR, et al. Brief report: newborn behavior differs with docosahexaenoic acid levels in breast milk. *J Pediatr Psychol.* 2006;31:221–226.

Hedberg-Nyqvist K, Ewald U. Successful breast feeding in spite of early mother–baby separation for neonatal care. *Midwifery.* 1997;13:24–31.

Hediger ML, Overpeck MD, Kuczmarski RJ, Ruan WJ. Association between infant breastfeeding and overweight in young children. *JAMA.* 2001;285:2453–2460.

Hegvik R, McDevitt SC, Carey W. The middle child-hood temperament questionnaire. *J Dev Behav Pediatr.* 1982;3:197–200.

Heinig MJ, Nommsen LA, Peerson JM, et al. Intake and growth of breast-fed and formula-fed infants in relation to the timing of introduction of complementary foods: the DARLING study. *Acta Paediatr.* 1993;82:999–1006.

Hurst N, Valentine CK, Renfro L. Skin-to-skin holding in the neonatal intensive care unit influences maternal milk volume. *J Perinatol.* 1997;27:213–217.

Immunization Action Coalition (IAC). *Needle Tips.* 2013;24(3). Available at: http://immunize.org. Accessed April 20, 2013.

Ismail I, Oppedisano F, Joseph SJ, et al. Reduced gut microbial diversity in early life is associated with later development of eczema but not atopy in high-risk infants. *Pediatr Allergy Immunol.* 2012;23:674–681.

Johnson DL, Swank PR, Howie VM, et al. Breast feeding and children's intelligence. *Psychol Rep.* 1996;79:1179–1185.

Joint Commission Release. Additional performance measurement requirements for general medical/surgical hospitals. 2012. Available at: http://www.jointcommission.org/assets/1/6/JCP1212_AddPerfMeasReq.pdf.

Julvez J, Ribas-Fito N, Forns M, et al. Attention behavior and hyperactivity at age 4 and duration of breast-feeding. *Acta Paediatr.* 2007;96:842–847.

Kaludjerovic J, Vieth R. Relationship between vitamin D during prenatal development and health. *J Midwifery Women's Health.* 2010:55(6):550–560.

Keane V, Chamey E, Strauss J, Roberts K. Do solids help baby sleep through the night? *Am J Dis Child.* 1988;142:404–405.

Kersey M, Lipton R, Sanchez-Rosado M, et al. Breast-feeding history and overweight in Latino preschoolers. *Ambulatory Pediatr.* 2005;5:355–358.

Klaus MH, Kennell JH. *Maternal–infant bonding: the impact of early separation and loss on family development.* St. Louis, MO: Mosby; 1975.

Kramer MS. Do breast-feeding and delayed introduction of solid foods protect against subsequent obesity? *J Pediatr.* 1981;98:883–887.

LactMed. United States National Library of Medicine (NLM). Toxicology Data Network (TOXNET). Vaccines. 2013. Available at: http://toxnet.nlm.nih.gov. Accessed September 17, 2013.

Lavie C, Lee J, Milani R. Vitamin D and cardiovascular disease. *J Am Coll Cardiol.* 2011;58(15):1546–1556.

Lawrence R, Lawrence RM. *Breastfeeding: a guide for the medical profession,* 6th ed. Philadelphia, PA: Mosby; 2005:634.

Li R, Fein SB, Grummer-Strawn LM. Do infants fed from bottles lack self-regulation of milk intake compared with directly breastfed infants? *Pediatrics.* 2010;125(6):e1386–e1393. doi: 1.1542/peds.2009-2549.

Li R, Magadia J, Fein SB, Grummer-Strawn LM. Risk of bottle-feeding for rapid weight gain during the first year of life. *Arch Pediatr Adolesc Med.* 2012;166(5):431–436. doi: 10.1001/archpediatrics.2011.1665.

Li L, Parsons TJ, Power C. Breastfeeding and obesity in childhood: cross sectional study. *BMJ.* 2003;327:904–905.

Lopez Del Valle L, Singh GD, Feliciano N, et al. Associations between a history of breast feeding, malocclusion and parafunctional habits in Puerto Rican children. *P R Health Sci J.* 2006;25:31.

Lorenz KZ. The companion in the environment of the bird. *J Ornithol.* 1935;83:137–215, 289–413.

Lucas A, Morley R, Cole TJ, et al. Breastmilk and subsequent intelligence quotient in children born preterm. *Lancet.* 1992;339:261–264.

Ludington-Hoe S, Johnson MW, Morgan K, et al. Neurophysiologic assessment of neonatal sleep organization: preliminary results of a randomized, controlled trial of skin contact with preterm infants. *Pediatrics.* 2006;117:e909–e923 doi: 10.1542/PEDS.2004-1422.

Ludington-Hoe S, Nguyen N, Swinth JY, Satyshur RD. Kangaroo care compared to incubators in maintaining body warmth in preterm infants. *Biol Res Nurs.* 2000;260–273.

Ludington-Hoe S, Swinth JY. Developmental aspects of kangaroo care. *JOGNN.* 1996;25:692–703.

Ludwig DS, Rouse HL, Currie J. Pregnancy weight gain and childhood body weight: a within-family comparison. *PLoS Med.* 2013;10(10):e1001521. doi: 10.1371/journal.pmed.1001521. Available at: http://www.plosmedicine.org/article/info%3Adoi/10.1371/journal.pmed.1001521. Accessed September 3, 2013.

Lunardelli SE, Peres MA. Breast-feeding and other mother–child factors associated with developmental enamel defects in the primary teeth of Brazilian children. *J Dent Child.* 2006;73(2):70–78.

Macknin ML, Medendorp SV, Maier MC. Infant sleep and bedtime cereal. *Am J Dis Child.* 1989;143:1066–1068.

Madhusmitam M, Pacaud D, Petryk A, et al. Vitamin D deficiency in children and its management: review of current knowledge and recommendations. *Pediatrics.* 2008;122:398–417.

Maffeis C. Childhood obesity: the genetic–environmental interface. *Endocrinol Metab.* 1999;13:31.

Maguire L, Lebovic G, Kandasamy S, et al. The relationship between cow's milk and stores of vitamin D and iron in early childhood. *Pediatrics.* 2012;131(1):e144–e151. Available at: http://pediatrics.aappublications.org/content/131/1/e144. Accessed March 22, 2013.

Makin JW, Porter RH. Attractiveness of lactating females' breast odors to neonates. *Child Dev.* 1989;60:803–810.

Malone R, Kessenich C. Vitamin D deficiency: implications across the lifespan. *J Nurs Pract.* 2008;4(6):448–456.

Mangels AR, Messina BV. Considerations in planning vegan diets: infants. *J Am Diet Assoc.* 2001;101:670–677.

Markowitz DL. Fluoride supplementation: the ongoing debate. *Medscape.* 2012. Available at: http://www.medscape.com/viewarticle/753193_2. Accessed August 12, 2014.

Marquis GS, Marquis GS, Brakohiapa L, et al. Breastmilk or animal-products foods improve linear growth of Peruvian toddlers consuming marginal diets. *Am J Clin Nutr.* 1997;66:1102–1109.

Martin RM, Goodall SH, Gunnell D, Davey Smith G. Breast feeding in infancy and social mobility: 60-year follow-up of the Boyd Orr cohort. *Arch Dis Child.* 2007;92:317–321.

Matee MIN, van't Hof M, Maselle S, et al. Nursing caries, linear hypoplasia, and nursing and weaning habits in Tanzanian infants. *Community Dent Oral Epidemiol.* 1994;22:289–293.

Matheson D, Robinson T. Obesity in young children. In: Birch L, Dietz W, eds. *Eating behaviors of the young child: prenatal and postnatal influences on healthy eating.* Elk Village, IL: American Academy of Pediatricians; 2008:33–58.

Maxwell C, Carbone E, Wood, R. Better newborn vitamin D status lowers RSV-associated bronchiolitis in infants. *Nutr Rev.* 2012;70(9):548–552.

McKenna J, Mosko S, Richard C. Bedsharing promotes breast-feeding. *Pediatrics.* 1997;100:214–219.

Mennella JA. Mothers' milk: a medium for early flavor experiences. *J Hum Lact.* 1995;11:39–45.

Mennella JA, Beauchamp GK. Mothers' milk enhances the acceptance of cereal during weaning. *Pediatr Res.* 1997;41:188–192.

Mennella JA, Jagnow CP, Beauchamp GK. Prenatal and postnatal flavor learning by human infants. *Pediatrics.* 2001;107:E88.

Mercer R. A theoretical framework for studying factors that impact on the maternal role. *Nurs Res.* 1981;30:73–77.

Morley R, Cole TJ, Powell R, Lucas A. Mother's choice to provide breastmilk and developmental outcome. *Arch Dis Child.* 1988;63:1382–1385.

Mosko S, Richard C, McKenna J. Infant arousals in the bedsharing environment: implications for infant sleep development and SIDS. *Pediatrics.* 1997;100:841–849.

Mosko S, Richard C, McKenna J, Drummond S. Infant sleep architecture during bedsharing and possible implications for SIDS. *Sleep.* 1996;19:677–684.

National Institutes of Health (NIH), Office of Dietary Supplements. Dietary supplement fact sheet. Revised June 2011. Available at: http://ods.od.nih.gov/factsheets/VitaminD-HealthProfessional/. Accessed September 3, 2013.

National Sleep Foundation. How sleep works. 2013. Available at: http://www.sleepfoundation.org/primary-links/how-sleep-works. Accessed April 3, 2014.

Nisbett RE, Aronson J, Blair C, et al. Intelligence: new findings and theoretical developments. *Am Psychol.* 2012;67(2):130–159. doi: 10.1037/a0026699.

Ogden, C., Caroll M, Kit BK, Flegal KM. *Prevalence of obesity in the United States, 2009–2010.* NCHS Data Brief no. 82. National Center for Health Statistics; January 2012.

Oulis CJ, Berdouses ED, Vadiakas G, Lygidakis NA. Feeding practices of Greek children with and without nursing caries. *Pediatr Dent.* 1999;21:409–416.

Owen CG, Martin RM, Whincup PH, et al. Does breastfeeding influence risk of type 2 diabetes in later life? A quantitative analysis of published evidence. *Am J Clin Nutr.* 2006;84:1043–1054.

Page-Goertz S. Breastfeeding beyond 6 months. *Adv Nurs Pract.* 2002;45–48.

Palmer B. The influence of breastfeeding on the development of the oral cavity: a commentary. *J Hum Lact.* 1998;14:93–98.

Piaget J. *The origins of intelligence in children.* Cook M, trans. New York: International Universities Press; 1952.

Piaget J, Inhelder B. *Psychology of the child.* New York: Basic Books; 1969.

Pickering LK, Baker CL, Kimberlin DW, et al., eds. *Red book: 2012 report of the Committee on Infectious Diseases,* 29th ed. Elk Grove Village, IL: American Academy of Pediatrics; 2012.

Pisacane A, Continisio P, Filosa C, et al. Use of baby carriers to increase breastfeeding duration among term infants: the effects of an educational intervention in Italy. *Acta Paediatrica.* 2012;101:e434–e438.

Pisacane A, De Vizia B, Valiante A, et al. Iron status in breast-fed infants. *J Pediatr.* 1995;127:429–431.

Pramyothin P, Hollick, M. Vitamin D supplementation: guidelines and evidence for subclinical deficiency. *Curr Opin Gastroenterol.* 2012;28(2):139–150.

Prechtl J, Beintema D. *The neurological examination of the full term infant* (Child Development Medical Series, 12). Philadelphia, PA: Lippincott; 1975.

Pridham KF, Chang AS. Transition to being the mother of a new infant in the first 3 months: maternal problem solving and self-appraisals. *J Adv Nurs.* 1992;17:204–216.

Prodromidis M, Field T, Arendt R, et al. Mothers touching newborns: a comparison of rooming-in versus minimal contact. *Birth.* 1995;22:196–2000.

Randle J. Starting solids. In *New beginnings.* La Leche League International; May–June 1999.

Rao MR, Hediger ML, Levine RJ, et al. Effect of breastfeeding on cognitive development of infants born small for gestational age. *Acta Paediatr.* 2002;91:267–274.

Riedl R, Javor A. The biology of trust: integrating evidence from genetics, endocrinology, and functional brain imaging. *J Neurosci Psychol Econ.* 2012;5(2):63–91.

Robertson J. *Young children in hospital.* New York: Basic Books; 1958.

Rogan WJ, Gladen BC. Breast-feeding and cognitive development. *Early Hum Dev.* 1993;31:181–193.

Rubin R. Attainment of the maternal role. *Nurs Res.* 1967;16:237–245.

Saalfield S, Jackson-Allen P. Biopsychosocial consequences of sweetened drink consumption in children 0–6 years of age. *Pediatr Nurs.* 2006;32:460–461.

Sachs H, Committee on Drugs. The transfer of drugs and therapeutics into breast milk: an update on selected topics. *Pediatrics.* Published online August 26, 2013. doi: 10.1542/PEDS.2013-1985. Available at: http://pediatrics.aappublications.org/content/early /2013/08/20/peds.2013-1985. Accessed September 16, 2013.

Sacker A, Quigley MA, Kelly Y. Breastfeeding and developmental delay: findings from the millennium cohort study. *Pediatrics.* 2006;111:3.

Sanger R, Bystrom E. Breastfeeding: does it affect oral facial growth? *Dent Hygiene.* 1982;56:44–47.

Schwarz, S. Obesity in children. *Medscape Reference.* December 12, 2012. Available at: http://emedicine.medscape. com/article/985333-overview. Accessed October 1, 2013.

Sears W. *Growing together.* Franklin Park, IL: La Leche League International; 1987:30, 71.

Servonsky J, Opas SR. *Nursing management of children.* Sudbury, MA: Jones and Bartlett; 1987.

Shur-Fen Gau S. Prevalence of sleep problems and their association with inattention/hyperactivity among children aged 6–15 in Taiwan. *J Sleep Res.* 2006;4:403–414.

Singhal A, Lanigan J. Breastfeeding, early growth and later obesity. *Obesity Rev.* 2006;8:51–54. Available at: http://www.blackwell-synergy.com. Accessed February 12, 2009.

Singhal A, Morley R, Cole TJ, et al. Infant nutrition and stereoacuity at age 4–6 years. *Am J Clin Nutr.* 2007;85:152–159.

Slykerman RE, Thompson JM, Becroft DM, et al. Breastfeeding and intelligence of preschool children. *Acta Paediatr.* 2005;94:832–837.

Smith PJ, Moffatt ME. Baby-bottle decay: Are we on the right track? *Int J Circumpolar Health.* 1998;57 (suppl 1):155–162.

Spitz AS, Weber-Gasparoni K, Kanellis MJ, Qian F. Child temperament and risk factors for early childhood caries. *J Dent Child.* 2006;73(2):98–104.

Spitz R. Anaclitic depression. *Psychoanal Study Child.* 1946;2:313–342.

Strathearn L. Maternal neglect: oxytocin, dopamine and the neurobiology of attachment. *J Neuroendocrinol.* 2011;23(1):1054–1065.

Strathearn L, Fonagy P, Amico J, Montague PR. Adult attachment predicts maternal brain and oxytocin response to infant cues. *Neuropsychopharmacology.* 2009;34:2655–2666. doi: 10.1038/npp.2009.103.

Strathearn L, Mamun AA, Najman JM, O'Callaghan MJ. Does breastfeeding protect against substantiated child abuse and neglect? A 15-year cohort study. *Pediatrics.* 2009;123:483–493. doi: 10.1542/peds.2007-3546.

Sugarman J, Kendall-Tackett KA. Weaning ages in a sample of American women who practice extended breastfeeding. *Clin Pediatr.* 1995;34:642–647.

Sullivan SA, Birch LL. Infant dietary experience and acceptance of solid foods. *Pediatrics.* 1994;93:271–277.

Syed A, Kohli A, Nadeau KC. Food allergy diagnosis and therapy: Where are we now? *Immunotherapy.* 2013;5(9):931–944.

Taheri S. The link between short sleep duration and obesity: we should recommend more sleep to prevent obesity. *Arch Dis Child.* 2006;11:881–888.

Tansky C, Lindberg C. Breastfeeding as a pain intervention when immunizing infants. *J Nurs Pract.* 2010;6(4):287–295.

Tarkka MT. Predictors of maternal competence by first-time mothers when the child is 8 months old. *J Adv Nurs.* 2003;41:233–240.

Temboury MC, Otero A, Polanco I, Arribas, E. Influence of breast-feeding on the infant's intellectual development. *J Pediatr Gastroenterol Nutr.* 1994;18:32–36.

Teti D, Kim BR, Mayer G, Countermine M. Maternal emotional availability at bedtime predicts infant sleep quality. *J Am Psychol Assoc.* 2010;24(3):307–315.

Thomas A, Chess S. *Temperament and development.* New York: Brunner/Mazel; 1977.

Tomlinson M, Landman M. It's not just food: mother–infant interaction and is better the wider context of nutrition. *MCN.* 2007;3:292–302.

Toschke AM, Vignerova J, Lhotska L, et al. Overweight and obesity in 6 to 14 year old Czech children in 1991: protective effect of breast-feeding. *J Pediatr.* 2002;141:764–769.

Trawitzki LV, Anselmo-Lima WT, Melchior MO, et al. Breastfeeding and deleterious oral habits in mouth and nose breathers. *Rev Bras Otorrhinolaryngol.* 2005;71:747–751.

Turner C, Lin H, Flores G. Prevalence of vitamin D deficiency among overweight and obese children. *Pediatrics.* 2013;131:e152; originally published online December 24, 2012. doi: 10.1542/PEDS.2012-1711.

USDHHS. Proposed HHS Recommendation for Fluoride Concentration in Drinking Water for Prevention of Dental Caries.Federal Register / Vol. 76, No. 9 / Thursday, January 13, 2011, 2383-2388. Accessed at http://www.gpo.gov/fdsys/pkg/FR-2011-01-13/pdf/2011-637.pdf

Uvnas-Moberg K. Physiological and endocrine effects of social contact. *Ann NY Acad Sci.* 1997;807(1):146–163.

Uvnas-Moberg K. Oxytocin may mediate the benefits of positive social interactions and emotions. *Psychoneuroendocrinology.* 1998;23(8):818–835.

Valaitis R, Hesch R, Passarelli C, et al. A systematic review of the relationships between breastfeeding and early childhood caries. *Can J Pub Health.* 2000;91:411–417.

Van Esterick P. Commentary: an anthropological perspective on infant feeding in Oceania. In: Marshall LB, ed. *Infant care and feeding in the South Pacific.* New York, NY: Gordon & Breach Science Publishers; 1985:331–343.

Vohr BR, Poindexter BB, Dusick AM et al. Beneficial effects of breast milk in the neonatal intensive care unit on the developmental outcome of extremely low birth weight infants at 18 months of age. *Pediatrics.* 2006;118:e115–e123.

von Knorring AL, Söderberg A, Austin L, Uvnäs-Moberg K. Massage decreases aggression in preschool children: a long-term study. *Acta Paediatr.* 2008;97(9):1265–1269. doi: 10.1111/j.1651-2227.2008.00919.x.

Wagner CL, Greer FR, American Academy of Pediatrics Committee on Nutrition and Section on Breastfeeding. Prevention of rickets and vitamin D deficiency in infants, children, and adolescents. *Pediatrics.* 2008;122(5):1142–1152.

Wagner C, Rosenkrantz T. Human milk and lactation. *Medscape Reference.* October 10, 2012. Available at: http://emedicine.medscape.com/article/1835675-overview. Accessed September 16, 2013.

Wang B, Brand-Miller J. The role and potential of sialic acid in human nutrition. *Eur J Clin Nutr.* 2003;57:1361–1369.

Weerheijm KL, Uyttendaele-Speybrouck BF, Euwe HC, Groen HJ. Prolonged demand breast-feeding and nursing caries. *Caries Res.* 1998;32:46–50.

Wigg NR, Tong S, McMichael AJ, et al. Does breastfeeding at six months predict cognitive development? *Aust N Z J Pub Health.* 1998;22:232–236.

Winberg J. Mother and newborn baby: mutual regulation of physiology and behavior—a selective review. *Dev Psychobiol.* 2005;47(3):217–229.

Woo T. Pharmacotherapy and surgery treatment for the severely obese adolescent. *J Pediatr Health Care.* 2009;23(4):206–212.

World Health Organization. Infant and young child feeding, Fact sheet, updated February 2014. Available at http://www.who.int/mediacentre/factsheets/fs342/en/. Accessed April 3, 2014.

Wrigley EA, Hutchinson SA. Long-term breastfeeding: the secret bond. *J Nurs Midwifery.* 1990;35:35–41.

Yoneyama K, Nagata H, Asano H. Growth of Japanese breastfed and bottle-fed infants from birth to 20 months. *Ann Hum Biol.* 1994;21:597–608.

Chapter 18

The Ill Child: Breastfeeding Implications

Sallie Page-Goertz

Breastfeeding is much more than nutrition—it is comfort and love shared between a mother and her baby. Babies born with congenital defects are less likely to ever be breastfed (Rendon-Macias et al., 2002). For ill or hospitalized children who have established breastfeeding, the breastfeeding relationship can be threatened. When illness or other health problems makes the breastfeeding relationship difficult or impossible, nurses and other healthcare providers help families by providing both practical and emotional support and encouragement to establish lactation, facilitate direct breastfeeding when possible, and prevent unnecessary weaning. This chapter presents strategies for helping parents of breastfeeding children who need special breastfeeding support due to health problems beyond the newborn period.

Team Care for the Child with Feeding Difficulties

A variety of healthcare specialists participate in assessment and treatment of a child who has ongoing feeding difficulties. This team might include a physical or occupational therapist, neurologist, developmental medicine specialist, lactation consultant, speech-language pathologist, dentist, social worker, psychologist, and dietitian. Box 18-1 describes the services that each has to offer the child and family. When several people are involved in the child's care, one of them should serve as the coordinator to facilitate communication with the family and the child's primary healthcare provider, and among the health team members themselves.

BOX 18-1 MEMBERS OF THE HEALTHCARE TEAM FOR THE BREASTFEEDING CHILD WITH SPECIAL HEALTHCARE PROBLEMS

Nurse

Assesses the global needs of child and family

Assists in identification of referral needs

Provides initial assessment of breastfeeding status

Ensures that the healthcare plan is implemented

Provides family education

Provides direct nursing care to the child as needed

(continues)

Box 18-1 (CONTINUED)

Lactation Consultant

Assesses the breastfeeding dyad

Identifies strengths and weaknesses

Identifies referral needs for the child with complex oral–motor difficulties

Develops a breastfeeding plan of care

Physician/Subspecialist

Diagnoses underlying illness/condition

Develops medical plan of care

Refers to other professionals as needed

Refers to neurologist or developmental specialist to assist in evaluation

Physical Therapist

Assesses gross motor capabilities

Develops plan of care to optimize baby's skills

Geneticist/Genetic Counselor

Provides risk counseling related to inherited conditions

Occupational Therapist

Assesses oral–motor/feeding capability as well as fine and gross motor skills as needed

Works with the mother to identify optimal positioning for the baby at breast

If breastfeeding is not possible, helps identify a preferred alternative feeding method

Develops plan of care to optimize baby's skills

Speech-Language Pathologist

Assesses oral–motor/feeding capabilities

May provide similar services to the OT related to oral–motor issues

Develops plan of care to optimize baby's skills

Dietitian

Assesses nutritional status of child

Develops plan of nutrition care

Identifies preferred supplements if needed

Mental Health Therapist

Assists families with the adaptation to a child with acute or chronic healthcare problem

Social Worker

Assesses family's needs for practical and psychosocial support

May provide counseling services

Families will need both verbal and written instructions, and they should be encouraged to perform return demonstrations of recommended feeding techniques. Videotaping the breastfeeding mother and child while teaching special techniques allows the family to have a customized teaching aid.

Feeding Behaviors of the Ill Infant/Child

A child who is not feeling well commonly has a diminished appetite. A breastfeeding infant may feed less vigorously, less often, or more frequently but in brief bouts. The magnitude of the change in feeding routine varies with the severity of the illness. The child's condition may impair ability to suckle vigorously or frequently enough to take in sufficient calories to meet requirements for growth. In the face of selected conditions, such as congenital heart defect, the metabolic needs of the child may increase beyond the normal recommended daily allowances for age and height (Ripmeester & Dunn, 2002).

Milk supply may diminish fairly quickly with waning demand. Mothers may have uncomfortable breast fullness if the child is breastfeeding less frequently or effectively. Anytime that a baby has diminished appetite or is unable to maintain normal weight gain with direct breastfeeding, the mother must augment breast stimulation by expressing breastmilk by hand or pump (see the *Breast Pumps and Other Technologies* chapter) to maintain her milk supply and to prevent engorgement. Milk obtained in excess of a baby's immediate need can be stored for use at a later date. Milk handling guidelines differ for patients in the neonatal intensive care unit (NICU), healthy term infants, and older children. It would seem prudent to follow NICU milk handling and storage guidelines for the hospitalized or fragile infant (see the *Donor Milk Banking* chapter); these guidelines are published by the Human Milk Banking Association of North America (Jones, 2011).

The infant who is unable to feed orally for prolonged periods of time (days, weeks, or months) needs oral stimulation by other means—typically a pacifier, despite the concern that sucking on an artificial teat may create problems in getting the baby back to the breast. If the infant is able to do so, suckling the empty breast is an alternative. The baby who experiences uncomfortable procedures in and around the mouth, such as suctioning, intubation, or operative intervention, may be reluctant to breastfeed and requires special attention.

Skilled feeding assessment of the child with special healthcare needs is vital. Assessment includes observation of at least one complete breastfeeding session and monitoring of the infant's weight to determine the adequacy of milk transfer and caloric intake. If the child is not gaining weight normally, the amount of milk ingested is inadequate, regardless of what that amount might be. Even if before- and after-feed weights indicate good intake for age (e.g., 3 oz/90 mL feeding in a 7 lb/3.2 kg infant), this volume may not be adequate for a daily weight gain of 0.5–1 oz (15–30 g), or 1% of the child's weight. An ill infant may have well-developed, effective oral–motor skills, yet lack the energy to maintain suckling long enough to obtain sufficient calories for normal weight gain, as in the case of complex congenital heart disease.

What to Do If Weight Gain Is Inadequate

If a child is not gaining sufficient weight, several strategies can be tried. General strategies are discussed in this section, and later condition-specific sections address specific strategies and techniques.

The first suggestion is to simply change the baby's position at the breast. The upright posture shown in Figure 18-1 increases the baby's alertness through stimulation of the vestibular system and may increase breastfeeding vigor. This position has recently been described as the koala hold (Thomson, 2013). Providing extra support for the baby's

Figure 18-1 UPRIGHT POSITIONING. EITHER (A) SIDE SITTING, OR (B) STRADDLING THE MOTHER'S THIGH MAY SERVE TO MAXIMIZE THE BABY'S BREASTFEEDING EFFICIENCY.

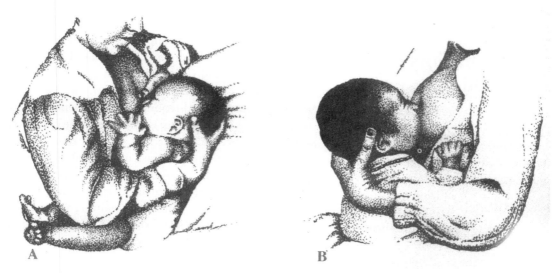

A   B

Source: Provided courtesy of the Cleft Palate Foundation, 1-800-24-CLEFT, http://www.cleftline.org

cheeks and jaw using the dancer-hand position (Figure 18-2) may also help. Other techniques for slow weight gaining infant are described in the *Low Intake in the Breastfed Infant: Maternal and Infant Considerations* chapter. Strategies for helping the child with abnormal tone (see Box 18-4 later in this chapter) are useful for a baby who is neurologically normal but has a weak suckle. Trying to feed a soundly sleeping baby usually results in frustration for both baby and mother, and is not recommended.

Supplementation with mother's milk, particularly high-calorie hindmilk, or calorie-enriched mother's milk may be needed to improve weight gain. For the child with greatly increased metabolic demands, such as the infant with congenital heart disease, continuous or intermittent feeding with higher-calorie milk through a nasogastric (NG) tube is often necessary to meet the increased caloric requirements for growth (Figure 18-3).

What to Do When Direct Breastfeeding Is Not Sufficient

When a child is incapable of breastfeeding, or does not thrive with direct breastfeeding, healthcare providers are faced with two challenges: (1) they must develop a feeding plan that will lead to optimal weight gain and (2) they must help a family come to a peaceful acceptance of at least a temporary change in their breastfeeding dreams. The health provider can make a difference in how a family comes to view these early experiences with their child. Some will remember brusque interactions and feelings that the provider had no understanding of the important nurturing aspect of breastfeeding. Other families may work with professionals who are so enthusiastic about breastfeeding that they lose sight of the importance of the infant's growth and development, even putting children at risk for severe dehydration or failure to thrive.

Figure 18-2 DANCER-HAND SUPPORT. DANCER-HAND POSITIONING PROVIDES STABILITY TO THE BABY'S JAW AND SUPPORT TO WEAK MASSETER MUSCLES. (A) THE HAND UNDER THE BREAST SLIDES FORWARD SO THAT THE BREAST IS SUPPORTED BY THREE FINGERS RATHER THAN FOUR. A "U" IS FORMED WITH THUMB AND INDEX FINGER. (B) THE BABY'S HEAD RESTS IN THE U WHERE THE JAW IS SUPPORTED AND CHEEKS ARE GENTLY SQUEEZED. (C) VIEW FROM OVER THE MOTHER'S SHOULDER SHOWS HOW THE HAND SUPPORTS BOTH THE MOTHER'S BREAST AND THE BABY'S HEAD. (D) A MODIFIED DANCER-HAND POSITION CAN PROVIDE JUST CHIN SUPPORT WITH THE INDEX FINGER APPLYING PRESSURE BEHIND THE MANDIBLE TO SUPPORT THE TONGUE.

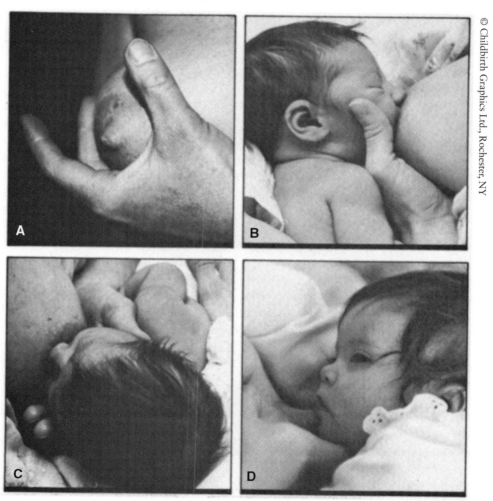

© Childbirth Graphics Ltd., Rochester, NY

Figure 18-3 BABY IS RECEIVING CALORIE-ENRICHED BREASTMILK VIA A SUPPLEMENTER MADE OF A 5 FR NASOGASTRIC TUBE AND A 60 ML SYRINGE. SHE IS SITTING UPRIGHT-STRADDLING HER MOTHER'S LAP TO MAXIMIZE SUCKLING EFFICIENCY.

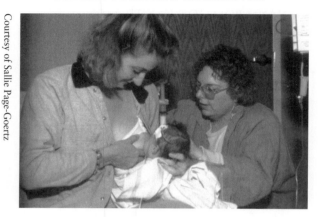

Courtesy of Sallie Page-Goertz

The fortunate family interacts with professionals who are skilled in feeding assessment, understand the importance of optimal growth, and know when the child needs something different than exclusive or direct breastfeeding—and who can communicate this information with sensitivity.

When families of children with chronic conditions are interviewed about their experiences, they express appreciation for advice that is straightforward and, most importantly, accurate. Mothers of babies with cleft palate report how frustrating it was to realize that the enthusiasm of the pamphlets and the professionals they spoke to about the possibility of exclusive breastfeeding was, in fact, extraordinarily misleading (Miller, 1998). These mothers experienced feelings of failure, because their babies did not breastfeed "like the story in the pamphlet." Such pressure often leads to unrealistic, exhausting breastfeeding efforts that undermine the developing relationship between mother and baby.

When it is evident that direct or exclusive breastfeeding is not working, the skilled lactation consultant needs to acknowledge the disappointment a mother may feel. Do point out other strengths that the child has—for example, "Look how the baby is watching you." "Isn't it wonderful how she follows your voice?" "What a wonderful snuggler you have." The goal is to reframe what is happening: mothers and babies are not breastfeeding failures, but rather are presented with a special challenge. It is also helpful to separate the two components of breastfeeding: the milk (nutrition) and the love (nurture) that happens with breastfeeding. The milk can continue to be offered, or saved until the baby can have oral feedings; the love continues on without interruption.

Alternative Feeding Methods

Breastfeeding specialists disagree about how to supplement children with special feeding needs. Unfortunately, there are insufficient data upon which to base the majority of recommendations, especially for infants and for children who are failing to thrive owing to a myriad of other underlying health problems or conditions. Lacking such evidence, we base the recommendations presented here on understanding the child's condition, the anatomy and physiology of breastfeeding, the occasional case report, discussions with colleagues, and one's best clinical judgment. Consultation with an occupational therapist, physical therapist, and speech-language pathologist, as well as a dietitian, should be considered when working with a child who is not thriving with direct breastfeeding. These professionals provide valuable input into the assessment of how a particular child's strengths and weaknesses determine a plan of care that will optimize feeding and growth. If the child is not taking in a sufficient volume of the mother's milk to thrive, the dietitian provides input as to the preferred way to enrich the milk's caloric content. Hindmilk or the addition of carbohydrate, fat, and/or protein supplements to breastmilk may be preferred, depending on the child's particular health condition.

Replacement feeding methods and supplementation devices such as cup-, finger-, and syringe-feeding are discussed in detail in the *Perinatal and Intrapartum Care* and *Low Intake in the Breastfed*

Infant: Maternal and Infant Considerations chapters. Although a supplementation device is suitable for a prolonged period, the infant must be able to generate sufficient negative intraoral pressure to pull milk from the device. If the reservoir of the device is flexible, the mother can squeeze it so that a bolus of milk goes directly into the child's mouth and normal suckling skills may not be needed to accomplish sufficient intake. If the baby can latch onto the breast, supplementing at the breast is always the preferred way to provide extra calories. If the child is unable to gain adequate weight, other feeding methods need to be explored. Neither cup-, nor finger-, nor syringe-feeding is conducive to long-term provision of large volumes of milk. Dowling et al. (2002) found that with cup-feeding, volumes of milk ingested were small and about one-third of the amount taken from the cup was recovered on the bib.

For some children, bottle-feeding may be the best alternative feeding method. The feeding bottle can be used in ways that help develop or mimic breastfeeding skills (Kassing, 2002; Noble & Bovey, 1997). Gromada and Sandora (2007) describe "paced feeding" techniques, an approach to bottle-feeding that assures the baby's feeding cues are respected and milk flow does not overwhelm the infant. With this strategy, the feeding bottle is held horizontally to reduce the speed of flow. When the baby exhibits stress cues, he is allowed to rest briefly, either by removing the nipple from the mouth or by leaving the nipple in place, but tipping the baby forward so that milk cannot flow into the mouth. A squeezable bottle allows the caregiver to deliver a milk bolus into the baby's oral pharynx for swallowing, even when the baby is unable to generate negative intraoral pressure to accomplish milk flow. Higher volumes of milk or normal volumes of calorie-enriched milk can be provided to maximize weight gain for many children who are not thriving with direct breastfeeding.

The choice of feeding bottle and teat depends on a particular infant's need. Some children will be successful with a standard baby bottle—a firm reservoir with a variety of teats. Figure 18-4 illustrates one such bottle, which has a teat with a very

Figure 18-4 THE AVENT BOTTLE HAS A WIDE-BASED TEAT TO ENCOURAGE A WIDE-OPEN MOUTH.

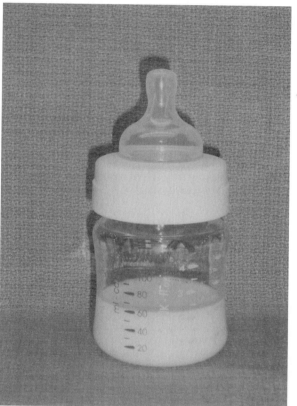

Courtesy of Sallie Page-Goertz

wide base that encourages a wide-open latch. In general, it is best to select a wide-based teat that encourages latch with a wide-open mouth, that has a soft texture like the breast, and that has a nipple length that goes deep into the child's mouth but does not cause the child to gag. Longer teats may be helpful for the child with cleft lip/palate to avoid milk going directly into the cleft. Bottles that have been recommended for children who are not thriving with direct breastfeeding or use of a traditional feeding bottle include the Haberman feeder and the Mead-Johnson cleft palate feeder (Figure 18-5). Each of these bottles has a flexible reservoir, allowing the caregiver to release a bolus of milk into the child's mouth. The Haberman feeder has a specially

Figure 18-5 BOTTLES RECOMMENDED FOR CHILDREN NOT THRIVING WITH DIRECT BREASTFEEDING. (A) THE HABERMAN FEEDER ALLOWS THE CAREGIVER TO ADJUST THE FLOW FOR THE BABY BY ALIGNING THE MARKS WITH THE BABY'S NOSE—THE LONGER LINE PROVIDES GREATER FLOW. THE ONE-WAY VALVE LIMITS THE NEGATIVE PRESSURE REQUIRED TO WITHDRAW MILK, AND THE FLEXIBILE NIPPLE RESERVOIR ALLOWS THE CAREGIVER TO SQUEEZE A BOLUS OF MILK INTO THE BABY'S MOUTH. (B) THE MEAD-JOHNSON CLEFT PALATE FEEDER HAS A FLEXIBLE RESERVOIR ALLOWING THE CAREGIVER TO SQUEEZE MILK INTO THE BABY'S MOUTH. THE NIPPLE IS SOMEWHAT FLATTENED AND LONG SO THAT MILK CAN BE RELEASED WELL INTO THE BABY'S ORAL CAVITY.

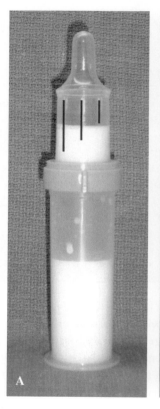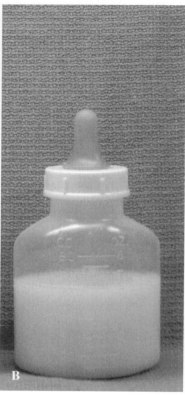

Courtesy of Sallie Page-Goertz

designed valve and teat that allows the feeder to adjust milk flow to suit the baby's needs. There is a slit in the nipple, rather than a hole, which closes when the baby is not compressing/sucking the teat, thereby preventing the flow of an unexpected bolus of milk into the mouth. The Pigeon nipple (Figure 18-6) has a flow valve that reduces the amount of negative intraoral pressure needed for milk transfer, similar to the Haberman feeder; the Pigeon nipple is softer and more flexible. It can be used on any standard infant feeding bottle.

The baby can be fed with a bottle in ways to maximize the closeness that naturally occurs with breastfeeding. Mothers and children need to be comfortable; babies can be in skin-to-skin contact with their mothers or other caregivers during

Figure 18-6 THE PIGEON NIPPLE HAS A ONE-WAY VALVE THAT DECREASES THE AMOUNT OF NEGATIVE PRESSURE REQUIRED TO WITHDRAW MILK. THE OUTLINED AREA OF THE NIPPLE IS SLIGHTLY FIRMER AND IS POSITIONED AGAINST THE ROOF OF THE MOUTH.

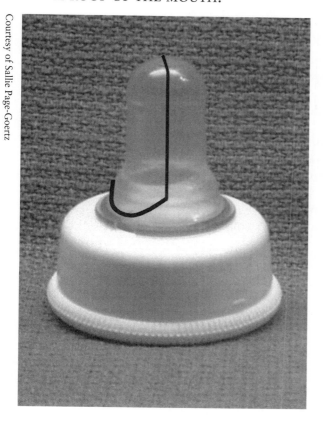

Courtesy of Sallie Page-Goertz

feeding. Eye contact, singing, and reading of stories are not precluded with bottle-feeding. Families should be taught to alternate holding the baby in the left and right arms to provide equal visual stimulation, as normally happens with breastfeeding. When presenting the bottle to the baby, touch the lips to stimulate root/gape, and if possible, allow the baby to draw the teat deeply into the oral cavity. If the baby is unable to draw in sufficient milk to form a bolus to stimulate swallowing, use a flexible bottle or feeders using nurser bags to squeeze intermittent small boluses into the baby's pharynx for swallowing.

If bottle-feeding, even with calorie-enriched milk, is insufficient for improving weight gain, more invasive feeding methods must be considered. Nasogastric feeding with a feeding tube, either by bolus or continuous drip for part or all of the day with regular or enriched milk, may need to be added to breast- or bottle-feedings. If oral feedings are not possible, enteral feedings can be given via gastrostomy or jejeunostomy tube.

Pain Management Concerns

Children with acquired or congenital conditions may be faced with pain related to their illness, surgery, or other procedures. Breastfeeding needs to be considered in the armamentarium of strategies for assisting with procedural pain. Infants who are breastfed during painful procedures appear to have less pain. A Cochrane review evaluated the effectiveness of breastfeeding in reducing procedural pain such as immunizations and heel sticks for blood sampling. Infants breastfed during such procedures had greater reductions in heart rate, duration of crying, and lower pain scores than did infants who were not breastfed during the procedure (Shah et al., 2006). However, it is not known to what extent breastfeeding might contribute to alleviating other types of pain.

Breastfeeding Care of the Hospitalized Infant

Families of breastfeeding children have a unique set of needs. Box 18-2 lists key characteristics of breastfeeding-friendly pediatric units. The American Academy of Pediatrics (AAP) breastfeeding policy statement includes a recommendation related to support of breastfeeding should hospitalization be necessary (Section on Breastfeeding, 2005). Spatz (2006) provides a clinical pathway designed to protect breastfeeding in the hospitalized infant, targeted at the readmitted newborn infant with complications of ineffective breastfeeding.

BOX 18-2 CHARACTERISTICS OF A BREASTFEEDING-FRIENDLY PEDIATRIC UNIT

- Has written breastfeeding policies in place.
- Employs or trains staff capable of skilled breastfeeding assessment and breastfeeding intervention when needed.
- Provides parents with written and verbal information about the benefits of breastfeeding and breastmilk.
- Facilitates unrestricted breastfeeding.
- Facilitates milk expression by mothers who wish to provide milk for infants who are unable to breastfeed. The following services should be available:
  - Breast pump and privacy for pumping.
  - Storage place for expressed milk.
  - Referral to lactation services and pump rental sources if needed.
- Provides breastfed children only age-appropriate or medically indicated supplementation of food or drink.
- Uses alternative feeding methods most conducive to successful breastfeeding and appropriate weight gain.
- Provides 24-hour rooming-in of parents and their children.
- Provides meals and snacks for the breastfeeding mother.
- Plans medication schedule and procedures to avoid interfering with the breastfeeding relationship.
- Provides information about breastfeeding support available in the hospital and the community.
- Assesses compliance with policies through quality assurance activities and research.

Data from Minchin et al., 1996 and Poipper, 1998.

This rubric can serve the bedside nurse as a guide for providing evidence-based patient care. It calls for breastfeeding assessment, use of before- and after-breastfeeding test weights, steps to assist women to increase their milk supply, and development of an alternative feeding plan for babies unable to take in sufficient volume and/or calories. As soon as it is noted that the infant's suckling abilities are not sufficient to maintain weight or when oral feedings are not possible, support for milk expression must be initiated. Healthcare providers are responsible for assuring that the mother has the education and equipment needed to maintain her milk supply. When the infant is ready to return to breastfeeding, mothers may need assistance in negotiating monitoring or therapeutic paraphernalia that are attached to her baby as she puts the child to breast (Figure 18-7).

For the child who is breastfed, feeding and nurturing patterns should approximate as closely as possible the normal home situation. Only by acquiring information can personalized and individualized care be given to families. Box 18-3 lists elements of the admission history that focus on breastfeeding issues. If the breastfeeding child is old enough to talk, the family may use a "code" word for breastfeeding, such as "nummies," "yum-yum," "nursie," "snugglies," "night-night," or "side." Acceptance of the normalcy of a walking and talking child who breastfeeds is discussed in the *Familial and Social Context of Breastfeeding* chapter.

Perioperative Care of the Breastfeeding Infant/Child

Perioperative issues include the preoperative fasting period and postoperative recovery. The purpose of fasting is to avoid pulmonary aspiration. The fasting period should be as short as physiologically appropriate for reducing anesthesia-related

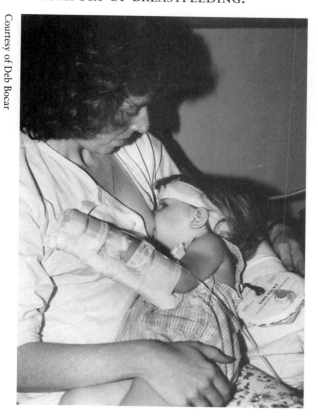

Figure 18-7 BREASTFEEDING WITH INTRAVENOUS INFUSION. MOTHER MAY NEED SOME HELP NEGOTIATING THE BABY'S EQUIPMENT AT FIRST SO BABY CAN SETTLE INTO THE COMFORT OF BREASTFEEDING.

Courtesy of Deb Bocar

risk due to aspiration, risk of dehydration, and risk of hypoglycemia. Cook-Sather and Litman (2006) report that the risk of aspiration in infants less than 6 months of age is 3:9266, using the "liberalized" fasting guidelines published in 1999 by the American Society of Anesthesiologists (ASA). These guidelines are as follows: clear liquids—2 hours; breastmilk—4 hours; formula, other nonhuman milks, or light meal—6 hours; full meal—8 hours (ASA, 1999, 2011). The preoperative patient who is breastfeeding does not need to be NPO (nothing by oral route) for as long as the formula-fed infant because human milk is digested more quickly. Kosko's (2006) meta-analysis summary states that for the infant at low risk for aspiration, there is no reason not to offer ad libitum clear fluids until 2 hours prior to surgery, and that there are insufficient data to comment on which period is safe for offering milk feedings or which period might be appropriate for high-risk infants. Although some feel even shorter fasting periods for breastfeeding infants are safe, the Academy of Breastfeeding Medicine's (ABM) Protocol #25, "NPO" guidelines, concurs with the ASA's recommendation. According to both ASA (2011) and ABM (2012) guidelines, a baby can be offered ad libitum clear fluids up to 2 hours before surgery, with water being least preferred due to its lack of calories.

Separation of child and family should be minimized to reduce stress on all parties. Anticipating ways to comfort a distressed breastfeeding baby

BOX 18-3 ADMISSION HISTORY FOR THE BREASTFEEDING PATIENT

- Are there any feeding concerns right now?
- Usual feeding routine
  - Frequency of breastfeeding
  - Length of breastfeeding
  - Behavior of the baby during and after feeding
  - Special equipment needs
  - Preferred positioning for feedings
  - Special words for breastfeeding
  - If parent not present, preferred alternative feeding method

(continues)

BOX 18-3 (*CONTINUED*)

- Use of supplements
  - How much is given per feeding and during a 24-hour period?
  - What is used for supplementation?
  - How is it given?
  - When is it given?
- Use of herbal or other complementary therapies for mother or baby
- Solid foods
  - Preferred foods
  - Schedule for solid foods
- Recent changes in feeding routine
- Recent changes in weight gain
- Other approaches to feeding that have been used
- Solitary or cosleeper

during the fasting period is important. If another family member can be with the baby, rather than the mother, this may reduce the child's desire for breastfeeding. A pacifier can be offered to soothe the baby during the preoperative fasting period. Following surgery, breastfeeding should resume as soon as the physician indicates oral feeds can safely begin. There is no need for a first glucose-water feeding. The mother may need to express milk until her infant is ready to resume breastfeeding.

Emergency Room

Nurses in the emergency room environment face the need to respond with split-second reactions and require a thorough background in a wide range of areas. Often, however, emergency room providers do not have basic knowledge regarding breastfeeding. We are frequently told of situations where mothers were advised to suspend or stop breastfeeding when there was, in fact, no medical indication to do so. For example, when the child presents with gastroenteritis, the typical advice is to suspend all milk feedings and begin an oral electrolyte solution, as the physicians may be unaware that guidelines recommend continuation of breastfeeding during diarrheal illness. In another scenario, a newborn with hematemesis (bloody vomit) may be given an

invasive gastrointestinal workup before someone thinks to ask whether the mother's nipples are sore and bleeding. Moreover, a breastfeeding mother may be prescribed pain medication or antibiotic and told that she needs to stop breastfeeding to protect the baby. Having a nurse in the emergency room who is aware of breastfeeding management concerns for the ill child or mother may prevent inappropriate treatment or unnecessary interruption of breastfeeding.

Care of Children with Selected Conditions

Infection

Numerous research studies demonstrate that breastfeeding, including short-term, nonexclusive breastfeeding, reduces the risk of a variety of infections, both minor and major (Duijts et al., 2009; Fisk et al., 2011). Protection from infection is afforded in a dose-response manner—the greater the dose, the greater the protection (Raisler et al., 1999; Scariati et al., 1997). The reduction in risk is most dramatic in resource-poor countries, but is also significant in developed countries. Nonetheless, any child may experience infection at some point during the breastfeeding period.

Breastfed children lose less weight during an infectious illness and are less likely to require hospitalization than if they are not breastfed. Lopez-Alarcon et al. (2004) postulate that DHA in human milk contributes to the decreased anorectic response of breastfed infants who have infection. There is no reason to interrupt breastfeeding during infectious illnesses. However, the infant occasionally may be so severely ill that feeding capability is temporarily impaired. In these situations, the mother can express her breastmilk and save it until the baby resumes breastfeeding. Expressed milk can be provided to the child via nasogastric feeding when appropriate or stored for use at a later date.

Gastroenteritis

Acute gastroenteritis (AGE) may be caused by a number of viral and bacterial pathogens. Symptoms include vomiting, diarrhea, fever, anorexia, and fussiness presumably due to nausea and abdominal cramping. Sometimes new parents mistakenly believe that the normally loose breastmilk stools they observe in their newborn or the normal spitting up that babies do are signs of illness. (The emergency room physician might think so as well!) Viral AGE is responsible for more than 1.5–2.5 million deaths annually worldwide, primarily in resource-poor areas; in the United States, it is estimated that there are about 5000 deaths and 600,000 hospitalizations for treatment of dehydration (Hall et al., 2011). Rotavirus, the most common cause of AGE, leads to an estimated 500,000 office or emergency room visits and 50,000 hospitalizations in the United States each year. Breastfeeding is associated with reduced hospitalization, with exclusive breastfeeding to 6 months providing the most potent benefit (Quigley et al., 2007). Risk factors for hospitalization for rotavirus infection in U.S. children include lack of breastfeeding, daycare attendance, siblings in the home, and economic disadvantage (Dennehy et al., 2006). In recent years, increased rotavirus vaccine uptake has dramatically reduced the incidence, hospitalization, and morbidity/mortality from rotavirus gastroenteritis in low-, middle-, and high-income countries (Patel et al., 2011).

The acute danger with AGE is dehydration, when the infant takes in less fluid than is lost through vomiting and diarrhea. With repeated gastrointestinal infections, the child also risks becoming chronically malnourished, increasing the likelihood of significant morbidity and mortality from other causes. Infants are at greater risk for dehydration than older children or adults due to their increased body surface area and therefore greater evaporative losses. Diarrhea and vomiting can also result in electrolyte imbalance caused by the losses of sodium and potassium. Electrolyte imbalance may be more severe if families have been supplementing the child's diet with either high-sodium fluids, such as broth, or very low-sodium fluids such as water or soda pop, thereby transforming a straightforward isotonic dehydration into a more complex hypotonic or hypertonic dehydration (Eliason & Lewan, 1998).

A review of the 2008 European Society for Paediatric Infectious Disease (ESPID) and the European Society for Paediatric Gastroenterology, Hepatology and Nutrition (ESPGHAN) guidelines and the National Institute for Health and Clinical Excellence guidelines noted agreement on the following key aspects of management of AGE: continuation of breastfeeding; rapid oral rehydration with hypotonic solutions; and rapid realimentation with normal feeding (Szajewska & Dziechciarz, 2010). The guidelines do not recommend use of antiemetics. However, subsequent to their publication, a meta-analysis revealed that use of ondansetron (Zofran) in children with persistent vomiting was associated with, and is highly recommended for, facilitation of rapid oral rehydration and reduced need for intravenous therapy and hospitalization (Carter & Fedorowicz, 2012); this antiemetic agent appears to be used widely in emergency departments.

Table 18-1 summarizes assessment and medical management of the child with AGE. Notably, babies with significant dehydration are listless; they look and act sick. The degree of dehydration is most accurately determined by the extent of weight loss. Dehydration is classified as none to minimal with 3% weight loss, mild with greater than 3% to 9% weight loss, and moderate to severe with

Table 18-1 ASSESSMENT AND MANAGEMENT OF GASTROENTERITIS IN CHILDREN

Signs/Symptoms	None to minimal < 3% weight loss	Mild to Moderate 3% to 9% weight loss	Severe > 9% weight loss
General Condition			
Infant	Alert, thirsty, restless	Drowsy, lethargic	Limp; cold, cyanotic extremities; may be unconscious; symptoms of shock with very severe dehydration
Child	Same	Alert, postural dizziness	Apprehensive; cold, cyanotic extremities; muscle cramps; symptoms of shock with very severe dehydration
Peripheral pulse	Normal	Thready, weak	Feeble, not palpable
Capillary refill	Immediate, no delay	Delayed ≤ 1.5 secs	Delayed ≥ 1.5–2 secs
Respiratory effort	Normal	Deep	Deep and rapid
Skin turgor	Pinch, immediate retraction	Pinch, retracts slowly	Pinch, retracts very slowly, > 2 secs (tenting)
Eyes	Normal	Sunken	Very sunken
Tears	Present	May be absent	Absent
Mucous membranes	Normal	Dry	Very dry
Urine output (by report)	Normal	Reduced	None for many hours
Treatment			
Rehydration	Not necessary	Oral rehydration solution (ORS), 50–100 ml/kg body weight over 3–4 hours	IV rehydration with lactated Ringer's or normal saline in 20 ml/kg boluses until perfusion, mental status improved; then ORS 100 ml/kg over 4 hours, or continued IV therapy with 5% dextrose ¼ normal saline at twice maintenance rates
Replacement of ongoing losses	ORS with each diarrheal or vomiting episode	Same	Same; if unable to drink, nasogastric tube administration of ORS or IV 5% dextrose 1/4 normal saline with 20 mEq/L potassium chloride
Nutrition during illness	Continue breastfeeding; age-appropriate normal diet	Continue breastfeeding; age-appropriate normal diet	Continue breastfeeding; age-appropriate normal diet

Data from Gorelick, Shaw, & Murphy, 1997, Armon et al., 1999, CDC, 2003, and Kleinman, 2009.

more than 9% loss (Centers for Disease Control and Prevention [CDC], 2003). However, the clinician rarely has access to a known pre-illness weight that is necessary to make this calculation and must depend on history and clinical findings. With just a clinical history of vomiting, the child has probably lost 3% of body weight and may be minimally dehydrated. Gorelick et al. (1997) found that the diagnosis of clinically important dehydration could be based on the presence of three of the following signs and symptoms: capillary refill greater than 2 seconds, absent tears, dry mucous membranes, and ill general appearance. Steiner et al.'s (2004) review noted that the most useful signs for predicting 5% dehydration were abnormal capillary refill time, skin turgor, and respiratory pattern. Normally, six to eight cloth diapers wet with urine in a 24-hour period is an indication of adequate hydration; however, frequent stools can confuse estimates of urine output.

The child with mild illness needs no special intervention other than increased frequency of breastfeeding and close monitoring for signs of dehydration, especially number of wet diapers. If the infant has fewer than four wet diapers in 24 hours, refuses to nurse, or becomes either inconsolable or somnolent (sleepy), evaluation by the medical care provider is necessary. (See Table 18-1 for indications for medical evaluation.) The child who has minimal dehydration may benefit from oral rehydration solution (ORS) to replace ongoing fluid losses (e.g., Pedialyte, Lytren, or the World Health Organization solution) in addition to continued breastfeeding (Kleinman, 2009). Even with moderate dehydration, oral rehydration therapy (ORT) is as effective as intravenous fluid therapy. ORS can be provided by mouth or via NG tube. Severe dehydration is a medical emergency and immediate rehydration with intravenous or intraosseous fluid is indicated.

There is no evidence that a period of gut rest contributes to improved outcomes for children with AGE. The BRAT diet (banana, rice, applesauce, toast) is too restrictive and should not be recommended. Children who are eating solids should continue to be offered age-appropriate diets including complex carbohydrates, meats, yogurt, fruits, and vegetables. Such intake reduces illness duration and improves nutritional outcomes (Kleinman, 2009). Foods that are high in simple sugars are to be avoided.

Breastfeeding Implications

It is never necessary to interrupt breastfeeding during either the rehydration or recovery phase of illness (CDC, 2003; Szajewska & Dziechciarz, 2010). Human milk is a very well-tolerated, easy-to-digest fluid. However, the nausea and abdominal cramping that accompany AGE may cause a period of anorexia and decreased interest in breastfeeding. If the youngster is reluctant to breastfeed for more than a couple of feedings, the mother might want to express her milk both for comfort and to protect her milk supply. If ORS is medically necessary for rehydration and replacement of excessive ongoing fluid losses, it can be given via spoon, tube at breast, or, if necessary, NG tube.

Respiratory Infections

Respiratory infections, the most common cause of illness in infancy and childhood, are usually caused by viral pathogens. Infants with few outside contacts develop fewer respiratory infections than do children in daycare settings. Breastfeeding has a protective effect against respiratory illness, even when important confounding variables (e.g., birth weight, number of siblings, maternal age, and smoking) are controlled (Ip et al., 2007). Quigley et al. (2007) report reduced hospitalization for respiratory illness associated with both partial and exclusive breastfeeding.

Symptoms of an upper respiratory tract infection include fever, rhinorrhea, cough, sneezing, hoarseness, sore throat, and dysphagia. Symptoms of lower respiratory tract infection are somewhat different and include fever, tachypnea, wheezing, rhonchi, rales, and hyperresonance. Nasal flaring, expiratory grunting, and cyanosis are worrisome signs that require emergency referral for medical evaluation. The intervention needed depends on the severity of symptoms.

Goldman (2011) reviewed management strategies for the common cold. Acetaminophen or ibuprofen will reduce the fever and make the child more comfortable. For infants older than 1 year, pasteurized honey may provide relief from cough. There is no evidence for effectiveness in children of other complementary therapies, including vitamin C, zinc, Echinacea, or humidifiers. Further, use of antihistamines and decongestants is not recommended due to lack of efficacy and the potential of dangerous side effects, including death. Both the U.S. Food and Drug Administration (FDA) and Health Canada have published warnings about these agents' use in children. The FDA warns against use in children younger than age 2 years and Health Canada in children younger than age 6 years. Many families and providers are unaware of or do not believe these warnings, so healthcare providers continue to see children with complications, including fatalities, from the use of over-the-counter cough and cold remedies.

Breastfeeding Implications

Breastfeeding difficulties commonly occur during both upper and lower respiratory tract infections because of the baby's difficulty in coordinating the suck, swallow, and breathe actions with nasal congestion, tachypnea (fast breathing), or pain of swallowing with pharyngitis. During coughing episodes, babies may gag and then vomit. Anorexia (loss of appetite) and vomiting are common. The child may be disinterested in breastfeeding, feed fretfully, or want frequent but short feedings. Pinnington et al. (2000) report that formula-fed infants with bronchiolitis had less effective coordination of breathing with swallowing, devoted less time to sucking, took in less volume per swallow, and had a total feeding volume that was about half that of well peers. It is not known if breastfeeding babies would demonstrate such dramatic differences in feeding. It is possible the differences might be less dramatic, in view of Mizuno et al.'s report (2002) that healthy children who were bottle-fed breastmilk had better coordination of suck–swallow–breathe patterns than did infants fed formula or water.

Symptoms of respiratory distress may worsen while feeding if the child is moderately to severely ill. If the child becomes hypoxic, has cyanotic episodes, or has other signs of worsening distress while feeding, oral feedings may need to be suspended until the child's condition improves. Caregivers should note oxygen status, respiratory rate, and pulse rate before and during feedings. If the child is extremely tachypneic (respiratory rates of 60 to 80 or more for a young infant), he may not be able to tolerate oral feedings.

To make it easier for the infant to breathe, the mother can feed the baby while he is held upright in a sitting position. Saline nose drops help thin the nasal secretions, which can then be aspirated with a bulb syringe before feedings. If oxygen is required, a low-flow nasal cannula can remain in place without interfering with breastfeeding. For the infant who refuses to keep a cannula or mask in place, a mist tent may be used. Although this imposes separation of the child from the parent, there is no reason for it to interfere with breastfeeding if the child is interested. The mother can join her baby under the tent if the child becomes hypoxic while feeding in the room-air environment—her presence may quickly quiet a crying, unhappy infant who has little energy to spare. Once the acute symptoms have passed, appetite will return, usually in a day or two. Until then, the mother should express her breastmilk to keep up her supply.

Pneumonia

Pneumonia is inflammation or infection of the lungs. Approximately 150 million cases of this infection occur annually worldwide, and it is the number one cause of mortality of children younger than age 5 years in the developing world (Fayade & Ayede, 2011), although mortality from this cause is rare in developed countries. Pneumococcal and pertussis vaccinations reduce the risks associated with these causes of pneumonia. Of recent concern is the resurgence of pertussis and pertussis-associated deaths, related to decreased uptake of the pertussis vaccine in selected communities, including in the United States. Increased efforts to vaccinate close contacts of newborns (known as cocooning) have been initiated, in an attempt to reduce risk in infants too young to be fully vaccinated (Wiley et al., 2013).

Common pathogens associated with community-acquired pneumonia vary according to age (Choi & Lee, 2012).

- Neonates: Group B streptococci, gram-negative enteric bacteria (*Escherichia coli*, *Haemophilus influenzae*), *Listeria*, anaerobes, and occasionally herpes simplex and cytomegalovirus.
- Age 3 weeks to 3 months: Bacterial agents include *H. influenzae*, *Moraxella catarrhalis*, *Staphylococcus aureus*, and *Bordatella pertussis*. Viral agents include *Chlamydia trachomatis*, respiratory syncytial virus (RSV), and parainfluenza.
- Age 4 months to 4 years: Viral agents are the most common causes, including RSV, human metapneumovirus (hMPV), and others. *Streptococcus pneumoniae* is the most common bacterial agent.

Infants with pneumonia develop signs of acute illness often abruptly—high fever, productive cough (with emesis after coughing bouts possible), and, in some instances, signs of systemic toxicity or sepsis (tachypnea, lethargy, delayed capillary refill). Investigators have not been able to identify a constellation of symptoms that would distinguish between bacterial and viral pneumonia. Several published guidelines outline the preferred management of infants and children with community-acquired pneumonia; they include criteria for obtaining chest radiographs, medications, and outpatient versus hospital management (Bradley et al., 2011; Principi & Esposito, 2012). Hospitalization may be necessary for closer monitoring, respiratory support, intravenous fluids, and antibiotics (Choi & Lee, 2012).

Bronchiolitis

Bronchiolitis is a lower respiratory tract infection caused by a number of viral pathogens. Globally, respiratory syncytial virus is the most common cause of bronchiolitis/acute lower respiratory infection,

with 99% of all deaths from this cause occurring in developing countries (Nair et al., 2010). Other causes include adenovirus, rhinovirus, enterovirus, influenza, parainfluenza, and human metapneumovirus (Manoha et al., 2007). Pertussis coinfection may occur in unvaccinated infants (Korppi & Hiltunen, 2007). Bronchiolitis occurs in epidemics in winter and early spring in temperate climates and during rainy season in tropical climates. Breastfeeding has a protective effect against RSV/bronchiolitis (Oddy, 2004; Quigley et al., 2007). Children with chronic lung disease of prematurity (CLD), congenital heart disease, and prematurity are at highest risk for complications. Other high-risk groups include those with cystic fibrosis and immunodeficiencies. Nevertheless, 80% of RSV-related deaths occur among children who do not have underlying high-risk conditions (Langley & Anderson, 2011). Infants and toddlers younger than 2 years with CLD and infants born before 32 weeks' gestation are advised to receive palivizumab to prevent RSV infection.

Symptoms of RSV infection include copious secretions and paroxysms of coughing that are sometimes severe. Infants will be tachypneic, have prolonged expiratory phase of respiration, and be in varying degrees of distress. Newborns and premature infants may not have the typical respiratory symptoms associated with RSV, but instead may present with lethargy, irritability, poor feeding, and apnea.

Medical treatment involves the provision of supportive care—ensuring hydration, providing supplemental oxygen, and implementing mechanical ventilation if needed. The use of heliox (a combination of helium and oxygen) inhalation for children with severe respiratory distress is being studied, but at this time its benefits are not clear (Liet et al., 2010). The use of nebulized 3% hypertonic saline has been reported to decrease length of stay for moderately ill hospitalized infants, with no adverse side effects (Hom & Fernandes, 2011). Current reviews and guidelines do not support the use of beta$_2$ agonists, such as albuterol, or corticosteroids, which are often prescribed, because neither has been proved effective, and both have significant side effects (Choi & Lee, 2012; Zorc & Hall, 2010).

Antibiotics are used only if a secondary bacterial infection develops. The use of ribavirin treatment is controversial due to conflicting reports about effectiveness, the high costs, and concerns about potential toxic effects to exposed personnel (Choi & Lee, 2012). Most cases of bronchiolitis are self-limiting, and hospitalization is not necessary unless the child is in severe respiratory distress with hypoxia. Feeding may be somewhat disrupted for a day or two due to the cough and respiratory distress.

Otitis Media

Otitis media (OM), inflammation of the middle ear, occurs most often in children between 6 months and 3 years of age. Common causative bacterial pathogens include *Streptococcus pneumoniae*, *H. influenzae*, and *M. catarrhalis*, in addition to viral pathogens. *S. pneumoniae* is the most common etiologic agent, and the least likely to resolve without treatment. Uptake of pneumococcal vaccine has resulted in decreased incidence of otitis media, as well as decreased incidence of antibiotic-resistant pneumococcal disease (Cohen et al., 2006). It is well established that breastmilk feeding decreases the risk of otitis media (Aniansson et al., 2002; Chantry et al., 2006); the greater the dose of breastfeeding, the greater the benefit. Harabuchi et al. (1994) suggested that one mechanism for the protective effects of human milk against otitis media may be the inhibition of nasopharyngeal colonization with *H. influenzae* by a specific secretory immunoglobulin A (IgA) antibody. Exposure to smoke and daycare attendance are the most significant risk factors (Rovers et al., 2008). OM prevention strategies include breastfeeding; pneumococcal vaccine; and avoidance of environmental smoke, pacifier use after 6 months of age, propped bottle-feeding of liquids other than breastmilk or water, and daycare attendance (Lieberthal et al., 2013).

OM generally occurs following an upper respiratory infection. The child begins to feel worse rather than better. Many, though not all, develop fever. Pain behaviors include refusal to suckle, crying when put in a supine position, and general fussiness. Some children pull on their ears only with an ear infection. Diagnosis of OM depends on the presence of moderate to severe bulging of the tympanic membrane (TM), or mild bulging of the TM with recent onset of pain symptoms and presence of effusion.

The AAP guideline for management of OM includes expectant monitoring depending on the age of the child and the severity of the symptoms. Children aged 6 to 23 months who have a body temperature less than 39°C, with pain symptoms for less than 48 hours, and only unilateral bulging TM may be monitored rather than prescribing antibiotic medication right away (Lieberthal et al., 2013). Children 24 months and older with unilateral or bilateral bulged TM and without severe signs or symptoms can be monitored. Analgesia should be prescribed, and parents instructed to call if pain symptoms persist more than 48 hours or other symptoms develop (Lieberthal et al., 2013). Anesthetic pain drops placed into the ear canal will numb the tympanic membrane and afford immediate pain relief. These drops can be given on an as-needed basis, particularly before feedings or bedtime, until the infection improves with time and/or antibiotic treatment. Oral analgesia such as acetaminophen or ibuprofen will help pain as well as fever. If the child continues to be symptomatic after 48 to 72 hours, antibiotic treatment needs to be implemented for the child who was being monitored, or reassessed for the child already on treatment. It is important that prescribed antibiotics be given as directed to reduce the risk of developing resistant organisms.

Breastfeeding Implications

An infant with otitis media may refuse to breastfeed or feed very briefly due to the discomfort caused by changes in middle ear pressure with suckling. This leads to more frequent requests for brief feedings until the ear pain subsides. The child will be more comfortable breastfeeding in an upright position to diminish pressure increases associated with supine positioning. Administering local anesthetic drops prior to feedings will help the child be more comfortable with feeds.

Meningitis

Meningitis is an acute inflammation of the meninges caused by viral or bacterial pathogens. The most common causative pathogens in infants and toddlers are pneumococci and meningococci. In areas where vaccination against *H. influenzae* and *S. pneumoniae* have high uptake, incidence of meningitis from these organisms has plummeted (Agrawal & Nadel, 2011), with disease from *H. influenzae* infection virtually eradicated. It is anticipated that with uptake of the new 13-valent pneumococcal vaccine, similar success will be observed. Meningitis is also associated with other viral diseases, such as enteroviruses, measles, mumps, and herpes.

The range of clinical symptoms linked to meningitis and their severity varies widely and may be sudden or gradual in onset, depending on the age of the child and the causative pathogen. In the youngest infants, symptoms may be very nonspecific—lethargy and poor feeding. Infants may not be febrile. Signs of meningeal irritation include changes in level of consciousness, nausea and vomiting, and a tense anterior fontanel. Another neurologic sign is pain with neck flexion. Infants may not exhibit positive Brudzinski or Kernig signs (see the *Infant Assessment* chapter).

One should suspect meningitis in the infant who prefers not to be held when ill (snuggling causes pain), and make urgent referral for medical evaluation. The child with meningitis requires emergent hospitalization. Lumbar puncture is done to culture cerebrospinal fluid. Intravenous antibiotics and corticosteroids are administered. The child is isolated until the causative organism is ascertained. The length of isolation will depend on which pathogen is identified.

Breastfeeding Implications

Infants with meningitis may be uninterested in breastfeeding for a day or two during the acute phase, but with effective treatment and recovery, they usually resume breastfeeding as eagerly as before. During the time the child is anorexic, mothers should be counseled to express their milk to keep their supply up. Children who have meningitis are at risk for a wide range of neurologic sequelae and require ongoing assessment to identify any deficits, which could include difficulty with reestablishing effective breastfeeding.

Alterations in Neurologic Functioning

The suck–swallow reflexes in a full-term, healthy infant are usually well developed at birth so the infant has little difficulty in establishing a pattern of effective suckling. This is not always true for children with neurologic impairment. Any deficit that affects neuromuscular function carries the risk of feeding difficulties. Sucking, swallowing, and breathing are integrated under medullary (brain stem) control. When this control is impaired, the normal muscle tension involved in these functions is affected. As a result, oral feeding can be difficult for both the baby and the caregiver. Children with neurologic impairment need careful assessment to determine the safety and the effectiveness of their feeding skills. The risks of oral feeds for the child with neurologic impairment include aspiration and failure to thrive. Swallowing coordination and safety may need to be assessed using videofluoroscopy or ultrasound. The overall muscle tone of the child will determine in part which interventions might be most helpful in facilitating oral feeding.

If breastfeeding is not going smoothly, it is important to seek expert intervention, calling on speech-language pathologists or occupational therapists to assist with the evaluation and treatment plan. Inappropriate oral exercises may not only be ineffective but actually exacerbate the child's difficulties (Bovey et al., 1999). Helpful techniques to improve suckling abilities in children with neurologic impairment are presented in Box 18-4.

Hypotonia and Hypertonia

Signs of hypotonia related to breastfeeding include weak suck, lack of effective tongue movement, poor lip seal, inability to generate adequate suction, and inability to keep the breast inside the oral cavity. Positioning, head support, maternal breast support,

---

BOX 18-4 BREASTFEEDING THE CHILD WITH ALTERED NEUROMUSCULAR TONE

Action	Rationale
Getting Started (both Hypo- and Hypertonia)	
• Arrange for a comfortable, quiet, lowlight environment for feedings.	• A comfortable mother will be able to attend to teaching more readily.
• Encourage the mother to find a comfortable position for herself first.	
• Teach her the dancer-hand position (see Figure 18-2).	• Enhances sucking efficiency with support of mandible (jaw) and masseter muscles (cheek) (Einarsson-Backes et al., 1994). • Shows the mother how to support her breast without interfering with latch-on.
• As with any special situation, ongoing assessment for breastfeeding effectiveness must be carried out.	• Feeding effectiveness may improve slowly for children with altered neuromuscular tone. Weight gain must be checked to ensure the baby continues to thrive while working on improving direct breastfeeding.
• If the following are not successful in moving a baby to effective breast-feeding, consider referral to a therapist (occupational therapist, speech language pathologist, or more experienced lactation consultant).	• Special diagnostic studies, such as a suck-swallow study, and special therapeutic measures may be needed to achieve improved breastfeeding.
• Provide the family with detailed written instructions, and observe return demonstration of prescribed techniques or devices.	• This assists the family's ability to replicate recommended strategies at home.
Baby with Hypotonia (Low Tone)	
• Help mother position the baby in an upright posture (Figure 18-1).	• Stimulates the arousal center. • Increases baby's ability to grasp the nipple.
• Teach mother how to tap gently and quickly around the baby's lips.	• Oral–motor stimulation may enhance latch and suckling ability.
• Provide support with a finger under the chin, behind the mandible, to support the tongue.	• This support may enhance suckling effectiveness.
• Try an extensor position with arms and legs extended if the upright position is not helpful.	• Some infants with low tone have more effective oral–motor function when positioned in extension.
• Massage the breast so that milk is available for the baby to swallow or use a supplementer at the breast.	• Milk flow into the oral pharynx stimulates swallow and subsequent suckling efforts.
• Use a nipple shield to facilitate latch-on and sustained suckling.	• Massage or use of the device helps to provide a liquid bolus with minimal suckling effort on the part of the infant. • The firmer texture of the nipple shield provides additional oral–motor stimulation, assists the mother to place the nipple over the baby's tongue, and in many cases stimulates more effective breastfeeding.

Baby with Hypertonia (High Tone)

- Provide smooth gentle massage around the lips prior to feeding.
- Help mother position the baby in an upright posture.

- Support the trunk in a more forward position, rather than perpendicular to the hips.

- Avoid direct pressure on the back of the baby's head by placing a cloth between the back of the baby's head and the supporting hand, or moving the hand down to support the upper trunk and neck to avoid direct pressure on the head.

- Use a nipple shield to help get the baby's tongue down from the palate.

- Prefeeding massage may help relax the baby's oral tone.
- Upright posture stimulates the arousal center, facilitates hip flexion, and helps drop the tongue to the floor of the mouth.
- Positioning with the head coming downward onto the breast may prevent rapid flow of milk directly into the oropharynx, which may cause the hypersensitive baby to gag and choke.
- Direct pressure on the occiput causes an infant to arch the head backward, toward the pressure, rather than bringing the head forward to the breast.

- The firmer nipple may facilitate moving the tongue to the floor of the mouth in the baby with increased oral–motor tone.

Compiled from Mohrbacher 2010, McBride and Danner, 1987; Danner, 1992; and assistance of the feeding team, Center for Child Health & Development, University of Kansas School of Medicine.

and easy milk flow may assist these children. If latch-on and sustained suckling are not progressing, a nipple shield might help. The firmer texture of this device provides a more dramatic stimulus for the baby compared with the nipple/areola. The use of a nipple shield to help infants achieve more effective milk transfer has been successful for premature infants and others (Bodley & Powers, 1996; Brigham, 1996; Meier, 2000). This is an area where there is very limited evidence to guide clinical practice. The Academy of Breastfeeding Medicine published a protocol regarding breastfeeding the hypotonic infant (Thomas et al., 2007) that emphasizes the importance of skin-to-skin care while providing good support for the infant's head and body, suggesting use of a sling or pillows to support the baby in a flexed posture to free the mother's hand's to use the dancer-hand position; use of a nipple shield; breast compression; and techniques for supplementation at breast. Growth assessment is obviously important. If the child has a specific syndrome, one should use the specific growth charts for that syndrome when they are available. (The

Internet site http://depts.ashington.edu/nutrpeds/fug/growth/specialty.htm provides links to various special growth charts for children.)

Babies with hypertonia may have a hypersensitive, "tight" mouth and an easy gag reflex. When feeding at the breast, they tend to arch backward, hyperextend their head, and thrust or retract their tongue. As with hypotonia, there is no literature to provide advice regarding facilitating breastfeeding. This baby will need help to come to a more flexed, relaxed posture to feed effectively. Swaddling or placing the baby in a sling to bring the shoulders forward and arms to midline helps accomplish this goal (Watson Genna, 2008). If the mother cannot get the baby's tongue down to the floor of the mouth for latch-on, a nipple shield may be of assistance.

Down Syndrome (Trisomy 21)

Down syndrome (DS; also known as trisomy 21) is the duplication of the 21st chromosome, resulting in a constellation of abnormalities. Worldwide, prevalence of DS is 1:1000 live births (Weijerman

& de Winter, 2010). Children with DS have characteristic physical features that include epicanthal folds, a flat nasal bridge, broad hands with shortened fingers, a simian crease (single crease across the upper palm), a flattened forehead, a small mouth, macroglossia (large tongue), and marked hypotonia. About half of DS children have congenital heart disease, some have anomalies of the gastrointestinal tract, and celiac disease occurs in as many as 7% (screening for this condition is recommended by age 3) (Weijerman & de Winter, 2010). Otitis media is more common in children with DS due to their anatomic differences; thus breastmilk feeding is particularly important. Most children with this condition have mild to severe developmental delays.

Breastfeeding Implications

Difficulties with feeding may be encountered for some children with DS, but this is not universal. A study of 59 breastfed infants with Down syndrome found that half had no difficulty in establishing suckling right after the birth. Four babies took less than 1 week to establish suckling, 8 took 1 week, and 16 took longer than 1 week to do so (Aumonier & Cunningham, 1983). Pisacane et al. (2003) report that children with DS were significantly more frequently bottle-fed than children who did not have DS (57% versus 24% and 15% in two non-DS control groups). The authors speculate that the health difficulties encountered by children with DS, as well as maternal–infant separation and lack of support, contributed to the low rates of breastfeeding.

Hypotonia, tongue protrusion, and significant congenital heart disease are among the factors that may affect the child's effectiveness at breast. Mizuno and Ueda (2001) documented sucking behavior in 14 children with DS, using sucking pressure waveform and ultrasonography during bottle-feeding. They concluded that the babies' sucking difficulties may have been in part due to deficiencies in the peristaltic movement of the tongue as well as to the hypotonicity of perioral muscles, lips, and masticatory muscles, and active tongue protrusion. The tongue was observed to fall to the back of the mouth and touch the posterior palate. It is not known if

these same sucking patterns are exhibited during breastfeeding. Oliveira et al. (2010) observed that children with DS were more likely to have open bite and cross-bite if they breastfed less than 6 months, were bottle-fed, or sucked on their fingers.

The same interventions used with the child with hypotonia (as discussed earlier) may help maximize the feeding skills of the child with DS. Very close monitoring is necessary to evaluate the child's ability to maintain a normal growth trajectory. As children with DS are shorter than the general population, a growth chart specifically for children with DS is the most accurate tool with which to assess the adequacy of their growth.

Neural Tube Defects

Neural tube defects are anatomic abnormalities that occur along the neural axis. They include encephalocele (protrusion of brain tissue), meningocele (protrusion of meninges), and myelomeningocele (protrusion of meninges and spinal cord) through bony defects of the skull or spine. The most common of these conditions is myelomeningocele (MM) or spina bifida, which typically occurs in the lumbosacral region. The infant may have variable neurologic deficits below the level of the lesion. Alteration in sensory–motor function of the lower extremities and altered bladder and bowel control are often observed in such cases. Causes of neural tube defects are multifactorial, including genetic factors, links to maternal obesity and diabetes, ethnicity (Hispanic, Irish), and insufficient dietary intake of folic acid prior to conception (Dunlap et al., 2011). Through aggressive campaigns regarding folic acid supplementation, the incidence of these defects has been reduced by 32% in the United States (National Center on Birth Defects and Developmental Disabilities, 2002).

Approximately 80% to 90% of MM-affected children with postnatal repair have hydrocephalus requiring a shunt. The goal of early care is to prevent infection and further loss of neuromuscular function. Surgical correction to repair the MM is performed as early as possible, preferably in the first 24 hours of life. If the defect is large, incisions lateral to the lesion will be made to allow the skin to cover the defect. Some centers perform fetal surgery for closure of MM at 24 to 30 weeks' gestation. A recent analysis of outcomes of the Management of Myelomeningocele Study showed that fetal closure of the defects resulted in improved ambulation, reduced risk of hindbrain herniation associated with Arnold-Chiari II malformation, reduced need for ventriculoperitoneal (VP) shunting, and improved distal neurologic function compared to children who had postnatal repair (Saadai & Farmer, 2012). With successful surgical interventions, most infants affected by neural tube defects are able to breastfeed.

Nearly all children with MM have a Chiari II malformation, a downward displacement of the brain into the neck. Anatomic differences in the whole brain accompany such a malformation. Affected infants are at risk for a Chiari crisis—a brain stem malfunction causing potentially life-threatening apnea and bradycardia. Nurses and lactation consultants need to be alert for symptoms of a Chiari crisis: weak or absent cry, stridor, apnea and associated color changes, feeding and swallowing problems, arching of the neck, gastroesophageal reflux, and failure to thrive. About one in three children with MM will have milder symptoms—typically related to feeding.

Breastfeeding Implications

Hurtekant and Spatz (2007) review a comprehensive approach to supporting breastfeeding for mothers expecting a child with spina bifida, beginning at the time of prenatal diagnosis. Feeding difficulties frequently encountered by infants with MM are due to oral hypersensitivity, poor oral–motor control, and a tendency to gag easily. These symptoms are probably attributable to the Chiari malformation that affects cranial nerves involved with sucking and swallowing (Sandler, 1997). When a baby is ready for oral feedings, the nurse can help with positioning to maximize breastfeeding effectiveness, while protecting the surgical site. A typical cradle hold can be used, taking care that the mother's arm does not put pressure over the defect/surgical site.

Postoperatively, a side-lying positioning of the mother and child may be the most comfortable.

Until the surgical site is healed, the infant cannot be burped by patting the back. Gently rubbing between the shoulders or rocking on a firm surface may help to release any air bubbles. Sandler (1997) suggests feeding the baby in a semi-reclined position (as with cradle hold) with good head support, avoiding neck extension. If significant brain stem impairment is involved, the baby may not be able to feed effectively by mouth for a long time, if ever, in which case the mother can be supported to express breastmilk for her infant.

Hydrocephalus

Hydrocephalus is the accumulation of fluid in the cerebral ventricles caused by interference in the flow or the absorption of cerebrospinal fluid. It may occur in isolation or along with myelomeningocele. As fluid accumulates within the ventricles, the infant's head enlarges to accommodate the increasing volume of fluid. With progressive hydrocephalus, sutures begin to separate and fontanels become distended. Children with marked hydrocephalus develop striking signs and symptoms, including the "setting sun" sign (the white of the eye showing above the iris and below the upper lid as a result of intracranial pressure), a high-pitched cry, muscle weakness, and severe neurologic defects. Diagnosis of hydrocephalus is confirmed by a variety of imaging techniques, including ultrasound, computerized axial tomography (CAT) scan, or magnetic resonance imaging (MRI). Surgery for placement of a ventricular shunt to decompress the ventricles is performed. The shunt drains the cerebrospinal fluid to another area, usually the peritoneum, where it is absorbed and finally excreted. Children are at increased risk for seizure disorder and meningitis.

Breastfeeding Implications

For the infant with advanced hydrocephalus (rarely seen in developed countries), care must be taken in positioning and supporting the infant's large, heavy head; a side-lying positioning with the infant's head supported by a pillow is probably the most comfortable. For the child who has had shunt placement, care with the incision sites is needed during the immediate postoperative period. If the tender site is pressed during a feeding, the pain experience may lead to breast aversion (Merewood & Philipp, 2002). The neurosurgeon will prescribe specific limits to head elevation in the immediate postoperative period. Usually the child is required to stay completely flat for a prescribed period of time postoperatively to avoid decompressing distended ventricles too rapidly. To prevent regurgitation due to increased intracranial pressure, feedings should be frequent and on demand. If there is severe brain damage associated with the hydrocephalus, effective breastfeeding may not be possible.

Congenital Heart Disease

Congenital heart disease (CHD) is the most common of structural birth defects. Symptoms range from none to severe, depending on the particular defect and the effectiveness of medical/surgical management. Presence of CHD does not preclude breastfeeding; however, children with critical CHD, associated with cyanosis/hypoxia or congestive heart failure, are likely to face challenges with feeding and normal growth. Recently, the AAP endorsed the U.S. Department of Health and Human Services' recommendations for performing pulse oximetry on all newborns prior to discharge to promote early detection of critical CHD (Mahle et al., 2012), but some infants with cardiac disease may still be missed. As a consequence, the nurse/lactation consultant who is assisting a newborn with breastfeeding difficulties should be very aware of the child who tires quickly, becomes tachypneic with feedings, or has color changes with feedings. Such a child may, in fact, have significant heart disease. The baby may begin with vigorous suckling, pulling away after a few minutes to rest, then again grasp the breast, and repeat the cycle. Feedings may become very lengthy, with limited intake due to the need for such frequent pauses to rest.

With selected defects, the infant may exhibit signs of congestive heart failure: tachypnea, initially effortless, then progressing to more labored respiratory effort; tachycardia; progressively more difficult feedings; and sweating. Some children may exhibit

hypoxic ("tet") spells during feeding—episodes of crying with intense cyanosis and deep and rapid breathing. Any of the symptoms described, along with auscultation of abnormal heart sounds, palpation of a thrill, or diminished femoral pulses, should lead the healthcare worker to suspect a cardiac defect. The child should be immediately referred for medical evaluation.

Breastfeeding Implications

Combs and Marino (1993) compared patterns of weight gain for 45 infants with CHD who had any breastfeeding to those who were exclusively formula-fed. The weight of the majority of infants in each group had dropped below their birth percentile at 5 months of age (66% of the breastfed infants versus 75% of the bottle-fed infants). More formula-fed infants significantly fell off their individual growth curves than did the breastfed infants. One-third of each group was below the fifth percentile in growth for age at 5 months. Contrary to conventional wisdom, the severity of the cardiac defect was not a predictor of the infant's ability to breastfeed or of the duration of breastfeeding; rather, it was the mother's commitment to continuing with breastfeeding that determined the duration of any breastfeeding. Mothers in this study reported that they spent 1 of every 2 to 3 hours feeding their babies. The authors hypothesized that babies who were breastfeeding had improved growth due to the fact that breastfeeding was less physiologically taxing to infants, the infants had less hypoxia, and they spent less energy during feedings. A later study of seven children confirmed this hypothesis. While breastfeeding, none of the children with CHD experienced a drop in their oxygen saturation level (SaO_2) to less than 90%, while the SaO_2 rates of four of the children dropped below 90% during bottle-feeding sessions (Marino et al., 1995). The volume of intake during breastfeeding or bottle-feeding was not reported.

Boctor et al. (1999) reported very different findings in their study of 24 infants who were also followed postoperatively. Exclusively breastfed infants lost a median of 49 g/day. Partially breastfed babies gained a median of 5 g/day, while exclusively bottle-fed infants gained a median of 20 g/day. Babies in the partial- and no-breastfeeding groups were supplemented with calorie-enriched milks. Rate of weight gain was not related to the particular cardiac lesion or hospital length of stay. Possibly, the difference in conclusions between the Boctor et al. (1999) study and the Combs and Marino (1993) study is that Boctor's group was able to look at exclusive breastfeeding, partial breastfeeding, and no breastfeeding patterns as distinct groups, while the Combs and Marino study looked at "any breastfeeding." Both of these studies make it clear that achieving normal weight gain in a child with CHD is a challenge, irrespective of feeding method.

Problems with weight gain stem from several issues. The child with congestive heart failure also has congestion of the gut, and may feel anorexic or nauseated because of the effects the congestion has on gut motility. Pressure on the gut from an enlarged liver or ascites may contribute to early satiety (Gervasio & Buchanan, 1985). Gastroesophageal reflux disease is common in children with heart failure. Medications given to treat congestive heart failure also may cause nausea and anorexia. In addition, the energy needs of a child with significant CHD frequently exceed the normal recommended daily allowance (RDA) of 100 to 110 kcal/kg/day of the breastfed infant. Some children may require as much as 140 to 160 kcal/kg/day to achieve positive weight gain (Gervasio & Buchanan, 1985). This incredible increase in metabolic demand is related to the extra energy required to support the child's increased respiratory rate and effort, and to the increase of circulating catecholamines (stress hormones). The healthy newborn that is breastfeeding perfectly could not achieve this degree of caloric intake—and it is certainly impossible to expect in the face of symptomatic heart disease.

Weight gain and sufficient protein calorie intake are important for minimizing operative risks related to malnutrition in the child with CHD. Thus every effort must be made to help the child achieve as normal a growth rate as possible. Currently, there are no consensus guidelines regarding nutrition for children with congenital heart disease, so each center may adopt different approaches to address preoperative and postoperative feeding recommendations (Medoff-Cooper et al., 2010). The youngster with severe cyanotic heart disease or with congestive heart failure often requires very invasive methods to facilitate growth. When the baby has significant heart failure, a more comfortable breast-feeding position is a more stretched-out posture, rather than a flexed one, as this avoids pressure on a distended and perhaps tender liver. Supplementation with hindmilk or calorie-enriched milk with a nursing supplementer during breastfeeding may be all that is required to push a baby into normal weight gain. However, other infants will require more intensive support with nasogastric feeding of calorie-enriched milk, with comfort time at the breast.

When fluid restrictions are imposed for children with congestive heart failure or during postoperative recovery, providing sufficient calories by any means—parenteral or enteral—becomes very challenging. Once the child's defect is repaired, a return to oral feeding is expected, but may take some time to achieve. Many children experience significant oral feeding difficulties; causes include injury to vocal cords, prolonged intubation, and surgery on or near the aortic arch (Kohr & Brudis, 2010). Children with hypoplastic left heart syndrome post Norwood operation, in particular, are known to have multiple challenges related to feeding, including dysphagia and necrotizing enterocolitis (Golbus et al., 2011). One-fifth of children in a recent study went home on nasogastric feeding (Kogon et al., 2007). Torowicz et al. (2012) describe the successful implementation of developmental care guidelines in a pediatric cardiac intensive care unit that incorporated kangaroo care and transition of infants to breastfeeding into its therapeutic approach. Consultation with an occupational therapist or speech-language pathologist is recommended.

Oral/Facial Anomalies

The majority of infants with oral/facial anomalies—cleft lip/palate or Pierre Robin sequence—require continuous feeding evaluation and support. Most are unable to gain weight or maintain hydration with only direct breastfeeding. Mothers will need continued support to maintain their breastmilk supply. Certain strategies can be implemented to maximize the child's capabilities to breastfeed, with the understanding that healthcare providers must frequently monitor growth, reevaluate feeding capability, and adjust feeding plans accordingly.

Cleft Lip and Palate

Cleft lip and palate are congenital malformations caused by incomplete fusion of the structures of the oral cavity and the palatine plates very early in gestation. This results in alteration in structure of the upper lip, maxilla, alveolar ridge, nose, and hard and soft palates. The clefting may involve only the lip, may extend into the hard and soft palates, and may be unilateral or bilateral. The general classifications include the following: lip only (CL); both the lip and the palate (CLP); and hard and/or soft palate only (CP). Cleft lip and cleft palate each account for 25% of the malformations; clefting of both structures is found in 50% of all cases. Approximately 15% to 76% of children with CL/CP have associated syndromes, depending on the anomaly definition. Across the literature, children with CP only are more likely to have associated anomalies compared to children with other types of clefting (Peterson-Falzone, 2011). Occasionally, small, isolated clefts of the soft palate are not identified until feeding difficulty becomes apparent. The lactation consultant may be the first to identify a problem during a feeding assessment.

One might think that children with CL would be at higher risk for parent–infant attachment disorders because of their unattractive appearance. However, Coy et al. (2002) found that this was not the case. In a sample of families whose babies had CLP, CP, and no clefts, it was found that the CL-affected babies demonstrated more secure attachment than those with CP or no cleft. The authors hypothesized that the perceived vulnerabilities of the children elicited extraordinary protectiveness and responsiveness in their mothers.

For the infant with CL/CP, a variety of preoperative orthopedic devices are used by some surgeons to help align the maxillary alveolar segments, decrease the width of the alveolar cleft, and improve cleft lip repair. These orthopedic interventions may be as low tech as the use of adhesive tape or steri-strips to approximate the lip segments, or they may involve splints or plates made of acrylic or soft dental material. Opinions vary as to the benefits of these devices. One recent meta-analysis did not indicate any long-lasting benefit from this approach (Uzel & Alparslan, 2011). However, use of the maxillary plates and other devices may improve long-term surgical outcomes, according to other sources (Choi & Lee, 2012; Hak et al., 2012; Shetye, 2012). Fabrication and fitting of these devices is labor intensive, is expensive, and requires professionals with very specialized expertise. Moreover, these devices are not universally available and, in particular, are less available in resource-poor countries.

Timing and approach to the surgical repair of cleft lip and palate partly reflect the preference of the surgeon or center, but the process normally takes place in stages. Typically lip closure is done at about 3 months of age, and palate repair at about 12 months. If the child has a complete cleft lip, a two-stage approach to lip closure may be done, with partial closure followed by conversion of the complete cleft lip to an incomplete deformity. Two authors (Denk, 1998; Hodges, 2010) have reported success in doing simultaneous repair of CL/CP in much younger infants, including neonates. Denk's group now has information on 241 infants and reports a 6% rate of complications among 241 children having definitive CLP repair in the first month of life (Sandberg et al., 2002). This approach is quite uncommon, in part due to the length of operative and anesthesia time, and the technical difficulties encountered with efforts to manipulate inside a small oral cavity.

Multiple prospective studies and case reports find that return to direct breastfeeding or bottle-feeding, rather than cup- or dropper-feeding, immediately following cleft lip repair is best for the baby (Cohen, 1997; Darzi et al., 1996). Furthermore, the former approach is more cost-effective, as hospitalization time is shorter and the need for intravenous fluids is reduced (Darzi et al., 1996). Babies having CP repair in the series reported by Sandberg et al. (2002) also went directly to breast-feeding or bottle-feeding without complications. However, most surgeons prefer to avoid having a teat inside the oral cavity following cleft palate repair. Ideally, babies will have been weaned from bottle- to cup-feeding prior to their palate surgery. There are very limited data regarding direct breast-feeding immediately following cleft repair.

Young et al. (2001) queried parents of 40 children with CL/CP, and as one would predict, found that they wanted basic information in the immediate newborn period, especially about feeding. Only half of the families recalled having specific feeding instruction, while 97% felt it was critical not only to be informed but also to be shown how to feed their babies and which difficulties to expect. Kuttenberger et al. (2010) interviewed 105 parents of children with CL/CP about their experience; they specifically wanted information about their child's surgery (80%) and feeding (63%). Feeding challenges are foremost on parents' minds and must be addressed very clearly.

Breastfeeding Implications

Breastmilk is particularly important for infants with CLP and Pierre Robin sequence as it reduces the risk of otitis media even beyond the time of weaning (Aniansson et al., 2002; Paradise et al., 1994). Newborns with clefts are interested in breastfeeding, approach the breast eagerly, and in many instances appear to latch on well. Their jaw movements appear effective, but usually swallows are very infrequent, particularly for the baby with cleft palate. Their sucking patterns are inefficient, explaining the high rate of failure to thrive observed in children with cleft palate (Pandya & Boorman, 2001). Masarei et al. (2007) and Reid et al. (2007) report that babies with CLP suck very differently than infants without CLP, based on bottle-feeding observations. Specifically, infants with CLP generate positive rather than negative pressure, "chomping" on the teat, and have more sucks per swallow.

The ease with which the baby takes the breast is related to the severity and extent of the defect. The child who has an isolated CL can usually breastfeed effectively with minimal intervention. Such a baby may, however, require some assistance from the mother in maintaining lip seal (Reid et al., 2007). Positioning the infant with the cleft as tightly to the breast as possible and placing the mother's thumb or index finger over the cleft can create sufficient closure for the infant to effectively milk the breast. According to Danner (1992, p. 625), the baby may do best if the breast enters the mouth from the side on which the defect is located: "An infant with a right-sided defect should be held so that the right cheek touches the breast . . . the mother can go from cradle-hold on one side, to the football or 'clutch' hold on the other."

CP causes more feeding challenges. In such a case, it is very unlikely that the child will ever achieve normal growth with exclusive breastfeeding. The opening in the palate dramatically alters suckling mechanics. Because the baby is unable to generate negative intraoral pressure, it is difficult to maintain breast tissue inside the oral cavity and impossible to generate the negative pressure that is a necessary part of milk transfer. As Wilson-Clay (1995) explained, "Try sucking on a straw with a hole in it." A review of pamphlets for parents and materials for health professionals noted that the information was unrealistically optimistic regarding the cleft-affected child's ability to thrive with exclusive breastfeeding (Miller, 1998). Miller interviewed several well-known clinicians and surveyed CLP centers in Canada and the United States. All respondents reported that their clinical experience revealed that it was exceedingly rare for the child with CP to accomplish normal weight gain with exclusive breastfeeding. Pandya and Boorman (2001) found that 32% of children with unilateral CL, 38% with bilateral CL, and 49% with CLP had failure to thrive in a retrospective review. Details of infant feeding methods were not described for this cohort. Babies with CLP who are not supplemented rarely grow well (Montagnoli et al., 2005). Oral feeding can be uncomfortable for the child due to regurgitation of the milk into the nostrils. Such regurgitation is minimized with upright positioning during feeding and with quick milk flow into the back of the oral cavity, where it can be swallowed rapidly (Reilly et al., 2007). A baby with a bilateral cleft suckles best when straddled on the mother's lap or sitting on one side of her body with his legs under her arm (see again Figure 18-1). The soft breast fills the alveolar-ridge defect as well as the palate defect and can be moved to one side or the other as needed. The author of this chapter has observed videos of babies at the breast who are drinking milk that the mother has hand-expressed into the baby's mouth. The baby is not at all an active participant in the milk transfer, but rather a passive recipient of expressed milk.

The use of a palatal obturator or maxillary plate is recommended by some cleft palate teams both to facilitate development of the oral cavity and to achieve suckling effectiveness. The dentist or plastic surgeon makes this appliance, which covers the cleft in the palate and may improve the infant's ability to suckle. An impression has to be made of the oral cavity to fabricate the device. The device then must be adjusted to accommodate the infant's growth, requiring repeated impressions. Anesthesia may be required to safely make the impression in the older baby—an issue that raises concerns about the effect of repeated anesthesia exposure on the infant's development. Several groups have reported

on outcomes of babies who had obturators or palatal plates that cover the cleft palate defect, with conflicting results being noted. Turner et al. (2001) report on eight infants who participated in a prospective feeding intervention study using a palatal obturator and Haberman feeders (see Figure 18-5). None of the babies in their cohort were able to achieve sustained effective breastfeeding with any of the interventions. The use of the palatal obturator and Haberman feeder allowed the children to drink larger volumes in less time and to achieve normal growth. Lactation support for the mothers facilitated continued milk expression, among a highly motivated group. A Cochrane review (Bessell et al., 2011) found no evidence that maxillary plates helped growth in cleft-affected infants. Watson Genna (2008) and Miller (2011) provide suggestions for optimizing feeding for children with craniofacial syndromes, including CL/CP (see Table 18-2).

While the parents and healthcare team are working to maximize the infant's capacity for breastfeeding, milk expression is critical to maintaining the mother's milk supply. The infant can be fed breastmilk by alternative methods. Some parents find that a small spouted cup works well. Others favor an eyedropper, a rubber-tipped syringe (Brecht feeder), or a pipette. Feeding-tube devices have been used successfully for the occasional

---

Table 18-2 FEEDING STRATEGIES FOR INFANTS WITH CLEFT PALATE

Positioning	Flexion, with neutral alignment of head and neck. Upright positioning to reduce nasopharyngeal reflux (see Figure 18-1).
Support of lip, chin, and cheeks	Use the dancer-hand positioning (see Figure 18-2) to support sucking movements.
Feeding	Breast compression, or squeezing of flexible infant feeder such as the Cleft Palate Feeder or Haberman Feeder (see Figure 18-5) in synchrony with child's sucking effort.
	Helps compensate for baby's inability to generate negative pressure.
Pacing	Impose pauses to allow child a rest for breathing, to help protect the airway.
Thickening feeds	Creates a bolus that moves more slowly, protecting the airway.

Note: Recent concerns have emerged regarding contamination of some commercially available thickeners.
Data from Miller, 2012; Watson Genna, 2008.

infant with cleft palates. Most children will do best with a flexible infant feeding bottle such as the Mead-Johnson cleft palate or Haberman feeders (Figure 18-5). Shaw et al. (1999) found that a squeezable bottle was more effective and better accepted than a rigid feeding bottle for providing supplement. As with any child having suckling difficulty, bottle-feeding is no guarantee of appropriate weight gain for the same reasons that breastfeeding is so difficult.

All babies with CLP must have expert breast-feeding assistance, a written feeding plan, a support phone number, and a follow-up outpatient appointment within 24 to 48 hours of dismissal from the newborn nursery. Continued frequent monitoring is a must. Some babies will benefit from calorie-enriched feedings. Box 18-5 discusses a typical case of a family whose 5-day-old baby with a CLP was extremely distressed.

Pierre Robin Sequence

Pierre Robin sequence is a complex of oral–facial abnormalities including micrognathia (small jaw) and glossoptosis (tongue with retropharyngeal placement). Micrognathia is the hallmark feature of Pierre Robin sequence. Most affected children also have clefts of the palate. As many as 80% have other associated anomalies.

Diagnosis is usually made very shortly after birth, when the child's respiratory distress is noted. The position of the tongue interferes with patency of the upper airway. Duskiness and apnea occur with feeding or supine positioning. The facial anatomy, particularly the placement of the tongue, leads to difficulties with airway obstruction and feeding, with or without presence of a cleft palate. The feeding problems, primarily caused by difficulties in maintaining the airway (Marcellus, 2001),

---

BOX 18-5 CASE STUDY—AN UNHAPPY BABY (AND FAMILY) WITH CLEFT LIP AND PALATE

History

Baby Anna and her parents came to the breastfeeding clinic on the child's fifth day of life. Her primary care physician referred them for assistance with breastfeeding. Anna was the couple's first child. Pregnancy, labor, and delivery were uneventful and she was healthy except for the unilateral CLP, which was unexpected. Birth weight was 3650 grams, dismissal weight was not known.

The family reported that during the newborn stay, the baby was nursed every 3 hours. They thought that nurses in the nursery might be supplementing the baby, but were not specifically told this. Dismissal instructions were to breastfeed on demand.

At 5 days of age, they reported that she was inconsolable, at the breast continuously, and had orange stuff in her diaper. They had been to the doctor's office, where her bilirubin was 17 mg/dl.

Observation

The baby was jaundiced down to her shins, crying, and slim. Her mucous membranes were moist, and her skin turgor was good. She had a wide, unilateral cleft lip and palate.

Her weight was 3190 grams—12% below birth weight. Breastfeeding was observed. In cradle hold, the baby eagerly rooted, but never latched onto the breast. She was placed in the upright position (see Figure 18-1) and latched onto the breast. Rhythmic jaw movements were noted. She did not demonstrate swallowing until the mother had let down, and then she lapped a little milk off the surface of the breast. No sustained suck-swallows were noted during 10 to 15 minutes of attempted breastfeeding. A tube at breast was attempted without success. Held in an upright position to avoid

(continues)

BOX 18-5 (*CONTINUED*)

nasal regurgitation, Anna's mother fed her with a Mead-Johnson cleft palate feeder (see Figure 18-5). Anna was able to take 3 oz in about 10 minutes and became relaxed, falling asleep in her mother's arms.

Assessment

Ineffective breastfeeding with resultant excessive weight loss, breastfeeding-associated jaundice, and mild dehydration based on history and weight loss.

Plan

Encourage breastmilk expression, feed Anna with cleft palate feeder on demand, follow up with primary provider in 24 hours. Parents were given an intake and output sheet to monitor hydration. Parents expressed relief at being able to satisfy their infant and anger at the nursing care they had received in the hospital—noting that their child had been put at risk. The baby gained 2 oz within the next 24 hours.

---

are complicated by difficulties in attaching to the breast and the presence of a cleft palate. A number of interventions may be required to prevent airway obstruction—ranging from prone positioning to prolonged nasopharyngeal intubation to glossopexy (in which the tongue is sutured so that it cannot occlude the airway) or tracheostomy for children who do not show clinical improvement with nasopharyngeal intubation (Marques et al., 2001). Nasopharyngeal intubation is preferred to glossopexy, as the child can then usually receive oral feedings.

Denny and Amm (2005) described a new surgical technique of progressive elongation of the mandible (distraction osteogenesis) to correct tongue ptosis, improve the airway, and correct micrognathia. At 1 month of age, 54% of the infants could feed orally, and at 2 years, 100% could do so. Five-year follow-up revealed no complications. Tracheostomy is avoided with this technique, and there is more rapid transition to oral feedings.

Breastfeeding Implications

Effective breastfeeding is possible in mild cases of Pierre Robin sequence, if the infant can maintain normal oxygenation. During initial feeding attempts, oxygen saturation should be monitored. To facilitate airway maintenance, the child may do better with upright positioning, rather than the cradle or football position, in terms of more forward tongue placement. Unfortunately, it is rare for babies with Pierre Robin sequence to be able to breastfeed or bottle-feed effectively in the first weeks of life owing to difficulties with airway, tongue placement, and receding mandible. In a prospective review of 35 children with Pierre Robin sequence, Baujat et al. (2001) found that 86% required nasogastric feedings to accomplish safe feeding and appropriate weight gain. None of the initially breastfed babies was able to feed effectively. In Baujat's series, 50% had abnormalities of esophageal motility that did not respond to standard gastroesophageal reflux treatment. In Smith and Saunders's (2006) series of 60 children, 95% of the infants who failed prone positioning for airway patency had feeding difficulties. In this study, 53% to 83% of the children required nasogastric or gastrostomy feeding from ages less than 3 months to more than 18 months. This information can help one guide the parents as to what to expect for their individual infant's capabilities of feeding orally.

Baudon et al. (2002) used electromyography and esophageal manometry to evaluate motor function of the upper digestive tract (tongue, pharynx, and esophagus) in a group of 28 neonates with Pierre Robin sequence during bottle-feeding. Their findings demonstrate that most had sucking–swallowing disorders along with abnormal esophageal peristalsis and abnormal lower esophageal sphincter pressures and relaxation—all of which may lead to difficulties with feeding. If a trial of breastfeeding fails, oral-feeding devices that are used for infants with clefts can be tried, although frequently nasogastric or gastrostomy feeding is required to ensure normal weight gain.

Parents of children with Pierre Robin sequence will need continued support to maintain breastmilk production for their baby. Over time, the micrognathia resolves, so that the older child has a nearly normal facial appearance and no longer has problems with airway maintenance. Feeding difficulties improve with age (Baujat et al., 2001; Smith & Saunders, 2006).

Choanal Atresia

Choanal atresia is the membranous or bony occlusion of the posterior nares, such that air cannot reach the pharynx via the nose. It may present as a component of the CHARGE syndrome (coloboma, heart disease, atresia choanae, retarded growth and development, genital hypoplasia, ear anomalies and/or deafness). Etiology in children who do not have associated syndromes is not understood. History of maternal hyperthyroidism treatment during pregnancy is seen in some cases, and a very recent reports link maternal residential exposure to atrazine, a commonly used pesticide, to increased incidence of choanal atresia (Agopian et al., 2013).

Complete bilateral atresia is a potentially life-threatening emergency in the affected neonate, who will develop respiratory distress with hypoxia within a few hours of birth. An oral airway must be placed securely to allow for breathing. Surgery is usually attempted early in the newborn period, depending on the condition of the infant. Repair of the blocked passageway creates a nasopharyngeal airway. Approaches to repair vary among surgeons and centers, with no approach preferred, as there have been no clinical trials to compare outcomes (Cedin et al., 2012). Depending on the characteristics of a particular child's anomaly and the surgical repair required, nasal stents may be in place for 24 hours up to 12 weeks postoperatively to maintain the integrity of the repair and to prevent restenosis of the tissue (Ramsden et al., 2009). Topical mitomycin C, a chemotherapeutic agent, when applied intraoperatively appeared to reduce the risk of scarring and restenosis (Rutter, 2006). Subsequent reports did not observe significant long-term differences in outcomes with and without mitomycin, and there have been no randomized trials to give definitive proof of this agent's effectiveness. In light of concerns over use of a potentially oncogenic medication in otherwise healthy infants and lack of definitive proof of efficacy, there is currently insufficient evidence to support the use of mitomycin (Ramsden et al., 2009).

Breastfeeding Implications

The baby with choanal atresia may resist taking any type of oral feeding until the problem is corrected. Initially, oral feeding is not usually possible with bilateral choanal atresia, as the baby is unable to suck, swallow, and breathe. Feeding requires oral-gastric tube placement until surgery is accomplished. With stents in the nasopharynx postoperatively, the baby will be able to feed orally, but the stent length may need to be adjusted to accommodate breastfeeding.

Gastrointestinal Anomalies and Disorders

Bloody Vomit or Bowel Movements

Blood in the vomit (hematemesis) or stool (hematochezia) is, of course, cause for alarm in any infant or child. It may signal a variety of medical or surgical problems of the gastrointestinal tract. One of the most common causes in the newborn is swallowed maternal blood, related either to delivery or to breastfeeding. When a young breastfed infant presents with blood in vomit or stool, it is possible that maternal blood was ingested with breastfeeding, even in the absence of obvious maternal nipple lesions. The Apt test can be performed on a sample of gastric material to distinguish between maternal and fetal hemoglobin. If more than 30 minutes has elapsed since the specimen was obtained, the test results are not reliable. If there is no maternal blood, then an appropriate workup is indicated. The test will not distinguish between infant and maternal blood if the baby is old enough to no longer have fetal hemoglobin, which occurs at around 6 to 12 months of age. If the newborn did not receive vitamin K, consider hemorrhagic disease of the newborn. Other causes of upper or lower gastrointestinal bleeding are much less common.

Other causes of hematochezia include anorectal fissures, allergic colitis, volvulus, and intussusception, among others. If the blood is due to swallowed maternal blood, the baby will not have pain or gastrointestinal symptoms, as would be expected with the other problems listed.

Esophageal Atresia/ Tracheoesophageal Fistula

Esophageal atresia/tracheoesophageal fistula (EA/TEF) occurs in about 1 in 3500 live births. In the most common form of EA/TEF, the upper end of the esophagus ends in a blind pouch, with a fistula connecting the lower segment of the esophagus to the trachea (Kunisaki & Foker, 2012). Only 10% to 40% of cases are identified prenatally: presence of polyhydramnios and the absence of a fetal stomach bubble observed during ultrasonography are poor predictors of EA (Kunisaki & Foker, 2012). About 50% of children will have other malformations seen with the VACTERL sequence (vertebral defects, anorectal malformation, cardiac anomalies, tracheoesophageal fistula, radial and renal dysplasia, and limb anomalies), CHARGE associations (coloboma, heart defects, atresia choanae, retarded development, genital hypoplasia, ear abnormalities), and trisomy 18.

Classic symptoms of esophageal atresia with tracheoesophageal fistula are evident shortly after

birth—copious, white frothy bubbles of mucus from the mouth, which return after suctioning. The child may have noisy respirations and experience coughing, choking, and cyanosis, which become worse with feeding. When an infant is symptomatic for EA/TEF, a nasogastric tube is passed into the esophagus to see whether gastric secretions can be aspirated. If gastric contents are not obtained and other symptoms are present, emergency medical attention should be obtained. X-ray and sonography will confirm the diagnosis.

Preoperatively the child is maintained with the head of the bed at 45-degree elevation, and continuous suction of the blind pouch is instituted to prevent aspiration. The infant is not fed by mouth and acid suppression medication may be prescribed (Kunisaki & Foker, 2012). Parenteral nutrition is provided until surgical correction is accomplished, usually in the first few days of life (Kunisaki & Foker, 2012). The premature or medically unstable baby will be provided with parenteral nutrition, along with gastrostomy and upper pouch to suction, until the child is stable enough for surgery. For children with more complex forms of EA/TEF, repair may be delayed, necessitating placement of a gastrostomy tube for enteral feedings. Postoperatively, enteral feeding typically begins on the second to third days for most infants. Minimally invasive surgical techniques are becoming more common, with more than 20% of pediatric surgeons reporting success using such procedures.

Common long-term problems for these children include difficulty with oral feeding and growth, respiratory difficulties associated with tracheomalacia and bronchomalacia, and recurrent respiratory infection. Although many will have gastroesophageal reflux, only 15% to 20% will require antireflux surgery (Kunisaki & Foker, 2012).

Breastfeeding Implications

As soon as a gastrostomy tube is in place, the infant can receive expressed human milk. Opportunities for oral feeding may not occur for weeks to months after birth, depending on the severity of the defect. It is very common for children with EA/TEF to demonstrate aversive behavior during feeding attempts. Consultation with a skilled occupational therapist or speech-language pathologist is recommended. Until oral feeding is allowed, a specific plan for providing nonaversive oral stimulation for the infant and supporting the mother's continued milk expression is required.

Gastroesophageal Reflux and Gastroesophageal Reflux Disease

Gastroesophageal reflux (GER) is the effortless regurgitation of gastric contents into the oral cavity or out of the mouth—commonly known as "spitting up" or "spilling." Relaxation of the lower esophageal sphincter allows this to happen. Infants with GER are happy, thriving infants, who spit up one or more times a day most days. Hegar et al. (2009) followed 180 infants from birth to age 12 months and found that most spit up one or more times per day from birth: 73% did so in the first month after birth, but this proportion decreased to 50% by 5 months, and to 4% at 12 months. Infants who were exclusively breastfed spit up less often than infants who received mixed feeding.

Only a fraction of these infants will develop gastroesophageal reflux disease (GERD). GERD is defined as symptoms or complications of GER— pain, respiratory disease, poor growth, Sandifer's syndrome (opisthotonic type of posturing with arched back and twisted neck), and, as a very late sign, hematemesis due to esophagitis (Malcolm & Cotten, 2012; Vandenplas et al., 2009). GERD is also associated with abnormal motility of the gut. Families of babies with GERD require reassurance that their infants are healthy and that the spitting will improve with time. Although Heacock et al. (1992) noted that breastfed newborns have shorter episodes of reflux and lower gastric pH values than formula-fed babies (only during active sleep), it is not uncommon for breastfed infants to have GERD.

GERD is not a common cause of apparent life-threatening events (ALTE), but may contribute to chronic respiratory disorders such as pneumonia and asthma. The link to chronic cough and stridor is not proven (Vandenplas et al., 2009). Parents may report that the child is happiest when prone (there is less reflux in this position). However, the prone position is no longer recommended in light of its link to sudden infant death syndrome (SIDS).

GERD is only one of many illnesses and conditions of infancy to present with vomiting. Children with projectile vomiting, those with persistent vomiting, and those who have additional signs and symptoms may have other problems, such as sepsis, meningitis, congenital metabolic or endocrine disorders, pyloric stenosis, malrotation of the bowel, intussusception, Hirschsprung's disease, or neurologic disorders that need to be considered in the medical evaluation (Sullivan & Sundaram, 2012). Children who have persistent symptoms affecting weight gain, feeding behavior, or happiness require referral for evaluation.

Contrary to many clinicians' and lactation consultants' opinions, the GER guidelines committee (Vandenplas et al., 2009) does not consider reflux to be a common cause of unexplained crying or irritability in otherwise healthy babies. Further, the guidelines state that the diagnosis of GERD in infants (as opposed to older children and adults) cannot be based solely on the clinical history, as there is no symptom or symptom complex that is definitively diagnostic, with the exception of Sandifer's syndrome. The I-GERQ-R questionnaire aids in diagnosis and subsequent assessment of effectiveness of therapy and has been found to be an effective tool to aid the clinician (Kleinman et al., 2006; Orenstein, 2010).

Diagnostic testing is appropriate for infants who have complications or in whom the diagnosis of GERD is uncertain (Sullivan & Sundaram, 2012; Vandenplas et al., 2009). A barium swallow is not useful for establishing the diagnosis of GERD, but will identify the rare anatomic anomaly that may cause the reflux (Vandenplas et al., 2009). The standard of care test for establishing the diagnosis of GERD in the infant is an esophageal pH probe (a probe inserted in the baby's esophagus to monitor the pH), which assesses frequency and duration of GER episodes. Results are not always easy to interpret given the frequency of infant feedings and inability to register episodes of nonacid reflux via an intranasal catheter. A newer technique is use of the multiple intraluminal impedance pH monitor, which measures fluid, air, and solids in the esophagus and detects acid and nonacid reflux via an intranasal catheter. The more detailed information obtained may be more helpful in establishing the diagnosis and tailoring medical management for the infant, but it is not yet considered the standard of care (Sullivan & Sundaram, 2012). An endoscopic examination establishes the presence of esophagitis, and allows for a biopsy of the esophagus if indicated. GERD is more common in children with neurologic impairments such as cerebral palsy, premature infants, and infants with other congenital gastrointestinal tract anomalies such as gastroschisis and EA/TEF.

If the child's symptoms are interfering with normal weight gain or causing pain behavior, medications may be prescribed that reduce the acidity of gastric secretions and promote gastric motility. Antacids offer short-term acid reduction and symptom relief. Aluminum-containing antacids must be used with caution in infants due to their side effects—neurotoxicities, anemia, and osteopenia—and should not be used for long-term treatment (Malcom & Cotten, 2012; Sullivan & Sundaram, 2012). Medications that reduce the acidity of gastric contents include histamine-2 receptor antagonists (H_2 blockers) such as ranitidine (Zantac), and proton pump inhibitors (PPIs). H_2 blockers generally are given twice daily, and have a very rapid onset of acid suppression. Proton pump inhibitors such as omeprazole (Prilosec), lansoprazole (Prevacid), and esomeprazole (Nexium) are FDA approved for infants older than 1 year, but are commonly prescribed for younger children. PPIs are usually given once daily before the first morning feeding, and take several days before maximal acid suppression is accomplished (Sullivan & Sundaram, 2012).

Agents that adhere to lesions in the esophagus, such as sucralfate (Carafate) or alginate (Gaviscon Infant), may be recommended to help with short-term pain management and healing of esophagitis. However, they must be used with caution in infants because some agents contain absorbable components that may be harmful with long term use (Vandenplas et al., 2009).

A recent review of research regarding GERD interventions concluded that the current data are insufficient to determine which treatments are most effective due to huge variations in measurement of confounders, methods used to establish the diagnosis of GERD, and definitions for outcome measures (Neu et al., 2012). Further, current GER clinical practice guidelines (Vandenplas et al., 2009) state that the adverse events associated with prokinetic medications (cisapride, domperidone, metoclopramide, and erythromycin) outweigh their benefits.

If medical management of GERD is not resulting in normal growth and development and resolution of associated complications, surgical intervention may be required, particularly for children with underlying neurologic impairment. The Nissen fundoplication and modified Nissen are the procedures most commonly used. These procedures wrap the antrum of the stomach around the esophagus to limit reflux of gastric contents into the esophagus. However, such surgery does not resolve the underlying gastrointestinal motility disorder, and it has significant morbidity.

Breastfeeding Implications

Typical challenges for parents include the symptomatic child's difficulty with feeding and sleeping. Mathisen et al. (1999) reported that infants with GERD aged 5 to 7 months in a case-match control study had significantly more feeding problems affecting behavior, swallowing, food intake, and mother–child interaction. Children with GERD wake at night and sleep more during the day (Ghaem et al., 1998). When mothers are faced with a very fussy baby, more feedings are offered. Thus one may see a chubby baby who is nearly continuously breastfeeding—and a vicious cycle quickly develops of fussing, short feeding, and more fussing that occurs with high-volume/high-lactose /low-fat foremilk feedings (Woolridge & Fisher, 1988). Encouraging several same-sided breastfeedings in a row may break the cycle of fussing associated with relative lactose intolerance observed in these breastfeeding situations.

When the infant is unable to gain appropriate weight with direct breastfeeding, supplemental calories can be provided with fortified mother's milk via a supplementation device or other method. Bottle-feeding may facilitate increased caloric intake, as it is not entirely dependent on the child's cooperation. Occasionally, nasogastric, gastrostomy, or jejunal feeding may be needed while fine-tuning medical management strategies to reduce discomfort with oral feedings. Box 18-6 presents interventions that may reduce the frequency and amount of gastroesophageal reflux.

Children with GERD need ongoing monitoring of growth. Breastfeeding does not need to be interrupted, but increased calories may be needed for normal growth. Some infants with GERD are found to have cow milk protein allergy, so the breastfeeding mother may be advised to try a dairy elimination diet to assess the effect on the child's symptoms. Occasionally, providers will suggest thickening feedings with cereal. When cereal is added to breastmilk, enzymes break it down very quickly, and it is an ineffective thickening agent. Furthermore, thickened feedings have not been found to be effective. The frequency of reflux episodes may be reduced, but exposure of the esophagus to acidic gastric material is increased, probably because thickened gastric contents do not clear as quickly (Bailey et al., 1987). In addition, use of cereal-thickened feedings is associated with coughing in infants with GERD (Orenstein et al., 1992). For the child who is the happy spitter and gaining weight well, no changes in routine are needed. Parents do need acknowledgment of their concerns, reassurance regarding how well their baby is doing, and sympathy for the increased laundry load.

Pyloric Stenosis

Pyloric stenosis (PS) is hypertrophy of the pyloric sphincter. The incidence varies with ethnicity and geography: it is estimated at 2–4:1000 live births in Western areas, but is significantly lower in Southeast Asia and China (Pandya & Heiss, 2012). This condition is seen more commonly in males than in females, at a 4:1 ratio. The relationship of feeding method to the incidence of pyloric stenosis is unclear (MacMahon, 2006).

Symptoms of progressively more severe projectile nonbloody and nonbilious vomiting develop at about 2 to 4 weeks of age. The typical clinical picture is of a hyperalert, emaciated baby who breastfeeds, promptly vomits a large amount, and then requests immediate refeeding. During and after a

---

BOX 18-6 INTERVENTIONS FOR THE INFANT WITH SYMPTOMATIC GASTROESOPHAGEAL REFLUX

- Feed the baby in a more upright position, avoiding abdominal compression.
- Use one breast per feeding to reduce the volume of each feeding and increase access to higher calorie hindmilk.
- Feed more frequently.
- Elevate the bed to a 30 to 45 degree angle. (A baby who is sleeping on the parent's chest is in this position.)
- Avoid placing child in an infant seat or car seat after feedings. This compresses the stomach, increasing reflux episodes.
- Avoid using cereal to thicken feedings, a commonly advised treatment that does not help (Bailey et al., 1987).
- Avoid prone positioning for sleep. Due to the association with increased risk of SIDS, this is not recommended by pediatric gastroenterologists (GER Guidelines Committee, 2001).
- Left-lateral positioning significantly reduces reflux frequency and duration (Tobin et al., 1997; Ewer et al., 1999).

feeding, it is possible to see peristaltic waves that pass from left to right. The experienced clinician can palpate an olive-shaped tumor (the hypertrophic pylorus) in the right upper quadrant of the abdomen, which is diagnostic in 99% of these patients (White et al., 1998). Current practice is to obtain an upper abdominal ultrasound to confirm the presence of a pyloric mass. Alternatively, an upper gastrointestinal study with barium swallow will demonstrate the elongated and narrowed pyloric canal (Pandya & Heiss, 2012).

With any delay in diagnosis, infants risk developing severe dehydration and electrolyte imbalance. Restoration of hydration and electrolyte balance via intravenous therapy is required prior to surgery. Pyloromyotomy is performed to widen the pylorus using one of three operative techniques: transumbilical (least preferred), open, or laparoscopic. Use of laparoscopic techniques is associated with quicker time to full feeds, shorter length of hospital stay, and no higher rate of complications than with the open technique (Oomen et al., 2012). Feeding resumes once the infant has recovered from anesthesia. Vomiting may occur irrespective of the postoperative feeding regimen, and families need to know to expect this (Pandya & Heiss, 2012).

Breastfeeding Implications

Lactation consultants should have PS on their list of concerns for any baby whom they see struggling with weight gain and spitting up—while remembering there are lots of causes for vomiting in infants in addition to GER. Ad libitum breastfeeding once the child has recovered from anesthesia is safe (Pandya & Heiss, 2012), decreases length of hospital stay, and saves an average of $400 per patient compared to a more lengthy fasting period with incremental feedings (Garza et al., 2002). Mothers will need to express their milk for the few feeds that are missed during the perioperative period.

Chylothorax

Chylothorax occurs when the lymphatic system becomes obstructed due to congenital anomalies in the development of the lymphatic system, or secondary to traumatic injury as a complication in

as many as 4.7% of children post thoracic surgery (Helin et al., 2006). Chylous fluid accumulates in the pleural space. This fluid consists of lymph and emulsified fat secreted from the intestine. Management includes drainage of the chest cavity via chest tubes, as well as dietary management including low-fat, high-protein oral feedings using special formulas with medium-chain triglycerides, or total parenteral nutrition. Octreotide, an intravenous medication, is the only agent that may hasten the resolution of a chylothorax. It reduces lymph fluid production by a number of mechanisms, including decreasing the volume of gastric, pancreatic, and biliary secretions so that the volume and protein content of fluid within the thoracic duct is reduced (Helin et al., 2006). Octreotide is being used more often, and is reported to reduce the number of days of chylous effusion and to have a relatively benign side-effect profile (Caverly et al., 2010).

Breastfeeding Implications

Previously, human milk was not given to infants with chylothorax because of its high long-chain fatty acid content. Chan and Lechtenberg (2007) reported the successful use of fat-free human milk in seven infants with chylous pleural effusion. The fat portion of the milk was skimmed off using a special centrifuging technique. The skim human milk then must be supplemented with calories, fats, and fat-soluble vitamins under the guidance of a pediatric dietitian. Once the drainage ceases, the baby will eventually be able to receive unaltered breastmilk/breastfeeding.

Imperforate Anus

Anorectal malformations are rare, occurring in 1 in every 4000 to 5000 live births. Imperforate anus ranges from no opening at all to a normal-appearing rectum that ends in a blind rectal pouch just above the opening. Presence of an imperforate anus is confirmed only by careful examination and by a diagnostic X-ray examination. Approximately two-thirds of all children with this condition have other congenital abnormalities. As with EA/TEF, there is an association between imperforate anus and a number of other VACTERL defects. Thus careful examination of the baby is critical to establish the presence of associated anomalies. Genitourinary and gynecologic anomalies are commonly found, so pre-surgical evaluation includes determining the presence and severity of these associated anomalies.

Depending on the severity of the defect and associated genitourinary anomalies, anal reconstruction may be done in the immediate newborn period. More commonly, a three-step approach is required—colostomy, anal reconstruction, and colostomy reversal (Herman & Teitelbaum, 2012). After colostomy placement surgery, feeding can begin as soon as bowel sounds are present, which usually occurs within 24 hours. When the colostomy is reversed, enteral feedings are suspended for 4 to 7 days—until nasogastric tube drainage is clear, and the child begins passing gastric secretions from the anus.

Breastfeeding Implications

The baby cannot have enteral feedings until there is either a reconstructed anus or a functioning colostomy. Parenteral nutrition is usually required for a period of time both preoperatively and postoperatively. Mothers will need to express their milk until the child can have oral feedings. The normally loose stools of the breastfed infant lessen the risk of constipation with subsequent breakdown of the surgical area and local infection.

Metabolic Dysfunction

More than 100 metabolic diseases can be detected in infancy. Diseases for which screening is performed vary from region to region, based in part on ethnic, financial, and political issues. Newborn screening for phenylketonuria (PKU) and congenital hypothyroidism is done in all 50 U.S. states and in most Western countries (Clague & Thomas, 2002). Other metabolic disorders for which screening is commonly performed include galactosemia, amino and organic acidemias, and cystic fibrosis. Private companies now make extensive newborn screening available directly to parents. Other acquired metabolic conditions such as diabetes are not screened for in the newborn period and may not become symptomatic until much later in infancy or childhood.

Rare Amino and Organic Acidemias

With the exception of PKU and galactosemia, there is very limited information regarding breastfeeding in the rare inborn metabolic diseases (IMDs). PKU is the only disorder for which there are consensus guidelines for including breastfeeding as part of the child's diet. Dietary control is critical to reduce the risk of the devastating permanent consequences of these disorders.

Gokcay et al. (2006) reported on a handful of infants with a variety of organic acidemias who were breastfed. Babies who received breastfeeding had fewer infections, metabolic episodes, and hospital admissions related to their metabolic disease. MacDonald et al. (2006) surveyed IMD centers worldwide regarding their experience with breastfeeding for their patients. In these centers, breastfeeding, in combination with special complementary formulas, was successful in a very small number of children with a variety of inborn errors of metabolism. Exclusive breastfeeding is rarely safe for children with these disorders, but combination of breastfeeding with a specifically prescribed formula can be accomplished and is recommended by some sources (Gokcay et al., 2006; MacDonald et al., 2006).

When a decision is made to include breastmilk in the diet, more frequent monitoring of clinical parameters and biochemistry is required. Huner et al. (2005) reported on another small group of breastfed children with a variety of inborn errors of metabolism. Not all of these children fared well with breastmilk as part of their diet, experiencing more frequent metabolic crises. Parents will need help to understand the balance of the risks versus the benefits of including breastmilk as part of their baby's diet. Close collaboration with the medical team is a must to avoid metabolic crises.

Phenylketonuria

Phenylketonuria is an autosomal recessive inherited metabolic disorder of phenylalanine (Phe) metabolism. Specifically, a defect in the enzyme phenylalanine hydroxylase decreases conversion of phenylalanine to tyrosine. Abnormal metabolites accumulate in blood and tissues, including the brain, interfering with central nervous system development. To prevent brain damage, the amount of dietary Phe must be strictly limited, beginning in the first days of life. Delay in dietary treatment is associated with developmental problems. Phe blood levels are monitored very closely, with the diet being adjusted accordingly. Current research concerns include the risk of micronutrient deficiency in children who are on the prescribed PKU diet; therefore, assessment of the effects of supplementation with specific nutrients is under way (Giovannini et al., 2007). Current thinking is that it is best to be on a special PKU diet for life.

Breastfeeding Implications

Ahring et al. (2009) surveyed European PKU centers and found that 80% recommend breastfeeding along with special Phe formulas as the standard of care. Human milk has lower levels of Phe than does any commercial infant formula. Infants with PKU who are breastfed, in addition to receiving special low-Phe or Phe-free formula, have significantly higher intelligence quotient scores—a 12.9-point advantage even after adjusting for social and maternal education status (Riva et al., 1996). McCabe et al. (1989) found that breastfed infants who received a daily amount of 362 mL (first month) to 464 mL (fourth month) of breastmilk each day,

in addition to supplemental Phe-free formula, had a lower Phe intake than did infants who were fed exclusively on low-Phe formula during their first 6 months of life. Thus fluctuations in the volume of breastmilk the baby takes are less worrisome than fluctuations in intake of formulas with higher Phe levels.

The lactation consultant needs to work closely with a physician and dietitian who specialize in metabolic disorders to manage the dietary plan for the breastfed infant with PKU. In the United States, there is at least one medical center in each state designated to serve as a consultant and treatment facility for children with metabolic defects, including PKU (Duncan & Elder, 1997).

Breastfeeding along with supplemental use of Phe-free formula is prescribed for infants with PKU. A number of approaches are available for manipulating the child's diet to maintain the low Phe levels required for normal brain development. Recommendations for incorporating breastfeeding into a PKU diet include weighing of infants before and after breastfeeding to ensure correct dietary intake—a time-consuming task that may not yield accurate results. Greve et al. (1994) developed a less cumbersome method of calculating the low-Phe dietary prescription (see Box 18-7). The child's healthcare provider uses this information to calculate the daily amount of Phe-free formula that is needed to keep the infant's Phe at the appropriate

---

BOX 18-7 CALCULATING BREASTMILK AND PHE-FREE FORMULA INTAKE FOR THE INFANT WITH PKU

Given: Maximum phenylalanine (PHE) intake allowed is 25 to 45 mg/kg/day depending on the age of the infant. Mature breastmilk has 0.41 mg/ml PHE.

Calculate the amount of PHE-free formula supplementation for the breastfed baby:

1. Find the estimated volume of daily milk intake in ml (110 kcal/kg/day): (Infant weight in kg) times 110 = total calories/day
   (Total calories) divided by 20 = total number of oz/day
   (Total number of oz) times 30 = total volume in ml/day
2. Calculate the maximum allowable PHE/day (breastmilk has 0.41 mg PHE/ml):
   45 mg times infant weight in kg = total number of mg PHE allowed
   Total mg divided by 0.41 = total volume in ml of breastmilk allowed

3. Calculate amount of replacement PHE-free formula required:
   Total daily volume minus maximum volume allowed = amount of replacement feeding needed

Below are the calculations for a 4.0 kg infant:

1. Estimate volume of daily intake in ml:
   110 kcal times 4.0 = 440 calories
   440 divided by 20 = 22 oz
   22 oz times 30 = 660 ml
2. Calculate maximum allowable breastmilk/24 hours:
   45 mg times 4.0 kg = 180 mg PHE maximum per day
   180 times 0.41 = 439 ml of breastmilk
3. Calculate amount of PHE-free replacement feedings needed in order for infant to not drink more breastmilk than allowed:
   660 ml minus 439 ml = 221 ml replacement PHE-free formula required daily

The PHE-free formula can be given via a nursing supplementer during breastfeeds or with a bottle prior to breastfeeding. The total daily amount needed can be divided into several aliquots. For example, the baby above needs about 220 ml/day of PHE-free formula. This could be given in 30 ml aliquots with each breastfeeding for approximately 8 feedings. The PHE-free formula should be offered prior to the breastfeeding, or along with the breastfeeding using a supplementer, rather than being offered after the breastfeeding.

level. The child receives the prescribed amount of Phe-free formula, along with breastfeeding. The Phe-free formula can be provided either via supplementation device at the breast or with some other alternative method prior to breastfeeding.

In 2003, van Rijn et al. reported on a series of nine infants fed with alternating breastfeeds and PKU formula-feeds. With each feeding, the baby was allowed to feed to satiety. Outcomes of these infants were compared with infants who had only formula-feeding. No differences in growth or Phe levels were noted between the groups. In a retrospective review of 97 infants with PKU, Banta-wright et al. (2012) found that infants who were breastfed (and also received Phe formula) were more likely to have normal mean Phe levels than exclusively formula-fed children.

Introduction of weaning foods must be undertaken very carefully, and includes introduction of special protein pastes used to provide appropriate amounts of Phe-free protein. MacDonald et al. (2011) suggest introducing weaning protein pastes and other solid foods beginning at 17 weeks of age, to reduce the risk of food refusal sometimes seen in older infants with PKU. However, there are no evidence-based guidelines for weaning at this time (MacDonald et al., 2011).

Women who have PKU should be on a diet prior to conception and throughout the pregnancy to reduce the chances of harming the developing fetus. Fox-Bacon et al. (1997) reported on the Phe levels in milk of identical twins with PKU and the Phe status of their infants. These researchers found that high maternal Phe serum levels and high milk Phe levels did not result in abnormal Phe levels in their breastfeeding infants who did not have PKU.

Galactosemia

Galactosemia is caused by deficiency of galactose-1-phosphate uridyltransferase (GALT), which is required for the metabolism of lactose. It is transmitted as an autosomal recessive trait, occurring in only 1 in about every 60,000 to 80,000 births.

There are several variants due to gene mutations. With "classic" galactosemia, any intake of galactose results in multiorgan dysfunction. Affected infants are at risk for sepsis and bleeding in the early newborn period. These neonates appear normal at birth but soon start having feeding difficulties. Other symptoms include vomiting, poor weight gain, jaundice, hepatosplenomegaly, and bleeding.

Untreated galactosemia leads to cognitive impairment and fatal liver disease. Treatment within the first 10 days of life is associated with the best neurodevelopmental outcomes; however, even when treatment is begun on day 1, individuals may have lifelong issues with cognition, speech, movement disorders, cataracts, and gonadal problems (Berry, 2012). Those with the variant types are much less likely to experience these difficulties.

Breastfeeding Implications

For infants with classic galactosemia, immediate, abrupt weaning is necessary due to the galactose content of human milk. Avoidance of all galactose is required to prevent irreversible damage to the infant (Berry, 2012). For those children found to have one of the variant forms, limited breastfeeding in combination with lactose-free formula may be possible, with very close monitoring of galactose-2-phosphate levels (Lawrence, 2013).

Positive newborn screening tests for galactosemia are not always accurate, so results should be confirmed before recommending that women stop expressing milk while awaiting confirmation. Nurses and lactation consultants working with babies that have jaundice and poor weight gain need to remember to check newborn screening results, as galactosemia as well as congenital hypothyroidism may cause these symptoms. If the diagnosis is confirmed, the mother will need instruction for relief of engorgement as well as emotional support for the loss of the breastfeeding relationship (see Box 18-8). If partial breastfeeding is allowed in the case of variant forms, very close collaboration with metabolic disease specialists is required. It is safe for women who have galactosemia to breastfeed. They need calcium and vitamin D supplements to support their own health (Lawrence, 2013).

Box 18-8 A Mother's Guide to Saying Goodbye to Breastfeeding/Milk Expression

- When the time comes to stop breastfeeding or milk expression, you may have very mixed emotions. The following are all normal responses when saying goodbye to breastfeeding.
- If you are not ready to give up breastfeeding or the hope for a breastfeeding relationship, you may feel regret or sadness.
- If you are tired, you may feel a bit glad that the time committed to milk expression is available for other demands.
- You may be glad to have your body back to yourself, but you may feel guilty that you have those feelings.
- Your hormones will also be changing, and that may affect your mood.
- As you stop breastfeeding/milk expression, you can express a small amount of milk to make yourself comfortable.

This will keep your breasts from being uncomfortably full, and reduce your risk of developing a breast infection.

- A firm, but not tight, bra may provide comfort.
- Cold compresses may be soothing, and pain medication such as acetaminophen or ibuprofen can provide pain relief if your breasts become uncomfortably engorged.
- If you find yourself feeling unbearably sad, please call on your healthcare provider for advice.
- Know that you gave your baby a wonderful gift of love.

Congenital Hypothyroidism

Congenital hypothyroidism (CH) is caused by a lack of thyroid secretion, either because the thyroid gland is absent or because there is an inborn enzymatic deficiency in the synthesis of thyroxine. Routine screening results show that rates of congenital hypothyroidism vary with geography: the incidence is as high as 1:800 in Greece, but on average ranges from 1:2000 to 1:4000 births worldwide, with increased rates noted in the United States (Rastogi & LaFranchi, 2010).

A transient form of hypothyroidism can occur from transfer in utero or during breastfeeding of antithyroid drugs or topical application of povidone-iodine on the mother at the time of delivery (Bartalena et al., 2001; Casteels et al., 2000). Prompt treatment in such cases is required to prevent irreversible developmental delay and growth problems. Hypothyroidism is rarely diagnosed based on clinical findings in the early weeks of life— yet this is when the child is most vulnerable to irreversible brain damage. In the early weeks, parents of an untreated infant may praise their "good baby" because he cries so little. Without treatment, the symptoms of hypothyroidism become noticeable in 3 to 6 months: coarse, brittle hair; anemia; a large, protruding tongue; a wide forehead; and lack of skeletal growth. Untreated cases result in severe mental retardation. Treatment for congenital hypothyroidism is daily thyroid replacement for life; synthetic levothyroxine sodium (levothyroxine or Synthroid) is prescribed. Blood levels are monitored periodically to adjust the dose as the child grows.

Breastfeeding Implications

Lactation consultants involved with newborns who are jaundiced or not thriving need to make sure that neonatal thyroid screening results are normal—as nonspecific early symptoms of CH may include feeding difficulties and hyperbilirubinemia.

Type 1 Diabetes

Protection from diabetes via breastfeeding is a controversial issue, as the data are conflicting. Proposed mechanisms for protection include the delayed exposure to cow milk protein provided with exclusive breastfeeding (Kimpimaki et al., 2001). In addition, gut permeability decreases faster with breastmilk feeding, and there is reduced risk of enteroviral infections during infancy, which in turn decreases risk of enterovirus-triggered B-cell autoimmunity (Knip et al., 2010). As the definitions and duration of breastfeeding along with timing of exposure to cow milk and complementary foods have not always been controlled for in existing research studies, more data are needed to confirm the role of breastmilk/breastfeeding in diabetes type 1 prevention.

It is very unusual for the onset of type 1 diabetes to occur during infancy. Diabetes management for the infant and toddler is challenging, as feeding schedules and activity level are not predictable, and the child is not able to communicate symptoms of low blood glucose to parents or caregivers. This increases the risk of severe hypoglycemia, which could result in coma, seizures, and subsequent learning and behavioral disorders. Target blood sugars are in the range of 100 to 200 mg/dL (5.56 to 11.11 mmol/L). Insulin administration is tailored to the child's feeding schedule—usually given 2 to 4 times per day. Insulin doses are quite low. Berhe et al. (2006) reported the effective use of insulin pumps in the diabetic management of toddlers and young children. The children had improved hemoglobin A_{1c} levels and fewer episodes of hypoglycemia, and parents felt much more confident in their ability to manage their child's diabetes.

Breastfeeding Implications

No research has been found that discusses breastfeeding and management of the infant with diabetes; however, the most important considerations for insulin dosing would be estimating the quantity of breastmilk the baby is taking. Night-time breastfeedings and demand breastfeedings are difficult to measure. Newer rapid-acting insulin can be given after feedings (contrary to the usual method of giving insulin prior to feedings), which facilitates incorporating breastfeeding into the diabetes management plan. If the healthcare team finds it critical to quantify the amount of breastmilk ingested per feeding to develop a treatment plan, the child could be weighed before and after feedings for a day or two using a rented scale. This would assist in estimating the contribution of breastmilk to the child's total caloric intake, as well as quantifying carbohydrate, fat, and protein points. Weaning would not be advised.

Celiac Disease

Celiac disease (CD) is an autoimmune condition triggered by gluten. Its incidence in Western populations is 1% to 2% (Ludvigsson & Fasano, 2012). Complete removal of gluten from the diet in a patient with celiac disease should result in symptomatic, serologic, and histologic remission. CD is characterized by changes in the intestinal mucosa or villi that prevent the absorption of foods, mainly fat. The mucosal damage appears to stem from sensitivity to gliadin, the protein fraction of gluten found in wheat, rye, barley, and other grains.

Nutrition during infancy appears to play an important role in the development of CD. Formula-feeding and the early introduction of solids accelerate the appearance of symptoms of celiac disease (Akobeng et al., 2006). The infant with this disorder is asymptomatic until solids containing gluten are introduced into the diet. Clinical symptoms are insidious and chronic. Fatigue, diarrhea, and failure to thrive are the most common presenting symptoms, with later onset observed in breastfed children (D'Amico et al., 2005). Because fat is not absorbed, the child's stools become frothy appearing, foul smelling, and excessive. Deficiencies of the fat-soluble vitamins (A, D, K, and E) appear. If the disease progresses without treatment, abdominal distension and general wasting are evident. The affected child's diet must be modified on a lifelong basis and vigorously maintained to exclude gluten, thus improving food absorption and preventing malnutrition.

Breastfeeding Implications

Most data show that breastfeeding at the time of gluten introduction reduces the risk to develop CD (Chertok, 2007; Ludvigsson & Fasano, 2012).

Ivarsson et al. (2013) found that children who had gradual introduction of gluten in small amounts during ongoing breastfeeding had significantly lower prevalence of CD at age 12 years. Introduction of gluten both before 3 months and after 7 months is associated with increased risk of symptoms in at-risk children (Norris et al., 2006). Farrell (2006) reminds us that it is not certain what the role of breastfeeding might be—is it the delay of exposure to glutens or the modulation of the child's immune response to gluten that is altered due to breastmilk's effect on the gut?

Cystic Fibrosis

Cystic fibrosis (CF) is an autosomal recessive genetic disorder affecting 1:3000 Caucasians, with lower incidence in other groups: Latino-Americans, 1:10,000; African Americans, 1:15,000; and uncommon in Africa and Asia, 1:35,000 to 1:350,000 (Antunovic et al., 2013). CF is caused by a defect in a single gene on chromosome 7. This mutation leads to abnormalities in the apical membrane of epithelial cells that line the airways, biliary tree, intestines, vas deferens, sweat ducts, and pancreatic ducts, producing generalized endocrinopathy. Secretions of these sites become more viscid and obstruct ducts, leading to dysfunction at the organ level. The exocrine glands of the affected child produce abnormally thick and sticky secretions that block the flow of pancreatic digestive enzymes, clog hepatic ducts, and impede the movement of cilia in the lungs. Approximately 20% to 30% of CF-affected young adults will develop diabetes mellitus.

Expanded newborn screening includes measurement of immunoreactive trypsinogen (IRT) to test for CF, resulting in early identification of and intervention with affected infants. The diagnosis is confirmed with a sweat test. Without newborn screening or meconium ileus, the average age at diagnosis is 14 months. The increased sodium chloride in the child's sweat provides an important diagnostic clue: the family reports that the child tastes salty when kissed. In the newborn, CF may present as a meconium ileus (intestinal obstruction caused by a plug of meconium) in 15% of affected newborns; 90% of infants who have meconium ileus have CF (Antunovic et al., 2013). Signs of intestinal obstruction—a surgical emergency—include abdominal distension, vomiting, and failure to pass stools.

At birth, some 85% to 90% of affected children are already pancreatic insufficient (Antunovic et al., 2013). Nutrient absorption—particularly of fat-soluble vitamins—is thus impaired from the beginning of life. Because of problems with fat absorption, the infant fails to gain weight, despite reports of a voracious appetite. When solid foods are introduced, the stools become bulky, more frequent, foul smelling, and frothy. Pulmonary complications are almost always present, and the child often has persistent, severe respiratory infections because of inability to clear thick secretions.

Prevention of respiratory complications and malnutrition is the mainstay of management for the child with CF. Protection from and aggressive treatment for respiratory infection is accomplished by airway clearance procedures (postural drainage and percussion, chest vest, and others), aerosol therapy, and medications, such as bronchodilators, hypertonic saline inhalation, inhaled corticosteroids, and antibiotics. The use of aerosolized recombinant human deoxyribonuclease to decrease the viscosity of secretions was a breakthrough in CF treatment and is found to reduce exacerbations and improve lung function (Antunovic et al., 2013).

Nutrition management includes promoting breastfeeding, providing fat-soluble vitamin supplements, and prescribing pancreatic enzyme replacement, known as pancrease (Antunovic et al., 2013). The enzyme microspheres are mixed in a tiny amount of applesauce. An acid food must be used to keep the enteric coating of the microspheres intact (O'Brien et al., 2012). The enzyme dose is based on estimated caloric intake, and adjusted according to symptoms of malabsorption or poor weight gain. Because salt content in the infant diet (whether breastmilk or formula) is very low, salt supplementation is usually recommended. This consideration is especially important during hot weather or periods of increased fluid losses (diarrheal illness, fever).

If the child is not gaining weight well, or presents with failure to thrive at the time of late diagnosis, calorie supplementation is needed. Extra calories may be added in a number of ways—for example, with glucose polymers or fat added to breastmilk. A dietitian should be included in decisions regarding alteration of breastmilk feedings to determine the best approach to boosting the caloric content. The child's medical provider will ensure that the enzyme replacement dose is sufficient. Other comorbid problems, such as GERD or cow milk protein allergy, may also interfere with weight gain.

Breastfeeding Implications

Breastfeeding offers protection from infection as well as easy digestibility of breastmilk—both considerations that are particularly important for this high-risk group. Babies with CF produce normal levels of gastric lipase, which is an important digestive enzyme. This enzyme, together with milk lipase in breastmilk, may help the infant with CF to absorb fat more efficiently. Human milk contains appreciably greater amounts of lipase than cow milk.

According to the Cystic Fibrosis Foundation (CFF), published CF guidelines from several groups support the importance of encouraging breastmilk feeding; the CFF cites evidence for improved growth and reduced pulmonary complications from this feeding practice (Borowitz et al., 2009). O'Brien et al. (2012) surveyed CF dietitians and found that most were following the CFF guidelines and recommending human milk for their patients with CF.

Allergies

The issue of the preventive nature of breastfeeding for allergic disease continues to be controversial (Lack, 2012). At present, there is no consensus about whether breastfeeding protects against the development of asthma and allergy. Several studies document that breastfeeding reduces risk, ameliorates severity, or delays onset of atopic conditions (Bloch et al., 2002; Tarini et al., 2006). However, others find that breastfeeding either has no effect on risk or even increases risk (Bergmann et al., 2002; Sears et al., 2002).

Allergic disease is multifactorial, with incidence being related to family history, sensitization, ethnicity, and geography (Lack, 2012). Family history has the best predictive value for identifying at-risk neonates who should be targeted for allergy prevention (Zieger, 2000). The atopy-prone infant is at increased risk to sensitization to allergens prior to birth and early after birth. Antigen exposure is evident as early as 22 weeks' gestation (Jones et al., 1996).

Food allergy is generally defined as hypersensitivity to any food accompanied by immunoglobulin E (IgE)– and non-IgE–mediated reactions (Greer et al., 2008). Incidence of food allergies is increasing, and researchers are uncertain as to why. Food allergy occurs in approximately 8% of children in the United States (Gupta et al., 2011). Some sources suggest that the many dietary changes associated with urbanized diets might explain the increased incidence; in turn, the issue of epigenetics is being explored (West et al., 2010). The most common offending foods in the United States are peanuts, cow milk, shellfish, tree nuts, chicken eggs, fin fish, strawberry, wheat, and soy (Gupta et al., 2011). The initial exposure is sensitization, which does not usually result in allergic symptoms. With a subsequent exposure, however, allergic symptoms may become evident.

"It was thought that the best strategy for preventing food allergy was to avoid exposure to common allergens, but this approach has been unsuccessful. [Recognizing] that oral tolerance is an antigen driven process, there is now focus on earlier, regular exposure to allergenic foods to promote tolerance" (West et al., 2010, p. 638). The 2013 recommendations from the American Academy of Allergy, Asthma and Immunology state that (1) avoidance diets are not advised during either pregnancy or lactation; (2) exclusive breastfeeding from 4 to 6 months is endorsed; (3) introduction of complementary foods should not be delayed beyond 4 to 6 months; and (4) most importantly, there has been a change regarding introduction of allergenic foods—rather than avoiding introduction, they should be introduced once a few typical complementary foods are tolerated (Fleischer et al., 2013).

For all infants, introduction of one food at a time is recommended (Fleischer et al., 2013; Kleinman, 2009).

Breastfeeding Implications

When someone asks if an infant can be allergic to breastmilk, the answer is a qualified "yes." Proteins of foods ingested by the mother pass into the breastmilk, where they may trigger an allergic response in the at-risk child who has been sensitized. Antigens in human milk have been detected for peanuts, lactoalbumin, and ovoalbumin (Casas et al., 2000; Vadas et al., 2001). Furthermore, cross-reactivity between cow milk and human milk proteins is possible (Bernard et al., 2000). The amount of allergen needed to sensitize or trigger symptoms is minute. For bovine beta-lactoalbumin, only 1 ng (one billionth of a gram!) is required for sensitization. The amount of bovine beta-lactoalbumin in mother's milk ranges from 0.5 to 32 ng/L. A 40-mL feeding of cow milk formula contains a concentration of bovine lactoalbumin equivalent to the amount found in 21 years of breastfeeding (Businco et al., 1999).

The list of symptoms caused by food allergy is long: vomiting, diarrhea, colic, colitis, bloody stools (hematochezia), eczema, urticaria, rhinitis, fussiness, and poor sleep patterns, among others. Two studies have reported on a series of children with proctocolitis during exclusive breastfeeding, which resolved within 48 to 72 hours with maternal dietary exclusion of cow milk protein (Patenaude et al., 2000; Pumberger et al., 2001). Some exclusively breastfed infants develop allergic symptoms following exposure to cow milk or other proteins because they have been sensitized to them transplacentally, through inadvertent exposure via supplementation, or through their own mother's milk (Fukushima et al., 1997). Individual infants may respond differently to allergenic foods. Cow milk protein allergy is the most common food allergy during infancy.

If the breastfed infant is thought to have food allergy, clinicians approach the problem in a variety of ways. One strategy is to have the mother begin an extreme diet, eliminating a list of common offenders. Food groups can then be reintroduced one at a time, from the least likely suspect to the most suspect food group. Other clinicians will have the mother begin with a more "simple" elimination diet (no elimination diet is really simple) of omitting all dairy products, as that is the most common offending food group. If the elimination diet is to be of any value, it must be carefully followed and clearly spelled out: written instructions are the most helpful, and scrupulous reading of labels on packaged foods helps to avoid inadvertent consumption of foods that should be eliminated. Especially if several foods are contributing to the baby's adverse reaction, the mother may find food-elimination plans difficult to implement (de Boissieu et al., 1997). It is necessary in some cases to remove all dairy foods. When the offending food is eliminated, symptoms typically improve within 48 to 72 hours, but some sources still recommend waiting a full 2 weeks to discover if eliminating a particular food is helpful (ABM, 2011).

Repucci (1999) and Schach and Haight (2002) reported success of a then-novel approach to helping the allergic breastfeeding dyad when the child's symptoms do not resolve with maternal elimination diets. Mothers of infants with severe bloody stools due to allergic colitis were prescribed pancrease MT4, digestive enzymes normally used in the treatment of cystic fibrosis for improving breakdown of foods in the gastrointestinal tract. With more thorough food digestion, fewer intact proteins would be available to enter the mother's milk. In these two reports, colitis symptoms in the infants resolved in most of the treated dyads. The Academy of Breastfeeding Medicine (2011) endorses this approach for infants with moderate to severe allergic proctocolitis that is not relieved by maternal elimination diet.

Occasionally, the healthcare provider recommends the interruption of breastfeeding, substituting a hypoallergenic formula for a short or long period of time to relieve severe symptoms (severe colic, significant gastrointestinal bleeding, severe eczema) before reintroducing breastfeeding. Soy-based formulas are not appropriate breastmilk substitutes for the atopic child (AAP & Kleinman, 2004).

Allergy prevention should be targeted to high-risk infants—those whose parents have allergies. Exclusive breastfeeding, with introduction of complementary foods between 4 and 6 months of life, is recommended. Maternal avoidance of common allergens is no longer recommended. If supplements are needed, use hydrolyzed or partially hydrolyzed breastmilk substitutes, although the data are not clear as to which of these options is the best choice (Fleischer et al., 2013).

Food Intolerance

Most children do not care at all what their mothers eat or drink. This is why it is not necessary to provide mothers with a list of foods to avoid. However, the occasional child may have a consistent uncomfortable response to the food ingested by the mother. Children who do not tolerate specific foods, but do not have true allergic responses, may have gastrointestinal and dermatologic symptoms that are difficult to distinguish from an allergic response. Typical offending foods, according to retrospective maternal reports, include chocolate, onion, and cruciferous vegetables such as broccoli or cauliflower (Lust et al., 1996). Some babies are sensitive to caffeine and become irritable when their mothers drink beverages containing too much of this substance. Mothers can be instructed to titrate their caffeine intake to their baby's behavior. If a mother notes that her baby is always excessively cranky after she has a huge serving of chocolate cake, then she can decide to reduce the size of the portion next time and see if the baby is happier.

Lactose Intolerance

Fortunately, primary lactase deficiency is an extremely rare problem in infancy, as lactose is the carbohydrate in human milk. Humans normally produce sufficient lactase for lactose digestion until age 3 to 7 years, which is when symptoms of lactose intolerance typically begin to emerge, more commonly in non-Caucasian groups (Kleinman, 2009). However, infants may experience symptoms related to secondary lactase deficiency following gastrointestinal illness or antibiotic use, or as a result of feeding mismanagement. Symptoms of lactose intolerance include escalating fussiness, excessive gassiness shortly after ingesting a lactose-containing meal, and bright green, irritating, slimy stools.

Woolridge and Fisher (1988) describe very clearly the problem of colicky symptoms and feeding mismanagement. When mothers rather than babies control the child's time at the breast, the child may receive high-volume, low-fat feedings that result in a higher than normal lactose load for the baby to digest. When a baby is allowed to nurse as long as desired on the first breast before being moved to the second, the feeding is more likely to have the appropriate balance of volume, fat, and lactose. Following gastrointestinal illness, or antibiotic administration, the brush border of the gastrointestinal tract where lactase is located may be damaged, leading to transient lactose intolerance.

Psychosocial Concerns

Anytime families face the unexpected with their children, the myriad of feelings and concerns that bombard them can be overwhelming. Nurses have an absolutely instrumental role in supporting a family's adaptation to whatever is facing them. Each family differs in their response to the birth of a child with a defect or who is diagnosed with a serious or chronic illness, and each will need support from their healthcare team. It is important for professionals to have a working knowledge of crisis and grief theories to support their clinical work with families.

Family Stress

Stressors related to a child's illness, new diagnoses, or hospitalization are added to daily life stressors. These stresses are not fixed or predictable (Burke et al., 1998). If there are underlying worries about finances, housing, relationships, or other concerns, a family's coping skills may be challenged. A thorough psychosocial assessment is important for identifying potential family needs. The provider needs to obtain this assessment, or review the history reported by others, as the degree of stress may relate more to issues of social support rather than to the specific health problem that the child faces (Smith et al., 2001; Visconti et al., 2002). Pelchat et al. (1999) compared parents of children with congenital heart disease, Down syndrome, cleft lip and palate, and children without disabilities. They discovered that parents of children with Down syndrome and congenital heart disease reported higher levels of parenting and psychological stress compared to parents of babies with cleft lip and palate and nondisabled children.

The family's response to a chronic illness involves their definition or perception of the event in the context of their cultural traditions, as well as the family's resources—social, financial, and emotional. A family with no health insurance and limited financial resources may perceive a child's chronic illness as more stressful than would a family with sufficient resources. Parents may harbor feelings of guilt for bringing on the illness or for not recognizing how sick the child was in early stages.

Stress of Hospitalization

Whether it is planned or emergent, hospitalization disrupts family equilibrium. Hospitalization brings about a disruption of lifestyle and environment to the family tantamount to culture shock. A barrage of unfamiliar stimuli is thrust upon them—for example, infusion pumps that periodically sound an alarm and a constantly rotating staff of new faces place tremendous stress on the family. Normally affable people can become demanding and even hostile as a by-product of their stress, guilt, and perceived or actual unmet needs. These defensive behaviors are part of the parents' coping strategies for managing their feelings and help to protect families from painful realities. They are not necessarily maladaptive. Sympathetic listening and simple, understanding statements, such as "I can see you are upset," or "This is such a difficult time," can help parents through this trying time.

Unexpected admission to a pediatric intensive care unit (PICU) of a previously healthy child causes parents to be near a panic level of anxiety

(Huckabay & Tilem-Kessler, 1999) and may result in post-traumatic stress disorder (PTSD) for a significant number of parents. In their study of 190 parents facing this situation, Bronner et al. (2010) found that 12% had clinical PTSD and 30% had subclinical PTSD. Meta-analysis of studies of parents' responses to their child's hospitalization found that the most severe parental stressor appeared to be role alteration (Shudy et al., 2006). Tomlinson et al. (1999) found that parents' uncertainties about their roles and responsibilities were lessened in an environment where the child was treated as a normal child and where the parents were free to continue to provide comfort care. Melnyk et al. (2004) implemented an educational behavioral intervention program within hours of PICU admission that taught families which specific behaviors to expect from their critically ill child and how to respond. Mothers and children in the treatment group demonstrated better outcomes than the group who did not receive the intervention.

Incorporating family-centered rounds (FCR) into hospital routines has been shown to enhance parents' satisfaction. FCR are multidisciplinary work rounds that occur at the bedside, with opportunities for interaction between the family and the health team, and the family sharing in the development of the plan of care for their child. Kuo et al. (2012) found that FCR resulted in higher parent satisfaction with their child's care, more consistent medical information and care plans, and no increased burden to the health system compared to situations in which families did not experience FCR. The Committee on Hospital Care of the AAP (2012) recommends incorporating FCR into care of the hospitalized child.

Parents who are far from home during their child's hospitalization must arrange for sleeping accommodations in the area if both are not allowed to stay overnight at the hospital. Fortunately, many hospitals have moved to rooms that accommodate both parents to reduce the stress of separation. Some hospitals and cities have housing specifically for families of hospitalized patients, such as Ronald McDonald Houses and others. Support groups of other parents experiencing a similar life crisis

may be helpful for some parents, because each person in the group understands the day-to-day issues and problems of caring for an ill child or rearing one with a chronic disease. Nevertheless, support groups are not for all parents; some are so overwhelmed by their own problems that they are not able to reach out and support others.

Home from the Hospital: The Rebound Effect

The child's reactions following hospitalization depend on the extent of trauma that was experienced and the availability of coping mechanisms for self-protection. When parents room-in with the child, very few behavior changes occur on returning home. In contrast, the young child who has experienced a painful separation may withdraw as a coping strategy, refusing to breastfeed and showing little interest in family members. The baby may cry a great deal and want to be held and breastfed exceptionally often, vigorously protesting having the mother out of sight for even a moment. For toddlers, emotional upheaval, including nightmares and insomnia, is common in the first few weeks following hospitalization. Helping parents to recognize their child's normal response to the stress of hospitalization and learn how to ameliorate their distress is a critical element of comprehensive nursing care.

Chronic Grief and Loss

When the breastfeeding child is chronically ill or has a disabling defect, the disappointment, sorrow, and frustration of parents can be overwhelming. Instead of the perfect child expected during the pregnancy, there is an intense feeling of loss. If the child requires indefinite special care and attention, there is a persistent effect that is described in Olshansky's classic work, "Chronic Sorrow" (1962). Unlike acute grief, which is limited in time, chronic sorrow is prolonged and recurrent. The onset of chronic sorrow is variable among families and sometimes difficult to identify; however, this condition is a natural outgrowth of parenting and is an adaptive response. Breastfeeding may have an ameliorating effect for both the child and the parents when chronic illness is involved. The mother of a breastfed baby has the satisfaction of giving something special to her child, which may help her deal with her feelings of loss.

The Empty Cradle: When a Child Dies— Caring for Bereaved Families

Health professionals may underestimate the depth of attachment that parents and other family members have to their fetus and newborn—dreaming about what the child will look like, what their relationship will be, what the child's future might bring. When families experience the death of their baby or child, all of those dreams are shattered. Parental (and grandparental/sibling) grief is often more intense and longer lasting than anyone would have expected (Wendler, 2012), and this is normal, although it certainly does not feel so. It is difficult to know how to best respond to families as they are grieving their loss, and there are limited data to guide one as to the best approaches. A meta-analysis of bereavement indicated that families appreciated the opportunity to have contact with their child's body. However, Hughes and Riches (2003) found that women who had contact with their deceased infant had more difficulty with grieving, and that the intensity of their difficulty was correlated with the "dose" of contact with their infant's body. This is clearly an area where we need more knowledge to guide our own actions as healers, as well as to provide counsel to the families we care for.

The assumption that mothers and fathers respond very differently to the death of their child is not validated by recent research. Seecharan et al. (2004) did not find significant differences in mothers' and fathers' responses to the death of their child. Mothers had more intense reactions when a death was unexpected (Seecharan et al., 2004). The breastfeeding mother may have to cope with the physical discomfort of breast fullness and leaking and needs advice for management of involution (see Box 18-8). Occasionally, a mother will continue to pump her milk, donating it to a milk bank so that other children may benefit from it. Doing so is her way of coping by maintaining visible evidence of the existence of the lost child. When she offers to do so, the best approach is to put the mother in touch with a milk bank whose staff members can assist her.

When an infant dies, memories that tie the parents to the child are very important to families. Parents should never be denied the right to their sorrow. Remarks such as "It just wasn't meant to be," or "You can always have another baby," are hurtful. They provide no consolation whatsoever regarding the loss of this baby. The following suggestions for healthcare providers who are assisting parents and families through the grief process are based on the authors' experiences as well as those of other healthcare professionals:

- Call the baby by name.
- Help parents anticipate how to share the bad news with other children and family members.
- Refer the parents to bereavement support groups such as AMEND (Aiding Mothers and Fathers Experiencing Neonatal Death), Compassionate Friends, Bereaved Parents, or Share (see the Internet Resources list).
- Programs that involve grandparents and siblings are helpful to the entire family (Roose & Blanford, 2011).
- Allow parents to verbalize feelings.
- Feel your way through the conversation, getting feedback from the parent; wait for him or her to lead the way. Most parents appreciate a chance to talk about their baby and their experience with someone who will understand. Ensure that they know you are available to talk whenever needed.
- Families should have the opportunity to participate in a post-death debriefing with the child's healthcare provider. Such a conference serves to review the events that led to the child's death and to respond to questions and concerns that the family may have about the events or about the medical care provided. Timing of such a conference is at the family's request, but it may be more helpful to wait weeks to months after the death, in addition to holding a conference at the time of death.

- Acknowledge the parents' loss by sending a card or calling. If you do not know the parents well, anything more may be too much.
- Attend the funeral if it seems like the right thing to do.

Lactation Care After the Death

Women have reported distress at the lack of lactation information provided to them at the time of their child's death (Cole, 2012). It is important that the plan of care for women include a post-death lactation plan. If the mother was lactating, help her to remain comfortable. Mothers who lose a baby after 20 weeks' gestation may become engorged. This sometimes comes as a complete shock to mothers. Often, women are reluctant to relieve their discomfort by expressing milk for fear of stimulating milk production.

Healthcare providers often assume that women will want to suppress lactation, but that may not be what they desire. One must first educate families about what to expect when breastfeeding or milk expression ceases, then provide information about a mother's options—for example, lactation suppression via comfort measures or continuing to express milk for donation. The tried-and-true comfort measures include cold compresses, anti-inflammatory medication, and minimal expression for comfort in decreasing frequency (see Box 18-8). A 2012 Cochrane review (Oladapo & Fawole, 2012) found that the quality of evidence for any methods of lactation suppression was poor. Bromocriptine trials reviewed did indicate the effectiveness of this medication for ensuring suppression in the immediate postpartum period. Although there were no reports of thromboembolic events in the small number of subjects studied, there is a black-box warning regarding risk of stroke for this medication. If a mother prefers to continue milk expression for some time, referral to milk banks to facilitate this desire should be made.

ACKNOWLEDGMENT

Jan Riordan, a pioneer in the world of breastfeeding, was the original author of this chapter. I was honored when she invited me to be her coauthor beginning with the third edition. For this fifth edition, as solo author, I made a number of changes in organizing and updating the material, but the content honors Dr. Riordan's initial work, in particular regarding the psychosocial concerns.

SUMMARY

There are unique considerations for helping the breastfeeding family when their infant or young child has special healthcare needs or illness. These special needs can be met by recognizing the developmental stage, assessing family lifestyle, reducing parental stress, involving parents in direct care of their child, and, most of all, minimizing separation of family members. Discontinuing breastfeeding is rarely necessary for the child with a health problem. However, feeding patterns may need to be modified. Too often, weaning from the breast is assumed to be necessary, when this is rarely the case.

Each family is unique. The experience of one situation can never be duplicated; therefore, care providers helping families must be versatile and have solid knowledge about the nature of the health problem so that the best possible care can be provided. First, competent care, and then, compassionate care, are the top priorities. Informing the parents about every aspect of the health problem, including them in decision making, and developing a working relationship between the healthcare team members and the family will create mutual respect and allow for effective breastfeeding problem management.

KEY CONCEPTS

- The health, nutrition, and growth of the infant with special healthcare needs are of primary concern.
- Breastfeeding may be adversely affected when a child is ill or has special healthcare needs.
- Infants with certain special healthcare needs may not thrive on only direct breastfeeding.
- Babies and their mothers can often experience a better breastfeeding experience with the help of competent nurses and lactation consultants.

- Supplementation and alternative feeding methods may be needed to provide optimal nutrition in selected situations.
- The use of adaptive devices and positioning techniques can maximize breastfeeding effectiveness.
- The milk supply can be maintained and supported until the child is able to breastfeed directly, or for as long as is necessary.
- Direct breastfeeding rarely requires suspension or cessation.
- Galactosemia is the only condition requiring complete cessation of human milk feeding.
- Children with other inborn errors of metabolism (phenylketonuria, and amino or organic acidemias) may have human milk in addition to special dietary formulas.
- Families who have a child with special healthcare needs face many stressful issues and may be chronically grieving for the loss of the healthy baby they dreamed of.
- The loss of a "normal" breastfeeding experience may add to family stress.
- The breastfeeding mother whose child has died requires sensitive support.
- Breastfeeding-friendly pediatric hospital units can ease the unique stresses of the breastfeeding family.

INTERNET RESOURCES

Parents and Families

International Birth Defects Information System (links to information and support about many congenital problems in multiple languages): www.ibis-birthdefects.org

March of Dimes Birth Defects Foundation (information and support about birth defects): www.modimes.org

Mothers Overcoming Breastfeeding Issues (MOBI; support and advice for women who are/were unable to breastfeed, feel unsuccessful in breastfeeding, are/were experiencing severe breastfeeding problems, or experienced untimely weaning): www.mobimotherhood.org

National Organization for Rare Disorders (information for families and professionals): www.rarediseases.org

Bereaved Families

Compassionate Friends (local support groups, some with sibling groups): www.compassionatefriends.org

Share (for families touched by miscarriage, stillbirth, or neonatal death): www.nationalshare.org

Bereaved Parents USA (support for parents, siblings, and grandparents): www.bereavedparentsusa.org

Allergies

Food Allergy Research & Education (information for families and professionals, recipes, support): www.foodallergy.org

Celiac Disease

Celiac Disease Foundation (family support, information for professionals and family): www.celiac.org

Celiac Support Association (family support and information): www.csaceliacs.org

Congenital Heart Disease

American Heart Association: (information for families; English/Spanish): www.americanheart.org

Congenital Heart Information Network (information, parent support): http://www.heart.org/HEARTORG/

Diabetes Mellitus

American Diabetes Association (information and support; English/Spanish): www.diabetes.org

Learning About Diabetes (information, patient education materials in English/Spanish): www.learningabout diabetes.org

Juvenile Diabetes Research Foundation International (information and support): www.jdrf.org

Down Syndrome

National Association for Down Syndrome (parent support and information; English/Spanish): www.nads.org

National Down Syndrome Congress (parent support; English /Spanish): www.ndsccenter.org

National Down Syndrome Society (parent support and information in English and Spanish): www.ndss.org

Gastrointestinal Disorders

Esophageal Atresia/Tracheoesophageal Fistula (child and family support connection): www.eatef.org

PAGER (Pediatric and Adolescent Gastroesophageal Reflux Association; information and support; English /Spanish): www.reflux.org

Metabolic Problems

Children Living with Inherited Metabolic Disease (information and support): www.climb.org.uk

Parents of Galactosemic Children (parent information and support): www.galactosemia.org

PKU News (information and support): www.pkunews.org

Neural Tube Defects

Hydrocephalus Association (information and support): www.hydroassoc.org

Spinal Bifida Association of America (information and support): www.sbaa.org

Oral–Facial Anomalies

Cleft Palate Foundation (information for families and professionals): www.cleftline.org

FACES (support group of the National Craniofacial Association): www.faces-cranio.org

Pierre Robin Network (connects families of children with Pierre Robin sequence): www.pierrerobin.org

REFERENCES

Academy of Breastfeeding Medicine (ABM). ABM clinical protocol #24: allergic proctocolitis in the exclusively breastfed infant. *Breastfeed Med.* 2011;6(6):435–440.

Academy of Breastfeeding Medicine (ABM). ABM clinical protocol #25: recommendations for preprocedural fasting for the breastfed infant: "NPO" guidelines. *Breastfeed Med.* 2012;7(3):197–202.

Agopian AJ, Cai Y, Langlois PH, et al. Maternal residential atrazine exposure and risk for choanal atresia and stenosis in offspring. *J Pediatr.* 2013;162:581–586.

Agrawal S, Nadel S. Acute bacterial meningitis in infants and children: epidemiology and management. *Pediatr Drugs.* 2011;13(6):385–400.

Ahring K, Belanger-Quintana A, Dokoupil K, et al. Dietary management practices in phenylketonuria across European centres. *Clin Nutr.* 2009;28:231–236.

Akobeng A, Ramanan AV, Buchan I, Heller RF. Effect of breast feeding on risk of coeliac disease: a systematic review and meta-analysis of observational studies. *Arch Dis Child.* 2006;91(1):39–43.

American Academy of Pediatrics Committee on Nutrition, Kleinman, RE. *Pediatric nutrition handbook.* Elk Grove, IL: AAP; 2004.

American Society of Anesthesiologists (ASA). Practice guidelines for preoperative fasting and the use of pharmacologic agents to reduce the risk of pulmonary aspiration: application to healthy patients undergoing elective procedure—a report by the American Society of Anesthesiologists. Task Force on Preoperative Fasting. *Anesthesiology.* 1999;90(3):896–905.

American Society of Anesthesiologists (ASA) Committee. Practice guidelines for preoperative fasting and the use of pharmacologic agents to reduce the risk of pulmonary aspiration: an updated report by the American Society of Anesthesiologists Committee on Standards and Practice Parameters. *Anesthesiology.* 2011;114:495–511.

Aniansson G, Svensson H, Becker M, Ingvarsson L. Otitis media with breast milk of children with cleft palate. *Scand J Plast Reconstr Surg Hand Surg.* 2002;36(1):9–15.

Antunovic SS, Lukac M, Vujovic D. Longitudinal cystic fibrosis care. *Clin Pharmacol Ther.* 2013;93(1):86–97. doi: 10.1038/clpt.2012.183. Epub November 14, 2012.

Armon K, Stephenson T, MacFaul R, et al. An evidence and consensus-based guideline for acute diarrhoea management. *Arch Dis Child.* 1999;85:132–142.

Aumonier ME, Cunningham CC. Breastfeeding in infants with Down's syndrome. *Child Care Health Dev.* 1983;9:247–255.

Bailey DJ, Andres JM, Danek GD, Pineiro-Carrero VM. Lack of efficacy of thickened feeding as treatment for gastro-esophageal reflux. *J Pediatr.* 1987;110:187–189.

Banta-wright SA, Shelton KC, Lowe ND, et al. Breast-feeding success among infants with phenylketonuria. *J Pediatr Nurs.* 2012;27:319–327.

Bartalena L, Bogazzi F, Braverman LE, Martino E. Effects of amiodarone administration during pregnancy on neonatal thyroid function and subsequent neurodevelopment. *J Endocrinol Invest.* 2001;24(2):116–130.

Baudon JJ, Renault F, Goutet JM, et al. Motor dysfunction of the upper digestive tract in Pierre Robin sequence as assessed by sucking–swallowing electromyography and esophageal manometry. *J Pediatr.* 2002;140:719–723.

Baujat G, Faure C, Zaouche A, et al. Oroesophageal motor disorders in Pierre Robin syndrome. *JPGN.* 2001;32:297–302.

Bergmann RL, Diepgen TL, Kuss O, et al. Breastfeeding is a risk factor for atopic eczema. *Clin Exp All.* 2002;32:205–209.

Berhe T, Postellon D, Wilson B, Stone R. Feasibility and safety of insulin pump therapy in children aged 2–7 years with type 1 diabetes: a retrospective study. *Pediatrics.* 2006;117(6):2132–2137.

Bernard H, Negroni L, Chatel JM, et al. Molecular basis of IgE cross-reactivity between human beta-casein and bovine beta-casein, a major allergy in milk. *Mol Immunol.* 2000;37:161–167.

Berry GT. Galactosemia: when is it a newborn screening emergency? *Mol Genet Metab.* 2012;106(1):7–11.

Bessell A, Hooper L, Shaw WC, et al. Feeding interventions for growth and development in infants with cleft lip, cleft palate or cleft lip and palate. Cochrane Database of Systematic Reviews 2011, Issue 2. Art. No.: CD003315. doi: 10.1002/14651858.CD003315.pub3.

Bloch AM, Mimouni D, Mimouni M, Gdalevich M. Does breastfeeding protect against allergic rhinitis during childhood? A meta-analysis of prospective studies. *Acta Paediatr.* 2002;91:275–279.

Boctor DL, Pillo-Blocka F, McCrindle BW. Nutrition after cardiac surgery for infants with congenital heart disease. *Nutr Clin Pract.* 1999;14:111–115.

Bodley V, Powers D. Long-term nipple shield use: a positive perspective. *J Hum Lact.* 1996;12(4):301–304.

Borowitz D, Robinson KA, Rosenfeld M, et al. Cystic Fibrosis Foundation evidence-based guidelines for management of infants with cystic fibrosis. *J Pediatr.* 2009;155(6):s73–s93.

Bovey A, Noble R, Noble M. Orofacial exercises for babies with breastfeeding problems? *Breastfeed Rev.* 1999;7(1):23–28.

Bradley JS, Byington CL, Shah SS, et al. The management of community-acquired pneumonia in infants and children older than 3 months of age: clinical practice guidelines by the Pediatric Infectious Diseases Society and the Infectious Diseases Society of America. *Clin Infect Dis.* 2011;53(7):e25–e76.

Brigham M. Mothers' reports of the outcome of nipple shield use. *J Hum Lact.* 1996;12(4):291–297.

Bronner MB, Peek N, Knoester H, et al. Course and predictors of posttraumatic stress disorder in parents after pediatric intensive care treatment of their child. *J Pediatr Psychol.* 2010;35(9):966–974.

Burke SO, Kauffmann E, Costello E, et al. Stressors in families with a child with a chronic condition: an analysis of qualitative studies and a framework. *Can J Nurs Res.* 1998;30:71–95.

Businco L, Bruno G, Giampietro PG. Prevention and management of food allergy. *Acta Paediatr Suppl.* 1999;88(430):104–109.

Carter B, Fedorowicz Z. Antiemetic treatment for acute gastroenteritis in children: an updated Cochrane systematic review with meta-analysis and mixed treatment comparison in a Bayesian framework. *BMJ Open.* 2012;2(4). doi: pii: e000622. 10.1136/bmjopen-2011-000622.

Casas R, Böttcher MF, Duchén K, Björkstén B. Detection of IgA antibodies to cat, beta-lactoalbumin and ovoalbumin antigens in human milk. *J Allergy Clin Immunol.* 2000;105:1236–1240.

Casteels K, Punt S, Bramswig J. Transient neonatal hypothyroidism during breastfeeding after post-natal maternal topical iodine treatment. *Eur J Pediatr.* 2000;159(9):716–717.

Caverly L, Rausch CM, daCruz E, Kaufman J. Octreotide treatment of chylothorax in patients following cardiothoracic surgery. *Gongen Heart Dis.* 2010;5(6):573–578.

Cedin AC, Atallah ÁN, Andriolo RB, et al. Surgery for congenital choanal atresia. *Cochrane Database Syst Rev.* 2012;2:CD008993. doi: 10.1002/14651858. CD008993.pub2.

Centers for Disease Control and Prevention (CDC). Managing acute gastroenteritis among children: oral rehydration, maintenance, and nutritional therapy. *MMWR.* 2003;52(16):1–16.

Chan GM, Lechtenberg E. The use of fat-free human milk in infants with chylous pleural effusion. *J Perinatol.* 2007;27(7):434–436.

Chantry C, Howard C, Auinger P. Full breastfeeding duration and associated decrease in respiratory tract infection in US children. *Pediatrics.* 2006;17(2):425–432.

Chertok I. The importance of exclusive breastfeeding in infants at risk for celiac disease. *MCN.* 2007;32(1):50–54.

Choi J, Lee GL. Common pediatric respiratory emergencies. *Emerg Med Clin North Am.* 2012;30:529–563.

Clague A, Thomas A. Neonatal biochemical screening for disease. *Clin Chim Acta.* 2002;315(1–2):99–110.

Cohen M. Immediate unrestricted feeding of infants following cleft lip and palate repair. *Br J Plast Surg.* 1997;50:143.

Cohen R, Levy C, de La Rocque F, et al. Impact of pneumococcal conjugate vaccine and of reduction in antibiotic use on nasopharyngeal carriage of nonsusceptible pneumococci in children with otitis media. *J Pediatr Infect Dis.* 2006;25(11):1001–1007.

Cole M. Lactation after perinatal, neonatal or infant loss. *Clin Lact.* 2012;3(3):94–99.

Combs VL, Marino BL. A comparison of growth patterns in breast and bottle-fed infants with congenital heart disease. *Pediatr Nurs.* 1993;19:175–179.

Committee on Hospital Care and Institute for Patient and Family-Centered Care. Patient and family-centered care and the pediatrician's role. *Pediatrics.* 2012;129(2):394–404.

Cook-Sather SD, Litman RS. Modern fasting guidelines in children. *Best Pract Res Clin Anaesthesiol.* 2006;20(3):471–481.

Coy K, Speltz ML, Jones K. Facial appearance and attachment in infants with orofacial clefts: a replication. *Cleft Palate Craniofac J.* 2002;39(1):66–71.

D'Amico M, Holmes J, Stavropoulos SN, et al. Presentation of pediatric celiac disease in the United States: prominent effect of breastfeeding. *Clin Pediatr.* 2005;44:249–260.

Danner SC. Breastfeeding the infant with a cleft defect. *Clin Issue Perin Women's Health Nurs.* 1992;3:634–639.

Darzi MA, Chowdri NA, Bhat AN. Breast feeding or spoon feeding after cleft lip repair: a prospective, randomized study. *Br J Plastic Surg.* 1996;49:24–26.

de Boissieu D et al. Multiple food allergy: a possible diagnosis in breastfed infants. *Acta Paediatr.* 1997;86:1042–1046.

Denk MJ. Advances in neonatal surgery. *Pediatr Clin North Am.* 1998;45(6):1479–1506.

Dennehy P, Cortese MM, Bégué RE, et al. A case-control study to determine risk factors for hospitalization for rotavirus gastroenteritis in U.S. children. *Pediatr Infect Dis J.* 2006;25(12):1123–1131.

Denny A, Amm C. New technique for airway correction in neonates with severe Pierre Robin sequence. *J Pediatr.* 2005;147:97–101.

Dowling D, Meier PP, DiFiore JM, et al. Cup-feeding for preterm infants: mechanics and safety. *J Hum Lact.* 2002;18(1):12–20.

Duijts L, Ramadhani MK, Moll HA. Breastfeeding protects against infectious diseases during infancy in industrialized countries: a systematic review. *Matern Child Nutr.* 2009;5:199–210.

Duncan LL, Elder SB. Breastfeeding the infant with PKU. *J Hum Lact.* 1997;13:231–235.

Dunlap B, Shelke K, Salem SA, Keith LG. Folic acid and human reproduction: ten important issues for clinicians. *J Exp Clin Assist Reprod.* 2011;8:2.

Eliason BC, Lewan RB. Gastroenteritis in children: principles of diagnosis and treatment. *Am Fam Physician.* 1998;58:1769–1776.

Einarsson-Backes LM, Deitz J, Price R, et al. The effect of oral support on sucking efficiency in preterm infants. *Am J Occup Ther.* 1994 Jun;48(6):490–8.

Ewer AK, James ME, Tobin JM. Prone and left lateral positioning reduce gastro-esophageal reflux in preterm infants. *Arch Dis Child Fetal Neonatal Ed.* 1999;81:F201–F205.

Farrell R. Infant gluten and celiac disease: too early, too late, too much, too many questions. *JAMA*. 2006;293(19):2410–2412.

Fayade AG, Ayede AI. Epidemiology, aetiology and management of childhood acute community-acquired pneumonia in developing countries: a review. *Afr J Med Sci*. 2011;40:293–308.

Fisk CM, Crozier SR, Inskip HM, et al. Southampton Women's Survey Study Group. Breastfeeding and reported morbidity during infancy: findings from the Southampton Women's Survey. *Matern Child Nutr*. 2011;7:61–70.

Fleischer DM, Spergel JM, Asaa'ad AH, et al. Primary prevention of allergic disease through nutritional intervention. *J Allergy Clin Immunol: In Practice*. 2013;1:29–36.

Fox-Bacon C, McCamman S, Therou L, et al. Maternal PKU and breastfeeding: case report of identical twin mothers. *Clin Pediatr*. 1997;36(9):539–542.

Fukushima Y, Kawata Y, Onda T, Kitagawa M. Consumption of cow milk and egg by lactating women and the presence of beta-lactoglobulin and ovalbumin in breast milk. *Am J Clin Nutr*. 1997;65:30–35.

Garza JJ, Morash D, Dzakovic A, et al. Ad libitum feeding decreases hospital stay for neonates after pyloromyotomy. *J Pediatr Surg*. 2002;37(3):493–495.

GER Guidelines Committee, North American Society for Pediatric Gastroenterology and Nutrition. Pediatric GE reflux clinical practice guidelines. *J Pediatr Gastoenterol Nutr*. 2001;32(suppl):2.

Gervasio MR, Buchanan CN. Malnutrition in the pediatric cardiology patient. *Crit Care Q*. 1985;8:49–56.

Ghaem M, Armstrong KL, Trocki O, et al. The sleep patterns of infants and young children with gastrooesophageal reflux. *J Paediatr Child Health*. 1998;34(2):160–163.

Giovannini M, Verduci E, Salvatici E, et al. Phenylketonuria: dietary and therapeutic challenges. *J Inherit Metab Dis*. 2007;30:145–152.

Gokcay G, Baykal T, Gokdemir Y, Demirkol M. Breast feeding in organic acidaemias. *J Inherit Metab Dis*. 2006;29:2–3, 304–310.

Golbus JR, Wojckik BM, Charpie JR, Hirsch JC. Feeding complications in hypoplastic left heart syndrome after the Norwood procedure: a systematic review of the literature. *Pediatr Cardiol*. 2011;32:539–552.

Goldman RD, Canadian Paediatric Society, Drug Therapy and Hazardous Substances Committee. Treating cough and cold: guidance for caregivers of children and youth. *Paediatr Child Health*. 2011;16(9):564–566.

Gorelick MH, Shaw KN, Murphy KO. Validity and reliability of clinical signs in the diagnosis of dehydration in children. *Pediatrics*. 1997;99(5):E6.

Greer FR, Sicherer SH, Burks AW, et al. Effects of early nutritional interventions on the development of atopic disease in infants and children: the role of maternal dietary restriction, breastfeeding, timing of introducing complementary foods and hydrolyzed formulas. *Pediatrics*. 2008;121(1):183–191.

Greve L, Wheeler MD, Green-Burgeson DK, Zorn EM. Breast-feeding in the management of the newborn with phenylketonuria: a practical approach to dietary therapy. *J Am Diet Assoc*. 1994;94:305–309.

Gromada K, Sandora L. *Safe and breastfeeding compatible oral behaviors for the infant receiving a bottle*. ILCA 2007 Conference. San Diego, CA, August 17, 2007.

Gupta RS, Springston EE, Warrier MR. The prevalence, severity, and distribution of childhood food allergy in the United States. *Pediatrics*. 2011;128(1):e9–e17. doi: 10.1542/peds.2011-0204.

Hak MS, Sasagari M, Sulaiman FK, et al. Longitudinal study of effect of Hotz's plate and lip adhesion on maxillary growth in bilateral cleft lip and palate patients. *Cleft Palate Craniofac J*. 2012;49(2):230–236.

Hall AJ, Rosenthal M, Gregoricus N, et al. Incidence of acute gastroenteritis and role of norovirus, Georgia, USA, 2004–2005. *Emerg Infect Dis* [serial on the Internet]. August 2011 [date cited]. Available at: http://dx.doi.org/10.3201/eid1708.101533.

Harabuchi Y, Faden H, Yamanaka N, et al. Nasopharyngeal colonization with nontypeable *Haemophilus influenzae* and recurrent otitis media. *J Infect Dis*. 1994;170(4):862–866.

Heacock HJ, Jeffery HE. Baker JL, Page M. Influence of breast versus formula milk on physiological gastroesophageal reflux in healthy, newborn infants. *J Pediatr Gastroenterol Nutr*. 1992;14:41–46.

Hegar B, Devanti NR, Kadim M, et al. Natural evolution of regurgitation in healthy infants. *Acta Paediatr*. 2009;98:1189–1193.

Helin R, Angeles ST, Bhat R. Octreotide therapy for chylothorax in infants and children: a brief review. *Pediatr Crit Care Med*. 2006;7(6):576–579.

Herman RS, Teitelbaum DH. Anorectal malformations. *Clin Perinatol*. 2012;39:403–422.

Hodges AM. Combined early cleft lip and palate repair in children under 10 months: a series of 106 patients. *J Plastic Reconstructive Surg*. 2010;63:1813–1819.

Hom J, Fernandes RM. When should nebulized hypertonic saline solution be used in the treatment of bronchiolitis? *Paediatr Child Health*. 2011;16(3):157–158.

Huckabay LM, Tilem-Kessler D. Patterns of parental stress in PICU emergency admission. *Dimens Crit Care Nurs*. 1999;18(2):36–42.

Hughes P, Riches S. Psychological aspects of perinatal loss. *Curr Opin Obstet Gynecol*. 2003;15(2):107–111.

Huner G, Baykal T, Demir F, Demirkol M. Breastfeeding experience in inborn errors of metabolism other than phenylketonuria. *J Inherit Metab Dis*. 2005;28:457–465.

Hurtekant K, Spatz D. Special considerations for breastfeeding the infant with spina bifida. *J Perinat Neonatal Nurs*. 2007;21(1):69–75.

Ip S, Chung M, Raman G, et al. *Breastfeeding and maternal and infant health outcomes in developed countries* [Evidence Report/Technology Assessment No. 153]. AHRQ

Publications No. 07-E007. Rockville, MD: Agency for Healthcare Research and Quality; 2007.

Ivarsson A, Myleus A, Norstrom F, et al. Prevalence of childhood celiac disease and changes in infant feeding. *Pediatrics.* 2013;131:687–694.

Jones AC, Miles EA, Warner JO, et al. Fetal peripheral blood mononuclear cell proliferative responses to mitogenic and allergenic stimuli during gestation. *Pediatr Allergy Immunol.* 1996;7:109–116.

Jones F. *Best practice for expressing, storing and handling human milk in hospitals, homes and child care settings.* Raleigh, NC: Human Milk Banking Association of North America; 2011.

Kassing D. Bottle-feeding as a tool to reinforce breastfeeding. *J Hum Lact.* 2002;18(1):56–60.

Kimpimaki T, Erkkola M, Korhonen S, et al. Short-term exclusive breastfeeding predisposes young children with increased genetic risk of type I diabetes to progressive beta-cell autoimmunity. *Diabetologia.* 2001;44(1):63–69.

Kleinman L, Rothman M, Strauss R, et al. The infant gastroesophageal reflux questionnaire revised: development and validation as an evaluative instrument. *Clin Gastroenterol Hepatol.* 2006;4(5):588–596.

Kleinman RE, ed. *Pediatric nutrition handbook.* Elk Grove Village, IL: American Academy of Pediatrics; 2009.

Knip M, Virtanen SM, Akerblom HK. Infant feeding and the risk of type 1 diabetes. *Am J Clin Nutr.* 2010;91(suppl):1506s–1513s.

Kogon BE, Ramaswamy V, Todd K, et al. Feeding difficulty in newborns following congenital heart surgery. *Congenital Heart Dis.* 2007;2:332–337.

Kohr LM, Brudis NJ. *Growth and nutrition in paediatric cardiology.* Philadelphia: Churchill Livingston; 2010.

Korppi M, Hiltunen J. Pertussis is common in nonvaccinated infants hospitalized for respiratory syncytial virus infection. *Pediatr Infect Dis J.* 2007;26(4):316–318.

Kosko J, EBCH European editorial base. Summary of preoperative fasting for preventing perioperative complications in children. *Evidence-Based Child Health: Cochrane Rev J.* 2006;1:281–284.

Kunisaki SM, Foker JE. Surgical advances in the fetus and neonate: esophageal atresia. *Clin Perinatol.* 2012;39:349–361.

Kuo DZ, Sisterhen LL, Siegrest TE, et al. Family experiences and pediatric health services use associated with family-centered rounds. *Pediatrics.* 2012;130:299–305.

Kuttenberger J, Ohmer JN, Polska E. Initial counselling for cleft lip and palate: parents' evaluation, needs and expectations. *Int J Oral Maxillofac Surg.* 2010;39(3):214–220.

Lack G. Update on risk factors for food allergy. *J Allergy Clin Immunol.* 2012;129(5):1187–1197.

Langley GF, Anderson LJ. Epidemiology and prevention of respiratory syncytial virus infections among infants and young children. *Pediatr Infect Dis J.* 2011;30:510–517.

Lawrence R. Circumstances where breastfeeding is contraindicated. *Pediatr Clin North Am.* 2013;60(1):295–318.

Lieberthal AS, Charroll AE, Chonmaitree T, et al. Diagnosis and management of acute otitis media. *Pediatrics.* 2013;131(3):e964–e999.

Liet JM, Ducruet T, Gupta V, Cambonie G. Heliox inhalation therapy for bronchiolitis in infants. *Cochrane Database Syst Rev.* 2010;4:CD006915.

Lopez-Alarcon M, Garcia-Zuñiga P, Del Prado M, Garza C. Breastfeeding protects against the anorectic response to infection in infants: possible role of DHA. *Adv Exp Med Biol.* 2004;554:371–374.

Ludvigsson JF, Fasano A. Timing of introduction of gluten and celiac disease risk. *Ann Nutr Metab.* 2012;60 (suppl 2):22–29.

Lust K, Brown JE, Thomas W. Maternal intake of cruciferous vegetables and other foods and colic symptoms in exclusively breast-fed infants. *J Am Diet Assoc.* 1996;96(1):46–48.

MacDonald A, Depondt E, Evans S, et al. Breastfeeding in IMD. *J Inherit Metab Dis.* 2006;29:299–303.

MacDonald A, Evans S, Cochrane B, Wildgoose J. Weaning infants with phenylketonuria: a review. *J Hum Nutr Diet.* 2011;25:103–110.

MacMahon B. The continuing enigma of pyloric stenosis of infancy: a review. *Epidemiology.* 2006;17(2):195–201.

Mahle WT, Martin GR, Beekman RH . Endorsement of Health and Human Services recommendation for pulse oximetry screening for critical congenital heart disease. *Pediatrics.* 2012;129(1):190–192.

Malcolm WF, Cotten CM. Metoclopramide, H_2 blockers and proton pump inhibitors: pharmacotherapy for gastroesophageal reflux in neonates. *Clin Perinatal.* 2012;39:99–109.

Manoha C, Espinosa S, Aho SL, et al. Epidemiological and clinical features of hMPV, RSV and RVs infections in young children. *J Clin Virol.* 2007;38:221–226.

Marcellus L. The infant with Pierre Robin sequence: review and implications for nursing practice. *J Pediatr Nurs.* 2001;15(1):23–33.

Marino BL, O'Brien P, LoRe H. Oxygen saturations during breast and bottle-feedings in infants with congenital heart disease. *J Pediatr Nurs.* 1995;10(6):360–364.

Marques IL, de Sousa TV, Carneiro AF, et al. Clinical experience with infants with Robin sequence: a prospective study. *Cleft Palate Craniofac J.* 2001;38(2):171–178.

Masarei A, Sell D, Habel A, et al. The nature of feeding in infants with unrepaired cleft lip and/or palate compared with healthy noncleft infants. *Cleft Palate Craniofac J.* 2007;44(3):21–28.

Mathisen B, Worrall L, Masel J, et al. Feeding problems in infants with gastrooesophageal reflux disease: a case controlled study. *J Paediatr Child Health.* 1999;35:163–169.

McCabe L, Ernest AE, Neifert MR, et al. The management of breastfeeding among infants with phenylketonuria. *J Inherit Metab Dis.* 1989;12:467–474.

Medoff-Cooper B, Naim M, Torowicz D, Mort A. Feeding, growth, and nutrition in children with congenitally malformed hearts. *Cardiol Young.* 2010;20(suppl 3):149–153.

Meier P. Nipple shields for preterm infants: effect of milk transfer and duration of breastfeeding. *J Hum Lact.* 2000;16(2):106–114.

Melnyk B, Alpert-Gillis L, Feinstein NF, et al. Creating opportunities for parent empowerment: program effects on the mental health and coping outcomes of critically ill young children and their mothers. *Pediatrics.* 2004;113(6):e597–e607.

Merewood A, Philipp BL. *Breastfeeding: conditions and diseases.* Amarillo, TX: Pharmasoft Publishing; 2002.

Miller CK. Feeding issues in children with craniofacial syndromes. *Semin Speech Lang.* 2011;32:115–126.

Miller JH. *The controversial issue of breastfeeding cleft-affected infants.* Alberta, Canada: InfoMed Publications; 1998.

Minchin M, Minogue C, Meehan M, et al. Expanding the WHO/Unicef baby friendly hospital initiative: eleven steps to optimal infant feeding in a pediatric unit. *Breastfeeding Rev.* 1996;4:87–91

Mizuno K, Ueda A. Development of sucking behavior in infants with Down's syndrome. *Acta Paediatr.* 2001;90:1384–1388.

Mizuno K, Ueda A, Takeuchi T. Effects of different fluids on the relationship between swallowing and breathing during nutritive sucking in neonates. *Biol Neonate.* 2002;81(1):45–50.

Mohrbacher N., Stock J. The Breastfeeding answer book. 3rd ed. Schaumburg, IL:La Leche League International 2003.

Montagnoli L, Barbieri MA, Bettiol H, et al. Growth impairment of children with different types of lip and palate clefts in the first 2 years of life: a cross-sectional study. *J Pediatr.* 2005;81(6):461–465.

Nair H, Nokes DJ, Gessner BD, et al. Global burden of acute lower respiratory infections due to respiratory syncytial virus in young children: a systematic review and meta-analysis. *Lancet.* 2010;375(0725):145–155.

National Center on Birth Defects and Developmental Disabilities, Centers for Disease Control and Prevention (CDC). Neural tube defects (NTDs) rates, 1995–1999. *Teratology.* 2002;66(suppl 1):s212–s217.

Neu M, Corwin E, Lareau SC, Marcheggiani-Howard C. A review of nonsurgical treatment for the symptom of irritability in infants with GERD. *J Spec Pediatr Nurs.* 2012;17(3):177–192.

Noble R, Bovey A. Therapeutic teat use for babies who breastfeed poorly. *Breastfeed Rev.* 1997;5(2):37–42.

Norris J, Barriga K, Hoffenberg EJ, et al. Risk of celiac disease autoimmunity and the timing of gluten introduction in the diet of infants at increased risk of disease. *JAMA.* 2006;293(19):2343–2351.

O'Brien CE, Harden H, Com G. A survey of nutrition practices for patients with cystic fibrosis. *Nutr Clin Pract.* December 6, 2012. [Epub ahead of print.]

Oddy W. A review of the effects of breastfeeding on respiratory infections, atopy and childhood asthma. *J Asthma.* 2004;4(6):605–621.

Oladapo OT, Fawole B. Treatments for suppression of lactation (review). *Cochrane Library.* 2012;9:DC005937. doi: 10.1002/14651858.

Oliveira AC, Pordeus IA, Torres CS, et al. Feeding and nonnutritive sucking habits and prevalence of open bite and crossbite in children/adolescents with Down syndrome. *Angle Orthodontist.* 2010;80(4):748–753.

Olshansky S. Chronic sorrow: a response to having a mentally defective child. *Soc Casework.* 1962;43:190–193.

Oomen MWN, Hoekstra LT, Bakx R, et al. Open versus laparoscopic pyloromyotomy for hypertrophic pyloric stenosis: a systematic review and meta-analysis focusing on major complications. *Surg Endosc.* 2012;26:2104–2110.

Orenstein SR. Symptoms and reflux in infants: Infant Gastro-esophageal Reflux Questionnaire Revised (I-GERQ-R): utility for symptom tracking and diagnosis. *Pediatr Gastroenterol.* 2010;12(6):431–436.

Orenstein SR, Shalaby TM, Putnam PE. Thickened feedings as a cause of increased coughing when used as therapy for gastroesophageal reflux in infants. *J Pediatr.* 1992;121:913–915.

Pandya AN, Boorman JG. Failure to thrive in babies with cleft lip and palate. *Br J Plast Surg.* 2001;54(6): 471–475.

Pandya S, Heiss K. Pyloric stenosis in pediatric surgery: an evidence-based review. *Surg Clin North Am.* 2012;92:527–539.

Paradise JL, Elster BA, Tan L. Evidence in infants with cleft palate that breast milk protects against otitis media. *Pediatrics.* 1994;94:853–860.

Patel MM, Steele D, Gentsch JR, et al. Real-world impact of rotavirus vaccination. *Pediatr Infect Dis J.* 2011;30 (1 suppl):S1–S5. doi: 10.1097/INF.0b013e3181fefa1f.

Patenaude Y, Bernard C, Schreiber R, Sinsky AB. Cow's milk-induced allergic colitis in an exclusively breast-fed infant: diagnosed with ultrasound. *Pediatr Radiol.* 2000;30:379–382.

Pelchat D, Bisson J, Ricard N, et al. Longitudinal effects of an early family intervention programme on the adaptation of parents of children with a disability. *Int J Nurs Stud.* 1999;36(6):465–477.

Peterson-Falzone SJ. Types of clefts and multianomaly craniofacial conditions. *Semin Speech Lang.* 2011;32:93–114.

Pinnington LL, Smith CM, Ellis RE, Morton RE. Feeding efficiency and respiratory integration in infants with acute viral bronchiolitis. *J Pediatr.* 2000;137:523–526.

Pisacane A, Toscano E, Pirri I, et al. Down syndrome and breastfeeding. *Acta Paediatr.* 2003;92;1479–1481.

Principi N, Esposito S. Management of severe community-acquired pneumonia of children in developing and developed countries. *Thorax.* 2012;66:815–822.

Pumberger W, Pumberger G, Geissler W. Proctocolitis in breast-fed infants: a contribution to differential diagnosis of haematochezia in early childhood. *Postgrad Med.* 2001;77(906):252–254.

Quigley M, Kelly Y, Sacker A. Breastfeeding and hospitalization for diarrheal and respiratory infection in the United Kingdom millennium cohort study. *Pediatrics.* 2007;119(4):e837–e842.

Raisler J, Alexander C, O'Campo P. Breastfeeding and infant illness: a dose-response relationship. *Am J Public Health.* 1999;89:25–30.

Ramsden JD, Campisi P, Forte V. Choanal atresia and choanal stenosis. *Otolaryngol Clin North Am.* 2009;42(2):339–352.

Rastogi MN, LaFranchi SH. Congenital hypothyroidism. *Orphanet J Rare Dis.* 2010;5:17.

Reid J, Reilly S, Kilpatrick N. Sucking performance of babies with cleft conditions. *Cleft Palate Craniofac J.* 2007;44(3):312–320.

Reilly S, Reid J, Skeat J. ABM clinical protocol #17: guidelines for breastfeeding infants with cleft lip, cleft palate, or cleft lip and palate. *Breastfeed Med.* 2007;2(4):243–250.

Rendon-Macias M, Castañeda-Muciño G, Cruz JJ, et al. Breastfeeding among patients with congenital malformations. *Arch Med Res.* 2002;33(3):269–275.

Repucci A. Resolution of stool blood in breast-fed infants with maternal ingestion of pancreatic enzymes. *J Pediatr Gastro Nutr.* 1999;84:353–360.

Ripmeester P, Dunn S. Against all odds: breastfeeding a baby with Harlequin ichthyosis. *JOGNN.* 2002;31:521–525.

Riva E, Agostoni C, Biasucci G, et al. Early breastfeeding is linked to higher intelligence quotient scores in dietary treated phenylketonuric children. *Acta Paediatr.* 1996;85:56–58.

Roose RE, Blanford CR. Perinatal grief and support spans the generations: parents' and grandparents' evaluations of an intergenerational perinatal bereavement program. *J Perinat Neonat Nurs.* 2011;25(1):77–85.

Rovers MM, Numans ME, Langenbach E, et al. Is pacifier use a risk factor for acute otitis media? A dynamic cohort study. *Fam Pract.* 2008;25(4):233–236.

Rutter M. Evaluation and management of upper airway disorders in children. *Semin Pediatr Surg.* 2006;15:116–123.

Saadai P, Farmer DL. Fetal surgery for myelomeningocele. *Clin Perinatol.* 2012;39:279–288.

Sandberg D, Magee W, Denk M. Neonatal cleft lip and cleft palate repair. *AORN J.* 2002;75(3):490–506.

Sandler A. *Living with spina bifida: a guide for families and professionals.* Chapel Hill, NC: University of North Carolina Press; 1997.

Scariati PD, Grummer-Strawn LM, Fein SB. A longitudinal analysis of infant morbidity and the extent of breastfeeding in the United States. *Pediatrics.* 1997;99:E5.

Schach B, Haight M. Colic and food allergy in the breast-fed infant: is it possible for the exclusively breast-fed

infant to suffer from food allergy? *J Hum Lact.* 2002;18(1):50–52.

Sears MR, Greene JM, Willan AR, et al. Long-term relation between breastfeeding and development of atopy and asthma in children and young adults: a longitudinal study. *Lancet.* 2002;360:901–907.

Seecharan G, Andresen EM, Norris K, Toce SS. Parents' assessment of quality of care and grief following a child's death. *Arch Pediatr Med.* 2004;158:515–520.

Section on Breastfeeding. Breastfeeding and the use of human milk. *Pediatrics.* 2005;115(2):496–506.

Shah PS, Aliwalas LI, Shah V. Breastfeeding or breast milk for procedural pain in neonates. *Cochrane Database Syst Rev.* 2006;3:CD004950.

Shaw WC, Bannister RP, Roberts CT. Assisted feeding is more reliable for infants with clefts: a randomized trial. *Cleft Palate Craniofac J.* 1999;36:262–268.

Shetye PR. Presurgical infant orthopedics. *J Craniofac Surg.* 2012;23(1):210–211.

Shudy M, de Almeida ML, Ly S, et al. Impact of critical illness and injury on families: systematic literature review. *Pediatrics.* 2006;118(S3):S203–S218.

Smith M, Saunders C. Prognosis of airway obstruction and feeding difficulty in the Robin sequence. *Int J Pediatr Otorhinolaryngol.* 2006;70:319–324.

Smith TB, Oliver MN, Innocenti MS. Parenting stress in families of children with disabilities. *Am J Orthopsychiatry.* 2001;71(2):257–261.

Spatz D. Preserving breastfeeding for the rehospitalized infant: a clinical pathway. *MCN.* 2006;31(1):45–51.

Steiner MJ, DeWalt DA, Beyerley JS. Is this child dehydrated? *JAMA.* 2004;291(22):2746–2754.

Sullivan JS, Sundaram SS. Gastroesophageal reflux. *Pediatr Rev.* 2012;33(6):243–254.

Szajewska H, Dziechciarz P. Gastrointestinal infections in the pediatric population. *Curr Opin Gastroenterol.* 2010;26:36–44.

Tarini B, Carroll AE, Sox CM, Christakis DA. Systematic review of the relationship between early introduction of solid foods to infants and the development of allergic disease. *Arch Pediatr Adolesc Med.* 2006;160:502–507.

Thomas J, Marinelli KA, Hennessy M, Academy of Breastfeeding Medicine Protocol Committee. ABM clinical protocol #16: breastfeeding the hypotonic infant. *Breastfeed Med.* 2007;2(2):112–118.

Thomson SC. The koala hold from down under: another choice in breastfeeding position. *J Hum Lact.* 2013;29(2):147–149.

Tobin JM, McCloud, P, Cameron DJS. Posture and gastroesophageal reflux: a case for left lateral positioning. *Arch Dis Child.* 1997;7:254–258.

Tomlinson PS, Swiggum P, Harbaugh BL. Identification of nurse–family intervention sites to decrease health-related family boundary ambiguity in PICU. *Issues Compr Pediatr Nurs.* 1999;22(1):27–47.

Torowicz D, Lisanti AJ, Rim JS, Medoff-Cooper B. A developmental care framework for a cardiac intensive care unit: a paradigm shift. *Adv Neonatal Care.* 2012;12(suppl 5):S28–S32.

Turner L, Jacobsen C, Humenczuk M, et al. The effects of lactation education and a prosthetic obturator appliance on feeding efficiency in infants with cleft lip and palate. *Cleft Palate Craniofac J.* 2001;38(5): S510–S524.

Uzel A, Alparslan ZN. Long-term effects of presurgical infant orthopedics in patients with cleft lip and palate: a systematic review. *Cleft Palate Craniofac J.* 2011;48(5):587–595.

Vadas P, Wai Y, Burks W, Perelman B. Detection of peanut allergens in breast milk of lactating women. *JAMA.* 2001;285:1746–1748.

Vandenplas Y, Rudolph CD, Di Lorenzo C, et al. Pediatric gastroesophageal reflux clinical practice guidelines: joint recommendations of the North American Society for Pediatric Gastroenterology, Hepatology, and Nutrition (NASPGHAN) and the European Society for Pediatric Gastroenterology, Hepatology, and Nutrition (ESPGHAN). *J Pediatr Gastroenterol Nutr.* 2009;49:498–547.

van Rijn M, Bekhof J, Dijkstra T, et al. A different approach to breastfeeding of the infant with phenylketonuria. *Eur J Pediatr.* 2003;162:323–326.

Visconti KJ, Saudino KJ, Rappaport LA, et al. Influence of parental stress and social support on the behavioral adjustment of children with transposition of the great arteries. *J Dev Behav Pediatr.* 2002;23(5): 314–321.

Watson Genna C. *Supporting sucking skills in breastfeeding infants.* Sudbury, MA: Jones and Bartlett; 2008.

Weijerman ME, de Winter, JP. Clinical practice: the care of children with Down syndrome. *Eur J Pediatr.* 2010;169:1445–1452.

Wendler E, Committee on Psychosocial Aspects of Child and Family Health. Supporting the family after the death of a child. *Pediatrics.* 2012;130:1164–1169.

West CE, Videky DJ, Prescott SL. Role of diet in the development of immune tolerance in the context of allergic disease. *Curr Opin Pediatr.* 2010;22:635–641.

White M, Langer JC, Don S, DeBaun MR. Sensitivity and cost minimization analysis of radiology versus palpation for the diagnosis of hypertrophic pyloric stenosis. *J Pediatr Surg.* 1998;33:913–917.

Wiley KE, Zuo Y, Macartney KK, McIntyre PB. Sources of pertussis infection in young infants: a review of key evidence informing targeting of the cocoon strategy. *Vaccine.* 2013;31(4):618–625. doi: 10.1016/j.vaccine .2012.11.052. Epub November 29, 2012.

Wilson-Clay B. *Clefts.* Personal communication, December 12, 1995.

Woolridge M, Fisher C. Colic, "overfeeding" and symptoms of lactose malabsorption in the breast-fed baby: a possible effect of feed management? *Lancet.* 1988;2(8605):382–384.

Young JL, O'Riordan M, Goldstein JA, Robin NH. What information do parents of newborns with cleft lip, palate, or both want to know? *Cleft Palate Craniofac J.* 2001;38(1):55–58.

Zieger RS. Dietary aspects of food allergy prevention in infants and children. *J Pediatr Gastroenterol Nutr.* 2000;30:S77–S86.

Zorc JJ, Hall CB. Bronchiolitis: recent evidence on diagnosis and management. *Pediatrics.* 2010;125(2):342–349. doi: 10.1542/peds.2009-2092. Epub January 25, 2010.

Chapter 19

Infant Assessment

Mary Koehn
Jolynn Dowling

Introduction

Breastfeeding is dependent not only on the mother, but also on the behaviors of the infant. In the normal, healthy, full-term infant, the reflexes needed for breastfeeding are strong and support the capability of the infant to obtain sufficient nutrition from the breast. Therefore, a complete infant assessment is critical to breastfeeding. The infant assessment includes evaluation of perinatal history, gestational age assessment, breastfeeding assessment, physical assessment, and behavioral assessment. Encouraging parent participation during the assessment promotes discussion about normal newborn characteristics as well as any variations or minor congenital anomalies that may require further evaluation (Askin, 2009; Cheffer & Rannalli, 2011; Creehan, 2008).

Perinatal History

A perinatal history is essential for a complete infant assessment. The perinatal history focuses on the preconception, prenatal, and intrapartum periods. This history provides the context for the physical and behavioral assessment of the infant and may be useful in determining normal physical variations versus existing infant problems. For example, exposure to certain teratogens, such as alcohol, may alert the

practitioner to the possibility of related congenital anomalies (Askin, 2009). However, it is important to remember that the presence of maternal obstetric and infant prenatal risk factors does not automatically indicate an infant problem. Table 19-1 summarizes the essential components of the perinatal history (Barron, 2008; Orr, 2011).

Gestational Age Assessment

Gestational age assessment determines the degree of maturity of the infant at birth. This assessment, recommended by the American Academy of Pediatrics and American College of Obstetricians and Gynecologists (2002), helps to identify potential infant mortality and morbidity risk. Because gestational age affects his ability to suckle, swallow, and breathe, this classification of the infant is useful in determining the infant's vulnerability to feeding problems (Table 19-2).

Historically, gestational age was based on the mother's estimated date of delivery and/or the infant's birth weight. However, these methods are unreliable, as the infant's maturity may be influenced by other factors, such as heredity, maternal nutritional status, maternal exposure to environmental hazards, maternal disease, and genetic disorders of the infant.

Table 19-1 ESSENTIAL COMPONENTS OF THE PERINATAL HISTORY

Component	Required Data
Family history	• Family history of genetic disorders such as cystic fibrosis, sickle cell anemia, trisomy, phenylketonuria • Family history of diseases such as diabetes, seizures, chronic disorders
Psychosocial history	• Marital status and support systems • Substance abuse • Tobacco use • Exposure to environmental hazards • Inadequate finances • Poor nutrition • Inadequate housing • Psychiatric history • Maternal age <16 or >35 years • Education <11 years • Domestic violence
Maternal medical history	• Surgical procedures, particularly involving reproductive organs • Hospitalizations • Endocrine disorders (diabetes, thyroid) • Cardiovascular disorders (hypertension, heart disease) • Respiratory disorders (asthma, pneumonia) • Renal (frequent infections, chronic kidney disease) • Hematologic (sickle, blood type and Rh factor, blood disorders, Rh isoimmunization)
Maternal reproductive history	• Cancer • Infections • Sexually transmitted diseases • Medications taken prior to pregnancy • Gravidity, parity • Infertility • History of abnormal Pap smear • Previous perinatal loss • Last birth <1 year before present conception • Previous cesarean birth • Infant with congenital anomaly, birth injury, neurologic deficit • Spontaneous or elective abortions • Malformations of cervix, uterus

Table 19-1 ESSENTIAL COMPONENTS OF THE PERINATAL HISTORY (*CONTINUED*)

Component	Required Data
Pregnancy history	• Last known menstrual period • EDC (estimated date of confinement) • Nutrition and general health • Prenatal care (when first obtained and frequency) • Prenatal laboratory tests (VDRL; screening for hepatitis B, HIV, STDs, rubella) • Weight gain during pregnancy • Results of prenatal testing (ultrasonography, amniocentesis, chorionic villus testing, alpha-fetoprotein, triple screen) • Medications (prescription, over-the-counter, recreational)
Intrapartum history	• Length of labor • Type of birth (vaginal or cesarean) • Rupture of membrane (spontaneous or artificial, time from rupture until birth) • Appearance of amniotic fluid • Complications • Instrumentation • Analgesia and anesthesia • Apgar scores and resuscitation of infant
Breastfeeding history	• Previous maternal breastfeeding experience • Desire to breastfeed • Anticipated duration of breastfeeding • Exposure to breastfeeding education • Cultural influences related to breastfeeding • Maternal support system

Data from Barron, 2008; Orr, 2004.

Table 19-2 PHYSIOLOGIC CHARACTERISTICS ASSOCIATED WITH GESTATIONAL AGE AND SIZE THAT AFFECT FEEDING/NUTRITION

Gestational Age/ Size Classification	Characteristic	Risk
Low birth weight Prematurity	• Coordination of sucking and swallowing not present until 32–34 weeks, full coordination after 36–37 weeks	Aspiration
	• Immature gag reflex <37 weeks	
	• Higher extracellular water content (90% vs. 70% in full-term infant)	Inadequate hydration
	• Poor muscle tone in the area of the lower esophageal sphincter <37 weeks	Regurgitation into the esophagus, which can cause vagal stimulation—apnea, bradycardia, aspiration
	• Limited stomach capacity	Over distention; compromises respiration
	• Carbohydrates and fat less tolerated	Inadequate nutrition

(continues)

Table 19-2 PHYSIOLOGIC CHARACTERISTICS ASSOCIATED WITH GESTATIONAL AGE AND SIZE THAT AFFECT FEEDING/NUTRITION (*CONTINUED*)

Gestational Age/ Size Classification	Characteristic	Risk
	• Secretion of lactase low < 34 weeks	
	• Inefficient in digesting and absorbing lipids—low levels of pancreatic lipase and low bile acid	
	• Low reserve of calcium, iron, phosphorus, proteins, and vitamins A and C	
	• Absent, weak, or ineffectual sucking	
	• Decreased muscle mass; decreased deposits of brown fat	Thermoregulation Hypoglycemia
	• Lack of subcutaneous fat	
	• Poor reflex control of skin capillaries	
Postmaturity	• Decreased efficiency of the placenta	Respiratory distress
	• Macrosomia	Hypoglycemia
	• Meconium aspiration	Hyperbilirubinemia
	• Polycemia	
LGA	Transient hyperinsulinism	Hypoglycemia
SGA	Intrauterine malnutrition	Hypoglycemia

Adapted from Wheeler (2013); McGrath & Hardy (2011).

The following classification terms are used to describe the developmental status of the newborn (Fraser, 2013):

- Classification according to size
  - ◀ Extremely low birth weight (ELBW): An infant whose birth weight is less than 1000 g (2.2 lb)
  - ◀ Very low birth weight (VLBW): An infant whose birth weight is less than 1500 g (3.3 lb)
  - ◀ Low birth weight (LBW): An infant whose birth weight is less than 2500 g (5.5 lb)
  - ◀ Small for date (SFD) or small for gestational age (SGA): An infant whose birth weight is below the 10th percentile on intrauterine growth curves
  - ◀ Appropriate for gestational age (AGA): An infant whose birth weight falls between the 10th and 90th percentiles on intrauterine growth curves
  - ◀ Large for gestational age (LGA): An infant whose birth weight is above the 90th percentile on intrauterine growth curves
  - ◀ Intrauterine growth restriction (IUGR): An infant whose intrauterine growth curve is retarded
- Classification according to gestational age
  - ◀ Preterm (premature): An infant born at less than 37 weeks' gestation, regardless of weight
  - ◀ Late-preterm infant: An infant born between 34 0/7 and 36 6/7 weeks of gestation regardless of birth weight
  - ◀ Full term: An infant born between 37 and 42 weeks' gestation, regardless of weight
  - ◀ Post-term (post-mature): An infant born after 42 weeks' gestation, regardless of birth weight

The New Ballard Score

The New Ballard Score (Ballard et al., 1991) continues as a commonly used objective tool that includes the assessment of six external physical characteristics and six neurologic signs to estimate the gestational age of the infant (Creehan, 2008). This scoring system has its highest reliability when performed within 48 hours of birth and is considered accurate within 2 weeks of actual gestation (Ballard et al., 1991). Although the New Ballard Score has been expanded to include extremely premature infants, the Donovan et al. (1999) study failed to demonstrate a close relationship between gestational age and fetal maturation, as measured by this scoring system, in infants less than 28 weeks' gestation. Thus possible inaccuracies in gestational age based on New Ballard Scores should be considered when implementing treatment for infants less than 28 weeks' gestation.

Other assessment tools for the preterm infant have also been developed. Noble and Boyd's (2011) systematic review of neonatal assessment for the preterm infant identified eight assessments that were the most suitable for preterm infants. These tools varied in time to administer, formal training, and cost.

Each item on the New Ballard Score is scored from –1 to 4 (or 5 with two of the signs) by comparing the infant with the descriptor on the scoring sheet (Figure 19-1). The numbers of points assigned per item are added to obtain a total score. The total score is then used to determine an estimate of gestational age in weeks by comparing the infant's score with the maturity rating score on the New Ballard Score. The following neuromuscular and physical signs are used for scoring (Cheffer & Rannalli, 2011; Creehan, 2008):

- Neuromuscular signs of maturity
  - ◄ Posture: Observe the posture when the infant is quiet. A term newborn's arms and legs are flexed with good body muscle tone. A preterm infant's arms and legs are extended with the body flaccid (Figure 19-2).
  - ◄ Square window: Flex the infant's wrist down toward the ventral forearm and estimate the angle between the hand and forearm. Do not rotate the wrist. Measure the degree of flexion against the New Ballard Score chart. There is no downward angle with the full-term infant (i.e., a score of 3 or 4). The angle decreases with decreasing gestational age.
  - ◄ Arm recoil: Fully flex the infant's arms for 5 seconds. Release. Score the degree of immediate return of arm flexion against the score sheet. A vigorous, fully flexed response is a score of 4. A slow response receives a lower score.
  - ◄ Popliteal angle: With the infant's hips flat on the examining table, place one of the infant's thighs on the abdomen. Slowly, attempt to straighten the leg toward the infant's head. Do not force. Stop when resistance is met. Score the angle of the flexed leg according to the chart. A full-term infant will usually score a 3 or 4.
  - ◄ Scarf sign: Pull the infant's arm across the chest and around the neck. Observe the infant's elbow in relation to the midline of the body. Score according to the chart. A full-term infant will usually score 2, 3, or 4.
  - ◄ Heel to ear: With the infant's hips on the examining table, slowly pull the heel toward the ear until resistance is felt. Observe the distance between the foot and the head as well as the degree of knee extension. Score according to the chart. A full-term infant will usually score 3 or 4.
- Physical signs of maturity
  - ◄ Skin: Observe the skin for color and texture. Observe the trunk area for opacity. With increasing gestational age, the skin becomes less transparent and develops more texture. Blood vessels are generally not visible on the trunk of a full-term infant. Some peeling of the hands and feet is common in full-term infants. A preterm infant's skin is thin and smooth with visible vessels. Score the infant according to the chart. A full-term infant will usually score a 3 or 4.
  - ◄ Lanugo: Observe the skin for this fine, downy hair. Lanugo covers the body of

the fetus from about 24 to 28 weeks' gestation. After 28 weeks, it begins to disappear. Score the infant according to the descriptors on the chart. Note that a very premature infant will have no lanugo or it is sparse, thus scoring a 0 or −1. A full-term infant will usually score 3 or 4.

◀ Plantar surface: Observe the soles of the feet for creases. The creases on the anterior surface of the foot begin to appear between 28 and 30 weeks' gestation. As gestational age increases, so do the number and depth of creases. Score according to the descriptors on the chart. A full-term infant will usually score a 3 or 4. Note that after 12 hours, the validity of plantar creases as an indicator of gestational age decreases because the skin begins to dry.

◀ Breast: Place two fingers of one hand on either side of the areola bud tissue. Measure (in millimeters) the diameter of the bud with a tape measure. Score according to the chart. A full-term infant will usually score a 3 or 4.

◀ Eye/ear: Prior to 26 to 30 weeks' gestation, the eyelids are fused. After the eyes are open, there is no maturity scoring on the New Ballard Score. The ears are assessed for formation and amount of cartilage that is present in the pinna. Examine the pinna between the thumb and forefinger for amount of cartilage that is present. Fold the ear anteriorly. After approximately 36 weeks' gestation when some cartilage has developed, the pinna will spring back from being folded. Score according to the chart. A full-term infant will usually score 3 or 4.

◀ Genitalia (male): Gently feel for the presence of the testes by examining the scrotum between the thumb and fingers of one hand. Observe the degree of descent into the scrotum and the development of rugae. The testes begin to descend at 28 weeks' gestation and descent is normally

complete by 40 weeks' gestation. The scrotum of a full-term infant is also covered with deep rugae.

◀ Genitalia (female): Observe the genitalia of the female infant without spreading the labia majora. At full term, the infant's labia majora covers the labia minora. The premature infant will have a more prominent clitoris with small, widely separated labia.

After these assessments, complete the scoring by adding the total neuromuscular maturity score to the total physical maturity score. Compare that score, found on the left side of the maturity rating scale, with the corresponding gestational age on the right side of the rating scale. To complete the assessment of gestational age, plot the infant's weight, length, and head circumference in relation to maturity rating from the New Ballard Score on the Classification of Newborn by intrauterine growth and gestational age (Figure 19-3). The infant's maturity level can then be classified according to the previously defined classification terms.

Using the initial assessment as a baseline, continue to monitor infant growth and development. The World Health Organization's (WHO, 2006) growth standards for continuing assessment of appropriate growth in the breastfed infant are recommended (Figure 19-4).

Indicators of Effective Breastfeeding and Assessment Scales

This section defines behaviors that indicate whether breastfeeding is going well and reviews several breastfeeding assessment scales.

Breastfeeding Behaviors and Indicators

Breastfeeding is not a single behavior of suckling, but rather a series of behaviors that can be

Figure 19-1 NEW BALLAD SCORE.

MATURATIONAL ASSESSMENT OF GESTATIONAL AGE (New Ballard Score)

NAME _____   DATE/TIME OF BIRTH _____   SEX _____

HOSPITAL NO. _____   DATE/TIME OF EXAM _____   BIRTH WEIGHT _____

RACE _____   AGE WHEN EXAMINED _____   LENGTH _____

APGAR SCORE: 1 MINUTE _____ 5 MINUTES _____ 10 MINUTES _____   HEAD CIRC. _____

EXAMINER _____

NEUROMUSCULAR MATURITY

NEUROMUSCULAR MATURITY SIGN	SCORE							RECORD SCORE HERE
	-1	0	1	2	3	4	5	
POSTURE								
SQUARE WINDOW (Wrist)	>90°	90°	60°	45°	30°	0°		
ARM RECOIL		180°	140°-180°	110°-140°	90°-110°	<90°		
POPLITEAL ANGLE	180°	160°	140°	120°	100°	90°	<90°	
SCARF SIGN								
HEEL TO EAR								

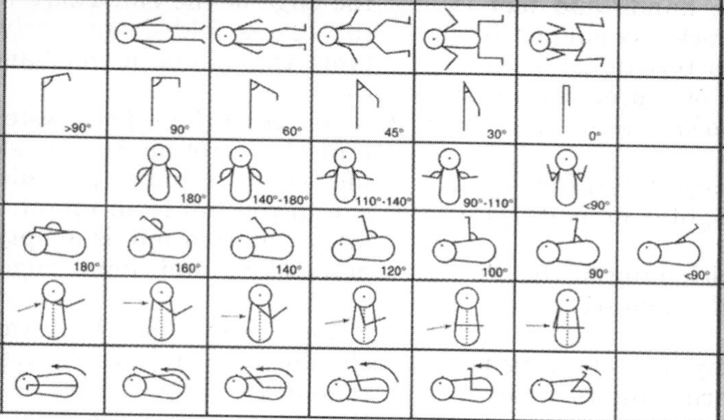

TOTAL NEUROMUSCULAR MATURITY SCORE

SCORE

Neuromuscular _____

Physical _____

Total _____

MATURITY RATING

score	weeks
-10	20
-5	22
0	24
5	26
10	28
15	30
20	32
25	34
30	36
35	38
40	40
45	42
50	44

GESTATIONAL AGE (weeks)

By dates _____

By ultrasound _____

By exam _____

PHYSICAL MATURITY

PHYSICAL MATURITY SIGN	SCORE							RECORD SCORE HERE
	-1	0	1	2	3	4	5	
SKIN	sticky friable transparent	gelatinous red translucent	smooth pink visible veins	superficial peeling &/or rash, few veins	cracking pale areas rare veins	parchment deep cracking no vessels	leathery cracked wrinkled	
LANUGO	none	sparse	abundant	thinning	bald areas	mostly bald		
PLANTAR SURFACE	heel-toe 40-50 mm:-1 <40 mm:-2	>50 mm no crease	faint red marks	anterior transverse crease only	creases ant. 2/3	creases over entire sole		
BREAST	imperceptible	barely perceptible	flat areola no bud	stippled areola 1-2 mm bud	raised areola 3-4 mm bud	full areola 5-10 mm bud		
EYE/EAR	lids fused loosely: -1 tightly: -2	lids open pinna flat stays folded	sl. curved pinna; soft; slow recoil	well-curved pinna; soft but ready recoil	formed & firm instant recoil	thick cartilage ear stiff		
GENITALS (Male)	scrotum flat, smooth	scrotum empty faint rugae	testes in upper canal rare rugae	testes descending few rugae	testes down good rugae	testes pendulous deep rugae		
GENITALS (Female)	clitoris prominent & labia flat	prominent clitoris & small labia minora	prominent clitoris & enlarging minora	majora & minora equally prominent	majora large minora small	majora cover clitoris & minora		

TOTAL PHYSICAL MATURITY SCORE

Source: Reprinted from Journal of Pediatrics, Vol. 119, No. 3, Ballard et al., "Maturational Assessment of Gestational Age (New Ballard Score)," pp. 417–423, Copyright 1991, with permission from Elsevier.

Figure 19-2 NEONATE POSTURE. (A) FULL-TERM INFANT. (B) PREMATURE INFANT.

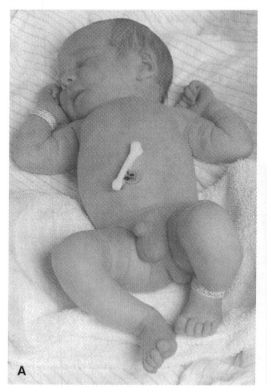

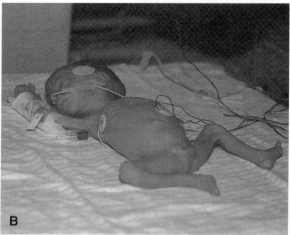

Source: Moore ML, Nichols FH, Zwelling E eds. Maternal-newborn nursing: theory and practice. Philadelphia: W. B. Saunders, 1080–1131, 1997. Reprinted with permission of Elsevier Publications.

described, assessed, and measured. Historically, a lack of consistency in defining breastfeeding behaviors resulted in difficulty comparing breast-feeding studies, thus limiting their use; however, generally speaking, breastfeeding infants who are feeding effectively spontaneously turn their mouth to the mother's nipple when put to breast, grasp the nipple firmly, suckle rhythmically, and pause to rest between bursts of suckling while continuing to hold the nipple in the mouth. Swallowing is observed during the first 3 days postpartum; swallowing is both observed and heard beginning 4 days postpartum or earlier for some mothers (Howe et al., 2008; Janke, 2008; Riordan et al., 2005).

A concept analysis is sometimes done for the development of a tool (Mulder, 2006). In the case of breastfeeding tools, agreed-upon operational definitions of interactive breastfeeding behaviors have not been clearly determined, yet they are needed before we can consistently evaluate relationships between breastfeeding behaviors and breastfeeding outcomes (Mulder, 2006). Mulder further points out that to be considered essential attributes or behaviors of effective breastfeeding the characteristics must occur and be present in all feedings and be required to achieve the transfer of milk between the mother and infant to meet both maternal and infant needs. As a starting point, the authors of this chapter define commonly used breastfeeding concepts.

Figure 19-3 INTRAUTERINE GROWTH GRIDS.

New gender-specific intrauterine growth curves for girls' weight for age (A), girls' length and HC for age (B), boys' weight for age (C), and boys' length and HC for age (D).

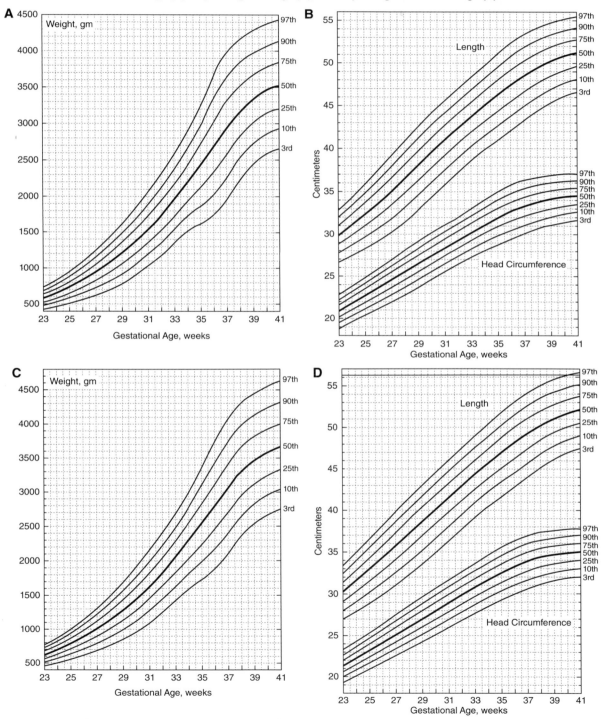

Source: Reproduced from Olsen IE, Groveman SA, Lawson ML, Clark RH, Zemel BS. New intrauterine growth curves based on United States data. Pediatrics. 2010;125:e214, DOI: 210.1542/peds.2009-0913.

Figure 19-4 WHO GROWTH CHARTS: GIRLS 0-6 MONTHS.

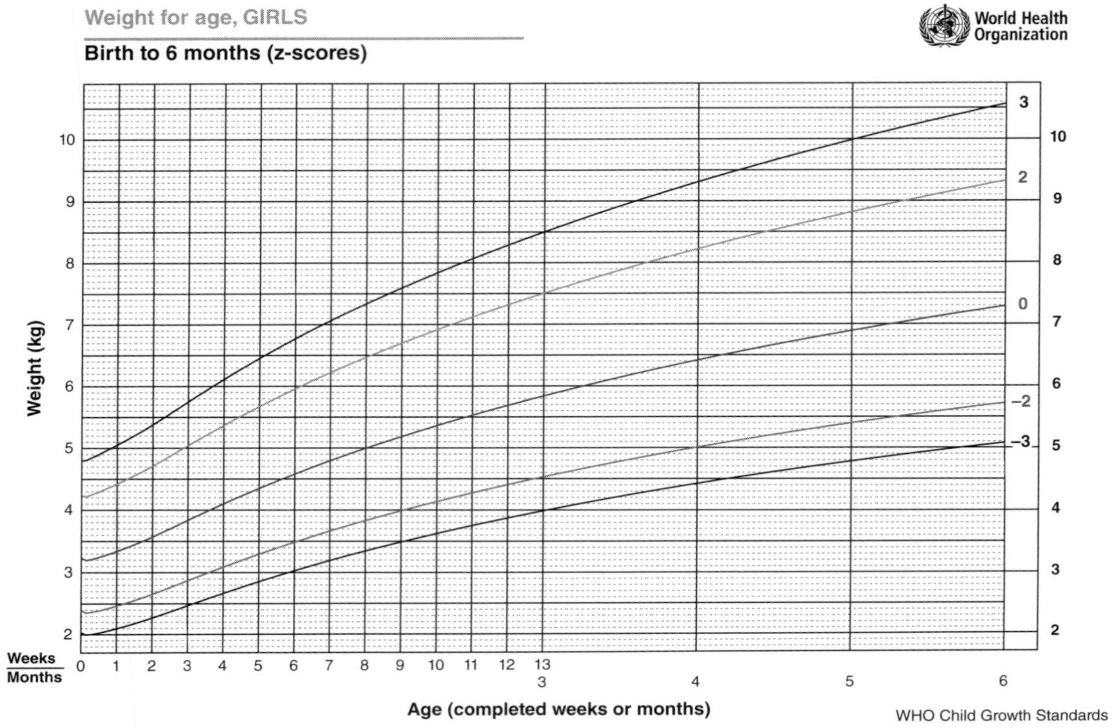

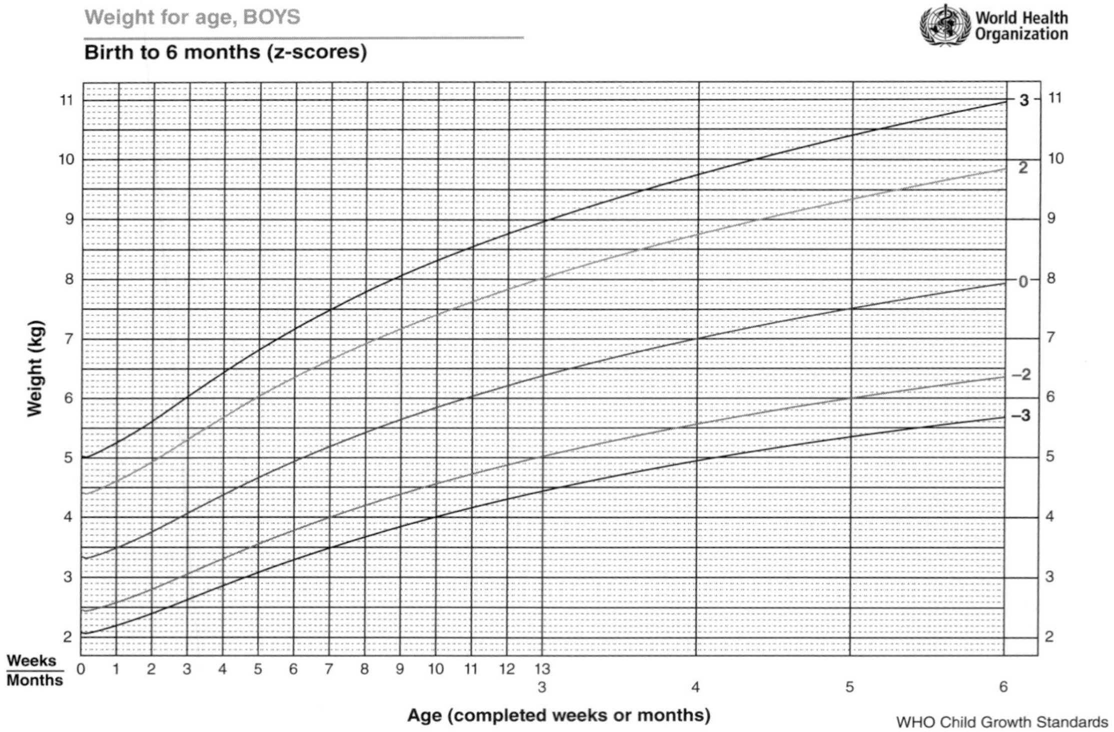

Weight for age, GIRLS

Birth to 6 months (z-scores)

World Health Organization

WHO Child Growth Standards

Weight for age, BOYS

Birth to 6 months (z-scores)

World Health Organization

WHO Child Growth Standards

Source: WHO Multicentre Growth Reference Study Group. WHO Child Growth Standards: Length/height-for-age, weight-for-age, weight-for-length, weight-for-height and body mass index-for-age: Methods and development. Geneva: World Health Organization;2006.

Rooting

Rooting is a reflexive behavior in which the infant turns his head in the direction of the stimulus and opens his mouth wide anticipating feeding. Rooting enables the infant to "catch" the mother's nipple and keeps the infant's tongue on the bottom of the mouth, important for compressing milk ducts (Figure 19-5). Licking movements typically precede and follow rooting in the early neonatal period.

Length of Time Before Latch-on

The time before latch-on is the amount of time in minutes before the infant latches on and remains on the breast.

Latch-on

Latch-on refers to the ability of the infant to grasp the nipple, flange the upper and lower lips outward against the breast areola, and remain firmly on the breast between bursts of suckling.

Suckling

Coordinated and rhythmic suckling, swallowing, and breathing is characterized by a pattern of

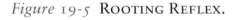

Figure 19-5 ROOTING REFLEX.

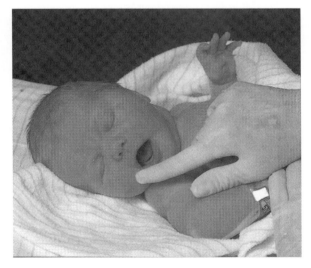

Source: Moore ML, Nichols FH, Zwelling E eds. Maternal-newborn nursing: theory and practice. Philadelphia: W. B. Saunders, 1080–1131, 1997. Reprinted with permission of Elsevier Publications.

suckling burst, pause, suckling burst, pause—that is, alternating between nutritive (milk ingested) and non-nutritive (no milk ingested) suckling. The infant's lips should be visibly flanged outward during suckling to prevent friction and abrasion of the mother's areolar tissue and to provide the seal that allows negative intra-oral pressure. During nutritive sucking, the suck cycle begins with the tongue compressing the nipple and resting it against the hard and soft palates. As the tongue lowers, milk flows into the intra-oral space. This cycle concludes with the mid-tongue rising back to contact with the palate. In contrast, during non-nutritive sucking, the tongue does not lower to the extent as in the nutritive sucking cycle and, therefore, does not result in milk entering the oral cavity (Sakalidis et al., 2012).

Swallowing

In swallowing, the back of the tongue elevates and presses against the posterior pharyngeal wall. The soft palate rises and closes off the nasal passageways. The larynx then moves up and forward to close the trachea and propels the milk into the esophagus, thus initiating the baby's swallow reflex. Afterward, the larynx returns to its previous position. A sufficient volume of milk is needed to trigger swallowing.

Swallowing can usually be observed during the first several days following birth and becomes audible following lactogenesis at approximately 4 days postpartum (or earlier). Swallowing produces observable movements of the infant's jaw (long, rhythmic jaw excursions) and throat muscles. To date, audible swallowing has been identified as the only significant predictor of how much breastmilk transfers from mother to baby at any feeding (Riordan et al., 2005).

Other Behaviors

Positioning or alignment is commonly named as an essential attribute for breastfeeding to be "correct" (Wheeler, 2013). A number of authors suggest that good positioning prevents breastfeeding problems and may be the only assistance the mother needs for optimal breastfeeding. However, there is a conspicuous lack of evidence and agreement on what constitutes optimal positions of the mother and baby during a feed despite considerable attention paid to this issue.

Four breastfeeding positions (Orr, 2011) are commonly used:

- Cradle hold
- Cross-cradle hold
- Football hold
- Side-lying

As an alternative, Colson (2012) describes biological nurturing with the mother in a laid-back position. In this position, the mother or the healthcare provider supports the infant as he discovers the breast on his own. According to Colson, the laid-back position "helps mothers tap into what they innately know and breastfeed easily without a lot of rules about how to do it or prescriptive advice."

Thus, since there is no definitive evidence regarding the best position, more research is needed before we reach an agreement about the attributes of positioning. Generally, experienced lactation specialists are able to quickly assess when the feeding is going well. A baby may not look technically perfect but if the sucking is strong and regular, there is audible swallowing, and the mother is pain free, chances are that the positioning is right for that mother and baby.

Breastfeeding Scales and Tools

Early feeding assessment scales were developed for and tested on infants who were bottle-fed. Because breastfeeding was less quantifiable, hospital nurses initially documented feedings with subjective phrases such as "breastfed well" or "breastfed poorly." Since then, breastfeeding assessment has evolved to use quantitative scales, to evaluate neonate breastfeeding activity. One of the earliest of these scales, developed by Matthews (1988), separated and labeled indicators of infant feedings at the breast into the first scored assessment tool for breastfeeding. Around the same time, Shrago and Bocar (1990) published a list of breastfeeding

behaviors for assessing feedings; however, they did not add a scoring system. Since then, numerous other assessment tools have been developed, including the IBFAT, the LATCH, the MBA, the PIBBS, and the NOMAS. Three of these tools are shown in Appendices 19-A through 19-C.

Howe et al. (2008) reviewed the psychometric properties of seven feeding assessment tools, including those noted previously. These researchers found that none of the seven tools identified in the study were psychometrically sound. Specifically, four overall general concerns were identified: (1) there was no consensus regarding successful feeding behaviors, (2) the studies all had small sample sizes, (3) the samples did not adequately represent the target population, and (4) the psychometric information was insufficient. Clinicians who use these tools should take these shortcomings into account; nevertheless, Howe and colleagues' findings provide the opportunity for further research. In spite of the psychometric issues, the breastfeeding scales are useful for documentation and communication among healthcare workers as well as for teaching mothers to show them normal breastfeeding patterns of their babies.

Infant Breastfeeding Assessment Tool (IBFAT)

A Canadian midwife developed the IBFAT (Appendix 19-A), the first such breastfeeding assessment scale, as her master's thesis (Matthews, 1988). The IBFAT has four indicators: (1) readiness to feed, (2) rooting, (3) fixing, and (4) sucking. A numerical score (0 to 3) is given for each indicator; the total score can range from 0 to 12. Breastfeeding is considered to be effective when scores range from 9 to 12.

Although the IBFAT has been used in numerous studies (Benson, 2001; Crowell et al., 1994; Matthews, 1993; Riordan et al., 2001), the results of reliability studies have been mixed. In support of the tool's utility, both Matthews (1990) and Riordan et al. (2001) found that the higher the score, the more pleased the mother was with the feeding.

Low IBFAT scores have been associated with the use of labor analgesia (Crowell et al., 1994; Matthews, 1993; Riordan et al., 2000) and significantly shorter periods of breastfeeding than medium or high scores ($P < 0.001$) (Riordan et al., 2000).

LATCH Assessment Tool

The LATCH tool (Jensen et al., 1994) evaluates five indicators of breastfeeding (Appendix 19-B). A numerical score (0, 1, or 2) is assigned to each measure, for a maximum possible total score of 10. Each letter of the acronym title denotes a category: "L" represents how well the infant latches onto the breast, "A" represents audible swallowing, "T" describes the mother's nipple type, "C" represents the mother's degree of breast or nipple comfort, and "H" evaluates the amount of help the mother needs to position her baby at breast. This tool can be helpful in identifying needed interventions and teaching (Howe et al., 2008).

When LATCH scores were compared with the overall duration of breastfeeding, women still breastfeeding at 6 weeks postpartum had significantly higher LATCH scores than those who had weaned (Riordan et al., 2001). Although this finding supports some overall validity for the breastfeeding scale, it should be noted that this prediction was due to the item "comfort of nipples." Mothers who had very sore nipples stopped breastfeeding early. Although Adams and Hewell (1997) found acceptable reliability, only poor to moderate predictive ability has been found for the LATCH assessment tool (Kumar et al., 2006; Riordan et al., 2001).

Via Christi Breastfeeding Assessment Tool

The Via Christi Breastfeeding Assessment Tool was modified from the LATCH and IBFAT scales. It is a combination of indicators from other assessment scales that were selected because they demonstrated positive correlations with the mother's evaluation and amount of breastmilk ingested during feedings—indicators of reliability and validity—in previous studies (Adams & Hewell, 1997; Riordan

et al., 2001; Riordan & Koehn, 1997; Schlomer et al., 1999). Mothers' evaluations of the feedings were added to the scale because of a high positive correlation with other indicators. Mothers can gauge the effectiveness of the feed; only they can feel the sensations of breastfeeding (e.g., the baby's firm latch on the breast, letdown, uterine contractions). Audible swallowing was included because it predicts the amount of breastmilk taken by the baby (Riordan et al., 2005). Morrison et al. (2002) reported a strong correlation between the LATCH and the next tool described here—the MBA.

Mother–Baby Assessment Tool (MBA)

The MBA scoring system (Appendix 19-C) divides the process of breastfeeding into five sequential behaviors of both the mother and the infant: (1) signaling, (2) positioning, (3) fixing, (4) milk transfer, and (5) ending (Mulford, 1992). For each step, both a maternal behavior and an infant behavior are scored. Ten is the highest possible feeding score: 5 for infant indicators and 5 for maternal indicators. The indicator associated with the greatest agreement was readiness of the baby and mother to feed (97%); the least agreement was found for the milk transfer indicator (37%) (Riordan & Koehn, 1997). As with the other tools, reliability and validity testing have mixed results.

Preterm Infant Breastfeeding Behavior Scale (PIBBS)

The Preterm Infant Breastfeeding Behavior Scale was developed as an observational tool to study preterm infant feeding behavior (Hedberg-Nyqvist & Ewald, 1999). However, this tool can be used to assess feeding readiness of both low-birth-weight and full-term babies (Hedberg-Nyqvist et al., 1996). Hedberg-Nyqvist, and colleagues (1996) found acceptable agreement of scores between nurses and raters but not as satisfactory agreement between nurses and mothers. The PIBBS tool has been shown to significantly predict the amount of breastmilk ingested by the infant during a feeding (Radzyminski, 2005).

Neonatal Oral–Motor Assessment Scale (NOMAS)

The NOMAS was originally developed to assess feedings in premature and medically compromised newborns (Palmer et al., 1999). This non-nutritive sucking assessment is done with the examiner's finger in the infant's mouth. The revised version has four parts that test normal and abnormal characteristics of the jaw and tongue. The examiner assesses and rates the newborn for these characteristics. The rating ranges from 0 to 16 (MacMullen & Dulski, 2000). Two studies have shown consistent support for the NOMAS's validity. Case-Smith and colleagues (1988) found support for construct validity of this tool in infants with a gestational age of 34 to 35 weeks, while Palmer and Heyman's 1999 study demonstrated its predictive validity. Overall, Howe and colleagues' (2008) study results showed that the NOMAS has two advantages over other scales: it demonstrates more consistent psychometric properties and it was the only tool out of the seven examined that could be used for assessment of both breastfed and bottle-fed infants.

Summary of Breastfeeding Assessment Scales

As more women choose to breastfeed and are discharged early with uncertain breastfeeding support, we need valid and reliable tools that measure breastfeeding. Because the scoring must take place quickly in busy maternity units, the scale should be short and easy to use. Which scales are best for assessing feedings of full-term babies? At the time of this writing, the following tools are all being successfully used in clinical settings: (1) the IBFAT, (2) the LATCH, (3) the Via Christi, and (4) the PIBBS. However, it is important to remember that evidence of validity and reliability are mixed (Howe et al., 2008). Again, it should be noted that the only single behavior found that predicts milk intake is audible swallowing (Riordan et al., 2005). Thus, the journey to find the "best" breastfeeding assessment scale continues. Existing tools will be revised and new tools developed as new knowledge becomes available.

Physical Assessment

Transitional Assessment

During the first 24 hours of life, the newborn undergoes a typical pattern of adjustment indicating normal adaptation to extrauterine life. The first several hours after birth are considered the first period of reactivity (Wheeler, 2013). During the first 30 minutes of this time, the healthy full-term newborn is alert (unless affected by maternal medication), cries spontaneously, and when put to the mother's breast will root, lick, and otherwise nuzzle the mother's breast. This behavior is followed by hand-to-mouth movements and later latching-on to the nipple and suckling. This is an ideal time to begin breastfeeding, as the newborn is wide-eyed, alert, and responsive to environmental cues.

Physiologic changes during this time include rapid respiration and heart rate, and increased mucus secretions. There may be a transient episode of tachypnea and nasal flaring, but this should resolve spontaneously within the first 30 minutes. The next phase of this period begins when the infant falls into a deep sleep. Heart and respiratory rate decrease, temperature continues to be unstable, and mucus production decreases. Stimulation of the newborn at this time usually results in little response. This is normal neonatal behavior but can be upsetting to parents and nurses who are anxious for the baby to breastfeed sooner than the baby is ready for it. Some acrocyanosis may still be evident, although it usually shows a steady improvement. Bowels sounds may become audible at this time.

The second stage of reactivity occurs when the newborn awakens from a deep sleep state, becoming alert and responsive (Wheeler, 2013). The newborn's heart and respiratory rate increase; however, the baby can have periods of apnea associated with a decrease in heart rate. Tactile stimulation is used to improve the heart and respiratory rate. When apneic periods are associated with skin color changes, further evaluation is necessary. It is not unusual for the newborn to gag, choke, and regurgitate as gastric and respiratory secretions increase. The gastrointestinal system is active, and most newborns will pass the first meconium stool within 8 to 24 hours of birth. Many newborns void immediately after birth. If the infant was not fed during the first period of reactivity, this is an ideal time to initiate a feeding.

When the healthcare provider is performing a head-to-toe physical assessment of the neonate (Table 19-3), a warm surface must be provided for the newborn. Exposing the newborn's body to uncontrolled temperatures increases the risk of hypothermia. Placing the baby in a radiant warmer for the initial examination after the birth avoids this problem. If there is no medical contraindication, it is important to consider delaying the first examination until after skin-to-skin holding and the mother's opportunity to breastfeed has occurred. If you notice the Moro or startle reflex during the examination, be aware that it is normal. The Moro or startle reflex is elicited by loud noise or sudden movement of the surface on which the infant is lying (Figure 19-6). Before assessing each body system, a description of the posture and general appearance of the infant should be noted. Full-term infants typically have a flexed posture consistent with the fetal position in utero.

Skin

Observe the condition of the skin for color, opacity, thickness, and consistency. Dryness, cracking, and peeling are signs of full- or post-term maturity. A full-term newborn is likely to have flaking skin in the major creases at the ankles. Vernix caseosa—a combination of discarded epithelial cells, lanugo, and sebaceous gland secretions—is evident on term newborns and usually becomes less visible after 40 weeks' gestation. Vessels should not be visible over the trunk of the body of the full-term newborn. Inspect the skin for color as well as bruises, lesions, rashes, or discolorations in natural light.

The skin should be warm, dry, and smooth. Skin color of the newborn will depend on the ethnicity of the parents. African American newborns may appear pink or yellow-brown. Asian-descent newborns may have a tan or rose color. Caucasian newborns are usually pink to red, and Hispanic newborns may have pink skin with an olive or yellow tint. Native American newborns may vary from pink to light brown or darker brown. Blanch the skin by gently pressing a finger over the chest or forehead. The skin should show its own color as the finger is removed.

The skin should not be jaundiced or yellow tinged during the first 24 hours of life. Jaundice usually appears on the head first and progresses to the lower portion of the body and extremities as the bilirubin level rises. This abnormal finding requires documentation and a report to the physician. In Hispanic and African American babies, the color of the mucous membranes is used to assess for jaundice.

The color of the skin changes with the activity state of the newborn. When the newborn is crying, the skin is likely to be darker in color. Within the first few hours of birth, the newborn may have brief periods of cyanosis, not associated with heart rate changes or apnea. Generally, this resolves within the first few hours of life. Transient mottling may be apparent, especially when the newborn is exposed to cool temperatures. A common variation in the first 24 to 48 hours of life is acrocyanosis, a bluish discoloration of the hands and feet. As peripheral circulation improves, this effect will resolve and disappear within a few days after birth.

Figure 19-6 **MORO REFLEX.**

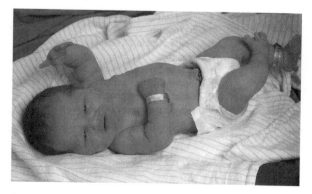

Source: Moore ML, Nichols FH, Zwelling E eds. Maternal-newborn nursing: theory and practice. Philadelphia: W. B. Saunders, 1080–1131, 1997. Reprinted with permission of Elsevier Publications.

Table 19-3 NEWBORN PHYSICAL ASSESSMENT

	Normal	Normal Variations	Abnormal
Vital Signs	• Temperature axillary 36.5–37.4°C (97.9–98°F) • Pulse 120–140 beats/minute	• Increased with crying • Decreased when sleeping	• <36.5°C • >37.4°C • Tachycardia • Bradycardia <80 to 100 • Associated with color changes
	• Respirations 30–60/minute	• Increased during first period of reactivity and with crying • Decreased when sleeping	
Measurement	• Head circumference 33–35 cm (13–14 in.) • Chest circumference 30.5–33 cm (12–13 in.) • Head-to-heel length 48–53 cm (19–21 in.) • Birth weight 2700–4000 gm (6–9 lb)	• Molding may decrease head circumference	• Head <10th or >90th percentile • Weight <10th or >90th percentile
Skin	• Bright red, smooth at birth • Vernix caseosa, lanugo	• Acrocyanosis • Cutis marmorata—mottling when exposed to low temperature, stress, or overstimulation • Milia • Erythema toxicum • Mongolian spots • Telangiectatic nevi • Harlequin color changes • Jaundice after first 24 hours	• Jaundice in the first 24 hours • Central or generalized cyanosis • Pallor • Mottling • Plethora • Persistent petechiae or hemorrhage or ecchymosis • Café au lait spots • Nervus flammeus • Fused sutures • Depressed or bulging fontanelles when quiet
Head	• Anterior fontanelle 2.5–4.0 cm (1–1.75 in.), diamond-shaped • Posterior fontanelle 0.5–1 cm (0.2–0.4 in.), triangular-shaped • Soft, flat fontanelles	• Molding after vaginal birth • Fontanelle bulging when crying • Caput succedaneum • Cephalhematoma	

Table 19-3 NEWBORN PHYSICAL ASSESSMENT (*CONTINUED*)

	Normal	Normal Variations	Abnormal
Eyes	• Edematous lids • Absence of tears • Slate gray, dark blue, or brown • Positive red, corneal, pupillary, and blink reflex • Fixes on objects, follows to midline	• Subconjunctival hemorrhages • Epicanthal folds in Asian newborns	• Purulent discharge • Upward slant of eyes • Iris pink color • Constricted or dilated pupil • Absence of red, corneal, papillary reflex • Inability to follow objects to the midline • Sclera yellow
Ears	• Pinna flexible, well formed level with outer canthus of the eye	• Pinna flat against the head • Irregular shape, size • Skin tags	• Low placement of ears
Nose	• Patent • Thin, white nasal discharge	• Flattened, bruised, or slightly deviated	• Nonpatent • Thick, bloody discharge • Nasal flaring
Mouth/Throat	• Intact, arched palate • Midline uvula • Tongue centered in the mouth • Reflexes: sucking, rooting, gagging extrusion • Vigorous cry	• Natal teeth • Epstein's pearls	• Cleft lip • Cleft palate • Large, protruding tongue • Drooling or copious salivation • Candidiasis– white, adherent, thick patches on tongue, palate, buccal surfaces • Weak, highpitched cry
Neck	• Short, thick • Tonic neck reflex	• Torticollis	• Extra skinfolds or webbing • Resistant to flexion • Absence of tonic neck reflex
Chest	• Equal anteroposterior and lateral diameter • Smooth clavicles • Breast enlargement	• Supernumerary nipples • Thin breast secretions	• Crepitus or asymmetry-over clavicle • Depressed sternum • Marked retractions • Asymmetrical expansion • Wide-spaced nipples

(*continues*)

Table 19-3   **Newborn Physical Assessment** (*continued*)

	Normal	Normal Variations	Abnormal
Lungs	• Bilateral bronchial breath sounds • Periodic breathing	• Crackles immediately after birth	• Inspiratory stridor • Expiratory grunting • Retractions • Unequal breath sounds • Apnea • Persistent fine crackles or wheezing • Peristaltic sounds
Abdomen	• Cylindrical shape • Soft to palpation • Umbilical cord bluish white at birth, with 2 arteries and 1 vein • Bowel sounds present • Femoral pulses equal bilaterally	• Firm to palpation when crying • Umbilical hernia • Diastasis recti	• Abdominal distension • Localized bulging • Absent bowel sounds • Drainage or blood at umbilical cord • Absent or unequal femoral pulses • Visible peristaltic waves
Genitalia	*Female* • Labia majora and clitoris edematous • Urethral meatus behind clitoris • Vernix caseosa between labia • Urination within first 24 hours	• Blood-tinged, mucous discharge • Hymenal tag	• Fused labia • Absence of vaginal opening • Masses in labia • Enlarged clitoris with urethral meatus at tip • Ambiguous genitalia • No urination within first 24 hours
	Male • Urethral opening at tip of penis • Palpable testes • Scrotum: rugae edematous, pendulous, deeply pigmented in dark-skinned newborns • Smegma • Urination within first 24 hours	• Nonretractable foreskin • Urethral opening covered by prepuce • Testes palpable in inguinal canal • Small scrotum	• Hypospadius • Epispadius • Chordee • Testes nonpalpable in scrotum or inguinal canal • Hypoplastic scrotum • Hydrocele • Masses in scrotum • Discoloration of testes • Ambiguous genitalia • No urination within first 24 hours

Table 19-3 Newborn Physical Assessment (CONTINUED)

	Normal	Normal Variations	Abnormal
Back/Rectum	• Spine intact, no deviations, openings, or masses • Trunk incurvation reflex • Patent anal opening • Anal reflex • Meconium passed within first 24 hours		• Anal fissures or fistulas • Imperforate anus • Absent anal reflex • No meconium within 36–48 hours • Pilonidal cyst or sinus • Tuft of hair • Spina bifida
Extremities	• Ten fingers and toes • Full range of motion • Pink nail beds • Creases on anterior two-thirds of sole • Symmetrical extremeties • Equal muscle tone bilaterally • Equal bilateral brachial pulses • Equal leg and gluteal folds	• Partial syndactyly between second and third toes • Second toe overlapping third toe • Wide gap between hallux and second toes • Asymmetric length of toes • Dorsiflexion and shortness of hallux	• Polydactyly • Syndactyly (webbing) • Persistent nail bed cyanosis • Nail beds yellowed • Transverse palmar crease • Fractures • Decreased or absent range of motion • Unequal leg or gluteal folds • Limited hip abduction • Audible click with abduction • Asymmetry

Acrocyanosis lasting longer than the first 48 hours after birth should be investigated.

Newborns with plethora, a ruddy color, have an excess of red blood cells contributing to the bright red skin color. This occurs more often in infants of diabetic mothers. Plethora is one sign of polycythemia; thus a complete blood count should be obtained. Polycythemia is defined as a hematocrit of 65% or higher. These infants should be monitored closely for other signs of polycythemia, which include peripheral cyanosis, respiratory distress, lethargy, hypoglycemia, and hyperbilirubinemia (McGrath & Hardy, 2011).

Pallor is most often associated with anemia, hypoxia, or poor peripheral perfusion, and needs to be evaluated. Harlequin color changes may occur as the result of the dependent half of the newborn's body reacting to a temporary autonomic imbalance of the cutaneous vessels. The skin on the dependent portion of the body becomes deep red, while the upper portion appears pale. When the newborn is turned to the opposite side, the color variation reverses. This benign condition occurs more often in low-birth-weight infants (Fraser, 2013).

Observe and note the location of petechiae, pinpoint superficial hemorrhages that occur due to pressure during descent and rotation through the birth canal. Petechiae are more likely to be seen if there has been a nuchal cord; they will usually fade within 24 to 48 hours after birth.

Skin turgor is the result of the outward pressure of interstitial fluid on the cells. Assess skin turgor by gently grasping and lifting the skin of the chest, abdomen, or thigh between the thumb and the finger. Skin that readily springs back to its original shape indicates the newborn has adequate skin turgor, a sign of appropriate hydration. Dimpling, wrinkling, or folding of the skin indicates possible dehydration.

Milia are common variations that may occur on the skin of the newborn, commonly visible over the nose, cheeks, and brow. Milia comprise sebaceous glands that have swollen under the influence of maternal hormones. Treatment is not required for milia, as they resolve spontaneously within the few weeks after birth.

A common rash seen in newborns is erythema toxicum. It consists of a pink, papular rash with vesicles occurring first on the face and then spreading to the chest, abdomen, back. and buttocks; it is often visible by the first or second day post birth. This rash will disappear within 1 week, but may reappear and dissipate spontaneously without treatment.

Birthmarks

A bluish-black area of pigmentation over the buttocks and back of the newborn with dark skin may be apparent. This can easily be confused with bruising, but is actually a common variation known as a Mongolian spot caused by a collection of melanocytes in the dermal layer (Figure 19-7). Mongolian spots are most often observed in African American, Asian, Hispanic, and other dark-skinned races (Cheffer & Rannalli, 2011). The macular lesion or patch may also be seen on the legs or flank of the newborn, appearing gray or blue-green; it usually fades over time.

Café-au-lait spots are light brown or tan macular areas with well-defined edges. As long as there are fewer than six spots, and they are less than 3 cm in length, they do not hold significance. Infants with larger or numerous spots may have cutaneous neurofibromatosis (Fraser, 2013).

Telangiectatic nevi ("stork bites") are flat, deep pink areas over the eyelids or on the forehead or

Figure 19-7 MONGOLIAN SPOT.

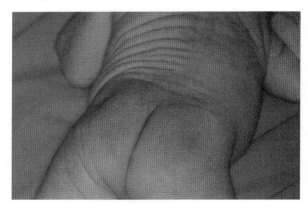

Source: Moore ML, Nichols FH, Zwelling E eds. Maternal-newborn nursing: theory and practice. Philadelphia: W. B. Saunders, 1080–1131, 1997. Reprinted with permission of Elsevier Publications.

bridge of the nose that blanch with pressure. Most nevi fade with time, although they may become brighter in color when the newborn is crying.

Nevus flammeus ("port wine nevus") is a reddish or flat pink lesion that does not blanch with pressure, caused by dilated capillaries below the epidermal surface. This lesion usually remains constant in size and does not fade with time. It often appears over the face, but may also be observed over the upper body.

Capillary hemangiomas, also known as strawberry hemangiomas, are benign cutaneous tumors that involve only capillaries. These soft, raised, lobed tumors have a bright red color and usually occur on the head, neck, trunk, or extremities. The red color is caused by the dilated mass of capillaries formed in the dermal and subdermal layers of the skin. Although spontaneous regression usually occurs, it may take several years. There will be no permanent scars if these lesions are left alone. Tumors that interfere with feeding, respiration, and vision require treatment. Infection, bleeding, ulceration, and compression of the vital organs are rare complications of strawberry hemangiomas.

Head

Observe the head for shape, symmetry, bruises, and lesions. Palpation of the head may reveal swelling, masses, or bony defects. Common variations are molding, caput succedaneum, and cephalhematoma. The negative pressure created when the amniotic sac ruptures and draws a portion of the scalp into the cervical os causes a caput succedaneum. Dilated capillaries cause the edema and bruising that occurs over the occipitoparietal area of the head. Swelling usually resolves within 24 hours after birth. Overriding suture lines are common in the infant born vaginally in a vertex position. This irregular shape resolves within a few days in the full-term infant and may persist for several weeks in premature infant. A soft area over the suture lines indicates the sutures are separated.

The intersections of the cranial sutures are called fontanels. The anterior fontanel, diamond in shape, is the largest and most important for assessment (Figure 19-8). The anterior fontanel is normally described as soft and flat but may appear to be bulging when the infant is crying vigorously, coughs, or vomits. Palpate the tension in the fontanel with the infant in an upright and a recumbent position. A soft sunken fontanel may indicate the newborn is dehydrated. The anterior fontanel usually closes

around 18 months of age. The posterior fontanel—triangular shaped at the junction of the sagittal and lambdoidal suture—is small, 0.5–1 cm (0.25–0.5 in.), and closes between 2 to 4 months of age (Wheeler, 2013).

Move the head through its full range of motion to assess flexion, extension, and rotation of the neck. The normal newborn's head is easily mobile in all directions, although the infant is not able to turn its head from side to side until 2 weeks of age. Assess for signs of torticollis, as this may contribute to feeding difficulties. Torticollis is present when the newborn holds the head to one side with the chin pointing to the opposite side and active range of motion is restricted (Wheeler, 2013).

Infants with mandibular asymmetry (crooked jaw) or receding chin (micrognanthia) may have difficulty with successfully latching onto the breast, with resultant excessive weight loss. Mothers of these infants frequently report nipple pain with breastfeeding attempts (Genna, 2013). Assessment techniques include the following:

- Positioning: Assess if the infant consistently turns to one side.
- Eyes: Assess for one eye that is smaller and higher.
- Ears: Assess for one ear that is cupped forward with the other ear flat.
- Lips: Assess for symmetry at rest, crying, or yawning.
- Gum lines: Assess for parallel upper and lower jaws.

Newborns have varying degrees of head control. When held in a supine position and pulled forward from the arms into a sitting position by the examiner, hyperextension and head lag are normal. While in a supported sitting position, the newborn may attempt to raise the head. The head will be in a straight line with the spine when the newborn is held in a ventral suspension position (Wheeler, 2013).

Ears and Eyes

Inspect facial features for symmetry, shape, bruising, or dysmorphic features. Asymmetry may result from compression of the fetal head in the uterus or

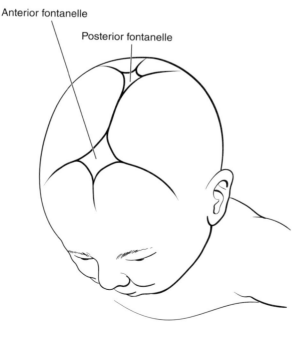

Figure 19-8 **FONTANELLES.**

Anterior fontanelle

Posterior fontanelle

from nerve injury related to birth trauma. The sclera of the eyes should be white and without drainage. The eyelids are usually edematous immediately after birth, with no tears present. Scleral and small conjunctival hemorrhages may be present.

The newborn is able to fix on objects and follow objects to the midline, and can focus on objects 8 to 10 inches (20 to 25 cm) away. This is the distance of the mother's face when the infant is at the breast. Immediately after birth, visual acuity ranges from 20/100 to 20/400. It is common in the newborn for the eyes to lag behind when the head is moved through full range of motion (doll's eye reflex). Persistence of doll's eye reflex beyond the newborn period may indicate neurologic dysfunction. By 4 weeks, the infant can intently watch when spoken to by the parent. Convergence on near objects begins at 6 weeks and is well established by 4 months of age (Wheeler, 2013).

The ear should be horizontal with the outer canthus of the eye. The pinna is flexible and well formed in the full-term infant. There should be no drainage from the ears. Fold the ear forward to examine the undersurface of the ear for skin tags. Assessment of hearing can begin early in the infant's life with simple observation of reaction to auditory stimuli. The newborn should respond with a startle reflex, head turning, eye blinking, and a pause in body movements, particularly when a familiar voice is heard. The degree of the infant's alertness will affect response; however, it is wise to be observant for signs of normal behavior. Practice standards vary by geographic area, although routine auditory screening of all newborns is common.

Nose

Inspect the nose for shape, symmetry, patency, and skin lesions. Observe each naris for a visual opening and gently occlude one side of the naris to observe breathing through the other side. Repeat the same process for the other naris. Newborns are obligatory nose breathers, but should be able to tolerate occluding one naris during assessment. Auscultation of nasal breathing using a stethoscope is helpful during this assessment. There should be no visible drainage from either naris. The nose may be misshapen at birth, due to uterine or vaginal compression, but resolves within a few days. Obstructions or deformities, such as choanal atresia, may indicate congenital syndromes or anatomic malformations. Since clefting of the oral area may include the nose, close assessment is necessary.

Mouth

Inspect the mouth for size, shape, symmetry, color, and presence of abnormal structures and masses when the newborn is both at rest and crying. Birth trauma may result in facial asymmetry due to nerve damage. The midline (vertical) region between the nose and the lips, known as the philtrum, should be well defined. The lips should be fully formed and the maxilla rounded. Newborns with at least two dysmorphological characteristics of the face may have fetal alcohol syndrome or effects: microcephaly (head circumference below the 10th percentile), short palpebral fissures, thinned upper lip, hypoplastic or smooth philtrum, or short, upturned nose (Fraser, 2013).

The sucking reflex, so important for breastfeeding, can be elicited right after birth by stimulating the mucous membranes of the mouth with a gloved finger (Figure 19-9). Assess the buccal pads on the sides of the mouth. A full-term newborn has adequate buccal pads that assist in creating the negative pressure observed when suckling at the breast. Preterm or malnourished newborns may not have full buccal pads. The mucous membranes and tongue should be pink and moist, and the tongue should protrude symmetrically over the alveolar ridge (gum line) when the mouth is open. The tongue should fit easily within the mouth when closed. Macroglossia, an abnormally large tongue, may be seen in some congenital syndromes such as Beckwith-Wiedeman syndrome and in hypothyroidism. Underdevelopment of the jaw, micrognathia, may be seen in certain malformation syndromes such as Pierre-Robin sequence.

The lingual frenulum has a consistency that may vary from thick and fibrous to very thin. The frenulum may be attached at the tip or midway

Figure 19-9 SUCKLING REFLEX.

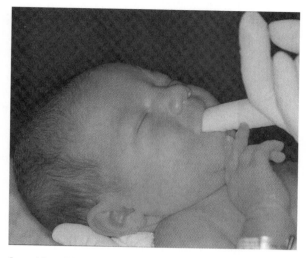

Source: Moore ML, Nichols FH, Zwelling E eds. Maternal-newborn nursing: theory and practice. Philadelphia: W. B. Saunders, 1080–1131, 1997. Reprinted with permission of Elsevier Publications.

along the undersurface of the tongue. Ankyloglossia (tongue-tie) occurs when the frenulum is unusually thick, tight, or short. Variations and differing degrees of severity occur. During breastfeeding, as opposed to bottle-feeding, the tongue is projected farther forward, causing the nipple to elongate. During normal feeding, the nipple, along with some of the breast tissue, is held in the mouth with the tongue covering the lower gum ridge. The infant's lower jaw elevates, compressing the breast behind the nipple, while the front of the tongue moves up to compress the milk ducts under the areola (Sakalidis et al., 2012). Ankyloglossia prohibits tongue extension beyond the lower gum and contributes to problems with latching on, nipple trauma, and continued breastfeeding. There is a lack of a uniform definition for ankyloglossia and, therefore, a lack of sufficient evidence to support the best treatment: intensive lactation support or frenotomy (Genna, 2013).

Along the gums—which should be smooth and raised—or the palate, there may be retention cysts known as Epstein's pearls, which are yellow or white in color and commonly found along the midline of the hard palate. They will resolve spontaneously within a few weeks after birth (Wheeler, 2013). Occasionally an infant will be born with supernumerary teeth that are soft with no enamel and are usually shed spontaneously. Primary teeth will normally erupt at a wide range of ages.

Palpate the soft and hard palates, which should be smooth, gently arched, and intact with the uvula in the midline. Assess for a cleft in the lip or palate by visual observation and palpation, taking care to assess the junction between the hard and soft palates. With a gloved finger in the mouth, assess the suck reflex. It should be strong and coordinated in the full-term newborn. The newborn should be able to completely form a seal around the examiner's finger. Saliva will be either minimal or absent. Excessive drooling or oral secretions indicate an inability to swallow, or the presence of a pharyngeal or esophageal obstruction.

Neck

The newborn's neck is short and thick, which makes it difficult to observe swallowing, a cardinal sign of breastmilk intake. Palpate the clavicles for crepitus or shortening, which may indicate fracture. The tonic reflex elicited by rotating the baby's head to one side (Figure 19-10) is seen as early as 35 weeks' gestation. Observe the neck for excess folds or webbing that may be indicative of congenital malformations.

Chest

Inspect the chest for size, symmetry, musculature, and bony structure. The chest should be barrel shaped, with the anteroposterior and lateral dimensions being equal. Chest circumference is approximately 2 cm smaller than head circumference. Newborn breast tissue is usually hypertrophied as a result of exposure to maternal hormones. Examination of the chest includes an assessment of the respiratory stability of the newborn necessary to initiate feedings. The respiratory rate is likely to be irregular and abdominal at 30 to 60 breaths per minute, with no retractions or signs of distress. The chest should rise equally on the right and left side during

Figure 19-10 TONIC NECK REFLEX.

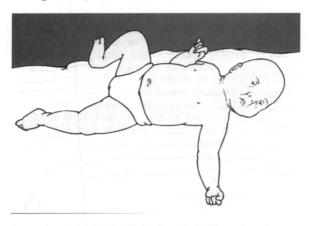

Source: Moore ML, Nichols FH, Zwelling E eds. Maternal-newborn nursing: theory and practice. Philadelphia: W. B. Saunders, 1080–1131, 1997. Reprinted with permission of Elsevier Publications.

inspiration. Auscultate the lung sounds bilaterally and in all lung fields. It is not unusual for the lungs to sound coarse immediately after birth. Respirations will usually be shallow and slow, alternating with rapid and deep respirations. When the infant's head is turned to one side, it is not unusual for lung sounds to be diminished on the side to which the head is turned.

Auscultate the heart at the point of maximum impulse (PMI), which is located at the left third or fourth intercostal space at the midclavicular line. If a murmur is heard, auscultate the heart at the second intercostal space, to the right of the sternum, for the aortic valve; auscultate at the second intercostal space, to the left of the sternum, for the pulmonic valve; auscultate at the fourth intercostal space, to the left of the sternum, for the tricuspid valve; auscultate at the fourth intercostal space, to the left of the midclavicular line, for the mitral valve. Murmurs heard during the first 48 hours after birth are often due to the transition from fetal circulation to neonatal circulation. These murmurs will be audible during the systolic phase and usually disappear spontaneously. Murmurs with high intensity and those that do not resolve within 48 hours need further investigation (Wheeler, 2013).

Abdomen

The abdomen should be rounded with no discoloration or visible bowel loops. Auscultate bowel sounds with the diaphragm of the stethoscope. Bowel sounds should be audible within the first hour after birth, and meconium is usually passed within the first 24 hours after birth. Observe the rise of the abdomen with the chest during respiration. Palpate the abdomen for consistency and masses. Using deep palpation, assess the abdominal organs. The liver is 1 to 3 cm below the right costal margin. The kidneys are 1 to 2 cm above and to both sides of the umbilicus. Observe the umbilical cord stump for drainage and bleeding. After the cord has been clamped for several hours, the vessels will no longer be visible. Prior to that time, observe for two umbilical arteries and one umbilical vein.

Genitalia

Male

Observe the penis on the male newborn for the urinary meatus in the midline and at the tip of the glans penis. Since the foreskin is tightly adhered to the glans penis, the best way to assess the meatal opening is by observing the stream of urine. An opening on the dorsal side of the penis is epispadius; an opening on the ventral side is known as hypospadius. The scrotum is large and edematous in the full-term newborn. African American and Hispanic newborns may have a deeply pigmented scrotum. Note the presence of rugae on the scrotal sac. Palpate the testes by placing one finger at the inguinal ring and pressing lightly; this prevents the testes from moving up into the inguinal canal while the examiner is palpating the scrotal sac. The testes should feel firm, about the size of a pea. The cremasteric reflex may be observed by stroking the upper thigh or the scrotal sac. When stimulated, the testes appear to recoil in toward the inguinal canal.

Female

The labia majora and the clitoris of the full-term female newborn are normally large and cover the labia minora, and may have a darker pigmentation. A small amount of white or blood-tinged discharge may be present at the vaginal opening. This is a response to the elevated estrogen levels to which the newborn has been exposed during development. Observe for the presence of hymenal tags. Tags usually disappear within the first few weeks and are of no great significance.

Back and Spine

Observe the back and spine for symmetry and closure. There should be no sign of openings, masses, curves, dimples, or hairy tufts. The anal opening should be visually patent and the gluteal folds even. A positive trunk incurvation reflex, the Galant reflex, is observed when suspending the newborn supine in the examiner's hand and stroking along the spine in a downward manner. The infant will curve the body inward to the side the examiner is stroking (Figure 19-11).

Extremities

The extremities of the full-term newborn are symmetrical and should remain flexed, yet straighten out easily when moved by the examiner. Ortolani's

Figure 19-11 TRUNCH INCURVATION (GALANT REFLEX).

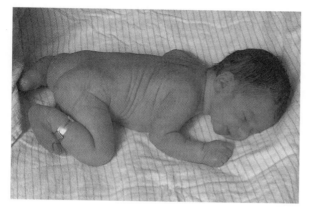

Source: Moore ML, Nichols FH, Zwelling E eds. Maternal-newborn nursing: theory and practice. Philadelphia: W. B. Saunders, 1080–1131, 1997. Reprinted with permission of Elsevier Publications.

and Barlow's maneuvers are used to assess the hips of the newborn for dislocation.

To perform the Ortolani's test, bend the knee and grasp the infant's thigh and lower leg between the thumb and fingers. The examiner's middle finger is placed over the greater trochanter. Flex the hip approximately 90 degrees while bending the infant's knee. This gently abducts the infant's leg. An audible click sound will be heard if the femoral head slides into the hip socket. Then adduct the hip. A second click will be heard as the femoral head is displaced out of the acetabulum.

Barlow's test is used to determine hip instability and will help to identify the hip that can be easily displaced with manipulation. Placing the middle finger over the greater trochanter, as with Ortolani's test, and the thumb placed over the medial aspect of the thigh, apply gentle pressure downward and out to the side. A dislocated hip will again make a click sound and the hip will be reduced as the examiner releases the thumb pressure. Further evaluation is necessary when a hip dislocation is suspected, although in many cases this condition is temporary and resolves without treatment.

The stepping reflex seen in Figure 19-12 is elicited by holding the infant upright so that the sole of a foot is in firm contact with a flat surface. This reflex appears at 34 weeks' gestation and disappears at approximately 1 to 2 months of age. Parents may mistakenly interpret this reflex for the ability of the baby to take his first steps.

Palpate the clavicle for any signs of fracture, which may be detected by crepitus. Rotate the arm through the full range of motion in the shoulder. At this time, observe under the arm for any skin tags. Palpate the humerus, radius, and ulna for symmetry. Compare the brachial pulses bilaterally; the right and left pulses should be equal. Compare the brachial pulse with the femoral pulse again for equality.

Spread the fingers, count, and observe for webbing and the presence of extra digits (polydactyly). Observe the color of the fingernails. Infants who have been in meconium-stained amniotic fluid may have yellow-stained fingernails. Long fingernails are an indication that the newborn may be full term or postmature.

Figure 19-12 STEPPING REFLEX.

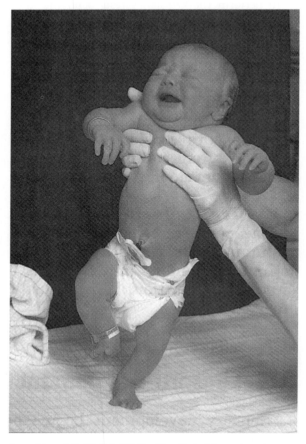

Source: Moore ML, Nichols FH, Zwelling E eds. Maternal-newborn nursing: theory and practice. Philadelphia: W. B. Saunders, 1080–1131, 1997. Reprinted with permission of Elsevier Publications.

Elimination

The urine of the newborn is pale yellow to clear in color and is odorless. The first urination should occur within the first 24 hours of life. The normal newborn will void 2 to 6 times per day for the first 2 days; up to 20 times per day after 2 days, owing to the kidneys' inability to concentrate urine; and later on 5 to 8 times per day. By the end of the first week, the newborn's output is approximately 200 to 300 mL per 24 hours (Wheeler, 2013). The presence of uric acid crystals, or pink or red stains in the diaper, may be insignificant during the first week of life; however, assessment of adequate hydration is important if this finding is noted.

Stool progression in the newborn follows a fairly predictable pattern relative to feedings. The first stool, meconium, usually occurs within the first 24 hours. Composed of intestinal secretions, mucosal cells, and other fluids, this stool will appear black, thick, and tarry. Within 2 to 3 days, the stools will transition to greenish black to greenish brown, then yellow or golden in color. These transitional stools may be watery or thick in texture, and they are odorless and less sticky than meconium.

Behavioral Assessment

The infant's behavior is a reflection of his capacity for self-regulation (Brazelton, 1984). Self-regulation refers to the infant's ability to communicate his needs through body movements, sounds, and visual responses (Salamat, 2010). Infants who demonstrate organized self-regulation are better equipped to successfully meet the challenge of feeding. Furthermore, an infant's reaction to stimuli affects how mothers as well as other caregivers react to the child. This has important implications for breastfeeding as well as parent–child relationships.

Infant state is the foundation for interpreting an infant's behavior. Initially, newborns exhibit a period of alertness (2 to 4 hours) followed by a longer period of sleep. A newborn may sleep most of the next 2 to 3 postbirth days, most likely to recover from the birth experience. Subsequently, infants will demonstrate more organization of behavioral states. Infant behavior is state dependent. Infant behaviors while feeding at the breast follow a pattern as the baby develops. Table 19-4 shows infant behaviors at certain points of development.

Karl and Keefer (2011) have developed an institutional training model using the Behavioral Observation of the Newborn Educational Trainer (BONET). Clinicians may find this model helpful in developing the skill needed to effectively differentiate between organized and disorganized infant self-regulation. The BONET contains 19 behavioral items and 8 newborn reflexes arranged in order of increasing behavioral maturity. Skill and confidence in assessing infant behavior are especially helpful when assisting and educating parents with beginning breastfeeding.

Table 19-4 Infant Psychosocial and Breastfeeding Behaviors by Age

Age	Psychosocial Behavior	Breastfeeding Behavior
First day postpartum	• Quiet alert state after birth, followed by long sleep.	• May or may not feed following delivery; sleepy; learning how to suckle.
1 month	• Follows objects with eyes; reacts to noise by stopping behavior or crying.	• Becoming efficient at suckling; feedings last approximately 17 minutes. • Feedings now 8–16 times per day.
2 months	• Smiles; vocalizes in response to interactions.	• Easily pacified by frequent breastfeeding.
3 months	• Shows increased interest in surroundings; voluntarily grasps objects. • Vocalizes when spoken to. • Turns head as well as eyes in response to moving objects.	• Will interrupt feeding to turn to look at father or other familiar person coming into room and to smile at mother.
4–5 months	• Shows interest in strange settings. • Smiles at mirror image.	• Continues to enjoy frequent feedings at the breast.
6 months	• Laughs aloud. • Shows increased awareness of caregivers versus strangers. • May become distressed if mother or caregiver leaves.	• Solids offered; fewer feedings. • Feeds longer before sleep for the night. • May begin waking to nurse more often at night.
7–8 months	• Imitates actions and noises. • Responds to name. • Responds to "no." • Enjoys peek-a-boo games. • Reaches for toys that are out of reach.	• Will breastfeed anytime, anywhere. • Actively attempts to get to breast (i.e., will try to unbutton mother's blouse).
9–10 months	• Distressed by new situations or people. • Waves bye-bye. • Reaches for toys that are out of reach.	• Easily distracted by surroundings and interrupts feedings frequently. • May hold breast with one or both hands while feeding.
11–12 months	• Drops objects deliberately to be picked up by other people. • Rolls ball to another person. • Speaks a few words. • Appears interested in picture books. • Shakes head for "no."	• Tries "acrobatic" breastfeeding (i.e., assumes different positions while keeping nipple in mouth).

(*continues*)

Table 19-4 INFANT PSYCHOSOCIAL AND BREASTFEEDING BEHAVIORS BY AGE (*CONTINUED*)

Age	Psychosocial Behavior	Breastfeeding Behavior
12–15 months	• Fears unfamiliar situations but will leave mother's side to explore familiar surroundings. • Shows emotions (e.g., love, anger, fear). • Speaks several words. • Understands meanings of many words.	• Uses top hand to play while feeding: forces finger into mother's mouth, plays with her hair, and pinches her other nipple. • Pats mother's chest when wants to breastfeed. • Hums or vocalizes while feeding. • Verbalizes need to breastfeed; may use "code" word.
16–20 months	• Has frequent temper tantrums. • Increasingly imitates parents. • Enjoys solitary play or observing others. • Speaks 6 to 10 words.	• Verbalizes delight with breastfeeding. • Takes mother by the hand and leads her to favorite nursing chair.
20–24 months	• Helps with simple tasks. • Has fewer temper tantrums. • Engages in parallel play. • Combines 2 or 3 words. • Speaks 15 to 20 words.	• Stands up while nursing at times. • Nurses mostly for comfort. • Feeding before bedtime is usually last feeding before weaning. • When asked to do so by mother, willing to wait for feeding until later.

Sleep–Wake States

The normal, healthy infant demonstrates six sleep–wake states (Table 19-5; Figure 19-13). The first two are sleep states. In the first, "deep sleep," the infant cannot be easily aroused even when stimulated. While in the second state, "quiet sleep," the infant exhibits some bodily movements and facial expressions. In this state, the infant is more easily aroused by stimuli, either internal or external. The newborn infant may spend as much as 18 hours per day in a combination of these sleep states. Consequently, the infant will not easily latch on to the breast when in one of these two sleep states.

The third state, "drowsy," is a transitional state. In this state, the infant is relaxed; he exhibits irregular breathing and his eyes are either open or closed. The infant is more reactive to stimuli and may either return to a sleep state or progress to one of the three awake states.

In the fourth state, "quiet alert," the infant is attentive to external stimuli but exhibits little

Table 19-5 **INFANT SLEEP–WAKE STATES WITH IMPLICATIONS FOR BREASTFEEDING**

Infant State	Description	Implications for Breastfeeding
Deep or quiet sleep	• Closed eyes with no eye movement; regular breathing • Relaxed • Absent body movements with occasional isolated startles	• Only intense stimuli will arouse • Do not attempt to feed
Light or active sleep	• Closed eyes with rapid eye movements • Irregular breathing • Sucking, smiling, grimacing, yawning • Some slight muscular twitching of the body • Most infant's sleep is in this state	• More easily aroused by stimuli • Not alert enough to feed
Drowsy	• May have eyes open • Irregular breathing • Variable body movements with mild startles • Relaxed	• Stimuli may arouse infant but may return to sleep • May enjoy non-nutritive sucking
Quiet alert	• Eyes bright and wide open • Responsive to stimuli • Minimal body activity	• Interacts with others • Excellent time to initiate breastfeeding before becomes fussy and agitated
Active alert	• Eyes open • Rapid and irregular breathing • More sensitive to stimuli and discomfort • Active	• Comfort (change diaper, hold, talk quietly) • Initiate breastfeeding before progression to crying
Crying	• Eyes open or tightly closed • Irregular breathing • Crying, very active • Uncoordinated, thrashing movements of extremities	• Comfort (hold, swaddle, talk quietly, rock) before attempting to breastfeed

Figure 19-13 INFANT STATES. (A) DEEP SLEEP. (B) LIGHT SLEEP. (C) DROWSY. (D) QUIET ALERT. (E) ACTIVE ALERT. (F) CRYING.

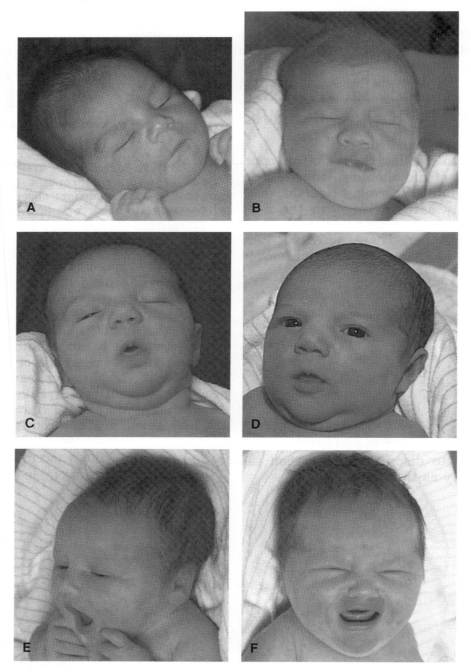

Source: Moore ML, Nichols FH, Zwelling E eds. Maternal-newborn nursing: theory and practice. Philadelphia: W. B. Saunders, 1080–1131, 1997. Reprinted with permission of Elsevier Publications.

bodily movement. Because the infant is calm in this state, this is an excellent time for breastfeeding. If a stimulus is presented at this point, such as the stroking of the cheek or the lips, the infant will become more alert and search for the stimulus. As the infant moves into the "active alert" state, he will become more sensitive to external stimuli, such as increased handling, diaper changing, or bathing, or internal stimuli such as hunger.

The last state, "crying," is a state of much activity with crying and color change (pink to red). The infant is highly sensitive to external and internal stimuli and may need to be calmed and comforted before he will latch on to the breast. Comforting interventions such as swaddling, rocking, and softly singing or talking may help the infant return to the quiet alert or active alert state.

As part of the complete infant assessment, assess the infant's ability to move from one state to another. Observe for any self-quieting activities, such as the infant sucking on his own hand. Also, observe the infant's response to a caregiver's voice or other calming interventions. Is the infant able to move from a crying state to one of the alert states? As the infant matures, he should show increasing ability to move from one state to another.

Neurobehavioral Cues

The cues that an infant gives about his self-regulation abilities assist the caregiver in recognizing the infant's readiness for interactions. Early and late cues that indicate the baby is hungry are seen in Table 19-6. For example, if the infant displays disengagement cues such as yawning, facial grimacing, arching, or rapid state change, he may be indicating a lack of self-regulation and the need for a period of rest. In this scenario, instead of playing with the infant or attempting to breastfeed, it may be better to swaddle, hold, rock, or otherwise provide comfort. In contrast, engagement cues such as alertness, sucking, mouthing, smiling, or smooth movements indicate good self-regulation and readiness for interaction or feeding (Wheeler, 2013) (Figure 19-14). Neonatal reflexes that have important implications for breastfeeding are listed in Table 19-7.

Table 19-6 Early and Late Feeding Cues

Early Feeding Cues	Late Feeding Cues
• Body wriggling	• Crying
• Hand and foot clasping	• Exhaustion
• Bringing hands to mouth or face	• Falls asleep
• Light sucking motions followed by more vigorous sucking	
• Rooting behavior	
• Tongue extension	
• Light sounds or whimpering	
• Body flexion	
• Turning head to the side	

Figure 19-14 INFANT BEHAVIORS. (A) SELF-CONSOLING. (B) SOCIAL. (C) DISENGAGEMENT.

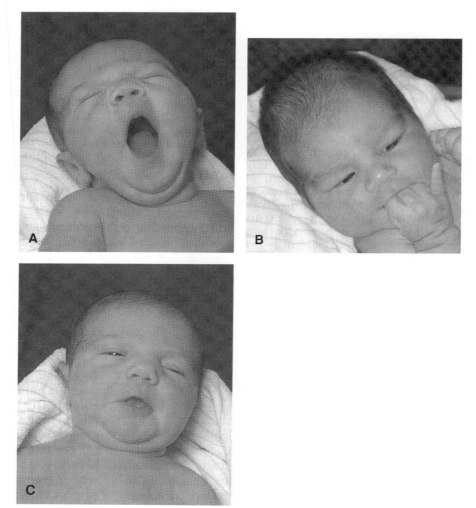

Source: Moore ML, Nichols FH, Zwelling E eds. Maternal-newborn nursing: theory and practice. Philadelphia: W. B. Saunders, 1080-1131, 1997. Reprinted with permission of Elsevier Publications.

Table 19-7 DEVELOPMENTAL INFANT REFLEXES AND IMPLICATIONS FOR
BREASTFEEDING

Reflex	Description	Implications for Breastfeeding
Moro (Startle)	• Elicited by any sudden noise or motion such as a handclap or jarring of the crib or cradle. • Extension of arm and opening of hands followed by flexion of arms on the chest and closing of hands. • Present by 34 weeks, gestation. • Disappears at approximately 6 months of age.	• If the infant is exhibiting the Moro reflex, handle the infant more gently. • Avoid exposure to sudden, loud noises.
Sucking	• Elicited by stimulating the mouth/lips. • Infant will open the mouth and begin to suck. • Appears at 28 weeks, gestation (weak and uncoordinated). • Mature at 34 weeks gestation. • Disappears at approximately 4 months of age.	• Cue for feeding (in quiet alert state). • Nutritive sucking: long, deep, suck-swallow-breathe pattern; audible. • Non-nutritive sucking: light, no audible sucking.
Rooting	• Elicited by lightly stroking the infant's cheek. • Infant will turn head in direction of stimulus. • Appears at 28 weeks, gestation (immature). • Mature at 34 weeks, gestation. • Disappears at approximately 4 months of age.	• May be difficult to elicit in a recently fed infant or one in a state of deep sleep. • Lightly stroking the mother's nipple on the center of the infant's lower lip will cause the infant to turn toward the breast. • Facilitates latch-on.

SUMMARY

A complete infant assessment includes the perinatal history, gestational age assessment, breastfeeding assessment, physical assessment, and behavioral assessment. The purpose is to identify prenatal influences on the health status of the infant, provide a baseline of the infant's health status, and provide early identification of actual or potential problems. Finally, a complete assessment is important when initiating breastfeeding, as well as educating and assisting the parents in understanding how to best meet the needs of their infant.

KEY CONCEPTS

• The perinatal history provides the context for the physical and behavioral assessment.

• The New Ballard Score has its highest reliability when assessed within 48 hours of birth.
• The infant's gestational age classification is useful for determining the infant's vulnerability to feeding or nutritional problems.
• The quiet alert state is the most appropriate time to initiate breastfeeding.
• Behavioral assessment is useful for helping families understand how to meet their infant's needs as well as how to foster positive attachment.
• Providing a warm surface when performing physical assessment is necessary to maintain thermoregulation.
• Inspect the mouth for size, shape, symmetry, color, and the presence of abnormal structures and/or masses when the newborn is both at rest and crying.

- The tongue should be pink and moist and protrude symmetrically over the alveolar ridge when the mouth is open.
- Bowel sounds should be audible within the first hour after birth.
- The first stool, meconium, usually occurs within the first 24 hours.
- Transitional stools may be watery or thick in texture, and are odorless and less sticky than meconium.

REFERENCES

Adams D, Hewell SD. Maternal and professional assessment of breastfeeding. *J Hum Lact.* 1997;113:279–283.

American Academy of Pediatrics, American College of Obstetricians and Gynecologists. *Guidelines for perinatal care,* 5th ed. Washington, DC: Author; 2002.

Askin DF. Physical assessment of the newborn: minor congenital anomalies. *Nurs Women's Health.* 2009;13(2):140–149.

Ballard J, Khoury JC, Wedig K, et al. New Ballard Score, expanded to include extremely premature infants. *J Pediatr.* 1991;119:417–423.

Barron ML. Antenatal care. In: Simpson KR, Creehan PA. *AWHONN's perinatal nursing,* 3rd ed. Philadelphia, PA: Wolters Kluwer/Lippincott Williams & Wilkins; 2008:88–124.

Benson S. What is normal? A study of normal breastfeeding dyads during the first sixty hours of life. *Breastfeed Rev.* 2001;9:1, 27–32.

Brazelton TB. *Neonatal Assessment Scale,* 2nd ed. Philadelphia, PA: JB Lippincott; 1984.

Case-Smith J, Cooper P, Scala V. Feeding efficiency of premature infants. *Am J Occup Ther.* 1988;43:245–250.

Cheffer ND, Rannalli DA. Transitional care of the newborn. In: Mattson S, Smith JE, eds. *AWHONN's core curriculum for maternal–newborn nursing,* 4th ed. St. Louis, MO: Saunders Elsevier; 2011:345–361.

Colson S. Biological nurturing: the laid-back breastfeeding revolution. *Midwifery Today.* 2012;66:9–11.

Creehan PA. Newborn physical assessment. In: Simpson KR, Creehan PA. *AWHONN's perinatal nursing,* 3rd ed. Philadelphia, PA: Wolters Kluwer/Lippincott Williams & Wilkins; 2008:546–579.

Crowell MK, Hill PD, Humenick SS. Relationship between obstetric analgesia and time of effective breastfeeding. *J Nurse Midwifery.* 1994;39:150–156.

Donovan EF, Tyson JE, Ehrenkranz RA, et al. Inaccuracy of Ballard scores before 28 weeks' gestation. *J Pediatr.* 1999;135:147–152.

Fraser D. Health problems of newborns. In: Hockenberry MJ, Wilson D, eds. *Wong's essentials of pediatric nursing,* 9th ed. St. Louis, MO: Elsevier Mosby; 2013:228–307.

Genna CW. The influence of anatomical and structural issues on sucking skills. In: Genna CW, ed. *Supporting sucking skills in breastfeeding infants,* 2nd ed. Burlington, MA: Jones & Bartlett Learning; 2013:197–238.

Hedberg-Nyqvist K, Ewald U. Infant and maternal factors in the development of breastfeeding behaviour and breastfeeding outcome in preterm infants. *Acta Paediatr.* 1999;88:1194–1203.

Hedberg-Nyqvist K, Rubertsson C, Ewald U. Development of the Preterm Infant Breastfeeding Behavior Scale (PIBBS): a study of nurse–mother agreement. *J Hum Lact.* 1996;12:207–219.

Howe T, Lin K, Fu C, et al. A review of psychometric properties of feeding assessment tools used in neonates. *JOGNN.* 2008;37(3):338-349.

Janke J. Newborn nutrition. In: Simpson KR, Creehan PA, eds. *AWHONN's perinatal nursing,* 3rd ed. Philadelphia, PA: Wolters Kluwer/Lippincott Williams & Williams; 2008:582–611.

Jensen D, Wallace S, Kelsay P. LATCH: a breastfeeding charting system and documentation tool. *JOGNN.* 1994;23:27–32.

Karl DJ, Keefer CH. Use of the behavioral observation of the newborn educational trainer for teaching newborn behavior. *JOGNN.* 2011;40(1):75–83.

Kumar SP, Mooney R, Wieser LJ, Havstad S. The LATCH scoring system and prediction of breastfeeding duration. *J Hum Lact.* 2006;22(4):391–397.

MacMullen NJ, Dulski LA. Factors related to sucking ability in health newborns. *JOGNN.* 2000;29:390–396.

Matthews MK. Developing an instrument to assess infant breastfeeding behaviour in the early neonatal period. *Midwifery.* 1988;4:154–165.

Matthews MK. Mothers' satisfaction with their neonates' breastfeeding behaviors. *JOGNN.* 1990;20:49–55.

Matthews MK. Assessments and suggested interventions to assist newborn breastfeeding behavior. *J Hum Lact.* 1993;9(4):243–248.

McGrath JM, Hardy W. The infant at risk. In: Mattson S, Smith JE, eds. *Core curriculum for maternal newborn nursing,* 4th ed. St. Louis, MO: Saunders Elsevier; 2011:362–414.

Morrison B, Anderson GC, Ludington-Hoe SM, et al. *Psychometric validation of the mother–baby assessment instrument.* Presented at State of the Nursing Science Congress, Washington, DC, September 29, 2002.

Mulder PJ. A concept analysis of effective breastfeeding. *JOGNN.* 2006;35:332–339.

Mulford C. The Mother–Baby Assessment (MBA): an "Apgar score" for breastfeeding. *J Hum Lact.* 1992;8:79–82.

Noble Y, Boyd R. Neonatal assessments for the preterm infant up to 4 months corrected age: a systematic review. *Develop Med Child Neurol.* 2011;54(2):129–139.

Olsen IE, Groveman SA, Lawson ML, et al. New intrauterine growth curves based on United States data. *Pediatrics.* 2010;125:e214. doi: 210.1542/peds.2009-0913.

Orr SS. Breastfeeding. In: Mattson S, Smith JE, eds. *AWHONN's core curriculum for maternal–newborn nursing*, 4th ed. St. Louis, MO: Saunders Elsevier; 2011: 315–334.

Palmer MM, Crawley K, Blanco IA. Neonatal oral–motor assessment scale. *J Perinatol*. 1999;13:28–34.

Palmer MM, Heyman MB. Developmental outcome for neonates with dysfunctional and disorganized sucking patterns: preliminary findings. *Infant–Toddler Intervention*. 1999;9(3):299–308.

Radzyminski S. Neurobehavioral functioning and breastfeeding behavior in the newborn. *JOGNN*. 2005;34: 335–341.

Riordan J, Gill-Hopple K, Angeron J. Indicators of effective breastfeeding and estimates of breast milk intake. *J Hum Lact*. 2005;21:406–412.

Riordan J, Gross A, Angeron J, et al. The effect of labor pain relief medication on neonatal suckling and breastfeeding duration. *J Hum Lact*. 2000;16(1):7–12.

Riordan J, Koehn M. Reliability and validity testing of three breastfeeding assessment tools. *JOGNN*. 1997;26:181–187.

Riordan J, et al. Predicting breastfeeding duration using the LATCH tool. *J Hum Lact*. 2001;17:20–23.

Sakalidis VS, Williams TM, Garbin CP, et al. Ultrasound imaging of infant sucking dynamics during the establishment of lactation. *J Hum Lact*. 2012. http://jhl.sagepub.com/content/early/2012 /09/08/0890334412452933.abstract. Accessed February 11, 2012.

Salamat A. Right on cue: interpreting infant self-regulation. *OT Practice*. 2010;15(18):13–16.

Schlomer JA, Kemmerer J, Twiss J. Evaluating the association of two breastfeeding assessment tools with breastfeeding problems and breastfeeding satisfaction. *J Hum Lact*. 1999;15:35–39.

Shrago LC, Bocar DL. The infant's contribution to breastfeeding. *JOGNN*. 1990;19:211–217.

Wheeler B. Health promotion of the newborn and family. In: Hockenberry MJ, Wilson D, eds. Wong's essentials of pediatric nursing, 9th ed. St. Louis, MO: Elsevier Mosby; 2013:185–227.

World Health Organization (WHO) Multicentre Growth Reference Study Group. WHO child growth standards: length/height-for-age, weight-for-age, weight-for-length, weight-for-height and body mass index-for-age: methods and development. Geneva, Switzerland: WHO; 2006. http://www.who.int /childgrowth/standards/Technical_report.pdf.

Infant Breastfeeding Assessment Tool (IBFAT)*

Indicator	3	2	1	0
Readiness to feed	No effort needed	Needs mild stimulation	Needs more stimulation to rouse	Cannot be roused
Rooting	Roots effectively at once	Needs coaxing, prompting, or encouragement	Roots poorly, even with coaxing	Did not root
Fixing/latch-on	Latches on immediately	Takes 3–10 minutes	Takes over 10 minutes	Did not latch on
Suckling	Suckles well on one or both breasts	Suckles on and off but needs encouragement	Weak suckle, suckles on and off	Did not suckle

*Scored 0–12.

Source: Reproduced from Matthews MK. Developing an instrument to assess infant breastfeeding behaviour in the early neonatal period. *Midwifery*. 1988;4:154–165.

LATCH Assessment Tool*

Indicator	0	1	2
Latch-on	Too sleepy, reluctant, no latch	Repeated attempts; holds nipple in mouth; needs stimulus to suck	Grasps breast; tongue down; lips flanged; rhythmic suckling
Audible swallowing	None	A few with stimulation	Spontaneous and intermittent, 24 hours old; spontaneous and frequent > 24 hours old
Type of nipple	Inverted	Flat	Everted after stimulation
Comfort (breast/nipple)	Engorged, cracked, bleeding, blisters, bruises	Filling; reddened; small blisters or bruises; moderate discomfort	Soft; tender
Hold (positioning)	Full assistance needed	Minimal assistance; teach one side, mother does other; staff holds, mother takes over	No assistance needed; mother able to position/hold infant

*Scored 0–10.

Source: Reproduced from Jensen D, Wallace S, Kelsay P. LATCH: a breastfeeding charting system and documentation tool. *JOGNN.* 1994;23:27–32.

Mother–Baby Assessment Scale

Indicator	Mother Score = 1	Baby Score = 1	Score 0–10
Signaling	Watches and listens for baby's cues; holds, strokes, rocks, talks to baby; stimulates baby if he is asleep, calms if he is fussy.	Gives readiness cues: stirring, alertness, rooting, suckling, hand-to-mouth, cries.	
Positioning	Holds baby in good alignment within latch-on range of nipple; body is slightly flexed; entire ventral surface facing mother's body; head and shoulders are supported.	Roots well; opens mouth wide, tongue cupped and covering lower gum.	
Fixing	Holds her breast to assist baby; brings baby in close when his mouth is wide open; may express drops of milk.	Latches on, takes all of nipple and about 2 cm (1 in.) of areola into mouth, then suckles, has burst-pause suckling pattern.	
Milk transfer	Reports feeling any of the following: uterine cramps, increased lochia, breast ache or tingling, relaxation, sleepiness; milk leaks from opposite breast.	Swallow audibly; milk is observed in baby's mouth; may spit up milk when burping. Rapid "call-up suckling" rate (2 suckles/second); changes to nutritive suckling, about 1 suckle/second.	
Ending	Breasts are comfortable; lets baby suckle until he is finished. After nursing, breasts feel softer; has no lumps, engorgement, or nipple soreness.	Releases breast spontaneously; appears satiated. Does not root when stimulated. Face, arms, and hands relaxed; may fall asleep.	

Source: Reproduced from Mulford C. The mother-baby assessment (MBA): an "Apgar Score" for breastfeeding. *J Hum Lact.* 1992;8:79–82.

Section Five

Sociocultural and Research Issues

CHAPTER 20   Research , Theory, and
              Lactation

CHAPTER 21   Breastfeeding Education

CHAPTER 22   The Cultural Context
              of Breastfeeding

CHAPTER 23   The Familial and Social
              Context of Breastfeeding

Breastfeeding exists within the constraints of each culture. Theoretical constructs that allow us to examine the family, its members, and their roles also enable us to identify issues around breastfeeding and to understand breastfeeding women of all cultures. Breastfeeding education, interwoven within the threads of a culture, leads to better care and a more satisfying experience.

As the trend continues toward evidence-based health care, caring for breastfeeding mothers and infants also means measuring clinical outcomes. Thus, lactation consultants need to know about research methods. In addition, they need more research to expand the knowledge of lactation and the variations in breastfeeding behavior. Only with such research will myths about breastfeeding be put to rest.

Chapter 20

Research, Theory, and Lactation

Karen Wambach

Introduction

For lactation consultants, and other healthcare professionals who work with breastfeeding mothers, basing their practice on evidence derived from research findings is the standard. Intuition, gut reaction, and use of traditional procedures are no longer a sufficient base for accountable and responsible professional practice. Practice and education are founded on knowledge generated or validated from data gathered and interpreted by systematic methods that practitioners continually question, study, and expand. Theories provide the structure for systematically organizing and synthesizing knowledge derived from many sources to facilitate its use in research and to guide clinical practice. Both a body of knowledge founded on research and a practice based on the best available evidence legitimize professional care.

The intent of this chapter is to assist lactation practitioners to develop an interest in—and understanding of—lactation research and theories that support them in their role as research consumers. This entails a complex process: reading articles to learn about current practices, understanding research methods to evaluate and determine whether study findings are relevant, incorporating appropriate findings into practice, and consistently

questioning practices to develop questions for further research.

Theories Related to Lactation Practice

Lactation consultant/specialist and other provider practice draws on an abundance of rich and diverse literature generated in the disciplines of anthropology, immunology, medicine, nursing, nutrition, psychology, and sociology, among others. This specialized and in-depth body of knowledge, which is increasingly based on scientific findings, serves as the foundation of lactation practice. Theories are constructions of concepts and their relationships that can be tested through research as well as act as a guide to practice. Theories provide structure for systematically organizing and synthesizing knowledge that may be derived from many sources, so as to facilitate its use in research and to guide clinical practice. As the specialty advances, assumptions about breastfeeding and lactation are tested using theoretical frameworks and theories to guide the studies.

A theoretical framework is a representation of the concepts and relationships inherent in the theory that is the underpinning of a study. Other terms used—often interchangeably, which can be confusing—are conceptual frameworks and models.

All are conceptual structures made up of concepts relevant to a phenomenon that are useful in organizing studies and that make research results more meaningful for application to clinical practice (Polit & Beck, 2012).

Theories range from those that are exceptionally broad in scope, such as grand theories, to those that are very narrow in scope, such as micro theories. The grand theories are complex, often comprising several smaller theories; micro theories are a limited set of propositions about a well-defined phenomenon (Butts, 2015). Theories in the middle range are considered to be most useful to both practice and research, and for highlighting the links between theory, practice, and research (Butts, 2015). The majority of the theories presented in this chapter are middle-range theories. Their selection is based on the interest they have generated among researchers and their historical relationship to lactation and the care of childbearing families.

Maternal Role Attainment Theory and Becoming a Mother

Rubin (1967a, 1967b) attempted to explain the process of taking on the maternal role as a learned rather than intuitive experience. Based on role theory described by Sarbin (1954) and Mead (1934) and observations of and interviews with women throughout pregnancy and the postpartum period, Rubin proposed two fundamental processes of maternal role attainment (MRA): (1) acquisition of the maternal role and (2) identification of the partner—the infant—through psychological processes such as mimicry, role-play, fantasy, introjection–projection–rejection, and the grief work of letting go of a former role until a new identity or sense of self in the maternal role is recognized. In 1984, Rubin updated her perspectives, replacing the term *maternal role attainment* with *maternal identity* and *maternal experience* and postulating that the maternal identity evolves and changes with the birth of each child.

Rubin's work provided a foundation for Mercer (1981, 1985, 2004), who developed a theoretical framework for studying maternal role attainment during the first year after delivery. Initially Mercer postulated that "maternal role attainment is a process by which mothers achieve competence in the mothering role, integrating their mothering behaviors into their established roles so that they achieve confidence and harmony with their new identities" (Mercer & Ferketich, 1994, p. 382). Findings from studies by numerous researchers (Koniak-Griffin, 1993; Martell, 2001; McBride & Shore, 2001; Nelson, 2003) have provided a base for expanding the theory of maternal role attainment to that of "becoming a mother," a concept that captures the ongoing advancement of the maternal self (Mercer, 2004). Maternal identity is associated with establishing intimate knowledge of the infant and feeling competent and confident in mothering activities, feeling love for the infant, and readjusting to changing relationships within the family and with friends. Mercer (2004) advocates that the ongoing transitions of motherhood (e.g., when children are school age, adolescents, and adults, and becoming a grandmother) should be investigated to expand the theory throughout a woman's life span. Studies conducted by Mercer and associates have shown that links between a mother's breastfeeding experience and maternal role attainment are highly relevant. For many women, successful breastfeeding is viewed as part of the mothering role; thus, when feeding problems occur, mothers may question their competence and mothering abilities.

Theory is always open to further development, testing, and evaluation for applicability to specific populations. Fouquier (2013), concerned with the relevance of maternal role attainment theory in describing African American motherhood, reviewed the literature on the theory using 25 studies published between 1975 and 2007. Most studies that used this theory or concepts relevant to MRA included predominantly white middle- and upper-class women or low-income, single, African American adolescents in the samples. Three qualitative studies of African American maternal transition provided description and amplified cultural and social differences of mothering in the

African American community. Fouquier concluded that the maternal role attainment theory was not totally applicable to African American mothers and suggested that further testing and research using the theory are needed to identify attributes influencing this theory, specifically among larger samples of African American women with demographics similar to those of the white populations that have been included in studies to date.

Parent–Child Interaction Model

Based on empirical research showing that mother–infant interactions influence the mother–child relationship and the psychosocial development of the child, and that characteristics of each of the interactive partners affect the interaction, the Barnard model was developed to represent the caregiver–infant interaction system (Barnard & Eyres, 1978; Sumner & Spietz, 1994). This interaction is influenced by characteristics of the caregiver and the infant. The early work done by Barnard evolved into a program of training for health professionals at the University of Washington School of Nursing, first provided using distance education via satellite—hence the name given to the Nursing Child Assessment Satellite Training (NCAST). This program has continued to grow over the years, and additional information can be found at the organization's website (see the Internet Resources at the end of the chapter).

Caregiver/parent/mother characteristics important for positive interactions include showing sensitivity to the infant's cues, acting to alleviate the infant's distress, and using strategies that provide experiences that foster growth for the infant. Important infant/child characteristics are clarity of cues and responsiveness to the caregiver or parent. Feeding is considered an excellent context for viewing mother–infant interactions. Practitioners throughout the world use the Nursing Child Assessment Feeding Scale (NCAFS; now known as the Parent–Child Interaction Scale—Feeding) and the Nursing Child Assessment Teaching Scale (NCATS) for assessing parent–child interactions during feeding and teaching (Sumner & Spietz, 1994). Certification,

earned through NCAST, is required to ensure that assessments and interpretations are correctly made.

The Child Health Assessment Interaction Model (Barnard & Eyres, 1978; Sumner & Spietz, 1994) is an overall framework that is exceptionally useful for practitioner assessments and as a guide for research. In this model, three concentric, overlapping circles represent the environment, the caregiver, and the infant/child. For use in breastfeeding assessments, the largest circle represents the environment, which can include breastfeeding support from family, friends, and health professionals as well as cultural influences, physical surroundings, and all other extrinsic factors influencing the breastfeeding dyad. The second largest circle, representing the mother, can include factors influencing breastfeeding such as maternal age, education, intent to breastfeed, physical attributes for breastfeeding, and postpartum depressive state. The smallest circle, which represents the infant, includes what the infant brings to the interaction, such as physical attributes and abilities for breastfeeding and interactional behaviors. A small area where all circles overlap represents the interaction of the infant, mother, and environment and the potential influence each has on the others.

Although numerous infant feeding studies using these conceptualizations have been undertaken, those specific to breastfeeding are few. Furr and Kiregis (1982) examined the quality of mother–infant interactions in an intervention study in which breastfeeding mothers received education on neonatal behaviors. Hewat (1998) examined and compared mother–infant interactions during breastfeeding for dyads whose infants were perceived as problem breastfeeders and dyads whose infants were perceived to feed well. Brandt and colleagues (1998) explored the relationship of early postpartum maternal–infant interactions with breastfeeding outcomes at 6 weeks postpartum in 42 Latina mothers in a Northern California setting in which participants were receiving benefits from the Women, Infants, and Children (WIC) program. Their findings indicated that optimal maternal–infant interactions, as evidenced by higher scores on Barnard's NCAFS measured at 28–90 hours postpartum, were related to longer breastfeeding duration. Lower scores on the NCAFS, suggesting difficulties in maternal–infant interaction, were related to weaning earlier than planned.

An ongoing multisite randomized control trial to reduce early childhood obesity is being conducted in Colorado and Michigan ($n = 372$) with economically and educationally disadvantaged African American, Hispanic, and Caucasian mothers and their infants using the Parent–Child Interaction Scale—Feeding (Horodynski et al., 2011). The intervention consists of six in-home visits by a trained paraprofessional instructor, followed by three reinforcement telephone contacts when the baby is 6, 8, and 10 months old. Main maternal outcomes include (1) maternal responsiveness, (2) feeding style, and (3) feeding practices. The major infant outcome is infant growth pattern.

Bonding and Attachment Theory

The concept of maternal attachment in healthcare literature is generally founded in the bonding theory proposed by Klaus and Kennell (1976). This theory attempts to explain maternal attachment to the infant as well as disruption in that attachment. In a study that compared women who had extended contact with their infant at birth and for the first 3 postpartum days with women whose contact with their infant was limited during this time, the researchers found that the mothers with greater access responded differently to their infants, having more eye contact and positive interactions with their infant. Klaus and Kennell postulated that close parent–infant contact soon after birth is critical for optimal child development. In 1982, these claims were modified to include the premise that attachment can occur at a later period because of the adaptability of humans.

In spite of critical reviews, this theory was the basis for recognizing the importance of parent–infant ties at delivery and in the early postpartum period (Klaus et al., 1995). This has led to the following changes in hospital practices that support breastfeeding and mother–infant attachment: mother and newborn skin-to-skin contact immediately following birth, keeping mother and infant together throughout hospitalization, and the practice of kangaroo care in neonatal intensive care nurseries (Kennell & McGrath, 2005; Moore et al., 2012).

Theory of Darwinian and Evolutionary Medicine

The tenets of Darwinian medicine are founded in the theory of natural selection postulated by Charles Darwin in his 1859 publication, *On the Origin of Species by Means of Natural Selection*. The process of natural selection occurs whenever genetically influenced variation among individuals affects their survival and reproduction. Darwinian medicine is the application of Darwin's theory of natural selection to the understanding of human diseases. Emerging in the early 1980s, this biomedical research approach aims at finding evolutionary explanations of vulnerabilities of disease such as infection, injuries and toxins, genetic factors, and abnormal environments (Williams & Nesse, 1991). Evolutionary medicine has the same underpinnings and beliefs, but allows for greater breadth in scope in application. For the breastfeeding dyad, it is the basis for focus on the uniqueness of the infant and the mother–infant dyad as the true unit of study (McKenna & Gettler, 2007). This view suggests that "many contemporary social, psychological, and physical ills are related to incompatibilities between the lifestyles and environments in which humans currently live and the conditions under which human biology evolved" (Trevathan et al., 1999, p. 1).

Evolutionary theory was the basis for a study conducted by McKenna, Mosko, and Richard (1999) on the association of sudden infant death syndrome (SIDS) and breastfeeding and mother–infant co-sleeping. Their findings suggest that the interactive responses between mother and infant throughout the night support optimal breastfeeding activities and are a protective mechanism for decreasing the occurrence of SIDS, although this latter finding remains controversial. McKenna et al. also concluded that the notion of infants sleeping alone meets the beliefs and values of Western culture rather than the biological needs of the infant.

Two other evolutionary explorations and interpretations of interest to the field of lactation are the questioning of whether neonatal jaundice is a disease or an adaptive process (Brett & Niermeyer, 1999) and the relationship between infant crying behavior and colic (Barr, 1999). The conclusions of these explorations question conventional knowledge and treatments for both conditions.

Self-Care Theory

Self-care is the basis of Orem's (1983) self-care deficit theory of nursing, which includes self-care requisites (a mother's abilities), self-care demand or measures of care required and acted on during times of transition or to maintain well-being, and actions taken by a nurse (or a health professional such as a lactation consultant) to assist the client in meeting self-care deficits. In the self-care approach to breastfeeding, the lactation consultant assists, encourages, and nurtures the mother and her family toward effective use of their own resources for achieving an optimal breastfeeding experience. Professional assistance is needed only when a problem prevents or hinders normal breastfeeding. This orientation is congruent with healthcare consumer participation. Self-care theory provides a framework that is especially appropriate for lactation practice where the clients are usually in a healthy state.

A qualitative study in Swedish neonatal intensive care unit used Orem's self-care theory in conjunction with two other theories to explore the experience of mothers receiving "hands-on-breast" assistance from nurses (Weimers et al., 2006). The authors contended that the theory was an appropriate underpinning for the study because Orem insists on actions

empowering parents, who then act as self-care agents for their dependent newborn.

Self-Efficacy Theory

The basic proposition of self-efficacy theory, derived from social learning theory (Bandura, 1977, 1982), is described as an ongoing cognitive process in which individuals determine their confidence or their perceived ability for performing a specific behavior. Factors influencing this ability consist of the individuals' motivation, emotional state, and social environment. For measuring self-efficacy, a behavior-specific, task-related approach is suggested.

Dennis and Faux (1999; Dennis, 1999) used this theory for developing a breastfeeding self-efficacy scale (BSES) that reflects maternal confidence in breastfeeding. In keeping with the theory, the researchers postulated that self-efficacy expectancies are based on the mother's previous breastfeeding experience, observations of successful breastfeeding, encouragement received from others, and the mother's state of wellness. The initial 40-item scale has since been shortened to 14 items (BSES-SF; Dennis, 2003), and both scales are internally consistent and have construct validity. For mothers completing the scale before hospital discharge, the scores on the scale were found to predict breastfeeding patterns, which were defined as exclusive breastfeeding, breastfeeding and bottle-feeding, and exclusive bottle-feeding at 6 weeks postpartum. The findings revealed that the scores for mothers who were exclusive breastfeeding were significantly different than those for mothers who were bottle-feeding. A study by Blyth et al. (2002) showed that mothers who scored high in the self-efficacy scale were significantly more likely to breastfeed and to breastfeed exclusively than were mothers with low breastfeeding self-efficacy, exemplifying the use of this theory and scale for predicting which mothers may terminate breastfeeding early because of lack of confidence in their ability to breastfeed. Continued use of Dennis's scale and self-efficacy theory is readily evident in the literature, with many examples of methodological, descriptive, and intervention research in several different cultures and maternal age groups demonstrating the concept and theory's applicability (Dennis et al., 2011; McQueen et al., 2013; Oliver-Roig et al., 2012; Tokat et al., 2010; Wutke & Dennis, 2007).

Theory of Planned Behavior and Theory of Reasoned Action

The origins of the theory of planned behavior (TPB) is an expansion of the theory of reasoned action (TRA) (Ajzen & Fishbein, 1980). TRA and TPB are a function of intention to perform a behavior, and the intention is the main factor in predicting behavior. The original theory (TRA) constructs are attitudes and social norms; control was added to the revised theory, TPB. Intention, as the antecedent to behavior, includes an individual's determination as to whether a behavior is worthwhile to perform (attitude), the perception about what others think one should do with respect to a certain behavior (social norm), and assessment as to whether a behavior is considered easy to perform (control). Both theories have been used to predict breastfeeding behavioral intentions.

TRA was used in a study that examined nurses' support of breastfeeding mothers (Bernaix, 2000). The findings showed that the nurses' knowledge and attitudes were the best predictors of the support they provided to mothers, but a relationship between intentions and behavior was not found. Thus the major premise of this theory was not supported in this study.

TPB has been used as the theoretical underpinning in several studies that have used different research methods. In studies of infant feeding decision making and breastfeeding experiences among economically disadvantaged pregnant and parenting adolescents, Wambach and Koehn (2004) and Wambach and Cohen (2009) used TPB to develop questions for focus groups and individual interviews. That research laid the foundation for a TPB-based randomized clinical trial in which pregnant adolescents were provided with peer counselor and lactation consultant education and support in an effort to increase breastfeeding initiation and duration (Wambach et al., 2011).

TPB is also the basis of the BAPT tool developed by Janke (1992, 1994), which was later revised by other researchers including Dick et al. (2002). Study results using the revised breastfeeding attrition and prediction tool (BAPT) indicated that it effectively predicted 78% of mothers who had stopped breastfeeding at 8 weeks and 68% of those who continued to breastfeed. The researchers concluded that BAPT is a useful tool for clinicians in determining which women are at risk for premature termination of breastfeeding.

Situation-Specific Theory of Breastfeeding

A situation-specific or micro theory is precisely defined for specific populations, desired situations, or fields of practice. Nelson (2006) developed a preliminary situation-specific theory of breastfeeding using an integrative, inductive approach suggested by Im and Meleis. Nelson's theory proposed that varying levels of conflict versus congruity exist within the mother–infant dyad, between a mother and her support networks, and both between and within the networks, all of which may either block or facilitate breastfeeding. To decrease conflict, lactation/health professionals need to carefully consider their approach to promoting and supporting breastfeeding so as to respect the right of maternal decision making and to avoid any semblance of coercion or paternalism. Nelson proposed the concept of *salutary breastfeeding* as an ideal breastfeeding experience that is positive, healthy, and fulfilling to the mother, and encompasses acknowledgment of diversity in maternal–infant dyads and the situational context. No further testing of the theory has been done to date.

In summary, theories that provide a base for lactation research and practice have been described by numerous authors. Incorporating theory into practice demonstrates cognitive awareness as to the meaning of the *what* and the *why* of practices used, which is a contributing factor to legitimizing a profession.

Origins of Research Methodologies

Research can be conducted in many ways, and the basis of these diversities is often referred to as research paradigms (Polit & Beck, 2012). Paradigms are worldviews that represent belief systems based on philosophical foundations and assumptions (Crotty, 1998). The type of research conducted by individuals is often closely linked to their beliefs, in that they frame research questions congruent with how they view the world. The associated assumptions guide investigators in the research methods used and establish the parameters for conducting the study and interpreting the findings. Perspectives used for developing knowledge in healthcare disciplines are the positivist and postpositivist perspective; the naturalistic, humanistic, or interpretive perspective; and the critical or emancipatory perspective (Gillis & Jackson, 2002; Jacox et al., 1999). Extending the kinds of research perspectives contributes to developing a broader knowledge base for providing relevant health care.

Positivist and Postpositive Perspective

Positivism is the foundation of traditional science methods that are based on objectivity, precision, and a search for accurate, valid, and absolute truth (Fawcett & DeSanto-Madeya, 2012). Often using quantitative research, the ascribed methods are characterized by objectivity, measurement, and control that are context free and void of investigator bias. Investigators use these methods to examine specific variables, control intervening variables, and determine associations or cause-and-effect relationships among variables using statistical procedures. The

goal is to explain, predict, and generalize. Scientists with this worldview claim that new knowledge is attained only through traditional methods.

As philosophers and social scientists challenged these claims during the 1900s, the postpositivist perspective emerged. Based on the same worldview and scientific principles, this perspective is tempered in that certainties have changed to probabilities, and truth seeking is approximate rather than a totality. Greater flexibility in use of methods and adherence to philosophical assumptions is evident, although the debate continues between scientists who hold on to the conservative view and those who accept multimethods as means to understand a phenomenon under study. This perspective dominated health science inquiry throughout the 1900s.

Naturalistic, Humanistic, or Interpretive Perspective

The constructivist paradigm, also referred to as the naturalistic, humanistic, or interpretive perspective, builds understanding of the meaning that human values, beliefs, practices, or life experiences and events have for individuals (Polit & Beck, 2012). Through interactions between the investigator and participants, new information or a new perspective of a phenomenon, and its meaning, is created. With studies generally being conducted in naturalistic settings, all possible variables that influence individuals' perspectives are considered data, and these data are broad and frequently complex. Often using qualitative research, this humanistic approach is congruent with a holistic philosophy of providing health care.

The outcomes of qualitative studies are mainly twofold: (1) theory generation and (2) rich descriptions that provide a deeper understanding of the meaning of experiences, events, or practices of individuals. Theory is generated primarily by the process of inductive reasoning, which means that specific ideas progress to more generalized statements. Thus, from the study of an everyday life phenomenon, variables and how they relate are identified.

Further interpretation of the data can lead to a conceptualization of an experience from which theories are developed (Morse & Field, 1995). In some studies, a rich, linguistic construction of the essence of a human experience showing meaning in a deeper manner can provide greater understanding of a phenomenon (van Manen, 1984).

Critical or Emancipatory Perspective

The critical or emancipatory perspective is based on both the postpositivist and the humanistic perspectives, as well as sociopolitical and cultural factors that influence experience (Jacox et al., 1999). It includes critical theory, action research, feminist research, and ethnocentric approaches of minority groups. The aim of emancipatory methods is to engender social change through or as a result of the research process for individuals or groups that are often unrecognized or considered oppressed. This perspective accentuates growth, change, and empowerment of individuals or groups as well as barriers that limit social change. Participant involvement and equity in every phase of the research process is critical. Research designs and methods may be combined and variable. The methods thought to have the greatest potential to generate the greatest amount of change for a particular group and situation are generally chosen.

Although it is important to understand and recognize these different perspectives as the underpinnings to research, the perspectives themselves are not necessarily method specific. Recently, there has been greater use of multimethods, particularly in large studies, to answer the research questions and study goals (Creswell, 2014). In addition, increasing numbers of studies have been undertaken by teams with representatives from different disciplines, academics to maintain the rigor of the research, and practitioners—and at times patients—to enhance clinical relevance. This trend of research teams conducting studies and the use of multimethods not only broadens the purpose and outcomes of studies, but also contributes to greater research complexity.

Types of Research Methods

Research methods are based on philosophical foundations. Quantitative methods emanate from the positivism and postpositivism paradigm and utilize the traditional scientific method. These methods consist of processes for controlling and systematically collecting, analyzing, and interpreting data about a topic of interest. In contrast, qualitative methods originate from the naturalistic paradigm or human science. The focus is on human experience that is holistic and occurs within a specific context. Collection of information, analysis, and interpretation is generally a concurrent process leading to emergence of new insights. Both qualitative and quantitative methods, as well as observational, historical, and feminist research that is suitable for breastfeeding research, are described in this section.

Qualitative Methods

The origins of qualitative methods are inherent in philosophy and the social sciences. Phenomenology, ethnography, and grounded theory are three methods commonly used, but studies using other methods—for example, discourse analysis, and narrative and interpretive descriptions—are increasing.

Phenomenology and grounded theory methods emanate from philosophy and sociology; ethnographic methods from anthropology; discourse analysis from sociolinguistics and cognitive psychology; and interpretive descriptions from nursing. Depending on the origin, variations of each method may exist as well as specific practices and procedures for conducting the research.

Phenomenology

Phenomenology is a philosophy, research method, and humanistic scientific approach. The objective is to understand the meaning or nature of everyday life experiences or events from the perspective of those living the experiences. As the science developed, variations in phenomenological methods emerged. An existential–phenomenological approach includes in-depth interviews with individuals who have lived the experience of interest, then reflection to grasp the essential meaning, followed by written articulation using the form and language specific to phenomenological writing. These rich descriptions attempt to show how these experiences are lived in the everyday world (Colaizzi, 1978; van Manen, 1990). Examples of studies using this approach are "Persistence in Breastfeeding: A Phenomenological Investigation" (Bottorff, 1990), "Living with an Incessantly Crying Infant" (Hewat, 1992), "Maternal–Newborn Nurses' Experiences of Inconsistent Professional Breastfeeding Support" (Nelson, 2007), and "Breastfeeding in Chronic Illness: The Voices of Women with Fibromyalgia" (Schaefer, 2004). The deeper understanding that practitioners gain from reading these studies should contribute to more humanistic care when they are working with individuals who are currently living these experiences.

A more structured process for conducting and analyzing phenomenological research has been proposed by Giorgi (1985), a psychologist. One study using this structured method addresses women's perceptions of the breastfeeding experience (Hewat & Ellis, 1984). The findings describe similarities and differences of women who breastfeed for short and long durations and discuss a conceptualization of the mother–infant breastfeeding relationship. The complexity of the breastfeeding experience is explained and direction is provided for breastfeeding practitioners.

Ethnography

Ethnography is a method used to explain the beliefs, practices, and patterns of behavior from the perspective of the individuals of a culture or subculture within the context of their environment. A traditional ethnography describes the many facets of an entire culture or subculture, whereas a focused ethnography portrays one aspect of a culture (Morse, 1991a). The purpose is to understand, from information provided by the study participants, the cultural meanings and perceptions they use to organize and interpret their experiences (Spradley, 1979).

Dykes (2005) conducted a focused ethnography that describes 61 women's breastfeeding experiences in hospital postpartum units in northern England, but whose findings are more broadly applicable to Western industrialized and medicalized countries. The identified themes of providing, supplying, demanding, and controlling are based on industrial-model, mechanistic illustrations of breastfeeding initiation within the context of the factory-like environment of many hospitals. Findings support the need to shift emphasis from the nutritional aspects of breastmilk to the relational importance of breastfeeding as well as the introduction of strategies that assist women to regain confidence in their bodies and abilities to breastfeed.

Grounded Theory

Grounded theory is a research method for "generating explanatory theory that furthers the understanding of social and psychological phenomena" (Chenitz & Swanson, 1986). Using a rigorous and structured process, data based on individuals' realities are simultaneously collected and analyzed to develop theoretical constructs (Glaser, 1978; Strauss & Corbin, 1990). The emerging theory represents reality because it is "grounded" in the data. From this new understanding, relevant interventions for clinical practice can evolve.

Using grounded theory, Leff, Jefferis, and Gagne (1994a) interviewed 26 mothers concerning successful and unsuccessful breastfeeding. The categories used to gauge successful breastfeeding were infant health, infant satisfaction, maternal enjoyment, desired maternal role attainment, and lifestyle compatibility. The overall theme or core concept was "working in harmony." The mothers described successful breastfeeding as a "complex interactive process resulting in mutual satisfaction of maternal and infant needs" (p. 99).

Nelson and Sethi (2005) also used this method to examine the breastfeeding experiences of Canadian teenage mothers. The core concept, "teenage mothers: continuously committing to breastfeeding" was supported by four categories described as deciding, learning, adjusting, and ending breastfeeding and the subcategories of vacillating between the good things and hard things about breastfeeding and social support and other social influences. The authors concluded that teenage mothers' breastfeeding experiences were similar to adult women's experiences but that teenage mothers need additional support.

Discourse Analysis

Discourse analysis examines language and how it is communicated in an effort to interpret and construct underlying meanings of participants' experiences, events, or practices (Potter & Wetherall, 1987). Accounts are critically analyzed to understand the social and cultural influences on the participants' perspectives and behaviors. Rich descriptions that are constructed to represent the meaning of the participants' dominant discourses lead to a deeper understanding of their experience.

This method was used by Schmied (1999) to examine the experiences of 25 women breastfeeding for 6 months following their infant's birth. The overall theme was that breastfeeding is an embodied experience, and 35% of the study participants' experience was "connected, harmonious, and intimate embodiment" (p. 328). Mixed feelings were revealed by 40% of the women, and the remaining 25% found breastfeeding to be "disrupted, distorted, and a disconnected experience" (p. 329). It was concluded that recognition of the variance of women's personal experiences is important for practitioners working with breastfeeding women.

In another study using discourse analysis, 76 midwives' interactions with 77 breastfeeding women in two Australian maternity units were observed, with audio of those encounters being recorded and analyzed (Burns et al., 2012). Mothers' milk was verbally and nonverbally referred to as "liquid gold," and the product often seemed to be more important than the process. The analysis showed that at times women were positioned as incompetent operators of their bodily "equipment," lacking knowledge and skill in breastfeeding. "In this context breastfeeding became constructed as a manufacturing process for

a demanding consumer" (p. 1737). The midwives' approach in communication was intensely focused on the nutrition of breastfeeding to the exclusion of relational communication and support.

Quantitative Methods

The major types of quantitative research are nonexperimental and experimental studies. Nonexperimental studies include descriptive and correlational studies that describe or compare conditions or relationships. Experimental and quasi-experimental studies focus on causal relationships and test interventions to determine whether an intervention causes a change in a specific outcome. The type of inquiry chosen depends on the current state of knowledge of the study topic and the purpose of the research.

Descriptive Studies

Descriptive studies are appropriate when there is little knowledge about a topic of interest and specific information is desired. For example, the research questions may address characteristics, influencing factors, or knowledge deficits related to a topic. Findings describe the studied phenomenon and may identify relationships among variables.

A study by Zimmerman and Guttman (2001) examined beliefs about breastfeeding and formula-feeding among 94 breastfeeding and 60 formula-feeding women. Major findings revealed that women in both groups rated breastfeeding higher than formula-feeding for health benefits, enhancement of the infant's development, and creation of a special bond between mother and infant, but breastfeeding was also viewed as restricting a mother's activity. Those who chose formula-feeding did so for lifestyle reasons in spite of their belief that breastfeeding is beneficial to an infant's health. The authors conclude that lifestyle issues should be part of breastfeeding promotion. The findings of some descriptive studies may identify relationships between variables that form the basis for further study.

Correlational or Association Studies

Correlational studies examine relationships between two or more variables and the type (negative or positive) and strength of the relationship(s). These studies require greater type of control than descriptive studies. The data collected are structured to allow for numerical representation for correlational analysis to determine whether the relationships between variables are statistically significant.

A study by Oddy et al. (2003) that illustrates this method was conducted prospectively to examine the association between the duration of full breastfeeding and the child's cognitive abilities measured by verbal IQ at 6 years of age and performance abilities at 8 years of age. Full breastfeeding was defined as breastfeeding "up to the introduction of milk other than breast milk and did not preclude the intake of solid foods" (p. 82). Data were categorized as never breastfed, full breastfeeding for less than 4 months, full breastfeeding from 4 to 6 months, and full breastfeeding for more than 6 months. Among the 2024 participants, longer periods of full breastfeeding were significantly associated with higher verbal IQ for children tested at 6 years and intellectual performance of children tested at 8 years. An interactive effect of longer breastfeeding and higher maternal education was seen with the verbal IQ score but not with the performance score. These study findings add to the growing evidence that breastfeeding is positively associated with children's intelligence in the early school years.

Experimental Studies

Experimental studies examine hypothesized relationships between variables to determine cause (often an intervention or treatment) and effect (the outcome). Rigorous control of variables is integral to conducting these studies. Several criteria are essential for a true experimental study:

- Manipulation of an experimental intervention or treatment (the independent variable) by the investigator
- Control of the experimental situation to eliminate interference or confounding effect of extraneous variables (additional influencing factors) on the outcome (dependent variable), which often includes devising an approximation of a counterfactual condition

(i.e., a control group that does not get an intervention)
- Randomization so that subjects are systematically allocated with all having an equal chance of participating in the experimental or control study groups (Polit & Beck, 2012)

Noel-Weiss et al. (2006) conducted an experimental study that was a randomized control trial to determine the effects of a prenatal breastfeeding workshop on maternal breastfeeding self-efficacy and breastfeeding duration. The 110 participants were randomly assigned to a control or an intervention group, and 92 completed the study. The intervention group attended a 2.5-hour prenatal breastfeeding workshop. A short form of the Breastfeeding Self-Efficacy Scale (BSES) was used to measure maternal self-efficacy both prenatally and at 4 and 8 months postpartum; the type of infant feeding, classified into eight categories, was assessed and compared at the same postpartum periods. Findings revealed that for mothers who attended the workshop, self-efficacy scores were significantly higher at 4 weeks postpartum and a higher proportion were exclusively breastfeeding at 8 weeks postpartum. The results of this study support home visits by peer counselors to increase exclusive breastfeeding rates for longer durations.

Intervention studies in breastfeeding have progressed to targeting vulnerable populations that have lower rates of breastfeeding. For example, Wambach and colleagues (2011) conducted a randomized clinical trial using a combination of peer counselor and lactation consultant education and support provided in person and by telephone with urban disadvantaged adolescents. Study participants (*n* = 289) were enrolled from multiple prenatal clinic and school settings, were 15 to 18 years of age, and were predominately African American, single, and primiparous. The intervention, which started in the second trimester of pregnancy and extended through 4 weeks postpartum, positively influenced breastfeeding duration ($p < 0.001$) within the experimental group, but not breastfeeding initiation or exclusive breastfeeding rates. Additional studies that are similar and have comparable outcomes are needed to confirm these findings. Research is an ongoing process, and many experimental studies about a topic are often necessary before conclusions will be accepted as definitive.

The involvement of human subjects does not always permit studies to enforce the rigor necessary for a true experiment. In many situations, it is not always practical, efficient, ethical, or feasible to randomly select subjects or to expose them to a specific treatment or experience. When an experimental method is used to study an intervention but only one of the two additional criteria for conducting a true experiment can be met, the research design is deemed quasi-experimental. A study by Martens (2000) to determine the effectiveness of a 1-hour breastfeeding education intervention provided to nursing staff in a small rural hospital illustrates this method. Another hospital in a community of similar size was selected as a control because of similarities to the intervention site but randomization of sites was not feasible. Hypothesized outcomes for the intervention site were to increase exclusive breastfeeding rates for infants at hospital discharge, positive beliefs and attitudes among nursing staff, and compliance with the 10 steps of the Baby-Friendly Hospital Initiative. In a 7-month period, the intervention hospital showed significant increases over the control site in all outcome measures except breastfeeding attitudes, demonstrating that a short and relatively inexpensive education session for nurses contributed to improved breastfeeding care and outcomes for mothers and infants.

Additional Methods and Approaches for Breastfeeding Research

Other research approaches suitable for breastfeeding studies that do not fit precisely into the qualitative or quantitative classification are observational, historical, participatory action, and feminist research. Either quantitative or qualitative methods, or a combination of the two, may be used to conduct these studies.

Observational Research

Observational research is important for studying human behavior or events that cannot be captured through interviews or self-report questionnaires. Originating in the discipline of biology and anthropology, ethology is an observational method that explores and examines animal behaviors within natural settings. Behavioristic psychology also contributes structured methods for conducting observational research. Study outcomes can include frequencies of behavioral occurrences, timing of specific behaviors, and sequences of behaviors. Types and timing of behaviors during experiences, practices, and events can add a new perspective on and greater understanding of a phenomenon.

Ethology was used in an observational study conducted by Hewat (1998). Videotapes examined and compared mother–infant interactions during breastfeeding between two sets of dyads: those whose infants were perceived by their mothers as problematic breastfeeders and those whose mothers perceived their infants as nonproblematic breastfeeders. From the initial assessment of the interactions, ethograms—detailed descriptions of behaviors and patterns—were created, hypotheses were generated, and a guide was developed for coding behaviors to further examine and compare the mother–infant interactions of the two groups. Differences in tempo and rhythm of the mother–infant interaction patterns were delineated as harmonic attunement, disharmonic attunement, and disattunement. The proportions of interactions that were disharmonically attuned or disattuned were significantly higher among the dyads whose infants were problematic breastfeeders. These findings provide insights for observing mother–infant interactions during breastfeeding and assisting mothers whose breastfeeding sessions are often active and disruptive rather than calm and restful.

Historical Research

Historical research methods are valuable for exploring past practices, examining patterns and trends during specific periods, discovering relationships, and drawing inferences. Past revelations can increase understanding of traditions and practices and guide decision making. Historical inquiry entails identifying, collecting, categorizing, and determining validity of evidence, critical analysis, synthesis, and writing to present meaningful discussion of the subject (Shafer, 1980).

Millard's work (1990) illustrates the value of historical research. Pediatric literature between 1897 and 1987 showed that although breastfeeding was advocated, advice centered on regimens and schedules. Even as flexibility in feeding times became more acceptable, advice including time limitations continued. Study findings suggest that emphasis on time in regard to breastfeeding and the allocation of control in breastfeeding to medical experts undermined breastfeeding during this 90-year period.

Participatory Action

Participatory action is a type of research method for conducting studies aimed at social action and change. It is based on a partnership between those individuals and groups most closely affected by and involved with the phenomenon under study. All participants contribute and work together through all stages of the research process. Recognition, increased knowledge, and empowerment for those most affected by an unacceptable or substandard situation contribute to eventual change. This method is often used for community development to establish programs with those who desire and will attend a service.

An example is an intervention study conducted in rural northeast Scotland, where breastfeeding rates were low (Hoddinott et al., 2006). In four geographical areas, group-based or one-to-one peer coaching breastfeeding interventions were provided that were specific to the needs of participants living in each area. Breastfeeding initiation and duration increased among participants. At 2 weeks postpartum, breastfeeding rates increased from 34.3% to 41.1%, and they remained higher at all time points examined (1, 2, and 6 weeks, and 4 and 8 months postpartum). Establishing working relationships

and "equal" partnerships with participants and community representatives is complex and challenging but often worthwhile in establishing meaningful programs in a community setting.

Feminist Research

Feminist research is an approach that is congruent with, but not overtly evident in, current breastfeeding research. Whether there is a "feminist method" or whether any research method can be conducted from a feminist perspective was at one time seen as questionable (Kelly et al., 1994). Feminist research is guided by the following principles: (1) it is about women, for women, and done with, not to, women; (2) it should be empowering for participants; (3) it is directed toward positive social change; and (4) it generally uses qualitative methods. A feminist perspective encourages the researcher to focus on women in a societal and political context and to consider cultural influences and attitudes within society as central to the experience of the women involved (Harding, 1987). Feminist researchers recognize the negotiated social act between the researcher and the participants. The researcher defines the study and interprets the findings and the participants decide which information they will share with the researcher (Maynard & Purvis, 1994).

An excellent example of qualitative research in which the participants were active participants in all phases was a study conducted by Spencer et al. (2014). Using black feminist thought and critical social theory as frameworks, Spencer explored the experiences of African American women who had successful breastfeeding experiences, as opposed to focusing on the negative experiences that are frequently focused on in this population. Sequential–consensual qualitative design (SCQD), a three-stage methodology, was used to explore the cultural, personal, and political context of African American women's breastfeeding experiences. Stage 1 included 4 individual interviews with key informants: African American women who assisted women with breastfeeding. Stage 2 included individual interviews with 17 African American women who breastfed at least one healthy baby. Stage 3 was accomplished through a focus group of 7 African American women who breastfed. Qualitative content analysis was used to analyze and code the interviews and focus group transcripts. Key informant interview data supported and mirrored the five key dimensions of black feminist thought, and provided cultural guidance in the development of the interview questionnaire for stage 2 of the study, accessing the personal voice. Themes from stage 2 included (1) self-determination and intrinsic motivation for breastfeeding, (2) breastfeeding as a spiritual tradition, and (3) empowerment through breastfeeding. Stage 3 focus group participants confirmed the stage 2 themes and discussed ideas for breastfeeding promotion. Themes from the focus group included (1) supportive spheres of influence surrounding African American women, (2) corporeal images of the sexual breast versus the nurturing breast, and (3) breastfeeding as activism and an act of resistance. Focus group participants recognized and recommended strengthening support systems to include healthcare providers, employers, faith communities, and family members as a necessary step to increase breastfeeding rates in the African American population.

Mixed Methods

Multimethod or mixed-methods studies that use both qualitative and quantitative approaches simultaneously are fast becoming an alternative research method. Those who support this approach argue that using several methods can enhance theoretical insights, facilitate incremental growth of knowledge, augment the validity of studies, and force investigators to reflect and find new views when, for example, findings from one method are incongruent with another method used. Challenges include the ability of the investigator(s) to reconcile differences in the philosophical underpinnings of the differing approaches; the expense involved in implementing such approaches; investigator knowledge about and skills for working with two approaches; analytic challenges; and the time-consuming nature of the

research (Polit & Beck, 2012). Studies using mixed methods are complex and should be conducted by an experienced researcher.

As an example, a mixed-methods study that used a phased quasi-experimental approach with concurrent qualitative data collection with key informants was conducted by Labbok and colleagues (2013). The purpose of the study was to examine the impact of a modified "Ten Steps" implementation approach relative to a control group. According to the researchers, the mixed-methods approach "intentionally integrated and combined these methods to draw on the strengths of each in our interpretation, both for the planned mid-project modifications and to help examine what worked and what did not work within the intervention elements" (p. 5). The intervention was carried out in hospitals where (1) the Baby-Friendly Hospital Initiative (BFHI) designation had not necessarily been under consideration and (2) the majority of the patient population was eligible for Medicaid benefits. Hospitals were systematically assigned to one of two groups: initial intervention or initial control/later intervention. Baseline findings included (1) a universal lack of consistent breastfeeding records and statistics for regular monitoring/review, (2) widespread misinterpretation of associated terminology, (3) healthcare providers' reported practices not necessarily being reflective of their knowledge and attitudes, and (4) specific steps found to be associated with hospital breastfeeding rates. Facilitators and obstacles to initiation of the "Ten Steps" were identified, and hospital-specific practice change challenges were also found. This study is ongoing and its final results pending.

Elements of Research

The elements of research are essential to writing proposals and reports, conducting research, and evaluating studies. The major elements include the research problem and purpose, the review of literature, the protection of human subjects, the method, the analysis, and the results and discussion. Although these elements are similar for both qualitative and quantitative research approaches, the content and processes vary. This section describes the elements and discusses the differences between qualitative and quantitative research methods.

Research Problem and Purpose

The research problem is a critical component of a study; it identifies what is studied and with whom. The purpose delineates why the study is conducted. There are many sources for generating research problems. For example, questioning clinical practice, observing clinical and societal patterns and trends, building on findings from previous studies, and examining theoretical propositions are all ways of developing research questions.

In the lactation/breastfeeding field, a problem that is suitable for study should be important to the topic of breastfeeding and amenable to investigation by scientific inquiry. It should be meaningful to many individuals or have a distinct influence on a few. A study examining the effect of labor pain relief medication on neonatal suckling and breastfeeding duration conducted by Riordan, Gross, et al. (2001) illustrates the importance of this investigation to all childbearing women and their infants. In contrast, a study about the effect of sequential and simultaneous breast pumping on milk volume and prolactin levels among women who express milk for a prolonged period of time (Hill et al., 1996) has important implications for a few women. Over time, however, extending the application of principles from a special population to a broader population can be explored. For example, Prime and colleagues (2012) examined sequential breast pumping in mothers of term infants, thereby expanding the principles found in earlier work to this larger group.

Criteria that render a problem appropriate for scientific inquiry include the following:

- Suitability of the research design for the research question
- Accessibility of study participants
- Feasibility of the study with regard to time, funding, and equipment

- Potentiality of adhering to ethical requirements throughout all study phases

Reviewing the literature about a study topic provides direction for asking a relevant question and selecting an appropriate method. A qualitative method is indicated when literature is limited about a phenomenon or when more in-depth knowledge is desired. When many studies about a topic have been undertaken, however, the findings often provide a base and focus for further study, and a quantitative method may be most appropriate.

Research problems can be written as questions or declarative statements. Clearly identifying the topic, population, and variables for study is essential for quantitative methods. In qualitative studies, less is known about the topic of interest; therefore, the research question is broader. The purpose in this case is to describe and interpret meanings of a phenomenon, to gain an in-depth understanding of an experience or situation, or to discover variables relevant to a topic rather than to examine variables previously identified. Examples of research questions that can be applied to specific methods are shown in Table 20-1. All of these questions pertain to breastfeeding following a cesarean birth. For quantitative methods, variables specific to breastfeeding duration and a scheduled lactation consultant visit have been specified.

Variables, Hypotheses, and Operational Definitions

Variables

A variable is defined as "an attribute that varies; that is, it takes on different values" (Polit & Beck, 2012, p. 745). Furthermore, variables are measurable and, in intervention research, can be manipulated. Qualitative studies may aim to discover indicators that influence the study phenomenon, whereas quantitative studies identify specific variables for investigation.

Experimental studies have at least one dependent variable and one independent variable. The dependent variable, also called the outcome variable, is what

---

Table 20-1 EXAMPLES OF RESEARCH QUESTIONS AND METHODS

Topic of Interest: Breastfeeding Following a Cesarean Birth

Questions for Qualitative Methods	Research Method	Variables for Study
What are mothers' experiences of breastfeeding following a cesarean birth?	Phenomenology	
What are the feeding patterns of Chinese women who experience a cesarean birth?	Ethnography	
What is the experience of learning how to breastfeed an infant following a cesarean birth?	Grounded Theory	
Questions for Quantitative Methods[1]		
What factors influence breastfeeding initiation among women who experience a cesarean birth?	Descriptive	Influencing variables
Is there a relationship between breastfeeding initiation and cesarean birth?	Correlational	Breastfeeding initiation Birth method
What is the effect on breastfeeding duration among women who experience a cesarean delivery and receive scheduled visits by a lactation consultant (LC) during the postpartum period?	Experimental	Scheduled LC visits (IV) Breastfeeding duration (DV)

[1]The topic and variables for study are more specifically identified in quantitative studies.

---

the investigator is most interested in understanding, explaining, or predicting. In the example of an experimental study cited in Table 20-1, the dependent variable is breastfeeding duration. The independent variable is thought to affect or change the dependent variable. It is the treatment or intervention that affects the outcome; in this example, it is the scheduled visits by a lactation consultant.

Uncontrolled, confounding, or extraneous variables are those elements in quantitative studies that may affect the dependent or outcome variable. Sometimes such variables come between the occurrence of the treatment (independent variable) and the measurement of the outcome variable. For example, if mothers experiencing a cesarean birth

view a television documentary on the advantages of breastmilk for infants following birth by cesarean section, the television program—rather than the scheduled visits by the lactation consultant—may be the motivating factor for prolonging breastfeeding. To "control" the effect of these variables on experimental study outcomes, subjects are randomly assigned either to an experimental group receiving visits by a lactation consultant or to a control group receiving existing care that does not include such visits. The random placement of subjects in each group is expected to ensure that each group is similar in regard to background characteristics, practices, and opportunities. Therefore, if the experimental group breastfeeds longer than the control group (as determined by statistical procedures), the increased breastfeeding duration may be attributed to the visits by the lactation consultant.

Hypotheses

A hypothesis is "a statement of predicted population parameters or relationships between variables" (Polit & Beck, 2012, p. 730). Qualitative studies may generate hypotheses, whereas correlational and experimental studies examine and test relationships between identified variables.

In experimental studies, a hypothesis represents a prediction of how an intervention will specifically influence an identified outcome. The written hypothesis includes these components as well as names the study groups. For the experimental study described in Table 20-1, a research hypothesis is written as follows: "Mothers who have had a cesarean birth and who have scheduled visits by a lactation consultant will breastfeed longer than mothers who do not have scheduled visits by a lactation consultant." In this statement of a hypothesis, the experimental and control groups, the dependent and independent variables, and the predictor (longer breastfeeding duration) are identified.

For statistical purposes, some investigators prefer to write hypotheses in the null form—for example, "There will be no difference in the duration of breastfeeding between mothers having a cesarean section who receive scheduled visits by a lactation consultant and mothers who do not receive scheduled visits by a lactation consultant." In using the null hypothesis, outcomes for the groups are considered the same until it is established that they are statistically different. When this occurs, the null hypothesis is rejected, and an inference is made— in the example, the inference that the visits by a lactation consultant are the reason for the different group outcomes. The visits are then considered an effective intervention.

Operational Definitions

Operational definitions are explicit descriptions of how the major variables are observed and measured—

and how they are integral to correlational and experimental studies. In the Noel-Weiss et al. (2006) study, the independent variable, the prenatal breastfeeding workshop, is described and the outcome variables are defined as (1) number of days and amount of breastfeeding post delivery and (2) maternal breastfeeding self-efficacy measured using the BSEF-SF questionnaire. Numerical comparisons can then be made between mothers receiving the intervention and those experiencing the usual postpartum care.

Operational definitions used in a study influence sample size, data collection, analyses, outcomes, interpretation, and the credibility of the study. In experimental studies and those examining breastfeeding relationships, the definitions of the major variables must be clearly and precisely described for findings to be considered accurate. Clear definitions are also necessary for comparing the results of studies that address similar topics, and they are essential for replication of a study. The number of categories included in a definition is a consideration; however, increasing the number of categories requires larger samples. Measurement of breastfeeding and/or breastmilk is determined differently in studies.

In the Noel-Weiss et al. (2006) experimental study, types of infant feeding over time were compared using the six categories identified by Labbok and Krasovec (1990)—exclusive, almost exclusive, high, partial, or token breastfeeding, and bottle-feeding—as well as two additional categories identified by the authors. Exclusive breastfeeding was defined as feeding only at the breast, and the added categories were exclusive feeding by breast with some expressed breastmilk (EBM) and exclusive feeding by EBM.

Breastmilk intake was measured in a study conducted by Haisma et al. (2003) to examine the extent to which breastmilk is replaced by intake of other liquids or foods and to estimate the energy intake of infants. A complex method called dose-to-the mother, deuterium oxide turnover technique consisted of mothers receiving deuterium oxide, followed by tests of maternal saliva and infant urine over a 14-day period. When infants were 4 months old, findings for the 70 mother–infant participants revealed that breastmilk intake was similar when infants were exclusively (EBF) or predominantly (PBF) breastfed, but those infants who were partially breastfed (PartBF) received significantly less breastmilk. Also, the mean intake of water from supplements was significantly higher among the PBF and PartBF infants than among the EBF infants. It was estimated that the energy intake for infants receiving the combination of breastmilk and formula was 20% higher than the 1996 World Health Organization recommendations.

Lack of consistency in how breastfeeding is defined and at which times data are collected is a problem for comparing individual studies and collecting data and comparing breastfeeding rates in different regions and countries. In 1988, the Interagency Group for Action on Breastfeeding (IGAB), an international organization, started developing standard definitions for breastfeeding patterns (Armstrong, 1991; Labbok & Coffin, 1997), but these were not precisely described and would not support rigorous investigations. Following this, the World Health Organization/United Nations Children's Fund (WHO/UNICEF) published breastfeeding definitions that are used for the global databank on breastfeeding (Labbok, 2000). These include exclusive, predominant, and full breastfeeding as well as complementary feeding and bottle-feeding. As suggested by Labbok, it is the responsibility of all readers of the literature to be aware of the many breastfeeding definitions used by writers and researchers and to "be diligent to ensure that our decisions are evidence based and our understanding reflects the definitions of breastfeeding used in the research" (p. 21).

The problem of breastfeeding definitions has continued into the second decade of this millennium. Labbok and Starling reviewed the breastfeeding research in major breastfeeding- and health-related journals in 2012 and conducted a descriptive analysis of breastfeeding terminology, descriptors (e.g., "exclusive," "partial"), and full definitions. Descriptors were used 68% of the time, and full definitions were given 28% of the time. Among

journals primarily dedicated to breastfeeding research, 43–64% of articles included descriptors, and 20–29% included definition of the descriptor. Among other journals, there was a wide range (0–60%) in terms of providing descriptors, but fewer articles provided definitions. Only 26 articles offered a definition; of these, 21 articles included a citation, mostly derived from the IGAB and WHO definitional schemas. Labbok and Starling called for continued attention by journals and researchers to this issue, and recommended reconfirmation and development of a set of consistently used definitions for the study of breastfeeding behaviors, support interventions, and maternal and infant health outcomes. To achieve this goal, they recommend using an inclusionary international working group process similar to that used in 1988.

Consistent definitions for databases and national surveys that could be used for comparing breastfeeding rates between regions and countries, however, have not been globally determined and remain an issue. In Canada, in 2006, the country's 10 provinces and 3 territories endorsed breastfeeding definitions developed by the Breastfeeding Committee for Canada (2006) that were based on the WHO definitions. The next stage was to have the definitions entered into all provincial and territorial government databases; only then would it be possible to compare breastfeeding rates across the country. In the United States, improvement in definitions for national surveys has occurred in recent decades in the measurement of exclusive breastfeeding and any breastfeeding, oftentimes using the American Academy of Pediatrics and WHO definitions for EBF (see information from the Centers for Disease Control and Prevention at http://www.cdc.gov/breastfeeding/data/index.htm). Examples of surveys using such definitions include the Pediatric National Nutrition Survey (PedNNS), National Immunization Survey (NIS), Infant Feeding Practices Survey II, and Maternity Care Practices Survey (mPINC) (also see the *Tides in Breastfeeding Practice* chapter). In addition The Joint Commission mandated use of the Perinatal Care Core Measure for Exclusive Breast Milk Feeding in January 2014 for hospitals with more than

1100 births per year (http://www.jointcommission.org/perinatal_care/). This measure uses a very specific definition of exclusive breastmilk-feeding, thereby providing movement toward national standards for measuring exclusive breastfeeding at hospital discharge.

Review of Literature

Reviewing literature on a study topic provides knowledge and understanding about the phenomenon. Findings from studies help to formulate the research problem and provide direction for research methods. The purpose of a literature review can be different for qualitative and quantitative approaches. In qualitative studies, an initial review of literature is done for investigator awareness and knowledge of the studies conducted. Because the goal of qualitative methods is discovery or a new view of a phenomenon, literature should not influence the mindset of the investigator during initial data collection. In the analysis stage, study findings reported in the literature are used to compare, contrast, and verify findings of the current study. Findings from a new study may also be combined with those from a previous study to identify new insights and expand current knowledge about a phenomenon.

In quantitative studies, the existing literature will help to clarify the research problem and identify theories or concepts on which the study is based. Identification of key concepts and their relationships provides a conceptual framework or structure for the study. Existing knowledge and gaps in knowledge can be determined using the literature. Literature is also useful in assisting with selection of a research design, providing strategies for data collection and analysis, and interpreting findings.

Protection of the Rights of Human Subjects

Most breastfeeding research involves human subjects. To protect the rights of study participants throughout the research process, investigators must adhere to ethical guidelines. The first international ethical standards were the Nuremberg Code, developed in 1949. This code is the basis of ethical standards developed by medicine and the behavioral science disciplines. The Declaration of Helsinki, adopted in 1964 and revised in 1975 by the World Medical Assembly, provides further guidelines for investigators conducting clinical research. Governments and institutions stipulate ethical requirements for research as well. In the United States, the National Commission for the Protection of Human Subjects of Biomedical and Behavioral Research adopted a code of ethics in 1978, issuing the Belmont Report, a model for many disciplinary guidelines and the regulatory basis for research sponsored by the U.S. government (Polit & Beck, 2012, p. 151). Individual codes of ethics have also been developed by professional associations for researchers within the discipline to adhere to when conducting human research.

The Belmont Report (National Commission for the Protection of Human Subjects of Biomedical and Behavioral Research, 1979) described three broad principles for ethical research conduct:

- Beneficence, which requires the researcher to minimize harm (physical, emotional, social) and maximize benefits to research participants
- Respect for human dignity, including the right to self-determination (voluntary participation and right to withdraw) and right to full disclosure (study purpose, procedures, time commitment)
- Justice, involving the right to fair treatment (equitable distribution of benefits and burdens of research to all meeting sampling criteria regardless of age, race, and income) and the right to privacy (confidentiality, anonymity)

Mechanisms developed to ensure that research is ethically conducted include the investigator's use of an informed consent document and review of the proposed study by ethical review boards. An informed consent document describes the study, addresses how the rights of subjects will be maintained, explains that the subject can withdraw from the study at any time without compromising health care, and provides a contact number for the investigator. This form is presented to subjects when they are recruited. A subject's signature on the informed consent document indicates an understanding of the study and willingness to participate. Ethical review boards—established by universities and many healthcare agencies, school boards, or organizations that are resources for human subjects—review study proposals to ensure that the research process protects the rights of study participants. The investigators are bound by the recommendations of these review boards during the research process.

Method

Each study method addresses setting, sample, data collection, and data analysis.

Setting

Setting is the location of the study or source of participating subjects or sample. In all studies, the setting must be clearly described.

Population

Population, which is often referred to as the target population, is the group of individuals in whom the researcher is interested. For example, it could be all breastfeeding mothers, primiparas who breastfeed, mothers who work and breastfeed, or mothers of preterm infants. Or, in some cases, an object, such as breastmilk, may be the phenomenon of interest rather than individuals. Because it is difficult to study an entire population, researchers generally study a sample of the larger population.

Sampling

Sampling is a process for selecting the sample from the population. The two basic types are probability and nonprobability sampling.

Probability sampling is specific to quantitative studies and is used when investigators want to generalize findings from the sample studied to larger populations. For these studies, it is important that the sample be representative of the target population. This is accomplished by the random selection of subjects from the population—a process requiring that every individual in the population of interest has an equal and independent chance of being chosen. There are several methods of probability sampling.

Simple random sampling is achieved by establishing a sampling frame, in which all members or elements of the population are listed and then numbered. Subjects are then selected by using a computer program or a table of random numbers available in many quantitative research books (Polit & Beck, 2012). Other procedures include drawing subjects' names from a hat or flipping a coin.

Systematic sampling follows the procedure of choosing every nth (e.g., every 8th, 10th, or 100th) subject from a list of individuals in the target population (Polit & Beck, 2012). To ensure that all possible subjects have an equal chance of being selected, the names on the list must not be grouped in any special way, such as by alphabetical order or age of subjects. For example, in a study of the effect of hospital practices on early breastfeeding experience, selecting every nth case from the list of mothers admitted to a particular postpartum unit would be an appropriate sampling technique.

Stratified random sampling is a process of identifying subgroups of a population and selecting numbers of subjects that represent the distribution of the subgroups in the population (Polit & Beck, 2012). For example, if a researcher wishes to study a population of all mothers giving birth in a specific geographic location and learns that the population distribution is 40% primiparas and 60% multiparas, then the investigator will randomly select the numbers for each subgroup or stratum that reflects the population distribution.

Multistage cluster sampling is used when it is impossible to establish a complete listing of all elements for simple or stratified random sampling (Polit & Beck, 2012). Thus this sampling method begins with clusters (broad groups) rather than individuals.

In a breastfeeding study, the first cluster might be a random sample of hospitals across a country, with a sample of mothers then being drawn from selected hospitals in different regions of the country.

In studies that involve human subjects, probability sampling is frequently not possible because all subjects in a population—for example, all breast-feeding mothers—cannot be identified. As a result, many breastfeeding studies utilize nonprobability sampling. Nonprobability sampling is the nonrandom selection of subjects or participants for a study. Methods for selecting the study participants depend on the type of study that is being conducted.

Convenience sampling, sometimes called accidental sampling, is often used for both qualitative and quantitative studies. In this case, the sample consists of consenting subjects from a readily available source (Polit & Beck, 2012). An example would be all mothers giving birth at a hospital or attending a particular clinic. For intervention studies measuring and comparing outcomes between groups, convenience sampling may be used, but random assignment of participants to groups is advocated and necessary for the experimental condition and the ability to make statements regarding causation (Polit & Beck, 2012).

Quota sampling is a nonprobability sampling method in which the researcher establishes quotas for specific characteristic(s) to increase the representativeness of the sample (Polit & Beck, 2012). Stratification is based on one or more variables that would reflect important differences in the dependent variable (e.g., parity, premature versus full-term birth, first-time breastfeeding or not). This type of sampling should not be confused with simple stratified random sampling as described previously.

Consecutive sampling involves soliciting all of the elements/persons from an accessible population who meet the sample criteria over a specific time interval or for a specified sample size (Polit & Beck, 2012). For example, in a study of breastfeeding initiation among WIC recipients, if the accessible population was mothers served by the WIC clinic of a specific city, a consecutive sample might consist of all eligible mothers enrolling in the WIC program

during their pregnancy over a 1-year period. This approach is considered better than convenience sampling, especially if the sampling period is long enough to deal with potential biases that reflect seasonal or other time-related fluctuations.

Network or snowball sampling is a strategy that bases recruitment on asking current study participants to identify other individuals similar to themselves, who may also consent to be study subjects (Polit & Beck, 2012). This method is useful in the study of an ethnic group or individuals with a specific condition for which a support group has been established, such as parents who have experienced a perinatal loss.

Solicited or volunteer sampling is used when the investigator wishes to broaden the sample. Advertisements in newspapers and notices on bulletin boards regarding the research often entreat interested participants to join the study (Morse, 1991b).

Purposive sampling occurs when the investigator selects participants "according to the needs of the study" (Morse, 1991b). Participants are selected either because they are thought to be knowledgeable about the study topic or because as much variation as possible is wanted for the sample.

Theoretical sampling is similar to purposive sampling but is utilized to support the development of a theory, as in grounded theory. As the study progresses, the investigator might determine that more information or greater diversity in views is needed to examine and represent categories and their relationships for expanding the theory (Polit & Beck, 2012).

Methods of Data Collection

Data are collected by asking questions, observing, and measuring key variables identified in the research question. The data collection method must be appropriate to the research method and the study population.

Self-report questionnaires are an effective and common way of obtaining specific information from a large sample. However, questionnaires that can be understood by all participants and are sufficiently broad in scope to reflect "true" meanings can be time consuming and expensive to develop. If they are too long or repeated frequently throughout a study, participants may not complete all questionnaires. This results in study attrition; in turn, if the sample size is sufficiently diminished, determination of statistically significant outcomes may be compromised.

Interviews elicit more in-depth information, but they are more time consuming and expensive to administer. A skilled interviewer is required to ensure explicit and valid collection of data. When more than one interviewer is used, varying degrees of bias on the part of the interviewer must be considered as a potential limitation of the data.

Observations are useful for collecting data about events, patterns of behavior, activities, or interactions. Observations can be unstructured and recorded as field notes. Participant observation is common in qualitative studies. Structured observations of behaviors specific for recording on checklists are used for quantitative studies. Developing a coding scheme that is congruent with the research question and specific to the level of behaviors that are of interest is essential. However, the process must be precise, and it is time consuming. Methods of recording data include paper and pencil, a digital data acquisition system such as a handheld keyboard for entering coded behaviors as they occur, or videotaping (Morse & Bottorff, 1990). The last technique is a means of recording observations that can then be coded more precisely and in greater detail at a later time. The widespread availability of digital video cameras and computer programs for making digitalized recordings has greatly enhanced the use of this method.

Biophysiological measurements—such as infant weight, length, head circumference, respirations, oxygen consumption, and heart rate, as well as the mother's temperature, prolactin levels, and milk composition—have been used in breastfeeding research. Such measurements are only as accurate as the equipment used and the investigator responsible for measuring and recording. Establishing sensitivity and specificity (analogous to reliability and validity) for biophysiological measures is a time-consuming

and exacting process for the researcher and takes special measurement expertise (Strickland, 2004a, 2004b).

Data Analysis

Data analysis is the process of examining, summarizing, and synthesizing the data collected to determine whether the study findings answer the research question. The appropriate strategies for data analysis depend on the research question, sample selection and size, and method and type of data collection.

Application of Methods to Qualitative Approaches

Specific methodological procedures, based on the philosophical foundations of each qualitative method, have been developed. Nevertheless, as qualitative research has become more common, the use of different kinds of methods has expanded and blending of methods has occurred. In the past, qualitative researchers debated whether these changes enhanced qualitative research or whether mixing methods transgressed assumptions of data collection procedures and analysis, thereby compromising the science (Morse, 1991a). It is inevitable that variation in method use will continue; indeed, the application of mixed methods (i.e., both quantitative and qualitative methods) has opened up even more possibilities in terms of methods choice.

Sampling

All nonprobability sampling methods are suitable for recruiting participants for studies utilizing qualitative designs. As the study progresses, theoretical sampling may be used, which will also help determine the appropriate number of participants. As data are simultaneously collected and analyzed from initial participants and as descriptions of experiences are revealed, additional informants may be recruited on the basis of expanding the developing knowledge base. Recruitment of new participants continues until no new information is disclosed and data are fully explored (data saturation) (Chenitz & Swanson, 1986; Glaser, 1978). Sample size depends on the scope of the topic, the method used, and the type of data collection, but most qualitative studies have relatively few participants. The number of study participants may range from 10 to 50.

Data Collection

Methods of data collection include interviews, field observations, and review of documents. In-depth, unstructured interviews, which explore participants' perceptions and in many studies validate the investigator's subjective interpretation of the data, remain the most common method among the qualitative approaches. The interviews are usually recorded and then transcribed for detailed analysis. Participant observation, another widely used method, is particularly suitable for ethnographic research. For the circumstance under study, the investigator observes the activities, people, and physical aspects of the situation while engaging, either passively or actively, in the activities (Spradley, 1980). Field notes of the observations are recorded for later analysis. In phenomenological studies, data resources may be expanded to include movies, pictures, poetry, stories, or any medium that portrays the nature of the meaning of the study topic. Focus groups are also used to augment data collection in some studies.

Data Analysis

Data analysis is ongoing throughout the period of data collection. Each piece of data, whether from transcriptions of interviews, detailed field notes, documents, or photographs, is compared and contrasted with the other bits of data. As the study progresses, the investigator makes interpretations of the data. Study participants validate the investigator's interpretations to ensure that they are congruent with the participants' experiences.

In phenomenological studies, several processes of analysis have evolved. For example, Giorgi (1985) outlines specific steps for data analysis: compiling and examining descriptions about the meaning of a phenomenon, identifying common elements or units of meaning, delineating themes, naming abstract meanings, and generating structural descriptions that embrace the meaning of the lived experience from the participants' perspectives. In contrast, van Manen (1990) describes methodological underpinnings of analysis as "the dynamic interplay of six research activities" (p. 30): selecting a phenomenon of great interest for study; investigating a lived rather than a conceptualized experience; reflecting on the themes representing the phenomenon; describing it through the art of writing and rewriting; maintaining a strong pedagogical orientation; and balancing the research context by considering parts and the whole (pp. 30–31). The lived experience is represented through language, a feat that is achieved by writing and rewriting until the written word portrays a deep understanding of the meaning of a lived experience.

In ethnographic studies, participant observation in the field is often an important component of data collection. In an attempt to understand the behaviors, activities, and experiences of individuals and how they interact with their environment, the investigator becomes an interactive group observer. The environment or culture of interest may be that of an ethnic group, a neonatal intensive care unit, or a breastfeeding support group, for example. In-depth interviews with participants and field note observations are qualitatively analyzed. Ethnographies may be descriptive or analytical. Descriptive ethnographies generally identify and describe social patterns or actions within a specific culture, whereas analytic ethnographies examine social meanings and cultural biases or norms that guide the actions of individuals within the identified culture (Morse & Field, 1995).

Grounded theory research follows an exceptionally systematic analytic process. Data from transcribed interviews are coded and categorized, and connections between categories are made; a tentative conceptualization or theory is formulated, and the examination continues until a core variable emerges that is the focus of the theory. Concept modification and integration continue through two processes called memoing and theoretical coding. The process of analysis is not linear. Throughout the course of the data analysis, codes, categories, conceptualizations, and theory are constantly compared, and the researcher moves between inductive and deductive reasoning. Conceptualizations of relationships are deductively proposed, and these are inductively examined for verification. The analytic process continues until a theory, substantiated by the data, is generated (Glaser, 1978; Strauss & Corbin, 1990).

Trustworthiness of Qualitative Research

Ensuring that study findings are trustworthy and reflect the truth is an essential component of qualitative research. This requires ongoing examination by the investigator throughout the research process. Sources of error may arise during sampling, data collection, and analysis. Factors to evaluate throughout the process include the integrity of key informants in providing accurate data, the interviewer's skill in obtaining the participants' true perspectives, the accuracy of field observations, the generation of codes or units of analysis that represent data accurately within a social context, and the interpretations of the data to determine whether they represent true meanings.

Criteria for assessing trustworthiness, as outlined by Lincoln and Guba (1985), include credibility, dependability, confirmability, and transferability. Credibility is achieved by implementing and demonstrating that the processes in conducting the research are plausible. Several practices demonstrate study credibility: engaging in data collection and analyses for a sufficient length of time to ensure the aspects of participants' experiences are understood; using multiple data sources; engaging others to read and interpret transcripts; involving participants to review data, interpretations, and emerging theories for correctness; and illustrating the experience of the research conducting the study. Dependability reflects the reality; that is, it ensures that the representations reflect the participants' views and situations. Dependability is shown through an inquiry audit, which entails having another researcher review the data, process, and rigor applied during analysis. Confirmability is achieved by developing an audit trail of the data and recording interpretations and their meanings for review by another person. Transferability is the extent to which findings can be transferred to another group or setting. Rich descriptions of the participants, settings, and experiences allow others to judge whether study findings can be transferred to similar settings or populations (Polit & Beck, 2012).

Application of Methods to Quantitative Approaches

Sampling and Sample Size

Probability sampling methods, particularly for correlational and experimental studies, are preferred, so that the study findings can be generalized to a larger population. However, as previously discussed, many studies involving human subjects must employ nonprobability sampling methods.

Deciding on the sample size is a critical issue in quantitative studies. Factors to consider include the study purpose, level of inquiry, design, and type of analysis, as well as the availability of subjects, research funds, and the time frame of the study. For descriptive studies that identify and describe characteristics of a population, sample size will generally not affect study outcomes to the same degree as it will for other quantitative methods. Recommendations are to recruit as large a sample as possible after considering the previously described factors.

Sample size is critical in experimental and quasi-experimental studies that statistically test hypotheses. If the sample size is too small, group differences may not be detected when they actually exist, and a null hypothesis (no difference between groups) is not rejected. The result is that an intervention or treatment that is effective is not recognized as making a difference—a situation referred to as a type II error (Polit & Beck, 2012).

For these kinds of studies, a sample size that is adequate to show true differences between groups can be estimated using a power analysis (Cohen, 1988; Kramer & Thiemann, 1987). Computer software programs are available for statistical computation of an adequate sample size, and investigators generally recruit additional participants to account for those who do not complete a study (i.e., subject attrition). When a research proposal is being developed, researchers frequently consult with a statistician to obtain advice about sample size, study design, and analysis procedures.

In experimental or quasi-experimental studies, random assignment of subjects to experimental and control groups is advised but should not be confused with random selection (previously discussed), which allows findings to be generalized to the population from which the sample was selected. A study that employs random assignment is called a randomized control trial (RCT). Random assignment has two purposes: (1) it ensures that all subjects have an equal and independent chance of receiving the treatment, and (2) it increases the probability that each group will be similar to the others in regard to background characteristics. The latter consideration serves as a means of controlling extraneous variables that may influence the effect of treatment. Many RCTs also use a procedure called intention to treat (ITT) in data analysis, which means that all participants are included in the analysis of the data even if they did not complete the study. Depending on the number of participants who are lost before the investigation is complete, study results may be compromised.

Correlational studies and those using survey questionnaires generally require large samples. The size depends on the number of variables to be examined and the number of subgroups to be compared. As each of these factors increases, so must the sample size. If sample sizes are insufficient, statistical analyses and study findings can be compromised.

Two types of epidemiological studies examine associations between variables such as exposure (risk factors) and a disease or health condition: (1) case-control studies and (2) cohort studies. In case-control studies, subjects with a specific condition are compared, generally retrospectively, with a control group whose members do not have the condition.

Differences between the two groups in the subjects' past experiences or life events are examined to identify factors that may lead to the onset of the condition (Polit & Beck, 2012). Cohort studies are similar except that they are generally follow-up studies of subjects who were exposed or not exposed to a risk factor that is assumed to be associated with the onset of an identified health problem. The subjects are followed prospectively to the presumed effect (Polit & Beck, 2012). For example, during the past decade or so, there has been increasing interest in the relationship of breastfeeding exclusivity and duration and diseases such as infant and childhood leukemia, diabetes, lower respiratory tract infections, and gastroenteritis, as well as the effect of breastfeeding on maternal risks of type 2 diabetes and breast and ovarian cancers. The review of these relationships carried out by Ip et al. (2007) included case-control and cohort studies, as well as systematic reviews and controlled trials to provide this information.

Data Collection

All of the methods of data collection described to this point are applicable to quantitative studies if they are applied consistently and objectively. Descriptive studies gather data that are broader in scope or more subjective than correlational or experimental studies. However, questionnaires, interview schedules, and observation criteria must be structured so that the same data are collected in the same manner from all subjects. Quantitative studies, such as correlational, quasi-experimental, and experimental studies, require data that can be reduced to numbers so that statistical procedures can be performed. Reliable and valid questionnaires and observation checklists used for measuring variable relationships often take years to develop. Once established, they may be used in numerous studies.

Reliability and validity estimates of the existing breastfeeding questionnaires and scales are widely available in the literature. Table 20-2 presents an overview of selected tools and what is known about their reliability and validity. Some of the tools can be found in the *Infant Assessment* chapter. For correlational and experimental studies, it is recommended that the questionnaires or measures used for data collection be both reliable and valid.

Reliability and Validity

Reliability and validity are central issues concerned with measurement error in research. Occurrence of error at any stage of the research process can affect study outcomes and limit the usefulness of the study

findings. Reliability refers to the accuracy, consistency, precision, and stability of measurement or data collection. Validity reflects the truth, accuracy, and reality of the data. To be valid, measures and methods of data collection must also be reliable.

Reliability

Accuracy and consistency in the way data are collected, as well as the tools or instruments used, are essential in quantitative studies. Several aspects of

Table 20-2 SELECTED BREASTFEEDING QUESTIONNAIRES AND ASSESSMENT TOOLS

Title	Purpose	Reliability (Original Testing and Selected Other Assessment)	Validity
Breastfeeding Attrition Prediction Tool (BAPT) (Janke 1992, 1994; Wambach et al., 2011) Modified BAPT Tool (Dick et al., 2002) Translation of BAPT: Spanish (Gill et al., 2007) Turkish (Karayağiz Muslu et al., 2011)	Based on the theory of planned behavior. To identify women at risk for early, unintended weaning. Four factors measure negative and positive breastfeeding attitude, perceived maternal control, and social and professional support.	Cronbach's alpha for all BAPT scales, 0.79–0.85 (Janke, 1992, 1994); 0.87–0.93 (Wambach et al. 2011). Modified BAPT 0.81–0.86 (Dick et al., 2002) Spanish BAPT: 0.78–0.86 (Gill et al., 2007) Turkish BAPT: 0.80–0.92 (Karayağiz Muslu et al., 2011)	Predictive validity: Three of four scales related to 8-week feeding outcome, and negative sentiment scale predicted early unintended weaning (Janke, 1992, 1994). Modified BAPT: Two scales predicted 78% women who discontinued breastfeeding at 8 weeks and 68% of those still breastfeeding (Dick et al., 2002). Turkish BAPT: Confirmatory factor analysis for construct validity confirmed 4 factors/subscales. Known group comparisons lent support for construct validity (Karayağiz Muslu et al., 2011).
Maternal Breastfeeding Evaluation Scale (MBFES) (Leff et al., 1994b; Riordan et al., 1994).	To measure a mother's overall evaluation of the breastfeeding experience using a 30-item Likert scale. Subscales include maternal enjoyment, role attainment, infant satisfaction/growth, and lifestyle/maternal body image.	Test–retest correlations: 0.82–0.93 Cronbach's alpha for subscales: 0.80–0.93 (Leff et al., 1994b) and 0.73–0.83 (Riordan et al., 1994)	Items developed from qualitative study (Leff et al., 1994a). Predictive validity: Significant positive correlation of total scale and subscales with maternal satisfaction and breastfeeding intent and duration (Leff et al., 1994b; Riordan et al., 1994).

Table 20-2 SELECTED BREASTFEEDING QUESTIONNAIRES AND ASSESSMENT TOOLS (*CONTINUED*)

Title	Purpose	Reliability (Original Testing and Selected Other Assessment)	Validity
Breastfeeding Self-Efficacy Scale (32 items) (BSES) (Dennis & Faux, 1999) Modified Short Form (14 items) (BSES-SF) (Dennis, 2003) Modified Short Form testing with adolescents (Dennis et al., 2011) Translation of BSES-SF: Turkish (Tokat et al., 2010)	To determine breastfeeding self-efficacy and to identify breastfeeding mothers at high risk, and assess breastfeeding behaviors and cognitions to individualize confidence-building strategies (Dennis, 2003).	Both forms, Cronbach's alpha: 0.96 (Dennis, 2003; Dennis & Faux, 1999) Adolescent testing: Prenatal 0.84; postnatal 0.93 (Dennis, 2003) Turkish BSES-SF: Prenatal 0.87; postnatal 0.86	Content validity. Predictive validity: Significant differences between breastfeeding and bottle-feeding at 4 and 8 weeks postpartum. Construct validity: contrasts and correlations with similar construct measures. Adolescent testing: Prenatal BSES-SF scores significantly predicted breastfeeding initiation, while prenatal and postnatal scores predicted duration and exclusivity to 4 weeks postpartum. Turkish BSES: Antenatal and postnatal BSES-SF scores were significant predictors of breastfeeding duration and exclusivity at 12 weeks (Tokat et al., 2010).
LATCH Breastfeeding Assessment Tool (Jensen et al., 1994) Testing the LATCH for use in telehealth assessment (Rojjanasrirat et al., 2012)	To assess effective breastfeeding in first week for latch-on, audible swallowing, nipple type, comfort of breast/nipple, and help needed to position baby.	Interrater reliability: Mothers' and nurses' total scores positively correlated (Riordan, Bibb, et al., 2001) Interrater reliability, percentage agreement between telehealth and home-visit International Board Certified Lactation Consultants (IBCLCs) for 2 visits on the 5 LATCH dimensions: 40–100% and 80–100%, respectively	Requires further testing, but mothers' total scores positively correlated with breastfeeding at 8 weeks postpartum (Kumar et al., 2006; Riordan, Bibb, et al., 2001).
Infant Breastfeeding Assessment Tool (IBFAT) (Matthews, 1988)	To assess and measure infant breastfeeding competence. Four subscales: readiness to feed, rooting, fixing, and sucking.	Interrater reliability: 1% agreement in coassessed feeds (Matthews, 1988) Pairwise correlations of raters .58 (Riordan & Koehn, 1997)	Content validity and observation in clinical practice (Matthews, 1988).

reliability should be addressed when designing and conducting such a study.

Interrater reliability refers to accuracy and consistency in data collection when more than one individual or instrument (such as a thermometer) is used for data collection (Waltz et al., 2010). In such instances the probability of error between the individuals or instruments increases. To control this aspect, checks are made. Similar instruments, or single instruments used across data collection periods with multiple respondents, should be calibrated until measurement is consistent. For individuals making similar observations, the degree of their accuracy can be statistically determined. Acceptable levels of reliability depend on the statistical method used—for example, for interobserver reliability, an agreement of 90% is adequate. When using the Cohen's kappa statistic, a procedure that corrects for level of chance agreement, an acceptable level is 0.70 (Bakeman & Gottman, 1986). For the Infant Breastfeeding Assessment Tool (IBFAT) described in Table 20-2, interrater reliability was determined by Matthews (1988, 1991) by comparing agreement of the mother's and the investigator's breastfeeding assessments. Overall, agreement was 91% accurate, although it was noted that infants who fed well or poorly were easier to assess than those who rated in the middle range and were classified as moderate feeders. Johnson, Mulder, and Strube (2007) report the percent agreement among three health professionals as follows: more than 90% for responsiveness to feeding cues, timing of feeding, and nutritive sucking bursts; 80% to 88% range for position and latch factors; and 79% agreement for maternal nipple trauma.

Intrarater reliability refers to the accuracy and consistency of observations made by one rater over time (Waltz et al., 2010). For example, when data are collected for more than 6 months, investigators may want to check the accuracy of the individual who is making the observations—and the instrument(s) used—every few months. Likewise, repeated observations over short periods of time by the same rater warrant assessment of intrarater reliability.

Calculations and acceptability are similar to interrater reliability.

Test–retest reliability indicates the stability of a measure, such as a questionnaire, over time (Waltz et al., 2010). Results of two questionnaire administrations to the same subjects, occurring approximately 2 to 3 weeks apart, are statistically compared. A coefficient reported as 0.80 or greater is generally acceptable for measurement questionnaires that reflect attitudes or feelings. In contrast, for some events, such as postpartum adjustment, a low correlation coefficient (such as 0.40 or 0.50) may be desired because differences in individual scores over a period of time reflect inconsistency and may indicate that the individual is changing or adjusting to a different lifestyle. In such a case, test–retest reliability would not be an appropriate measure of reliability. The Maternal Breastfeeding Evaluation Scale (MBFES), as described in Table 20-2, is highly reliable over time.

Internal consistency refers to the statistical agreement of several items on a questionnaire that reflect the meaning of a concept. Generally, we would expect respondents to answer items consistently if we are measuring a single concept—for example, satisfaction with breastfeeding (Waltz et al., 2010). Similarity in meaning or internal consistency of the items can be statistically determined. Cronbach's alpha, based on the average correlation among items and the number of items, is a reliability coefficient that is frequently computed to determine internal consistency. A coefficient of 0.70 to 0.80 is generally acceptable for a questionnaire measuring a construct (Nunnally, 1978). Values greater than 0.80 are preferable for scales that have been used over time, that is, are more mature. And when scores are being used to make decisions about individuals, scores at 0.90 are desirable (Waltz et al., 2010). It should be noted that the alpha coefficient is sensitive to the number of items on a scale; the more items, the higher alpha. Thus the Breastfeeding Attrition Prediction Tool (BAPT), the MBFES, and the Breastfeeding Self-Efficacy Scale (BSES), as described in Table 20-2, are all internally consistent questionnaires for data collection.

Validity

Validity addresses the extent to which a questionnaire or measurement instrument reflects the meaning of the concept that is being measured or does what it is intended to do (Waltz et al., 2010). Facets of validity referred to in quantitative studies are content, criterion, and construct validity. Questionnaires and interview schedules used for descriptive studies should have content validity, which means that the questions or items adequately represent the study concepts. In developing questionnaires, investigators review the literature to include dimensions of the concept being studied and then submit the questionnaire to individuals who are considered experts on the research topic for review. This validation of content with literature and experts leads to the characteristic known as content validity. Formalized procedures for assessing content validity and calculation of a content validity index (CVI) of measures have come to be an expected and very important part of the overall instrument development process (Polit & Beck, 2006).

Criterion-related validity is of importance when we want to infer from a measure an individual's probable standing on some other outside measure, generally a higher-order operationalization of the construct (Waltz et al., 2010). Predictive validity, a form of criterion-related validity, ascertains whether a measure at one time can predict future outcomes. Concurrent validity, another form of criterion-related validity, determines whether a measure may be used to estimate present standing on the criterion.

Construct validity assesses the degree to which a tool measures what it is intended to measure and does so in the context of the theoretical basis of the measure (Waltz et al., 2010). In Table 20-2, the BAPT, MBFES, and BFES-SF all show evidence of predictive validity for breastfeeding outcomes, as well as construct validity based on the support of theoretical relationships undergirding the concepts. The use of questionnaires and tools demonstrating these types of validity enhances the credibility of study findings.

Data Analysis

Data analysis is the process of organizing, summarizing, examining, and synthesizing the data collected so as to reach conclusions about the research question. Numerical analysis of data is central to quantitative studies. The data collected are converted to numerical values in a variety of ways. Table 20-3 defines levels of measurement and provides examples. The level of measurement has implications for the statistical procedures applied.

Two classes of statistical procedures are distinguished: parametric and nonparametric (Polit &

Table 20-3 LEVELS OF MEASUREMENT

	Nominal	Ordinal	Interval/Ratio
Definitions	Discreet categories of data that do not have any implied order.	Assigned categories of data that can be ranked in order; intervals between categories are not equal.	Categories of data that are ordered and are equal distances apart. Ratio also has a known zero point.
Examples	Gender: male/female Breastfed/not breastfed Marital status	Most Likert-type scales BAPT, MBFES, BSES, and IBFAT scales (see Table 20-2)	Body temperature Blood pressure Weight or length Duration of breastfeeding measured in specified days, weeks, months, or years.

Beck, 2012). Parametric tests are more powerful and preferred because they permit inferences to be made from findings of the study sample to the larger population. The use of parametric procedures requires that certain assumptions be met, including normal distribution of the variable responses and measurement of the dependent variable(s) at an interval level. Nonparametric statistics are more suitable for situations in which the distribution of variable responses in the sample cannot be assumed to be normal, the parameters of the population are unknown, and the level of measurement of variables is at a nominal or ordinal level.

The selection of an appropriate statistical procedure is dependent on the type of study, sample size, sampling procedure, and level or type of data to be analyzed. Table 20-4 identifies commonly used procedures based on the study type and level of data. In experimental or quasi-experimental studies, the level of data of the dependent variable dictates the type of statistical testing that can be done. Table 20-4 is intended to assist research novices in recognizing the appropriate use of statistics for reviewing studies. Extensive information about statistical procedures is beyond the scope of this chapter.

The choice of interval versus ordinal data is controversial. Human feelings and perceptions do not fit the interval scale, and most psychosocial variables can only be superimposed on an ordinal scale. Therefore, statistical procedures that traditionally require interval data are sometimes used with ordinal data based on human responses.

Descriptive Studies

Data collected to describe variables and their relationships are generally subjected to content analysis and descriptive statistics. Content analysis consists of examining the data, identifying similar content or meanings, and classifying those that are identified into mutually exclusive categories. These nominal data can then be used with the descriptive statistics identified in Table 20-4. Findings may be reported as frequencies, percentages, or modes; they may be displayed as bar graphs, pie charts, or contingency tables.

Correlational Studies

Correlation coefficients are the outcomes of statistical procedures for determining the relationship between two variables. The type of relationship is reported as positive (as one variable increases, so does the other), negative (variables both decrease), or inverse (as one variable increases, the other decreases). The strength of the relationship is reported as a number between 0 and +/−1; stronger relationships are near 1 (positive or negative), and 0 indicates no relationship.

Associations in epidemiological studies are estimated using the relative risk (or risk ratio; RR) and odds ratio (OR). Studies in which a subpopulation is followed and examined in regard to specific health factors can determine the probability or rate of incidence of developing a specific condition for a group exposed to an identified factor. An example is the rate of incidence of infants developing otitis media among those exclusively breastfed compared to those who are fed breastmilk substitutes. The incidence rate for one group (breastfed infants) is divided by the incidence rate for the other group (infants fed breastmilk substitutes) to determine the relative risk (Polit & Beck, 2012). In some types of studies, such as case-control studies, it is not possible to determine the incidence rate, but an odds ratio can be estimated by calculating the ratio of the odds of exposure among the cases (e.g., the exclusively breastfed infants) to that among the control group (e.g., infants fed breastmilk substitutes) (Hennekens et al., 1987). A relative risk or odds ratio of 1.0 suggests that the incidence rate of disease is the same for both the exposed and nonexposed groups. However, a value greater than 1—for example, 1.5—indicates an increased risk of 1.5 times or 50% higher among those exposed to the factor. Ratios less than 1 indicate decreased risk among those exposed. Odds ratios are often reported with confidence intervals, which "represent the range within which the true magnitude of effect lies with a certain degree of assurance" (Hennekens et al., 1987).

Table 20-4 STATISTICAL TESTS APPROPRIATE FOR LEVEL OF MEASUREMENT: A BASIC GUIDE

Numerical Descriptors for Univariate Analysis (One Variable)

Descriptors or Measures of Central Tendency

Numerical Descriptor	Function	Level of Measurement
Mode	Indicates most common value/score	Nominal
Median	Indicates value that is the middle position of a distribution of values	Ordinal
Mean	Indicates the average score	Interval or ratio

Descriptors or Measures of Variability

Range	Shows values/scores in a distribution; highest to lowest	
Standard Deviation	Indicates average deviation values from the mean	Interval or ratio

Descriptors for Bivariate Studies or Two Variables

Contingency table	Shows cross-tabulation of frequency distributions of two variables	Nominal or ordinal (two variables)

Commonly Used Statistical Tests for Bivariate Analysis (Two Variables)

Nonparametric Tests

Test & Test Statistic	Test Function	Measurement Level of IV	Measurement Level of DV
Chi square (χ^2)	Differences in proportions (frequency data) between two or more independent groups	Nominal or ordinal*	Nominal
Fisher exact test	Differences in proportions between two or more independent groups—used when samples sizes are small or <5 per cell	Nominal	Nominal
Median test (χ^2)	Differences between medians of two independent groups	Nominal	Ordinal
Mann-Whitney U (U)	Differences in ranks of scores/values of two independent groups	Nominal	Ordinal
McNemar's test (χ^2)	Differences in proportions within paired samples	Nominal	Nominal
Wilcoxon paired signed-rank test	Differences in ranks of scores within two dependent groups	Nominal	Ordinal
Kruskal Wallis	Differences in ranks of scores of three or more independent groups	Nominal	Ordinal
Spearman's rho (ρ)	Determines correlation between two variables	Ordinal	Ordinal
Kendall's tau (τ)	Determines correlation between two variables	Ordinal	Ordinal

(continues)

Table 20-4 STATISTICAL TESTS APPROPRIATE FOR LEVEL OF MEASUREMENT:
A BASIC GUIDE (*CONTINUED*)

Parametric Tests

Pearson's product moment correlation (*r*)	Determines correlation between two variables	Interval or ratio	Interval or ratio
t-test (*t*)	Differences between two independent group means	Nominal	Interval or ratio
t-test, pooled (*t*)	Differences between two related group means	Nominal	Interval or ratio
Analysis of variance (ANOVA) (*F*)	Differences between three or more independent groups	Nominal	Interval or ratio
Repeated measures ANOVA (*F*)	Differences between three or more related groups or scores	Nominal	Interval or ratio

Commonly Used Statistical Tests for Multivariate Analysis

Test	Test Function	Measurement Level and Number of IDs	Measurement Level and Number of DVs
Analysis of covariance (ANCOVA)	Differences between means of two or more groups and controls for one or more covariates	Nominal, one or more variables	Interval or ratio, one variable
Multivariate analysis of variance (MANOVA)	Differences between means of two or more groups for two or more dependent variables	Nominal, one or more variables	Interval or ratio, two or more variables
Multivariate analysis of covariance (MANCOVA)	Differences between means of two or more groups for two or more DVs. Controls for one or more covariates	Nominal, one or more variables	Interval or ratio, two or more variables
Multiple regression	Determine relationship between two or more IVs and one DV	Nominal, interval, or ratio, two or more variables	Interval or ratio, one variable
Canonical correlation	Determine relationship between two sets of variables	Nominal, interval, or ratio, two or more variables	Nominal, interval, or ratio, two or more variables
Logistic regression	Determine relationship between two or more IVs and one DV	Nominal, interval, or ratio, two or more variables	Nominal, one variable
Discriminant function analysis	Determine relationships between two or more IVs and one DV and identify group membership	Nominal, interval, or ratio, two or more variables	Nominal, one variable
Factor analysis	Examines interrelationships among numerous variables to identify clusters of variables that are similar		

Experimental and Quasi-experimental Studies

The statistical procedure used to determine differences between groups depends on the number of groups and the level of measurement of the dependent variable, as shown in Table 20-4. Statistical differences are calculated using probability theory. Before conducting the analysis, the investigator decides on a level of significance—or a *P* value—that will be used as a cutoff for accepting that a statistically significant result indicates true differences between groups. The *P* value reflects the probability that the statistical result can occur by chance, and it establishes the risk of the investigator making a type I error. This means that a null hypothesis is rejected when in reality the hypothesis is true, leading to an incorrect interpretation that an intervention was successful. Conversely, a type II error is the acceptance of a null hypothesis when it is actually false; in this situation, an intervention that is successful is not recognized as such.

In research, *P* values of 0.01 or 0.05 are most commonly used. A 0.01 *P* value means that there is 1 chance out of 100 that a type I error could occur; a 0.05 *P* value means that there are 5 chances out of 100 that a type I error could be made. Reducing the chance of a type I error, however, increases the probability of a type II error (Polit & Beck, 2012). For this reason, most investigators conducting breastfeeding research elect to use a *P* value of 0.05.

As well as a *P* value, differences between groups, such as the outcomes of two groups exposed to different care interventions, are based on a critical value of the statistical procedure used. Results may be reported numerically as a confidence interval (CI), which comprises a range of values and shows that an investigator is either 95% or 99% confident that values for a population falls within the specified range. A CI that is small in range is more precise than a CI with a wide range of values (Polit & Beck, 2012).

Multivariate Analysis

Multivariate analysis is the concurrent analysis of three or more variables to determine patterns of relationships between variables. These advanced statistical procedures are suitable for analyzing data from complex correlational and experimental studies that have several independent and/or several dependent variables (Tabachnick & Fidell, 2007). Generally, large sample sizes are required to accommodate analysis of increasing numbers of variables. The procedures commonly used include multiple regression, path analysis, analysis of covariance (ANCOVA), factor analysis, discriminate analysis, canonical correlation, and multivariate analysis of variance (MANOVA) (see Table 20-4). As research becomes more sophisticated, the use of multivariate statistics in studies increases. This is a dilemma for beginning researchers and research consumers because studies using complex analytic procedures may be more difficult to evaluate.

Results, Discussion, Conclusions, and Dissemination

Study results or findings should be clear, concise, and congruent with the research question(s) asked and the methods used. The presentation of results varies for the type of study conducted. Qualitative studies are descriptive narratives, which include participants' verbatim accounts that provide evidence of the researcher's data interpretations. The results may be rich descriptions or new constructions of the study phenomenon, hypothetical propositions generated from the data, or a proposed theory.

Quantitative studies frequently use tables and graphs to display results. Variables examined in descriptive studies should be precisely described, and responses should be numerically reported. The relationships of variables investigated in correlational studies and the procedures used to determine relationships must be clear. In studies that test hypotheses, the statistical procedures used, the results, and the decision of whether there is support for the hypothesized relationships must be evident for each hypothesis stated. Significant, nonsignificant, and unexpected results must be reported. Findings in studies that are not what the investigator anticipates also contribute knowledge about the study topic; they can be an impetus for asking more relevant or more detailed research questions in future studies.

Interpreting study results is an intellectual process that gives meaning to the study and addresses the implications of the study outcomes. The investigator considers the study results with regard to the study process as well as findings from other studies that either support or contradict results of the current study. These relationships can be addressed with the presentation of the results or separately in a section discussing the findings.

Limitations of a study acknowledge factors that may affect study outcomes. Compromises are often necessary in the study process for pragmatic and ethical reasons. These can create weaknesses in design, sampling process, sample size, methods of data collection, or data analysis techniques, and should be reported. The extent to which study findings can be generalized to populations beyond the study sample should also be discussed. Stating limitations assists readers in evaluating the scientific merits of the study and enhances the credibility of the investigator.

Conclusions are concise statements that synthesize the findings; they provide an overall account of the importance of the study and an understanding of the phenomenon in question. The conclusions must be pertinent to the findings and not expanded beyond the study parameters. Following the conclusions, implications of the findings for clinical practice are generally described, and suggestions for further research are identified.

Communicating the results of the study is the final step of conducting research. This may be done through research reports, journal articles, and presentations at conferences, workshops, and educational rounds in institutions. Dissemination of research solicits review by peers and facilitates the likelihood of study findings contributing to improved clinical practice.

Evaluating Research for Use in Practice

Evaluation is an analytical appraisal that makes judgments about the scientific merits of a study. The analysis objectively addresses the study's strengths and weaknesses, poses questions about the research, and makes constructive recommendations. Purposes for evaluating studies include determining whether study findings are useful to clinical decision making, contributing to knowledge that could change clinical practice, or concluding whether further study of a topic is indicated.

Evaluation begins with reading the research report or journal article several times to become familiar with the study. Analysis of the research elements can then proceed. This chapter can serve as a base for understanding the research process as well as expectations for research approaches and specific methods. A key issue in reviewing a study is congruency. All elements—the research question, purpose, design, sampling procedures, methods of data collection, analysis, interpretation of the findings, and discussion—should be consistent with one another. Table 20-5 lists questions to ask when evaluating qualitative and quantitative studies. Although not exhaustive, these guidelines will assist in the systematic review of studies. Research textbooks include additional description of the process and criteria used in conducting a comprehensive research study critique and should be consulted by the interested reader (e.g., Polit & Beck, 2012).

Following examination of the research elements, the reviewer identifies the strengths and weaknesses of the study. All studies have limitations; therefore, weaknesses are considered in relation to how they affect outcomes and the overall meaning of the study. Judgments are made regarding the relevancy of knowledge generated and the usefulness of findings for clinical practice. Legitimate criticisms of a study should be presented with rational and constructive recommendations. Evaluating studies is a skill that develops with practice, increased knowledge and understanding of the research process, and an awareness of the studies related to a specific topic.

Research articles published in professional journals are the most common source of research reports. The limitations, particularly the length of the report, must be considered in the appraisal. Journal articles lack the detail of full research

Table 20-5 GUIDELINES FOR EVALUATING QUANTITATIVE AND QUALITATIVE STUDIES

General Guidelines	Quantitative Studies	Qualitative Studies
1. Problem and purpose • Clearly stated? • Amenable to scientific investigation? • Significant to breastfeeding knowledge?	• Provides direction for study?	• Broadly stated? • Exploratory
2. Review of literature • Pertinent? • Well organized?	• Includes recent and classic references? • Theoretical base or conceptual framework evident?	• Acknowledges the existence of (or lack of) literature on the topic?
3. Protection of human rights • Subject's protection from harm ensured? • Subject suitably informed by a written informed-consent? • Reviewed by an ethics board? • Means for ensuring privacy, confidentiality, or anonymity are explained?		
4. Method • Design congruent with research question? • Sampling procedure appropriate for research method? • Method of data collection relevant for design?	• Deductive approach? • Variables identified and defined? • Sample representative of population and adequate size? • Measuring tools suitable, reliable, and valid? • Control of extraneous variables is evident?	• Inductive approach used? • Key informants and theoretical sampling addressed? • Data collection and analysis concurrent? • Process for data collection and analysis described? • Data saturated? • Credibility, dependability, confirmability, and transferability are evident?
5. Results and discussion • Analysis suitable for method and design? • Results clearly presented? • Interpretations clear and based on data? • Research question answered? • Limitations of study identified? • Conclusions based on results? • Implications for practice and research described?	• Statistical procedures used suitable for data and sample size? • Tables clear and represent the data? • Successful and unanticipated results reported?	• Examples of informants' accounts displayed? • Rich descriptions or theory presented? • Findings compared with literature? • Theory logical and complete?

reports. Studies in refereed journals are subject to review before publication. Members of journal review boards, generally regarded as experts in the field, critique articles to judge them for their scientific merit and make recommendations regarding whether they should be published.

Breastfeeding encompasses many disciplines in the natural, social, and health sciences; therefore, breastfeeding practitioners must consult numerous and varied journals to remain current with new knowledge. Although a challenging task, keeping up-to-date with the literature is essential for professional practice.

Using Research in Clinical Practice

Bridging the gap between generating and utilizing knowledge is an ongoing process that takes motivation, commitment, persistence, and patience. Implementing research findings into clinical practice is a challenge for researchers and practitioners alike. This process is facilitated when researchers and practitioners work together to achieve the goal of implementing evidence-based practice.

Researchers have the following responsibilities in assisting this process:

- Disseminating study findings directly to practitioners as soon as a study is completed through informal discussions; local, regional, and national presentations; and publications.
- Replicating studies that may improve clinical practice. (Changes are seldom made following the outcomes of one small study.)
- Encouraging and assisting practitioners to participate in research to develop their interest and awareness
- Listening to concerns about practice so as to generate problems for study that are relevant to a particular practice area; collaborating with practitioners in research projects.
- Assisting practitioners with evaluation of research articles so they may increase their

knowledge and competence in judging research findings.

Practitioners have the following responsibilities in translating research findings to the practice field:

- Developing a questioning attitude and openness to change
- Sharing concerns about practice with researchers to develop pertinent clinical studies
- Collaborating with researchers and participating in research projects
- Critically reading and evaluating research articles and using relevant findings in practice
- Attending professional conferences where research is presented and discussed
- Telling other clinicians about study findings that reflect, assist, or may alter practice

Evidence-based practice (EBP) is endorsed as the gold standard for care for healthcare professionals. It is the practice of making clinical decisions that are based on the best research evidence available, as well as the clinical knowledge and expertise of the practitioner, and in consultation with the individual receiving care (Sackett et al., 2000). Findings from studies provide the research evidence, which can be arranged into a hierarchy on the basis of which study design is used and whether single or multiple studies are available to provide evidence (Polit & Beck, 2012). Although references for EBP may vary in their hierarchy schema, generally systematic reviews of randomized clinical trials are placed at the pinnacle of the hierarchy, given that they summarize multiple RCT results. Subsequent levels of the hierarchy include (in order) systematic reviews of nonrandomized trials; single RCT and single nonrandomized trial reports; systematic review of correlational or observational studies; single correlational or observational study reports; systematic reviews of descriptive, qualitative, or physiologic studies; single descriptive, qualitative, or physiologic study reports; and opinions of authorities or expert committees.

Changes in clinical practice are not generally made on the basis of findings from one study.

This should happen only if the study is exceptionally large and the findings are definitive regarding improved practice. Instead, preprocessed or preappraised evidence, which "is evidence selected from primary studies and evaluated for use by clinicians" (Polit & Beck, 2012, p. 29), is increasingly being used by clinicians in practice to assist in changing practice based on evidence. According to Dicenso et al. (2004), a hierarchy of preappraised evidence includes single studies at the bottom of the hierarchy, with synopses of single studies, systematic reviews, and synopses of systematic reviews on successive ascending rungs of the hierarchy. Included in preappraised evidence are meta-analysis and meta-synthesis studies.

There are several resources available from which to obtain systematic reviews. The Cochrane Collaboration (http://www.cochrane.org) of systematic reviews of the effects of healthcare interventions is internationally recognized and increasingly used by healthcare professionals in making decisions to change practice. This type of review is updated regularly—a significant benefit. The Cochrane Collaboration has conducted several breastfeeding-related systematic reviews, including those addressing skin-to-skin contact, antibiotic use in mastitis, use of prenatal education for promoting breastfeeding, and effects of pacifier use on duration of breastfeeding.

Finally, evidence-based clinical practice guidelines (CPG) are developed by groups of researchers, clinicians, and other experts in the field. Clinical practice guidelines are recommendations for practice based on evidence of all levels, including expert opinion when evidence in an area is lacking. Oftentimes, professional organizations develop such guidelines. For example, the International Lactation Consultant Association (2014) recently published the third edition of the *Clinical Guidelines for the Establishment of Exclusive Breastfeeding*. This important document is used by lactation specialists and International Board Certified Lactation Consultants (IBCLC) in practice to support and promote exclusive breastfeeding; it is largely based in research evidence, a significant improvement from the earliest edition of the document.

A broad base of scientific evidence from studies using different approaches and methods is relevant and can expand scientific knowledge related to breastfeeding to optimal practice that benefits mothers, infants, families, and society.

SUMMARY

Research is a process, and theory is a base for developing knowledge that serves as a foundation for accountable and responsible practice. The approaches and methods involved in conducting research originate from various philosophical systems: the positivist/postpositivist perspective; the natural science, human science, and interpretation perspective; and the critical and emancipatory perspective. These perspectives give rise to research approaches and methods used in qualitative, quantitative, observational, historical, and feminist research. The research question asked—and whether knowledge is generated inductively or deductively—directs the approach used.

The qualitative approach generates an understanding of the "meaning" that reflects human values, beliefs, practices, and life experiences or events. The three qualitative methods commonly used are phenomenology, ethnography, and grounded theory. The quantitative approach is characterized by objectivity, measurement, and control. The quantitative methods commonly used are descriptive, correlational, experimental, and quasi-experimental studies. The simultaneous use of qualitative and quantitative methods in the same study is an increasing trend.

The major elements of research are the problem and purpose, review of literature, protection of human subjects, method, and results and discussion. The research problem identifies what is studied and with whom, and the purpose delineates why the study is conducted. Research questions for quantitative methods are more specific than those asked in qualitative studies. In quantitative studies, variables are delineated and operationally defined. How breastfeeding and the duration of breastfeeding are defined is of particular importance when conducting or evaluating studies related to lactation and breastfeeding.

Reviewing literature about a study topic assists in formulating the research problem and directs the research method. Qualitative methods are frequently used when little is known about a topic.

Research that involves human subjects must ensure that the basic rights of the study participants are respected. Ethical review boards or committees help protect subjects by reviewing the informed consent document and evaluating the study before it is conducted.

Study methods address setting, sample, data collection, and data analysis. The setting indicates the location of the study or the source of the participants. The sample is a subset of a larger population or group of individuals in whom the investigator is interested. Sampling is a process for selecting the sample from the population; the two types of sampling are probability and nonprobability. Nonprobability sampling is used in qualitative studies. Probability sampling is preferred in quantitative studies because findings can then be generalized from the study sample to the target population. This method requires random selection of subjects, which is not always possible; therefore, many quantitative studies involving human subjects use nonprobability sampling.

Data are collected when the researcher asks questions, makes observations, and measures key variables identified in the research question. In-depth interviews and observations are the methods most commonly used in qualitative studies, and data collection and analysis occur simultaneously. Systematic and rigorous methods for collecting and analyzing data are developed for all qualitative methods. Methods for data collection in quantitative studies are highly structured and must be the same for every subject.

Reliability and validity issues must be addressed for all research. Reliability refers to accuracy, consistency, precision, and stability of data collected; validity reflects the true meaning of data. In qualitative studies, this aspect is referred to as trustworthiness. Ensuring it is present includes building in checks in the data collection and analysis process. In quantitative studies, reliability of measurement tools and investigators collecting data can be statistically estimated, as can the validity of the measurements used.

Data analysis is the process of organizing, summarizing, examining, and synthesizing the data collected to identify study findings. Qualitative studies generate rich descriptions and posit hypotheses and theories. Descriptive narratives of participants' verbatim accounts support the investigator's interpretations of the data. In quantitative studies, data are translated into numerical terms for statistical analysis. Depending on the type of study and the level of measurement of the data collected, a variety of statistical procedures can be employed. Results are displayed in tables and graphs.

Study results should be clear, concise, and congruent with the method used, and they should answer the research question(s). All results—whether significant, nonsignificant, or unexpected—should be reported. Limitations of the study and the extent to which findings can be generalized to additional populations must also be addressed. Study conclusions should reflect only the study findings.

Research reports or articles are evaluated to make judgments about their scientific merit and the usefulness of findings for clinical practice. A key issue in evaluation is study congruency.

Implementing research findings into clinical practice is a challenge for researchers and practitioners alike, but this process can be expedited when both work together. Although findings from current studies are not generally definitive and further study is frequently recommended, using relevant findings in practice often serves to question effects and generate new studies. Breastfeeding research is an ongoing process that expands knowledge and facilitates evidence-based practice in this area. The beneficiaries of health professionals who draw from a scientific body of knowledge and establish practices based on best evidence are mothers, children, families, and society.

KEY CONCEPTS

- Research is the systematic and logical inquiry into a phenomenon to discover new knowledge or to validate existing knowledge.
- Theory is a conceptual construction of a view of reality that describes, explains, or predicts something. It includes concepts and their relationships.
- Middle-range theories include well-defined concepts and relationships, but the propositions are more easily tested than those of grand theories. They are amenable to theories used in clinical practice.
- Inductive reasoning is the process of reasoning from specific observations or abstractions to a general premise.
- Deductive reasoning is the process of reasoning from a general premise to the concrete and specific.
- A conceptual framework is a basic structure representing concepts and relationships; it is not a specific theory that explains these relationships.
- A theoretical framework is a basic structure representing theories, concepts, and propositions that are the underpinnings of a study and in which the propositions can be tested.
- A core concept is the overall theme of a grounded theory study. It is central to and interrelates the themes and categories identified in the study.
- A key informant is an individual who is most knowledgeable and who best articulates the meaning of the phenomenon under study.
- Bias is any factor, action, or influence that distorts the results of a study.
- Control is specific to quantitative research. It is the process of eliminating the influence of confounding variables that could compromise the research findings.
- An operational definition is an explicit description of a concept or variable of interest. For quantitative studies, operational definitions are expressed in measurable terms.
- The dependent or outcome variable is the variable the investigator measures in response to a change in the independent or treatment variable; the outcome variable is affected by the independent variable.
- The independent variable is the treatment or invention that is manipulated by the investigator to influence the dependent variable.
- Power is the probability that a statistical test will reject a null hypothesis when it should be rejected—in other words, that it will detect a significant difference that does exist.
- Reliability is the degree to which collected data are accurate, consistent, precise, and stable over time.
- Validity is the degree to which collected data are true and represent reality, and a measuring instrument reflects what it is intended to measure.
- Trustworthiness is the process of establishing the credibility of qualitative research.

ACKNOWLEDGMENT

I wish to recognize and thank Dr. Roberta Hewat, the original author of this chapter. I have revised and updated the chapter but the original content remains largely unchanged.

INTERNET RESOURCES

Theory-Related Resources

Nursing Child Assessment Satellite Training: http://www.ncast.org/index.cfm?fuseaction =page.display&page_id=29

Nursing Theories: http://currentnursing.com /nursing_theory/nursing_theorists.html

Clinical Practice Guidelines

Canadian Medical Association Infobase (Canada)—Clinical practice guidelines produced or endorsed in Canada by a national, provincial/territorial, or regional medical or health organization, professional society, government agency or expert panel: https://www.cma.ca/En/Pages/clinical-practice-guidelines.aspx

National Guideline Clearinghouse: http://www.guideline.gov/

Preappraised Evidence Resources

The Cochrane Collaboration—Cochrane database of systematic research reviews: http://www.cochrane.org

Agency for Healthcare Research and Quality (AHRQ)—Evidence-based practice centers that issue evidence reports: http://www.ahrq.gov/research/findings/evidence-based-reports/index.html

Federal US health databases and research articles (PubMed): http://www.ncbi.nlm.nih.gov/pubmed

REFERENCES

Ajzen I, Fishbein M. *Understanding attitudes and predicting behavior.* Englewood Cliffs, NJ: Prentice Hall; 1980.

Armstrong HC. International recommendations for consistent breastfeeding definitions. *J Hum Lact.* 1991;7:51–54.

Bakeman R, Gottman JM. *Observing interaction: an introduction to sequential analysis.* Cambridge, UK: Cambridge University Press; 1986.

Bandura A. Self-efficacy: toward a unifying theory of behavioural change. *Psych Rev.* 1977;84:191–215.

Bandura A. Self-efficacy mechanism in human agency. *Am Psychol.* 1982;37:122–147.

Barnard K, Eyres S. Overview of the nursing child assessment project. In: Barnard K, ed. *Nursing child assessment training learning resource manual.* Seattle, WA: University of Washington School of Nursing; 1978: 16–21.

Barr RG. Infant crying behavior and colic: an interpretation in evolutionary perspective. In: Trevathan WO, Smith EO, McKenna JJ, eds. *Evolutionary medicine.* Oxford, UK: Oxford University Press; 1999:27–51.

Bernaix LW. Nurses' attitudes, subjective norms, and behavioural intentions toward support of breastfeeding mothers. *J Hum Lact.* 2000;16:201–209.

Blyth R, Creedy DK, Dennis CL, et al. Effect of maternal confidence on breastfeeding duration: an application of breastfeeding self-efficacy theory. *Birth.* 2002;29: 278–284.

Bottorff J. Persistence in breastfeeding: a phenomenological investigation. *J Adv Nurs.* 1990;15:201–209.

Brandt K, Andrews C, Kvale J. Mother–infant interaction and breastfeeding outcome 6 weeks after birth. *JOGNN.* 1998;27:169–174.

Breastfeeding Committee for Canada. Breastfeeding definition and algorithms. 2006. Available at: http://breastfeedingcanada.ca/BCC. Accessed December 27, 2007.

Brett J, Niermeyer S. Is neonatal jaundice a disease or an adaptive process? In: Trevathan WR, Smith EO, McKenna JJ, eds. *Evolutionary medicine.* Oxford, UK: Oxford University Press; 1999:7–25.

Burns E, Schmied V, Fenwick J, Sheehan A. Liquid gold from the milk bar: constructions of breastmilk and breastfeeding women in the language and practices of midwives. *Soc Sci Med.* 2012;75:1737–1745. doi: 10.1016/j.socscimed.2012.07.035.

Butts JB. Components and levels of abstraction in nursing knowledge. In: Butts JB, Rich KL, eds. *Philosophies and theories for advanced nursing practice,* 2nd ed. Burlington, MA: Jones & Bartlett Learning; 2015: 87–105.

Chenitz WC, Swanson JM. *From practice to grounded theory.* Menlo Park, CA: Addison-Wesley; 1986: 96–98.

Cohen J. *Statistical power analysis for the behavioural sciences,* 2nd ed. New York, NY: Academic Press; 1988.

Colaizzi P. Psychological research as the phenomenologist views it. In: Valle R, King M, eds. *Existential phenomenological alternative for psychology.* New York, NY: Oxford University Press; 1978:48–71.

Creswell, JW. *A concise introduction to mixed methods research.* Thousand Oaks. CA: Sage; 2014.

Crotty M. *The foundations of social research.* Thousand Oaks, CA: Sage; 1998.

Dennis CL. Theoretical underpinnings of breastfeeding confidence: a self-efficacy framework. *J Hum Lact.* 1999;15: 195–201.

Dennis CL. The breastfeeding self-efficacy scale: psychometric assessment of the short form. *JOGNN.* 2003;32: 734–744.

Dennis CL, Faux S. Development and psychometric testing of the breastfeeding self-efficacy scale. *Res Nurs Health.* 1999;22:399–409.

Dennis CL, Heaman M, Mossman M. Psychometric testing of the breastfeeding self-efficacy scale—short form among adolescents. *J Adolesc Health.* 2011;49: 265–271.

Dicenso A, Guyatt G, Ciliska D. *Evidence-based nursing: a guide to clinical practice.* Philadelphia, PA: Mosby; 2004.

Dick MJ, Evans ML, Arthurs JB, et al. Predicting early breastfeeding attrition. *J Hum Lact.* 2002;18: 21–28.

Dykes F. "Supply and demand": breastfeeding as labour. *Soc Sci Med.* 2005;60:2283–2293.

Fawcett J, DeSanto-Madeya S. *Contemporary nursing knowledge: analysis and evaluation of nursing models and theories.* Philadelphia, PA: F. A. Davis; 2012.

Fouquier KF. State of the science: does the theory of maternal role attainment apply to African American motherhood? *J Midwifery Women's Health.* 2013;58(2): 203–210. doi: 10.1111/j.1542-2011.2012.00206.x.

Furr PA, Kiregis CA. A nurse–midwifery approach to early mother–infant acquaintance. *J Nurs Midwifery* 1982;27:10–14.

Gill SL, Reifsnider E, Lucke JF, Mann A. Predicting breastfeeding attrition: adapting the breast-feeding attrition prediction tool. *J Perinat Neonatal Nurs.* 2007;21: 216–224.

Gillis A, Jackson W. *Research for nurses: methods and interpretation.* Philadelphia, PA: F. A. Davis; 2002.

Giorgi A. Sketch of a psychological phenomenological method. In: Giorgi A, ed. *Phenomenology and psychological research.* Pittsburgh, PA: Duquesne University Press; 1985:8–22.

Glaser BG. *Theoretical sensitivity.* Mill Valley, CA: Sociology Press; 1978.

Haisma H, Coward WA, Albernaz E, et al. Breast milk and energy intake in exclusively, predominantly, and partially breast-fed infants. *Eur J Clin Nutr.* 2003:57(12); 1633–1642.

Harding S, ed. *Feminism and methodology.* Bloomington, IN: Indiana University Press; 1987.

Hennekens CH, Buring JE, Mayrent S. *Epidemiology in medicine.* Boston, MA: Little, Brown; 1987.

Hewat RJ. Living with an incessantly crying infant. *Phenomenology Pedagogy.* 1992;10:160–171.

Hewat RJ. *Mother–infant interaction during breastfeeding: a comparison between problematic and nonproblematic breastfeeders* [dissertation]. Edmonton, AB: University of Alberta; 1998.

Hewat RJ, Ellis DJ. Breastfeeding as a maternal–child team effort: women's perceptions. *Health Care Women Int.* 1984;5:437–452.

Hill PD, Aldag JC, Chatterton RT. The effect of sequential and simultaneous breast pumping milk volume and prolactin levels: a pilot study. *J Hum Lact.* 1996;12: 193–199.

Hoddinott P, Lee AJ, Pill R. Effectiveness of a breastfeeding peer coaching intervention in rural Scotland. *Birth.* 2006;33:27–33.

Horodynski MA, Olson B, Baker S, et al. Healthy babies through infant-centered feeding protocol: an intervention targeting early childhood obesity in vulnerable populations. *BMC Public Health.* 2011;11: 868.

International Lactation Consultant Association. *Clinical guidelines for the establishment of exclusive breastfeeding,* 3rd ed. Morrisville, NC: International Lactation Consultant Association; 2014.

Ip S, Chung M, Raman G, et al. *Breastfeeding and maternal and infant health outcomes in developed countries.* Evidence Report/Technology Assessment No. 153. Rockville, MD: Agency for Health Care Research and Quality; 2007. AHRQ Publication No. 07-E007.

Jacox A, Suppe F, Campbell J, Stashinko E. Diversity in philosophical approaches. In: Hinshaw AS, Feetham SL, Shaver JIF, eds. *Handbook of clinical nursing research.* Thousand Oaks, CA: Sage; 1999:3–17.

Janke J. Prediction of breast-feeding attrition: instrument development. *Applied Nurs Res.* 1992;5:48–63.

Janke J. Development of the Breastfeeding Attrition Prediction Tool. *Nurs Res.* 1994;34:100–104.

Jensen D, Wallace S, Kelsay P. LATCH: a breastfeeding charting system and documentation tool. *JOGNN.* 1994;26: 181–187.

Johnson TS, Mulder PJ, Strube K. Mother–infant breastfeeding progress tool: a guide for education and support of the breastfeeding dyad. *JOGNN.* 2007;36: 319–327.

The Joint Commission. Perinatal care core measures. 2014. Available at: http://www.jointcommission.org /perinatal_care/.

Karayağiz Muslu G, Basbakkal Z, Janke J. The Turkish version of the Breastfeeding Attrition Prediction Tool. *J Hum Lact.* 2011;27:350–357. doi: 10.1177/ 0890334411410692.

Kelly L, Burton S, Regan L. Researching women's lives or studying women's oppression? Reflections on what constitutes feminist research. In: Maynard M, Purvis J, eds. *Researching women's lives from a feminist perspective.* London, UK: Taylor and Francis; 1994:27–48.

Kennell J, McGrath S. Starting the process of mother-infant bonding. *Acta Paediatr.* 2005;94:775–778.

Klaus MH, Kennell JH. *Maternal–infant bonding,* St. Louis, MO: Mosby; 1976.

Klaus MH, Kennell JH. *Maternal–infant bonding,* 2nd ed. St. Louis, MO: Mosby; 1982.

Klaus M, Kennell JH, Klaus PH. *Bonding: building the foundations of secure attachment and independence.* New York, NY: Addison Wesley; 1995:54–92.

Koniak-Griffin D. Maternal role attainment image. *J Nurs Sch.* 1993;25:257–262.

Kramer HC, Thiemann S. *How many subjects? Statistical power analysis in research.* Newbury Park, CA: Sage; 1987.

Kumar SP, Mooney R, Wieser LJ, Havstad S. The LATCH scoring system and prediction of breastfeeding duration. *J Hum Lact.* 2006;22:391–397.

Labbok M. What is the definition of breastfeeding? *Breastfeeding Abstracts.* 2000;19:19–21.

Labbok MH, Coffin CJ. A call for consistency in definition of breastfeeding behaviors. *Soc Sci Med.* 1997;44: 1931–1932.

Labbok M, Krasovec K. Toward consistency in breastfeeding definitions. *Stud Fam Plann.* 1990;21:226–230.

Labbok MH, Starling A. Definitions of breastfeeding: call for the development and use of consistent definitions in research and peer-reviewed literature. *Breastfeed Med.* 2012;7(6):397–402. doi: 10.1089/bfm.2012.9975.

Labbok MH, Taylor E, Nickel N. Implementing the ten steps to successful breastfeeding in multiple hospitals serving low-wealth patients in the US: innovative research design and baseline findings. *Int Breastfeed J.* 2013;8:5. Available at: http://www.internationalbreastfeedingjournal.com/content/8/1/5.

Leff EW, Jefferis SC, Gagne MP. Maternal perceptions of successful breastfeeding. *J Hum Lact.* 1994a;10: 99–104.

Leff EW, Jefferis SC, Gagne MP. The development of the maternal breastfeeding evaluation scale. *J Hum Lact.* 1994b;10:105–111.

Lincoln YS, Guba EG. *Naturalistic inquiry.* Newbury Park, CA: Sage; 1985.

Martell LK. Heading toward the new normal: a contemporary postpartum experience. *JOGNN.* 2001;30:496–506.

Martens PJ. Does breastfeeding education affect nursing staff beliefs, exclusive breastfeeding rates, and baby-friendly hospital initiative compliance? The experience of a small, rural Canadian hospital. *J Hum Lact.* 2000;16:309–318.

Matthews MK. Developing an instrument to assess infant breastfeeding behavior in the early neonatal period. *Midwifery.* 1988;4:154–165.

Matthews MK. Mothers' satisfaction with their neonates' breastfeeding behaviors. *JOGNN.* 1991;20:49–55.

Maynard M, Purvis J. *Researching women's lives from a feminist perspective.* London, UK: Taylor and Francis; 1994.

McBride AB, Shore CP. Women as mothers and grandmothers. *Annu Rev Nurs Res.* 2001;19:63–85.

McKenna JJ, Gettler LT. Mother–infant cosleeping with breastfeeding in the Western industrialized context: a bio-cultural perspective. In: Hale TW, Hartmann P, eds. *Textbook of human lactation.* Amarillo, TX: Hale Publishing; 2007;271–302.

McKenna J, Mosko S, Richard C. Breastfeeding and mother–infant cosleeping in relation to SIDS prevention. In: Trevathan WR, Smith EO, McKenna JJ, eds. *Evolutionary medicine.* Oxford, UK: Oxford University Press; 1999:53–74.

McQueen KA, Montelpare WJ, Dennis CL. Breastfeeding and Aboriginal women: validation of the breastfeeding self-efficacy scale—short form. *Can J Nurs Res.* 2013; 45(2):58–75.

Mead GH. In: Morris CW, ed. *Mind, self and society.* Chicago, IL: University of Chicago Press; 1934.

Mercer RT. A theoretical framework for studying factors that impact on the maternal role. *Nurs Res.* 1981;30: 73–77.

Mercer RT. The process of maternal role attainment over the first year. *Nurs Res.* 1985;34:198–204.

Mercer RT. Becoming a mother versus maternal role attainment. *J Nurs Sch.* 2004;36:226–232.

Mercer RT, Ferketich SL. Predictors of maternal role competence by risk status. *Nurs Res.* 1994;43:38–43.

Millard AV. The place of the clock in pediatric advice: rationales, cultural themes, and impediments to breastfeeding. *Soc Sci Med.* 1990;31:211–221.

Moore ER, Anderson GC, Bergman N, Dowswell T. Early skin-to-skin contact for mothers and their healthy newborn infants. *Cochrane Database Syst Rev.* 2012;5: CD003519. doi: 10.1002/14651858.CD003519.pub3.

Morse JM. Qualitative nursing research: a free-for-all? In: Morse JM, ed. *Qualitative nursing research: a contemporary dialogue.* London, UK: Sage; 1991a:14–22.

Morse JM. Strategies for sampling. In: Morse JM, ed. *Qualitative nursing research: a contemporary dialogue.* London, UK: Sage; 1991b:127–144.

Morse JM, Bottorff JL. The use of ethology in clinical nursing research. *Adv Nurs Sci.* 1990;12:53–64.

Morse JM, Field PA. *Qualitative research methods for health professionals.* 2nd ed. London, UK: Sage; 1995.

National Commission for the Protection of Human Subjects of Biomedical and Behavioral Research. Ethical principles and guidelines for the protection of human subjects of research. 1979. Available at: http://www.hhs.gov/ohrp/humansubjects/guidance/belmont.html.

Nelson AM. Transition to motherhood. *JOGNN.* 2003;32: 465–477.

Nelson AM. Toward a situation-specific theory of breastfeeding. *Res Theory Nurs Pract.* 2006;20(1):9–27.

Nelson AM. Maternal–newborn nurses' experiences of inconsistent professional breastfeeding support. *J Adv Nurs.* 2007;60:29–38.

Nelson A, Sethi S. The breastfeeding experiences of Canadian teenage mothers. *JOGNN.* 2005;34:615–624.

Noel-Weiss J, Rupp A, Cragg B, et al. Randomized controlled trial to determine effects of prenatal breastfeeding workshop on maternal breastfeeding self-efficacy and breastfeeding duration. *JOGNN.* 2006;35:616–624.

Nunnally JC. *Introduction to psychological measurement.* Toronto, ON: McGraw-Hill; 1978:245.

Oddy WH, Kendall GE, Blair E, et al. Breast feeding and cognitive development in childhood: a prospective birth cohort study. *Birth.* 2003;17:1–90.

Oliver-Roig A, d'Anglade-González ML, García-García B, et al. The Spanish version of the breastfeeding self-efficacy scale—short form: reliability and validity assessment. *Int J Nurs Stud.* 2012;49(2):169–173. doi: 10.1016/j.ijnurstu.2011.08.005.

Orem DE. The self-care deficit theory of nursing: a general theory. In: Clements I, Roberts F, eds. *Family health: a theoretical approach to nursing care.* New York, NY: John Wiley & Sons;1983:205–217.

Polit DF, Beck CT. Content validity index: are you sure you know what's being reported? *Res Nurs Health.* 2006;29:489–497.

Polit DF, Beck CT. *Nursing research: generating and assessing evidence for nursing practice,* 9th ed. Philadelphia, PA: Wolters Kluwer/Lippincott, Williams & Wilkins; 2012.

Potter J, Wetherall M. *Discourse and social psychology: beyond attitudes and behavior.* London, UK: Sage; 1987.

Prime DK, Garbin CP, Hartmann PE, Kent JC. Simultaneous breast expression in breastfeeding women is more efficacious than sequential breast expression. *Breastfeed Med.* 2012;7:442–447.

Riordan J, Bibb D, Miller M, Rawlins T. Predicting breastfeeding duration using the LATCH breastfeeding assessment tool. *J Hum Lact.* 2001;17:20–23.

Riordan J, Gross A, Angeron J, et al. The effect of labor pain relief medication on neonatal sucking and breastfeeding duration. *J Hum Lact.* 2001;16:7–12.

Riordan JM, Koehn M. Reliability and validity testing of three breastfeeding assessment tools. *JOGNN.* 1997;26:181–187.

Riordan JM, Woodley G, Heaton K. Testing validity and reliability of an instrument which measures maternal evaluation of breastfeeding. *J Hum Lact.* 1994;10:231–235.

Rojjanasrirat W, Nelson EL, Wambach KA. A pilot study of home-based videoconferencing for breastfeeding support. *J Hum Lact.* 2012;28(4):464–467. doi: 10.1177/0890334412449071. [Epub July 16, 2012].

Rubin R. Attainment of the maternal role: part I. *Nurs Res.* 1967a;16:237–245.

Rubin R. Attainment of the maternal role: part II. *Nurs Res.* 1967b;16:342–346.

Rubin R. *Maternal identity and the maternal experience.* New York, NY: Springer; 1984.

Sackett DL, Straus SE, Richardson WS, et al. *Evidence-based medicine: How to practice and teach EBM.* Edinburgh, UK: Churchill Livingstone; 2000.

Sarbin TR. Role theory. In: Lindzey G, ed. *Handbook of social psychology.* Reading, MA: Addison-Wesley; 1954:223–258.

Schaefer KM. Breastfeeding in chronic illness: the voices of women with fibromyalgia. *Am J Matern Child Nurs.* 2004;29:248–253.

Schmied V. Connection and pleasure, disruption and distress: women's experience of breastfeeding. *J Hum Lact.* 1999;14:325–334.

Shafer RJ. *A guide to historical method,* 3rd ed. Belmont, CA: Wadsworth; 1980.

Spencer BS, Wambach K, Domian E. African American women's breastfeeding experiences: cultural, personal, and political. *Qual Health Res.* 2014. doi:10.1177/1049732314554097

Spradley JP. *The ethnographic interview.* New York, NY: Holt, Rinehart, and Winston; 1979:3–5.

Spradley JP. *Participant observation.* New York, NY: Holt, Rinehart, and Winston; 1980.

Strauss A, Corbin J. *Basics of qualitative research: grounded theory procedures and techniques.* Newbury Park, CA: Sage; 1990:24–32.

Strickland O. Ensuring the credibility of physiological measurements: assessing error variability. *J Nurs Measurement.* 2004a;12:91–93.

Strickland O. Factors that can affect the accuracy and precision of physiological measurements. *J Nurs Measurement.* 2004b;12:163–167.

Sumner G, Spietz A. *NCAST caregiver/parent–child interaction feeding manual.* Seattle, WA: NCAST Publications; 1994.

Tabachnick BG, Fidell LS. *Using multivariate statistics,* 5th ed. New York, NY: HarperCollins College; 2007.

Tokat MA, Okumuş H, Dennis CL. Translation and psychometric assessment of the breast-feeding self-efficacy scale—short form among pregnant and postnatal women in Turkey. *Midwifery.* 2010;26:101–108.

Trevathan WR, Smith EO, McKenna JJ. *Evolutionary medicine.* Oxford, UK: Oxford University Press; 1999:27–51.

van Manen M. Practicing phenomenological writing. *Phenomenology Pedagogy.* 1984;2:37–69.

van Manen M. *Researching lived experience: human science for an action sensitive pedagogy.* Ann Arbor, MI: Althouse Press; 1990.

Waltz CF, Strickland OL, Lenz ER. *Measurement in nursing and health research,* 4th ed. New York, NY: Springer; 2010.

Wambach K, Aaronson L, Breedlove G, et al. A randomized controlled trial of breastfeeding support and education for adolescent mothers. *W J Nurs Res.* 2011;33: 486–505. PMID: 20876551.

Wambach KA, Cohen SM. Breastfeeding experiences of urban adolescent mothers. *J Pediatr Nurs.* 2009;24: 244–254.

Wambach KA, Koehn M. Experiences of infant-feeding decision-making among urban economically disadvantaged pregnant adolescents. *J Adv Nurs.* 2004;48: 361–370.

Weimers L, Svensson K, Dumas L, et al. Hands-on approach during breastfeeding support in a neonatal intensive care unit: a qualitative study of Swedish mothers' experiences. *Int Breastfeed J.* 2006;1:20. doi: 10.1186/1746 -4358-1-20.

Williams GC, Nesse RM. The dawn of Darwinian medicine. *Q Rev Biol.* 1991;66:1–22.

Wutke K, Dennis CL. The reliability and validity of the Polish version of the breastfeeding self-efficacy scale— short form: translation and psychometric assessment. *Int J Nurs Stud.* 2007;44:1439–1446.

Zimmerman DR, Guttman N. "Breast is best": knowledge among low-income mothers is not enough. *J Hum Lact.* 2001;17:14–23.

Chapter 21

Breastfeeding Education

Barbara Morrison

Introduction

Education is the cornerstone supporting the framework of lactation and breastfeeding. This chapter describes the transitions occurring in healthcare provider education to provide a consistent knowledge base so that effective protection, promotion, and support of breastfeeding and lactation throughout pregnancy, birth, and the first years of an infant's life occur. In addition, the elaboration of breastfeeding education for parents presented here aims to assist families in having a positive breastfeeding experience. The chapter ends by describing strategies and tools to assist educators in fashioning meaningful educational experiences for families and colleagues. Addressed throughout the chapter are a broad range of educational issues, from theory to practical application, geared toward maximizing educational experiences for adult learners.

Factors Creating the Need for Breastfeeding and Lactation Education

Over the last several centuries, the need for breastfeeding and lactation education has changed dramatically. In traditional societies, breastfeeding "education" involved lifelong immersion in a culture where seeing a baby at breast for multiple years was normal. When a woman was with child, immediate and extended family members and women of the community provided emotional support and education during pregnancy, birth, and breastfeeding. Now, even though formal breastfeeding and parental education is common in many parts of the world, it is simply a replacement for a time-honored function of female family and community members—that is, women being with women (Kitzinger, 1995; Zareai et al., 2007). Cultural beliefs and practices continue to be a strong influence on breastfeeding and lactation experiences and, therefore, are central to promoting breastfeeding (Reinsma et al., 2012).

The dramatic decrease in breastfeeding in industrialized societies during the first half of the 1900s reduced the number of mothers and grandmothers who could share their breastfeeding experiences, rapidly changing expectations from breastfeeding as the norm to a custom of bottle-feeding. Over time, expectant mothers were less likely to see an infant breastfed or to know someone who could provide practical assistance with breastfeeding. Geographical mobility further isolated young families from their traditional support networks. Into the vacuum came alternative support systems for the few women who chose to breastfeed. Self-help groups such as La Leche League International, Australian Breastfeeding Association, and childbirth education groups began to organize. They flourished worldwide, providing accurate information, practical assistance, and emotional support for breastfeeding families using a mother-to-mother approach.

Today, as we work to reestablish a culture where breastfeeding, especially exclusive breastfeeding, is the norm (Shortt et al., 2013), education is available from a multitude of venues. Self-help groups continue to be a common source of education and support. Many healthcare systems now have lactation clinics that offer breastfeeding classes prenatally as well as individual counseling, classes, and support groups after mother–infant dyads leave the hospital or birth center. Lactation consultants, doulas, and peer or mother-to-mother counselors provide one-to-one and in-home educational opportunities. Additionally, breastfeeding education programs, advice websites, and blogs have inundated the Internet and YouTube as demonstrated by the number of hits found with a quick search one evening (Box 21-1). While the creators of Internet offerings undoubtedly have good intentions, it becomes the mothers' or parents' task to distinguish what is current, appropriate, and correct (Shaikh & Scott, 2005) (Figure 21-1).

The Changing Landscape for Breastfeeding Education

In 1984, in growing recognition of the multitude of benefits from breastfeeding, U.S. Surgeon General

Figure 21-1 SEEKING INFORMATION FROM THE INTERNET.

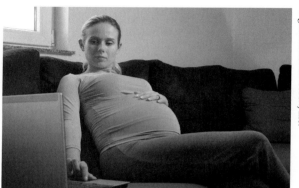

© grufnar/ShutterStock, Inc.

C. Everett Koop convened the Workshop on Breastfeeding and Human Lactation to develop a plan for enhancing the promotion and rate of breastfeeding across the United States. A focus of the primary interventions was improving the quality and availability of didactic and clinical education in breastfeeding and lactation for healthcare providers (HCPs) (see Box 21-2). This education needed to include development of skills in patient education and breastfeeding management.

BOX 21-1 BREASTFEEDING RESOURCES AVAILABLE ON THE INTERNET, OCTOBER 29, 2013: SEARCH TERM "BREASTFEEDING"

Search Engine Hits

Google	39,300,000
Bing	18,500,000
Yahoo	17,900,000
YouTube.com	396,000

Electronic Databases: New Scientific Articles in 2013 (Searched "breastfeeding" in title, not "cancer")

CINAHL (Cumulative Index of Nursing and Allied Health Literature)	413
PubMed (National Library of Medicine)	518
Google Scholar	882

**BOX 21-2 PROVIDERS WHO SHOULD HAVE SOME PROFICIENCY IN BREASTFEEDING
AND LACTATION COUNSELING AND SUPPORT**

- Lactation consultants (U.S. Department of Health and Human Service [USDHHS], 2011)
- Lactation educators/counselors
- Peer counselors/mother-to-mother
- WIC staff (Reidsnider et al., 2003)
- Nurses and nursing staff (Kaewsarn et al., 2003)
  - ◄ Outpatient offices and clinics (Register et al., 2000)
  - ◄ Antepartum/high-risk pregnancy
  - ◄ Labor and birth
  - ◄ Postpartum (Bernaix et al., 2010)
  - ◄ Nursery
  - ◄ Neonatal and pediatric intensive care units
  - ◄ Pediatrics (Karipis & Spicer, 1999)
  - ◄ Public health
  - ◄ Emergency room personnel

- Primary care providers (USDHHS, 2011)
  - ◄ Obstetrician/gynecologists
  - ◄ Pediatricians
  - ◄ Perinatologists
  - ◄ Neonatologists
  - ◄ Nurse–midwives (Hellings & Howe, 2000)
  - ◄ Midwives (Ward & Byrne, 2011)
  - ◄ Nurse practitioners (Hellings & Howe, 2004)
  - ◄ Physician assistants (Meusch et al., 2013)
- Dietitians and nutritionists (USDHHS, 2011)
- Social workers (USDHHS, 2011)
- Pharmacists (Edwards, 2013b)
- Physical therapists
- Emergency Medical Technicians (EMTs)
- Childcare providers (USDHHS, 2011)

In 1989, under the leadership of UNICEF and the World Health Organization (WHO), the *10 Steps to Successful Breastfeeding* (WHO, 1998)—a global effort to decrease formula use and increase breastfeeding rates—was initiated. Breastfeeding and lactation education became a priority around the world, and with the *Baby-Friendly Hospital Initiative* (BFHI) came a requirement for 20 hours of breastfeeding and lactation education for all HCPs (Table 21-1) (WHO, UNICEF, & Wellstart International, 2009). In 2000, under the auspices of U.S. Surgeon General David Satcher, the *Blueprint for Action on Breastfeeding* (USDHHS, 2000) reiterated the strong emphasis on education. However, rather than primarily focusing on HCP education, actions proposed training, awareness, support, research, and collaboration for and among all stakeholders.

One collaboration emerging from the *Blueprint for Action* was the United States Breastfeeding Committee (USBC), a coalition of professional organizations and state breastfeeding coalitions. "The mission of the United States Breastfeeding Committee (USBC) is to improve the Nation's health by working collaboratively to protect, promote, and support breastfeeding" (USBC, 2009). The USBC has become a leader in promoting breastfeeding and facilitating educational opportunities for HCPs. Recently, USBC recognized the need for consistent competencies in breastfeeding care and services across healthcare professions. Thus the *Core Competencies* were developed, providing definitions of basic breastfeeding knowledge, skills, and attitudes needed by all HCPs. Additional competencies needed by those providing direct care to pregnant and breastfeeding women were also established (Box 21-3) (USBC, 2010). Endorsed by at least 43 breastfeeding and women's healthcare professional organizations, the USBC has challenged these groups to develop curricula based on the core competencies to be included in all educational programs.

As we left the 20th century and moved through the first decade of the 21st century, breastfeeding rates started to climb, especially breastfeeding

Table 21-1 COMPARISON OF BREASTFEEDING CONTENT OF THE *BREASTFEEDING PROMOTION AND SUPPORT IN A BABY-FRIENDLY HOSPITAL: A 20-HOUR COURSE FOR MATERNITY STAFF* AND CONTENT IN MEDICAL SCHOOL AND RESIDENCY CURRICULA, AN ELECTIVE NURSING COURSE, AND NUTRITION/DIETETIC CURRICULA

A 20-Hour Course for Maternity Staff* (Step of the 10 Steps)	Medical School and Residency Curricula#	Elective Nursing Lactation Course$	Nutrition/Dietetic Breastfeeding Curricula+
• BFHI: A part of the global strategy • Promoting breastfeeding during pregnancy (Step 3) • Protecting breastfeeding	• The impact doctors have on breastfeeding initiation and duration • Members of the breastfeeding support team • The effect of breastfeeding at a community level • Benefits of breastfeeding for infant, mother, and community at large • Factors contributing to the breastfeeding decision • Cultural and psychosocial factors that have an impact on breastfeeding rates • Common barriers to successful breastfeeding	• Historical overview • Policy implication • Role of culture and families	• Importance of breastfeeding • Key guidelines, policies, and recommendations • Infant feeding practices and recommendations
• Communication skills • Talking with a pregnant woman (clinical practice)			• Counseling skills
• How milk gets from breast to baby	• Breast anatomy and physiology • Mammary structures in milk production and transfer • Process of milk production and removal • Nipple types • Relevant past medical history • Past breastfeeding history	• Anatomy and physiology: maternal–infant roles	• Anatomy and physiology of breastfeeding

- Maternal health concerns

- The effect of breastfeeding on the health of the mother and infant
- Unique properties of human milk

- Biologic specificity of human milk and benefits of breastfeeding

- Breastfeeding process: antepartum, intrapartum, and postpartum

- Management and support

- Birth practices and breastfeeding (Step 4)
- Helping with a breastfeed (Step 5)
- Practices that assist breastfeeding (Steps 6–9)
- Observing and assisting breastfeeding (clinical practice)

- Impact of intrapartum and immediate postpartum/medications on lactation
- Supportive measures that address common issues/concerns in breastfeeding
  - ▼ During the initial postpartum period
  - ▼ At 24 hours postpartum
  - ▼ At newborn follow-up
- Proper latch-on/attachment
- Effective suckling at the breast
- Signs of adequate milk supply
- Normal breastfeeding behaviors
- Ways of suckling and
- How suckling differs between breastfeeding and bottle-feeding
- Normal growth pattern of breastfed infants
- Introduction of solids and weaning

(continues)

Table 21-1 COMPARISON OF BREASTFEEDING CONTENT OF THE *BREASTFEEDING PROMOTION AND SUPPORT IN A BABY-FRIENDLY HOSPITAL: A 20-HOUR COURSE FOR MATERNITY STAFF* AND CONTENT IN MEDICAL SCHOOL AND RESIDENCY CURRICULA, AN ELECTIVE NURSING COURSE, AND NUTRITION/DIETETIC CURRICULA (*CONTINUED*)

A 20-Hour Course for Maternity Staff** (Step of the 10 Steps)	Medical School and Residency Curricula#	Elective Nursing Lactation Course$	Nutrition/Dietetic Breastfeeding Curricula+
• Milk supply	• Concerns mothers have with breastfeeding and strategies they may use to overcome them	• Maternal issues	• Relevant issues
• Breast and nipple conditions	• Causes and management of common breastfeeding problems	• Maternal issues panel (guest mothers and infants)	• Influential factors
• Ongoing support for mothers	▼ Sore/damaged nipples	• Infant issues	• Recommended interventions
• If baby cannot feed at the breast (Step 5)	▼ Engorgement		
	▼ Perception of not producing enough milk		
	▼ Candidiasis		
	▼ Plugged ducts		
	▼ Low milk supply		
	▼ Breast infections		
	• Maintaining lactation during separation		
	• Referral pathways in the local community		
	• Maternal nutrition	• Maternal nutrition	
	• Contraceptive advice	• Contraception	
	• Medication use in breastfeeding women	• Drugs and viruses in human milk	
	• Treatments compatible with breastfeeding		
	• Reputable sources of drug information		

- Infants with special needs

- Observing hand expression and cup-feeding (clinical practice)

- Making your hospital Baby-Friendly

- Medical conditions and contra-indications to breastfeeding
- Breastfeeding abilities of infants with special healthcare needs

- List types of breast pumps
- Identify appropriate indications for use of breast pumps

- Hospital policies supporting breastfeeding
- Means by which the community can support breastfeeding

- Use of human milk and breast-feeding for preterm or other hospitalized infants
- Human milk banking

- Technology to support breastfeeding

- Translation of lactation research into clinical practice

*Data from WHO, UNICEF, & Wellstart International, 2009. (Outlines and powerpoint slides for each presentation can be found at the UNICEF website http://www.unicef.org or the World Health Organization website at www.who.int/nutrition.)

#Data from Brodribb, 2012 and Ogburn, Espey, Leeman, & Alvarez, 2005.

$Data from Spatz, Pugh and the American Academy of Nursing Expert Panel on Breastfeeding, 2007.

†Data from Radcliff & Payne, 2011.

Box 21-3 Core Competencies in Breastfeeding Care and Services for All Health Professionals from the United States Breastfeeding Committee

Competence in the following areas represents the *minimal* knowledge, skills, and attitudes necessary for health professionals from *all* disciplines to provide patient care that protects, promotes, and supports breastfeeding.

At a minimum, *every* health professional {not just HCPs specializing in maternal–child care} should understand the role of lactation, human milk, and breastfeeding in:

- The optimal feeding of infants and young children
- Enhancing health and reducing:
  - ◄ Long-term morbidities in infants and young children
  - ◄ Morbidities in women

All health professionals should be able to facilitate the breastfeeding care process by:

- Preparing families for realistic expectations
- Communicating pertinent information to the lactation care team
- Following up with the family, when appropriate, in a culturally competent manner after breastfeeding care and services have been provided

USBC proposes to accomplish this by recommending that health professional organizations:

- Understand and act upon the importance of protecting, promoting, and supporting breastfeeding as a public health priority
- Educate their practitioners to:
  - ◄ Appreciate the limitations of their breastfeeding care expertise
  - ◄ Know when and how to make a referral to a lactation care professional
- Regularly examine the care practices of their practitioners and establish core competencies related to breastfeeding care and services

Knowledge

All health professionals should understand the:

1.1 Basic anatomy and physiology of the breast
1.2 Role of breastfeeding and human milk in maintaining health and preventing disease
1.3 Importance of exclusive breastfeeding, and its correlation with optimal health outcomes
1.4 Impact of pregnancy, birth, and other healthcare practices on breastfeeding outcomes
1.5 Role of behavioral, cultural, social, and environmental factors in infant feeding decisions and practices
1.6 Potentially adverse outcomes for infants and mothers who do not breastfeed
1.7 Potential problems associated with the use of human milk substitutes
1.8 Few evidence-based contraindications to breastfeeding
1.9 Indications for referral to lactation services
1.10 Resources available to assist mothers seeking breastfeeding and lactation information or services
1.11 Effects of marketing of human milk substitutes on the decision to breastfeed and the duration of breastfeeding

Skills

All health professionals should be able to:

2.1 Practice in a manner that protects, promotes, and supports breastfeeding

2.2 Gather breastfeeding history information sufficient to identify mothers and families who would benefit from specific breastfeeding support services

2.3 Seek assistance from and refer to appropriate lactation specialists

2.4 Safeguard privacy and confidentiality

2.5 Effectively use new information technologies to obtain current evidence-based information about breastfeeding and human lactation

Attitudes

All health professionals should:

3.1 Value breastfeeding as an important health promotion and disease prevention strategy

3.2 Recognize and respect philosophical, cultural, and ethical perspectives influencing the use and delivery of breastfeeding care and services

3.3 Respect the confidential nature of the provision of breastfeeding care and services

3.4 Recognize the importance of delivering breastfeeding care and services that are free of commercial conflict of interest or personal bias

3.5 Understand the importance of tailoring information and services to the family's culture, knowledge, and language level

3.6 Seek coordination and collaboration with interdisciplinary teams of health professionals

3.7 Recognize the limitations of their own lactation knowledge and breastfeeding expertise

3.8 Recognize when personal values and biases may affect or interfere with breastfeeding care and services provided to families

3.9 Encourage workplace support for breastfeeding

3.10 Support breastfeeding colleagues

3.11 Support family-centered policies at federal, state, and local levels

All health professionals do not need to have the level of competence expected of those practitioners who care for childbearing women, infants, and young children. Health professionals who care for childbearing women, infants, and young children can be further divided into two groups:

1. Those who provide *primary care* are front-line practitioners who care for women of childbearing age and/or infants and young children.
2. Those who provide *secondary care* may be front-line practitioners or practitioners with enhanced knowledge and skills specifically referable to the use of human milk and breastfeeding.

Those health professionals who provide primary and secondary care for childbearing women, infants, and young children should be able to:

4.1 Understand the evidence-based *Ten Steps to Successful Breastfeeding*

4.2 Obtain an appropriate breastfeeding history

4.3 Provide mothers with evidence-based breastfeeding information

(continues)

BOX 21-3 (CONTINUED)

4.4   Use effective counseling skills
4.5   Offer strategies to address problems and concerns to maintain breastfeeding
4.6   Know how and when to integrate technology and equipment to support breastfeeding
4.7   Collaborate and/or refer for complex breastfeeding situations
4.8   Provide and encourage use of culturally appropriate education materials
4.9   Share evidence-based knowledge and clinical skills with other health professionals
4.10 Preserve breastfeeding under adverse conditions

In addition, those health professionals who provide secondary or more direct "hands-on" care for childbearing women, infants, and young children should also be able to:

5.1   Assist in early initiation of breastfeeding
5.2   Assess the lactating breast
5.3   Perform an infant feeding observation
5.4   Recognize normal and abnormal infant feeding patterns
5.5   Develop and appropriately communicate a breastfeeding care plan

Source: Reproduced from United States Breastfeeding Committee. (2010). Core Competencies in Breastfeeding Care and Services for All Health Professionals. Rev ed. Washington, DC: United States Breastfeeding Committee. Retrieved from http://www.usbreastfeeding.org/core-competencies

initiation rates. For the first time in several decades, the *Healthy People 2020* objectives for breastfeeding rates increased (USDHHS, 2010). More and more hospitals are working toward achieving the Baby–Friendly designation (Baby-Friendly USA, 2013). One of the new Joint Commission perinatal core measures is changing practice to increase the rate of exclusive breastmilk feeding during the first days of a newborn's life (The Joint Commission, 2013). Yet in 2011, when U.S. Surgeon General Regina Benjamin released the *Call to Action to Support Breastfeeding* (USDHHS, 2011), education was still a top priority. Indeed, 13 of the 20 action steps either directly require or intimate the need for broader breastfeeding knowledge and education among numerous audiences and constituencies (Box 21-4). Significantly, the list of health professionals (see again Box 21-2) who should be competent in breastfeeding and lactation promotion and support for women as well as health promotion education to other constituencies broadened.

While it is clear from a health policy standpoint that more education is needed for HCPs, customers are also requesting more education on breastfeeding.

Research over several decades has documented the significantly positive influence that HCPs have on a mother's decision to breastfeed (Renfrew et al., 2012) and confirmed that antenatal breastfeeding education increases commitment to breastfeeding and, therefore, the duration of breastfeeding (Lumbiganon et al., 2012; Noel-Weiss et al., 2006). Nevertheless, when asked, pregnant and new mothers complain that they are uncertain about breastfeeding because they receive minimal and inconsistent information on this topic from their healthcare providers (Archabald et al., 2011; Cricco-Lizza, 2006a; Gill, 2001; Monzingo et al., 2000).

Indeed, their observations are correct. Many HCPs have neutral or perhaps even negative attitudes toward breastfeeding (Brewer, 2012; Brodribb et al., 2008; Cricco-Lizza, 2006b) and, therefore, are reluctant to educate mothers-to-be about breastfeeding or pass the responsibility for infant feeding education to specialists (Miller et al., 2007). Lack of didactic and clinical preparation regarding the protection, promotion, and support of breastfeeding and lactation has been recognized by many professional organizations and programs as a significant

Box 21-4 ACTION STEPS IN THE *SURGEON GENERAL'S CALL TO ACTION TO SUPPORT BREASTFEEDING* CALLING FOR OR INTIMATING A NEED FOR FURTHER EDUCATION AND SUPPORT AMONG ALL CONSTITUENCIES

Action 1. Give mothers the support they need to breastfeed their babies.

- Help pregnant women to learn about the importance of breastfeeding for their babies and themselves.
- Teach mothers to breastfeed.
- Encourage mothers to talk to their maternity care providers about plans to breastfeed.
- Support mothers to have time and flexibility to breastfeed.
- Encourage mothers to ask for help with breastfeeding when needed.

Action 2. Develop programs to educate fathers and grandmothers about breastfeeding.

- Launch or establish campaigns for breastfeeding education that target a mother's primary support network, including fathers and grandmothers.
- Offer classes on breastfeeding that are convenient for family members to attend.

Action 3. Strengthen programs that provide mother-to-mother support and peer counseling.

Action 4. Use community-based organizations to promote and support breastfeeding.

- Support and fund small nonprofit organizations that promote breastfeeding in communities of color.
- Integrate education and support for breastfeeding into public health programs that serve new families.
- Ensure around-the-clock access to resources that provide assistance with breastfeeding.

Action 7. Ensure that maternity care practices throughout the United States are fully supportive of breastfeeding.

- Accelerate implementation of the Baby-Friendly Hospital Initiative.
- Establish a new advanced certification program for perinatal patient care.

Action 8. Develop systems to guarantee continuity of skilled support for lactation between hospitals and healthcare settings in the community.

Action 9. Provide education and training in breastfeeding for all health professionals who care for women and children.

- Improve the breastfeeding content in undergraduate and graduate education and training for health professionals.
- Establish and incorporate minimum requirements for competency in lactation care into the health professional credentialing, licensing, and certification process.
- Increase opportunities for continuing education on the management of lactation to ensure the maintenance of minimum competencies and skills.

Action 10. Include basic support for breastfeeding as a standard of care for midwives, obstetricians, family physicians, nurse practitioners, [physician's assistants, nurses, and pediatricians.

(continues)

BOX 21-4 (*CONTINUED*)

Action 11. Ensure access to services provided by International Board Certified Lactation Consultants.

Action 14. Ensure that employers establish and maintain comprehensive, high-quality lactation support programs for their employees.

Action 16. Ensure that all childcare providers accommodate the needs of breastfeeding mothers and infants.

Action 18. Strengthen existing capacity and develop future capacity for conducting research on breastfeeding.

Action 20. Improve national leadership on the promotion and support of breastfeeding.

Modified from: USDHHS. (2011). The Surgeon General's call to action to support breastfeeding. Washington, DC: USDHHS, Office of the Surgeon General.

---

reason for the reluctance to educate mothers and inconsistent advice (Ouyang et al., 2012; Payne et al., 2007; Whelan et al., 2011).

Recognizing the need to correct the paucity of breastfeeding and lactation content within curricula, courses (Spatz, 2005), curriculum revisions (Feldman-Winter et al., 2010; Radcliffe & Payne, 2001), and educational interventions within healthcare facilities (Bernaix et al., 2010; Rempel & McCleary, 2012; Shinwell et al., 2006) have been piloted. The outcomes of these projects have been very positive, changing attitudes and improving breastfeeding and lactation knowledge and skills. After the educational offerings, participants express a greater belief in the importance of breastfeeding and their intentions to promote and support breastfeeding with mothers and within the community (Grossman et al., 2009).

Breastfeeding Programs for Healthcare Professionals

Lactation Consultants

An early endorser of the USBC core competencies, the International Board of Lactation Consultant Examiners (IBCLE) has recently changed the requirements to apply for admission to the lactation consultant certification examination to promote mastery of the core competencies. Now candidates must complete education in 14 health science subjects (natural and social sciences) as well as a minimum of 90 hours of instruction in human lactation and breastfeeding in combination with at least 300 hours of lactation-specific clinical experience (Lactation Education Accreditation and Approval Review Committee [LEAARC], 2013a). Another feature to assure consistency among breastfeeding and human lactation programs is accreditation. To this end, the Lactation Education Accreditation and Approval Committee (www.LEAARC.org) was created. LEAARC has published guidelines to facilitate the development of breastfeeding and human lactation degree programs at universities and colleges. In late 2013, only four degree or certificate programs were offered in academic institutions (IBCLE, 2012). However, at least 25 academic institutions offer lactation courses approved by LEAARC (LEAARC, 2013b), including the human lactation course developed by Dr. Jan Riordan and offered at Wichita State University (WSU) School of Nursing. In 1997, it was the first breastfeeding course offered completely online

(Riordan, 2000) and in 2012 received LEAARC approval. Now there are residency (on campus) and online lactation courses (see http://www.ilca.org/files/education_and_research/courses_and_clinical_experience/Directory_Lactation_Management_Courses.pdf), offering interested students a variety of options to suit their unique situations.

Physicians

Medical schools and residency programs have also identified the needed for curricula content on breastfeeding and human lactation. In 2011, the Academy of Breastfeeding Medicine (ABM) published breastfeeding educational objectives and skills for physicians and suggested three levels of expertise:

- Awareness (undergraduate medical education): basic knowledge, skills, and supportive attitudes attained by all physicians. While many physicians may not typically provide care for breastfeeding mother–infant dyads, they comprehend breastfeeding as a health promotion measure and could counsel or treat a patient if necessary.
- Generalist (graduate medical education): to be achieved by physicians specializing in an aspect of maternal and child health. Course work includes more interactive opportunities in both the classroom and clinical settings. The aim is for residents to become confident and competent in providing routine lactation management and support, and to know when and how to seek lactation specialist assistance.
- Specialist: practicing physicians who continue education in breastfeeding and human lactation (postgraduate/in-service/continuing medical education) not only to maintain competence but also to enhance expertise and skills (ABM, 2011; Ogburn et al., 2005).

The American Academy of Pediatrics (AAP), with the guidance of its Section on Breastfeeding, is becoming more definitive regarding its protection, promotion, and support for breastfeeding. This evolution is demonstrated in revisions to the policy statement *Breastfeeding and the Use of Human Milk* (AAP Section on Breastfeeding, 2005, 2012; AAP Work Group on Breastfeeding, 1995), development of a sample hospital breastfeeding policy for newborns (AAP Section on Breastfeeding, 2009), and the newest publication *Ten Steps to Support Parents' Choice to Breastfeed Their Baby* (AAP Section on Breastfeeding, 2014). These 10 steps are much like a pledge for pediatricians and other health providers to become ardent advocates for breastfeeding and to create a breastfeeding friendly and supportive office and community environment.

Additionally, the AAP Section on Breastfeeding has developed a *Breastfeeding Residency Curriculum* (http://www2.aap.org/breastfeeding/curriculum/). Designed for incorporation into existing curricula for pediatric, family medicine, preventive medicine, internal medicine, and obstetrics/gynecology residency programs, the AAP website includes implementation and evaluation strategies, useful tools, and many other resources. Based on the Accreditation Council for Graduate Medical Education Core Competencies, the curriculum itself includes goals and objectives, planning, teaching and evaluation tools, prepared cases and presentations, and suggested resources for each section (AAP, n.d.).

Several medical and residency programs have incorporated breastfeeding and human lactation content into their curricula with positive results. Topics are presented through didactic sessions, clinical rounds, self-study modules (Lewin & O'Connor, 2012; O'Connor et al., 2011), and hands-on clinical experience (Saenz, 2000). In one study, a majority of the residents and medical students in pediatrics, family medicine, and obstetrics and gynecology attended two or more of the education sessions. Residents and medical students indicated their knowledge about breastfeeding increased and they were better able to support and educate their breastfeeding mothers/patients (Ogburn et al., 2005). In an evaluation of implementation of the AAP curriculum, the participants reported improved knowledge, practice patterns, and confidence in breastfeeding management and increased rates of exclusive breastfeeding among the new mothers in their care (Feldman-Winter et al., 2010).

Nurses

In 2007, the American Academy of Nursing Expert Panel on Breastfeeding published content on human milk and breastfeeding that should be integrated into nursing curricula (Spatz & Pugh, 2007). A comparison of the suggested nursing content and curriculum topics for the BFHI 20-hour course, medical residency, and nutrition/dietetic programs appears in Table 21-1. However, breastfeeding and lactation are only one of a multitude of topics covered in maternal–child and advanced practice nursing courses and frequently are allotted only 1 to 2 hours of class time (Bozzette & Posner, 2013). Therefore, the recommended content with sufficient time to adequately cover the material has not been incorporated into nursing curricula or textbooks (Boyd & Spatz, 2013; Phillipp et al., 2007). Some nursing programs offer an elective course in breastfeeding and human lactation, but they are few and far between (Spatz, 2005; Watkins & Dodgson, 2010).

Given that many healthcare facilities offer only minimal breastfeeding and bottle-feeding instruction for maternal–child staff during new-hire orientation, nurses tend to learn about breastfeeding from their colleagues and their personal, work, and family experiences. Knowledge gained in these ways may or may not be accurate or evidence based (Smith et al., 2009); thus mothers may, in turn, receive inconsistent or conflicting information and breastfeeding support. Because nurses do not graduate from their degree programs with a foundation in breastfeeding basics, it is their passion about and devotion to breastfeeding and lactation that leads them to become specialists through personal experiences, continuing education, and perhaps certification as a lactation consultant.

Other Healthcare Providers

Hospitals seeking the Baby–Friendly Hospital designation require their maternal–child nursing staff to complete 20 hours and their primary care staff to complete 3 hours of breastfeeding education to meet the BFHI requirements. With this education,

breastfeeding counseling and support is more consistent and mothers more satisfied with their experiences—a component of the evaluation for BFHI (Mellin et al., 2011). Unfortunately, many other HCPs (Box 21-2) who may care for breastfeeding dyads are unprepared to assess, treat, counsel, support, or refer the pair (Dytrych et al., 2013). This is an example of how breastfeeding education for HCPs is siloed by professional and disciplinary boundaries. In reality, mothers need a team approach to breastfeeding education and support as they progress through pregnancy, birth, and the postpartum period.

The Breastfeeding Team

Because breastfeeding protection, promotion, and support are the responsibility of multiple healthcare disciplines, interprofessional education breaks down disciplinary barriers and enriches the content presentation when examined from multiple perspectives. Then, when HCPs come together as a team, the childbearing families are the winners, as their learning experiences are enhanced with such a comprehensive approach. Consistent information shared by a variety of providers on multiple occasions strengthens the impact of each breastfeeding education encounter. Additionally, the breastfeeding team's exposure to current information (e.g., workshops, articles) strengthens consistency of education. Clear, detailed documentation with teaching checklists, care maps, and narrative notes allows HCPs to build on previous education sessions and to reinforce key points.

Childbirth Educators

Childbirth educators have promoted and supported breastfeeding for decades. During their multisession classes, childbirth educators develop rapport with expecting families. They provide invaluable anticipatory guidance by including breastfeeding information in general childbirth education programs. Following childbirth, families frequently seek breastfeeding assistance from their childbirth instructors.

Nurses

Although many nurses are also lactation consultants, all nurses within healthcare facilities and in the community should be able to provide breastfeeding education and support, especially as breastfeeding is initiated (Box 21-4, Action 10). In addition, they should be able to recognize and correct common problems related to breastfeeding. Lactation consultants or breastfeeding specialists can utilize their advanced education to manage the more complex cases.

Other groups of nurses need to be included in the breastfeeding team. For example, it is common for breastfed neonates to be admitted with dehydration, hyperbilirubinemia, or other concerns. Frequently, the admitted mother–neonate dyad is breastfeeding, but having difficulties. However, most pediatric nurses are not breastfeeding savvy, but instead need education (Brewer, 2012). Similarly, breastfeeding dyads may present in the emergency room where and when no breastfeeding experts are available. Again, as recommended, if all nurses master the core breastfeeding competencies, healthcare efficiency would be increased and premature cessation of breastfeeding prevented (Box 21-4, Action 8).

Lactation Consultants

Lactation consultants (LCs) are persons who have received certification from the International Board of Lactation Consultant Examiners (International Board Certified Lactation Consultant [IBCLC]) or other certification in lactation management (e.g., Certified Lactation Counselor® [CLC]). Certification indicates a person has received training and competency verification in breastfeeding and human lactation support and assistance. LCs provide a variety of specialized services, including individual consultations for unusual breastfeeding situations, care plan development in collaboration with other healthcare providers, breastfeeding class sessions, and instruction in the use of specific breastfeeding products. They also serve as a resource for information and data, develop special programs or projects related to breastfeeding, provide continuing education programs for healthcare providers, and conduct research (Box 21-4, Action 11).

Breastfeeding Educator/Lactation Counselors

Breastfeeding educators and lactation counselors are persons who have completed a study of breastfeeding basics (Box 21-4). These persons maybe peer counselors or on the path to becoming LCs.

Doulas

Doulas are laywomen experienced (and usually certified) in providing emotional and physical support during labor and childbirth. Generally, they are strong breastfeeding advocates as well. Doula care has been shown to increase satisfaction with the childbirth experience, increase the likelihood of a vaginal birth, decrease the use of analgesia and anesthesia (Hodnett et al., 2013), and enhance breastfeeding success with timely onset of lactogenesis (within 72 hours of birth), and extended duration of breastfeeding (Kozhimannil et al., 2013; Nommson-Rivers et al., 2009). The breastfeeding results occur either indirectly, as the doula helps reduce maternal stress and promotes more natural birth outcomes, or directly, as the doula encourages and facilitates immediate skin-to-skin contact and early breastfeeding after birth. Doula care is especially beneficial to low-income and African American mothers' breastfeeding efforts (Mottl-Santiago et al., 2008). In addition to intrapartum care, doulas provide support and education to expectant parents during pregnancy and the postpartum, further enhancing positive breastfeeding outcomes.

Primary Care Providers: Physicians, Nurse–Midwives, Midwives, Nurse Practitioners, and Physician Assistants

Primary care providers (PCPs) can serve as powerful breastfeeding promoters (Kornides & Kitsantas, 2013) (Box 21-4, Action 10). Their support of breastfeeding can be a potent force in a family's decision to begin and continue breastfeeding (Odom et al., 2013). Many PCPs are young women who are likely to choose to breastfeed for their own personal health benefits (Riggins et al., 2012) and who later become strong advocates for breastfeeding. PCPs often refer families to lactation consultants for time-intensive treatment of breastfeeding difficulties or follow-up. Some PCPs are certified as lactation consultants and may have practices that are limited to breastfeeding families.

Nutritionists and Dietitians

The responsibilities of nutritionists or dietitians, many of whom are certified lactation consultants, include nutritional counseling for childbearing families. These providers can describe the influence of breastfeeding on maternal and infant nutrition needs. Many dietitians working with breastfeeding families are employed by Women, Infants, and Children (WIC) programs and in other community health settings.

Pharmacists

Pharmacists are a largely untapped resource for breastfeeding education and support (Edwards, 2013a, 2013b). As highly visible members of the community, they routinely see expectant and new parents. Their counseling regarding use of medications during pregnancy and lactation is invaluable. In addition, pharmacists can provide health promotion and public awareness campaigns regarding breastfeeding. They can also assist with purchase of breastfeeding items and pumps, and give advice on formulas. Finally, pharmacists can be a referral resource when mothers present with commonly encountered breastfeeding difficulties (Schaffar et al., 2012).

Social Workers

In many different ways, social workers have contact with families and mothers of childbearing age. Thus social workers are ideally positioned to promote and support breastfeeding. They can provide best practice information prenatally and postnatally, as well as being aware of breastfeeding resources within the community and making referrals as appropriate. Because social workers tend to work on a one-to-one basis with mothers and young families, they have a golden opportunity to provide individualized support and to listen to mothers' stories, concerns, and subjective meanings attached to breastfeeding, so as to promote personal growth and empowerment (Hurst, 2007).

Community Support Groups

Mother-to-mother support groups create an invaluable social support network for breastfeeding families (Figure 21-2). Practical tips and much incidental learning about parenting are derived from these important support groups. The largest and most effective self-care group for breastfeeding support is La Leche League International (LLLI). Founded in 1956, LLLI's core service is mother-to-mother support and information provided through small neighborhood-based groups.

Le Leche League leaders are available between meetings for individual assistance and problem solving. The relaxed, friendly interchange between women with common interests in breastfeeding, childbearing, and childrearing is a basic strength

Figure 21-2 LA LECHE LEAGUE MEETING. ADULT LEARNING IN ACTION.

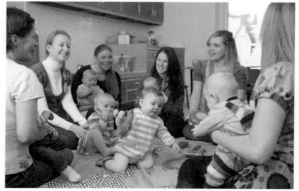

© MachineHeadz/iStockphoto

of this highly successful organization. LLLI is effective in meeting the educational and support needs of breastfeeding women worldwide.

The *Call to Action to Support Breastfeeding* identifies a number of other breastfeeding team members (Box 21-4). As the breastfeeding and human lactation landscape changes, the roles and responsibilities of the various team members are expanding. Some LCs and nurses are now working in physicians' office or clinics where they provide antenatal education, postpartum support, and advice for resolution of breastfeeding problems (Witt et al., 2012). Other LCs are opening independent practices. As the Affordable Care Act of 2010 is implemented on a practical level, insurance coverage will include prenatal and postnatal breastfeeding counseling and comprehensive lactation support by a trained provider as well as breastfeeding supplies such as a breast pump at no or low cost to the consumer (AAP Section on Breastfeeding, 2013). With assurance of reimbursement, opportunities for LCs and other breastfeeding team members abound.

Parent Education

The emphasis on provider education is intended to ensure that HCPs are competent, confident, and able to promote, protect, and support breastfeeding with those seeking care, including both expectant and new parents. It takes a village to assure all newborns get what is best for them and parents feel supported and able to do their best. If HCPs provide consistent messages regarding the significance of breastfeeding to mother, infant, and society, eventually a breastfeeding culture will be reestablished.

Prenatal Education

Most mothers make decisions about how they will feed their baby before or during their pregnancy. Pregnancy is an appropriate time to support a mother's decision to breastfeed, to correct inaccurate information, to add to the information she already has about breastfeeding, and to encourage undecided expectant mothers to consider breastfeeding. Infant feeding should be discussed before mothers start feeling the baby's movements (quickening usually occurs around the fifth month of pregnancy). When mothers begin to perceive their babies as separate beings, they start making concrete plans for care, including how they will feed their babies. Mothers need information about infant feeding, the short- and long-term benefits of breastfeeding for mother and infant, and concerns regarding bottle-feeding. With the renewed and growing emphasis on breastfeeding and, especially, on exclusive breastfeeding for 6 months, the assumption should be that all mothers will breastfeed. Therefore, the question "How are you going to feed your baby?" can be removed from our vocabulary and charting forms because frequently the expectation and advice of primary care providers can strongly influence behavior.

Preparing to Breastfeed

Toward the end of pregnancy, the focus of breastfeeding education changes to concentrate on the "how to" of breastfeeding initiation and management. Parents can be encouraged to attend breastfeeding classes offered by institutions and healthcare professionals in the community, such as hospitals, clinics, libraries, childbirth education programs, breastfeeding support groups, and lactation consultants. Classes should be accessible (with parking) and offered at times convenient to families.

To reinforce content learned in classes, expectant parents can read pamphlets and view videos while waiting for appointments. Additionally, healthcare providers can assess and add to the patients' knowledge, bringing up topics, such as appropriate nursing bras, not discussed in classes. It is generally better to have frequent, short discussions about breastfeeding throughout the course of prenatal care rather than to attempt to convey everything a mother may need to know in one breastfeeding talk.

Breastfeeding Education Topics

The content of breastfeeding classes and one-to-one discussions offered during prenatal care should include information necessary for a mother to feel confident with her decision to breastfeed as well as convinced that together baby and mother can successfully breastfeed (see Box 21-5). As birth day approaches, it is important that parents know what to expect during labor, birth, and the immediate postpartum (see Box 21-5). Some mothers might also benefit from a class providing very specific content on the "how to" of breastfeeding (see Box 21-6). A variety of teaching and learning techniques can be used to accomplish breastfeeding education, including formal or informal classes, videos, and printed materials (see the discussion later in this chapter). Nevertheless, education programs, however well developed, augment rather than replace the responsibility of healthcare providers for individualized assessment and one-to-one teaching specific to each family.

Early Postpartum Education

Parents need to appreciate the "work" and learning occurring immediately after birth and during the first 48 to 72 hours of the neonate's life and plan accordingly. The early postpartum is the babymoon (like honeymoon)—prime time for parents to get to know their newborn, and vice versa. It is also a time when neural synapses are being created in a newborn's brain exceedingly quickly, so every action and activity become learning experiences. To make the learning permanent, actions need to be repeated. For example, when infants are in kangaroo care (Figure 21-3), they are connecting to their mothers as they learn her smell, hear familiar sounds, and know they have ready access to food. Therefore, when developing their birth plan, parents need to include their desires for the first days and weeks after birth, making sure quiet, uninterrupted, relaxed time is available for the priorities—establishing breastfeeding, creating parent–infant attachments, and morphing into a parent.

As parents gain hands-on experience with their infants, many of the breastfeeding topics discussed during the pregnancy will be reinforced. When providing education, HCPs must remember new mothers have limited stamina and are unable to retain large quantities of new information (Eidelman

et al., 1993; Workman et al., 2012). Therefore, providing education in small segments with return demonstrations over the course of the postpartum stay enhances learning and retention (see Box 21-6), Additionally, parents' questions need to be addressed first, because parents will not attend to other information presented by HCPs until their own concerns are addressed. Finally, postpartum content needs to be prioritized from most important to least important. For example, information that relates to continuing breastfeeding and ensuring infant well-being is most important, whereas information pertaining to returning to employment and weaning is better presented closer to the time of occurrence.

When special circumstances, such as prematurity, multiple births, congenital anomalies, or

Figure 21-3 MOTHER PROVIDING KANGAROO CARE DURING POSTPARTUM STAY.

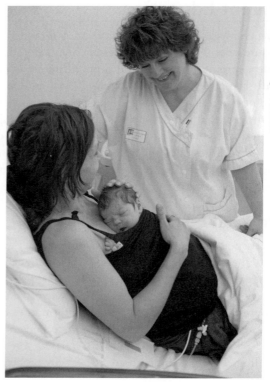

© CHASSENET/age fotostock

BOX 21-5 RECOMMENDED TOPICS FOR PRENATAL BREASTFEEDING CLASSES

Early Pregnancy

- Assess knowledge and perceptions regarding breastfeeding
- Explore and identify concerns
  - ◄ Personal feelings
  - ◄ Families' feelings (including partner/significant other, grandmothers)
  - ◄ Dealing with disapproval
- Acknowledge and validate feelings
- Breastfeeding as a public health issue
  - ◄ First immunization
  - ◄ Illness prevention
  - ◄ Obesity risk reduction
  - ◄ Chronic illness risk reduction for mother and infant
- Short-term advantages of breastfeeding and skin-to-skin care
  - ◄ For infant
  - ◄ For mother
- Long-term advantages of breastfeeding, kangaroo care, and holding
  - ◄ For infant
  - ◄ For mother
- Cons and pros of formula-feeding
- Other topics
  - ◄ Primary care provider (physician/midwife) recommendations
  - ◄ Ease of breastfeeding
  - ◄ Breastfeeding with modesty
  - ◄ Family involvement
  - ◄ Nutrition and lifestyle
  - ◄ Breastfeeding and work/school
  - ◄ Available people to assist
- Resource and support network
  - ◄ Family and friends
  - ◄ Healthcare providers
  - ◄ Mother-to-mother support group

Later Pregnancy

- Influences on breastfeeding
  - ◄ Labor and birth practices
  - ◄ Analgesia and anesthesia
  - ◄ Cesarean birth
- Birth and first breastfeeding
  - ◄ Immediate skin-to-skin contact and early breastfeeding
  - ◄ Abilities of newborn: breast crawl
  - ◄ Delay of measurements, eye treatment, first shots
- First postpartum days
  - ◄ Baby-lead, laid-back breastfeeding
  - ◄ 24 hour rooming-in
  - ◄ Importance of frequent breastfeeding: on demand and cluster feeds
  - ◄ Continuing kangaroo care
  - ◄ Rest
  - ◄ Visitors and interruptions
- Assessment of adequate milk intake
- Lactogenesis and engorgement
- Milk expression and engorgement
- Prevention of nipple trauma
- Establishing, maintaining, and increasing milk supply
- Nursing bras and clothing for discreet breastfeeding
- Choosing and obtaining a breast pump
- Follow-up for lactation concerns
- Significance of continuing breastfeeding, kangaroo care, and holding

BOX 21-6 SAMPLE CONTENT FOR "HOW-TO" BREASTFEEDING CLASS (BASED ON COMMON CONCERNS OF MOTHERS)

How Do I Get Off to a Good Start?

- Begin skin-to-skin contact immediately after birth
    - Baby, mother, and significant other time
    - Allow newborn to progress through the nine phases of adaptation to extrauterine life
    - Allow the newborn to crawl to the breast, latch on, and suckle at its own pace
    - Maintain skin-to-skin contact through the first breastfeeding, usually 60–90 minutes after birth
    - Delay of measurements, eye treatment, first shots
- 24 hour rooming-in
- Kangaroo care as much as possible or desired
- What if separation is medically necessary?
    - Initiate pumping within 6 hours of birth
    - Start kangaroo care as soon as medically possible
- How often to breastfeed
    - Baby-led feeding/on demand
    - If newborn is in kangaroo care (skin-to-skin on mother's chest/abdomen), allow him to crawl to the breast
    - Laid-back breastfeeding: recline at a 25- to 45-degree angle so infant is fully supported by mother's body, and can crawl and use primitive neonatal reflexes to reach the breast
    - Identify early feeding cues
    - Frequent feeding, at least 8–12 times/24 hours
    - Alternate breasts when starting a feeding
    - Allow newborn to suckle as long as desired
    - Listen for swallowing
    - Avoid clock watching

Will I Have Enough Milk?

- What causes decreased milk production?
    - Infrequent feedings during first 48–72 hours
    - Long intervals between feedings
    - Formula or water supplementation
    - Pacifier use
    - Smoking
- Do I have to change my lifestyle?
- Nutrition, fluids, and rest
    - Listen to your body
    - Eat when hungry
    - Drink when thirsty
    - Rest when tired
- Medications, drugs, alcohol, and nicotine
- If the mother gets a cold

Will Breastfeeding Hurt?

- Do I have to prepare my nipples?
  - ◄ Check for nipple protrusion
- Do I need special supplies or equipment?
- Kangaroo care for better newborn sleep and early recognition when ready to feed
- Positioning and latch-on
  - ◄ Find a comfortable, supportive place for laid-back nursing
  - ◄ Place the neonate on the chest/abdomen so he is completely supported, with head on the mother's chest where the mother can see and kiss the baby's face
  - ◄ Allow the neonate to crawl to the breast in his own time
  - ◄ Neonate will find asymmetrical position (not in cradle or football position, body at angle across maternal abdomen or perpendicular to breast)
  - ◄ Neonate will latch on; wide-open mouth will come over the nipple and areola, in the correct latch
  - ◄ Once breastfeeding is established, can use alternative positions: cradle hold, football hold, side-lying
  - ◄ Demonstrate with visual aids, doll
- What is a good latch?
  - ◄ Wide-open mouth
  - ◄ Lips flanged
  - ◄ Nose and chin to breast
  - ◄ No sharp pain
- Can I prevent sore nipples?
  - ◄ Break latch if it hurts
  - ◄ Breastfeed frequently
  - ◄ Start on less sore side
  - ◄ Creams and ointments (not always helpful)

Where Can I Get Help?

- Father/significant other's special role
- Types of help
  - ◄ Practical help
  - ◄ Emotional help
  - ◄ Skilled assistance
- Dealing with advice and opinions
- Sources for expert help with breastfeeding
- How do I know if the baby is getting enough?
  - ◄ Can hear baby swallowing regularly
  - ◄ Bowel movements (at least 4/24 hours)
  - ◄ Satisfied between feedings
  - ◄ Feeding at least 8 times/24 hours
- Family life with baby
  - ◄ Enjoying baby
  - ◄ Consoling baby
  - ◄ Fear of "spoiling" baby
- When to call for help
  - ◄ Baby feeding every hour (unless cluster feeding for growth spurt)
  - ◄ Feedings last more than 1 hour
  - ◄ Baby sleeping for more than 4–5 hours more than once/24 hours
  - ◄ Baby feeding fewer than 7 times/24 hours
  - ◄ Baby has fewer than 4 bowel movements/24 hours
  - ◄ Severe nipple pain
  - ◄ Tender swollen area in breast (mastitis)
- Learn and respond to baby's cues
- Use expert resources

(continues)

BOX 21-6 (CONTINUED)

Will Breastfeeding Hurt?	Where Can I Get Help?
• What is engorgement? How do I manage engorgement?	
◀ Breastfeed frequently	
◀ Cold packs/heat to breasts	
◀ Express or use breast pump to remove some milk if necessary	
◀ Softer, smaller breasts (after engorgement) do not mean lost milk supply	

---

infant neurologic impairment, affect the initiation of breastfeeding, the emotional ramifications of the experience complicate parents' learning. A family with special needs will benefit from individualized teaching and assistance and from ongoing group support. It is hard for parents to retain information when they are under stress. Prioritize content so that information is given when it is pertinent and is repeated frequently.

Continuing Support for Breastfeeding Families

Although mothers may have a positive breastfeeding experience at the birth setting, breastfeeding continuance is influenced by situations they encounter after they return home. The sharp decline in breastfeeding in the early weeks postpartum demonstrates the need mothers have for assistance and follow-up (Brand et al., 2011). A systematic program to ensure contact with the new breastfeeding mother can be a powerful influence on breastfeeding duration (Renfrew et al., 2012). Where feasible, telephone contact (Carlsen et al., 2013), home care, or early return visits to a clinic are ideal. Each mother should be able to identify at least one resource person for information, support, and assistance.

In addition to needing information and assistance with solving breastfeeding challenges, mothers need support and encouragement to continue

breastfeeding (see Box 21-7) (Renfrew et al., 2012). Family, peers, and community resources are often their primary sources of support. However, HCPs have a role to play in assessing and augmenting or creating support systems as well.

Adult Learning Principles and Education

We are born to learn. Learning is innately social and happens within a social context, referred to as situated learning (Hansman, 2001). It is the intersection of the interactions among learners, the tools used within the interaction, and the learning activity. Learning takes place in a context of practice where both mastery of practice and the process of gaining mastery are modelled. Thus learning is both cognitive and experiential (Sternberg & Zhang, 2000).

However, whether students are HCPs, parents, or community members, they are all adult learners. Adults are self-directed when they choose to attend educational activities (Knowles, 1980). Adults perceive time as one of their most valued and scarce assets, and they are not willing to spend it in meaningless activity. Education programs, therefore, must demonstrate a clear applicability to the adult's everyday life. For example, discussion of the anatomy of the breast and the physiology of breastfeeding is more meaningful when related directly

---

BOX 21-7 RECOMMENDED TOPICS FOR AN ONGOING BREASTFEEDING SUPPORT CLASS

Newborn Adjustment

- Parental fatigue, time management
- Physical changes during postpartum
- Maternal mood changes
- Management of fussiness, crying
  - ◀ Concerns about "spoiling" infants
  - ◀ Consoling techniques
  - ◀ Infant's need for holding/kangaroo care
- Infant sleeping issues, nighttime parenting
  - ◀ Sleep in mother/parent's room for first year
  - ◀ Safe sleep
- Transition of the family from two to three (feeling left out)
  - ◀ Being a person, a partner, and a parent
  - ◀ Sexuality and contraception
- Dealing with unsolicited advice
- Blended families
  - ◀ Sibling adjustments
  - ◀ Pet adjustments

Breastfeeding Concerns

- Milk supply concerns
- Assessing adequacy of infant intake
- Strategies to increase milk supply
- Appetite and growth spurts
- Frequency of breastfeeding as baby gets older
- Involving family members
- Obstructed ducts and mastitis
- Weaning

Returning to an Employment/School Setting

- Feasibility of combining breastfeeding and employment outside the home
- Feeding options
- Childcare considerations
- Time management
- Selecting a breastmilk expression technique (hand expression and breast pump options)
- Expression and storing breastmilk
- Maintaining milk supply
- Maintaining the baby's interest in breastfeeding
- Keeping breastfeeding in perspective

---

to practical skills, such as latch-on techniques and how often to feed baby.

Adult learners have a rich variety of backgrounds and motivations for participating in educational programs. They appreciate and expect respect as unique individuals. If the instructor identifies what these personal learning needs are and fulfills them, learning occurs quickly and easily. Adult learning should be self-directed and provide feedback about the learner's progress toward achieving these goals (Figure 21-4). Parents should be considered co-learners in that they teach each other as well as the instructor, who will invariably learn at least one new piece of information at every class—an exchange of who is the master and who is mastering.

Figure 21-4 ADULTS ARE
SELF-DIRECTED AND HAVE
INDIVUDAL LEARNING NEEDS.

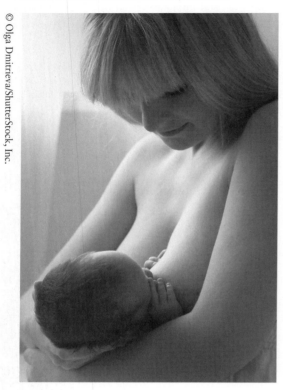

© Olga Dmitrieva/ShutterStock, Inc.

Learning is most effective when individuals are ready to learn. It comes at "teachable moments," those periods when learners perceive the need for information and skills that are relevant to their day-to-day lives. Motivation is further enhanced when the material to be learned is organized in a manner that makes it meaningful to the learner. Activities that are novel, creative, inventive, and challenging encourage learning. In addition, active, rather than passive, participation leads to more meaningful and permanent learning. Finally, as the facilitator, demonstrating enthusiasm and passion for the subject and for teaching it can be contagious, again increasing motivation and learning (Nilson, 2010).

Learning can be divided into three domains, and breastfeeding education incorporates all three (Bloom, 1956):

- Cognitive skills: Gathering information, linking concepts, problem solving
- Psychomotor skills: Listening to instructions, observing skills, repetitive practice, and mastery of skill performance
- Affective learning: Modifying attitudes, values, and preferences

Creating instructional activities that incorporate all three domains within a session or class will also enhance learning.

When planning teaching strategies, individual learning styles need to be considered (Lauwers & Shinskie, 2011). Some participants learn primarily through auditory perceptions; they listen intently and remember what they hear. Others learn best visually and retain information about what they see. These learners benefit from visual aids and printed materials. A third mode of learning is kinesthetic, or psychomotor, learning. Kinesthetic learners benefit from touching and handling equipment and models. Most learners use all three modalities. Therefore, in teaching about breast pumps, learning is strengthened by discussion coupled with showing slides that demonstrate how pumps work and having the learners manipulate the equipment.

Because success is predictably more motivating than failure, dividing tasks and information into easily mastered segments keeps the adult learners motivated to continue the program. Learners respond to specific descriptions of their positive performance. Praise enhances feelings of self-confidence and conveys respect for the learner.

Thus principles of adult education are applicable to breastfeeding education using these approaches:

- Ensure that content and timing of teaching coincide with parents' readiness to learn (prior to conception, during pregnancy, immediately postbirth, and later postpartum).
- Prioritize and present information in easily understood and easily mastered segments.
- Organize activities in increments to increase the likelihood of success.
- Give explicit instructions so that participants clearly understand what they are asked to do.
- Provide specific, immediate feedback following each activity.

- Recognize the importance of body language and nonverbal communication.
- Use handouts, DVDs, and other media to reinforce and augment rather than to replace individualized assessment and teaching. Repeating new material in different ways reinforces learning.
- Identify breastfeeding support resources, including telephone numbers of local resources.

Several factors enhance a positive learning climate. Lighting, temperature, seating, the availability of writing surfaces furnished with paper and pencils, and the ability to view materials comfortably have a tremendous impact on learning. Adults appreciate physical comfort and knowing where drinks, food, and restroom facilities are located.

Adult education programs need to be a social as well as a learning activity, because they afford opportunities to become acquainted with other adults. Greet each person warmly; demonstrate genuine concern for each one as an individual. It is a good idea to structure break periods with refreshments to encourage socializing. Adults enjoy sharing informal learning activities with others, and successful programs encourage adults to have fun as they learn. Adults also expect teachers to value students' opinions about the usefulness of learning activities. One way to find out which areas of the program were helpful is to request informal verbal feedback or formal written evaluations. Evaluations are important data to modify and improve programs.

Curriculum Development

Assessing Learning Needs

Assessing learning needs is mandatory when working with adult learners regardless whether the students are HCPs, parents, policy makers, church groups, or undergraduate or high school students. There must be a match between what the learner needs to know and what the teacher presents. If the teacher erroneously assumes that learners already possess a high level of knowledge, learners can be frustrated because the information is too complex. Conversely, learners may be offended if the instructor assumes they have minimal knowledge.

To assess levels of knowledge when working with small groups, the facilitator can ask nonthreatening questions, such as "What are some of the myths about breastfeeding you have heard?" In larger class settings, the content cannot be easily personalized. Therefore, asking participants at the beginning of class which specific topics they would like to discuss helps assess their learning needs and involves them in establishing the curriculum. If invited to speak to a group with which you are unfamiliar, ask the person extending the invitation about the group and specifics about the topics that he or she would like addressed. Ultimately, the time given to a topic is a reflection of its importance, taking into consideration how frequently the information will be used. For example, in a breastfeeding class, positioning and latch-on are fundamental to breastfeeding, so they deserve a more thorough discussion than adoptive nursing, which is relevant to a much smaller group of learners.

Too much information at one time is overwhelming, and prioritizing teaching is critical. For example, with pregnant mothers who plan to breastfeed, basic physiologic requirements, such as adequacy of the infant's nutrient intake, help guide prioritization. For nursing and medical students, basic physiologic requirements may include supplementation with vitamins and iron, along with signs of dehydration. The time span over which information can be conveyed needs to be considered, ensuring that information is given in smaller, time-appropriate chunks. Thus, when a family is in the birth setting, the HCP may share with the mother that breastfeeding can continue when she returns to work. However, explaining specific techniques for breastfeeding while working can wait until after breastfeeding is established and closer to when mother will be returning to work.

Attitudes Related to Breastfeeding

The types of attitudes and beliefs about breastfeeding that students bring with them when they enter the classroom will determine what and how breastfeeding information is received and shared with others (Juliff et al., 2007). For example, graduate students who take an elective lactation course will likely have a more positive attitude about breastfeeding than students who are taking a mandatory maternal–child or obstetric course (Froehlich et al., 2013). When Cricco-Lizza (2006b) studied the attitudes of entering nursing students, she uncovered and described students' vivid accounts of shocked reactions to women breastfeeding. Students generally believed that breastfeeding offered benefits for babies and mothers, but these beliefs were stronger for those individuals who grew up where breastfeeding was the norm. Additionally, many students considered formula to be equivalent to human milk. Most students were ambivalent about whether promoting breastfeeding would be forcing their personal views upon mothers and felt that nurses had more of an educational role with patients (Ahmed & El Guindy, 2011). By exploring these concerns about ambivalence and past experiences at the beginning of a course, it becomes less likely that they will negatively influence students' ability to choose to breastfeed or to promote breastfeeding.

Objectives and Outcomes

Whether for a single class or a semester-long course, it is useful to clearly identify what the learner is expected to master. Writing behavioral objectives is one concrete way of identifying learning goals. A behavioral objective states what the student will be able to do at the end of the session. Table 21-2 offers examples of the correct and incorrect way to write behavioral objectives.

Program outcomes are different from objectives. Objectives have to do with what a learner is able to do as a result of an education program, whereas outcomes are the results of clinical practice that may be an indirect outgrowth of educational programs. An example is staff nurses who become more knowledgeable about breastfeeding initiation after attending a series of continuing-education programs, with this new knowledge ultimately resulting in a practice change, such as putting newborns in skin-to-skin contact with their mothers immediately after birth for at least an hour, with breastfeeding being initiated during that time. Outcomes must be relevant, measurable, and a logical result of clinical practices or of institutional effort. Examples of breastfeeding outcomes are listed in Box 21-8.

All of the outcomes in Box 21-8 are relevant and measurable, and they reflect parent, staff, and institutional knowledge and effort. While clinical outcomes are monitored monthly or quarterly in most institutions, they also provide data for Joint Commission reports and national surveys like the Maternity Practices in Infant Nutrition and Care (mPINC; http://www.cdc.gov/breastfeeding /data/mpinc/index.htm). Additionally, outcomes, especially improving outcomes, reflect the effect of educational programs, thereby documenting the importance and effectiveness of continued learning.

Table 21-2 EXAMPLES OF BEHAVIORAL OBJECTIVES AND TERMS

Incorrect Objective	Correct Objective
The participant will understand the relationship between breastfeeding and jaundice.	The learner will list the types of neonatal jaundice.
(Note: The student's "understanding" is not observable.)	The learner will describe the relationship of each type of jaundice to breastfeeding.
Terms Not Observable or Measurable	**Observable/Measurable Terms for Objectives**
Understand, know, appreciate, learn, perceive, recognize, be aware of, comprehend, grasp the significance of, gain a working knowledge of	State, list, define, identify, describe, compare, critique, rate, demonstrate, plan, design, choose, discuss, match, relate, categorize, distinguish between (among), locate

---

BOX 21-8 EXAMPLES OF BREASTFEEDING OUTCOMES

- Number (percentage) of newborns placed skin-to-skin within 5 minutes of birth
- Duration of skin-to-skin contact immediately after birth
- Number (percentage) of newborns initiating breastfeeding within the first 2 hours after birth
- Number (percentage) of mothers who exclusively breastfeed (or breastmilk-feed) during their newborn's first 2 days of life
- Duration (weeks or months) of exclusive breastfeeding
- Rate of ER visits (or readmissions) for breastfed infants with dehydration
- Cost savings to the managed care organization due to the better health of infants because they were breastfed

---

Teaching Strategies

Good teaching or class facilitation involves organizing learning experiences that keep the participants' interest and use the facilitator's time efficiently. For example, the lecture format is an efficient use of the instructor's time; however, participants remain passive, which is associated with decreased retention. A more effective strategy is to vary the teaching format. Team presentations, small-group discussions, demonstrations, role playing, question-and-answer sessions with teacher-led or student-led questioning, observations and comments by participants, group projects, and individualized instruction modules are effective ways to break the monotony of lecture presentations (Nilson, 2010).

Each teaching session should include an introduction, learning experience, and conclusion or summary. A fundamental axiom is to "Explain what you're going to teach, teach, and then describe what you have taught."

Small-Group Dynamics

Formal classes and educational media might provide information to large numbers of people, but teaching small groups is a much more powerful method for behavioral change. Group discussions enhance peer support, facilitate decision making, and decrease dependence on healthcare professionals. A group is two or more people who interact and influence each other, accomplish common goals, and derive satisfaction from maintaining membership in the group. The ideal group size ranges from 8 to 12 people. In general, having more than 10 people in a group decreases productivity (Nilson, 2010).

Small-group interaction has the advantages of stimulating a free flow of information and encouraging participation as different questions are asked and new topics are raised. Small groups meet human needs for companionship, knowledge, and identity. Discussion in a small group is more likely to satisfy participants' information needs, because they usually feel more comfortable asking questions and changing the topic than when they are in a large group. An informal, relaxed setting also encourages participation.

The group leader needs to be an expert in the subject content area and skilled in group dynamics. Familiarity with the different roles played by group members will enhance the group leader's effectiveness in moving the group in a fruitful direction. Although the group leader initially may actively guide the discussion, the goal is to act as a resource for information, encouraging participants to develop their own creative and problem-solving abilities (Nilson, 2010). When participants share their personal experiences, it enhances learning and increases self-worth as individuals' efforts are reinforced and supported by the group.

Multimedia Presentations

Education programs must compete with television, videos/DVDs, smart phones, tablets, YouTube, and the Web. Consequently, visual enhancements are almost mandatory for educational programs. However, they should not lead to the lecture trap.

Generating a presentation via computer is now routine. Most persons are familiar with Power-Point®, Keynote®, or similar packages that are a standard component of office software packages. In addition, newer ways of creating presentations are emerging:

- Prezi© (Prezi.com): Prezi is an online tool that allows the creation of visual, interactive mindmaps. Prezi is nonlinear. Whereas slides are characterized by their static nature, with Prezi the "big picture" can be presented and then the user can zoom in to interact with different elements on the virtual canvas, always with the option of zooming out to see the big picture again.
- Google docs allows the creation of presentations and documents in the "cloud," where others can collaborate in their creation or access and view a presentation on their own time.
- Webinars (Web-based seminars) comprise a presentation, lecture workshop, or seminar transmitted over the Web. Webinars are interactive, allowing participants to both give and receive information discussed. For continuing-education offerings or online courses, webinars offer a means of reaching a diverse audience locally, regionally, nationally, or internationally. By archiving webinars, individuals who are unable to attend a live presentation can "attend" at their own convenience.

It is possible to make presentations truly multimedia experiences by embedding video clips within the presentation. Video clips are excellent means of demonstrating live-action psychomotor skills such as positioning mother and baby for breastfeeding. Videos and DVDs are also great for presenting content that is more commanding in real time, such as seeing newborns use their primitive neonatal reflexes to crawl to the breast. Similarly, using movies or movie segments, like *The Business of Being Born*, is a great way to introduce controversial topics and spur discussion or to compare cultural practices, as in *Babies*. DVDs can also allow education to occur wherever mothers might be: in a waiting room, on hospital networks, or at home. Many DVDs and YouTube videos with breastfeeding information are now available. The *Journal of Human Lactation* regularly publishes reviews of such breastfeeding-related visual presentations.

Case Studies

Case studies are an effective way to integrate experiences and knowledge, especially in professional education (Spatz, 2005). With case studies, real-life situations are analyzed by applying course knowledge and formulating solutions that can then be tested in a safe environment and revised with or validated by others in the course. Case studies help develop problem-solving and higher-level cognitive skills such as application, analysis, synthesis, and evaluation. Effective case studies can improve students' perceptions of and confidence in their learning as well as enhance faculty's sense of student achievement (Nilson, 2010).

Workbooks and Textbooks

Students benefit from exposure to content in multiple ways. Parents may find workbooks a great way to review topics covered in class, especially when so much material is presented at a time. Participants in continuing-education events appreciate receiving handouts, reference lists, and resource materials from speakers. These materials may be used later to develop class content for parent education, to develop policies, or to share with work colleagues in support of practice changes. Some courses provide more extensive workbooks or manuals, such as the *Skin-to-Skin Certified Kangaroo Caregiver Learner's Program Manual*, which was developed by members of the United States Institute of Kangaroo Care for the *Kangaroo Care Certification Course* (Ludington-Hoe et al., 2012). Within the manual are detailed summaries of all the evidence related to kangaroo care (more than 1000 published research studies) as well as a module on implementation and numerous other resources; the manual is a coveted take-home reference.

When teaching a course, it is always nice to find a textbook to reinforce and supplement the content. Fortunately, there are a number of texts on breastfeeding and human lactation, such as this one, written for a variety of audiences. As the breastfeeding and human lactation literature expands, some of the texts are focusing on special issues such as suckling skills (Genna, 2013), the impact of birthing practices on breastfeeding, and legal and ethical issues for lactation consultants (Brooks, 2013).

Faculty teaching breastfeeding and human lactation content in programs geared toward non-specialist health professionals are not as fortunate as faculty preparing lactation consultants. Breastfeeding information in maternal–child and obstetric textbooks needs to be critically reviewed before selecting these resources as course texts to confirm that the information is consistent, accurate, and evidence based. Unfortunately, recent studies found information in textbooks used by specialties such as nursing (Phillipp et al., 2007), midwifery (Kaso et al., 2011), pediatrics (Phillipp et al., 2004), obstetrics and gynecology (Ogburn et al., 2011), and pharmacy (Amir et al., 2013) to be highly variable and at times inaccurate and inconsistent with significant omissions. To provide some consistency within textbooks, WHO (2009) has developed a model breastfeeding chapter for medical students and allied health professionals.

Educational Materials

People retain new information for a shorter period when they are under stress. After the physical and emotional stress of pregnancy and childbirth, families will benefit from written materials that reinforce (not replace) one-on-one individualized teaching and class content provided throughout pregnancy and during the postpartum (Curro et al., 1997). Box 21-9 contains suggestions for creating effective printed materials.

BOX 21-9 SUGGESTIONS FOR CREATING AND USING WRITTEN MATERIALS

- Adults retain about 30% of the information they hear.
  - ◀ Multimodal approaches (seeing and hearing) increase retention to 50%.
  - ◀ Example: If a mother practices positioning at the breast or assembles a breast pump in addition to reading printed matter, her retention is improved.
- Scrutinize materials closely for accuracy and most current, evidence-based information (Box 21-10).
  - ◀ Conflicting, inconsistent recommendations frustrate new parents.
  - ◀ Ensure an unbiased presentation of benefits and risks to help parents make an informed feeding decision.
- Materials should not focus on management of every potential breastfeeding difficulty or complication, as these may frighten mothers, discouraging breastfeeding.
- Materials should always include a local resource telephone number.
- Printed matter should be attractively packaged, inviting parents to read it.
  - ◀ Easy to read (see Box 21-10).
  - ◀ Generous amounts of white space, as too much content on a page can be overwhelming.
- Pictorial learning is superior to verbal learning for recognition and recall. Pictures and drawings make materials more interesting.
- Assess the mother's interest in reading before making recommendations about written materials.
  - ◀ Women who do not like to read books or do not speak English may think that if they have to read a book, breastfeeding may be too difficult for them.

More is not always better when presenting printed materials. Bombarding families with thick stacks of pamphlets and materials decreases the likelihood of their use. By comparison, providing a few carefully selected pamphlets can convey the idea that breastfeeding is uncomplicated and enjoyable. Pamphlets and short audiovisual programs are preferable to lengthy materials that attempt to cover the gamut of breastfeeding experiences.

Brief, focused materials should address the issues that the family perceives as meaningful and that they are motivated to learn. This concept applies especially to mothers and families in special circumstances (such as prematurity, birth anomalies, and re-lactation). Books that are divided into small segments with detailed indices will help families locate needed information. Visual materials are more effective if they depict parents with ethnic, socioeconomic, and cultural backgrounds that are similar to the target audience. For example, teenage mothers respond most favorably to visual representations of adolescent mothers. Maintaining a lending library of books and videotapes conveys a commitment to empowering families.

When evaluating educational materials, the source of the information needs to be considered. Organizations whose purpose is to promote and sell formula cannot be expected to genuinely promote breastfeeding (Valaitis & Shea, 1993). Underlying messages may communicate that bottle-feeding is the cultural norm and that breastfeeding is difficult, complicated, uncomfortable, immodest, and inconvenient (Valaitis et al., 1997). There is often an explicit message that when families begin using formula, the product of that company is the optimal choice.

The target audience should also be considered when evaluating educational information. Materials must be written at a reading level that the reader can understand (Dollahite et al., 1996). Most word-processing programs can calculate the reading level of material with a simple click of a button. Box 21-10 lists the criteria for evaluation of education materials.

BOX 21-10 CRITERIA FOR EVALUATING EDUCATIONAL MATERIAL

Content

- Specific to family's needs
- Accurate, reliable, evidence-based information
- Accepted principles of anatomy and physiology
- Up-to-date recommendations
- Consistency between narrative and visual aids
- Simple, uncomplicated approach
- Avoids dwelling on difficulties or potential complications

Presentation

- Attractive, inviting
- Organized for easy scanning
  - ◀ Bold headings
  - ◀ Short paragraphs
  - ◀ Ample white space

Promotional Materials

- Enthusiastically discusses benefits of breastfeeding
- Includes risks of bottle-feeding
- Culturally appropriate breastfeeding modeled
- Includes practical tips for successful breastfeeding
- Provides information for additional resources

Source of Materials

- No underlying or hidden messages about the use of formula
- Breastfeeding presented as complicated, uncomfortable, immodest, and inconvenient
- Complies with WHO Code, which precludes healthcare providers from distributing materials provided by formula companies

Content	Promotional Materials
Appropriate reading level ◀ *Less than high school education (grade 3):* Need more visuals, less narrative. ◀ *High school graduate (grades 5–7):* Newspapers are written at this level. ◀ *College graduation (grades 12–13):* Professional journals are written at this level. • Generous use of appropriate pictures, drawings, and graphs consistent with narrative • Visual aids depict families from similar backgrounds as audience • Appropriate length to maintain interest	

SUMMARY

National and international policies and numerous healthcare professional organizations' recommendations strongly endorse exclusive breastfeeding for 6 months, with continued breastfeeding as complementary foods are introduced. However, it is recognized that most healthcare providers receive minimal breastfeeding content or hands-on experience during their educational programs. Therefore, to prepare healthcare providers as active breastfeeding advocates, provider education needs to be enhanced.

Educational programs for HCPs who assist breastfeeding families are being developed and implemented. As providers gain more expertise in this area, the ripple effect of the enhanced knowledge will benefit enormous numbers of breastfeeding families. A successful educational program—regardless of its subject matter—entails positive experiences for learners and educators. Identifying the components of effective breastfeeding education programs can assist faculty and teachers who are involved in planning, implementing, and evaluating breastfeeding services.

Breastfeeding families are empowered and gain self-confidence when healthcare providers furnish consistent, evidence-based information in an accurate, well-organized manner. Presenting good information with multiple modalities and addressing identified family goals enhances parents' confidence in their ability to breastfeed their newborn. Reinforcing the education with breastfeeding initiation and providing support throughout the postpartum increases the likelihood of exclusive breastfeeding for a longer duration.

KEY CONCEPTS

• Protecting, promoting, and supporting breastfeeding is component of public health policy and programs nationally and internationally.

• The lack of significant breastfeeding content within the curricula of healthcare providers' educational programs is a barrier to meeting breastfeeding goals.

• Breastfeeding curricula, core competencies, and recognition of levels of expertise in breastfeeding and human lactation are being proposed and verified.

• The breastfeeding team is expanding, which in turn increases the need for consistent, evidence-based, pertinent education for all healthcare providers.

• Many parents look to healthcare providers for information and advice on the best practices related to caring for their newest family member.

- There are six time periods to consider for breastfeeding and lactation education:
  1. Preconception: Introduce healthy lifestyle and possible changes to maximize personal health in preparation for pregnancy and breastfeeding.
  2. Early pregnancy: Promote breastfeeding. Provide information on breastfeeding and bottle-feeding so parents can make an informed choice about infant feeding.
  3. Late pregnancy: Discuss the "how-to" of breastfeeding and what to expect immediately after birth (skin-to-skin contact and breastfeeding) and during the postpartum stay (frequent breastfeeding, attachment, and rest).
  4. Immediate postpartum: Support and encourage families while initiating breastfeeding and prepare them for continuing breastfeeding.
  5. Postpartum: Offer continued support and encouragement regarding resolving breastfeeding difficulties and complications, preparing to return to work, and weaning.
  6. Continuous: Promote breastfeeding to mothers of all ages to create a breastfeeding culture (Giles et al., 2013; Howett et al., 2006; Kavanagh et al., 2012; November, 2013).
- Assessing learning needs of adults is mandatory. There must be a match between what the learner needs to know, what the teacher presents, and how much time is devoted to important topics.
- Learning is most effective when individuals are ready to learn (the teachable moment) and educational material is organized in a manner that makes it meaningful to the learner.
- Learning is divided into three domains: cognitive skills, psychomotor skills, and affective learning. Breastfeeding education for HCPs and parents addresses all of these domains.
- Knowledge retention increases when multiple instructional methods involving several senses are used.

- Adults retain only about 30% of the information they hear but 50% percent of a multimodal approach (both seeing and hearing).
- Education programs must demonstrate a clear applicability to adult learners' everyday life so they do not see it as a meaningless activity and a waste of time.
- To facilitate the learning experience for parents requires understanding the tasks of adulthood—that is, acquisition of the parental role.
- Families with special needs will benefit from individualized teaching, assistance, and ongoing group support.
  ◄ Individualize the content based on family concerns and not what healthcare providers think they should learn.
- When special circumstances, such as prematurity, multiple births, congenital anomalies, or neurological impairment, affect the initiation of breastfeeding, the learning needs of parents are complicated by the emotional ramifications of the experience.
  ◄ It is hard for parents to retain information when they are under stress.
  ◄ Prioritize content so that only important information is given and repeated.
- Numerous studies show that education and professional interventions extend the length of breastfeeding.
- The Internet and social media are now major sources for health education, including breastfeeding information, especially for the younger generations (Heinig, 2009).
  ◄ Evaluate websites before recommending them to parents.
- Online courses for continuing education and for college credit are available, and more offerings in this area are planned (O'Connor et al., 2011).
- Using case studies is an effective method for students to integrate knowledge and clinical experience in graduate-level courses.
- Small-group teaching is a powerful method for changing behavior. The ideal small-group size is 8 to 12 people.

- Create and deliver presentations to capture and maintain the audience's interest.
  - ◀ Develop an outline or story board of key concepts.
  - ◀ Sequence the main points and secondary points: one idea and six points per slide.
  - ◀ Include pictures or videos that illustrate the point on the slide.
  - ◀ Keep lectures to 15 to 20 minutes before doing another activity.
- A fundamental axiom is to "Explain what you're going to teach, teach, and then describe what you have taught."

RESOURCES

For a list of lactation management courses, see the International Lactation Consultant Association's website: http://www.ilca.org/i4a/pages/index.cfm?pageID=3353.

REFERENCES

Academy of Breastfeeding Medicine. Educational objectives and skills for the physician with respect to breastfeeding. *Breastfeed Med.* 2011;6(2):99–105. doi: 10.1089/bfm.2011.9994.

Ahmed A, El Guindy SR. Breastfeeding knowledge and attitudes among Egyptian baccalaureate students. *Int Nurs Rev.* 2011;58:372–378.

American Academy of Pediatrics (AAP). Breastfeeding residency curriculum. n.d. Available at: http://www2.aap.org/breastfeeding/curriculum/.

American Academy of Pediatrics (AAP) Section on Breastfeeding. Policy statement: breastfeeding and the use of human milk. *Pediatrics.* 2005;115(2):496-5-6. doi: 10.1542/peds.2004-2491.

American Academy of Pediatrics (AAP) Section on Breastfeeding. *Sample hospital breastfeeding policy for newborns.* Oak Grove Village, IL: AAP; 2009. Available at: http://www2.aap.org/breastfeeding/curriculum/documents/pdf/Hospital%20Breastfeeding%20Policy_FINAL.pdf.

American Academy of Pediatrics (AAP) Section on Breastfeeding. Policy statement: breastfeeding and the use of human milk. *Pediatrics.* 2012;129:e827. doi: 10.1542/peds.2011-3552. Available at: http://pediatrics.aappublications.org/content/129/3/e827.full.html.

American Academy of Pediatrics (AAP) Section on Breastfeeding. *Federal support for breastfeeding.* Elk Grove Village, IL: AAP; 2013. Available at: http://www2.aap.org/breastfeeding/.

American Academy of Pediatrics (AAP) Section on Breastfeeding. *Ten steps to support parents' choice to breastfeed their baby.* Oak Grove Village, IL: AAP; 2014. Available at: http://www2.aap.org/breastfeeding/files/pdf/tenstepsposter.pdf.

American Academy of Pediatrics (AAP) Work Group on Breastfeeding. Policy statement: breastfeeding and the use of human milk. *Pediatrics.* 1995;100(6):1035–1039.

Amir LH, Raval M, Hussainy, SY. Breastfeeding information in pharmacology textbooks: a content analysis. *Breastfeed Rev.* 2013;21(2):31–37.

Archabald K, Lundsberg L, Triche E, et al. Women's prenatal concerns regarding breastfeeding: are they being addressed. *J Midwifery Women's Health.* 2011;56:2–7.

Baby-Friendly USA. (2013). Find facilities. Available at: http://www.babyfriendlyusa.org/find-facilities.

Balmes T. (Director). *Babies.* 2010. Universal City, CA: Focus Features, A Division of NBC Universal.

Bernaix LW, Beaman ML, Schmidt CA, et al. Success of an educational intervention on maternal/newborn nurses' breastfeeding knowledge and attitudes. *JOGNN.* 2010;39:658–666. doi: 10.1111/j.1552-6909.2010.01184.x.

Bloom BS. *Taxonomy of educational objectives.* New York, NY: David McKay; 1956:7–8.

Boyd AE, Spatz DL. Breastfeeding and human lactation: education and curricular issues for pediatric nurse practitioners. *J Pediatr Healthcare.* 2013;27(2):83–90. doi: 10.1016/j.pedhc.2011.03.005.

Bozzette M, Posner T. Increasing student nurses' knowledge of breastfeeding in baccalaureate education. *Nurs Educ Pract.* 2013;13(3):228–233. doi: 10.1016/j.nepr.2012.08.013.

Brand E, Kothari C, Stark MA. Factors related to breastfeeding discontinuation between hospital discharge and 2 weeks postpartum. *J Perinatal Educ.* 2011;20(1):36–44. doi: 10,1891/1058-1243,20,1,36.

Brewer T. Pediatric nurses' knowledge and attitudes regarding the provision of breastfeeding support in a pediatric medical center. *Clin Lact.* 2012;3(2):64–68.

Brodribb WE. Breastfeeding: a framework for educating the primary care medical workforce. *Breastfeed Rev.* 2012;20(2):25–30.

Brodribb W, Fallon A, Jackson C, Hegney D. The relationship between personal breastfeeding experience and the breastfeeding attitudes, knowledge, confidence and effectiveness of Australian GP registrars. *Matern Child Nutr J.* 2008;4(4):264–274. doi: 10.1111/j/1740-8709.2008.00141.x/.

Brooks EC. *Physical and ethical issues for the IBCLC.* Burlington, MA: Jones and Bartlett; 2013.

Carlsen EM, Kyhnaeb A, Renault KM, et al. Telephone-based support prolongs breastfeeding duration in obese women: a randomized trial. *Am J Clin Nutr.* 2013. Epub ahead of print. doi: 10.3945/ajcn.113.059600.

Cricco-Lizza R. Black non-Hispanic mothers' perceptions about the promotion of infant-feeding methods by nurses and physicians. *JOGNN.* 2006a;35:173–180. doi: 10.1111/J.1552-6909.2006.0033.x.

Cricco-Lizza R. Nursing student attitudes and beliefs about breastfeeding. *J Prof Nurs.* 2006b;22:314–321.

Curro V, Lanni R, Scipione F, et al. Randomised controlled trial assessing the effectiveness of a booklet on the duration of breastfeeding. *Arch Dis Child.* 1997;76:500–504.

Dollahite J, Thompson C, McNew R. Readability of printed sources of diet and health information. *Patient Educ Counsel.* 1996;27:123–134.

Dytrych CJ, Krodstrand KS, Albrecht JA. Dieticians' problem solving knowledge to promote and support breastfeeding. *J Acad Nutr Diet.* 2013;113(9 suppl): A-26.

Edwards RA. Expanding pharmacists' roles in breastfeeding support: a pilot study of an online breastfeeding tutorial for student pharmacists. *Curr Pharm Teach Learn.* 2013a;8(2):129–133.

Edwards RA. Pharmacists as an underutilized resource for improving community-level support of breastfeeding. *J Hum Lact.* 2013b.

Eidelman A, Hoffmann N, Kaitz M. Cognitive deficits in women after childbirth. *Obstet Gynecol.* 1993;81: 764–767.

Feldman-Winter L, Barone L, Milcarek B, et al. Residency curriculum improves breastfeeding care. *Pediatrics.* 2010;126(2):289–297. doi: 10.10.1542/peds. 2009-3250.

Froehlich J, Boivin M, Rice D, et al. Influencing university students' knowledge and attitude toward breastfeeding. *J Nutr Educ Behav.* 2013;54(3):282–284.

Genna CW. *Supporting sucking skills in breastfeeding infants,* 2nd ed. Burlington, MA: Jones & Bartlett Learning; 2013.

Giles M, Millar S, Armour C, et al. Promoting positive attitudes to breastfeeding: the development and evaluation of a theory-based intervention with school children involving a cluster randomised controlled trial. *Matern Child Nutr.* 2013. doi: 10.1111/mcn.12079.

Gill SL. The little things: perception of breastfeeding support. *JOGNN.* 2001;30:401–409.

Grossman X, Chaudhun J, Feldman-Winter L, et al. Hospital education in lactation practices (Project HELP): does clinician education affect breastfeeding initiation and exclusivity in the hospital? *Birth.* 2009;36(1): 54–59.

Hansman CA. Context-based adult learning. *New Direct Adult Contin Educ.* 2001;89:43–51.

Heinig MJ. Breastfeeding promotion for Generation X and Y: why the old ways won't work. *J Hum Lact.* 2009;25(3):263–265. doi: 10.1177/0890334409341450.

Hellings P, Howe C. Assessment of breastfeeding knowledge of nurse practitioners and nurse-midwives. *J Midwifery Women's Health.* 2000;45(3):264–270.

Hellings P, Howe C. Breastfeeding knowledge and practice of pediatric nurse practitioners. *J Pediatr Health Care.* 2004;18(1):8–14. doi: 10.1016 /50891-5245(03)00108-1.

Hodnett ED, Gates S, Hofmeyr GJ, Sakala C. Continuous support for women during childbirth. *Cochrane Database Syst Rev.* 2013;7:CD003766. doi: 10.1002 /14651858.CD003766.pub5.

Howett M, Spangler A, Cannon RB. Designing a university-based lactation course. *J Hum Lact.* 2006;22(1): 104–107. doi: 10.1177/0890334405283668.

Hurst CG. Addressing breastfeeding disparities in social work. *Health Soc Work.* 2007;32(3):207–210.

International Board of Lactation Consultant Examiners (IBLCE). *Pathway 2 academic program list.* Raleigh, NC: IBLCE; 2012.

The Joint Commission. PC-05a exclusive breast milk feeding considering mother's choice. 2013. Available at: http:// manual.jointcommission.org/releases/TJC2014A /MIF0170.html.

Juliff D, Downie J, Rapley P. Knowledge and attitudes of secondary school students to breastfeeding. *Neonatal Pediatr Child Health Nurs.* 2007;10(3):13–18.

Kaewsarn P, Moyle W, Creedy D. Thai nurses' beliefs about breastfeeding and postpartum practices. *J Clin Nurs.* 2003;12:467–475.

Karipis TA, Spicer M. A survey of paediatric nurses' knowledge about breastfeeding. *J Pediatr Nurs.* 1999;14(3):193–200.

Kaso M, Miyamoto K, Koyama E, Nakayama T. Breastfeeding information in midwifery textbooks in Japan: content analysis with evaluation based on Delphi Method. *J Hum Lact.* 2011;27:367–377. doi: 10.1177/0890334411409751.

Kavanagh KF, Lou Z, Nicklas JC, et al. Breastfeeding knowledge, attitudes, prior exposure, and intent among undergraduate students. *J Hum Lact.* 2012;28:256–264.

Kitzinger S. *Ourselves as mothers: the universal experience of motherhood.* Reading, MA: Addison-Wesley; 1995.

Knowles M. *The modern practice of adult education.* New York, NY: Cambridge University Press; 1980.

Kornides M, Kitsantas P. Evaluation of breastfeeding promotion, support, and knowledge of benefits on breastfeeding outcomes. *J Child Health Care.* 2013;17:264–273. doi: 10.1177/1367493512461460.

Kozhimannil KB, Attanasio LB, Hardeman RR, O'Brien M. Doula care supports near-universal breastfeeding initiation among diverse, low-income women. *J Midwifery Women's Health.* 2013;58:378–382. doi: 10.1111/jmwh.12065.

Lactation Education Accreditation and Approval Review Committee (LEAARC). *Curriculum for a lactation program.* Morrisville, NC: LEAARC; 2013a. Available at: http://www.leaarc.org/download/LEAARC _Curriculum.pdf.

Lactation Education Accreditation and Approval Review Committee (LEAARC). *LEAARC approved courses.* Morrisville, NC: LEAARC; 2013b. Available at: http:// www.leaarc.org/download/LEAARC_ApprovedCourses .pdf.

Lake R (Executive Producer), Epstein A (Director). *The business of being born.* 2007. Los Angeles, CA: Millennium Films.

Lauwers J, Shinskie D. *Counseling the nursing mother,* 5th ed. Sudbury, MA: Jones and Bartlett; 2011.

Lewin LO, O'Connor ME. "Breastfeeding basics": web-based education that meets current knowledge competencies. *J Hum Lact.* 2012;28(3):407–413. doi: 10.1177/0890334411435990.

Ludington-Hoe S, Morrison B, Morgan K, Anderson GC. *Skin-to-skin certified kangaroo caregiver learner's program manual.* Cleveland, OH: USIKC; 2012.

Lumbinganon P, Martis R, Laopaiboon M, et al. Antenatal breastfeeding education for increasing breastfeeding duration [Review]. *Cochrane Library.* 2012;6.

Mellin PS, Poplawski DT, Gole A, Mass SB. Impact of a formal breastfeeding education program. *MCN.* 2011;36(2):82–88. doi: 10.1097/NMC .0b013e318205589e.

Meusch SM, Elliott EP, Fasser CE. Physician assistant students' perceived breastfeeding knowledge and counselling skills before and after web-based curriculum and lactation shadowing experience. *J Phys Assist Educ.* 2013;24(3):31–33.

Miller LC, Cook JT, Brooks CW, et al. Breastfeeding education: empowering future health care providers. *Nurs Women's Health.* 2007;11(4):374–380. doi: 10.1111/j.751-486X.2007.00193.x.

Monzingo JN, Davis MW, Droppleman PG, Merideth A. "It wasn't working": women's experiences with short-term breastfeeding. *MCN Am J Matern Child Nurs.* 2000;25(3):120–126.

Mottl-Santiago J, Walker C, Ewan J, et al. A hospital-based doula program and childbirth outcomes in an urban, multicultural setting. *Matern Child Health J.* 2008;12:372–377. doi: 10.1007/s10995-007-0245-9.

Nilson LB. *Teaching at its best: a research-based resource for college instructors,* 3rd ed. San Francisco, CA: Jossey-Bass; 2010.

Noel-Weiss J, Rupp A, Cragg B, et al. Randomized controlled trial to determine effects of prenatal breastfeeding workshop on maternal breastfeeding self-efficacy and breastfeeding duration. *JOGNN.* 2006;35:616–624.

Nommson-Rivers LA, Mastergrove AM, Hansen RL, et al. Doula care, early breastfeeding outcomes, and breastfeeding status at 6 weeks postpartum among low-income primiparae. *JOGNN.* 2009;38:157–173. doi: 10.111/j.1552-6909.2009.01005.x.

November L. Baby milk challenge: changing secondary school students' attitudes to breastfeeding. *Br J Midwifery.* 2013;21(11):775–781.

O'Connor ME, Brown EW, Lewin L O. An Internet-based education program improves breastfeeding knowledge of maternal–child healthcare providers. *Breastfeed Med.* 2011;8(6):421–427. doi: 10.1089/bfm.2010.0061.

Odom EC, Li R, Scanlon KS, et al. Association of family and health care provider opinion on infant feeding with mother's breastfeeding decision. *J Acad Nutr Diet.* 2013. doi: 10.1016/j.jand.2013.08.001.

Ogburn T, Espey E, Leeman L, Alvarez K. Breastfeeding curriculum for residents and medical students: a multidisciplinary approach. *J Hum Lact.* 2005;21(4): 458–464. doi: 10.1177/089033440520990.

Ogburn T, Phillipps BL, Espey E, et al. Assessment of breastfeeding information in general obstetrics and genecology textbooks. *J Hum Lact.* 2011;27(1):58–62. doi: 10.1177/0890334410375960.

Ouyang Y, Xu Y, Zhang Q. Survey on breastfeeding among Chinese female physicians and nurses. *Nurs Health Sci.* 2012;14:268–303. doi: 10.1111 /j.1442-2018.2012.00699.x.

Payne J, Radcliffe B, Blank E, et al. Breastfeeding: the neglected guideline for future dietitian-nutritionists? *Nutr Diet.* 2007;64:93–98. doi: 10.1111/j.1747-0080 .2007.00094.x.

Phillipp BL, McMahon MJ, Davies S, et al. Breastfeeding information in nursing textbooks needs improvement. *J Hum Lact.* 2007;23(4):345–349. doi: 10.1177/0890334407307576.

Phillipp BL, Merewood A, Gerendas EJ, Bauchner H. Breastfeeding information in pediatric textbooks needs improvement. *J Hum Lact.* 2004;20(2):206–210. doi: 10.1177/089033440426321.

Radcliffe B, Payne J. Heart and Minds Project: a breastfeeding curriculum intervention to improve the education outcomes for nutrition and dietetics graduates. *Nutr Diet.* 2001;68:201–207.

Register N, Eren M, Lowdermilk D, et al. Knowledge and attitudes of pediatric office nursing staff about breastfeeding. *J Hum Lact.* 2000;16(3):210–215.

Reinsma K, Bolima N, Fonteh F, et al. Incorporating cultural beliefs in promoting exclusive breastfeeding. *Afr J Midwifery Women's Health.* 2012;6(2):65–70.

Rempel LA, McCleary L. Effects of the implementation of breastfeeding best practice guidelines in a Canadian public health agency. *Res Nurs Health.* 2012;35: 435–449. doi: 10.1002/nur.21495.

Renfrew MJ, McCormick FM, Wade A, et al. Support for healthy breastfeeding mothers with healthy term babies [Review]. *Cochrane Collaboration.* 2012;5.

Riggins C, Rosenman MB, Szucs KA. Breastfeeding experiences among physicians. *Breastfeed Med.* 2012;7(3):151–154. doi: 10.1089/bfm.2011. 0045.

Riordan J. Teaching breastfeeding on the web. *J Hum Lact.* 2000;16:231–234.

Saenz RB. A lactation management rotation for family medicine residents. *J Hum Lact.* 2000;16(4): 342–345.

Schaffar A, Huyqhe AS, Suriez P, et al. Breastfeeding: opinion and knowledge of pharmacists: a study in a semi-urban territory. *Arch Pediatr.* 2012;19(5):476–483. doi: 10.1016/j.arcped.2012.02.020.

Shaikh U, Scott BJ. Extent, accuracy, and credibility of breastfeeding information on the Internet. *J Hum Lact.* 2005;21:175–183.

Shinwell ES, Churgin Y, Shlomo M, et al. The effect of training nursery staff in breastfeeding guidance on the duration of breastfeeding in healthy term infants. *Breastfeeding Med.* 2006;1:247–252.

Shortt E, McGorrian C, Kelleher C. A qualitative study of infant feeding decisions among low-income women in the Republic of Ireland. *Midwifery.* 2013;29:435–460.

Smith J, Dunstone M, Elliott-Rudder M. Health professional knowledge of breastfeeding: are the health risks of infant formula feeding accurately conveyed by the titles and abstracts of journal articles. *J Hum Lact.* 2009;25(3):350–358. doi: 10.1177/0890334409331506.

Spatz DL. The breastfeeding case study: a model for educating nursing students. *J Nurs Educ.* 2005;44:432.

Spatz DL, Pugh LC. The American Academy of Nursing Expert Panel on Breastfeeding. The integration of the use of human milk and breastfeeding in baccalaureate nursing curricula. *Nurs Outlook.* 2007;55:257–263. doi: 10.1016/j.outlook.2007.07.003.

Sternberg RJ, Zhang LF (Eds). Perspectives on cognitive, learning, and thinking styles. NJ: Lawrence Erlbaum, 2000.

United States Breastfeeding Committee (USBC). Strategic plan: 2009–2013. 2009. Available at: http://www.usbreastfeeding.org/Portals/0/USBC-Strategic-Plan-2009-2013.pdf.

United States Breastfeeding Committee (USBC). *Core competencies in breastfeeding care and services for all health professionals,* rev ed. Washington, DC: USBC; 2010. Available at: http://www.usbreastfeeding.org/Portals/0/Publications/Core-Competencies-2010-rev.pdf.

U.S. Department of Health and Human Services (USDHHS). *HHS blueprint for action on breastfeeding,* Washington, DC: USDHHS, Office on Women's Health; 2000.

U.S. Department of Health and Human Services (USDHHS). Healthy people 2020. 2010. Available at: http://www.healthypeople.gov/2020/topicsobjectives2020/overview.aspx?topicid=26.

U.S. Department of Health and Human Services (USDHHS). *The Surgeon General's call to action to support breastfeeding.*

Washington, DC: USDHHS, Office of the Surgeon General; 2011.

Valaitis RK, Shea E. An evaluation of breastfeeding promotion literature: does it really promote breastfeeding? *Can J Public Health.* 1993;84:24–17.

Valaitis RK, Stieesi-ka JD, O'Brien MF. Do consumer infant feeding publications and products available in physicians' offices protect, promote, and support breastfeeding? *J Hum Lact.* 1997;13:203–208. doi: 10.1177/089033449701300308.

Ward KN, Byrne JP. A critical review of the impact of continuing breastfeeding education provided to nurses and midwives. *J Hum Lact.* 2011;27(4):381–393. doi: 10.1177/0890334411052.

Watkins AL, Dodgson JE. Breastfeeding educational interventions for health professionals: a synthesis of intervention studies. *J Specialists Pediatr Nurs.* 2010;15(3):223–232. doi: 10.1111/j.1744-6155.2010.00240.x.

Whelan B, McEvoy S, Eldin N, Kearney J. What primary health professionals need to promote breastfeeding. *Pract Nurs.* 2011;22(1):35–39.

Witt AM, Smith S, Mason MJ, Flocke SA. Integrating routine lactation consultant support into a pediatric practice. *Breastfeed Med.* 2012;7(1):38–42. doi: 10.1089/bfm.2011.0003.

Workman JL, Barha CK, Galea LAM. Endocrine substrates of cognition and affective changes during pregnancy and postpartum. *Behav Neurosci.* 2012;126(1):54–72.

World Health Organization (WHO), Division of Child Health and Development. *Evidence for the ten steps to successful breastfeeding.* Geneva, Switzerland: WHO; 1998.

World Health Organization (WHO). *Infant and young child feeding: model chapter for textbooks for medical students and allied health professionals.* Geneva, Switzerland: WHO Press; 2009.

World Health Organization (WHO), UNICEF, & Wellstart International. *Baby-friendly hospital initiative: revised, updated and expanded for integrated care. Section 3, Breastfeeding promotion and support in a baby-friendly hospital: A 20-hour course for maternity staff.* Geneva, Switzerland: WHO Press; 2009.

Zareai M, O'Brien ML, Fallon AB. Creating a breastfeeding culture: a comparison of breastfeeding practises in Australia and Iran. *Breastfeed Rev.* 2007;15(2):15–24.

Chapter 22

The Cultural Context of Breastfeeding

Karen Wambach

Introduction

Culture exerts a major influence on a mother's attitude toward breastfeeding that crosses the boundary between private and public. Attitudes and patterns of infant feeding cannot be understood without placing them in their specific cultural context. In this chapter, we look at breastfeeding as a human behavior that is sensitive to cultural influence and social change.

The fastest growing segments of the U.S. population are minorities. Non-European ethnic minorities are fast becoming an aggregate majority. For example, Hispanics compose the fastest-growing minority population in the United States (U.S. Census Bureau, 2011). According to the 2010 U.S. census, Hispanics/Latinos make up 16% of the total population of the United States, and between 2000 and 2010 they accounted for more than half of the country's population growth. The Hispanic growth rate (43%) was more than four times the growth rate of the total population (10%) (U.S. Census Bureau, 2011). The increase in the U.S. Hispanic population is driven by high fertility rates, although they have declined drastically over the past decade. In 2012, the fertility rate for Hispanic women was 74.4 births per 1000 women aged 15–44, compared with 60.3 births per 1000 non-Hispanic women (Martin et al., 2013). In 2012, 907,677 of the 3,952,841 U.S. births were to Hispanic women, accounting for about 1 in every 4.4 live births. Fortunately, according to the 2007 National Immunization Survey (NIS), the rate of breastfeeding among Hispanic women (80%) is higher than that among non-Hispanic black (58.9%) or white women (75.2%) in the United States (Allen et al., 2013), but this also magnifies the need for support from lactation professionals.

Culture is defined as the values, beliefs, norms, and practices of a particular group, which are learned and shared, and which guide thinking, decisions, and actions in a patterned way (Leininger, 1985). Culture provides implicit and explicit codes of behavior:

- It is learned through language and socialization.
- It is shared, often unconsciously, by all members of a cultural group who are then bound together under one identity.
- It is an adaptation to specific conditions related to environmental and technical factors and to the availability of natural resources.
- It is a dynamic, ongoing process.

From a practical standpoint, a society's culture consists of whatever one has to know or believe to operate in a manner acceptable to the culture's members. Culture is a blueprint for human behavior—a guide that helps us to gain a clearer understanding of individual behaviors. The new mother is the product of all of her history: what she has learned about infants and infant feeding, and what she has seen. If she grows up in a breastfeeding culture, she has

Figure 22-1 EXPECTATIONS ABOUT BREASTFEEDING. EACH FAMILY HAS ITS OWN IDEAS, WHICH ARE BASED IN PART ON CULTURE.

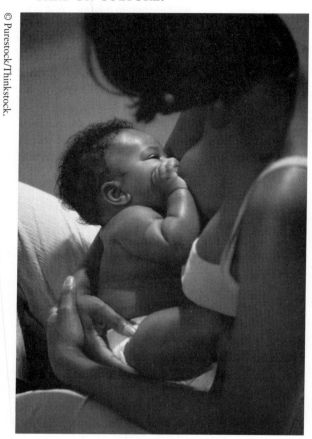

© Purestock/Thinkstock.

many opportunities to observe how infants are fed and knows that her female relatives and neighbors with breastfeeding experience will support her when she becomes a mother (Mulford, 1995; Purdy, 2010). Women and their families have a right to expect that their cultural needs will be met as they are helped with breastfeeding and lactation. Without an understanding of a mother's cultural practices, the care and intervention of healthcare professionals can do more harm than good (Figure 22-1). In the current U.S. healthcare delivery system, the expectation is that healthcare professionals, including lactation consultants/specialists, will be culturally competent and base their practice in evidence that incorporates cultural factors that can influence breastfeeding initiation

and continuation (Feldman-Winter, 2013; Noble et al., 2009).

The Dominant Culture

Every society has a dominant culture, the values of which are shared by the majority of its members as a result of early common experiences. There are approximately 100 ethnic groups in the United States and as an aggregate, ethnic minorities are growing rapidly—so much so that it is predicted that ethnic minorities will make up half of the U.S. population in 2050 (U.S. Census Bureau, 2011). Nevertheless, the dominant cultural group in the United States currently consists of white, middle-class Protestants, descendants of northern Europeans who immigrated to the United States several generations ago. Norms characteristic of this group are a conservative value system, family orientation, commitment to higher education for one's children, a work ethic, materialism, a personal faith in God, the quest for physical beauty, cleanliness, use of high technology, punctuality, independence, and support for free enterprise. Given these prevailing values, it may be relevant to consider women's roles, their contribution to the economy, and the extent to which breastfeeding is perceived to hinder this engagement.

Although changing slowly, the dominant health culture in the United States views birth as dangerous for the mother and neonate. Breastfeeding is seen as the optimal method of infant feeding, but some view it as difficult to accomplish and as a private act not to be practiced in public. These norms are slowly changing as waves of immigrating Asians and Hispanics become the "new" Americans. In the United States, Western allopathic medicine is viewed as "professional" health care; any medical tradition outside this system is considered traditional folk medicine with its accompanying connotations of primitive, useless, lay, and outdated. The dominant U.S. health system marketplace is composed of the hospital, the health worker's office, and the community health department. The folk belief system marketplace centers on the home of the clients or of their extended kin.

The role of women in a culture may also define the experience of breastfeeding. In some societies, male control (male physicians, for example) over breastfeeding serves to weaken the woman's role as mother and to emphasize her role as wife. Rather than viewing insufficient milk supply and early weaning as problems in themselves, these factors could be interpreted as reflecting insecurity about the abilities of women's bodies and the precariousness of their lives and as a symptom of broader self-questioning (Obermeyer & Castle, 1997). In 2002, Dykes echoed that sentiment based on her phenomenological study of 10 women's breastfeeding experience, noting that Westernized medicine and a preoccupation on breastmilk as a product undermined women's confidence in their ability to breastfeed. She cautioned healthcare providers not to rely solely on empirical parameters of success in breastfeeding such as infant weight gain, but rather to treat breastfeeding as a holistic process and relationship between mother and child.

Ethnocentrism Versus Relativism

Ethnocentrism may be defined as being centered in one's ethnic or cultural system (i.e., judging the world by one's standards or in the vernacular believing that "my group is best"). When caring for culturally diverse groups, nurses and healthcare workers at first tend toward ethnocentricity, believing that their professional, scientifically based practices are superior. Many healthcare workers have been socialized into their profession within the framework of a Western healthcare system that emphasizes the biomedical model and is based on the white, working- and middle-class value system. If this system is the only model used to evaluate and implement care, the nurse or lactation consultant is ethnocentric. When healthcare workers are exposed to other cultures, they may begin to appreciate why certain behaviors and values are effective in that culture, and the healthcare worker may move beyond ethnocentric behaviors.

The opposite of ethnocentrism is cultural relativism, in which the healthcare provider recognizes and appreciates cultural differences and treats individual clients with deference to their cultural backgrounds—building on and using cultural variations rather than seeing them as obstacles. Similar to cultural relativism is the concept of cultural sensitivity. To provide optimal assistance, caregivers must

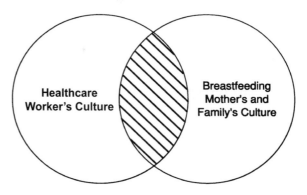

Figure 22-2 SHARED VALUES AND BELIEFS.

Healthcare Worker's Culture

Breastfeeding Mother's and Family's Culture

Source Adapted from Orque, Block, & Monrroy, 1983.

first understand their personal reactions to cultural differences and then appreciate how these cultural values affect the lives of their clients. By discovering areas of commonality between themselves and their patients, nurses and other care providers will be better able to recognize and deal with cultural similarities and variations between the clients and themselves. This process is illustrated in Figure 22-2.

Cultural relativism likewise recognizes variation within cultures, such as within the diverse ethnic groups in the United States. At one time, people expected and hoped that these ethnic and cultural groups would blend into one common whole, in what was called the melting-pot approach. History has not worked out that way; many third- and fourth-generation Americans proudly claim and identify with their original ethnic heritage. The tendency to label subpopulations to explain behaviors is responsible for many myths about new Americans.

Cultural Competence

Because of the great cultural diversity in the United States and other countries around the world, emphasis on cultural competence in clinical/healthcare practice has come to the fore (Purnell, 2002). Culturally competent care is defined as "the adaptation of care in a manner that is consistent with the culture of the client" (Purnell, 2002, p. 193). This process is conscious and nonlinear, and it involves the provider developing an awareness of his or her existence, sensations, thoughts, and environment without letting these factors have an undue effect on the care he or she provides. According to Purnell and Paulanka (as cited in Purnell, 2002), the healthcare provider develops competence along a continuum ranging from unconscious incompetence (not being aware that one is lacking knowledge about another culture), to conscious incompetence (being aware that one is lacking knowledge), to conscious competence (learning about the culture, verifying generalizations, and providing culturally specific interventions), to unconscious competence (automatically providing culturally competent care). Schools of medicine, nursing, and allied health professions are increasingly focusing on and providing education and training in cultural sensitivity, diversity, and competence (Harris et al., 2013; Isaacson, 2014; MacNamara et al., 2014; Roberts et al., 2014; Sasnett, 2010). Therefore, the practicing lactation consultant/specialist needs education and training in providing culturally competent care.

Noble et al. (2009) examined the general cultural competence of healthcare providers who cared for breastfeeding mothers in New York City, where approximately 52% of new mothers are foreign born. Among the 128 providers (physicians, nurses, allied health), the majority (77%) did not achieve a score representing cultural competence. Participants who had attended continuing education on cultural diversity scored higher on competence. This research suggests that there is much room for improvement in the provision of culturally competent care in the United States.

Assessing Cultural Practices

A cultural assessment elicits shared beliefs and customs that affect how nursing care is given (Mattson, 2000). When a nurse or lactation consultant examines cultural traditions, it is helpful to ask questions that indicate respect for cultural practices. A practice that seemingly does not provide any immediately visible benefit may be important to the mother, and its value should be acknowledged. Nurses and lactation consultants who show that they respect a mother's practices will gain respect and, in turn, better adherence to teaching.

The following three questions can be used to examine cultural values:

- Are they helpful? All cultures have beliefs, myths, and rituals that may help breastfeeding. For example, the Lusi people in Papua New Guinea prohibit the lactating mother from having intercourse because it is believed that semen poisons her breastmilk (Maher, 1992). One result of this practice is elimination of the likelihood of a superimposed pregnancy. Such beliefs ensure that infants continue to be breastfed and are well nourished and nurtured. Cultural practices such as carrying a baby close, breastfeeding on demand, and spacing children by long-term breastfeeding are likewise considered beneficial.

- Are they harmless? Placing an amulet or charm of garlic around the baby's neck to protect him from harm or pinning a bellyband around his abdomen to prevent an umbilical hernia are harmless practices, assuming that such items are kept clean. If the mother eats garlic to prevent illness, the practice is harmless to her baby even though her milk will be garlic flavored (Mennella & Beauchamp, 1991).

- Are they harmful? Unlike most of the rest of the world's people, white Europeans put mother and baby in separate sleeping rooms, sometimes even in the hospital, which hinders the establishment of breastfeeding. In rural southern Senegal, the mother expresses and discards her colostrum and the infant is fed only water with sugar or honey until the "true" milk comes in, thereby depriving the baby of the concentrated immune properties of colostrum (Whittemore & Beverly, 1996).

Language Barriers

When working with families who speak a different language, the healthcare provider ideally can understand and speak that language. If she cannot, she should study the language spoken by the breastfeeding families whom she frequently serves.

Rapport is difficult when language differences create a barrier.

Healthcare workers who can speak Spanish are desperately needed in the southwestern United States and in many other large cities where Hispanics/Latinos are fast becoming ethnic majorities (Mattson, 2000). Health agencies with large Hispanic/Latino populations should provide courses in Spanish for their employees (Berry, 1999; Hernandez, 2006). In towns with a large population of Hmong women, Hmong nurses are needed. In the northeast Canadian-border area, French is appropriate.

When it is necessary to find someone fluent in a language, a trained interpreter is best able to rephrase words so that they are understandable and more acceptable to the member of the culture. When a translator is available, care providers should speak slowly in a normal voice and should avoid using slang and subjectives (e.g., "would" and "if"). It may also be wise to record the discussion with the mother, so that the discussion may be referred to again. Even with a translator, there may be problems, because different dialects exist within some countries. Vietnamese, for example, is a language with many regional dialects. Also, a word may have different shades of meaning in different regions of the country.

Most people who are new to a culture are shy. Out of respect for the people with whom they are dealing, they may nod their head and say "yes" even though they may disagree or not understand what is being said. Whenever possible, printed materials regarding breastfeeding should be written in the family's language. Information sheets on breastfeeding in many different languages may be ordered from La Leche League International. Phrases that are frequently used when helping Spanish-speaking mothers breastfeed are provided in Table 22-1.

The Effects of Culture on Breastfeeding

Immigrants tend to adopt the cultural practices of their new country; in years gone by, for newcomers to the United States, adaptation meant bottle-feeding instead of breastfeeding. Today, the overall rate of breastfeeding in the United States is approximately 75% and many efforts are under way to improve maternity practices in hospitals to promote and support breastfeeding (e.g., the Baby-Friendly Hospital Initiative). Thus, newly immigrated women in the United States who come from a country where breastfeeding was the norm may not be influenced to formula-feed as they often were 15 to 20 years ago. In the past, the longer a newly immigrated woman had lived in the United States, the more likely she was to choose to formula-feed, even though she came from a country where the breastfeeding rate was high. Mexican women in the United States were an example—the least acculturated were more likely to breastfeed than the more acculturated (Libbus, 2000).

This phenomenon of taking on the dominant culture's way was seen in the 1990s when U.S. and Australian care providers worked increasingly with Asian families who immigrated in search of a new life and opportunities. Few of the women chose to breastfeed (Rasbridge & Kulig, 1995; Rossiter, 1994). These mothers were breastfed as infants, and they breastfed those children born in their native land. However, in a move attributed to their eagerness to acculturate, these women turned away from their cultural heritage of breastfeeding. A local community health nurse asked a Vietnamese mother, "But didn't your mother breastfeed you?" The woman replied, "Yes, but that's the old way. We're in a new land now." More recent research with Vietnamese immigrants in Quebec, Canada, also found that few of the women initiated breastfeeding, and none of the primiparae in the sample breastfed (Groleau et al., 2006). However, acculturation to a formula-feeding culture was not the reason for formula-feeding. Rather, women's narratives revealed that their new home and separation from family prevented them from engaging in the traditional support and rituals that nurture the new mother, restore her health, and promote healthy breastmilk production. Culturally competent care may have assisted in changing this unfortunate situation.

An example of this was demonstrated by Galvin and colleagues (2008), who were anxious to get to the root of the low rate of breastfeeding initiation among Cambodian women in Lowell, Massachusetts

Table 22-1 Commonly Used Phrases When Speaking with Spanish-Speaking Women About Breastfeeding

Spanish	English
Leche materna	Breastmilk
Calostro	Colostrum
Madre	Mother
Bebé	Baby
Consultor de lactancia	Lactation consultant
Consejera	Nurse
Masaje del pecho	Breast massage
Expresión manual	Hand expression
No usar chupetes	Do not use pacifiers
No usar biberones	Do not use bottles
Succionar los pechos	Pump breasts
Alimentación suplementaria	Supplemental feeding
Alimentación de pecho	Breastfeeding
Amamantar a su bebé	Breastfeeding
Pecho	Breast
Pezón	Nipple
Ya puede amammantar a su niño(a).	You can breastfeed your baby now.
¿Le va bien cuando da pecho?	How is breastfeeding going?
¿Cada cáundo el niño come cada ves que le da pecho?	How often does the baby breastfeed each day?
¿Esta recibiendo suficiente? Cinco a seis pañales mojados al día?	Getting enough? Five or six wet diapers each day?
¿Esta recibiendo suficiente? Cuatro o más deposiciónes al día?	Getting enough? Four or more bowel movements a day?
¿Cuantas veces hace pupu el niño al día?	How many dirty diapers does the baby have each day?
Le da pecho las veces que el niño quiere, usualmente ocho a doce veces al día.	Breastfeed as often as the baby wants, usually eight to twelve times a day.
Usted puede comer lo que quiera al menos que el niño se ponga malo después de que come algo en particular.	You can eat what you want unless you notice the baby is fussy after you eat certain foods.
Sus pezónes van a estar un paquito enflamados. Pero en unos cuantos dias se le va a quitar.	Your nipples may be sore for a few days. But the soreness will go away.

(35% versus 76.6% in the state overall). According to these authors' research report, breastfeeding rates in Cambodia were 96%, so the low initiation rates in U.S. residents were particularly alarming. The traditional Cambodian "yin/yang" belief system dictates that in the "cold" postpartum period, "hot" foods are required for at least 6 weeks. If the mother does not get the proper diet, her milk will not be suitable and can result in health and character problems in the child. In the United States, the hospital postpartum diet was an "insurmountable barrier to breastfeeding" among Cambodian immigrants

(p. 546). A culturally acceptable Cambodian post-partum meal plan was initiated, after which breast-feeding initiation rates more than tripled, to the point that differences in breastfeeding rates were no longer significantly different between Cambodian (66.7%) and non-Cambodian women (68.9%). This evidence demonstrates the importance of cultural sensitivity and cultural competence to effect change in a health-related behavior such as breastfeeding.

Indeed, cultural awareness has grown in the United States overall and has helped to bring recognition to the disparities that exist in breastfeeding rates among different cultural groups. Breastfeeding rates among African American women remain the lowest. According to the 2008 National Immunization Survey (NIS), black women currently have the lowest rates of breastfeeding in the United States (58.9%), compared to white (75.2%) and Hispanic women (80%). Fortunately, like the rest of the United States in general, breastfeeding rates have increased among black women, rising from 47.4% in 2000 to 59.7% in 2008 (Allen et al., 2013).

Why do African American women choose to breastfeed less often? Research to explore breastfeeding beliefs among African American women has been conducted in an effort to understand and potentially identify ways to improve rates of breastfeeding. In a qualitative study carried out by Corbett (2000), an African American woman described the curiosity of friends who wanted to watch her feed her baby because they had never seen a woman breast-feed. Breastfeeding seemed to be an unfamiliar and uncertain activity, as is reflected in the lower rate of breastfeeding in African Americans than among other groups.

In another study, when African American women were asked why they chose formula-feeding, they acknowledged that breastfeeding is more health-ful than formula-feeding (Riordan & Gill-Hopple, 2001), but they offered many reasons for not doing so: "If you've got a job you've got to pump," "It ties women down," "You've got formula given to you from WIC [Women, Infants, and Children program]," "It hurt too much and I couldn't take the pain," and "I thought it was just a turn-off." Others said they chose not to breastfeed because they believed that the baby would be "spoiled" and that the baby would not receive enough milk.

Are there other, deeper, unstated reasons why African American women turn away from breast-feeding? Blum (1999) thinks so, and attributes these women's reluctance to breastfeed to their history of slavery and the common practice of Southern black women wet-nursing white infants—a legacy of embodied exploitation where their sexuality and reproduction were appropriated by white men. Such breastfeeding, in which the black baby was denied its mother's milk as she nursed the white infant, is a particularly charged symbol (Blum, 1999).

The baby's grandmother plays a key role in an African American woman's decision to breastfeed and in the timing of introducing complementary foods and replacement feedings. Younger mothers in urban settings are often single and living at home with their own mother. The grandmother, who serves as the decision maker in the family, wields the authority and experience (Bentley et al., 2003; Masvie, 2006). For any breastfeeding promotion in these groups to be successful, it must first educate and convince the grandmothers.

Newer research indicates that origin of birth (outside the United States) is predictive of breastfeeding intention among black and Hispanic women in New York City (Bonuck et al., 2005). In contrast to previous research, the researchers found that black (non-Hispanic) and Hispanic women's breastfeeding plans were similar. This shift was attributed to a dramatic increase in the study locale of blacks from West Indian countries in which breastfeeding is the norm. The research highlights the importance of subcultural differences among ethnic minority groups.

Healthcare provider influence is also important to black women's decision making regarding infant-feeding method. Cricco-Lizza (2006), in her ethnographic investigation of 11 black women enrolled in WIC clinics, found that healthcare providers offered limited breastfeeding education and support during pregnancy, childbirth stay in neonatal intensive care unit, postpartum, and recovery in the community. The participants in this study also expressed trust/distrust concerns and varying degrees of anxiety about the ways they were treated by nurses and physicians. The researcher concluded that healthcare professionals can improve disparities in breastfeeding rates among blacks, but their efforts in education and support must be coupled with development of trusting relationships and continuity of care.

Cricco-Lizza (2005), in the same sample of women used for the 2006 study, found that when the WIC clinic environment set a positive tone for service, WIC employees treated the women with caring and respect, and in general the women believed that WIC was a source of support in time of need, personalized breastfeeding promotion with trusting relationships influenced the breastfeeding decisions for about half of the women. However, the availability of free formula in the WIC clinic facilitated bottle-feeding. Thus, social institutions and healthcare providers do have influence on breastfeeding decisions, and cultural awareness is important in working with ethnic groups that traditionally have lower rates of breastfeeding.

The U.S. view of the breast as erotic and society's notion that motherhood is incompatible with sexuality also have negative ramifications for breastfeeding among immigrants or ethnic minority groups. For example, native Ojibwe women in Canada expressed a belief that breastfeeding is the "right way to feed the baby," yet they were uncomfortable about breastfeeding owing to their view of the breast as sexual (Dodgson et al., 2002).

Breastfeeding in a public place or in the presence of friends is an activity that is extremely sensitive to cultural norms (Figure 22-3). For instance, in Saudi Arabia it is not uncommon to see a totally veiled woman baring her breast to feed her infant in public with no one taking notice—except, perhaps, a foreigner. In France, women in topless swimsuits are perfectly acceptable on certain beaches. However, a French woman would hesitate, or at least cover herself carefully, while breastfeeding in public, even in a restaurant near the "topless" beach. Modesty is important for the Mexican American mother and may be viewed as inconsistent with breastfeeding in public. Breastfeeding in public is becoming a more accepted practice in the United States and other countries of the world. In the United States, there are laws in 46 states, the

Figure 22-3 WELL-NOURISHED WOMAN AND BREASTFEEDING INFANT IN SEARO. BREASTFEEDING IS A BASIC PART OF THE LIFE PROCESS IN THIS PART OF THE WORLD.

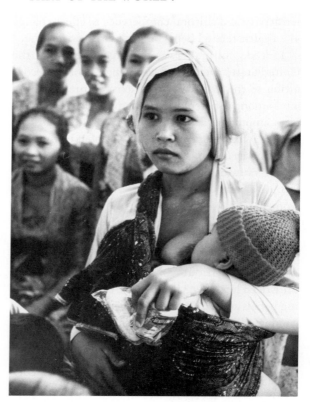

Courtesy of the World Health Organization.

District of Columbia, and the Virgin Islands that allow women to nurse their infants in public; moreover, 29 states exempt breastfeeding from public indecency laws (National Conference of State Legislatures, 2014).

Rituals and Meaning

Rituals and cultural meanings associated with infant feeding are critical elements in assessing the culture's infant-feeding practices. Unfortunately, the word *ritual* has come to connote a meaningless ceremonial act. Actually, rituals can have a significant effect if the individual believes in them. Eating a special food or praying to a patron saint to increase the milk supply are cultural rituals that work for some people, just as taking a pill on the advice of a Western-trained doctor may have a positive effect, even if the medicine is a sugar pill. Researchers call the latter relationship the placebo effect, which is based on the observation that if one believes that a particular action will have a desired effect, it will.

In the Philippines, the ritual of *lihi* ensures a good flow of rich milk. This ceremony involves stroking the mother's breasts with broken papaya leaves and stalks of sugar cane. The white sap of the papaya ensures that the mother's milk will be copious, thick, and white, whereas the cane guarantees that it will be sweet. In certain rural areas of Japan, figurines and paintings depicting a woman with a bounteous milk supply are displayed in the belief that they increase the mother's milk (Figure 22-4). A picture of a breastfeeding mother seated in front of a waterfall has been used in the United States

for similar effect. The use of nipple creams, popular in some Western countries, could be considered a ritual that is a comfort measure, even if it is not necessary from a physiological point of view.

Colostrum

In many cultures throughout the world, colostrum is accepted and encouraged as the first food for infants. In other cultures, colostrum is considered to be "old" milk that has been in the breasts for months and is unfit for the newborn; thus it should be expressed and thrown away until the "true" milk appears on the second or third day (Conton, 1985; Fishman et al., 1988). In many developing countries, mothers do not give their babies this first milk because they fear it to be pus or poison. This belief exists among people in countries thousands of miles apart, including the native peoples of Guatemala and Korea, and Africans in Sierra Leone and Lesotho. Lactation consultants have the opportunity and responsibility to encourage women to breastfeed their baby early by explaining that colostrum is "special" early milk made just for their baby and will help keep their baby healthy.

Sexual Relations

We are sexual beings, and the breastfeeding woman is no exception. Although breastfeeding is usually a rich meaningful experience, its effect on a woman's sexuality is generally ignored. Historically, sex during the lactation period has been fraught with myths and prescribed behaviors. For example, the notion that semen contaminates breastmilk—a vestige of medieval European thought—is still widely accepted in many developing countries. This myth assumes that there is a physiological connection between the uterus and the breast and that the mother's milk may become contaminated by sexual contact. Negative results of a taboo against having sexual intercourse while lactating are that men may pressure women to shorten breastfeeding so they can resume sexual relations, and that women, concerned that their milk may be "contaminated" by sperm, are more likely to wean early (Maher, 1992).

Figure 22-4 VOTIVE PICTURE (*EMA* IN JAPANESE). THIS WOODEN PLAQUE IS GIVEN TO THE BREASTFEEDING MOTHER BY THE TEMPLE. SHE IN TURN PRAYS TO THE PLAQUE FOR SUFFICIENT MILK. IF HER WISH IS FULFILLED, SHE WRITES HER NAME AND AGE ON THE PLAQUE AND DEDICATES IT TO THE TEMPLE.

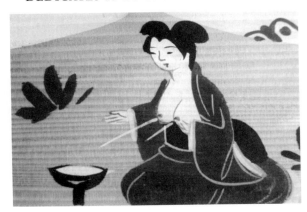

Courtesy of K. Sawada

On the positive side, this taboo is an effective means of birth spacing.

When Avery, Duckett, and Frantzich (2000) surveyed 576 breastfeeding women in Minnesota about their sex life, overall they reported that breastfeeding had a slightly negative impact on some aspects of sexuality but did not greatly affect the woman's sexual relationship with her partner. The striking thing was their wide range of experiences. When asked if the sensations of suckling elicited arousal, most of the women (60%) reported negatively. Based on the information from this study, caregivers can help mothers deal with sexuality during the breastfeeding by doing the following:

- Teaching normal (and wide) variations of experiences of sexuality
- Discussing resumption of intercourse when the woman feels ready
- Providing good information about safe and efficacious contraceptives
- Describing methods of reducing perineal pain, such as vaginal lubricants
- Emphasizing that a priority should be placed on time for sleep
- Reminding couples that the window of time devoted to breastfeeding is relatively short compared to their total life together

Wet-Nursing

Wet-nursing, a historical practice worldwide, may provide for a child whose mother has died or who is otherwise unable to breastfeed. Among Japanese, Chinese, and Thai mothers, breastmilk can be shared between infants of the same sex but not those of the opposite sex. Infants who had the same wet nurse cannot marry in Arabic Moslem countries. In cultures that view breastmilk as a conduit for ancestral power, it is not unusual for wet nurses to be restricted to women from the mother's or father's clan or lineage (van Esterik & Elliott, 1986). Americans practiced wet-nursing up until recent times; for example, Southern women sometimes used black slaves to wet-nurse their babies. Wet-nursing is now discouraged because of concerns about AIDs transmission. However, a few women

still practice wet-nursing; for example, mothers in Northwest Indian tribes, especially sisters, regularly practice wet-nursing secretly.

The practice of wet-nursing by sisters is more accurately labeled cross-feeding or cross-nursing, according to Thorley (2008). She described cross-feeding as the practice of informal sharing of breastfeeding between equals, which is often of a reciprocal nature. Describing the practice within the context of Australia, Thorley reviewed the literature and found only sporadic written reports of the practice in the 1900s, due to the informal nature of the practice and public sentiment against the practice. She did, however, point out that there had been "popular press and media" reports about cross-nursing in the United States, the United Kingdom, and Canada, with women reporting satisfaction with the experience. Anecdotally, she reported that lesbian couples practice cross-nursing, and advised that lactation consultants inquire sensitively about both partners breastfeeding.

Other Practices

A seclusion period of about 40 days after giving birth is common in many cultures. This time of support from female kin and seclusion for the mother and baby varies according to the culture. Generally, it permits a mother to become acquainted with her baby, to establish her milk supply, and to reduce both her own and her infant's exposure to infectious disease. In Bedouin Arab society, female relatives visit the new mother and baby and bring small gifts of money to mark the birth of the baby (Forman et al., 1990).

In Korea, the mother's mother-in-law traditionally takes care of her after the child's birth and serves as her "doula." During pregnancy, Korean women undergo *Thae Kyo*—that is, education-teaching of the fetus. In this ancient tradition, a mother-in-law trains her daughter-in-law to be a mother. *Thae Kyo* instructs the expectant mother that to avoid bad luck in having her baby, she should not see fires or fights, she must think pure thoughts and eat "pretty" foods, and she must always walk in a straight line. During the postpartum period, which lasts about 3 to 4 weeks, the woman is also cared for by her own mother and her husband. This perception that the mother is "sick" and requires care runs counter to the expectations of U.S.-trained nurses and the trend to discharge new mothers and their babies early from the hospital.

Contraception

Methods of contraception used by breastfeeding mothers of any culture should not interfere with lactation. Nurses who advise women in community family planning services play a key role in monitoring the type of oral contraceptive dispensed. Combination hormonal contraceptives (patch, pill, injectable, ring) that contain both progesterone and estrogen should be avoided for at least 4 weeks postpartum due to the risk of blood clots and theoretical risks related to decreased milk production (World Health Organization [WHO], 2008). Progesterone-only pills, rings, patches, injection, or implants may inhibit milk production when initiated before lactogenesis II occurs, and both WHO (2008) and the Centers for Disease Control and Protection (CDC, 2013) suggest delaying initiation of such contraceptive methods for at least 4 weeks. The lactational amenorrhea method (LAM) is 98% effective in preventing pregnancy during the first 6 months postpartum if the mother is exclusively or almost exclusively breastfeeding, the interval between feedings is less than 6 hours, and the mother has not resumed menstruation (WHO, 2009). Barrier devices are also options for contraception.

Infant Care

Swaddling or bundling is an ancient practice still used today to soothe the infant and maintain his body temperature. Swaddling and carrying the baby on the mother's side or back also frees her hands for other tasks. In many parts of rural Nigeria, an infant is wrapped on the mother's back all day and sleeps with her at night. During the first 40 days, the baby is snugly wrapped, a practice that ensures that the infant stays warm and reduces his energy requirements (Omuloulu, 1982).

In parts of the world that do not have intensive care nurseries, premature infants who are clinically stable go directly to the mother as early as 2 to 3 hours after birth. By being held in an upright position, in skin-to-skin contact between their mother's breasts, they are kept warm (Anderson, 1992; Anderson et al., 1986). This practice spread to intensive care units worldwide in many countries and is now known as "kangaroo care" (Figure 22-5). Of course, this practice is now recognized as an important facilitator of breastfeeding and is recommended in full-term newborns as well (Moore et al., 2012).

In any culture, swaddling and carrying the baby close typifies mothers who practice unrestricted breastfeeding. As early as 24 hours after delivery, the Zambian infant is secured to his mother's body with a dashica, or long piece of cloth. The baby rides on the mother's hip in the dashica, and his head is not supported. As a result, the Zambian infant maintains a strong shoulder girdle to keep his head steady and thereby develops early head control. The aquawo—a specially woven, strong cotton cloth folded in a special way—is the infant carrier in Bolivia. The aquawo

Figure 22-5 A PREMATURE INFANT IN BOGOTA GOES HOME. TWELVE HOURS AFTER BIRTH, THE BABY CRADLED SKIN-TO-SKIN WITH HIS MOTHER.

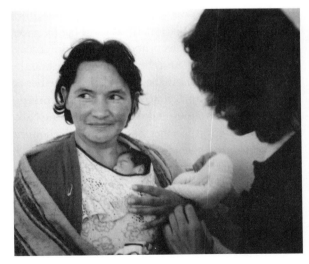

can be turned around to several positions to facilitate breastfeeding. In Mexico, a woman uses a long, wide shawl called a rebozo for carrying her infant while she goes about her daily activities.

Many different types of baby carriers are used worldwide. Mothers and fathers, regardless of their cultural backgrounds, recognize and enjoy the convenience these carriers afford. Carrying the infant swaddled to his mother's body develops the child's muscle tone and seems to encourage alertness. Being carried about during daily activities offers many opportunities for tactile, visual, and social stimulation.

Babies in the Dominican Republic are not secured to their mother in any fashion but are carried in their arms in a horizontal position until they are old enough to sit up by themselves. Because it is believed that a baby can break his or her neck easily if the head is not held, a mother often will become visibly anxious when the nurse assesses her baby's head control.

Diseases recognized only in a particular culture may affect an infant. In Spanish-speaking cultures, the most common is *mollera caida* (fallen fontanel). The health professional interprets a depressed fontanel in the baby as a symptom of dehydration, whereas a Hispanic mother may see it as curable illness caused by removing her nipple while the baby is still suckling or by the baby falling.

Another Hispanic and Puerto Rican folk disease is *mal de ojo*, or evil eye, which is presumably caused by someone casting very strong glances at the baby or by someone who admired the baby but did not touch him. Symptoms of *mal de ojo* are sometimes vague, but the baby is usually very unhappy, cries continuously, cannot sleep, and may even die (Lacay, 1981). The cure is to find the person who is thought to have given the infant the evil eye and have her or him touch the baby. Lactation consultants working with such clients should take care to touch the baby when admiring him or her to avoid being thought of as the cause of a later case of *mal de ojo*.

Babies often are outfitted with special ornaments or bands that have a specific purpose. Hispanic grandmothers often worry a great deal about the infant's umbilicus and may insist that the baby wear a belly-band (*fajita*) to prevent an umbilical hernia. A traditional necklace protects the Laotian newborn. Babies

in Papua New Guinea are protected from disease by special rituals, such as blackening the top of the baby's head with burnt coconut husk (Lepowsky, 1985).

Maternal Foods

Whether she lives on a mountaintop in remote Tibet, in a dusty Mexican village, or in an American suburb or urban high-rise apartment, the lactating woman produces milk that is amazingly homogeneous in composition, despite the wide diversity of foods she consumes. Only the milk of a woman who is severely malnourished will be measurably diminished in its nutrient content and volume because body nutrients are depleted before the milk suffers.

Part of understanding a culture involves becoming acquainted with its foodways—the way in which a distinct group selects, prepares, consumes, and otherwise uses portions of the available food supply. For more than half the inhabitants of this planet, including lactating women, beans, rice, and grains are daily fare. Fruits and vegetables appear seasonally, and meat is found in the family cooking pot only on special occasions. When it does appear, it is usually poultry, goat, horse, or dog, rather than beef. In most cultures, meat plays a minor part in flavoring rice, beans, and vegetables—not the major role it has served in affluent Western industrialized countries.

The daily food pattern of a breastfeeding Mexican mother who eats very little meat might concern us if we did not have a basic knowledge of amino acids and complementary proteins. Beans, a staple item in Mexican foodways, provide an incomplete protein when served alone, because they are low in methionine, an essential amino acid. This deficiency is completely corrected when beans are served with a food high in methionine, such as whole-grain breads or cereals. Complementary proteins can be obtained by numerous combinations. For example, eggs or a milk product will balance the protein and amino acids of a meal consisting primarily of plant proteins. However, two protein foods cannot complement each other if they have similar amino acids in their composition. For this reason, nuts and black-eyed peas are not complementary proteins, because both legumes lack the same amino acids.

"Hot" and "Cold" Foods

For many cultural groups, foods involve a balance that must be maintained to sustain health or be restored when illness occurs. Balance between opposing energy forces is based on the Greek theory of body humors. After centuries of dissemination throughout the world, this theory now appears as the hot (*caliente*) and cold (*frio* or *fresco*) system in Hispanic cultures. Other peoples, such as the Cambodian, Vietnamese, Chinese, East Indians, and Arabs, also use a hot–cold designation to some extent. Classifying foods as hot or cold in a given culture has little to do with their form, color, texture, or temperature, although hot foods are believed to be more easily digested than are cold foods. Instead, the classification is based on the food's effect on an illness or condition, which is itself categorized as hot or cold. During the last trimester of pregnancy, the unborn child is believed to be hot; therefore the mother is in a hot state. Once the child is born, accompanied by a loss of blood, a cold condition exists for both mother and infant. To correct this imbalance, women believe that they need hot drinks and foods and to keep warm to replace heat and energy (Davis, 2001). Baths are taboo, as exposure to water cools the body. Birthing in a hospital where postpartum showers are expected poses serious concerns for these mothers.

Traditional Chinese consider chicken, squash, and broccoli to be hot. Cold foods include melon, fruits, soybean sprouts, and bamboo shoots. In India, milk may be hot or cold, depending on where a person lives. In Hispanic cultures, cold foods include most fresh vegetables, tropical fruits, dairy products, beans, squash, and some meats. Hot foods—cereal grains, chili peppers, temperate-zone fruits, goat's milk, oils, and beef—serve to balance the cold foods. Because the potential listing of hot and cold foods in any particular culture is almost endless, health providers must do their ethnographic homework regarding the belief system of the cultures with whose members they are working. Among Southeast Asian women who delivered infants in the United States in the late 1990s, foods restricted after childbirth included all fruit. Postpartum foods are mainly rice and some boiled chicken. Garlic, black pepper, and ginger create warmth in the body and are encouraged (Davis, 2001).

Another belief system concerning food balance is the Chinese yin–yang theory. In America, people who use macrobiotics practice this system. Like the hot–cold theory, the basis of the yin–yang belief rests on a proper balance between opposing energy forces. On one side, yin represents "female," a negative force (cold, emptiness, darkness); on the other side, yang represents "male," a positive force (warmth, fullness, light). Too much of either yin or yang food is considered threatening to health. Whether a food is considered yin or yang depends on the effect it is thought to have on the body; the designation is not associated with color, texture, or other obvious characteristics.

Herbs and Galactagogues

Almost all cultures abound with an array of certain foods for lactating women. In the past, beer and brewer's yeast have been touted as galactagogues—foods that are thought to increase milk secretion and improve let-down. Rice, gruel, soup, vegetables, and medicinal herbs may be used extensively by many cultures during the immediate postpartum period to promote the secretion of milk. Fenugreek tea is a popular galactagogue in the United States but is also used in many other parts of the world. Northern Mexicans make special teas from "hot" plants such as sesame and absinthe, and in some parts of Latin America herbal teas are drunk in the evening to stimulate milk for the morning (Baumslag, 1987).

The lack of evidence for the safety and effectiveness of galactagogues has raised concerns about the use of herbs (Budzynska et al., 2013). The Academy of Breastfeeding Medicine does not have recommendations for use of galactagogues. A recent systematic review by Mortel and Mehta (2013) included trials involving shatavari, torbangun, fenugreek, milk thistle, and a Japanese herbal medication. Five trials found an increase in breastmilk production. Several limitations were identified that affected the validity of the trial results, including small sample sizes, insufficient randomization methods, poorly defined eligibility criteria, use of poly-herbal interventions, and variable breastfeeding practices among enrolled subjects. The authors cited the insufficiency of evidence from the trials and made no recommendation for the use of herbs as galactagogues.

Lactation specialists should be aware that safety and efficacy evidence is lacking and inform their clients of this situation. However, if the mothers within a particular ethnic group believe that certain foods can promote lactation, and the safety of these foods is known, encourage these women to eat those foods. This practice gives a clear signal that the healthcare system supports breastfeeding and respects these cultural beliefs.

Weaning

Weaning is a time when childhood illness and death are more likely in developing countries; thus it is a key issue in studies of cross-cultural childcare practices. Cultural assessment includes the timing of feeding, types of foods given to infants, and weaning practices. When a substantial proportion of dietary intake comes from food other than breastmilk, growth rates falter and the effects of morbidity come into play. Woolridge (1991) suggests, as a rule of thumb, that when 25% to 50% of a baby's kilocalories come from breastmilk, the milk will protect the baby from environmental pathogens. At the same time, every breastfed infant reaches a point at which breastmilk alone can no longer meet its nutritional needs and solid foods are necessary.

Early solid and semisolid infant foods given by mothers vary widely across cultures, as does the timing of their introduction. Worldwide, there is a high rate of both the initiation of breastfeeding and early supplementation with other foods, even in maternity units certified as Baby-Friendly (Alikasifoglu et al., 2001). Although infants in Papua New Guinea are not introduced to supplemental foods until 6 months (Lepowsky, 1985)—an optimal age—this is not a usual pattern. In a comparison study of how mothers feed their infants in four diverse countries, Winikoff, Castle, and Laukaran (1988) noted that early introduction of other foods is common. The majority of Kenyan babies are given foods other than breastmilk before they are 4 months old (Dimond & Ashworth,

1987; van Esterik & Elliott, 1986); in East Java, force-feeding by hand is a common practice from as early as few days after birth (van Steenbergen et al., 1991). Clearly, much work remains to be done before the goal of exclusive breastfeeding is achieved.

Types of Weaning

Weaning from the breast is a process during which mothers gradually introduce their babies to culturally assigned foods as they continue to breastfeed. Weaning begins with the introduction of sources of food other than breastmilk and ends with the last breastfeeding. Three types of weaning have been described:

- Gradual weaning that takes place over several weeks or months
- Deliberate weaning, a conscious effort initiated by the mother to end breastfeeding at a particular point
- Abrupt weaning, an immediate cessation of breastfeeding, which may be forced on the baby by the mother or on the mother and baby by others

Examples of gradual, deliberate, and abrupt weaning may be found in any culture. Gradual weaning, however, is the least traumatic, to both the infant and the mother.

Weaning practice can affect infant health, particularly in developing countries or in inner-city areas in which weaning diarrhea is prevalent. In cultures in which food is available sporadically or is meager, *kwashiorkor*—a severe form of protein deficiency—appears during the transition from breastmilk to other foods. In Ga, the language of Ghana, the term *kwashiorkor* means "the disease of the deposed baby." Identifying the reasons for women weaning early sheds considerable light on the beliefs and attitudes that influence the continuation of breastfeeding.

Various stages in infant development are sometimes used as cues to begin deliberate weaning. A common belief among African cultures is that the child should be walking before weaning is attempted. Some kind of independence is implicit in the concept of weaning, so it seems reasonable that the child be self-sufficient in locomotion before leaving the dependency of his mother's breast. In many Western cultures, teething is a developmental reference point thought to signal readiness to wean. In others, subsequent pregnancy signals the time to wean (Bohler & Ingstad, 1996). Usually a toddler or child will spontaneously wean with a new pregnancy. The reasons include a diminished milk supply, changes in the milk composition, and a less desirable taste.

For mammals, the length of lactation is positively correlated with adult female mass. Generally, larger mammals have long lactation periods (Hayssen, 1993). What is the "natural" age for weaning in humans? Dettwyler (1995) suggests four criteria associated with age at weaning in primates that range from 27 months to 7 years:

- Weaning according to tripling or quadrupling of birth weight: Using U.S. data, male infants quadruple their birth weight by about 27 months and female infants by around 30 months.
- Weaning according to attainment of one-third adult weight: Weaning for the human would be predicted at between 4 and 7 years of age.
- Weaning according to adult body size: Using this comparison predicts the age for weaning in humans at between 2.8 and 3.7 years, with larger-bodied populations breastfeeding for the longest time.
- Weaning according to time of dental eruption of permanent molars: Modern humans' first molar eruption occurs around 5.5 to 6.0 years of age (the same time as that for adult immune competence).

Some rather harsh techniques have been used to bring about abrupt weaning. One time-honored method calls for pepper, garlic, ginger, or onion to be applied to the mother's breasts to discourage the baby from breastfeeding. In the Fiji Islands, weaning of *kali* ("to separate") is a 4-day period during which the breast is denied to the infant and the baby's food is specially cooked in a separate pot. The infant is not allowed to sleep with the mother until after weaning and is sometimes cared for by one of the mother's female relatives in another household for this period.

In cultures in which early weaning is a common practice, a minority of people accept long-term breastfeeding. The sight of a walking child calmly sliding onto the mother's lap for milk and deftly opening her buttons to gain access to her breasts is considered shocking and subject to ridicule in some cultures. The term *closet nursing* describes a practice that has evolved in the United States in response to criticism of breastfeeding that extends beyond the culture's expectations. In closet nursing, breastfeeding continues by mutual consent of mother and child, but only in secret. The mother and baby usually have a code word for breastfeeding that can be used in public (Wrigley & Hutchinson, 1990). In many Western cultures, teething is a developmental reference point thought to signal readiness to wean. In others, subsequent pregnancy signals the time to wean. As noted earlier, many toddlers will spontaneously wean with a new pregnancy because of a diminished milk supply and a less desirable taste (Bohler & Ingstad, 1996). Regardless of the culture, weaning is ideally a collaborative effort in which both the mother and the baby reach a state of readiness to begin weaning.

Implications for Practice

Every culture has its visible elements (e.g., housing, clothing, food) and its invisible elements (attitudes, tradition, values); an understanding of both contributes significantly to communication between the breastfeeding client and the healthcare provider. Some Spanish-speaking folkways and strategies to handle them are identified in Box 22-1. Immigrant mothers may be served foods that traditionally are forbidden to postpartum women, such as raw vegetables and fruit for Vietnamese mothers. Lactation consultants working in these birthing areas can make sure that alternative foods are provided to these women.

Many Indochinese women living in the United States formula-feed their infants, at least while in the hospital, and then both breastfeed and bottle-feed after leaving the hospital; therefore, formula

---

Box 22-1   Specific Folkways and Ways to Handle Them

- Touching the baby of a Spanish-speaking family while admiring him helps avoid giving the baby *mal de ojo*—the evil eye.
- An anemic breastfeeding mother who is not vegetarian believes that anemia is a yin condition. Suggest that she consume more meat, a yang food, to improve her iron status.
- A Korean mother refuses a cold pack for engorged breasts or for pain resulting from an episiotomy. Offer her cool water from a washcloth or from a peri bottle.
- A mother expects a 40-day period of special care postpartum. Respect the tradition and help her through early discharge with one or more home visits.
- A baby burps during feedings. According to some Hispanic mothers, this air goes to the breast and stops the flow of milk, causing her milk duct to become plugged. Ask her to switch to the other breast and then back to the first breast to release the "air."
- A mother believes that colostrum is "bad." Suggest that she express the first few drops of "impure" milk and discard it before putting the baby to breast, then say, "the sooner you breastfeed, the better the milk."
- Avoid serving ice water or cold drinks to a new mother from Southeast Asia.

---

discharge packs are not appropriate. It is advisable to have women health workers care for these mothers, because they regard it as improper for men to touch a woman's body (especially the breasts). If mothers in any culture believe that certain foods can promote lactation, these women should be encouraged to bring these foods to the postpartum unit. This practice will enhance breastfeeding and provide a clear signal that the healthcare system supports breastfeeding and is respectful of these cultural beliefs.

Regardless of the culture, weaning is ideally a collaborative effort in which both mother and baby reach a state of readiness to begin weaning. In a culture in which unrestricted breastfeeding is practiced and in which the child breastfeeds for a prolonged period, the mother has very little ambivalence when she decides to wean and says, "You, child, have had enough milk!" (Mead & Newton, 1967).

Although weaning practices vary from culture to culture, weaning is thought to be the least traumatic when it is slow, gradual, and related to the needs of the child. It is essential to identify factors that influence continuation or early termination of breastfeeding so as to develop appropriate programs to assist the mother who wishes to maintain breastfeeding. Women involved in long-term breastfeeding develop

a special bond with their baby. The mother's choice of how long she wishes to breastfeed is an individual right that may not mesh with others' expectations. All breastfeeding families deserve to be treated in a nonjudgmental manner that accepts the cultural diversity that they represent.

Summary

The study of child-rearing patterns of a given culture is crucial to all healthcare professionals who work with new and growing families. The seeds of a culture are planted, grow, and thrive in child-rearing patterns. Cultural awareness provides liberation from egocentric views in which one looks at the universe and sees only one's beliefs in the center. The study of any culture begins with critical self-reflection and awareness of the differences between one's cultural values and those of other people. By becoming aware of these differences, we begin a process of partnership in which all groups have something to contribute and something to learn. Although acculturation to the United States generally has a negative effect on breastfeeding, that influence can be offset if the mother receives support from healthcare providers, friends and family, and other social institutions (Cricco-Lizza, 2005; Thiel de Bocanegra, 2008).

Analysis of infant feeding within its cultural context is critically linked to social action and policy decisions regarding breastfeeding promotion and teaching. For those who examine cultural issues carefully, so-called cultural obstacles to solving problems usually include the solutions, too. Within the cultural context of underlying infant-feeding problems, solutions must ultimately emerge. If changes are to last, they must originate from within a culture, rather than being imposed from without.

KEY CONCEPTS

- Culture is a blueprint for human behavior, one that helps us to gain a clearer understanding of individual behaviors. The new mother is the product of all of her history: what she has learned about infants and infant feeding, and what she has seen.
- Culture is defined as the values, beliefs, norms, and practices of a particular group, which are learned and shared and guide thinking, decisions, and actions in a patterned way.
- Ethnocentrism—being centered in one's ethnic or cultural system (i.e., believing that "my group is best")—is the opposite of cultural relativism—the recognition and appreciation of cultural differences and backgrounds.
- Culturally competent care is defined as the adaptation of care in a manner that is consistent with the culture of the client.
- A nonjudgmental way to assess a cultural practice is to ask certain questions: Is it helpful? Is it harmless? Is it harmful?
- Ideally, the care provider can understand and speak the language of the mother and her family. When it is necessary to translate a conversation, a trained interpreter should be used.
- Breastfeeding in public, time of weaning, and giving the neonate colostrum are all practices that are extremely sensitive to cultural norms.
- If a cultural ritual is important for a new mother and causes no harm to either her or her baby, the lactation consultant should respect

the mother's wishes regardless of whether the ritual has been scientifically tested.

INTERNET RESOURCES

- Collection of papers in different languages (also artworks, stamps, and paintings): http://global-breastfeeding.org
- EthnoMed (cultural beliefs, medical issues, and other related topics pertinent to the health care of recent immigrants to Seattle, specifically, or to the United States): http://ethnomed.org
- La Leche League International (breastfeeding printed information and visuals in many languages): http://www.llli.org
- Office of Minority Health (established in 1986 to improve the health of racial and ethnic minority populations through the development of health policies and programs that will help eliminate health disparities; OMH was reauthorized by the Patient Protection and Affordable Care Act of 2010): http://www.minorityhealth.hhs.gov/
- Online guide to breastfeeding and baby care from India (including links, discussion forum, and photo album): http://www.breastfeedingindia.com/home.html
- San Diego County Breastfeeding Coalition (breastfeeding information in Spanish and English): http://www.breastfeeding.org

REFERENCES

Alikasifoglu M, Erginoz E, Gur ET, et al. Factors influencing the duration of exclusive breastfeeding in a group of Turkish women. *J Hum Lact.* 2001;17:220–225.

Allen JA, Li R, Scanlon KS, et al. Progress in increasing breastfeeding and reducing racial/ethnic differences — United States, 2000–2008 births. *MMWR.* February 8, 2013;62(05);77–80.

Anderson GC. Current knowledge about skin-to-skin (kangaroo) care for preterm infants. *J Perinatol.* 1992;11:216–226.

Anderson GC, Marks EA, Wahlberg V. Kangaroo care for premature infants. *Am J Nurs.* 1986;86:807–809.

Avery M, Duckett L, Frantzich CR. The experience of sexuality during breastfeeding among primiparous women. *J Midwifery Women's Health.* 2000;45:227–237.

Baumslag N. Breastfeeding: cultural practices and variations. *Adv Int Matern Child Health.* 1987;7:36–50.

Bentley ME, Dee DL, Jensen JL. Breastfeeding among low income African-American women: power, beliefs and decision making. *J Nutr.* 2003;133:S305–S309.

Berry AB. Mexican American women's expressions of the meaning of culturally congruent prenatal care. *J Transcultural Nurs.* 1999;10:203–212.

Blum L. *At the breast: ideologies of breastfeeding and motherhood in the contemporary United States.* Boston, MA: Beacon Press; 1999.

Bohler E, Ingstad B. The struggle of weaning: factors determining breastfeeding duration in East Bhutan. *Soc Sci Med.* 1996;43:1805–1815.

Bonuck KA, Trombley M, Freeman K, McKee D. Randomized controlled trial of a prenatal and postnatal lactation consultant intervention on duration and intensity of breastfeeding up to 12 months. *Pediatrics.* 2005; 116(6):1413–1426.

Budzynska K, Gardner ZE, Low Dog T, Gardiner P. Complementary, holistic, and integrative medicine: advice for clinicians on herbs and breastfeeding. *Pediatr Rev.* 2013;34:343–352. doi: 10.1542/pir.34-8-343.

Centers for Disease Control and Protection. U.S. Selected Practice Recommendations for Contraceptive Use, 2013. *MMWR.* 2013;62:1–60.

Conton L. Social, economic and ecological parameters of infant feeding in Usino, Papua New Guinea. *Ecol Food Nutr.* 1985;16:39–54.

Corbett KS. Explaining infant feeding style of low-income Black women. *J Pediatr Nurs.* 2000;15:73–81.

Cricco-Lizza R. The milk of human kindness: environment and human interactions in a WIC clinic that influence infant-feeding decision in Black women. *Qual Health Res.* 2005;15:525–538.

Cricco-Lizza R. Black non-Hispanic mothers' perceptions about the promotion of infant-feeding methods by nurses and physicians. *JOGNN.* 2006;35:173–180.

Davis RE. The postpartum experience for Southeast Asian women in the United States. *Matern Child Nurs.* 2001; 26(4):208–213.

Dettwyler KA. A time to wean: the hominid blueprint for the natural age of weaning in modern human populations. In: Stuart-Macadam P, Dettwyler KA, eds. *Breastfeeding: biocultural perspectives.* New York, NY: Aldine De Gruyter; 1995:39–72.

Dimond HJ, Ashworth A. Infant feeding practices in Kenya, Mexico, and Malaysia: the rarity of the exclusively breast-fed infant. *Hum Nutr Appl Nutr.* 1987;41A: 51–64.

Dodgson JE, Duckett L, Garwick A, Graham BL. An ecological perspective of breastfeeding in an indigenous community. *J Nurs Scholarship.* 2002;34:235–241.

Dykes F. Western medicine and marketing: construction of an inadequate milk syndrome in lactating women. *Health Care for Women Int.* 2002;23:492–502.

Feldman-Winter L. Evidence-based interventions to support breastfeeding. *Pediatr Clin North Am.* 2013;60(1): 169–187. doi: 10.1016/j.pcl.2012.09.007.

Fishman C, Evans R, Jenks E. Warm bodies, cool milk: conflicts in postpartum food choice for Indochinese women in California. *Soc Sci Med.* 1988;26:1125–1132.

Forman MR, Hundt GL, Towne D, et al. The forty-day rest period and infant feeding practices among Negev Bedouin Arab women in Israel. *Med Anthropol.* 1990;12: 207–216.

Galvin S, Grossman X, Feldman-Winter L, et al. A practical intervention to increase breastfeeding initiation among Cambodian women in the US. *Matern Child Health J.* 2008;12(4):545–547.

Groleau D, Souliere M, Kirmayer LJ. Breastfeeding and the cultural configuration of social space among Vietnamese women. *Health Place.* 2006;12:516–526.

Harris MS, Purnell K, Fletcher A, Lindgren K. Moving toward cultural competency: DREAMWork online summer program. *J Cult Divers.* 2013;20(3):134–138.

Hayssen V. Empirical and theoretical constraints on the evolution of lactation. *J Dairy Sci.* 1993;76:3213–3233.

Hernandez IF. Promoting exclusive breastfeeding for Hispanic women. *MCN.* 2006;31:318–324.

Issacson M. Clarifying concepts: Cultural humility or competence. *J Prof Nurs.* 2014; 30:251–258.

Lacay GI. The Puerto Rican in mainland America. In: Clark A, ed. *Culture and childrearing.* Philadelphia, PA: F. A. Davis; 1981:211–227.

Leininger M. *Qualitative research methods in nursing.* Orlando, FL: Grune and Stratton; 1985.

Lepowsky MA. Food taboos, malaria and dietary change: infant feeding and cultural adaptation of a Papua New Guinea island. *Ecol Food Nutr.* 1985;16:105–126.

Libbus MK. Breastfeeding attitudes in a sample of Spanish-speaking Hispanic American women. *J Hum Lact.* 2000;16:216–220.

MacNamara M, Wilhelm A, Dy G, et al. Promoting quality care for recently resettled populations: curriculum development for internal medicine residents. *J Grad Med Educ.* 2014;6(2):310–314. doi: 10.4300/JGME-D-13-00170.1.

Maher V. Breastfeeding in cross-cultural perspectives, paradoxes and proposals. In: Maher V, ed. *The anthropology of breastfeeding.* Oxford, UK: Berg; 1992:1–32.

Martin JA, Hamilton BE, Osterman MJK, et al. Division of Vital Statistics. Births: final data for 2012. *National Vital Statistics Report.* 2013;62(9).

Masvie H. The role of Tamang mothers-in-law in promoting breast feeding in Makwanpur District, Nepal. *Midwifery.* 2006;22:23–31.

Mattson S. Striving for cultural competence. *AWHONN Lifelines.* 2000;4(3):48–52.

Mead M, Newton N. Cultural patterning of perinatal behavior. In: Richardson SA, Buttmacher AF, eds.

Childbearing: its social and psychological aspects. Baltimore, MD: Williams & Wilkins; 1967:142–143.

Mennella JS, Beauchamp GK. Maternal diet alters the sensory qualities of human milk and the nursling's behavior. *Pediatrics.* 1991;88:737–744.

Moore ER, Anderson GC, Bergman N, Dowswell T. Early skin-to-skin contact for mothers and their healthy newborn infants. *Cochrane Database of Systematic Reviews* 2012, Issue 5. Art. No.: CD003519. 10.1002/14651858. CD003519.pub3.

Mortel M, Mehta SD. Systematic review of the efficacy of herbal galactogogues. *J Hum Lact.* 2013;29:154–162. doi: 10.1177/0890334413477243.

Mulford C. Swimming upstream: breastfeeding care in a non-breastfeeding culture. *JOGNN.* 1995;24:464–473.

National Conference of State Legislatures. Breastfeeding state laws. 2014. Available at: http://www.ncsl.org/research/health/breastfeeding-state-laws.aspx.

Noble LM, Noble A, Hand IL. Cultural competence of health-care professionals caring for breastfeeding mothers in urban areas. *Breastfeed Med.* 2009;4:221–224. doi: 10.1089/bfm.2009.0020.

Obermeyer CM, Castle S. Back to nature? Historical and cross-cultural perspectives on barriers to optimal breastfeeding. *Med Anthropol.* 1997;17:39–63.

Omuloulu A. Breastfeeding practice and breastmilk intake in rural Nigeria. *Hum Nutr Appl Nutr.* 1982;36:445–451.

Orque MS, Block B, Monrroy LS. *Ethnic nursing care: a multi-cultural approach.* St. Louis, MO: Mosby; 1983:19.

Purdy IB. Social, cultural, and medical factors that influence maternal breastfeeding. *Issues Ment Health Nurs.* 2010;31:365–367. doi: 10.3109/01612840903359757.

Purnell L. The Purnell model for cultural competence. *J Transcult Nurs.* 2002;13(3):193–196; discussion 200–201.

Rasbridge LA, Kulig JC. Infant feeding among Cambodian refugees. *Am J Matern Child Nurs.* 1995;20:213–218.

Riordan J, Gill-Hopple K. Breastfeeding care in multicultural populations. *JOGNN.* 2001;30:216–223.

Roberts SG, Warda M, Garbutt S, Curry K. The use of high-fidelity simulation to teach cultural competence in the nursing curriculum. *J Prof Nurs.* 2014;30:259–265. doi: 10.1016/j.profnurs.2013.09.012.

Rossiter JC. The effect of a culture-specific education program to promote breastfeeding among Vietnamese women in Sydney. *Int J Nurs Stud.* 1994;31:369–379.

Sasnett B, Royal PD, Ross T. Introduction of a cultural training experience into interdisciplinary health science education program. *J Allied Health.* 2010;39(2): e55–e60.

Thiel de Bocanegra H. Breast-feeding in immigrant women: the role of social support and acculturation. *Hispanic J Behav Sci.* 2008;20(4):448–467.

Thorley V. Sharing breastmilk: wet-nursing, cross-feeding, and milk donations. *Breastfeed Rev.* 2008;16:25–29.

U.S. Census Bureau, U.S. Department of Commerce, Economics and Statistics Administration. The Hispanic population: 2010. 2011. Available at: http://www.census.gov/prod/cen2010/briefs/c2010br-04.pdf.

van Esterik P, Elliott T. Infant feeding style in urban Kenya. *Ecol Food Nutr.* 1986;18:183–195.

van Steenbergen WM, Kusin JA, Kardjati S, Renqvist UH. Nutritional transition during pregnancy in East Java, Indonesia: I. A longitudinal study of feeding pattern, breastmilk intake and the consumption of additional foods. *Eur J Clin Nurs.* 1991;45:67–75.

Whittemore RD, Beverly EA. Mandinka mothers and nurslings: power and reproduction. *Med Anthropol Q.* 1996; 10:45–62.

Winikoff B, Castle MA, Laukaran VH, eds. *Feeding infants in four societies: causes and consequences of mothers' choices.* New York, NY: Greenwood Press; 1988:187–201.

Woolridge M. *Breastfeeding in the US and Thailand* [presentation]. Miami, FL: International Lactation Consultant Association; 1991.

World Health Organization. Selected practice recommendations for contraceptive use. 2008 update. Geneva, Switzerland: World Health Organization; 2008. Available at: http://whqlibdoc.who.int/hq/2008/WHO_RHR_08.17_eng.pdf.

Wrigley EA, Hutchinson S. Long-term breastfeeding: the secret bond. *J Nurs Midwifery.* 1990;35:35–41.

Chapter 23

The Familial and Social Context of Breastfeeding

Karen Wambach

When healthcare professionals help a breastfeeding mother and baby, they help a family. The breastfeeding family exists in a social context; therefore, care providers must recognize "family" as a group that is variously defined and experienced. They need to know about the family from which the mother comes and into which her child will be born and reared. Although every family is expected to perform similar functions, the ways in which those functions are recognized and accomplished will vary.

In this chapter we will examine the family from a developmental perspective. The birth of a baby has rightly been described as a crisis because it forces new ways of behavior on all family members. We also will describe issues pertaining to the development of spousal–partner and parent–child attachment, paying particular attention to the father's role as a helpmate and supporter of his partner's role as mother and as breastfeeding woman. We also address the special needs of the adolescent mother, the adoptive mother and family, and women living in poverty. Finally, we consider certain negative family experiences, including violence against women and children.

Family Forms and Functions

Every individual experiences many family forms during a lifetime. Each form meets different needs and serves different functions. Historically, the traditional family has been one in which the mother is a full-time homemaker and primarily responsible for rearing the children, while her husband is a full-time worker outside the home. He is committed to seeing that the children are raised to adulthood, but his role in child rearing is seen as secondary to that of his wife. Although this form has often been viewed as ideal, it is experienced by a much smaller percentage of families today than it was in the mid-1900s (U.S. Department of Labor, 2013). A nuclear family includes one or both parents and their children, either born to or adopted by them. An extended family usually contains lateral kin (such as aunts, uncles, or cousins), who occupy the same generational status as the parents and children in a nuclear family, or vertical kin (such as grandparents or grandchildren), who represent generations different from the parents and children in the nuclear family. In some cases, an extended family may include "fictive" kin—that is, individuals who cannot trace lineage through blood or marriage ties to the nuclear family members but who act, and are treated, as if they were related (Friedman et al., 2003).

Examining how different family forms are likely to be experienced throughout an individual's lifetime can provide insight into the stresses that an individual is likely to encounter. It also reveals the people on whom an individual will lean as he or she attempts to cope with those stresses.

Today's families increasingly recognize that child rearing will occupy only a portion of the entire life experience of a couple (regardless of the number of relationships experienced). Although a baby may be the outcome and reflection of the love its parents feel for one another, the presence of a baby nearly always adds stress to the new family unit (Cox et al., 1999; Fonseca et al., 2013; Rovine & Belsky, 1990; St. John et al., 2005; Twenge et al., 2003).

One way to identify how babies represent potential and ongoing stress for the couple is to recognize how family interaction patterns are affected by the addition of a new member. The couple's relationship is easy to understand. Each member of this pair relates to the other. Add one child and two new relationships are added: one linking mother to child, and one linking father to child. In addition, the couple is now both husband and wife and mother and father. In assuming these roles, each partner may view the other in new ways that are not always supportive of a continued spousal role. When another child is added, the relationships become even more complex. The mother and the father each have a new relationship with the new baby, but a sibling relationship is added as well. Thus, in a two-person household, two relationships exist; in a three-person household, three relationships exist; and in a four-person household, six relationships exist (Figure 23-1). With each new person added to the family, more than one new relationship is added, because each person interacts with all other family members.

Family Theory

Numerous types of theories have been applied to understanding how families work, what influences them to work effectively, and how best to offer assistance when they do not. Examples of theories or theory classes used to examine and assist new families include family systems theories, Roy's adaptation model, role theories, family stress theories, social support theories, and social exchange theory. A developmental approach seems particularly appropriate to healthcare providers assisting families, in that it recognizes that families expand and contract at different times, based on the addition or launching of children (Rodgers & White, 1993). Thus, over time and based on a stage approach, a given family is likely to experience a couple stage, an expansion stage, a stable stage, and a launching stage.

Most families begin as couples and then move to the expansion stage, which begins with the first pregnancy and continues until the birth of the last child. In some families, this stage may be very brief—the duration of one pregnancy only. In other families, it might last more than two decades as new infants are added to the family. The stable stage occurs when members are neither added nor taken away. This stage is followed by the launching stage, which begins when the oldest child leaves home, and continues until the only individuals remaining in the home are the original couple or their replacements in the family (if one or both of the original couple has remarried). However one views the family from a developmental perspective, the number of stages identified is not nearly as important as the tasks expected of the family at different times in the family career or family life course.

The healthcare worker assisting breastfeeding mothers is most likely to interact with members of families during the expansion phase of the family's life course. It is important to recognize that varying

Figure 23-1 HOW RELATIONSHIPS CHANGE WITH THE ADDITION OF A NEW FAMILY MEMBER.

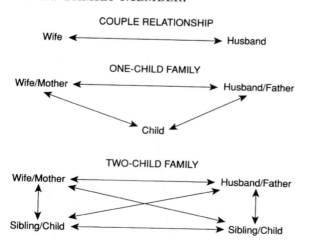

tasks characterize this phase of the family so as to identify how those tasks will influence decision making and behavior related to infant feeding and other aspects of the early mother–child relationship.

Social Factors That Influence Breastfeeding

The role of supportive significant others in the breast-feeding mother's life cannot be overemphasized. Social support is the mobilization and access to inter-personal resources that occurs when an individual attempts to deal with the stress and strains of life. Social support includes emotional support, instru-mental support, appraisal support, and informational support (House, 1981; Hughes, 1984). Choices regarding infant-feeding decisions are always couched in terms of the social context in which they occur. For example, in a family in which extended breastfeeding is viewed as aberrant behavior, it is unlikely that the mother will choose to continue breastfeeding unless she receives a preponderance of positive, or at least neutral, reactions from her significant others. In another family in which breastfeeding is viewed as just another activity of 2- or 3-year-olds, extended breastfeeding is far more likely to occur. The interaction of mother and baby with significant others and their acceptance and/or approval of such breastfeeding behavior must be taken into account when determining how best to assist the woman (Hills-Bonczyk et al., 1994; Rempel, 2004).

Table 23-1 summarizes some of the other variables, in addition to social support, that affect breastfeeding and can be influenced by the healthcare provider.

Table 23-1 How Healthcare Providers Can Influence Factors That Affect Breastfeeding

Factor	Influence	Studies
Social support/social approval/social stigma	Women with greater access to support choose to breastfeed more frequently and breastfeed longer. Support is manifested differently across ethnic and social groups. Support and social approval decrease and social stigma increases with long-term breastfeeding in Western societies.	Balcazar et al., 1995; Bar-Yam & Darby, 1997; Hills-Bonczyk et al. 1994; Kaufman & Hall, 1989; Kendall-Tackett & Sugarman, 1995; Kessler et al., 1995; Rempel, 2004
Intention to breastfeed	The majority of pregnant women decide how they will feed their baby before or early in pregnancy. A consistent positive association exists between intended and actual duration of breastfeeding.	Blyth et al., 2004; Chapman & Perez-Escamilla, 2000; Grossman et al., 1990; Losch et al., 1995; Rempel, 2004; Wambach, 1997, 2011
Attitude toward breastfeeding	There is increased breastfeeding initiation and duration by women with a positive attitude.	Avery et al., 1998; Janke, 1994; Rempel, 2004; Tarkka et al., 1999
Mother's confidence/ breastfeeding self-efficacy/ perceived behavioral control	Women with high confidence breastfeed longer than women with low confidence.	Blyth et al., 2004; Boettcher et al., 1999; Chezem et al., 2003; Dennis & Faux, 1999; Glassman et al., 2014; O'Campo et al., 1992; Rempel, 2004
Staff knowledge and attitudes toward breastfeeding	Lack of appropriate breastfeeding knowledge in hospital staff is a barrier to assistance from nurses and breastfeeding support.	Augustin et al., 2014; Balcazar et al., 1995; Bernaix, 2000; Coreil et al., 1995; Freed et al., 1996; Lazzaro et al., 1995; Li et al., 2014; Merten et al., 2005

The results of numerous studies have consistently revealed that the mother's intention to breastfeed is the single most important factor in determining whether she will start breastfeeding and how long she will continue to breastfeed. Research findings have also shown that intention is linked to social support and influence, the mother's attitude, and her confidence in herself regarding breastfeeding. For example, most lactation consultants can report that they have worked with women whose firm intention to breastfeed resulted in their overcoming all types of adversity to continue nursing; conversely, lactation consultants can also describe cases where a mother has plenty of breastmilk and the baby is gaining weight well, yet for no obvious reason she weans the baby. We might possibly assume that her intention was not to breastfeed (at least not for very long). Intention is invisible, but it can be measured with research tools (see the *Research, Theory, and Lactation* chapter).

Coupled with intention to breastfeed and maternal attitude toward breastfeeding, support systems influence choices (Kessler et al., 1995; Wade et al., 2009). In an older study, Kaufman and Hall (1989) found that women who gave birth to preterm babies and who identified no source of support were six times more likely to stop breastfeeding than were women with a support system. Those most likely to continue breastfeeding could identify several persons who supported their feeding decision. Like mothers of preterm infants, teenage mothers tend to breastfeed longer when they have a support system whose members affirm, aid, and affect in specific practical ways their mothering behavior, including breastfeeding (Nelson & Sethi, 2005; Wambach & Cole, 2000).

Social support also influences the timing of weaning the baby from the breast (Kendall-Tackett & Sugarman, 1995; Morse & Harrison, 1987; Rempel, 2004; White, 2009). Usually pressure from family members to wean and others is more likely as the baby approaches or exceeds the age of 12 months. The support of others moves gradually from actively supporting breastfeeding in the first few months of the baby's life, to tolerating breastfeeding, to ignoring breastfeeding, to actively encouraging weaning.

This last stage usually is manifested sometime after the baby reaches 6 months of age and may grow markedly stronger after the baby's 12th month in the developed world, when others view the baby as too old to breastfeed. Healthcare providers and lactation consultants can offer anticipatory guidance to women as they navigate the experience of breastfeeding beyond 6 months (Page-Goertz, 2002).

Social support is especially important in the period immediately following any life stress. As noted previously, one such stress, insofar as it necessitates changes in relationships and life patterns, is childbirth. Another is breastfeeding, particularly if the mother has not breastfed an older child, or if she is the first in her family or group of friends to do so. Very often, mothers and others assume that the mode of feeding is the cause of other infant behaviors. Lower-income, first-time mothers are more likely to breastfeed, and to keep feeding the baby mother's milk, when they receive support and information before, during, and after the baby's birth. Disadvantaged and younger U.S. mothers tend to follow the advice of their own mothers, especially if the two live in the same house (Bica & Giugliani, 2014; Grassley & Eschiti, 2008; Nunes et al., 2011; Wiemann et al., 1998). Healthcare workers should recognize the grandmother as a key informant and network person and involve her in health care and advice giving.

Mothers who choose to combine breastfeeding and bottle-feeding have not been studied extensively but may make this choice to reap the infant health benefits of breastfeeding and to avoid embarrassment if they are not able to provide sufficiently for their infants (Boettcher et al., 1999); this combination may also reflect ambivalence associated with their own developmental or confidence levels, as in teenage mothers (Wambach & Koehn, 2004). More recently, Nommsen-Rivers and colleagues (2010) studied the relative contributions of breastfeeding and formula-feeding psychosocial factors in explaining disparities in breastfeeding intentions. They found that comfort with the idea of formula-feeding mediated 37% of the disparity in breastfeeding intentions between African American and non–African American women.

Lactation consultants may have the greatest influence on the mother who is undecided about infant feeding. Early studies indicated that health-care workers are not viewed as consistent support resources for breastfeeding. However, newer research and secondary analysis of these older data found that prenatal education was a strong predictor of intention to breastfeed (Dennis, 2001).

The racial or ethnic group with which the mother identifies influences whose advice she seeks and follows relating to childbearing and breastfeeding. For example, among low-income Anglo-American women, the male partner, the mother's own mother, the grandmother, and the best friend tend to support breastfeeding. This pattern, with the exception of the best friend, is also seen among Mexican Americans. However, in a study of 100 breastfeeding and 100 bottle-feeding women, Giugliani et al. (1994) concluded that, regardless of maternal age, education level, ethnicity, and marital status, women who indicated that their partners preferred breastfeeding were significantly more likely to initiate breastfeeding when compared with women whose partners were ambivalent or preferred bottle-feeding (odds ratio [OR], 32.8; 95% confidence interval [CI], 6.7–159.5).

In contrast, some evidence indicates that black women choose breastfeeding because of the information and encouragement they receive from their physician during prenatal care (Bentley et al., 1999). Alternatively, they may choose bottle-feeding because of lack of encouragement from healthcare providers (Wiemann et al., 1998). In many cases, they report minimal support from family members.

In a qualitative study based on interviews (Corbett, 2000), an African American woman told of the curiosity of friends who wanted to watch her because they had never seen a woman breastfeed. Breastfeeding seemed to them to be an unfamiliar and uncertain activity. Recently, researchers in Memphis, Tennessee, conducted focus-group interviews to explore perceived barriers to breastfeeding, especially among African American women, and also to gather potential solutions from the target population (Ware et al., 2014). Focus groups were conducted in nine community settings. They primarily consisted of women of childbearing age, but other groups included men, grandmothers, and teens. Common breastfeeding barriers included pain, embarrassment with public nursing, going back to work, concern about "partying" and breastfeeding, and "just not wanting to" breastfeed. There was also significant concern about sexuality and breastfeeding. Participants recommended placing breastfeeding educational materials widely across the county in many venues to provide more education on breastfeeding.

Another study in the southern United States validated the influence of family and personal experiences on the choice to initiate and continue breastfeeding (Meyerink & Marquis, 2002). Among a random sample of 150 mothers (93% African American) at a county health clinic in Birmingham, Alabama, only 41% of women initiated breastfeeding, 24% breastfed for at least 1 month, and 8.3% breastfed for 3 months or more. Initiation of breastfeeding was positively associated with the mother having been breastfed herself and having breastfed a previous infant. Breastfeeding at and beyond 1 month was more likely among older women and women with close relatives who breastfed, and when the mother had been breastfed herself and had breastfed a previous infant. These findings highlight that family influence and role modeling are important to choices, and that such support could potentially come from a peer counselor or "surrogate mother" as suggested by these researchers.

For many Southeast Asian women, the mother-in-law is traditionally the person who makes decisions and gives advice about childbearing and child rearing, including breastfeeding (Schneiderman, 1996). Most of the Vietnamese women in one study who chose to breastfeed were encouraged by the experiences of significant others: "My mum breastfed all her nine children in Vietnam. She said breastmilk is good for a baby," and "My mother-in-law and my husband both wanted me to breastfeed, particularly because this is our first child" (Rossiter & Yam, 2000, p. 273).

Generally, the more support a mother has for breastfeeding, the more likely she is to initiate and continue this feeding practice. Healthcare workers should make clear their support of breastfeeding and encourage other family members to support this choice as well. After discharge from the hospital, the degree of support that new mothers have at home is critical. It is imperative that the healthcare provider learns whether the new mother will have someone to whom she can turn once she is at home. If she does not, steps need to be taken to provide follow-up support or to arrange for home visitation by a hospital or social service organizations that provide such assistance. Many hospitals today provide outpatient support for lactation in the form of breastfeeding clinics or warm-lines to call for assistance with breastfeeding problems or questions. These services and support groups are considered very important to initiation and continuation of breastfeeding and are part of the World Health Organization's (WHO) *Ten Steps to Successful Breastfeeding* and the Baby-Friendly Hospital Initiative (https://www.babyfriendlyusa.org/about-us/baby-friendly-hospital-initiative/the-ten-steps). In the United States, state-level programs are available to train hospital staff in supportive maternity practices, including ensuring that mothers have accessible support after hospital discharge (e.g., Kansas High Five for Mom and Baby; see http://www.high5kansas.org/).

Given the short hospital stays for childbirth that are common today, much of the teaching that is viewed as appropriate during the postpartum period may have to be shifted to a prenatal setting to free what little time is available at discharge for key planning issues.

Research indicates that healthcare providers have no control over certain characteristics associated with breastfeeding, although it is helpful for providers to be knowledgeable about their effects. Furthermore, these characteristics are often associated with vulnerable populations and can be targeted for breastfeeding promotion and support efforts (Table 23-2). When attempting to provide ongoing information and help, particularly when that help is offered outside an institutional setting, the healthcare provider and lactation consultant need to be aware of the social support system, whether familial or community based, that the mother can tap.

Fathers

Fathers are often the most influential support persons prior to birth in feeding decisions and throughout the breastfeeding period (Bar-Yam & Darby,

Table 23-2 FACTORS THAT AFFECT BREASTFEEDING OVER WHICH HEALTHCARE PROVIDERS HAVE NO INFLUENCE

Factor	Influence	Studies
Maternal age	Older women are more likely to choose to breastfeed and to breastfeed for a longer period.	Callen & Pinelli, 2004; Chapman & Perez-Escamilla, 2000; Forster et al., 2006; Nolan & Goel, 1995
Socioeconomic status	Varies by culture; women in higher socioeconomic status levels in United States are more likely to breastfeed.	Callen & Pinneli, 2004; Kelly & Watt, 2005; Raisler, 2000
Maternal education	Women with more education are more likely to breastfeed; varies according to culture.	Callen & Pinneli, 2004; Glassman et al., 2014; Nolan & Goel, 1995
Maternal employment	Although not associated with breastfeeding initiation, employment is likely to shorten breastfeeding duration.	Arthur et al., 2003; Augustin et al., 2014; Chapman & Perez-Escamilla, 2000; Dodgson & Duckett, 1997; Fein & Roe, 1998; Kimbro, 2006; Novotny et al., 2000; Roe et al., 1999; Ryan et al., 2006; Visness & Kennedy, 1997
Previous breastfeeding experience	Experienced breastfeeders are more likely to breastfeed longer than those without previous experience.	Boettcher et al., 1999; Glassman et al., 2014; Meyerink & Marquis, 2002; Wambach, 1997

1997; Giugliani et al., 1994; Gorman et al., 1995; Pavill, 2002; Rempel & Rempel, 2011). In a study of culturally diverse fathers, 81% wanted their babies to be breastfed; more African American men indicated they preferred their infants to be breastfed than had been reported in any previous study (Pollock et al., 2002). Similarly, Preston (2004), in her qualitative study of infant feeding among African American teenage mothers, reported that the adolescent fathers were pleased with the participants choosing to breastfeed their infants. Sipsma et al. (2013), in their sample of adolescent and young adult pregnant women and their partners, also found that 80% of males wanted their partners to breastfeed because they viewed this practice as a healthier and natural feeding choice.

When helping to care for a family breastfeeding a new baby, the healthcare provider or lactation consultant can gather information by paying attention to the father. Fathers' reactions to their breastfeeding babies vary a great deal. Some will enthusiastically participate in putting the baby to breast, making suggestions, and generally helping. Others, often first-time fathers, will hang back and observe but not interact. A few of these first-time fathers look shell-shocked with the first few breastfeedings—perhaps partly due to the unfamiliarity of having their wife's breasts exposed. Alternatively, fathers may feel like they have little control in the situation in which mothers and infants are the focus of attention. In a study of the transition to first-time fatherhood, it was suggested that early postpartum experiences, with the aforementioned focus on mother and infant, could compound feelings of inadequacy in new fathers (Buist et al., 2003). Indeed, studies of fathers' role in the breastfeeding experience speak to fathers feeling left out of the breastfeeding relationship (Brown & Davies, 2014; Mitchell-Box & Braun, 2012). Conversely, Rempel and Rempel (2011) describe fathers as members of the "breastfeeding team." In their study, fathers identified their unique roles as ensuring that their babies received the benefits of breastfeeding by supporting breastfeeding "by becoming breastfeeding savvy, by using their knowledge to encourage and assist mothers in breastfeeding, by valuing the breastfeeding mothers,

and by sharing housework and child care" (p. 115). Thus, informing expectant and new fathers of their expected roles relative to the care of the infant, as well as support of the mother, is important to their feelings of adequacy, paternal role development, and subsequent mental well-being.

When fathers enter into caregiving roles immediately after the birth of their infants, they are more likely to feel that they are an important part of the baby's life and have bonded more readily (Goodman, 2005; Pavill, 2002) (Figure 23-2). When teaching the mother how to put the baby to breast, the healthcare provider should involve the father by asking him to help with the breastfeeding—meaning placing the baby, helping to control the baby's hands and arms, burping, and so on. Likewise, when giving discharge instructions, address the father as well as the mother. The mother, already overloaded with

Figure 23-2 A FATHER ATTACHES TO HIS BABY IN MUCH THE SAME WAY AS THE MOTHER.

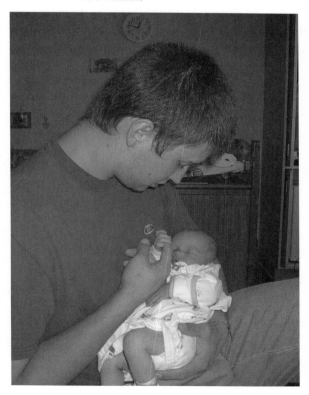

stress, may not remember what the provider is saying, but fathers often pay close attention to what is said, sometimes adding questions of their own to the mother's questions.

Examinations of the ways in which men evolve into fathers suggests that the role remains relatively invisible to others; it is a relatively passive reflection of what is happening to the pregnant wife until after the baby's birth. When the baby begins to interact with the father directly, the father's role becomes more explicit—in his own mind as well as in the awareness of others (Goodman, 2005; Jordan & Wall, 1993; Rempel & Rempel, 2011). Nurturing is a fundamental human quality that need not be gender specific. That many view it as feminine must be seen as a cultural artifact rather than a reflection of inherent differences between males and females.

Fathers play a vital role as a supporter of breastfeeding, particularly when they have a positive mind-set regarding breastfeeding (Earle, 2000; Pavill, 2002; Rempel & Rempel, 2011). Thus prenatal discussions of infant feeding in childbirth and breastfeeding classes are effective in allaying concerns and dispelling myths. Prenatal classes are also ideal for teaching fathers the benefits of breastfeeding and the physiology of lactation, and for informing a father about how he can help his breastfeeding wife without having to feed the baby. Jordan and Wall (1993) suggested father-only classes in which fathers could communicate openly with one another and have experiences in practicing skills that would be important for them in the care of their infants. Indeed, recent research on father support of breastfeeding asserts that fathers desire "father-specific" information on breastfeeding and ways to support the breastfeeding mother (Brown & Davies, 2014; Mitchell-Box & Braun, 2012; Sherriff et al., 2014).

Intervention research aimed at fathers as supporters of breastfeeding is still limited, but a systematic review of four intervention studies indicated that education for fathers was effective in improving at least one breastfeeding outcome (Mitchell-Box & Braun, 2013). More recently, a randomized clinical trial in Western Australia, known as the Fathers Infant Feeding Initiative (FIFI) study, used a short educational intervention during the pregnancy and postnatal support to fathers to enhance duration of breastfeeding (Maycock et al., 2013). The "any breastfeeding" rate for the intervention group was significantly greater at 6 weeks: 81.6% in the intervention group compared to 75.2% in the control group (OR, 1.46; 95% CI, 1.01–2.13). Cumulatively, this evidence clearly indicates that prenatal providers and lactation specialists can positively influence breastfeeding outcomes with simple interventions aimed at fathers.

The early days of fathering can be stressful and disruptive to the father, just as mothering is to the mother (St. John et al., 2005). A synthesis of qualitative study findings indicated that the birth of an infant strains the couple relationship (Goodman, 2005). Furthermore, some fathers report jealousy of the physical and emotional closeness of mother and infant, feelings of uselessness during breastfeeding, sexual frustration, and repulsion from the sight of full, dripping breasts. Some fathers feel ashamed of these emotions and tend not to talk about them, or they may joke about being jealous of the new baby (Brown & Davies, 2014; Gamble & Morse, 1993; Jordan & Wall, 1990).

The most comfortable place for fathers to express these feelings is with other new fathers, many of whom may conceal the same feelings. Childbirth education classes, La Leche League groups, and online discussions for fathers (see the "Other Resources" section at the end of the chapter) provide communication outlets in which new fathers can openly share their feelings and perceptions about the realities of parenthood in an atmosphere of unconditional acceptance. Experienced fathers can help new fathers realize that they are not alone in having ambivalent feelings about the closeness between their breastfeeding wives and babies and about giving up certain pleasures in exchange for new responsibilities. One such father offered this description:

> If I'd been more prepared that they would be this complete unit unto themselves, it would have been easier. For a while I felt left out, like I was around only to bring home the money and wasn't a part of it. I felt bad, then guilty about feeling bad. Before the baby came, my wife really spoiled me, you know, really adored and lavished attention on me. Then, whammo, she was pregnant 3 months after we were married and I wasn't getting that kind

of treatment anymore. I resented it. Things really broke loose and we had a showdown; I finally had to open up and let her know how I really felt. After that, when it was all in the open, things got better. With the next baby, I don't think I'll go through those feelings again.

Support groups for new fathers validate a commitment to recognize the needs of new fathers—to help them develop coping strategies for optimal and involved parenting of their breastfed baby. These father groups tend to attract men who are having more difficulty or who are more open in admitting to feeling stressed by making adjustments. These actions can potentially strengthen family relationships in the years ahead.

Implicit in the notion that breastfeeding prevents father–child closeness is acceptance of the assumption that the most (perhaps the only) significant way in which a father can interact with his child is by feeding her or him. Encourage the father to consider the many ways in which he can interact with the baby, particularly during the very early period when artificial feeding may increase the risk of breastfeeding failure (Figure 23-3). Several options are available, and some are supported by research in which fathers described their role in the breastfeeding team (Rempel & Rempel, 2011):

- Burping the baby after a feeding: The necessity of burping is less an issue than is the opportunity to frequently hold the baby when the infant is likely to be relaxed and somnolent; if a burp is obtained, the father also gains a sense of having accomplished something tangible that can be translated to mean "I am a good father."
- Changing the baby's wet diapers: This activity occurs frequently.
- Changing the baby's soiled diapers: This, too, occurs frequently and, in breastfed infants, is far less unpleasant because the odor is less noxious than are the soiled diapers of a formula-fed baby.
- Giving the baby a massage: Fathers who massage their babies often find that they can put a baby to sleep with little effort; such activity can assist an overstimulated or colicky baby to relax sufficiently to fall asleep.
- Bathing the baby: Assisting with the baby's bath is usually most happily accomplished after the baby begins to enjoy the bath.
- Rocking the baby: The father's involvement with the baby frees the mother to engage in other activities.
- Singing or reading to the baby: This activity can begin as soon after birth as the father wishes. Often, repeating the same songs that were played during the pregnancy will result in clear signals of recognition by the baby.
- Playing with the baby: Generally occurs as the infant ages and is more alert and receptive to interaction.
- Giving the mother a break from the baby and other children at the grandparents' house.

The Adolescent Mother

Adolescent motherhood presents many social and personal challenges to the individual mother, her family, and society. Although the rate of adolescent pregnancy in the United States is currently at a historical low, U.S. rates remain higher than many other industrialized countries (McKay & Barrett, 2010). Breastfeeding initiation rates among adolescent mothers, although improving according to recent surveys, generally are lower than those among adult women, and breastfeeding duration is shorter

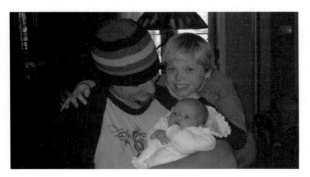

Figure 23-3 ONE OF THE MANY WAYS A DAD HELPS WITH THE CARE OF A NEW BABY.

in such young mothers (Centers for Disease Control and Prevention [CDC], n.d.).

Many caregivers assume that the young mother is neither interested in giving nor ready to give to another person by breastfeeding. On the contrary, a significant percentage of adolescents consider breastfeeding an option even if they ultimately bottle-feed (Leffler, 2000; Wambach & Koehn, 2004; Wiemann et al., 1998). Many of those who breastfeed make their decision before pregnancy or in the early stages of pregnancy, which suggests that adolescent mothers may be responsive to prenatal intervention to promote breastfeeding (Wambach & Cohen, 2009; Wambach & Cole, 2000).

Role modeling and peer influence are powerful tools for altering adolescent behavior. Not surprisingly, Wiemann, DuBois, and Berenson (1998) found that using a breastfeeding video geared toward teens was a key intervention to help adolescents overcome perceived barriers to breastfeeding. Likewise, when Volpe and Bear (2000) started a Breastfeeding Educated and Supported Teen (BEST) Club, more teenagers subsequently breastfed than did teenage mothers preceding the implementation of the club. Martens (2001) randomized breastfeeding education sessions that included a video to Canadian Ojibwa adolescents whose beliefs about breastfeeding subsequently improved. In another study, almost all (82%) participants in an Australian program for pregnant teenagers decided to breastfeed after attending prenatal classes (Greenwood & Littlejohn, 2002). Recently, Wambach and colleagues (2011) completed the first randomized control trial in the United States of an intervention to promote and support breastfeeding in 15- to 18-year-old mothers by using education and support from a lactation consultant and peer counselor team. They found significant differences in duration of breastfeeding between the experimental and control group subjects. Median breastfeeding duration was 177, 42, and 61 days for the experimental, the attention control, and the usual care groups respectively ($\chi 2(df = 2) = 16.26$, $p < 0.001$).

Concern about keeping their figure and not gaining weight is common among new mothers of all ages, but it is particularly intense among adolescents (Wambach & Cole, 2000). A study of Korean adolescents tested an intervention using a video that explained misconceptions about breastfeeding including body changes. Apparently the video did not positively impact the adolescents' views; they reported that breastfeeding might make them gain weight and "lose" their figure (Kim, 1998). As in other studies (Hannon et al., 2000; Wambach & Koehn, 2004; Wood et al., 2013), these adolescents indicated that "embarrassment" was a major barrier to breastfeeding. Fear of pain related to breastfeeding is another major factor in deciding whether to breastfeed. Wambach and Koehn (2004) encouraged healthcare providers to assist pregnant teens with the overall decision-making process by evaluating the developmental level of the teen as well as her knowledge level. These are important aspects of adolescent decision-making processes (Mann et al., 1989).

Teen mothers, when asked to identify their needs after the birth of their baby, identified the infant's health and medical needs first, followed by daily physical care of the infant, psychosocial needs of mothers and babies, and, finally, the mother's physical care. Mothers rated information about how to breastfeed and care for the breasts as important or very important. This high level of interest in meeting their baby's needs suggests that teen mothers are likely to be motivated to follow advice when it is offered. However, because many teenage mothers often share social characteristics that are linked with the choice not to breastfeed—such as lower educational attainment, low income, and unmarried status—fewer of these young women will choose to breastfeed (Peterson & Da Vanzo, 1992).

Usually, questions asked by new adolescent mothers who initiate breastfeeding are no different from those posed by older, more experienced women, except for concerns about embarrassment with public exposure (Hannon et al., 2000; Wambach & Cohen, 2009; Wood et al., 2013). Most new mothers, no matter what their age, are concerned about how to help a baby grasp the breast, how to avoid sore nipples, and how to provide sufficient milk. The kind of assistance offered to teens, however, depends on their life situation. The teen mother who is living alone may need more frequent assistance and referral to a breast-feeding support group. The teenage mother who is living with her own mother—who may be caring for the baby while the teen is in school—may need to know about resources on which she can draw for additional information and support about breastfeeding. The teen mother living with the baby's father or another male adult needs to know how to balance her baby's needs and the needs associated with the couple relationship. The familial context of breastfeeding is important to all nursing mothers, but may be acutely important for adolescent mothers.

All breastfeeding mothers need support. In general, support needs of teenage mothers are as great as, or greater than, those of older mothers, and developmental and social status may impede the teen's ability to reach out for assistance when needed (Dykes et al., 2003; Nelson & Sethi, 2005; Wambach & Cohen, 2009). Therefore, the healthcare provider or lactation consultant must anticipate needs more accurately and efficiently and also teach the teen how to solicit help when needed. Grassley (2010) conducted a systematic review of the literature to identify and define breastfeeding social support needs of adolescent mothers. Eighteen studies illuminated four social support dimensions that mimic House's (1981) conceptualization of informational, instrumental, emotional, and appraisal support and Sarafino's network support. Nurse behavior (and by extension, behavior of the lactation specialist) was defined for each type of support. Subsequently, Pentecost and Grassley (2014) investigated adolescents' needs for nurses' support in the hospital when initiating breastfeeding. Their results indicated that adolescent mothers wanted informational, instrumental, emotional, and appraisal support.

Table 23-3 provides descriptions and definitions of the types of support and examples of questions

Table 23-3 BREASTFEEDING SUPPORT FOR ADOLESCENT MOTHERS WHO BREASTFEED

Support Type and Definition	Verbal Examples	Behavioral Examples
Informational support: Offers to the mother information, ideas, instructions, or guidance	What have you heard about breastfeeding? What are your biggest concerns about breastfeeding now and later as you prepare to return to school or work?	Provides the mother with written breastfeeding information that is culturally appropriate and at a reading level consistent with her age.
Instrumental support: Provides useful and concrete help to the mother	Your baby is showing signs of hunger. Would you like me to assist you in getting the baby positioned for feeding?	Provides the mother with privacy during breastfeeding by asking visitors to step out of the room.
Emotional support: Conveys to the mother understanding, compassion, trust and concern	I understand that you may feel like there is a lot to learn about breastfeeding and that might be overwhelming to you. What can I do to help you sort through your questions and feelings?	Calls the mother and baby by name. Sustains eye contact during conversation.
Esteem/appraisal support: Offers encouragement to the mother via affirmation and feedback	Your baby looks like he is very comfortable on your chest while skin-to-skin. How do you think breastfeeding is going so far?	Provides one-to-one time with the mother during breastfeeding.
Network support: Identifies who will provide support for the mother	Who will help you with breastfeeding when you are at home? Would you like for them to be present when I help you with breastfeeding so they can learn more?	Encourages identified support persons to be involved in breastfeeding sessions in the hospital.

Source: Adapted from Grassley (2010) and Pentecost and Grassley (2014).

and behaviors that nurses and lactation specialists can use with adolescent mothers as they initiate and maintain breastfeeding. To facilitate longer duration of breastfeeding and to promote exclusive breastfeeding (e.g., continued breastfeeding after return to school and/or work), identification of resources for obtaining a breast pump is an important way the healthcare provider can assist the adolescent mother (Hannon et al., 2000; Wambach et al., 2011; Wood et al., 2013). The breastfeeding experience of the teenage mother, of whatever duration, helps her to progress toward adulthood with a stronger and more positive sense of self and motherhood and will likely influence a repeat breastfeeding decision for future children.

The Adoptive Mother and Family

Induced lactation is the process of stimulating lactation in nonpuerperal women, mainly in the context of adoption of a newborn or surrogate pregnancy. In the United States 136,001 children were adopted in 2007 and 135,813 children were adopted in 2008 (Child Welfare Information Gateway, 2011). The latter figure represents a 6% increase in total adoptions from 2000, when 127,985 children were adopted. Given this increase in adoptions, coupled with the emphasis on the benefits of breastfeeding, induced lactation is becoming more common in the United States. However, relatively little research has focused on the breastfeeding experiences of adoptive mothers who induce lactation (Cheales-Siebenaler, 1999; Szucs et al., 2010) or the intended mothers of surrogate pregnancies (Biervliet et al., 2001). Most of the literature in this area takes the form of case studies. Furthermore, there is little research evidence to describe these experiences on a larger scale.

Auerbach and Avery's (1981) study is the largest known research study on women's experiences of induced lactation. Through various means of primary and secondary recruitment, these researchers studied 240 American and British Commonwealth women using retrospective survey methods. Women who volunteered to participate in the study were categorized into three groups: those who had

never had a pregnancy or lactated prior to inducing lactation ($n = 83$), those who had been pregnant before but had not lactated ($n = 55$), and those who had breastfed one or more infants prior to inducing lactation ($n = 102$). The major reasons for inducing lactation included building the mother–infant relationship, providing emotional benefits for the baby, experiencing body contact with the baby, providing nutritional benefits for the baby, and fostering nurturing or the mother. Factors of lesser importance were the ability to produce milk, expression of femininity, the quantity of milk produced, and any physical changes the mother might experience (such as regulation of menstrual cycling, increased size of her breasts, or protractility of nipple tissue). Women who had lactated before (group 3) considered quantity of milk produced to be a more important factor than women who had never lactated (groups 1 and 2). Women prepared for lactation by reading information on induced lactation, improving their nutrition, performing nipple stimulation before and after the baby arrived, and taking hormones to simulate pregnancy for breast preparation (only 6% used hormones prenatally), and/or helping the milk-ejection reflex. Nearly all of the women used supplements to their own milk for feeding their baby, with those who had lactated previously reporting less supplementation across time.

With an increased knowledge base, protocols for inducing lactation have been developed based on the principles of preparing the breasts anatomically prior to beginning lactation, continued stimulation and emptying of the breast with suckling by the infant and/or pumping, and building the milk supply using medications and galactogogues. Drs. Jack Newman and Lorraine Goldfarb (2002) developed protocols for inducing lactation and have assisted more than 500 women in inducing lactation or relactation. Information on the various protocols can be found at the AskLenore website (http://www .asklenore.info/breastfeeding/induced_lactation /protocols_intro.shtml). There is also a decision tool available to assist in choosing the protocol based on the estimated date of the baby's arrival and the functionality of the woman's ovaries (http://www .asklenore.info/breastfeeding/induced_lactation

/ilca2007decision_tool.pdf). A regular, accelerated, or menopausal protocol can be chosen based on these criteria. Phase II involves building the mother's milk supply, and breastfeeding and/or pumping begins based on the baby's estimated date of arrival and whether the protocol has been completed.

Despite the progress made in protocols for inducing lactation, some women may not know that induced lactation is a possibility. In describing her experience with nursing her adoptive daughter, Lorraine Hawke commented that initially she did not know about induced lactation and actually questioned its naturalness (Hawke et al., 2005). However, knowing the nutritional benefits of human milk for the infant convinced this 40-year-old woman that it was the right thing to do. Family support was necessary for her decision:

> My husband said he would fully support whatever I decided. My brothers' and sisters' responses differed from disbelief, to thinking I was nuts, to wondering how it would work and why I would want to do it, to excitement. In the end, they all supported my actions. Afterwards, the key response was fascination that I really could breastfeed without having been pregnant. (p. 18)

Hawke's story further describes the challenges of inducing lactation beginning one month before the birth using breast stimulation via pumping and use of domperidone and oxytocin spray. A lactation consultant, a midwife, and the birth mother, who was a relative, supported this mother during the rigorous process. The benefits of nursing proved to be much more than nutritional for this mother. Like birth mothers who breastfeed, Hawke described the development of a deep bond through breastfeeding with her adopted daughter. Lactation consultants play an important role in supporting the adoptive mother in this important process.

The Low-Income Family

In the United States and other developed countries, fewer low-income mothers than their more affluent countrywomen choose to breastfeed. Poor women, whose babies most need the benefits of human milk, including its far lower production cost and its marked safety as compared to artificial baby milk, are least likely to breastfeed. As more women in the developing world seek to emulate women in the developed world, the cost to these women and the countries in which they live will be even higher.

Background variables can predict whether a low-income woman will breastfeed. Grossman et al. (1989) found that if a poor woman was married, if she had at least a high school education, if she began prenatal care in the first trimester, and if she was white or Hispanic, she was more likely to breastfeed. Libbus and Kolostov (1994) reported that if the maternal grandmother breastfed and if the male partner endorsed breastfeeding, the low-income women in their study were more likely to intend to breastfeed and to view it as a positive experience. As described elsewhere in this chapter, role modeling and the mother's own previous breastfeeding experiences are very strong predictors of breastfeeding among low-income African American women (Meyerink & Marquis, 2002).

Environmental efforts to support low-income women's efforts to breastfeed are important to decreasing breastfeeding disparities across race and income levels. Cricco-Lizza (2005) interviewed 109 low-income black women enrolled in a Women, Infants, and Children (WIC) Nutritional Supplemental Program clinic in New York City and found that trusting and respectful relationships between WIC personnel and these women influenced their breastfeeding decision positively.

Lack of Information

Sometimes the reasons for not breastfeeding are related to lack of information. In fact, the major assumption behind providing childbirth and breastfeeding education classes prenatally is that women and families need information regarding these events to make informed choices (i.e., knowledge is power). However, research has indicated that low-income women do not attend childbirth education classes as much as higher-income women, and that childbirth education classes are highly associated with breastfeeding initiation (Lu et al., 2003). Kistin et al. (1990) studied low-income black women in the United States and found that prenatal education sessions that included in-depth discussions about breastfeeding not only increased the likelihood that the women would choose to breastfeed, but also boosted the likelihood that they would act on their choice when the baby was born. In addition, these sessions positively influenced the duration of breastfeeding. Brent, Redd, and Dworetz (1995) found that prenatal and postpartum instruction from a lactation consultant resulted in more low-income women choosing breastfeeding. One-on-one intervention by a lactation consultant has a positive impact on breastfeeding for mothers of all income levels (see *The Lactation Consultant: Roles and Responsibilities* chapter).

Hospital Practices

Sometimes the reasons for choosing not to breastfeed are related to hospital factors. Overall, hospital practices concerning breastfeeding have improved in the last decade. Much of this improvement comes from two sources: consumer demand and the Baby-Friendly Hospital Initiative (BFHI), an international program created by WHO and UNICEF. BFHI has successfully inculcated practices that support breastfeeding into hundreds of hospitals across the world (Turner-Maffei, 2002). As noted in the *Tides in Breastfeeding Practice* chapter, the Baby-Friendly Hospital Initiative highlights 10 steps by which any institution caring for new postpartum mothers and their neonates can assist the initiation of breastfeeding. Baby-Friendly USA, the certifying body for BFHI in the United States, reports that 189 U.S. hospitals and birthing centers have achieved Baby-Friendly Hospital designation, representing approximately 7.7% of the approximately 5000 hospitals in the United States. Administrators' concerns about the added cost of buying formula (a hospital cannot receive free formula and qualify for Baby-Friendly designation) and lack of professional support from community physicians and nursing staff present barriers to pursuing Baby-Friendly certification.

When the 10 steps recommended by the BFHI are part of the caregiving offered in a given institution, the mothers who give birth and begin breastfeeding

there are more likely to have an optimal experience. Three studies in particular have identified the ways in which implementation (or the failure of implementation) of these 10 steps has influenced the breastfeeding experiences of the mothers who gave birth and subsequently received care in the hospitals whose care patterns were examined.

The PROBIT study was a large randomized trial carried out in Belarus. In this study, hospitals and clinics were randomized into two groups: an intervention group where the Baby-Friendly 10 steps were implemented and a control group where no practice changes were made. Infants ($n = 17,000$) born at the intervention sites were breastfed significantly more often and had fewer gastrointestinal infections and atopic eczema than infants at the control sites (Kramer et al., 2001).

Merewood and Philipp (2001) overcame numerous obstacles in an inner-city teaching hospital in Boston to become the first Baby-Friendly hospital in Massachusetts. Receiving free formula was a major roadblock to achievement of this designation. After 2 years of work, 9 of the 10 steps were in place except for dealing with the estimated cost ($72,000) for buying formula instead of receiving it free. Further investigation showed that the quantity of formula listed by the formula company was far in excess of the amount actually used by the hospital. Using a standard figure of 20 cents per bottle of formula, the estimated annual cost of formula came to only $20,000—a far cry from the original $72,000 figure and a proportionately small amount of money for a large hospital with 1800 births per year.

Merewood and colleagues (2005) conducted a large U.S. survey of all Baby-Friendly hospitals in the United States in 2001. They determined that breastfeeding initiation (83.8% versus 69.5%) and exclusivity rates (78.4% versus 46.3%) were higher in these facilities than the national rates at the time, providing further evidence of the impact of the BFHI.

Which of the 10 steps have the greatest impact on breastfeeding? Wright, Rice, and Wells (1996) compared the effects of these steps on the likelihood that the women were fully breastfeeding at 4 months postpartum. The duration of breastfeeding and the duration of exclusive breastfeeding were longer for women who did not receive formula in the hospital, who were not given discharge packs or coupons, who roomed-in more than 60% of the time, who gave no pacifiers, and who received referral to breastfeeding support organizations. Further validation of these practices, with the exception of discharge packs distribution, as predictors of longer breastfeeding duration was found by Murray and colleagues (2007). In their population-based study using data from the Pregnancy Risk Assessment Monitoring System (PRAMS), the following practices were significant predictors of breastfeeding duration:

- Breastfeeding within the first hour
- Breastfeeding only (no formula in the hospital)
- Infant rooming-in
- No pacifier use
- Receipt of a telephone number for support after discharge

The Importance of Peer Counselors

The availability of an outside source of support in the first 6 weeks postpartum nearly always lengthens breastfeeding duration in a group of low-income women. Generally, the more breastfeeding friends the mother has, the longer she is likely to breastfeed.

Peer counseling programs, in which breastfeeding support is given by trained lay female advisors knowledgeable about breastfeeding, is an effective intervention (Anderson et al., 2005; Bronner et al., 2001; Campbell et al., 2014; Dennis, 2001; Martens, 2002; Rozga et al., 2014; Wambach et al., 2011). Women who receive support from trained peer counselors are more likely to initiate breastfeeding and to breastfeed longer than those who do not. Peer counselors know current information; establish supportive personal relationships with low-income women, many of whom are enrolled in the WIC program; refer women to breastfeeding specialists for problems; show enthusiasm; and facilitate breastfeeding (Raisler, 2000). Studies addressing the effectiveness of peer counseling are listed in Table 23-4.

The message that "Breast Is Best" has reached most low-income mothers. Regardless of how they choose to feed their baby, low-income women

acknowledge the health benefits from breastfeeding. The choice not to breastfeed can be accompanied by a nagging feeling of guilt (Guttman & Zimmerman, 2000). Younger low-income women may believe that their community views breastfeeding as the optimal feeding method, however, they report that friends and peers perceive it as "nasty." In addition, some low-income mothers associate breastfeeding with socioeconomic privilege. When poor women do breastfeed, the empowerment these women gain from the breastfeeding experience is an overlooked secondary effect that has potentially long-term impacts on other aspects of these women's lives (Locklin, 1995). These programs should be supported and expanded.

The Downside of Family Experience

Not all families meander into the sunset "happily ever after." When a marriage dies, the death of that relationship affects not only the spouses but also any children they may have, as well as other relatives and friends. When the mother is breastfeeding, issues surrounding custody may be colored by the fact that she feels (rightly or wrongly) that the court should take her feeding method into consideration in deciding on custody arrangements and contacts of her children with her soon-to-be former husband.

The role of the lactation consultant in such a situation must necessarily be limited to advocacy for breastfeeding. Unless the lactation consultant is an attorney, points of law are not her concern. Instead, she can perform a valuable service by educating the judge and the mother's (and perhaps the father's) attorney about the importance of breastfeeding for the child's continued physical and psychological health (Suhler et al., 1991). Questions may surface pertaining to how the father's attachment to the child is enhanced when breastfeeding is protected. Questions relating to the frequency of breastfeeding may not arise. In most cases, if the child is older than a few months, short periods of time with the father (away from the mother) are unlikely to place the breastfeeding relationship at risk. In addition, maintaining the child's attachment with both

Table 23-4 STUDIES OF PEER COUNSELORS

Arlotti et al. (1998) (*n* = 36)	Women in Florida WIC program contacted by telephone, by letter, or in person 5 times postpartum. Significant difference between groups in breastfeeding exclusivity but not in overall duration.
Anderson et al. (2005) (*n* = 162)	Randomized, controlled trial in low-income, mainly Hispanic, pregnant women in Hartford, Connecticut. Exclusive breastfeeding peer-counseling support was offered through 3 prenatal home visits, daily perinatal visits, 9 postpartum home visits, and telephone counseling as needed. The likelihood of nonexclusive breastfeeding throughout the first 3 months was significantly higher for the control group than the peer-counseling group. The likelihood of having one or more diarrheal episode in infants was cut in half in the peer-counseling group.
Campbell et al. (2014) (*n* = 3070)	Retrospective cross-sectional study of data from 2009 Texas Department of State Health Services (DSHS) WIC Infant Feeding Practices Survey (IFPS) in 73 WIC agencies. Women who had peer-counselor contact during pregnancy, in the hospital, and after delivery were more likely to initiate breastfeeding than women without such contacts, (OR = 1.36, 2.06, and 1.85, respectively).
Caulfield et al. (1998) (*n* = 548)	Low-income pregnant women in Baltimore WIC program. Prenatal and postnatal weekly contact. Peer support associated with breastfeeding initiation but not duration at 7 to 10 days postpartum.
Dennis et al. (2002) (*n* = 256)	Randomized trial of primiparous postpartum women near Toronto. Telephone contact occurred within 48 hours post discharge and as needed. Significant statistical difference between groups in breastfeeding duration and exclusivity at 12 weeks.
Gross et al. (1998) (*n* = 115)	African American WIC recipients in four Baltimore, Maryland, clinics. Two-by-two factorial design. Interventions: video and/or peer counseling versus control group. Higher proportion of breastfeeding in intervention groups versus control.
Grummer-Strawn et al. (1997)	1989–1993 Pediatric Nutrition Surveillance System data were analyzed to compare breastfeeding rates in Mississippi WIC clinics with and without peer-counseling programs. The peer-counseling program significantly increased the incidence of breastfeeding, particularly in clinics with lactation specialists and consultants.
Haider et al. (2000) (*n* = 720)	Prenatal and postnatal home visits for pregnant women in Bangladesh. Significant differences between initiation and duration of exclusive breastfeeding (70% versus 6%).
Kistin et al. (1990) (*n* = 102)	Low-income U.S. women who received support from peer counselors had significantly greater breastfeeding initiation, exclusivity, and duration than those who did not.
Long et al. (1995) (*n* = 141)	Pregnant Native American women in Utah WIC program. Prenatal and postpartum contact by home and clinic visits and by telephone. Significantly higher breastfeeding initiation (84% versus 70%) in the intervention group but not at the 12-week duration point (49% versus 36%).
Martens (2002) (*n* = 283)	Non-WIC Canadian Sankeeng First Nation community. Prenatal community health nurse and postpartum peer-counseling approach at breastfeeding education and support. Designated points of contact by the peer counselor were once a week for the first month, and once every 2 weeks for months 2 and 3 (at weeks 1, 2, 3, 4, 6, 8, 10, and 12 postpartum). Clients who received peer counseling were half as likely to wean, with 61% still breastfeeding at 2 months (versus 48% of nonclients) and 56% at 6 months (versus 19%). Clients who received peer counseling had fewer problems and greater satisfaction with breastfeeding.

Table 23-4 STUDIES OF PEER COUNSELORS (CONTINUED)

Mongeon & Allard (1995) (*n* = 194)	Prenatal and postnatal telephone contact with 194 pregnant women in Montreal. No significant difference between control and intervention groups in breastfeeding duration.
Morrow et al. (1999) (*n* = 130)	Low-income women in Mexico City. Prenatal and postnatal home visits. One control and two intervention groups (Group 1: 6 home visits; Group 2: 3 home visits). Significant difference between groups in breastfeeding exclusivity (6 visits = 67%; 3 visits = 50%; control = 12%) and duration at 12 weeks.
Pugh et al. (2002) (*n* = 41)	Community health nurse and peer counselor support starting during postpartum hospitalization. Randomized trial. The intervention group received visits from the team including daily hospital visits; visits at home during weeks 1, 2, and 4; and peer-counselor telephone support twice weekly through week 8 and weekly through month 6. Breastfeeding duration was longer among the experimental group.
Rozga et al. (2014) (*n* = 5886)	Secondary data analysis of the Michigan Breastfeeding Initiative Peer Counseling Program. For each additional home, phone and other peer-counseling contact, there was a significant reduction in the hazard of discontinuing any breastfeeding by 6 months (hazard ratio [HR] = 0.90, 95% CI, 0.88–0.92; HR = 0.89; 95% CI = 0.86–0.90; HR = 0.93, 95% CI = 0.90–0.96, respectively) and exclusive breastfeeding by 3 months (HR = 0.92, 95% CI = 0.89–0.95; HR = 0.90, 95% CI = 0.88–0.91; HR = 0.93, 95% CI = 0.89–0.97, respectively).
Schafer et al. (1998) (*n* = 134)	Prenatal and postnatal face-to-face and telephone contact for rural, low-income women in Iowa. Significant differences between intervention and control groups in breastfeeding initiation (82% versus 32%) and duration.
Shaw & Kaczorowski (1999) (*n* = 192)	Prenatal clinic visit and postnatal phone contact for low-income women in Tennessee WIC program. Significantly higher breastfeeding initiation and duration for the intervention group.
Wambach et al. (2011) (*n* = 289)	Randomized clinical trial in Midwestern United States. Three-group longitudinal design focusing on urban disadvantaged teenagers (15–18 years old). Experimental interventions: Two prenatal breastfeeding education classes facilitated by lactation consultant (LC) and peer counselors (PC); PC prenatal telephone support; inpatient/postbirth PC and LC support; and postpartum telephone support by PC and LC through 4 weeks. Significantly longer duration of breastfeeding in experimental group (*p* < 0.001).

parents requires that child and parent are together as often (as much as possible) as they would have been if the marriage and joint parenting experience had remained intact. Prior to her death, Elizabeth Baldwin, a family lawyer, assisted many lactation consultants and their clients in custody and breastfeeding cases (Neely, 2003). The La Leche League International (LLLI) website offers resources regarding breastfeeding in child custody situations such as divorce, many from the late Elizabeth Baldwin. Also on the LLLI website is information on state legislation that has been enacted in Hawaii,

Maine, Michigan, and Utah regarding custody and breastfeeding.

When the mother is seeking to maintain breastfeeding beyond the time when most people in her society—including the judge and the attorneys—are likely to find it acceptable, the lactation consultant can provide information that again focuses on the health-preserving aspects of breastfeeding (Wilson-Clay, 1990). Such longer-term breastfeeding does not necessarily limit reasonable visitation periods with the noncustodial parent, nor does it prevent periods of separation of the child from the mother. It does place the issue squarely where the focus must remain: preserving the best interests of the child.

Violence

The lactation consultant may become involved if a woman wishes to breastfeed or is breastfeeding and living in a situation in which she or her children are being threatened or assaulted. Whenever the lactation consultant believes that such violence is occurring, she has a legal responsibility to report this suspicion to relevant authorities who are in a position to intervene and to provide a safe haven for the mother and her children if the mother chooses to use it. Assisting with breastfeeding in abusive households need not be any different from assisting any other woman, although sensitivity to the abuse situation is necessary.

The number of breastfeeding women who are in homes in which they are being abused is not known. However, in the United States and the world, estimates of violence against women and girls are high. The National Intimate Partner and Sexual Violence Survey (NISVS) is an ongoing, nationally representative, random-digit-dial telephone survey that collects information about experiences of intimate-partner violence (IPV), sexual violence, and stalking from non-institutionalized English- and/or Spanish-speaking women and men aged 18 or older in the United States (Breiding et al., 2014). Data from this survey collected in 2010 suggested that 1 in 10 women had experienced IPV in the form of rape; an estimated 16.9% had experienced other non-rape sexual violence. The lifetime prevalence of severe physical violence by an intimate partner was estimated at 24.3%, and approximately 2.7% of women had experienced severe physical violence in the year preceding the survey.

What is the impact of violence on women's choice to breastfeed? Research evidence on this question from the United States has been inconsistent over time. Acheson (1995) reported that lack of breastfeeding was associated with physical and sexual abuse of the woman or her children, or both. In her retrospective review of 800 pregnancies and births in one family practice, Acheson also noted that postpartum depression occurred more frequently in the absence of breastfeeding, as did marital problems and domestic violence. This author suggested that the striking 38-fold decrease in frequency of violence against women or their children (or both) when breastfeeding is practiced warrants careful scrutiny.

Bullock et al. (2001) examined whether there were differences between women who had experienced IPV versus those who had not experienced IPV (measured with the Abuse Assessment Screen [AAS]) based on data obtained through collection of breastfeeding vouchers as opposed to formula vouchers from the WIC Nutritional Supplemental Program (n = 221). There was no significant difference in breastfeeding initiation or duration between abused and nonabused women.

Using a large sample of 118,579 women, Silverman et al. (2006) investigated the relationship between IPV prior to pregnancy only, during pregnancy, or during both periods with breastfeeding. The researchers found that 5.8% of participants were abused by a partner before pregnancy, during pregnancy, or both. Breastfeeding was initiated by 71% of the sample, and 18.3% ceased breastfeeding before 4 weeks postpartum. Adjusting for socioeconomic characteristics and smoking status, there was no significant association between IPV and breastfeeding initiation or cessation.

In contrast to U.S. research evidence, researchers in other countries have found IPV to negatively impact breastfeeding choice or duration. In Brazil, Moraes et al. (2011) randomly sampled 800 women with children younger than 5 months of age from five public clinics. They found exclusive breastfeeding cessation was 31% more likely in women who had experienced severe physical violence during pregnancy after controlling for socio-economic, demographic, reproductive, and lifestyle variables. In China, Lau and Chan (2007) found that those women who did not experience IPV during pregnancy were significantly more likely to initiate breastfeeding (adjusted OR, 1.84; 95%

CI, 1.16–2.91) after adjusting for demographic, socioeconomic, and obstetric variables.

Childhood Sexual Abuse

A history of abuse during childhood, including sexual abuse, is likely to result in a variety of reactions to the breastfeeding experience. For example, if a mother wishes to breastfeed but cannot bring herself to allow the baby to latch onto the breast, and if issues such as breast tenderness are not immediately evident, the consultant should consider the possibility that the breast area may have been involved in sexual abuse that the mother may have suffered years earlier.

An international review of 38 articles (involving 39 prevalence studies) of childhood sexual abuse (CSA) demonstrated that CSA is a continuing problem throughout the world (Pereda et al., 2009). According to the review, in the 6 U.S. studies including only women (sample size range, 65–654; mean = 332), prevalence rates ranged from 18 to 50.8 per 100 (mean = 32.1/100 or 32%). Given such a high incidence of abuse, beliefs surrounding the breasts' function and emotions pertaining to these beliefs are very likely to include fears that stem from experiences outside the realm of most lactation consultants' field of expertise.

Sexual abuse can have both short-term and long-term effects on the victim. Those effects may be expressed in various ways, including symptoms of posttraumatic stress disorder, cognitive distortions, emotional distress, impaired sense of self, interpersonal difficulties, health problems, and numerous kinds of avoidance behavior (including amnesia for the abuse-related events, dissociation, and self-destructive behaviors such as drug abuse) (Kendall-Tackett, 1998, 2007; Leeners et al., 2006). Sometimes pregnancy (Grant, 1992), childbirth (Courtois & Riley, 1992; Grant, 1992; Kitzinger, 1992; Rose, 1992), or breastfeeding (Kendall-Tackett, 1998; Klingelhafer, 2007) may trigger recall of memories that had previously been suppressed. One woman first regained memories of her abuse when she tried to breastfeed her infant. Because she was so unprepared for the sensations and the accompanying memories, she was unable to tolerate putting the baby to breast (Heritage, 1998). Coping mechanisms will vary from one woman to the next and may or may not be manifested during pregnancy, childbirth, or breastfeeding (Kendall-Tackett, 1998).

When she has established rapport with the lactation consultant and feels safe, the mother may disclose that she has been a victim of childhood abuse. In many cases, however, she may be unaware of the reason for her extreme discomfort, owing to brain changes that occur as a result of abuse and the coping mechanisms, including amnesia relating to the abusive events, that she may have practiced for years to maintain a facade of normalcy (Mukerjee, 1995). Additionally, if the mother recalls the abuse, she may or may not view it as being connected in any way with her current situation, including difficulties she may be having with breastfeeding.

Bowman (2007) conducted a review of the literature on the mental health impact of CSA on breastfeeding decision making in adolescent mothers and concluded that healthcare providers need to be aware that a history of CSA may affect the decision to breastfeed in the teenage mother. She pointed out that CSA victims are more likely than non-CSA victims to become sexually active earlier and more likely to become pregnant as a teenager. These mothers are more likely to have issues with establishing an intimate relationship with their infants, and breastfeeding may be considered an intimate parenting behavior. Therefore the provider needs to be sensitive to the possibility of CSA in the pregnant teenager, but should not assume that all teenage mothers have been victims of CSA as demonstrated in some research (Romano et al., 2006). In fact, Bowman and colleagues (2009) went on to explore CSA further in Mexican American mothers (*n* = 78) between 15 and 19 years of age in the southwestern United States. Approximately one-third of this sample (*n* = 24; 30.77%) reported CSA histories. The researchers found no correlation between CSA history and intimate parenting anxiety, there was no difference between breastfeeding and formula-feeding mothers in CSA severity, and

---

BOX 23-1 INTERVENTIONS FOR HELPING SEXUAL ABUSE SURVIVORS

- Be gentle and respectful when asking questions about sexual abuse. Whether the LC should ask directly depends on the rapport established with the mother.
- Teach the normal course of lactation, including the normalcy of pleasurable aspects of breastfeeding. Offer suggestions to make breastfeeding more comfortable.
- Suggest that the mother express her milk if she is unable or unwilling to feed at breast. This may be the most comfortable way for the mother to provide her milk to her baby while protecting herself from what she perceives emotionally (consciously or unconsciously) as an assault on her person.
- Make a referral to a mental healthcare provider. Be cautious about becoming the main source of emotional support.

Source: Adapted from Kendall-Tacket, 1998.

---

intimate parenting anxiety did not predict dissociation. The researchers postulated that supportive resources may have played a role in adolescent mothers' responses to CSA.

Survivors of past sexual abuse may have symptoms of posttraumatic stress disorder. These survivors frequently reexperience the traumatic event through nightmares or intrusive thoughts, such as sudden flashbacks of the abuse experience. If breastfeeding triggers sudden recall, nurturing her baby in this manner may be frightening to the mother. Box 23-1 offers suggestions on how to deal with a new mother who may have been sexually abused.

One mother had no recall of being abused until she put her baby to her breast for the first time. This action triggered a flashback so frightening to her that she screamed and immediately dropped the baby onto her bed. By the time hospital staff reached her, she was weeping and begged them to take the baby to the nursery. She subsequently cried uncontrollably each time she attempted to put her baby to her breast. The staff began helping her by giving her permission to pump her breasts to give her baby her milk. This action was something she could completely control. Being able to determine the degree of suction the pump exerted was important to her. After a week of pumping, during which time she gradually increased the pump pressure, she was willing to "try the baby again." She gradually was able to tolerate feedings without fearing that she would harm her baby.

Despite incidents such as these, the evidence is actually contrary to what may be expected. At least one research group (Prentice et al., 2002) found that mothers who self-identify sexual abuse as a child are more likely—not less likely—to initiate breastfeeding than women who report no such abuse. In fact, in their study of 1220 biological mothers of children younger than 3 years of age, 7% of the participants reported experiencing CSA; those mothers were more than twice as likely to initiate breastfeeding compared to their counterparts who had not experienced CSA. Could it be possible that women who were sexually abused as children are more concerned about parenting? If this is true, then these women may be more likely to breastfeed because it is a healthier way to feed a baby. Coles (2009), in her descriptive study of 11 successful Australian breastfeeding women who had experienced childhood sexual assaults, discovered four theses that reflected the challenges, requirements, and rewards of breastfeeding: (1) enhancement of the mother–baby relationship, (2) validation of the maternal body, (3) splitting of the breasts' dual role as maternal and sexual objects, and (4) exposure and control when breastfeeding in public. Women had to overcome intrusive and negative feedings and memories to establish and maintain the breastfeeding relationship with their infants.

One qualitative, participatory study that used in-depth interviews to explore the experiences of 6 Canadian mothers who had experienced CSA offers more information for lactation consultants and healthcare providers to consider as they work with this special group of mothers (Wood & Van Esterik, 2010). The women in this study all believed that breastfeeding was the best infant feeding choice for them and went on to breastfeed, albeit with problems. The themes that emerged from the women's accounts included shame, touch, breasts, dissociation, medical care, and healing;

- Shame was felt by each woman and, in turn, impacted her breastfeeding experience.
- Three kinds of touch were identified as difficult for the women: self-touch due to negative body image, infant touch (too much), and medical touch (too much and without warning or permission).
- Breasts were seen as the cause of abuse by some and in one case as positive due to an increase in breast size and a wonderful milk supply.
- Dissociation was one way that these women coped with CSA and for some with breastfeeding. Separating themselves from the physical sensations of breastfeeding actually allowed breastfeeding but not the emotionality of the process.
- Women experienced medical care in various ways—including some that was seen as unsupportive, inconsistent, or incorrect in the information given; because of their issues with authority, the women were unable to challenge providers.
- Two women felt they were able to transform and heal from the effects of CSA through their birth and breastfeeding experience.

Thus, although each woman's experience of breastfeeding was unique, some similarities were seen among the women and reflect what has been reported in previous studies.

Although these studies provide some evidence related to the CSA victim's breastfeeding experience, Kendall-Tackett (2007) cautioned that more research is needed to accurately describe the breastfeeding experiences and outcomes of women with a history of physical or sexual abuse. Cortisol levels are known to be higher or lower in abuse victims.

Does the response to current stressors, such as those following birth, impact lactogenesis? Do perceptions of insufficient milk supply hamper breastfeeding success? Prentice et al. (2002) found that at 1 month after birth, more mothers without CSA histories (82%; $n = 517$) were breastfeeding than mothers with CSA histories (73%; $n = 41$), but the difference was not statistically significant. Clearly, more research is needed in this area.

Acceptance of each woman's decision to breastfeed—however that is defined at a given time—may enable her to move closer to a full breastfeeding relationship with her baby and to further cement a healthy ongoing relationship with all of her children, something she may not have enjoyed in her family of origin.

Summary

Different family forms reflect different members' needs. Family developmental theories enable the healthcare worker to identify specific family functions throughout the life cycle. The goal of the healthcare provider should be to help the family to meet its own needs without her or his assistance. Key issues related to family functioning are the family's place within the support system and larger community. The early parenting period is characterized by patterns of attachment behavior and ways that these reflect the growing competence of the parents as parents. In some cases, the father may be the mother's single and most constant supporter; in other situations, he may be less involved in the family and unlikely to support breastfeeding.

Key Concepts

- Examining how different family forms and relationships are likely to be experienced throughout a lifetime can provide insight into the stresses that a family with a new baby is likely to encounter.
- How families interact with healthcare workers in a hospital or clinic setting often is related to the family structure, stage, and tasks related to childbearing.

- A mother's intention to breastfeed is the single most important factor in deciding whether she will start breastfeeding and how long she will continue to breastfeed. In turn, her intention in regard to breastfeeding is influenced by her attitude and her confidence in herself and the social support she receives. The more support she has for breastfeeding, the more likely she is to continue.
- The racial or ethnic group with which the mother identifies has a major influence on her infant-feeding choices.
- Fathers are often the most influential support persons in the early breastfeeding period.
- When fathers are involved with taking care of their new baby, they are more likely to have positive feelings that they are an important part of the baby's life.
- Experienced fathers can help one another realize that they are not alone in having ambivalent feelings about the closeness between their breastfeeding wives and babies and about giving up pleasures in exchange for new responsibilities.
- Role modeling and peer influence are powerful tools in teaching breastfeeding to pregnant adolescents, especially when these young mothers' concerns about keeping their figure and embarrassment are addressed.
- Adoptive mothers require support of family and healthcare providers to make the decision to induce lactation and carry out this challenging process.
- Imparting information about the benefits and importance of breastfeeding through classes and other educational means increases the likelihood that women with a low income will choose to breastfeed.
- Peer counselors have a powerful effect on promoting and maintaining breastfeeding through one-on-one contact and support.
- Several studies have demonstrated the positive impact of changes in hospital practices on breastfeeding initiation and duration because of the influence of the Baby-Friendly Hospital Initiative.

- The number of hospitals designated as Baby-Friendly in the United States has grown over the last 5 years. One major obstacle U.S. hospitals encounter when seeking to comply with the Baby-Friendly 10 steps is paying for formula used in the hospital, rather than receiving it free from formula companies.
- Women who experience physical and/or sexual abuse may experience difficulty in breastfeeding initiation and continuation. Lactation specialists and healthcare providers should treat each abuse survivor as an individual but recognize that the previous trauma can impact women physically and emotionally and deserves special care.

INTERNET RESOURCES

Academy of Pediatrics, information on breastfeeding: http://www.AAP.org/family/brstguid.htm

Adult Survivors of Child Abuse: http://www.ascasupport.org

Baby-Friendly USA: https://www.babyfriendlyusa.org/

Induced Lactation Protocol, Newman-Goldfarb Protocols: http://www.asklenore.info/breastfeeding/induced_lactation/gn_protocols.shtml

La Leche League stories by fathers: http://www.llli.org/nb/nbfathers.html

Legal issues such as employment and breastfeeding, and breastfeeding in child custody cases: http://www.llli.org/law/familylaw.html

Rape, Abuse, and Incest National Network: https://www.rainn.org/

OTHER RESOURCES

Breastfeeding father. La Leche League International. Pamphlet provides an introduction to breastfeeding for fathers, and explains why a father's support is critical to a successful breastfeeding experience. Set of 10 pamphlets. $9.95. Available at: http://store.llli.org/public/product/116.

National Domestic Violence Hotline: 1-800-799-SAFE

Sears W. *Becoming a father* (rev. ed.). La Leche League International; 2003.

REFERENCES

Acheson L. Family violence and breastfeeding. *Arch Fam Med.* 1995;4:650–652.

Anderson A, Damio G, Young S, et al. Randomized trial assessing the efficacy of peer counseling on exclusive breastfeeding in a predominantly Latina low-income community. *Arch Pediatr Adolesc Med.* 2005;159: 836–841.

Arlotti J, Cottrell BH, Lee SH, Curtin JJ. Breastfeeding among low-income women with and without peer support. *J Comm Health Nurs.* 1998;15:163–178.

Arthur CR, Saenz RB, Replogle WH. The employment-related breastfeeding decisions of physician mothers. *J Miss State Med Assoc.* 2003;44(12):383–387.

Auerbach KG, Avery JL. Induced lactation: a study of adoptive nursing by 240 women. *Am J Dis Child.* 1981; 135(4):340–343.

Augustin AL, Donovan K, Lozano EA, et al. Still nursing at 6 months: a survey of breastfeeding mothers. *MCN Am J Matern Child Nurs.* 2014;39(1):50–55. doi: 10.1097/01.NMC.0000437534.99514.dc.

Avery M, Duckett L, Dodgson J, et al. Factors associated with very early weaning among primiparas intending to breastfeed. *MCN Am J Matern Child Nurs.* 1998;2(3): 167–179.

Balcazar H, Trier CM, Cobas JA. What predicts breastfeeding intention in Mexican-American and non-Hispanic white women? Evidence from a national survey. *Birth.* 1995;22:74–80.

Bar-Yam NB, Darby L. Fathers and breastfeeding: a review of the literature. *J Hum Lact.* 1997;13:45–50.

Bentley ME, Caulfield LE, Gross SM, et al. Source of influence on intention to breastfeed among African-American women at entry to WIC. *J Hum Lact.* 1999;15: 27–33.

Bernaix LW. Nurses' attitudes, subjective norms, and behavioral intentions toward support of breastfeeding mothers. *J Hum Lact.* 2000;16:201–219.

Bica OC, Giugliani ER. Influence of counseling sessions on the prevalence of breastfeeding in the first year of life: a randomized clinical trial with adolescent mothers and grandmothers. *Birth.* 2014;41:39–45.

Biervliet FP, Maguiness SD, Hay DM, et al. Induction of lactation in the intended mother of a surrogate pregnancy: case report. *Hum Reprod.* 2001;16:581–583.

Blyth RJ, Creedy C, Dennis CL, et al. Breastfeeding duration in an Australian population: the influence of modifiable antenatal factors. *J Hum Lact.* 2004;20: 30–38.

Boettcher JP, Chezem JC, Roepke J, Whitaker TA. Interaction of factors related to lactation duration. *J Perinat Educ.* 1999;8:11–19.

Bowman KG. When breastfeeding may be a threat to adolescent mothers. *Iss Ment Health Nurs.* 2007;28: 89–99.

Bowman KG, Ryberg JW, Becker H. Examining the relationship between a childhood history of sexual abuse and later dissociation, breast-feeding practices, and parenting anxiety. *J Interpers Violence.* 2009;24(8):1304–1217. doi: 10.1177/0886260508322196.

Breiding MJ, Chen J, Black MC. *Intimate partner violence in the United States—2010.* Atlanta, GA: National Center for Injury Prevention and Control, Centers for Disease Control and Prevention; 2014.

Brent NB, Redd B, Dworetz A. Breastfeeding in a low-income population: program to increase incidence and duration. *Arch Pediatr Adolesc Med.* 1995;149:798–803.

Bronner Y, Barber R, Vogelhut J. Breastfeeding peer counseling: results from the National WIC Survey. *J Hum Lact.* 2001;17:135–139.

Brown A, Davies R. Fathers' experiences of supporting breastfeeding: challenges for breastfeeding promotion and education. *Matern Child Nutr.* April 10, 2014. E-pub ahead of print. doi: 10.1111/mcn.12129.

Buist A, Morse CA, Durkin S. Men's adjustment to fatherhood: Implications for obstetric health care. *JOGNN.* 2003;32:172–180.

Bullock LF1, Libbus MK, Sable MR. Battering and breastfeeding in a WIC population. *Can J Nurs Res.* 2001;32: 43–56.

Callen J, Pinelli J. Incidence and duration of breastfeeding for term infants in Canada, United States, Europe and Australia: a literature review. *Birth.* 2004;31:285–292.

Campbell LA, Wan J, Speck PM, Hartig MT. Women, Infant and Children (WIC) peer counselor contact with first time breastfeeding mothers. *Public Health Nurs.* 2014; 31(1):3–9. doi: 10.1111/phn.12055.

Caulfield LE, Gross SM, Bentley ME, et al. WIC-based interventions to promote breastfeeding among African-American women in Baltimore: effects on breastfeeding initiation and continuation. *J Hum Lact.* 1998;14: 15–22.

Centers for Disease Control and Prevention (CDC). Breastfeeding among U.S. children born 2000–2010. CDC National Immunization Survey. n.d. http://www.cdc.gov/breastfeeding/data/NIS_data/index.htm.

Chapman DJ, Perez-Escamilla R. Maternal perception of the onset of lactation is a valid, public health indicator of lactogenesis stage II. *J Nutr.* 2000;130:2972–2980.

Cheales-Siebenaler NJ. Induced lactation in an adoptive mother. *J Hum Lact.* 1999;15:42–43.

Chezem J, Friesen C, Boettcher J. Breastfeeding knowledge, breastfeeding confidence and infant feeding plans: effects on actual feeding practices. *JOGNN.* 2003;32: 40–47.

Child Welfare Information Gateway. *How many children were adopted in 2007 and 2008?* Washington, DC: U.S. Department of Health and Human Services, Children's Bureau; 2011.

Coles J. Qualitative study of breastfeeding after childhood sexual assault. *J Hum Lact.* 2009;25(3):317–324. doi: 10.1177/0890334409334926.

Corbett KS. Explaining infant feeding style of low-income black women. *Pediatr Nurs.* 2000;15:73–81.

Coreil J, Bryant CA, Westover BJ, Bailey D. Health professionals and breastfeeding counseling: client and provider views. *J Hum Lact.* 1995;11:265–271.

Courtois CA, Riley CC. Pregnancy and childbirth as triggers for abuse memories: implications for care. *Birth.* 1992; 19:222–223.

Cox MJ, Paley B, Burchinal MR, Payne CC. Marital perceptions and interactions across the transition to parenthood. *J Marriage Fam.* 1999;61:611–625.

Cricco-Lizza R. The milk of human kindness: environmental and human interactions in a WIC clinic that influence infant-feeding decisions of black women. *Qual Res.* 2005;15:525–538.

Dennis C. Breastfeeding initiation and duration: a 1999–2000 literature review. *JOGNN.* 2001;31:12–32.

Dennis CL, Faux S. Development and psychometric testing of the breastfeeding self-efficacy scale. *Res Nurs Health.* 1999;22:399–409.

Dennis CL, Hodnett E, Gallop R, Chalmers B. A randomized controlled trial evaluating the effect of peer support on breastfeeding duration among primiparous women. *Can Med Assoc J.* 2002;166:21–28.

Dodgson JE, Duckett L. Breastfeeding in the workplace: building a support program for nursing mothers. *AAOHN J.* 1997;45:290–298.

Dykes F, Moran VH, Burt S, Edwards J. Adolescent mothers and breastfeeding: experiences and support needs an exploratory study. *J Hum Lact.* 2003;19:391–401.

Earle S. Why some women do not breastfeed: bottle-feeding and father's role. *Midwifery.* 2000;16:323–330.

Fein S, Roe B. The effect of work status on initiation and duration of breastfeeding. *Am J Pub Health.* 1998;88:1042–1046.

Fonseca A, Nazaré B, Canavarro MC. Parental psychological distress and confidence after an infant's birth: the role of attachment representations in parents of infants with congenital anomalies and parents of healthy infants. *J Clin Psychol Med Settings.* 2013;20(2):143–155. doi: 10.1007/s10880-012-9329-9.

Forster DA, McLachlan HL, Lumley J. Factors associated with breastfeeding at six months postpartum in a group of Australian women. *Int Breastfeed J.* 2006;1:18.

Freed GL, Clark SJ, Harris BG, Lowdermilk DL. Methods and outcomes of breastfeeding instruction for nursing students. *J Hum Lact.* 1996;12:105–110.

Friedman M, Bowden VR, Jones E. *Family nursing: research, theory and practice,* 5th ed. Norwalk, CT: Appleton-Century-Crofts; 2003.

Gamble D, Morse J. Fathers of breast-fed infant: postponing and types of involvement. *JOGNN.* 1993;22:358–365.

Giugliani ER, Caiaffa WT, Vogelhut J, et al. Effect of breastfeeding support from different sources on mothers' decisions to breastfeed. *J Hum Lact.* 1994;10:157–161.

Glassman ME, McKearney K, Saslaw M, Sirota DR. Impact of breastfeeding self-efficacy and sociocultural factors on early breastfeeding in an urban, predominantly Dominican community. *Breastfeed Med.* 2014;9:301–307. doi: 10.1089/bfm.2014.0015.

Goodman JH. Becoming an involved father of an infant. *JOGNN.* 2005;34:190–200.

Gorman T, Byrd TL, VanDerslice J. Breastfeeding practices, attitudes, and beliefs among Hispanic women and men in a border community. *Fam Commun Health.* 1995;18: 17–27.

Grant LJ. Effects of childhood sexual abuse: issues for obstetric caregivers. *Birth.* 1992;19:220–221.

Grassley J. Adolescent mothers' breastfeeding social support needs. *JOGNN.* 2010;39:713–722. doi: 10.1111/j.1552-6909.2010.01181.x.

Grassley J, Eschiti V. Grandmother breastfeeding support: what do mothers need and want? *Birth.* 2008;35: 329–335.

Greenwood K, Littlejohn P. Breastfeeding intentions and outcomes of adolescent mothers in the Starting Out program. *Breastfeed Rev.* 2002;10(3):19–23.

Gross SM, Caulfield LE, Bentley ME, et al. Counseling and motivational videotapes increase duration of breastfeeding in African-American WIC participants who initiate breastfeeding. *J Am Diet Assoc.* 1998;98: 143–148.

Grossman LK, Fitzsimmons SM, Larsen-Alexander JB, et al. The infant feeding decision in low and upper income women. *Clin Pediatr.* 1990;29:30–37.

Grossman LK, Larsen-Alexander JB, Fitzsimmons SM, Cordero L. Breastfeeding among low-income, high-risk women. *Clin Pediatr.* 1989;28:38–42.

Grummer-Strawn LM, Rice SP, Dugas K, et al. An evaluation of breastfeeding promotion through peer counseling in Mississippi WIC clinics. *Matern Child Health J.* 1997; 1:35–42.

Guttman N, Zimmerman DR. Low income mothers' views on breastfeeding. *Soc Sci Med.* 2000;50:1457–1473.

Haider R, Ashworth A, Kabir I, Huttly SR. Effect of community-based peer counselors on exclusive breastfeeding practices in Dhaka, Bangladesh: a randomized controlled trial. *Lancet.* 2000;356:1643–1647.

Hannon PR, Willis SK, Bishop-Townsend V, et al. African-American and Latina adolescent mothers' infant feeding decisions and breastfeeding practices: a qualitative study. *J Adolesc Health.* 2000;26:399–407.

Hawke L, Falloon M, Parsons S. Adopted, embraced and nurtured. *Kai Tiaki Nurs N Z.* 2005;18–20.

Heritage C. Working with childhood sexual abuse survivors during pregnancy, labor, and birth. *JOGNN.* 1998;27: 671–677.

Hills-Bonczyk SG, Tromiczak KR, Avery MD, et al. Women's experiences with breastfeeding longer than 12 months. *Birth.* 1994;21:206–212.

House JS. *Work stress and social support.* Reading, MA: Addison-Wesley; 1981.

Hughes R. Development of an instrument to measure perceived emotional, instrumental, and informational support in breastfeeding mothers. *Iss Compr Pediatr Nurs.* 1984;7:357–362.

Janke JR. Development of the breastfeeding attrition prediction tool. *Nurs Res.* 1994;43:100–104.

Jordan PL, Wall VR. Fathers' experiences with breastfeeding: illuminating the dark side. *Birth.* 1990;17(4): 210–213.

Jordan PL, Wall VR. Supporting the father when an infant is breastfed. *J Hum Lact.* 1993;9:31–34.

Kaufman KJ, Hall LA. Influences of the social network on choice and duration of breastfeeding in mothers of preterm infants. *Res Nurs Health.* 1989;12:149–159.

Kelly YJ, Watt RG. Breast-feeding initiation and exclusive duration at 6 months by social class: results from the Millennium Cohort Study. *Public Health Nutr.* 2005; 8(4):417–421.

Kendall-Tackett K. Breastfeeding and the sexual abuse survivor. *J Hum Lact.* 1998;14:125–130.

Kendall-Tackett KA. Violence against women and the perinatal period: the impact of a lifetime of violence and abuse on pregnancy, birth, and breastfeeding. *Trauma Violence Abuse.* 2007;8:344–353.

Kendall-Tackett KA, Sugarman M. The social consequences of long term breastfeeding. *J Hum Lact.* 1995;11: 179–183.

Kessler LA, Gielen AC, Diener-West M, Paige DM. The effect of a woman's significant other on her breastfeeding decision. *J Hum Lact.* 1995;11:103–109.

Kim Y. The effects of a breastfeeding campaign on adolescent Korean women. *Pediatr Nurs.* 1998;24:235.

Kimbro RT. On-the-job moms: work and breastfeeding initiation and duration for a sample of low-income women. *Matern Child Health J.* 2006;10:19–26.

Kistin N, Benton D, Rao S, Sullivan M. Breast-feeding rates among black urban low-income women: effect of prenatal education. *Pediatrics.* 1990;86(5):741–746.

Kitzinger JV. Counteracting, not reenacting, the violation of women's bodies: the challenge for perinatal caregivers. *Birth.* 1992;19:219–220.

Klingelhafer SK. Sexual abuse and breastfeeding. *J Hum Lact.* 2007;23(2):194–197.

Kramer MS, Chalmers B, Hodnett ED, et al. Promotion of breastfeeding intervention trial (PROBIT): a randomized trial in the Republic of Belarus. *JAMA.* 2001;285: 413.

Lau Y, Chan KS. Influence of intimate partner violence during pregnancy and early postpartum depressive symptoms on breastfeeding among Chinese women in Hong Kong. *J Midwifery Women's Health.* 2007;52(2):e15–e20.

Lazzaro DE, Anderson J, Auld G. Medical professionals' attitudes toward breastfeeding. *J Hum Lact.* 1995;11: 97–101.

Leeners B, Richter-Appelt H, Imthurn B, Rath W. Influence of childhood sexual abuse on pregnancy, delivery, and the early postpartum period in adult women. *J Psychosom Res.* 2006;61(2):139–151.

Leffler D. United States high school age girls may be receptive to breastfeeding promotion. *J Hum Lact.* 2000;16:36–40.

Li CM, Li R, Ashley CG, et al. Associations of hospital staff training and policies with early breastfeeding practices. *J Hum Lact.* 2014;30(1):88–96. doi: 10.1177/ 0890334413484551.

Libbus MK, Kolostov LS. Perceptions of breastfeeding and infant feeding choice in a group of low-income mid-Missouri women. *J Hum Lact.* 1994;10:17–23.

Locklin MP. Telling the world: low income women and their breastfeeding experiences. *J Hum Lact.* 1995;11: 285–291.

Long DG, Funk-Archuleta MA, Geiger CJ, et al. Peer counselor program increases breastfeeding rates in Utah Native American WIC population. *J Hum Lact.* 1995; 11:279–284.

Losch M, Dungy CI, Russell D. Impact of attitudes on maternal decision regarding infant feeding. *J Pediatr.* 1995; 126:507–514.

Lu MC, Prentice J, Yu SM, et al. Childbirth education classes: sociodemographic disparities in attendance and the association of attendance with breastfeeding initiation. *Matern Child Health J.* 2003;7:87–93.

Mann L, Harmoni R, Power C. Adolescent decision-making: the development of competence. *J Adolesc.* 1989;12: 265–278.

Martens PJ. The effect of breastfeeding education on adolescent beliefs and attitudes: a randomized school intervention in the Canadian Ojibwa community of Sagkeeng. *J Hum Lact.* 2001;17:245–255.

Martens PJ. Increasing breastfeeding initiation and duration at a community level: an evaluation of Sagkeeng First Nation's community health nurse and peer counselor programs. *J Hum Lact.* 2002;18:236–246.

Maycock B, Binns CW, Dhaliwal S, et al. Education and support for fathers improves breastfeeding rates: a randomized controlled trial. *J Hum Lact.* 2013;29(4):484–490. doi: 10.1177/0890334413484387.

McKay A, Barrett M. Trends in teen pregnancy rates from 1996–2006: a comparison of Canada, Sweden, USA and England/Wales. *Can J Hum Sexuality.* 2010;19 (1–2):43–52. Available at: http://www.thefreelibrary. com/Trends+in+teen+pregnancy+rates+from+1996 -2006%3A+a+comparison+of...-a0229542649.

Merewood A, Philipp BL. Implementing change: becoming Baby-Friendly in an inner city hospital. *Birth.* 2001;28: 36–40.

Merewood A, Mehta SB, Chamberlain LB, et al. Breastfeeding rates in United States Baby-Friendly hospitals: results of a national survey. *Pediatrics.* 2005;116:628–634.

Merten S, Dratva J, Ackermann-Liebrich U. Do Baby-Friendly hospitals influence breastfeeding duration on a national level? *Pediatrics.* 2005;116(5):e702–e708.

Meyerink RO, Marquis GS. Breastfeeding initiation and duration among low-income women in Alabama: the importance of personal and familial experiences in making infant-feeding choices. *J Hum Lact.* 2002;18:38–45.

Mitchell-Box K, Braun KL. Fathers' thoughts on breastfeeding and implications for a theory-based intervention. *J Obstet Gynecol Neonatal Nurs.* 2012;41(6):E41–E50. doi: 10.1111/j.1552-6909.2012.01399.x.

Mitchell-Box KM, Braun KL. Impact of male-partner–focused interventions on breastfeeding initiation, exclusivity, and continuation. *J Hum Lact.* 2013;29(4):473–479. doi: 10.1177/0890334413491833.

Mongeon M, Allard R. Controlled study of a regular telephone support program given by volunteers on the establishment of breastfeeding [French]. *Can J Public Health.* 1995;86:124–127.

Moraes CL, de Oliveira AS, Reichenheim ME, Lobato G. Severe physical violence between intimate partners during pregnancy: a risk factor for early cessation of exclusive breast-feeding. *Public Health Nutr.* 2011;14(12): 2148–2155. doi: 10.1017/S1368980011000802.

Morrow A, Guerrero ML, Shults J, et al. Efficacy of home-based peer counseling to promote exclusive breastfeeding: a randomized controlled trial. *Lancet.* 1999;353: 1226–1231.

Morse JM, Harrison MJ. Social coercion for weaning. *J Nurs Midwifery.* 1987;32:205–210.

Mukerjee M. Hidden scars: sexual and other abuse may alter a brain region. *Sci Am.* 1995;273(5):14–15.

Murray E, Ricketts S, Dellaport J. Hospital practices that increase breastfeeding duration: results from a population-based study. *Birth.* 2007;34:202–211.

Neely AM. A tribute to Elizabeth Baldwin. *J Hum Lact.* 2003; 19:267.

Nelson A, Sethi S. The breastfeeding experiences of Canadian teenage mothers. *JOGNN.* 2005;34:615–624.

Newman J, Goldfarb L. Origins of the protocols. 2002. Available at: http://www.asklenore.info/breastfeeding/induced_lactation/intro.shtml.

Nolan L, Goel V. Sociodemographic factors related to breastfeeding in Ontario: results from the Ontario health survey. *Can J Public Health.* 1995;86:309–312.

Nommsen-Rivers LA, Chantry CJ, Cohen RJ, Dewey KG. Comfort with the idea of formula feeding helps explain ethnic disparity in breastfeeding intentions among expectant first-time mothers. *Breastfeed Med.* 2010;5(1): 25–33. doi: 10.1089/bfm.2009.0052.

Novotny R, Hla MM, Kieffer EC, et al. Breastfeeding duration in a multiethnic population in Hawaii. *Birth.* 2000;27:91–96.

Nunes LR, Giugliani ER, Santo ET, de Oliveira LD. Reduction of unnecessary intake of water and herbal teas on breast-fed infants: a randomized clinical trial with adolescent mothers and grandmothers. *Jrnl Adol Health.* 2011;49:258–264.

O'Campo P, Faden RR, Gielen AC, Wang MC. Prenatal factors associated with breastfeeding duration: recommendations for prenatal interventions. *Birth.* 1992;19: 195–201.

Page-Goertz S. Breastfeeding beyond 6 months: practical support and solutions. *Ad Healthcare for NPs and PAs.* 2002; 10(2):45. Available at: http://nurse-practitioners-and-physician-assistants.advanceweb.com/Article/Breastfeeding-Beyond-6-Months.aspx.

Pavill BC. Fathers and breastfeeding. *Lifelines.* 2002;6:324–331.

Pentecost R, Grassley JS. Adolescents' needs for nurses' support when initiating breastfeeding. *J Hum Lact.* 2014;30(2):224–228. doi: 10.1177/0890334413510358.

Pereda N, Guilera G, Forns M, Gómez-Benito J. The international epidemiology of child sexual abuse: a continuation of Finkelhor (1994). *Child Abuse Negl.* 2009;33(6): 331–42. doi: 10.1016/j.chiabu.2008.07.007.

Peterson CE, Da Vanzo J. Why are teenagers in the United States less likely to breastfeed than older women? *Demography.* 1992;29:431–450.

Pollock CA, Bustamante-Forest R, Giaratano G. Men of diverse cultures: knowledge and attitudes about breastfeeding. *JOGNN.* 2002;31:673–679.

Prentice JC, Lu M, Lange L, Halfon N. The association between reported childhood sexual abuse and breastfeeding initiation. *J Hum Lact.* 2002;18:219–226.

Preston JAM. *The experience and perceptions of African-American adolescent mothers regarding infant feeding* [abstract]. Dissertation; University of Virginia; 2004.

Pugh A, Milligan RA, Frick KD, et al. Breastfeeding duration, costs, and benefits of a support program for low-income breastfeeding women. *Birth.* 2002;29:95–100.

Raisler J. Against the odds: breastfeeding experiences of low income families. *J Midwifery Women's Health.* 2000;45: 253–263.

Rempel LA. Factors influencing the breastfeeding decisions of long-term breastfeeders. *J Hum Lact.* 2004;20: 306–318.

Rempel LA, Rempel JK. The breastfeeding team: the role of involved fathers in the breastfeeding family. *J Hum Lact.* 2011;27(2):115–121. doi: 10.1177/0890334410390045.

Rodgers R, White JH. Family development theory. In: Boss P, Doherty W, LaRossa R, et al., eds. *Sourcebook of family theories and methods: a contextual approach.* New York, NY: Plenum; 1993:225–254.

Roe B, Whittington LA, Fein SB, Teisl MF. Is there competition between breast-feeding and maternal employment? *Demography.* 1999;36:157–171.

Romano E, Zoccolillo M, Paquette D. Histories of child maltreatment and psychiatric disorder in pregnant adolescents. *J Am Acad Child Adolesc Psychiatry.* 2006;45(3):329–336.

Rose A. Effects of childhood sexual abuse on childbirth: one woman's story. *Birth*. 1992;19:214–218.

Rossiter JC, Yam BMC. The perceptions of Vietnamese women in Australia. *J Midwifery Women's Health*. 2000;45: 271–276.

Rovine M, Belsky J. Patterns of marital change across the transition to parenthood: pregnancy to three years postpartum. *J Marriage Fam*. 1990;52:9–15.

Rozga MR, Kerver JM, Olson BH. Impact of peer counseling breast-feeding support programme protocols on any and exclusive breast-feeding discontinuation in low-income women. *Public Health Nutr*. May 8, 2014:1–11.

Ryan AS, Wenjun A, Arensberg MB. The effect of employment status on breastfeeding in the United States. *Women's Health Issues*. 2006;16:243–251.

Schafer E, Vogel MK, Viegas S, Hausafus C. Volunteer peer counselors increase breastfeeding duration among rural low-income women. *J Hum Lact*. 1998;25:101–106.

Schneiderman JU. Postpartum nursing for Korean mothers. *Am J Mat Child Nurs*. 1996;21:155–158.

Shaw E, Kaczorowski J. The effect of a peer counseling program on breastfeeding initiation and longevity in a low-income rural population. *J Hum Lact*. 1999;15:19–25.

Sherriff N, Panton C, Hall V. A new model of father support to promote breastfeeding. *Community Pract*. 2014;87(5): 20–24.

Silverman JG, Decker MR, Reed E, Raj A. Intimate partner violence around the time of pregnancy: association with breastfeeding behavior. *J Women's Health (Larchmt)*. 2006;15(8):934–940.

Sipsma HL, Divney AA, Magriples U, et al. Breastfeeding intentions among pregnant adolescents and young adults and their partners. *Breastfeed Med*. 2013;8(4):374–380. doi: 10.1089/bfm.2012.0111.

St. John W, Cameron C, McVeigh C. Meeting the challenge of new fatherhood during the early weeks. *JOGNN*. 2005; 34:180–189.

Suhler AM, Bornmann PG, Scott JW. The lactation consultant as expert witness. *J Hum Lact*. 1991;7:129–140.

Szucs KA, Axline SE, Rosenman MB. Induced lactation and exclusive breast milk feeding of adopted premature twins. *J Hum Lact*. 2010;26(3):309–313. doi: 10.1177/0890334410371210.

Tarkka M, Paunonen M, Laippala P. Factors related to successful breast feeding by first-time mothers when the child is 3 months old. *J Adv Nurs*. 1999;29:113–118.

Turner-Maffei C. Using the Baby-Friendly Hospital Initiative to drive positive change. In: Cadwell K, ed. *Reclaiming breastfeeding in the United States*. Sudbury, MA: Jones and Bartlett; 2002:23–73.

Twenge JM, Campbell WK, Foster CA. Parenthood and marital satisfaction: a meta-analytic review. *J Marriage Fam*. 2003;65:574–583.

U.S. Department of Labor. *Employment characteristics of families*. Washington, DC: Author; 2013. Available at: http://www.bls.gov/news.release/famee.nr0.htm.

Visness C, Kennedy K. Maternal employment and breastfeeding. *Am J Public Health*. 1997;87:945–950.

Volpe EM, Bear M. Enhancing breastfeeding initiation in adolescent mothers through the Breastfeeding Educated and Supported Teen (BEST) Club. *J Hum Lact*. 2000; 16:196–200.

Wade D, Haining S, Day A. Breastfeeding peer support: are there additional benefits? *Community Practitioner*. 2009; 82(12):30–33.

Wambach KA. Breastfeeding intention and outcome: a test of the theory of planned behavior. *Res Nurs Health*. 1997; 20:51–59.

Wambach K, Aaronson L, Breedlove G, et al. A randomized controlled trial of breastfeeding support and education for adolescent mothers. *West J Nurs Res*. 2011;33: 486–505. PMID: 20876551.

Wambach KA, Cohen SM. Breastfeeding experiences of urban adolescent mothers. *J Pediatr Nurs*. 2009;24:244–254. doi:10.1016/j.pedn.2008.03.002.

Wambach KA, Cole C. Breastfeeding and adolescents. *JOGNN*. 2000;29:282–294.

Wambach KA, Koehn M. Experiences of infant-feeding decision making among urban economically disadvantaged pregnant adolescents. *J Adv Nurs*. 2004;48:361–370.

Ware JL, Webb L, Levy M. Barriers to breastfeeding in the African American population of Shelby County, Tennessee. *Breastfeed Med*. June 27, 2014. E-pub ahead of print.

White J. Weaning: what influences the timing? *Community Practitioner*. 2009;82(12):34–37.

Wiemann C, DuBois J, Berenson A. Strategies to promote breast-feeding among adolescent mothers. *Arch Pediatr Adolesc Med*. 1998;152:862–869.

Wilson-Clay B. Extended breastfeeding as a legal issue: an annotated bibliography. *J Hum Lact*. 1990;6:68–71.

Wood NK, Chesser AK, Wipperman J. Describing adolescent breastfeeding environments through focus groups in an urban community. *Jrnl Pri Care Comm Health*. 2013;4:307–310. doi:10.1177/2150131913487380.

Wood K, Van Esterik P. Infant feeding experiences of women who were sexually abused in childhood. *Can Fam Physician*. 2010;56(4):e136–e141.

Wright A, Rice S, Wells S. Changing hospital practices to increase the duration of breastfeeding. *Pediatrics*. 1996; 97:669–675.

Index

Note: Page numbers followed by *b*, *f*, and *t* indicate material in boxes, figures, and tables, respectively.

A

abdomen, assessment of newborn, 798
ABM. *See* Academy of Breastfeeding Medicine
ABM Protocol, general management recommendations, 259*b*
abrupt weaning, 908
abscesses, of breast, 328
Academy of Allergy, Asthma and Immunology (AAAA), 703
Academy of Breastfeeding Medicine (ABM), 398, 873
Academy of Breastfeeding Medicine's Protocol Committee, 597
accessibility, research participants', 828
accessory nipples, 85
accommodation, 679
Accreditation Council for Graduate Medical Education Core Competencies, 873
ACEIs. *See* angiotensin-converting enzyme inhibitors
acetaminophen, 237
acetylsalicylic acid, 184
acrocyanosis, 788, 789, 793
across-the-lap (feeding) position, 238, 239*f*
ACTH. *See* adrenocorticotropic hormone
acupuncture, for mastitis, 325
acute gastroenteritis (AGE), 729
acute illness, maternal, 588–603
   dysfunctional uterine bleeding, 578–581
   group B *streptococcus*, 491, 590
   tuberculosis, 592–593
acute lymphoblastic leukemia (ALL), 144
acute myeloblastic leukemia (AML), 144
acyclovir, 214
adaptation, cultural, 897
adenitis, of breasts, 326
"adequate" infant weight gain, 372
adolescents, as mothers, 924–927
adoptive mother and family, 926–927
adoptive nursing, 581–582, 929

feeding-tube devices and, 455
   galactagogues and, 582
   protocol, 583*b*
adrenocorticotropic hormone (ACTH), 606
adult conditions, response to donor milk, 541
adult education
   principles of, 884
   programs, 885
advanced beginner lactation consultants, 16
AEDs. *See* antiepileptic drugs
Affordable Care Act (ACA), 423, 477, 877
African-American women, breastfeeding perceptions of, 903, 920
AG. *See* areolar glands
AGE. *See* acute gastroenteritis
agricultural revolution, hand-fed foods and, 49–50
Aiding Mothers and Fathers Experiencing Neonatal Death (AMEND), 764
AIDS
   donor milk banking and, 527
   wet-nursing and transmission of, 906
alcohol drinking, low intake in breastfed infant and, 386
ALL. *See* acute lymphoblastic leukemia
allergies
   breastmilk and, 157
   breastmilk protection from, 144–145
   to cow's milk, 298
      gastroesophageal reflux and, 751
      low intake and, 379–380
   Internet resources, 766
alpha-lactalbumin-oleic acid, 541
Alternate Suck-Training Technique, 114
aluminum, in breastmilk, 136
alveolar cells, 86*f*
alveolar epithelial cells, 173*f*
alveoli, 80
AMA. *See* American Medical Association
Ameda One-Hand breast pump, 433*f*
   flanges, 441*t*

shields, 451*t*
AMEND. *See* Aiding Mothers and Fathers Experiencing Neonatal Death
amenorrhea, factors related to duration of, 560*b*
American Academy of Nursing Expert Panel on Breastfeeding, 874
American Academy of Pediatric Dentistry (AAPD), 697
American Academy of Pediatrics (AAP), 364, 371, 469, 641, 678, 705, 725, 734, 740, 763, 873
   on donor milk banking, 527
American Academy of Pediatrics' Committee on Nutrition, 700
American Academy of Pediatrics Policy Statement on Breastfeeding, 655
American Business Collaboration (ABC), 640
American Medical Association (AMA), 526
American Public Health Association (APHA), 641
American Society of Rheumatology, 609
amino acidemias, 753
AML. *See* acute myeloblastic leukemia
Ammehjelpen of Sweden, 68
amylase, 154
analgesics, 183–185, 184*t*, 233
Anderson behavioral state scale, 677*b*
Anderson, Gene Cranston, 101
androgens, low intake and, 385
anemia, 389
angiotensin-converting enzyme inhibitors (ACEIs), 188–189
angiotensin receptor blockers (ARBs), 189
animal milks, history of use, 50
ankyloglossia, 381–384, 382*f*, 383*t*, 797
   studies of, 382*t*
annualized relapse rate (ARR), 612
anti-infective properties of breastmilk, 137–146

anti-inflammatory components, breastmilk, 152–153
antibiotics, 185–188, 186*t*, 589, 601, 734
antibodies, in breastmilk, 149–150
antibody to HBsAg (anti-HBsAg), 218
antibody to hepatitis B core antigen (anti-HBcAg), 218
antidepressants, 192–193
antiepileptic drugs (AEDs), 616–617
antifungals, 185–188, 186*t*, 333, 334, 334*t*
antihypertensives, 188–189
antimanics, 193–194
antiplatelet and anticoagulant therapy, 189
antipsychotics, 194
antiretroviral therapy (ART), 208
anus, imperforate, 752–753
anxiety, 368
APHA. *See* American Public Health Association
apnea, feeding-induced, 105, 106*f*
appropriate for gestational age (AGA), classification of, 778
Apt test, 748
arachidonic acid (AA), in breastmilk, 130–132, 667
ARBs. *See* angiotensin receptor blockers
area under the curve (AUC) value, for medication, 177
areola, 80, 82–83
areolar compression, 255, 256
areolar glands (AG), 84–85
aripiprazole, 194
arm recoil (New Ballard Score), 779
arousal, levels of, 676
ARR. *See* annualized relapse rate
ART. *See* antiretroviral therapy
arthritis, maternal rheumatoid, 612–613
ASD. *See* autism spectrum disorder
aspirin, 183–184
assimilation, 679
association studies, 824
asthma
    breastmilk protection from, 146
    maternal, 594
atopic dermatitis, food allergies and, 759
atopic disease, breastmilk protection from, 144–145
attachment
    components of, 687*f*
    father-infant, 931
    milk transfer for preterm infants at breast in NICU, 501–504
Australian Breastfeeding Association, 641
autism spectrum disorder (ASD), 696
autocrine control, of lactation, 94
autoimmune diseases, maternal, 608–613
    multiple sclerosis, 611–612
    rheumatoid arthritis, 612–613
    systemic lupus erythematosus, 609–610

automatic electric breast pumps, 425*b*, 436, 437
autonomy, as ethical principle, 26
availability of donor milk, 532–533
Avent feeder, 723*f*
Avent Isis breast pump, 431
Avent squeeze-handle manual pump, 431, 433*f*
axillary enlargement, for breast augmentation, 341
axillary tail, of breast, 82, 83*f*
azithromycin, 187, 325
AZT, 209

B

B cells, 147, 148, 148*f*
babbling, language and communication development and, 681
baby carriers, 908
Baby-Friendly Hospital Initiative (BFHI), 45*b*, 67–68, 689, 825, 828, 863, 930
    for preterm infant, 475–476
baby watching, 236, 237*b*
baby's cheeks, 100
baby's tongue, dysfunctional, suck training with, 119
Bacillus Calmette-Guérin (BCG), 593
back, assessment of newborn, 799
"Back to Sleep" campaign, 278
bacteria, in breastmilk, 132, 137
bacterial infections, breast pain and, 335–336
Balancing Act, The (La Leche League International), 641
BALT. *See* bronchus-associated lymphoid tissue
"Band-Aid therapy," 454
BAPT. *See* Breastfeeding Attrition Prediction Tool
Barlow's maneuver, 799
basal metabolic index (BMI), 602
Basic Suck-Training Technique, 117–118, 118*f*
bathing babies, father's role in, 925
battery-operated breast pumps, 425*b*, 430, 434–435
BCG. *See* Bacillus Calmette-Guérin
Beckwith-Wiedeman syndrome, 796
bed sharing, safety issues for, 305–307, 306*f*, 308*t*
Bedouin Arab society, 906
behavioral state scale (Anderson), 677*b*
behavioristic psychology, 826
Bellagio consensus, 563–565, 563*b*
Belmont Report, 834
beneficence, as ethical principle, 26
BEST Club. *See* Breastfeeding Educated and Supported Teen Club
"BEST Program," 475

beta agonists, 594
beta-endorphins, 155
beta-glucuronidase, 407
BFHI. *See* Baby-Friendly Hospital Initiative
bicycle horn hand breast pumps, 433
bifidus factor, 151–152
bilirubin
    enterohepatic circulation of, 407, 413
    intestinal metabolism of, 407
    neonatal jaundice and, 406–407
bilirubin encephalopathy, 410–412, 416
bilirubin glucuronide, 407
bilirubin metabolism, 407
bioactive components, breastmilk, 153–156
bioavailability, of medications, 176–177
bioethics, principles of, 26–27
biophysiological measurements, for research, 836
biopsy, breast lump, 343
bipolar syndrome, treatment of, 193
birth
    hand-feeding from, 52
    injuries, 278
    libido-enhancing factors related to, 568–569
    social support after, 920
birthmarks, 794, 794*f*
bleeding, from breast, 345–346
blocked ducts, mastitis and, 323
blood donations, maternal, 619
bloody vomit or stool, 747–748
Blueprint for Action on Breastfeeding, U.S., 656
BMI. *See* basal metabolic index
body size, weaning and, 911
bonding and attachment theory, 818
borrowed breast pumps, 444
Boston Milk Bank, 527
bottle-feeding
    for ill children, 723, 725, 743, 745, 746
    nursing-bottle caries, 698
bottle nipples, as nipple shields, 451
bras, postpartum care and, 293
BRAT diet, 731
Brazil, donor milk banking in, 527–528, 532
breast(s). *See also* breast-related problems
    abscess, 328
    assessment of
        inspection, 95–96
        latch-on difficulty and, 244–245
        palpation, 96
    augmentation, 340–342, 340*f,* 341*f*
    baby's seal on, 277*f*
    breastmilk differences between, 126–128, 127*f*
    cancer, 346–350
        axillary breast enlargement and, 341
        lactation following, 348–349
        mastitis *vs.* inflammatory, 328
        screening for, 349–350

development, 79–83
edema, 255–256, 286, 286*t*
engorgement, 254–255, 285–286
   breast augmentation, 342
   breast pain and, 335–336
   mastitis, 323–324
   secondary, milk expression with pump
    and, 426
hypertrophy (gigantomastia), 336–337
infant (New Ballard Score), 780
insufficient glandular development, 387
large, feeding positions with, 244–245
leaking, postpartum, 293
lumps and surgery, 342–343
marked asymmetry in, 95
massage, 291, 395
   milk-ejection reflex and, 422
   techniques, 292*t*–293*t*
painful, 335–336
rashes and lesions, 328, 329*b*
reduction, 337–339, 338*f*
refusal, 245
structure, 80–83, 81*f*, 83*f*
   pregnancy and, 85–86
   variations in, 85
breast-nonfeeding jaundice, 406, 409
breast pads
   candidiasis and, 335
   postpartum care and, 293
breast pumps, 419–462
   breast shells, 449*f*, 454
   cleaning, 443
   clinical implications, 426–427
   comparison of, 430–437
    battery-operated, 434–435
    electric, 442, 443
    hand pumps, 433–434
    studies, 431
   compression, 430
   evolution, 430
   feeding-tube devices, 454–457
   flanges, 439, 441, 441*t*
   historical examples, 419
   hormonal considerations, 425–428
   Internet resources, 461–462
   manual, mastitis and, 324
   mothers' concerns, 421–424
   nipple shields, 447–454
   pedal models, 441
   problems, 444
    reporting, 444
   recommendations on use, 424*b*–425*b*
   sample guidelines, 444–446
   selection of, 477–478
   sequential, 423, 437
   simultaneous, 437
   stimulating milk-ejection reflex, 421–422
   third-party payment request, 478*f*
   used, FDA policy on, 445*b*

breast-related problems, 319–353
   abscess, 328
   bleeding from breast, 345–346
   breast lumps and surgery, 342–343
   breast pain, 335–336
   cancer, 346–350
   candidiasis (thrush), 330–335
    diagnosis, 331–332
    treatment for, 333–335, 334*t*
   clinical implications, 350
   Internet resources, 353
   mammoplasty, 336–342
   mastitis, 323–328
   milk blister, 336
   nipple variations, 319–321
   plugged ducts, 321–323, 322*b*
   rashes and lesions, 328, 329*b*
breast shells, 449*f*, 453, 454
breast shields, silicone, 85
breast surgery, 386–387
breastfed infants, low intake in, 359–401
   abnormal growth patterns with healthy
    appearance, 373–384
    ankyloglossia, 381–384, 382*f*, 382*t*
    cow milk allergy, 379–380
    gastroesophageal reflux, 379–380
    inadequate first month weight gain,
     373
    late-preterm infants, 373, 378
    nonspecific neurological problems,
     380–381
    oral-motor dysfunction, 376*t*, 378–379,
     380*f*
    oversupply, 379–380
   abnormal growth patterns with obvious
    illness, 384
   assorted schema for, 362*t*
   case study, 381*b*
   clinical management of, 390–394
   definitions and incidence of occurrence
    confusing terminology and nonstan-
     dard research, 371–373
    infant's presentation, 372
   growth variations in newborn and young
    infants, 372*t*
   history and physical for evaluation, 375*t*,
    389–390
   hormonal alterations, 385
   infant and maternal conditions for, 374*b*
   infant factors, 376*t*–377*t*
   Internet resources, 400–401
   intervention for, 391–394
    family and peer support, 394
    flowchart, 392*f*
    homemade and commercial feeding-
     tubes, 391*f*
    measures encouraging increased milk,
     393*b*
    supplementation reduction, 394

    when maternal milk does not increase,
     394
   management, 395–399
    breast massage, 395
    feeding-tube devices, 395, 396*b*
    galactagogues, 398–399
    hindmilk, 399
    switch nursing, 395
    test weighing, 395–396, 397*b*
   maternal factors, 377*t*–378*t*
   mother with healthy appearance, 384–389
    breast surgery, 386–387
    delayed lactogenesis, 384
    insufficient glandular development, 387
    inverted nipples, 385
    maternal nutrition, 388–389
    medications and substances, 386
    nipple shields, 385
    psychosocial factors, 388
    stress, 387–388
   mother with obvious illness, 389
   negative cycle of milk intake and weight
    gain, 361*f*
   positive cycle of milk intake and weight
    gain, 360*f*
   U.S. growth charts, 362, 364
    birth to 2 years (boys), 365*f*
    compared to WHO charts, 363*f*, 364*f*,
     366*t*
   WHO child growth charts, 362–367,
    363*f*–365*f*, 366*t*
    birth to 6 months (boys), 363*f*
    birth to 2 years (boys), 364*f*
    compared to CDC charts, 365*f*, 366*t*
breastfeeding, 41–70, 606, 610, 717
   admission history for, 727*b*–728*b*
   after breast biopsy, 343
   archeological evidence for, 47
   assessment of, 278*t*–279*t*, 651*t*
   attitudes related to, 883–884
   basic techniques guidelines, 258
   breast cancer risk and, 346–347
   characteristics of, 726*b*
   child with altered neuromuscular tone,
    736*b*–737*b*
   common situational factors unrelated to,
    565–566
   computer modeling of breast pumps and,
    429
   concepts to practice, 97
   cost of artificial, 59–62
   defining, 362
   demographic impact of, 556–557
   in developing regions, 58–59
   doulas and childbirth educators, 228
   drugs to avoid during, 179*t*
   evidence about, 41–47
   flow chart, 242*f*
   frequency, 107–108, 107*f*

breastfeeding (*contd.*)
goals and prevalence, U.S., 63*t*
HSV and, 213
infant reflexes and implications for, 807*t*
interruption after drug abuse, 196*t*
long-term, 706–707
maternal employment and, 635–660
    clinical implications, 658–660
    community strategies, 654–655
    effect on breastfeeding, 636–637
    historical perspective, 635–636
    Internet resources, 661–662
    national and international strategies, 655–658
    strategies, 638–642
and maternal health outcomes, 555*b*
mothering and, 227
mother's guide to, 756*b*
nipple pain after, 284–285
nursing caries, 698
oxytocin and, 672–673
as pain management technique, 725
perioperative care, 726–728
positioning/alignment, 785
positions used, 786
practices for, 48–49
during pregnancy, 304–305
preparation for, 227–228
preterm infants, in NICU, 469–476, 479, 482, 483, 485, 486*f*, 489, 498, 501, 503–506
    milk transfer during, 497–504
    non-nutritive suckling, 491–497, 492*f*
    physiology research on, 494*t*–495*t*
    progression of, 496–497
prevalence of, 57–59
promotion of, 62–68
questionnaires and assessment tools, 840*t*–841*t*
reverse-cycle, 649
social support for, 920
surveys, 42*b*–46*b*
Ten Steps to, 67*b*
in U.S., England, and Europe, 52, 57, 58
viral infections and. *See* viruses
women interested in, 68
Breastfeeding Abstracts, 4
Breastfeeding and Lactation, The Pediatrician's Pocket Guide to Coding, 31
breastfeeding and perceived fatigue, relationships between, 648–649
Breastfeeding Atlas, The (2005), 129
Breastfeeding Attrition Prediction Tool (BAPT), 820, 840*t*, 843
breastfeeding care, core competencies in, 868*b*–870*b*
breastfeeding clinic, 9*f*, 12*f*
Breastfeeding Committee for Canada, 833

Breastfeeding Educated and Supported Teen (BEST) Club, 924
breastfeeding families, continuing support for, 882
Breastfeeding Friendly Workplace program, 654
breastfeeding jaundice, 409
Breastfeeding Residency Curriculum, 873
Breastfeeding Resource Nurse (BRN) model, 475
Breastfeeding Self-Efficacy Scale (BSES), 819, 825, 841*t*, 843
breastmilk, 121–157
    anti-infective properties of, 137–146
        controversies and claims, 143
        gastroenteritis and diarrhea, 139–140
        respiratory illness, 140, 143
    breast storage capacity, 125, 127, 128
    caloric density of, 124
    cells, 147–149, 148*f*
    chronic disease protection and, 143–144
    color of, 129
    components and function of, 138*t*–139*t*
    composition of, 124, 129, 156
        bioactive components, 153–156
        during breast infection, 327, 327*t*
        during first month of lactation, 133*t*
    disease amelioration by, 141*t*–142*t*
    immune system and, 146–153
    implications for practice, 156–157
    infant growth and, 128–129
    intakes during established lactation, 125
    jaundice, 405, 408–409
    kilocalories ingested per kilogram by infant age, 124*t*
    lactoengineering own mother's, 488
    lactogenesis and sodium levels of, 86, 88
    letdown, 92–93
    low intake and oversupply of, 371–373
    lymphocytes, 147–148
    massage to increase volume and fat content of breastmilk, 395
    mastitis and ample supply of, 323
    measures encouraging increased production, 393*b*
    milk synthesis and maturational changes in, 122–123
    mother's guide to ending, 756*b*
    nutritional values of, 129–137
        fat, 130
        lactose, 132
        minerals, 135–137
        nonprotein nitrogen, 132–133
        nucleotides, 133
        preterm, 137
        protein, 132
        vitamins and micronutrients, 133–135
    phagocytes, 147
    physiological principles of, 126*b*

production of, 93–94, 287–291
    cluster pumping, 446
    concerns/worries, 287*t*–288*t*
    delayed lactogenesis, 288–289
    drugs that inhibit, 180–182, 180*b*
    drugs that stimulate, 182–183
    herbs for, 183, 582
    latch-on difficulties and, 243–244
    late-preterm infants, 246–247, 247*f*
    maternal employment and, 643
    oversupply/overproduction, 289–291
    pharmaceutical agents for, 290–291, 291*t*
    strategies to increase, 289*t*
    strategies to reduce, 291*t*
    prolactin in, 89–91, 89*f*
    retention of (stasis), 285
    types of, by day, 123*f*
    volume of, 123–125
        differences between breasts, 126–128, 127*f*
    when measures to increase fail, 394
breastmilk jaundice, 405, 408–409
breastmilk storage
    guidelines for preterm infants, 484*b*
    for maternal employment, 647–648
breathing, coordinated with suckling, 103–106
BRN model. *See* Breastfeeding Resource Nurse model
bromocriptine, 386
bronchiolitis, 733–734
bronchus-associated lymphoid tissue (BALT), 150
Brown-Séquard-plus syndrome (BSPS), 614
BSES. *See* Breastfeeding Self-Efficacy Scale
BSPS. *See* Brown-Séquard-plus syndrome
bubble palate, 99
budesonide, 195
Buppert, Carolyn, 31
bupropion (Wellbutrin, Zyban), 193
burping, father's role in, 923
Business Case for Breastfeeding, 17, 650, 652, 654

C

C-hold, 235, 235*f*
C-section. *See* cesarean section
cabbage compresses, breast engorgement and, 255
cabergoline, 386
Cadogan, William, 55
café-au-lait spots, 794
calcium-channel blockers, 189
calcium in breastmilk, 136
calibration stage, of lactation, 427
cancer, breast, 346–350
    axillary breast enlargement and, 341

lactation following, 348–349
mastitis *vs.* inflammatory, 328
screening for, 349–350
cancer, childhood, 144
candidiasis *(Candida albicans)*, 187–188,
330–335
diagnosis, 331–332
treatment for, 333–335, 334*t*
"canker sores," 212
caput succedaneum, 795
car seats, gastroesophageal reflux and, 751*b*
carbimazole, 195
cardiovascular disorder, 705
carrying infants, swaddling and, 907
CCK. *See* cholecystokinin
CDC. *See* Centers for Disease Control
*CDC Guide to Strategies to Support Breastfeeding
Mothers and Babies, The,* 649
celiac disease (CD), 758
Internet resources, 766
cells, in breastmilk, 147–149
cellulitis, of breasts, 326
Center for Devices and Radiological Health,
U.S. FDA, 444, 459
Centers for Disease Control (CDC)
breastfeeding surveys sponsored by,
42*b*–44*b*
U.S. growth charts, 362, 364
birth to 2 years (boys), 365*f*
compared to WHO charts, 363*f,* 364*f,*
366*t*
Vaccine Adverse Event Reporting System
(VAERS), 695
worksite lactation program tool kit,
650–653
central nervous system active drugs,
lipophilicity and, 176
cephalhematoma, 795
cereal, gastroesophageal reflux and, 751,
751*b*
cesarean births, 253–254
cesarean section (C-section), 368
CHARGE syndrome, 747
charting, 19
narrative example for, 19*b*
CHD. *See* congenital heart disease
cheeks, infant, 100
chemokines, 145, 152
chemotherapy, 347–348
chest, assessment of newborn, 797–798
Chiari II malformation, 739
chickenpox, 214–215
Child care decisions, maternal employment
and, 640–642
child health, 667–709
clinical implications, 691–692
dental health and orofacial development,
697–699
development theories, 678–691, 679*t*

Erikson's psychosocial theory, 678–679,
679*t*
nature *vs.* nurture, 678–679, 681
Piaget's cognitive theory, 679, 679*t,*
681
developmental outcomes and infant feeding, 667, 672
growth and development, 673–678
levels of arousal, 676–678
physical, 673, 674*f*
senses, 675–676
weight and length, 673–675
immunizations, 692–696
implications for practice, 707–708
Internet resources, 709
language and communication, 681–684
long-term breastfeeding, 706–707
obesity, 704–706
social development, 681, 682*f*
attachment and bonding, 684–689,
687*f*
separation anxiety, 691
stranger distress, 691
temperament, 689–690, 690*t*
solid foods, 699–704
delaying, 703–704
diet choices, 700–703
feeding location selection, 703
introducing, 699–700, 701*t*–702*t*
quick, easy to prepare, 703*b*
studies on breastfeeding and intelligence,
668*t*–672*t*
vitamin D and rickets, 696–697
weaning, 707
Child Health Assessment Interaction Model,
817
Child Nutrition and WIC Reauthorization
Act (1989), 64
Child Wellbeing study, 653
childbirth educators, breastfeeding, 228, 874
childhood sexual abuse, 935–937, 936*b*
Children's Hospital of Philadelphia (CHOP),
475
chimpanzees, breastfeeding practices by, 49
chlorpromazine, 194
choanal atresia, 747, 796
cholecystokinin (CCK), 155, 157
cholesterol, in breastmilk, 131
CHOP. *See* Children's Hospital of
Philadelphia
chromium, in breastmilk, 136
chronic diseases, breastmilk protection from,
143–144
chronic lung disease of prematurity (CLD),
733
chronic social stress, 573
Chronic Sorrow (Olshansky), 763
chronic stress, 673
Church of Latter-Day Saints (LDS), 346

chylothorax, 752
ciprofloxacin ophthalmic products, 187
Circadian rhythms, 677
citalopram, 192
CL/CP. *See* cleft lip and palate
CLD. *See* chronic lung disease of prematurity
cleaning breast pumps, 443
cleft lip and palate (CL/CP), 379, 742–745
case study, 745*b*–746*b*
Mead-Johnson feeder, 723, 724*f*
palatal obturator, 744
Pierre Robin sequence and, 745–747
clindamycin, 325
clinical care plans, 21, 22*b*
clinical issues, infant gastroenteritis, 731
clinical practice guidelines (CPG), 854
clopidogrel, 189
closet nursing, 911
clothing, postpartum, 293
clotrimazole, for candidiasis, 333, 334*t*
cluster pumping, 446
clutch (feeding) position, 238, 239*f,* 240*t,*
254
CMV. *See* cytomegalovirus
Cochrane Collaboration, 854
Cochrane review, 540
of LC effectiveness, 4
Code of Professional Conduct (CPC), IBLCE,
23–24
cognitive theory of development (Piaget),
679, 679*t,* 681
Cohen's kappa statistic, 842
cohort studies, sampling and sample size for,
839
coital frequency, studies of, 569
cold treatments, breast engorgement and,
255
colds, maternal, breastfeeding and, 600
colic, 297–299
Collaborative Group on Hormonal Factors in
Breast Cancer, 346
colonial empires, breastfeeding in developing
regions and, 58–59
color, breastmilk, 129
colostrum, 122, 228, 905
comfort breastfeeding, 707
community, economic costs of manufactured
infant milks to, 61–62
community strategies for breastfeeding and
work, 654–655
community support groups, breastfeeding
education by, 876–877
competent lactation consultants, 16
conceptual frameworks, 815
concurrent validity, for quantitative research,
843
confidentiality, by lactation consultant, 23
confirmability, of research, 838
congeners, 185

congenital abnormalities, heart disease, 740–741
congenital heart disease (CHD), 740–741
congenital hypothyroidism (CH), 757
congenital varicella syndrome, 214
conjugated bilirubin, 407
consecutive sampling, 835
construct validity, for quantitative research, 843
content validity, for quantitative research, 843
content validity index (CVI), 843
continuation, lactation, 94
continuing education, 888
    examples of behavioral objectives for, 886t
    programs, 886
contraception
    cultural differences in, 907
    women's health, 556
contractile cells, of breast, 80
contracting stage of families, theory on, 918
controls, in experimental studies, 825
convenience sampling, 835
cooing, language and communication development and, 681
Coombs' test, 413
cooper's ligaments, 82, 82f
coordination of breathing and suckling, 103–106
copper, in breastmilk, 136
correlation coefficients, 842, 849
correlational studies, 824
    appropriate statistics for, 844t–847t
    data analysis, 849–850
    sampling and sample size for, 839
corticosteroids, 194–195, 613
cortisol, 91, 155
costs of not breastfeeding, 59–62
    economic costs of manufactured infant milks, 60–62
    health risks of manufactured infant milks, 60
countries, economic costs of manufactured infant milks to, 61–62
couples, family theory on, 918
cow's milk, infant's allergies to, 298, 759–761
    gastroesophageal reflux and, 751
    low intake and, 379–380
CPC. See Code of Professional Conduct
CPG. See clinical practice guidelines
cracked/fissured nipples, 282
    mastitis and, 323
cradle-clutch position, 300f
cradle (feeding) position, 238, 239f, 240t
cranial nerves, 105, 105f
creams, nipple, 283
credibility, for research, 838
cremasteric reflex, 798
criterion-related validity, 843
critical research perspectives, 821–822

Crohn's disease, 595, 608
Cronbach's alpha, 842–843
cross-cradle position, 238, 239f, 240t
crying
    language and communication development, 681
    latching on, 236
    postpartum care, 297–299
cues, neurobehavioral, 805, 805t, 806f, 807t
cultural relativism, 899
culture, 897–913
    assessing practices of, 900
    breastfeeding perceptions, 901–908
        for African-American women, 903, 920
        colostrum, 905
        contraception, 907
        for immigrants, 901
        infant care, 907–908
        in public places, 904
        rituals and meaning, 904–905
        seclusion period, 906
        sexual relations, 905–906
        wet-nursing, 906
    definition of, 897
    dominant, 898–899
    ethnocentrism vs. relativism, 899
    Internet resources, 913
    language barriers, 900–901
    maternal foods, 908–910
        herbs and galactagogues, 909–910
        "hot" and "cold," 909
    practice implications, 911, 912b
    weaning and, 910–911
cup-feeding, 247–249, 248f, 391
    for ill children, 723
    as nipple shield alternative, 506
curriculum development in breastfeeding education, 885–887
CVI. See content validity index
cyanosis, 789, 793
cylinder hand breast pumps, 424b–425b, 434
CYP3A4 enzyme inhibitors, 398
cystic fibrosis
    infant, 758–759
    maternal, 601–602
cysts
    milk-filled lacteal, 342
    theca lutein, 603
cytokines, 152, 472
cytomegalovirus (CMV), 215–216, 490, 527

D

D-MER. See dysphoric milk-ejection reflex
dancer-hand position, 719–720, 721f, 736b
Darwin, Charles, 818
Darwinian theory, 818
data analysis, 836–837

appropriate statistics for study type and data level, 844t–847t
    levels of measurement for, 844t–847t
    for qualitative research, 837–838
    for quantitative research, 843–850
data collection methods, 836
    breastfeeding questionnaires and assessment tools, 840t–841t
    for qualitative research, 837
    for quantitative research, 840–842
day care decisions, maternal employment and, 640–642
death
    of child, 764–765
    lactation care after, 765
Declaration of Helsinki, 834
decline stage, of lactation, 427
dehydration, 727, 729
delayed lactogenesis, 288–289, 359, 384
delayed secretory activation, 359
deliberate weaning, 910
Demographic and Health Surveys (WHO/UNICEF), 46b
denial stage, of separation anxiety, 691
Dennis's scale, 819
dental caries, 699
dental fluorosis, 698
dental health, orofacial development and, 697–699
dependability, of research, 838
dependent variables, for research, 829
depression, postpartum (PPD), 603–608
    clinical care plan, 607t
    support for, 608
dermatitis
    atopic, breastmilk protection from, 145
    of breast, 328–330, 329b
descriptive studies, 824, 844t–847t, 849
despair stage, of separation anxiety, 691
desvenlafaxine, 193
detachment stage, of separation anxiety, 691
developing regions
    colonial empires and, 58–59
    current breastfeeding practices in, 58, 59
    infant feeding and infant mortality in, 59
DHA. See docosahexaenoic acid
diabetes, 595–598
    gestational, 595–596
    Internet resources, 766
    type I
        infant, 757–758
        maternal, 596–598
diagnostic mammogram, breast cancer, 347
diaper changing, father's role in, 925
diaper rash, candidiasis and, 331
diarrhea, breastmilk protections from, 139–140
diazepam, 191
dietitians, breastfeeding education by, 876

dilemmas, moral and ethical, 26

diphtheria, tetanus, pertussis (DTaP) vaccine, 692

direct-reacting bilirubin, 407

discharge from hospital
neonatal weight loss at, 258, 263*b*
planning for, 259–260
preterm infants, 504–506
post-discharge rebound, 763

discharge packs, of formula, 260–261

discipline committee, IBCLE, 27

discourse analysis, 823–824

disease-modifying therapies (DMTs), 611

disorganized sucking and suckling, 106, 106*f*, 107

divorce, breastfeeding, custody arrangements and, 933

DMTs. *See* disease-modifying therapies

docosahexaenoic acid (DHA) in breastmilk, 130–132, 667, 668*t*

documentation
of donor human milk, 524–525
of interventions, 19

documented hypoglycemia, management of, 262*b*

dominant culture, 898–899

"domino" effect, epidurals, 233

domperidone (Motilium), 182, 398
induced lactation and, 290, 582

donor milk banking, 523–545
availability, 532–533
bank in 2012, 524*f*
case studies, 541, 542*b*–544*b*
diagnoses for milk orders, 524*f*, 525*t*
for-profit *vs.* not-for-profit, 539
history of, 526–527
Internet resources, 545
medical indications, 524–525
nonmedical indications, 525–526
outside North America, 526
procedures for, 533–536
processing of milk, 534
recall procedures, 536
record keeping, 533
screening donors, 534, 535, 539
storage and handling of milk, 534
research on donor milk, 539–541
safety, 532, 533*t*
today, 527, 528, 532
use of, 523

dopamine agonists, 600

dopamine antagonists, 182

dose-to-the mother, 831

doubel cradle position, 300*f*

double clutch position, 300*f*

doulas educators, breastfeeding, 228

Down syndrome, 737–738
Internet resources, 766

Dr. Brown's double electric pump, 430, 431*f*, 439

drastic hormonal changes postpartum, 566

dropper-feeding, 456

drug abuse, 195–196, 196*t*

drug metabolites, 177

drug therapy, 171–198
alveolar subunit and, 172–173, 172*f*, 173*f*
analgesics, 183–185, 184*t*
antibiotics, 601
and antifungals, 185–188, 186*t*
for mastitis, 324*t*
antihypertensives, 188–189
antiplatelet and anticoagulant therapy, 189
for breast engorgement, 254–255
calculating infant exposure, 177–180
maternal factors, 178, 180
minimizing risk in, 180
unique factors, 177–178, 179*t*
contraindicated during breastfeeding, 179*t*
corticosteroids, 194–195
galactagogues, 398–399
milk production and
herbs for, 183
inhibition of, 180–182, 180*b*
stimulation of, 182–183
psychotherapeutic agents, 190–194, 190*t*–191*t*
radioactive agents, 197, 198*t*
radiocontrast agents, 197, 198*t*
radioisotopes, 197
thyroid and antithyroid, 195
transfer into human milk, 174–177
bioavailability, 176–177
drug metabolites, 177
ion trapping, 174
lipophilicity, 175–176
maternal plasma levels, 176
milk/plasma ratio, 176
molecular weight, 175
passive diffusion, 174, 175*f*
vaccines, 188, 188*b*

DTaP vaccine. *See* diphtheria, tetanus, pertussis vaccine

duct pore openings, absence of, 321

ducts, plugged, 321–323, 322*b*

ductules, 80

duloxetine, 193

dynamics, cultural, 897

dysfunctional uterine bleeding, 578, 581

dysphoric milk-ejection reflex (D-MER), 291

E

EA/TEA. *See* esophageal atresia/tracheoesophageal fistula

early feeding cues, 805*t*

early-onset nipple pain, 280–284

early postpartum education, 878–882

early term infants, 246

ears
assessment of newborn, 795–796
infections, breastmilk protections from, 143
New Ballard Score, 780

EBM. *See* expressed breastmilk

EBP. *See* evidence-based practice

echinacea, 325

eczema, of breast, 328–330, 329*b*

edema, breast, 255–256, 286, 286*t*

Edinburgh Postnatal Depression Scale (EPDS), 605

education, breastfeeding, 859–891
adult education, 882–883
adult learning principles and, 882–885
changing landscape for, 860–870
childbirth educators, 872
community support groups, 874–875
continuing education, 886
continuing postpartum support, 876–880
recommended topics for, 881*b*
curriculum development, 883–885
doulas, 873
early "how to," 876–880
sample content for, 878*b*–880*b*
factors creating need for, 859–860
for fathers, 924
healthcare professionals, breastfeeding programs for, 870–872
Internet resources, 891
LCs, 873
learning principles, 880–883
materials for, 887–888
evaluation criteria, 888*b*–889*b*
multimedia presentations, 885–886
nurses, 873
nutritionists, 874
outcomes of, 884*t*
parent education, 875–880
pharmacists, 874
prenatal, 875
recommended topics for, 877*b*
primary care providers, 873–874
programs, 859–860
small group dynamics, 885
social workers, 874
teaching strategies, 885–887

education programs, 641, 880

educational materials, evaluating, 888, 888*b*–889*b*

EGF. *See* epidermal growth factor

Egnell's pump, 428

EHR. *See* electronic health records

ELBW infants. *See* extremely low birth weight infants

electric breast pumps, 430, 435–437, 442, 443

electronic health records (EHR), 20–21

elimination (infant), assessment of, 800
elongated nipples, 321
emancipatory research perspective, 821–822
emergency room, 728
EMM. *See* expressed mothers milk
emotional care, milk expression with pump
        and need for, 444
Employer Support for Breastfeeding
        Questionnaire (ESBQ), 654
Employer's perspective on breastfeeding,
        653–654
encephalocele, 738
encephalopathy, bilirubin, 410–412, 416
endocrine and metabolic functioning, mother
    cystic fibrosis, 601–602
    diabetes, 595–598
    pituitary dysfunction, 600–601
    polycystic ovarian syndrome, 602–603
    theca lutein cysts, 603
    thyroid disease, 598–600
endocrine control, of lactation, 94
endocrine disorder, 705
Endocrine Society Guidelines, 600
endogenous opioids, 553
energy density of breastmilk, 125*f*
England, breastfeeding in, 52
enteral feeds, initiation of, 483
enterohepatic circulation of bilirubin, 407,
        413
entrapment, 306
Environment requirements for workplace
        breastfeeding support, 653
enzymes, in breastmilk, 153
EPDS. *See* Edinburgh Postnatal Depression
        Scale
epidemiological studies, sampling and sample
        size for, 839
epidermal growth factor (EGF), 154
epidurals, neonatal sucking and, 232–233
epiglottis, infant, 99–100
epilepsy (seizure disorders), maternal,
        616–617, 617*b*
Epstein's pearls, 797
ergotamine alkaloids, 594
Erikson, Eric, 678, 679*t*
Erikson's psychosocial theory, 678–679,
        679*t*
erythema toxicum, 794
erythromycin, 187
erythropoietin, 406
ESBQ. *See* Employer Support for
        Breastfeeding Questionnaire
Escherichia coli, maternal urinary tract
        infections and, 589
escitalopram (Lexapro), 192–193
esophageal atresia/tracheoesophageal fistula
        (EA/TEF), 748–749
estrogen-positive breast cancer, 349
estrogens, 180

ETCOc for ambient air. *See* exhaled end-tidal
        carbon monoxide corrected for ambi-
        ent air
ethical issues for lactation consultants, 24–27
ethnicity, breastfeeding and childbearing, 921
ethnocentrism, cultural relativism *vs.,* 897
ethnography, 822–823
    data analysis for, 837–838
ethology, 826
Europe, breastfeeding in, 58–59
European Milk Banking Association, 532
evidence-based medicine, research
        foundations for, 850
evidence-based nursing, 850
evidence-based practice (EBP), 850
evolutionary theory, 818
"excess weight loss," 367
excessive postpartum bleeding, nonpharmaco-
        logic interventions for, 578
exchange transfusion, guidelines for, 415
exclusive breastfeeding, 505
    HIV and, 210
    prevalence of (U.S.), 52, 57–58
    stooling patterns and, 295*t,* 296
exhaled end-tidal carbon monoxide corrected
        (ETCOc) for ambient air, 413
existential-phenomenological approach, 822
expansion stage of families, theory on, 916
experimental or quasi-experimental studies,
        824–825
    appropriate statistics for, 844*t*–847*t*
    data analysis, 849
    sampling and sample size for, 838–839
expressed breastmilk (EBM), 831
expressed mothers milk (EMM), 283
    creamatocrit readings and lipid/caloric
        content of, 488
    guidelines for collection and storage, 484*b*
    guidelines to minimize/prevent bacterial
        growth in, 484*b*
    mother's guide to ending, 756*b*
    preparation for preterm infant feeding
        quality control, 483
        warming, 490
    special issues for preterm infant feeding
        commercial nutritional additives,
            487–488
        delivery methods, 489–491
        hindmilk feeding, 488–489
        maternal medication use, 490
        volume restriction status, 486
    virus and pathogen transmission via,
        490–491
expression, 285–286
expressive language, 681
extended families, 915
extremely low birth weight (ELBW) infants,
        778
extremities, assessment of newborn, 799, 800*f*

eyes
    assessment of newborn, 795–796
    New Ballard Score, 780

F

FA. *See* food allergy
Fair Labor Standards Act (FSLA), 639, 650,
        652
families, 915–935
    adolescent mothers, 923–926
    adoptive, 926–927
    caring for bereaved, 764–765
    childhood sexual abuse, 933–935, 934*b*
    costs of manufactured infant milks and,
        60–62
    divorce, 931
    fathers' support for breastfeeding, 920–923
    forms and functions of, 915–916
    Internet resources, 766, 938
    low-income, 927–929
        hospital practices, 928–929
        lack of information, 927–928
        peer counselors for, 929
    relationship changes with addition to, 916*f*
    social factors influencing breastfeeding,
        917–920, 920*t*
        health-care providers and, 920*t*
    theories, 916–917
    violence, 932–933
family-centered rounds (FCR), 763
Family Medical Leave Act (FMLA), 655, 656
fathers, 920–923
Fathers Infant Feeding Initiative (FIFI), 922
fatigue, 581, 609
    mastitis and, 323
    maternal employment and, 648–649
fat(s) in breastmilk, 130
    refrigeration and, 648
FCR. *See* family-centered rounds
feasibility, research problem, 829
feedback inhibitor of lactation (FIL), 94
feeding behaviors of ill infant/child, 719
feeding cues, 805*t*
feeding-induced apnea, 105, 106*f*
feeding methods, alternate, 247–249. *See also*
        specific methods
    ill children, 722–725
    infant with CL/CP, 744
feeding positions, 238, 238*f*–240*f*, 240*t*
    CL/CP, 742
    for multiple newborns, 300*f*
    sandwich analogy, 239
    women with large breasts, 244–245
feeding problems, postpartum, 276–278,
        277*f*
feeding-tube devices, 395, 454–457,
        744–745
    amount of supplement to use in, 393*b*

guidelines for using, 396*b*
homemade and commercial, 390*f*–391*f*
feeding vessels, history of, 50
feminist research, 827
"hot" and "cold," 907
fentanyl, 185, 237
fertility
Bellagio consensus, 563–565
breastfeeding, demographic impact of, 556–557
lactational amenorrhea, 557–558
menstrual cycle, 557
repetitive nature of the recovery of, 561–563
suckling stimulus, 558–561
supplemental feeding, 561
women's health, 556
fetal alcohol syndrome, 796
"fever blisters," 212
fevers, mother's, breast engorgement and, 255
fibrocystic changes (FCCs), of breast, 344–345
FIFI. *See* Fathers Infant Feeding Initiative
FIL. *See* feedback inhibitor of lactation
finger-feeding, 249, 249*b*–250*b*, 249*f*, 391, 503, 722, 723
fingernails, assessment of newborn, 799
fingers
extra, 799
suck training with, 116–117
flanges, breast pump, 439, 441, 441*t*
flat nipples, 85, 228, 319–321
breast shells, 454
fluconazole, 325
for candidiasis, 333, 334*t*
fluorine, in breastmilk, 136
fluoxetine (Prozac), 192
fluticasone, 195
FMLA. *See* Family Medical Leave Act
follicle-stimulating hormone (FSH), 90, 91*f*
fontanelles, 795, 795*f*
food allergy (FA), 703, 760
Food and Drug Administration, U.S.
policy on used breast pumps, 445*b*
Vaccine Adverse Event Reporting System (VAERS), 695
foods
hand-fed, history of, 49–50
intolerance, 761
football position, 238, 239*f*, 240*t*
for-profit milk banking, 539
foremilk, 399
composition of, 125*f*. *See also* breastmilk, composition of
formal stage, parent education and, 876
formula. *See also* bottle-feeding
discharge packs of, 260–261
feeding-tube devices and, 456
phenylalanine-free, 754–755, 754*b*

postpartum feeding, 279–280
safety, 533*t*
Fragile Families and Child Wellbeing study, 653
free bilirubin, 411
free-nipple technique, for breast reduction, 337
frenulum, 100
FSH. *See* follicle-stimulating hormone
FSLA. *See* Fair Labor Standards Act
full-term infant, 778

G

galactagogues, 398–399, 582, 584*t*–587*t*, 587–588, 909–910
galactoceles, 343–344
galactopoiesis, 79, 94–95
galactorrhea, 95
galactose-1-phosphate uridyltransferase (GALT), 755
galactosemia, 755–756
Galant reflex, 799, 799*f*
GALT. *See* galactose-1-phosphate uridyl-transferase; gut-associated lymphoid tissue
gastric function, neonatal, 274
gastroenteritis
infant, 729–731
assessment and management, 730*t*
breastfeeding implications, 731
breastmilk protections from, 139–140
maternal, breastfeeding and, 588
gastroesophageal reflux (GER), 379–380, 749–751, 751*b*
gastroesophageal reflux disease (GERD), 379, 741, 749–751
gastrointestinal anomalies and disorders, 749–751
bloody vomit or bowel movements, 747–748
CHD and, 741
EA/TEF, 748–749
gastroesophageal reflux, 749–751, 751*b*
GER and GERD, 749–751
imperforate anus, 752–753
Internet resources, 766
pyloric stenosis (PS), 751–752
gastrointestinal disorder, 705
GBS. *See* Group B *streptococcus*
"genital herpes," 212
genitalia
assessment of newborn, 798–799
New Ballard Score, 780
gentian violet, for candidiasis, 334*t*, 335
GER. *See* gastroesophageal reflux
GERD. *See* gastroesophageal reflux disease
"German measles." *See* rubella
gestational age, 775, 777*t*–778*t*, 778–780

New Ballard Score, 778–780, 781*f*–784*f*
physiologic characteristics affecting feeding/nutrition, 778*t*
gestational diabetes, 595–596
gestational weight gain (GWG), 369
gigantomastia, 336–337
Gilbert's syndrome, 405, 409, 412
glands of Montgomery, 84–85
GLAT. *See* glatiramer acetate
glatiramer acetate (GLAT), 612
Global Data Bank on Infant and Young Child Feeding, 45*b*
Global Program for Vaccines and Immunization, 593
Global strategies for breastfeeding and work, 655–658
gonadotropin-releasing hormone (GnRH), 557
gooing, language and communication development and, 681
G6PD deficiency, 412
gradual weaning, 910
grand mal epilepsy, 616
Graves's disease, 599, 600
grief, chronic, 763–765
grounded theory, 823, 838
data analysis for, 838
group B *streptococcus* (GBS), 491, 590
growth curves
U.S. growth charts, 362, 364
birth to 2 years (boys), 365*f*
compared to WHO charts, 363*f*, 364*f*, 366*t*
WHO child growth charts, 362–367, 363*f*–365*f*, 366*t*
birth to 6 months (boys), 363*f*
birth to 2 years (boys), 364*f*
compared to CDC charts, 365*f*, 366*t*
growth factors, in breastmilk, 154–156
gruels, history of use, 50
Guidelines for Establishment and Operation of a Donor Human Milk Bank, 533
gut-associated lymphoid tissue (GALT), 150
Gyne-Lotrimin, 333

H

Haberman feeder, 723–724, 724*f*, 745
Haemophilus influenzae, 733–735
Haemophilus influenzae type b vaccine, 694
haloperidol, 194
HAMLET. *See* human alpha-lactalbumin made lethal to tumor cells
hand breast pumps, 430, 433–434
cylinder models, 434
rubber bulb models, 433
squeeze-handle models, 433–434, 433*f*
hand expression, 256, 257*f*
to avoid milk stasis, 285–286
maternal employment and, 643–647

hand-feeding, introduction of, 51
hard palate, infant, 98–99
Harlequin color, in newborns, 793
Hartmann Human Lactation Group, 379
HB-DNA. *See* hepatitis B DNA
HBeAg. *See* hepatitis B e antigen
HBsAg. *See* hepatitis B surface antigen
HCPs. *See* healthcare providers
head, assessment in newborns, 794–795, 795*f*
headaches, maternal, 593–594
Health Information Technology Institute, 655
Health Insurance Portability and
    Accountability Act (HIPAA), 23, 25
health organizations statements, 65
health professional curricula, 868*b*–870*b*
healthcare professionals, breastfeeding
    programs for, 872–874
healthcare providers (HCPs), 539, 862, 870,
    877
HealthStyles Survey, 45
Healthy Eating and Activity Together (HEAT),
    706
Healthy People statements, U.S., 62–63
hearing, assessment of newborn, 796
hearing tests, 234
heart disease
    congenital, 740–741
    Internet resources, 766
HEAT. *See Healthy Eating and Activity Together*
heel to ear (New Ballard Score), 779
Helicobacter pylori infection, 298
heliox inhalation, use of, 733
Helsinki, Declaration of, 834
hematemesis, 747–748
hematochezia, 748
heme oxygenase, 406
hemolysis, 411, 412
heparin, 189
hepatitis A, immunization, 695
hepatitis B DNA (HB-DNA), 218
hepatitis B e antigen (HBeAg), 217
hepatitis B, immunization, 693
hepatitis B surface antigen (HBsAg), 217
hepatitis B virus (HBV), 217–218
hepatitis C virus (HCV), 218–219
herbal galactogogues, 584*t*–587*t*
herbs
    galactagogues and, 907–908
    to induce lactation, 582
    to stimulate milk production, 183
heroin, in breastfeeding mothers, 196
herpes simplex virus (HSV), 212–214, 328
    and breastfeeding, 213
    counseling, 213
    outcomes, 213
    treatment/interventions, 213–214
herpetic gingivo-stomatitis, 212
Hib (*Haemophilus influenzae* type b) vaccine,
    692

hindmilk
    collection of, 399
    composition of, 125*f*. *See also* breastmilk,
        compostion of
    feeding for preterm infants, 488–489
Hinson, Pardee, 12
HIPAA. *See* Health Insurance Portability and
    Accountability Act
historical research, 826
HIV. *See* human immunodeficiency virus
HMAs. *See* human milk nutrient analyzers
HMBANA. *See* Human Milk Banking
    Association of North America
HMF. *See* human milk fortifier
HMGF. *See* human growth factors
holophrasing, language and communication
    development and, 681
home, working at, 640
Horlick's Malted Milk, 53
hormonal alterations, low intake in breastfed
    infant and, 385
hormones, 705
    in breastmilk, 154–156
    during lactation, 89–93, 89*f*
        cortisol, 91
        oxytocin, 92–93
        progesterone, 89
        prolactin, 89–91
        prolactin-inhibiting factor, 92
        thyroid-stimulating hormone, 92
    during pregnancy, 89*f*
hospital-based lactation support services,
    models for, 475–476
hospitalization
    maternal, 619–620
    stress of, 762–763
hospitals
    care for breastfeeding ill children,
        725–726
        admission history, 727*b*–728*b*
        program characteristics, 726*b*
    lactation programs in, 8, 9*f*
        development of, 8–11
        staffing needs, 12, 13*b*
    post-discharge rebound effect, 763
"hot" and "cold" foods, 907
hot treatments, milk-ejection reflex and, 421
HPV vaccines. *See* human papillomavirus
    vaccines
HSV. *See* herpes simplex virus
HTLV-1. *See* human T-cell lymphotrophic
    viruses
human alpha-lactalbumin made lethal to
    tumor cells (HAMLET), 541
human growth factors (HMGF), 154
human immunodeficiency virus (HIV),
    208–212
    breastmilk transmission risks of, 208
    counseling, 211–212

    donor milk banking and, 527
    healthcare practitioners, 211
    interventions/treatments, 208–209
    maternal/infant antiretroviral treatment/
        prophylaxis, 209–211
    outcomes, 208
human milk
    drug transfer into, 174–177
        bioavailability, 176–177
        drug metabolites, 177
        ion trapping, 174
        lipophilicity, 175–176
        maternal plasma levels, 176
        milk/plasma ratio, 176
        molecular weight, 175
        passive diffusion, 174, 175*f*
    for feeding, 486–489
    general guidelines for storing, 647*b*
    management, 482–486
    optimization, 489
Human Milk Banking Association of North
    America (HMBANA), 527
    centers that ordered milk from, 524*f*
    diagnosis codes for milk orders, 525*t*
    *Guidelines for Establishment and Operation of
        a Donor Human Milk Bank,* 533
    International Milk Banking Initiative
        (IMBI), 532
    member banks in North America, 525*t*,
        529*f*, 529*t*–531*t*
    milk banking procedures, 533–536
        processing of milk, 534
        recall procedures, 536
        record keeping, 533
        screening donors, 533–535
        storage and handling of milk, 534
human milk fortifier (HMF), 487
human milk nutrient analyzers (HMAs), 489
human papillomavirus (HPV) vaccines, 695
human sexual expression, 568
human subjects' rights, protection of,
    833–834
human T-cell lymphotrophic viruses
    (HTLV-1), 219
humanistic research perspective, 821
hunter-gatherers, breastfeeding practices
    by, 47
hydralazine, 189
hydrocephalus, 739–740
hygiene hypothesis, 145, 704
hymenal tags, 799
hyperbilirubinemia, 296–297, 297*f*,
    405–407, 408*f*, 410
hyperthyroidism, maternal, 599
hypertonia, 735–737
hypertonic glucose infusions, 253
hypertrophy, breast, 336–337
hypnotics, 190–191
hypoglycemia, 251–253, 252*t*

management of documented, 262*b*
hypopituitarism, 385
hypoplasia, of breast(s), 95
hypothalamic-pituitary-ovarian axis, 558
hypotheses, for research, 829–832
hypothyroidism, 388, 757, 797
  congenital, 757
  maternal, 599
hypotonia, 735–737

I

IBCLCs. *See* International Board Certified
  Lactation Consultants
IBD. *See* inflammatory bowel disease
Ibero-American Network of Human Milk
  Banks, 532
IBFAT. *See* Infant Breastfeeding Assessment
  Tool
IBLCE. *See* International Board of Lactation
  Consultant Examiners
ibuprofen, 237
ICD-10. *See* International Classification of
  Diseases
icterus. *See* jaundice
IgA antibodies, 149–150
IGAB. *See* Interagency Group for Action on
  Breastfeeding
IgD levels, 149–150
IgE levels, 145, 149–150
IGF-I. *See* insulin-like growth factor
ILCA. *See* International Lactation Consultant
  Association
ill children, 717–767
  allergies, 761
  altered neuromuscular tone, 735
  bronchiolitis, 733–734
  CHD, 740–741
  death of, 764–765
  dehydration, 729
  diseases specific to particular cultures, 906
  emergency room care, 728
  feeding behaviors of, 719
  food intolerance, 761
  gastroenteritis, 729–731
    assessment and management, 730*t*
  gastrointestinal anomalies and disorders,
    749–751
    EA/TEF, 748–749
    gastroesophageal reflux, 749–751, 751*b*
    imperforate anus, 752–753
    pyloric stenosis (PS), 751–752
  hospitalized, 725–726
    admission history, 727*b*–728*b*
    program characteristics, 726*b*
  hypertonia, 735–737
  hypotonia, 735–737
  inadequate weight gain strategies,
    719–720

alternate feeding methods, 722–725
  nasogastric tube feeding, 722*f*
  when direct breastfeeding is insuffi-
    cient, 720–722
infections, 728–729
Internet resources, 766–767
meningitis, 735
metabolic defects, 753–759
  celiac disease, 758
  congenital hypothyroidism, 757
  cystic fibrosis, 758–759
  galactosemia, 755–756
  phenylketonuria, 753–755
  rare amino and organic acidemias, 753
  type I diabetes, 757–758
neurological impairment, 735–740
  breastfeeding with, 736*b*–737*b*
  Down syndrome, 737–738
  hydrocephalus, 739–740
  neural tube defects, 738–739
oral/facial anomalies, 741–747
  choanal atresia, 747
  CL/CP, 742–745, 745*b*–746*b*
  Pierre Robin sequence, 745–747
otitis media, 734
pneumonia, 732–733
psychosocial concerns, 762
  chronic grief and loss, 763–765
  family stress, 762
  rebound effect, 763
  stress of hospitalization, 762–763
respiratory infections, 731–732
RSV, 733
surgery for oral/facial anomalies, 743
team care for feeding difficulties in,
  717–719, 717*b*–718*b*
IMBI. *See* International Milk Banking
  Initiative
IMDs. *See* inborn metabolic diseases
immigrants, breastfeeding perceptions of, 899
immune-modulating therapies (IMTs), 611
immune system, 152–153
  breastmilk and, 146–153
immunity
  active *vs.* passive, 146–147
  breastfeeding and, 692
immunizations, 589*t*
  childhood, 692
  maternal, 588
immunoglobulins, in breastmilk, 149–150
immunomodulating components, breastmilk,
  152–153
IMTs. *See* immune-modulating therapies
in-hospital breastfeeding, progression of,
  496–497
inactivated viral polio vaccine (IPV), 694
"inadequate" infant weight gain, 373
inborn metabolic diseases (IMDs), 753
"Incident to" billing, 31

independent variables, for research, 829
India, discard of colostrum in, 51
indirect-reacting bilirubin, 407
induced lactation, 581–582
  galactogogues and, 582
  protocol, 583*b*
infant(s)
  breastmilk kilocalories ingested per
    kilogram by age of, 124*t*
  feeding, biological norm in, 47
  health risks of manufactured infant milks
    for, 60
  low milk supply conditions and, 374*b*
infant assessment, 775–807
  behavioral
    infant states, 800, 801*t*–803*t*
    neurobehavioral cues, 805, 805*t*, 806*f*,
      807*t*
    psychosocial and breastfeeding behav-
      iors by age, 801*t*–802*t*
    sleep–wake states, 803, 803*t*, 804*f*, 805
  effectiveness of breastfeeding
    behaviors and indicators, 780, 782,
      785–786
    scales and tools, 786–788
  gestational age, 775, 777*t*–778*t*, 778–780
    New Ballard Score, 778–780,
      781*f*–784*f*
    physiologic characteristics affecting
      feeding/nutrition, 778*t*
  perinatal history, 775, 776*t*–777*t*
  physical, 788–800, 790*t*–793*t*
    abdomen, 798
    back and spine, 799
    birthmarks, 794, 794*f*
    chest, 797–798
    ears/eyes, 795–796
    elimination, 800
    extremities, 799, 800*f*
    genitalia, 798–799
    head, 794–795, 795*f*
    mouth, 796–797, 797*f*
    neck, 797
    nose, 796
    skin, 789, 793–794
    transitional, 788–789
Infant Breastfeeding Assessment Tool
  (IBFAT), 786–787, 810, 841*t*, 842
infant concerns, postpartum, 294–299
  crying and colic, 297–299
  hyperbilirubinemia, 296–297, 297*f*
    testing, 412
  pacifiers, 294–295
  regurgitation, 299
  stooling patterns, 295–296, 295*t*
infant feeding
  developmental outcomes and, 667, 672
  technological innovations in, 52–53
Infant Feeding Practices Study (IFPS II), 641

Infant Feeding Practices Survey II, 42*b*
infant milk manufacturers, medical
    community and, 54*f*, 57
infant seats, gastroesophageal reflux and, 751*b*
infant states, 800, 801*t*–803*t*
infants
    feeding positions, positive and negative
        elements, 240*t*
    suckling reflex, 230
infection, maternal, 588–603
    dysfunctional uterine bleeding, 578–581
    group B *streptococcus,* 491, 590
    tuberculosis, 592–593
infectious illnesses, 728–729
    protective properties of breastmilk, 136–146
infectious mastitis, 327
inflammatory bowel disease (IBD), 608–609
influenza vaccine, 694–695
informal stage, parent education and, 878
informed decision, 469–472
    lactation support for preterm infants, 474
informed decision making on donating
    breastmilk, 536–537
inframammary procedure, for breast augmen-
    tation, 341
initiation, lactation, 94
    milk expression with pump and, 426
Innocenti Declaration (1990), 66–67
insufficient milk production, 372, 373, 373*t*,
    376*t*–378*t*, 386
insulin-like growth factor (IGF-I), 154–155
insurance
    for lactation consultants, 27, 30–31
    liability, for lactation consultants, 23
    request for breast pump reimbursement,
        478*f*
intellectual property rights, 23–24
intention to breastfeed, 920
intention to treat (ITT), 839
Interagency Group for Action on
    Breastfeeding (IGAB), 832
internal consistency, in quantitative research,
    842–843
International Board Certified Lactation
    Consultants (IBCLCs), 5–6, 5*t*, 854
    staffing, 12, 13*b*
International Board of Lactation Consultant
    Examiners (IBLCE), 5–6, 5*t*, 872
    CPC, 23–24
    examination, 5
    intellectual property rights, 23–24
International Classification of Diseases
    (ICD10), 31, 32*b*
International Code of Marketing Breast-Milk
    Substitute, 25–27, 65–68, 65*b*
    ethics and discipline committee, 27
International Labour Organization, 657–658
International Lactation Consultant
    Association (ILCA), 3, 6, 854

International Milk Banking Initiative (IMBI),
    532
Internet resources
    breast pumps, 461–462
    breast-related problems, 353
    breastfeeding education, 893
    breastfeeding networks, 18
    child health, 709
    cultural context, 913
    donor milk banking, 545
    families, 938
    jaundice, 416
    lactation education, 862
    low intake in breastfed infants, 400–401
    maternal employment, 661–662
    perinatal and intrapartum care, 265
    postpartum care, 244
    preterm infants, 508
    research and theory, 856
    suck training, 116–120
    viruses, 222
    women's health, 623
interpretive research perspective, 821
interrater reliability, in quantitative research,
    842
intervention by lactation specialists, impact
    of, 4*t*–5*t*
intervention signs, perinatal, 259
interviews, for research, 836
intestinal metabolism of bilirubin, 407
intestine, neonatal, 123
intimate partner violence (IPV), 934
intrapartum management, neonate glucose
    level, 253
intrarater reliability, in quantitative research, 842
intrauterine devices (IUDs), 557
intravenous infusion, breastfeeding baby
    with, 727*f*
inverted nipples, 85, 97*t*, 228
    breast shells, 454
    low intake in breastfed infant and, 385
    management of, 319–321
involution, 79, 87*t*, 88, 285–286, 426, 427
    edema, 286, 286*f*
    milk stasis, 285–286
ion trapping, medications and, 174
IPV. *See* inactivated viral polio vaccine;
    intimate partner violence
iron, in breastmilk, 136
Isis breast pump, 431
ITT. *See* intention to treat
IUDs. *See* intrauterine devices

J

*JAMA. See Journal of the American Medical
    Association*
Japan, breastfeeding rituals in, 903, 903*f*
jaundice, 405–416

assessment of, 407–408
bilirubin encephalopathy, 410–412
diagnostic assessment, 412–413
evaluation of, 412
evolutionary medicine theory on, 818
hyperbilirubinemia, 296–297, 410
Internet resources, 416
management of, 413–415
neonatal, 406–407
postnatal pattern of, 408–412
job sharing, 640
Journal of Human Lactation, 3, 4, 6, 12
*Journal of the American Medical Association
    (JAMA),* 526
justice, as ethical principle, 27

K

Kaiser Permanente health system, 261
Kalahari Desert, breastfeeding practices in, 48
kangaroo (skin-to-skin) care, 301, 606, 907,
    907*f*
    after cesarean birth, 232, 232*f*
    breastfeeding promotion, 230–231, 232*f*
    newborn stabilization, 228–230, 228*f*,
        229*f*
    non-nutritive suckling, 491–497, 492*f*
    for preterm infants, mother's milk volume
        and, 483, 485–486
    risks of *not* using, 229*b*
kernicterus. *See* bilirubin encephalopathy
ketoconazole, for candidiasis, 334, 334*t*
kinesthetic learners benefit, 884
Korea, pregnancy and birth rituals in, 906

L

La Leche League groups, 924
La Leche League International (LLLI), 68,
    654–655, 876, 933
    breastfeeding education by, 876
La Leche League leaders, 5, 7, 8
    suck training technique, 119
Lact-Aid (USA) feeding-tube device, 455
lactating breasts, 538
lactation, 828
    anatomy and physiology
        autocrine *vs.* endocrine control, 94
        breast structure, 80–83, 81*f*, 83*f*
        breathing and suckling, 103–106
        concepts to practice, 97
        frequency of feedings, 107–108, 107*f*
        hormonal influences, 89–93, 89*f*
        lactogenesis, 86–88
        mammogenesis, 79–80
        milk production, 93–94
        newborn oral development, 97–100
        pregnancy, 85–86
        suckling, 101–108

breast cancer and, 348
galactopoiesis, 94–95
galactorrhea, 95
induced, 581–582
libido-enhancing factors related to, 568–569
libido-inhibiting influences of, 567–568
sexual behavior during, 569–570
stages of, 79–80, 87t, 427
women's health, 556
lactation care, after death, 765
Lactation Consultant Department, 4
lactation consultant education by, 3
Lactation Consultant in Private Practice, The: The ABCs of Getting Started (Smith), 33
lactation consultants (LCs), 3, 873
assisting during first breastfeeding, 232f
breastfeeding education by, 870–871
certification, 5–6
clinical care plans, 21, 22b
clinical issues
culture, 911
low intake in breastfed infants, 388
maternal employment, 658–660
postpartum depression, 608
prolactin and mechanically expressed milk, 426
in community settings, 16–17
education, 8
effectiveness, 4–5
expert, 16
gaining clinical experience as, 6–7
history of, 3–4
legal and ethical considerations, 21–27
in medical offices, 17
mentoring and precepting, 7b
networking and mentoring, 18
optimizing first breastfeeding, 231, 232f
postpartum care, 299
in private practice, 33–34
reimbursement for, 27–28, 28b–30b
reporting and charting, 19
role development stages, 16
roles and responsibilities, 15–16
unique characteristics, 15
viruses, 220
volunteer counselors and, 17–18
at worksites, 17
Lactation Education Approval and Accreditation Review Committee (LEAARC), 8, 872
lactation education, factors creating need for, 861–862
lactation programs, 8
development of, 8–11
staffing needs, 12, 13b, 14t
hospital, 8, 9f
marketing for, 13–15

resources needed for, 11–12
at worksites, 17, 650–653
lactational amenorrhea method (LAM), 557–558, 564, 907
lactational infertility, physiological mechanisms in, 558f
LACTNET, 18
Lactobacillus bifidus, 132, 151
Lactococcus lactis, 325
lactocytes, 172
lactoengineering own mother's milk, 488
lactoferrin, 151
lactogenesis. *See also* breastmilk
delayed in, 288–289, 359, 384
risk factors for delayed, 369b
stage I, 79, 86
markers of, 122
stage II, 79, 86, 87t
delay in, 88t
markers of, 122
tight junctions of, 87f
lactogenesis II, 359
lactoperoxidase, 152
lactose, 597. *See also* diabetes
in breastmilk, 132
intolerance, 761–762
LAM. *See* lactational amenorrhea method
Lamictal (lamotrigine), 193–194
language and communication, child development of, 681–684
language barriers, cultural differences and, 900–901
lanugo (New Ballard Score), 780
large for gestational age (LGA), classification of, 778
large nipples, 321
larynx, infant, 100
LATCH Assessment Tool, 787, 811, 841t
latch-on, 236f, 238–240
breastfeeding effectiveness and, 785
difficulties, 240–246
assessment of mother's breast and nipples, 244–245
baby problems in, 245–246
establishing milk supply, 243–244
length of time before, 785
planning for, 242–243, 243t
positioning and, 238–240, 239f, 240t
late feeding cues, 805t
late-onset nipple pain, 284
late-preterm infants, 373, 378, 778
perinatal and intrapartum care, 246–247, 247f
latent TB infection (LTBI), 592
latex nipple shields, 451
LCs. *See* lactation consultants
LDS. *See* Church of Latter-Day Saints (LDS)

LEAARC. *See* Lactation Education Approval and Accreditation Review Committee
leaking (breast), postpartum, 293
learned cultural values and beliefs, 895
left breast, milk volume of, 126–127, 127f
legal issues for lactation consultants, 21–23
legislation, U.S., 64–65, 655–657
length. *See also* weight gain (infant)
infant growth in, 673–675
leptin, 154, 706
lesions, breast, 328–330, 329b
letdown, 92–93
leukemia, 144
leukocytes, 147–148
Lexapro (escitalopram), 192–193
LGA infants. *See* large for gestational age infants
LH. *See* luteinizing hormone
liability insurance, for lactation consultants, 23
liability issues for lactation consultants, 21–23
libido
breastfeeding woman's partner, factors related to, 569
common situational factors unrelated to breastfeeding, 565–566
libido-enhancing factors related to pregnancy, birth, and lactation, 568–569
libido-inhibiting influences
of lactation, 567–568
related to parturition, 566–567
Liebig's Food, 53
limbic-cortical loops, 578
lipase, 153
lipophilicity, medications and, 175–176
literature, review of, 833
on breastfeeding practices, 47
lithium, 193
LLLI. *See* La Leche League International
LLLI Mother-to-Mother Forums, 655
LMWHs. *See* low-molecular-weight heparins
lobes, mammary, 81f, 82, 83f
long-term breastfeeding, 706–707
lorazepam, 191
loss, feelings of, 762, 764
loss of sleep, maternal employment and, 648–649
low birth weight (LBW) infants
classification of, 778
Harlequin color, 793
low-molecular-weight heparins (LMWHs), 189
low-progestin contraceptives, 56
LTBI. *See* latent TB infection
lupus erythematosus, maternal systemic, 609–610
luteinizing hormone (LH), 91f, 557

lymph drainage therapy, 291, 292t
lymphocytes, 147–148
lysozyme, 153

M

macrolide antibiotics, 187
macrophages, 147
magazine illustrations of breastfeeding, 55
magnesium in breastmilk, 136
magnetic resonance imaging (MRI) for breast
    cancer screening, 349
maintenance stage, of lactation, 427
mammalian evolution, 48
mammary papilla, 83
mammogenesis, 79–80, 87t
mammograms, 349
mammoplasty, 336–342
    augmentation, 340–342, 340f, 341f
    gigantomastia, 336–337
    mastopexy, 339–340, 340f
    reduction, 337–339, 338f
managed care organizations (MCOs), 30
Manager's Attitude Toward Breastfeeding
    Support Questionnaire, 654
manganese, in breastmilk, 137
manipulation, in experimental studies, 824
MANOVA. See multivariate analysis of
    variance
manufactured infant milks, 60–62
marijuana, 196
Marmet, Chele, 345
mass media, influence of, 56
massage, breast, 395
massage of babies, by fathers, 925
masseter, 100
mastitis, 285, 323–328
    selected antibiotics for, 324t
    teaching plan, 326t
    treatment for, 324–326, 324t, 326t
    types and severity of, 326–328, 327t
mastopexy, 339–340, 340f
maternal bonding, 688
Maternal Breastfeeding Evaluation Scale
    (MBFES), 840t, 842
maternal cigarette smoking, 594
maternal employment and breastfeeding,
    635–660
    clinical implications, 658–660
    community strategies, 654–655
    effect on breastfeeding, 636–637
    historical perspective, 635–636
    Internet resources, 661–662
    national and international strategies,
        655–658
        International Labour Organization,
            657–658
        legislative support and public advocacy,
            655–657

strategies, 638–642
    community strategies, 654–655
    individual strategies, 638–642
    national and international strategies,
        655–658
    returning to work, 642–649
    workplace strategies, 649–654
maternal experience, theoretical framework
    of, 816
maternal health outcomes, breastfeeding and,
    555b
maternal identity, theoretical framework of,
    816
maternal nutrition, 388–389
maternal role attainment theory, 816–817
Maternity Care Practices Survey, 42b–43b
MBA. See Mother–Baby Assessment Tool
MBFES. See Maternal Breastfeeding
    Evaluation Scale
McGill pain questionnaire, 580t
MCOs. See managed care organizations
MCV vaccines. See meningococcal virus
    vaccines
Mead-Johnson cleft palate feeder, 723, 724f,
    745
meaning, cultural, 902–903
measles, mumps, rubella (MMR) vaccine, 695
mechanical milk expression
    at maternal workplace, 644
    for preterm infants, 445
        breast pump selection, 477–478
        principles of, 476–477
        schedule, 479
        technique, 478–479
        written pumping records, 479, 480f
mechanical milk removal, 428–430
mechanical nipple pain, 282–284
meconium, 789, 800
Medela breast pumps, 426, 432, 434, 435f,
    441
    flanges, 441t
    pedal pumps, 441
    shields, 451t
    Supplemental Nutrition System (USA), 455
Medela Symphony pump, 422, 436, 436f
media, influence of, 56
Medicaid programs, 30–31
medical clinics, 17
medical community
    breastfeeding regulation by, 54
    childbirth regulation by, 54
    contraception regulation by, 56–57
    infant milk manufacturers and, 54f, 57
    regulation and industrialization of, 56
Medicare programs, 30–31
medications
    expressed mothers' milk for preterm
        infants and maternal use, 490
    low intake in breastfed infant and, 386

medium-chain fatty acid concentrations, 472
MedWatch (medical device reporting pro-
    gram), 444
Mellin's Food, 53
memoing, in grounded theory, 838
meningitis, 735
meningocele, 738
meningococcal virus (MCV) vaccines,
    695–696
menstrual cycle, 557
mentoring, 18
meperidine, 185, 237
MER. See milk-ejection reflex
metabolic and endocrine function, mother
    cystic fibrosis, 601–602
    diabetes, 595–598
    pituitary dysfunction, 600–601
    polycystic ovarian syndrome, 602–603
    theca lutein cysts, 603
    thyroid disease, 598–600
metabolic defects
    celiac disease, 758
    congenital hypothyroidism, 757
    cystic fibrosis, 758–759
    galactosemia, 755–756
    infant, 753–759
    Internet resources, 766
    phenylketonuria, 753–755
    rare amino and organic acidemias, 753
    type I diabetes, 757–758
metabolic function, neonatal, 274
metabolism, bilirubin, 407
metformin, 602
methadone, 184–185
methicillin-resistant Staphylococcus aureus
    (MRSA), 491, 591–592
method of study, for research, 834–836
methotrexate therapy, 613
methyldopa, 189
metoclopramide (Reglan), 182, 398
    induced lactation and, 290, 584t
MGRS. See Multicenter Growth References
    Study
miconazole, for candidiasis, 334t, 335
microcephaly, 796
micrognathia, 745
micronutrients in breastmilk, 133–135
midazolam, 191
midwives, primary care providers, 875–876
migraine, maternal, 593–594
milia, 794
milk blister, 336
milk delivery, methods of, 489–491
milk ducts, 83
milk-ejection reflex (MER)
    breast pump
        problems and, 446–447
        recommendations, 421–422
    forceful, breast pain and, 335–336

full breasts and, 427
oxytocin and, 92–93
milk expression
    methods of, 438*t*–439*t*
    principles of, 476–477
    schedule of, 479
    technique of, 478–479
milk/plasma (M/P) ratio, of medications, 176
milk stasis, 285–286
milk supply, postpartum, 287–291
    cluster pumping, 446
    concerns/worries, 287*t*–288*t*
    delayed lactogenesis, 288–289
    maternal employment and, 643
    oversupply/overproduction, 289–291
    pharmaceutical agents for, 290–291, 291*t*
    strategies
        to increase, 289*t*
        to reduce, 291*t*
milk transfer, preterm infants at breast in NICU
    algorithm of essential components in, 499*t*
    estimating methods for, 499, 501
    facilitation strategies, 501
    factors influencing, 497–499
    sustaining attachment for, 501–504
minerals in breastmilk, 135–137
mist tents for respiratory infections, 732
mixed feeds, history of, 52
MMR vaccine. *See* measles, mumps, rubella
        vaccine
models, 815
modified clutch position, 239*f*
molding, of newborn head, 795
Mongolian spots, 794, 794*f*
Montgomery's tubercles, 84
mood disorders during lactation
    autoimmune diseases, 608–613
    epilepsy (seizure disorders), 616–617
    physically challenged mothers, 613–616
    PPD, 603–608
morality and ethics, 26
morbidity, 61
Mormons, breast cancer and, 346
Moro reflex, 789, 789*f*, 807*t*
morphine, 185, 237
mother-baby dyad care, 247
mother-to-child transmission (MTCT), 207
mother-to-mother support groups, 874
Mother–Baby Assessment Tool (MBA), 787,
        812
mothercraft manuals, 55
mothers
    dietary intake, breastmilk and, 131
    health risks of manufactured infant milks
        for, 60
    illness
        breastfeeding and, 588–589
        hospitalization, breastfeeding and,
            619–620

low intake in breastfed infants and
        obvious, 389
    intention to breastfeed, 920
    low intake in breastfed infants and,
        384–389
        breast surgery, 386–387
        delayed lactogenesis, 384
        hormonal alterations, 385
        insufficient glandular development, 387
        inverted nipples, 385
        medications and substances, 386
        nipple shields, 385
        psychosocial factors of, 388
        stress, 387–388
    low milk supply conditions of, 374*b*
    nutrition
        cultural influences on choices for, 908
        low intake in breastfed infants and,
            388–389
    surgery for, 618–619
Motilium (domperidone), 182
mouth, assessment of newborn, 796–797,
        797*f*
MRI. *See* magnetic resonance imaging
MRSA. *See* methicillin-resistant
        Staphylococcus aureus
MTCT. *See* mother-to-child transmission
Multicenter Growth References Study
        (MGRS), 362, 363*b*
multimedia presentations, 885–886
    slides, 886
    television, videotapes, and DVDs, 886
    visual formatting, 886
multiple infants, 299–304
    full-term twins/triplets, 300–301
    managing breastfeeding for, 301–303
    partial breastfeeding and human milk
        feeding, 303–304
    preterm/ill, 301
multiple newborns, 300*f*
multiple sclerosis, maternal, 611–612
multiples, postpartum care for, 300
multistage cluster sampling, 835
multivariate analysis of variance (MANOVA),
        847
Munchausen syndrome, 388
myelomeningocele (MM), 738
myoepithelial cells, of breast, 80
MyPlate, 700

N

naftifine, for candidiasis, 335
nails, assessment of newborn, 799
NAPNAP. *See* National Association of Pediat-
        ric Nurse Practitioners
narrative charting, 19, 19*b*
nasogastric tube feeding, 722*f*
    infant with CHD, 741

infant with gastroesophageal reflux, 751
    Pierre Robin sequence, 745–747
nasopharyngeal intubation
    choanal atresia and, 747
    Pierre Robin sequence and, 745–747
National Association of Neonatal Nurses, 483
National Association of Pediatric Nurse
        Practitioners (NAPNAP), 706
National Birth Certificate Data, 43*b*
National Breastfeeding Center, 477
National Health and Nutrition Examination
        Survey (NHANES) data, 43*b*, 704
National Immunization Survey (NIS), 43*b*,
        636, 656, 897, 903
National Intimate Partner and Sexual
        Violence Survey (NISVS), 932
national strategies for breastfeeding and work,
        655–658
National Survey of Family Growth, 43*b*
naturalistic research perspective, 821
nausea while breastfeeding, 291
NCAFS. *See* Nursing Child Assessment
        Feeding Scale
NCAST. *See* Nursing Child Assessment
        Satellite Training
NCATS. *See* Nursing Child Assessment
        Teaching Scale
NCPAP. *See* Neonatal Continuous Positive
        Airway Pressure
near-term infants, late-preterm infants,
        246–247, 247*f*
NEC. *See* necrotizing enterocolitis
neck, assessment of newborn, 797
necrotizing enterocolitis (NEC), 540
negative pressure, oral, 241
Nelson's theory, 820
Neonatal Continuous Positive Airway
        Pressure (NCPAP), non-nutritive
        suckling and, 492, 492*f*
neonatal intensive care units (NICUs), 442,
        523, 524, 539
    breastfeeding preterm infants in, 469–476,
        479, 482, 483, 485, 486*f*, 489, 498,
        501, 503–506
    milk transfer during, 497–504
    non-nutritive suckling, 491–497,
        492*f*
    physiology research on, 494*t*–495*t*
    progression of, 496–497
neonatal jaundice, 406–407
Neonatal Oral–Motor Assessment Scale
        (NOMAS), 101, 788
neonates, feeding, sleeping, and behavior
        patterns of, 274–275, 275*t*
Nestlé's Milk Food, 53
network sampling, 836
networking, 18
neural tube defects, 738–739
    Internet resources, 766

Neurodevelopmental Effects of Antiepileptic Drugs, 617
neurofibromatosis, cutaneous, 794
neurological abnormality
    nonspecific, low breastmilk intake and, 380–381
    oral-motor dysfunction and, 378–379
    suck training, 120
nevi, 794
nevus flammeus, 794
New Ballard Score, 778–780, 781*f*–784*f*
    intrauterine growth and, 778, 783*f*
    neuromuscular signs of maturity, 779
    physical signs of maturity, 779–780
newborns
    C-hold, 235, 235*f*
    drugs to avoid in breastfeeding mothers of, 179*t*
    early feedings, 228–232
    oral development of, 97–100
    physical, 788–800, 790*t*–793*t*
        abdomen, 798
        back and spine, 799
        birthmarks, 794, 794*f*
        chest, 797–798
        ears/eyes, 795–796
        elimination, 800
        extremities, 799, 800*f*
        genitalia, 798–799
        head, 794–795, 795*f*
        mouth, 796–797, 797*f*
        neck, 797
        nose, 796
        skin, 789, 793–794
        transitional, 788–789
    physiologic jaundice of, 407
    problems causing latch-on difficulties for, 245–246
    sleep and eating patterns, 234–237, 234*t*
    sleep cycle, 274–275
Newman's (Jack) All Purpose Nipple Ointment, 334, 334*t*
NHANES data. *See* National Health and Nutrition Examination Survey data
NICUs. *See* neonatal intensive care units
nifedipine, 189, 610
nipple(s), 83*f*
    absence of duct pore openings, 321
    accessory, 85
    functional classification of, 96–97, 97*t*, 98*f*
    inverted/flat, 228, 319–321
    large/elongated, 321
    latch-on difficulty and, 244–245
    pain, 280–285
        after breastfeeding, 284–285
        early-onset, 280–284
        mastitis and, 323
        sudden (late-onset), 284
        treatment for, 282–285

pinch test of, 85, 96, 98*f*
postfeed appearance, 281*f*
pregnancy and, 80
prenatal nipple changes, 228
rashes of, 328, 329*b*
Raynaud's phenomenon of, 330
size of, 83–84
stimulation of, 230
structure of, 80, 96
nipple confusion, 506
nipple enhancers/everters, 320
nipple glasses, 454
nipple shields, 249–250, 251*f*, 282, 320, 447–454, 448*f*
    breast shells, 449*f*, 453, 454
    low intake in breastfed infants and, 385
    professional responsibilities with, 452, 454
    quick guide to, 452*b*–453*b*
    research, 450*t*–451*t*
    selection and use, 451–452
    silicone, 449*f*, 451, 451*t*
    types, 450–451
    weaning from, 460
NIS. *See* National Immunization Survey
nisin, 325
NISVS. *See* National Intimate Partner and Sexual Violence Survey
nitrogen, nonprotein, in breastmilk, 132–133
NNS. *See* non-nutritive suckling
NOMAS. *See* Neonatal Oral–Motor Assessment Scale
non-A hepatitis. *See* hepatitis C virus (HCV)
non-immune healthcare workers, 215
non-nutritive suckling (NNS), 101, 378–379, 395, 491–497, 492*f*
non-steroidal anti-inflammatory agents (NSAIDs), 183–184, 613
non-tricyclic compounds, 607
nonantibody antibacterial protection, 150–152
nondrug therapies, 707
noninfectious mastitis, 327
nonmaleficence, as ethical principle, 26–27
nonparametric statistical procedures, 843, 844*t*–847*t*
nonprobability sampling, 834, 835
North America, prevalence of, 58–59
not-for-profit milk banking, 539
novice lactation consultants, 16
NSAIDs. *See* non-steroidal anti-inflammatory agents
nuclear families, 917
nucleotides, in breastmilk, 133
null hypothesis, 831
numerous scientific reports, 469
Nuremberg Code, 834
nurse behavior, 927
nurse-midwives, primary care providers, 873–874

nurse practitioners
    primary care providers, 873–874
    U.S., 31
Nurse Practitioner's Business Practice and Legal Guide, 31
nurses, breastfeeding education by, 874
nursing-bottle caries, 698
Nursing Child Assessment Feeding Scale (NCAFS), 817
Nursing Child Assessment Satellite Training (NCAST), 817
Nursing Child Assessment Teaching Scale (NCATS), 817
nursing diagnosis and nursing care plan, 21, 22*b*
Nursing Mothers' Association of Australia, 68
Nurture III breast pump, 435, 436*f*
nutrition
    dairy products, 299
    maternal, 388–389
"nutritional programming" for preterm infants, 472
nutritionists, breastfeeding education by, 874
nuts allergy, 760
nystatin, for candidiasis, 333, 334*t*

O

obesity, childhood, 704–706
object permanence, 681
observational research, 826
observations, for data collection, 836
octreotide, 752
odds ratio (OR), 844
ointments, nipple, 282
Oketani massage, 291
olanzapine, 194
oligosaccharides, 152
on-site lactation programs, 650–653
On the Origin of Species by Means of Natural Selection (Darwin), 818
operational definitions, for research, 832
OR. *See* odds ratio
oral analgesia, 734
oral/facial anomalies, 741–747
    Internet resources, 766–767
oral-motor dysfunction, 379, 380*f*
oral polio vaccine, 188
oral rehydration solution (ORS), 731
oral rehydration therapy (ORT), 731
oral suctioning, 233
Orem's self-care theory, 819
organ transplants, maternal, 619
organic acidemias, 753
oro-motor skills, 248
orofacial development, 697–699
ORS. *See* oral rehydration solution
ORT. *See* oral rehydration therapy
orthopedic disorder, 705

Ortolani's maneuver, 799
otitis media (OM), 143, 734
outcome variables, for research, 829
oversupply, feedback inhibitor and, 94
own mother's milk, lactoengineering, 488
oxiconazole, for candidiasis, 335
oxycodone, 237
oxygen saturation measures, 493
oxygenation
    early breastfeeding and, 493–496
    Pierre Robin sequence and, 746
    respiratory infections and, 732
oxytocin, 92–93, 325, 422, 672–673
    milk expression with pump and, 427–428,
        446
    nasal spray, 446
    release and effect of, 93*f*

P

pacifiers, 294–295
pacing feedings, 103–106
packaging of donor human milk, 537*f*
pain management, breastfeeding as, 725
pain, oral-motor dysfunction and, 376*t,* 379
pain, postpartum period, 573, 574*t*–577*t,*
    578
paladai, for cup feeding, 248
palate, infant, 98–99
pallor, in newborns, 793
panhypopituitarism, 600
Papua New Guinea, breastfeeding practices
    in, 48
Papyrus Ebers, 47
parametric statistical procedures, 843,
    844*t*–847*t*
parametric tests, 843
parent-child interaction model, 817–818
Parent Child Interaction Scale-Feeding,
    817–818
parent education, 875–880
paroxetine (Paxil), 192, 622
partial breastfeeding, multiple infants,
    303–304
participatory action, 826–827
partnerships, lactation consultant, 33
passive language, 681
pasteurized human donor milk (PHDM),
    523–525, 533–535, 536*f,* 541
PATH. *See* Program for Appropriate
    Technology in Health
pathogens in expressed mother's milk,
    488–491
Patient Protection and Affordable Care Act,
    650, 655
pause (suckling assessment), 103
Paxil (paroxetine), 192, 622
PCOS. *See* polycystic ovarian syndrome
PCPs. *See* primary care providers

PCV vaccines. *See* pneumococcal virus
    vaccines
peanut allergy, 760
pedal breast pumps, 441
Pediatric Nutrition Surveillance System,
    43*b*–44*b*
pedicle technique, for breast reduction, 337
peer counseling programs, 931
peer counselors, 931, 932*t*–933*t*
perceived fatigue, relationships between
    breastfeeding and, 648–649
perceived insufficient milk supply (PIMS),
    359
periareolar technique, for breast
    augmentation, 341
perinatal and intrapartum care, 227–263
    baby-friendly hospital initiative, 261–262
    basic feeding techniques guidelines, 258
    breast edema, 255–256
    breast engorgement, 254–255
    breastfeeding assessment, 258, 258*t*
    breastfeeding flow chart, 242*f*
    cesarean births, 253–254
    clinical implications, 256–261
    commercial formula advertisement,
        260–261
    digital examination, 241, 242*b,* 242*f*
    discharge planning, 259–260, 504–506
    early feedings, 228–232
        C-hold, 235, 235*f*
    feeding methods
        cup-feeding, 247–249, 248*f*
        finger-feeding, 249, 249*b*–250*b,* 249*f*
    feeding positions, 238, 238*f*–240*f,* 240*t*
    hand expression, 256, 257*f*
    hypoglycemia, 251–253, 252*t*
    internet resources, 265
    intervention signs, 259
    latch-on difficulties, 240–246
    late-preterm infants, 246–247, 247*f*
    nipple shields, 249–250, 251*f*
    pain medications, 237
    preparation for breastfeeding, 227–228
    sleep and eating patterns, 234–237,
        234*t*
    written instructions, for community
        support, 260
perioperative care, 726–728
peripartum depression, 604
periumbilical (superior) umbilical incisions,
    for breast augmentation, 341
personnel requirements for workplace breast-
    feeding support, 650
petechiae, in newborns, 793
pewter breast pump, 419, 420*f*
PGL. *See* plasma glucose level
phagocytes, in breastmilk, 147
pharmacists, breastfeeding education by,
    874

pharmacokinetic parameters, safe and unsafe
    medications, 172
pharmacologic galactogogues, 584*t*–587*t*
pharynx, infant, 99, 100
PHDM. *See* pasteurized human donor milk
phenomenology, 822
    data analysis, 837
phenylalanine-free (PHE-free) formula,
    754–755, 754*b*–755*b*
phenylketonuria (PKU), 753–755
Philippines, breastfeeding rituals in, 903
phototherapy, for jaundice, 414, 414*f*
physical assessment of newborn, 788–800,
    790*t*–793*t*
    abdomen, 798
    back and spine, 799
    birthmarks, 794, 794*f*
    chest, 797–798
    ears/eyes, 795–796
    elimination, 800
    extremities, 799, 800*f*
    genitalia, 798–799
    head, 794–795, 795*f*
    mouth, 796–797, 797*f*
    neck, 797
    nose, 796
    skin, 789, 793–794
    transitional, 788–789
physically challenged mothers, 613–616
    baby care guidelines, 615*b,* 617*b*
    breastfeeding and physical challenges,
        614–615
    seizure disorders, 616–617
    spinal cord injury, 613–614
physician assistants, primary care providers,
    873–874
physicians
    breastfeeding education by, 873
    primary care providers, 875–876
physiologic jaundice of newborn, 407
Piaget, Jean, 679, 679*t*
Piaget's cognitive theory, 679, 681
PIBBS. *See* Preterm Infant Breastfeeding
    Behavior Scale
Pierre Robin sequence, 745–747, 796
PIF. *See* prolactin-inhibiting factor
Pigeon nipple, 724, 725*f*
PIMS. *See* perceived insufficient milk supply
pituitary dysfunction, 600–601
pituitary hormone prolactin, 182
PJ's Comfort pump, 430, 430*f,* 432, 439
PKU. *See* phenylketonuria
placebo effect, 903
planned behavior, theory of (TPB), 820
planning teaching strategies, 884
plantar surface (New Ballard Score), 780
plasma glucose level (PGL), 252*t*
playing with babies, father's role in, 923
plethora (skin color), 793

plugged ducts, 321–323, 322b
  breast cancer and, 347
  galactoceles, 344
  mastitis and, 323
  milk blister and, 336
pneumococcal virus (PCV) vaccines, 694
Pneumococcus, 152
pneumonia, 732–733
PNI framework. *See* psychoneuroimmunology
        framework
policy requirements for workplace
        breastfeeding support, 650
polio vaccine
  inactivated, 694
  oral, 188
polycystic ovarian syndrome (PCOS),
        602–603
polydactyly (extra digits), 799
polyethylene bags, 647
polymastia, 85
popliteal angle (New Ballard Score), 779
population, for research, 834, 843
port wine nevus, 794
positivism, 821
post-term infant, 778
post-term infants, classification of, 778
post-traumatic stress disorder (PTSD),
        762–763
postbirth care, of newborn, 233–234
postdischarge breastfeeding
  discharge planning for, 504–506
  management, 506
postnatal pattern of jaundice, 408
  bilirubin encephalopathy, 410–412
  breastmilk jaundice, 408–409
  hyperbilirubinemia, 410
  starvation jaundice, 409–410
postpartum care, 273–310
  bedsharing, 305–307, 306f
  breast massage, 291
    techniques, 292t–293t
  breastfeeding during pregnancy, 304–305
  clinical applications, 307–308
  clothing, leaking, bras, and breast pads,
        293
  early days and weeks
    latching, sucking/feeding problems,
        276–278, 277f
    torticollis, 278, 278t–279t
  fathers and, 922–925
  immediate postbirth, 273
  infant concerns
    crying and colic, 297–299
    hyperbilirubinemia testing, 296–297,
        297f, 412
    pacifiers, 294–295
    regurgitation, 299
    stooling patterns, 295–296, 295t
  Internet resources, 244

involution, 285–286
  edema, 286, 286f
  milk stasis, 285–286
milk supply, 287–291
  concerns/worries, 287t–288t
  delayed lactogenesis, 288–289
  maternal employment and, 643
  oversupply/overproduction, 289–291
  pharmaceutical agents for, 290–291,
        291t
  strategies to increase, 289t
  strategies to reduce, 291t
multiple infants, 299–304
  full-term twins/triplets, 300–301
  managing breastfeeding for, 301–303
  partial breastfeeding and human milk
        feeding, 303–304
  preterm/ill, 301
nausea while breastfeeding, 291
nipple pain, 280–285
  clinical care plan for, 283t–284t
  sudden (late-onset), 284
  treatment for, 282–285
principles and expectations, 273–275
returning to work, 642–649
  fatigue and loss of sleep, 648–649
  hand-expressing and pumping,
        643–647
  milk storage, 647–648
  milk supply, 643
seclusion period, 906
SIDS, 305–307
sleeping, 305–307
  safety issues, 308t
  smothering, 305–307, 306f
social support, 922
supplementation guidelines and cautions,
        279–280
tandem nursing, 304–305
postpartum depression, 603–608
  clinical care plan, 607t
  support for, 608
postpartum health and care, 553–555
postpartum hemorrhage, 578, 581
postpartum maternal thyroid disease, 390
postpartum psychosis, 604
postpartum thyroid dysfunction, 598
postpartum thyroiditis, 385, 599–600
postpartum well-being and sexual health
  libido, 565–569
  sexual behavior during lactation, 569–570
postpositivism, 822
posture (New Ballard Score), 779, 782f
potentiality, research problem, 829
power analysis, sample size using, 839
power pumping, 446
PPD test. *See* purified protein derivative test
PRAMS. *See* Pregnancy Risk Assessment
        Monitoring System

prebiotic bacteria, 132, 137
predictive validity, for quantitative research,
        843
pregnancy, 589t
  breast development and, 80, 85–86
  HIV and, 210
  hormones during, 89f, 91f
  libido-enhancing factors related to,
        568–569
Pregnancy Discrimination Act, 636
Pregnancy Risk Assessment Monitoring
        System (PRAMS), 44b, 931
prelacteal feeds, history of, 51
prenatal breastfeeding classes, 639, 879b
prenatal classes, 924
prenatal education, 877
prenatal planning for maternal work, 638–639
preparing for maternal work, 638–639
preterm breastmilk, 137
Preterm Infant Breastfeeding Assessment
        Scale, 787
Preterm Infant Breastfeeding Behavior Scale
        (PIBBS), 498
preterm infants, 469–508
  assessment document for, 500f
  breastfeeding in NICU, 469–476, 479,
        482, 483, 485, 486f, 489, 498, 501,
        503–506
    milk transfer during, 497–504
    non-nutritive suckling, 491–497, 492f
    physiology research on, 494t–495t
    progression of, 496–497
  breastfeeding initiation and duration rates,
        473
  classification, 778
  commercial nutritional additives, 487–488
  delivery methods, 489–491
  discharge planning for postdischarge
        breastfeeding, 504–506
  drugs to avoid in breastfeeding mothers,
        179t
  expressed mothers' milk, 486
    collection and storage guidelines, 482t
    commercial nutritional additives,
        487–488
    delivery methods, 489–491
    hindmilk feeding, 488–489
    maternal medication use, 490
    warming for feeding, 490
  hindmilk feeding, 488–489
  human milk suitability for, 469–472, 470t
  Internet resources, 508
  maternal milk volume maintenance,
        479–482
    guidelines for, 479–480
    preventing/increasing low volume,
        481–482, 481t
    skin-to-skin (kangaroo) care, 483,
        485–486

written pumping records, 479, 480*f*
mechanical milk expression, 446
    breast pump selection, 477–478
    principles of, 476–477
    schedule, 479
    technique, 478–479
    mothers of, 472–473
    with neural tube defects, 738–739
    research-based lactation support services, 474–476
        alternatives to exclusive, long-term breastfeeding, 474
        decision to breastfeed, 474
        facilitating an informed decision, 476
        models for hospital-based, 475–476
    volume restriction status, 486
    warming for feeding, 490
Prezi©, 886
primary care providers (PCPs), 875–876
primary progressive MS (PPMS), 611
priming stage, of lactation, 427
private lactation consultant practice, 20, 23, 33–34
    business of, 33
    do's and dont's of, 34*b*
    partnerships in, 33
    payments and fees for, 33
probability sampling, 834
probiotic bacteria, 132, 137
PROBIT study, 928
problem-oriented charting, 19–20
problem, research, 828–829
processing of donor human milk, 534
production, 359
    of breastmilk, 93–94, 287–291
        cluster pumping, 446
        concerns/worries, 287*t*–288*t*
        delayed lactogenesis, 288–289
        drugs that inhibit, 180–182, 180*b*
        drugs that stimulate, 182–183
        herbs for, 183, 582
        maternal employment and, 643
        oversupply/overproduction, 289–291
        pharmaceutical agents for, 290–291, 291*t*
        strategies to increase, 289*t*
        strategies to reduce, 291*t*
proficient lactation consultants, 16
progesterone, lactation and, 89, 89*f*
progesterone-positive breast cancer, 349
progestin-only hormonal contraception, 56
Program for Appropriate Technology in Health (PATH), 532
progressive relapsing MS (PRMS), 611
prolactin
    lactation and, 89–91, 89*f*
    milk expression with pump and, 425–426
        clinical implications, 426–427
    during pregnancy and lactation, 91*f*
    release and effect of, 93*f*

prolactin-inhibiting factor (PIF), 92
prolactin receptor theory, 91
prolactinomas, 600
prostaglandins, 155–156
protein in breastmilk, 125*f*, 132
protest stage, of separation anxiety, 691
protraction, of nipples, 85, 97*t*, 98*f*
Prozac (fluoxetine), 192
pseudoephedrine, 386
pseudomembranous colitis, 187
psychoneuroimmunology (PNI) framework, 605
psychosocial disorder, 705
psychosocial factors
    ill children, 762–765
    low intake in breastfed infants, 388
psychosocial theory of development (Erikson), 678–679, 679*t*
psychotherapeutic agents, 190–194, 190*t*–191*t*
    antidepressants, 192–193
    antimanics, 193–194
    antipsychotics, 194
    sedatives and hypnotics, 190–191
PTSD. *See* post-traumatic stress disorder
public breastfeeding, cultural perceptions of, 902
Puerto Rican folk disease, 906
purified protein derivative (PPD) test, 593
purpose, research, 828–829
purposive sampling, 835
pyloric stenosis (PS), 751–752
pyloromyotomy, 752

Q

qualitative research, 822–824
    applications of methods to, 837–838
        data analysis, 837–838
        data collection, 837
        sampling, 837
        trustworthiness of, 838
    discourse analysis, 823–824
    ethnography, 822–823
    grounded theory, 823
    guidelines for evaluation of, 852*t*
    phenomenology, 822
    questions for, 830*t*–831*t*
quantitative research, 824–825
    applications of methods to, 838–851
        data analysis, 843–850
        data collection, 840–842
        reliability and validity, 842–843
        results, discussion, conclusions, and dissemination, 850–851
        sampling and sample size, 838–839
    correlational studies, 824
    descriptive studies, 824
    experimental studies, 824–825

    guidelines for evaluation of, 852*t*
    questions for, 830*t*–831*t*
quasi-experimental approach, 826
questionnaires, breastfeeding, 840*t*–841*t*
quetiapine, 194
quota sampling, 835

R

race, breastfeeding and childbearing, 927
radioactive agents, 197, 198*t*
radiocontrast agents, 197, 198*t*
radioisotopes, 197
RADS2 gene, 130
random assignment, of samples, 839
randomization
    in experimental studies, 825
    for parametric statistical procedures, 843
randomized control trial (RCT), 839
rashes, of breast, 328, 329*b*
Raynaud's phenomenon (RP), 609, 610
    of the nipple, 330
RCT. *See* randomized control trial
reading to babies, father's role in, 923
reasoned action, theory of (TRA), 820
rebound effect, 763
recall procedures for donor milk, 536
receptive language, 681
records of donor human milk, 536
reflexes, child
    cremasteric, 798
    development of, 676
    Galant, 799, 799*f*
    Moro/startle, 789, 789*f*, 807*t*
    neurobehavioral cues, 805, 805*t*, 806*f*, 807*t*
    rooting, 100, 235, 807*t*
        as breastfeeding effectiveness indicator, 785, 785*f*
    stepping, 799, 800*f*
    suck-swallow, 735
    sucking, 796, 807*t*
    suckle, 100, 101
    tonic neck, 797, 798*f*
refusal of breast, 245
Reglan (metoclopramide), 182
regurgitation, 299
reimbursement, for lactation consultants, 27–28, 28*b*–30*b*
rejection of billing, 31
relactation
    feeding-tube devices and, 455
    women's health and, 581–582
relapsing-remitting MS (RRMS), 611
relative infant dose (RID), 177
relative risk (RR), 844
relativism, ethnocentrism *vs.* cultural, 897
reliability, for quantitative research, 842–843
    breastfeeding questionnaires and assessment tools, 840*t*–841*t*

research. *See also* research methods
  clinical practice use of, 853–854
  elements of, 828–837
    data analysis, 836–837
    data collection methods, 836
    hypotheses, 829–832
    operational definitions, 832
    problem and purpose, 828–829,
      830*t*–831*t*
    protection of human subjects' rights,
      833–834
    review of literature, 833
    study method, 834–836
    variables, 829
  evaluation for use in practice, 851–852, 852*t*
  Internet resources, 856
research methods, 822–828
  breastfeeding questionnaires and
    assessment tools, 840*t*–841*t*
  feminist, 827
  historical, 826
  observational, 826
  participatory action, 826–827
  perspectives, 821–822
  qualitative, 822–824
    applications of methods to, 837–838
    discourse analysis, 823–824
    ethnography, 822–823
    grounded theory, 823
    phenomenology, 822
    questions for, 830*t*–831*t*
  quantitative, 824–825
    applications of methods to, 838–851
    correlational studies, 824
    descriptive studies, 824
    experimental studies, 824–825
    questions for, 830*t*–831*t*
respiratory disorder, 705
respiratory illness
  breastmilk protections from, 140, 142
  infant, 731–732
  maternal infections, breastfeeding and, 594
respiratory syncytial virus (RSV), 733
retention of breastmilk, 285
retracted nipples, 96, 97*t*, 98*f*
  breast shells, 454
returning to work while breastfeeding,
    642–649
  fatigue and loss of sleep, 648–649
  hand-expressing and pumping, 643–647
  milk storage, 647–648
  milk supply, 643
reverse-cycle breastfeeding, 649
reverse-cycle nursing episode, 660
reverse pressure softening, for breast edema, 256
rheumatoid arthritis, maternal, 612–613
ribavirin treatment, use of, 734
rickets, vitamin D and, 696–697
RID. *See* relative infant dose

right breast, milk volume of, 126–127, 127*f*
risk ratio (RR), 849
risperidone, 194
rituals, cultural meaning and, 904–905
rocking babies, father's role in, 923
rollover concerns (smothering), 305–307,
    306*f*
rooting reflex, 100, 235, 807*t*
    as breastfeeding effectiveness indicator,
      785, 785*f*
Ross Mothers Survey, 44*b*
rotavirus vaccine, 693
Rotch, Thomas, 53, 55
RP. *See* Raynaud's phenomenon
RR. *See* relative risk; risk ratio
RRMS. *See* relapsing-remitting MS
RSV. *See* respiratory syncytial virus
rubber bulb hand breast pumps, 433
rubber nipple shields, 450
rubella, 216–217
Rush-Presbyterian Hospital program, 475,
    476
rusty pipe syndrome, 129, 345

S

safety of donor milk, 532, 533*t*
sale of milk, 537–539
saline, breast implants, 341
saltation, 367
salutary breastfeeding, 820
sampling, 834–836
    parametric *vs.* nonparametric analysis and,
      843
    for qualitative research, 837
    for quantitative research, 838–839
sandwich analogy, 239
scarf sign (New Ballard Score), 779
SCI. *See* spinal cord injury
Scott, JoAnne, 5
SCQD. *See* sequential-consensual qualitative
    design
screening for HIV, 210
screening human milk donors, 533–535
screening mammogram, breast cancer, 347
seal, breast, 277*f*
secondary progressive MS (SPMS), 611
secretory IgA (sIgA), 150
secretory immune system, 146
sedatives, 190–191
seizure disorders, maternal, 616–617, 617*b*
seldane, antifungal drugs contraindications
    for, 334
selective serotonin reuptake inhibitors
    (SSRIs), 192, 607
    for postpartum depression, 607
selenium, in breastmilk, 136
self-care teaching, 598
self-care theory, 818–819

self-efficacy theory, 819
self-help groups, 859
self-limiting, infections, 588
self-report questionnaires, 836
semi-automatic breast pumps, 425*b*, 435
senses, development of, 675–676
Sensorial Oral Stimulation technique, 119
sentences, complete, language and communi-
    cation development and, 681, 682
separation anxiety, 691
sequential-consensual qualitative design
    (SCQD), 827
sequential pumping, 423, 437
serotonin and norepinephrine reuptake
    inhibitors (SNRIs), 193
Serratia marcescens infection, 442
sertraline (Zoloft), 192, 622
serum glucose concentration, 252
setting, research, 834
"setting sun" sign, 739
sexual abuse, childhood, 935–937, 936*b*
sexual abuse survivors, interventions for
    helping, 936*b*
sexuality
    behavior during lactation, variations in
      cultural beliefs about, 904
    women's health, 556
sexually transmitted infections (STIs), 212
shadowing, 18
shared cultural values and beliefs, 895, 897*f*
sharing bed with infant, 308*t*
Sheehan's syndrome, 385, 600
shingles, 214–215
shipping of donor human milk, 534, 537*f*
short sucking bursts, 105, 106*f*
SHRM. *See* Society for Human Resource
    Management
sialic acid, in breastmilk, 672
SIBB. *See* suboptimal infant breastfeeding
    behavior
side-lying (feeding) position, 238, 240*f*, 240*t*
    infant with hydrocephalus, 739
    infant with neural tube defects, 739
    left-lateral, gastroesophageal reflux and,
      751*b*
SIDS. *See* sudden infant death syndrome
significant hyperbilirubinemia, 407
silicone breast implants, 340
silicone nipple shields, 451, 451*t*
simple random sampling, 835
simultaneous pumping, 437
singing to babies, father's role in, 925
sinuses, breast structure and, 80
size, nipple, 83–84
skill acquisition model, 16
skin
    New Ballard Score, 779
    newborn assessment, 789, 793–794
skin-to-skin (kangaroo) care, 301, 907, 907*f*

after cesarean birth, 232, 232f
breastfeeding promotion, 230–231, 232f
newborn stabilization, 228–230, 228f, 229f
non-nutritive suckling, 491–497, 492f
for preterm infants, mother's milk volume and, 483, 485–486
risks of *not* using, 229b
skin turgor, 794
SLE. *See* systemic lupus erythematosus
sleep deprivation, 648
sleep, levels of, 676–678
sleeping patterns, postpartum, 305–307
crying and, 681
safety issues, 308t
smothering, 305–307, 306f
sleeping position, gastroesophageal reflux and, 751b
sleep–wake states, 803, 803t, 804f, 805
small for gestational age (SGA), classification of, 778
small-group dynamics, 887
Smillie, Christina, 335
Smith, Hugh, 55
Smith, Linda, 5, 33
smoking, maternal, 386, 594–595
smothering, 305–307, 306f, 308t
snowball sampling, 836
SNRIs. *See* serotonin and norepinephrine reuptake inhibitors
SOAP or SOAPIE method, 19, 20b
social context for infant feeding, 52–53
social development, 681
social workers, breastfeeding education by, 876
Society for Human Resource Management (SHRM), 652
sodium, in breastmilk, 135
soft palate, infant, 99
solicited sampling, 835
solid foods, 699–704
delaying, 703–704
diet choices, 700–703
feeding location selection, 703
introducing, 699–700, 701t–702t
quick, easy to prepare, 703b
Soranus, 47
space requirements for workplace breastfeeding support, 650
Spanish-speaking women
breastfeeding phrases for use with, 902t
lactation support for, 901
Special Supplemental Nutrition Program for Women, Infants, and Children, 642
specialty medical clinics, 17
spina bifida, 738
spinal cord injury (SCI), 613–614
maternal, 613–614
syndrome, 614

spine, assessment of newborn, 799
SPMS. *See* secondary progressive MS
spoon-feeding, 456
square window (New Ballard Score), 779
squeeze-handle hand breast pumps, 433–434
SSRIs. *See* selective serotonin reuptake inhibitors
stable stage of families, theory on, 918
staffing, hospital lactation programs, 12, 13b
stair-step pattern, infant, 367
Staphylococcus aureus, 187
mastitis and, 324
methicillin-resistant (MRSA), 591–592
startle reflex, 789, 789f, 807t
starvation jaundice, 406, 409–410
state, economic costs of manufactured infant milks to, 61–62
State-Trait Anxiety scores, 605
stem cells, 148–149, 149f
stepping reflex, 799, 800f
steroids, breastmilk and, 195
STIs. *See* sexually transmitted infections
stooling patterns (infant), 295–296
assessment of, 800
bloody stool, 747–748
breastfeeding and infant, 295t
storage of donor human milk, 534
"stork bites," 794
stranger distress, development of, 690–691
stratified random sampling, 835
strawberry hemangiomas, 794
Streptococcus group B, maternal, 491, 590
Streptococcus mutans, 698
Streptococcus pneumoniae, 733, 734
stress
family, ill children and, 762
of hospitalization, 762–763
low intake in breastfed infants and, 387–388
mastitis and, 323
and stressors, 571–573
stress-induced COR elevation, 673
subclinical lactation mastitis, 326
suboptimal infant breastfeeding behavior (SIBB), 368
suck, definition of, 101
suck-swallow reflex, neurological impairment and, 735
suck training, 116–120
sucking, 100–108
postpartum problems, 276–278, 277f
sucking glasses, 419, 419f
sucking reflex, 796, 807t
suckle, definition of, 101
suckle reflex, 100, 101
suckling, 101–108
as breastfeeding effectiveness indicator, 785

breathing and, 103–106
ineffective, 378–379, 395
neural control of, 105
"pause" during, 101
suckling reflex, infants, 230
suckling stimulus, 558–561
suctioning, oral, 233
sudden infant death syndrome (SIDS), 294, 305–307, 678, 818
"Back to Sleep" campaign, 278
sudden unexplained infant death (SUID), 305–307, 306f
sufficient milk production, 372
SUID. *See* sudden unexplained infant death
suitability, research problem, 828
sulfisoxazole milk, 187
sulfonamides, 187
sulpride, induced lactation and, 585
super pumping, 446
superior pedicle technique, for breast reduction, 338
supernumerary breasts, 85
Supplemental Nutrition System (USA) (feeding-tube device), 455
supplements, dietary with postpartum care, 279–280
supply-demand response, 94
support groups, 925
support systems
for breastfeeding, 918
for fathers, 924
Supporting Nursing Moms at Work: Employer Solutions, 652
Supporting Working Moms Act, 657
surgery (mother's breast)
breast lumps and, 342–343
FCCs, 344–345
galactoceles, 344
feeding-tube devices and, 455
Internet resources, 353
low intake in breastfed infants and, 386–387
suspensory ligaments, 82
swaddling and carrying infants, 905
swallowing
as breastfeeding effectiveness indicator, 785
neural control of, 105
switch nursing, 395
syringe- or spoon-feeding, 391
systematic sampling, 835
systemic immune system, 146
systemic lupus erythematosus (SLE), 609–610

T

T cells, 147, 148, 148f
tandem nursing, 304–305
tardive dyskinesia, 398

taurine, 156
Taylor's model, 572
team care, child with feeding difficulties, 717–719
technological context for breastfeeding, history of, 53
teen mothers, 924
teeth
    supernumerary, 797
    weaning and permanent molars, 911
teething, weaning and, 911
TEF. See tracheoesophageal fistula
telangiectatic nevi, 794
telegraphic speech, language and communication development and, 682
temperament, child, 689–690, 690t
TennesSee, breastfeeding protection legislation, 636
terfenadine, antifungal drugs contraindications for, 334
term infants, classification of, 778
test-retest reliability, in quantitative research, 842
test weighing, 395–396, 397b
textbooks in breastfeeding education, 888–889
thalamocortical loops, 578
The Joint Commission (TJC), 21
theca lutein cysts, 603
theophylline, 594
theoretical coding, in grounded theory, 838
theoretical models, 815–820
    bonding and attachment, 818
    Darwinian and evolutionary medicine, 818
    Internet resources, 856
    maternal role attainment, 816–817
    parent-child interaction, 817–818
    planned behavior, 819–820
    reasoned action, 819–820
    self-care, 818–819
    self-efficacy, 819
theoretical sampling, 836
thermography imaging, 349–350
thiazide diuretics, low intake in breastfed infant and, 386
third-party payments, for lactation consultants, 30–31
34 to 36 "weekers"
    breastfeeding, 247f
    perinatal and intrapartum care for, 246–247, 247f
thyroid and antithyroid medications, 195
thyroid disease, 598–600
thyroid screening tests, 598
thyroid-stimulating hormone (TSH), 92
thyrotropin-releasing hormone (TRH), 155, 598
thyroxine, 155
tight junctions, 87f, 87t

time requirements for workplace breastfeeding support, 649–650
TJC. See The Joint Commission
tongue dysfunction, suck training with, 119–120
tongue-tie/ankyloglossia, 281
tonic neck reflex, 797, 798f
torticollis, 278, 278t–279t
tracheoesophageal fistula (TEF), 748–749
traditional families, 917
transabdominal insertion, for breast augmentation, 341
transareolar incisions, for breast augmentation, 342
transferability, of research, 838
transitional milk, 122
transplants, maternal, 619
TRH. See thyrotropin-releasing hormone
Trisomy 21, 737–738
trunk incurvation reflex, positive, 799, 799f
TSH. See thyroid-stimulating hormone
tuberculosis, maternal, 592–593
twins
    feeding positions for, 300f
    maternal phenylketonuria and, 755
type 1 diabetes, 596–598
type 2 diabetes, 595, 598

U

UGT1A1. See uridine diphosphate glucuronyl transferase
UKAMB. See United Kingdom Association of Milk Banks
ultrasound
    for breast cancer screening, 349
    for breast engorgement, 255
unconjugated bilirubin, 407
undersupply
    feedback inhibitor and, 94
    pharmaceutical agents for, 290–291, 291t
    strategies to increase supply, 289t
United Kingdom Association of Milk Banks (UKAMB), 532
United States
    breastfeeding in, 57–58
    breastfeeding legislation in, 655–657
    breastfeeding promotion in, 62–65, 63t
    breastfeeding rituals in, 904
    Recommended Childhood Immunization Schedule, 692
United States Breastfeeding Committee (USBC), 64, 656, 657, 863
upper respiratory tract infections (maternal), breastfeeding and, 588
upright feeding position, 719, 720f
    CL/CP, 744
    gastroesophageal reflux, 751b
    neurological impairment, 736b–737b

Pierre Robin sequence, 746
    respiratory infections, 732
uridine diphosphate glucuronyl transferase (UGT1A1), 407, 409, 413
urinary tract infections (UTIs), maternal, breast-feeding and, 589
U.S. Breastfeeding Committee (USBC), 656
U.S. Department of Agriculture's Food and Nutrition Service, 655
U.S. Department of Health and Human Services (USDHHS), 650, 652, 656, 697–698
U.S. Department of Labor, 640
U.S. Food and Drug Administration, 645
U.S. growth charts, 362, 364
    birth to 2 years (boys), 365f
    compared to WHO charts, 363f, 364f, 366t
U.S. hispanic population, 897
USBC. See U.S. Breastfeeding Committee
USDHHS. See U.S. Department of Health and Human Services
used breast pumps, 445b
uterine bleeding, dysfunctional, 578–581
uterine contractions, 304

V

Vaccine Adverse Event Reporting System (VAERS), 695
vaccines, 188, 188b
VACTERL defects, 748, 752
vacuum, 429
    extraction, 233
VAERS. See Vaccine Adverse Event Reporting System
vaginal delivery, 212
validity, for quantitative research, 843
    breastfeeding questionnaires and assessment tools, 840t–841t
valproic acid, 193
variables, for research, 829
    parametric vs. nonparametric analysis and, 843
varicella, 214–215
varicella-zoster virus (VZV), 214–215
venlafaxine, 193
verapamil, 189
vernix caseosa, 789
very low birth weight (VLBW) infants, 778
Via Christi Breastfeeding Assessment Tool, 787
violence, 934–935
viral AGE, 729
viruses, 207–222
    cytomegalovirus, 215–216
    hepatitis B, 217–218

hepatitis C, 218–219
HIV
  breastmilk transmission risks of, 208
  counseling, 211–212
  healthcare practitioners, 211
  interventions/treatments, 208–209
  maternal/infant antiretroviral treatment/prophylaxis, 209–211
  outcomes, 208
HSV
  and breastfeeding, 213
  counseling, 213
  outcomes, 213
  treatment/interventions, 213–214
HTLV-1, 219
implications for practice, 220
Internet resources, 222
mother-to-child transmission, 207
rubella, 216–217
transmitted via expressed mother's milk, 490–491
VZV, 214–215
WNV, 219–220
vitamin A, in breastmilk, 134
vitamin B_6, in breastmilk, 135
vitamin B_{12}, in breastmilk, 135
vitamin D
  in breastmilk, 134
  deficiency, 705
  rickets and, 696–697
vitamin E
  in breastmilk, 134
  fed to cows, 325
vitamin(s), in colostrum and breastmilk, 133–135
vitamin K, in breastmilk, 134–135
VLBW infants. *See* very low birth weight infants
volunteer sampling, 836
vomit, bloody, 747–748
VZV. *See* varicella-zoster virus

W

WABA. *See* World Alliance for Breastfeeding Action
warming expressed milk, 490
weaning, 707
  age of, historically, 48–49
  culture and, 910–911
  infants, 304
  mother's guide to ending expression, 756*b*
  social support and, 920
  types of, 910–911
webinars, 888
weight gain (infant), 673–675
  inadequate first month, 373
  negative cycle of milk intake and, 361*f*
  positive cycle of milk intake and, 360*f*

U.S. growth charts, 362, 364
  birth to 2 years (boys), 365*f*
  compared to WHO charts, 363*f,* 364*f,* 366*t*
  as weaning criteria, 911
WHO child growth charts, 362–367, 363*f*–365*f,* 366*t*
  birth to 6 months (boys), 363*f*
  birth to 2 years (boys), 364*f*
  compared to CDC charts, 365*f,* 366*t*
weight loss (infant), 258, 263*b,* 370*b*
Wellbutrin (bupropion), 193
West Nile virus (WNV), 219–220
wet-nursing, 537–539
  history of, 49
  variations in cultural beliefs about, 906
whey-casein ratio of human milk, 296
Whisper Wear breast pump, flanges, 441*t*
white blood, 137, 147*f*
white cells, 147*f*
  lymphocytes, 147–148
  phagocytes, 147
WHO Code, 25–27
WIC Program. *See* Women, Infants, and Children Program
Wichita State University School of Nursing breast-feeding education course, 872
WNV. *See* West Nile virus
Women, Infants, and Children (WIC) Program, 7, 63–64, 817, 876
  breastfeeding surveys sponsored by, 44*b*
  peer counseling, 931
women's health, 553–620
  across childbearing years, 570–571
    galactogogues, 587–588
    immediate postpartum concerns, 573–581
    measures to initiate and enhance lactation, 588
    re-lactation and induced lactation, 581–587
    stress and stressors, 571–573
  acute illness and infections, 588–603
    CF, 601–602
    chronic illnesses, 594–595
    dysfunctional uterine bleeding, 578–581
    endocrine and metabolic functioning, alterations in, 595–601
    gestational ovarian theca lutein cysts, 603
    group B *streptococcus,* 590
    headaches, 593–594
    MRSA, 591–592
    PCOS, 602–603
    tuberculosis, 592–593
  asthma, 594

autoimmune diseases, 608–613
  multiple sclerosis, 611–612
  rheumatoid arthritis, 612–613
  systemic lupus erythematosus, 609–610
blood donations, 619
endocrine and metabolic functioning, 595–603
  cystic fibrosis, 601–602
  diabetes, 595–598
  pituitary dysfunction, 600–601
  polycystic ovarian syndrome, 602–603
  theca lutein cysts, 603
  thyroid disease, 598–600
fertility
  Bellagio consensus, 563–565
  breastfeeding, demographic impact of, 556–557
  lactational amenorrhea, 557–558
  menstrual cycle, 557
  repetitive nature of recovery, 561–563
  suckling stimulus, 558–561
  supplemental feeding, 561
group B *streptococcus,* 491
headaches, 593–594
illness and hospitalization impact, 619–620
immunizations, 588
induced or adoptive lactation, 581–582
Internet resources, 623
lactation, fertility, sexuality, and contraception, 556
mood disorders during lactation
  autoimmune diseases, 608–613
  epilepsy (seizure disorders), 616–617
  physically challenged mothers, 613–616
  PPD, 603–608
physical challenges, 613–616
  baby care guidelines for, 615*b*
postpartum depression (PPD), 603–608, 607*t*
postpartum health and care, 553–555
postpartum well-being and sexual health libido, 565–569
  sexual behavior during lactation, 569–570
relactation, 581–582
smoking, 594–595
surgery, 618–619, 618*b*
transplants, 619
workbooks in breastfeeding education, 888–889
workplace
  breastfeeding in, 638
  lactation program, 653

workplace strategies to support breastfeeding,
    649–654
  employer's perspective, 653–654
  lactation programs, worksite,
    650–653
worksite lactation programs, 17, 650–653
World Alliance for Breastfeeding Action
    (WABA), 66, 656
World Health Organization/UNICEF, 560,
    675, 863, 922
  Baby-Friendly Hospital Initiative, 67–68
  breastfeeding definitions for databank of,
    832

breastfeeding surveys sponsored by,
    42b–46b, 45–46, 45b–46b
child growth charts, 362–367, 363f–365f,
    366t
  birth to 2 years (boys), 365f
  U.S. growth charts vs., 362, 364
Innocenti Declaration (1990),
    66–67
International Code of Marketing
    Breast-Milk Substitute, 25–27,
    65–68, 65b
  ethics and discipline committee,
    27

Y

"yin/yang" belief system, 900
yin-yang theory, maternal nutrition and, 907

Z

"zero-risk" approach, 211
zidovudine, 209
zinc, in breastmilk, 135–136
Zoloft (sertraline), 192, 622
zoster, 214–215
Zyban (bupropion), 193

9386487359